Visual Guide to Neonatal Cardiology

Visual Guide to Neonatal Cardiology

Edited by

Ernerio T. Alboliras, Ziyad M. Hijazi, Leo Lopez, and Donald J. Hagler

WILEY Blackwell

This edition first published 2018

Registered Office(s)
John Wiley & Sons, Inc., 111 River Street, Hoboken, NJ 07030, USA
John Wiley & Sons Ltd, The Atrium, Southern Gate, Chichester, West Sussex, PO19 8SQ, UK

Editorial Office
9600 Garsington Road, Oxford, OX4 2DQ, UK

For details of our global editorial offices, customer services, and more information about Wiley products visit us at www.wiley.com.

Wiley also publishes its books in a variety of electronic formats and by print-on-demand. Some content that appears in standard print versions of this book may not be available in other formats.

Library of Congress Cataloging-in-Publication Data

Names: Alboliras, Ernerio T., editor. | Hijazi, Ziyad M., editor. | Lopez, Leo, editor. | Hagler, Donald J., editor.
Title: Visual guide to neonatal cardiology / edited by Ernerio T. Alboliras, Ziyad M. Hijazi, Leo Lopez, and Donald J. Hagler.
Description: Hoboken, NJ : Wiley, 2018. | Includes bibliographical references and index. |
Identifiers: LCCN 2017054083 (print) | LCCN 2017054741 (ebook) | ISBN 9781118635346 (pdf) | ISBN 9781118635223 (epub) | ISBN 9781118635148 (hardback)
Subjects: | MESH: Heart Diseases | Infant, Newborn, Diseases | Fetal Diseases | Infant, Newborn
Classification: LCC RJ421 (ebook) | LCC RJ421 (print) | NLM WS 290 | DDC 618.92/12–dc23
LC record available at https://lccn.loc.gov/2017054083

Cover Design: Wiley
Cover Image: © garymilner/Gettyimages

Set in 10/12pt WarnockPro by SPi Global, Chennai, India
Printed and bound in Singapore by Markono Print Media Pte Ltd

10 9 8 7 6 5 4 3 2 1

We would like to dedicate this book to our spouses, families, colleagues, trainees both past and present, sonographers, and friends. We would also like to thank the international group of notable authors of this book for their exceptional scholarly contributions to the understanding of the complexity of neonatal heart disease.

Contents

Preface

Majority of cardiac defects manifest themselves in the neonate. The uniqueness of their cardiovascular issues and the complexities of the spectra of cardiac defects in this age group necessitate that this teaching medium be made available. This book is the product of the cumulative efforts of 103 pediatric cardiologists, cardiac surgeons, pathologists, radiologists, sonographers, scientists, and others who are authorities in the care of newborns with heart disease.

This book discusses all aspects of neonatal heart disease in a comprehensive, clear, and succinct way. Each section will be valuable, not only for its textual content but also for the use of figures, charts, plates, graphs, illustrations, and tables. The use of these visual aids will make it easier for the reader to understand the corresponding topic. In many sections, the written text may be juxtaposed with illustrations, photographs of a patient, chest roentgenograms, electrocardiograms, echocardiograms, angiograms, computed tomography, magnetic resonance imaging, pathologic specimens, and other relevant visual aids.

The 71 chapters have been grouped into seven major parts. The first part, **Prenatal and Perinatal Issues**, includes new principles in cardiac embryogenesis and embryopathy and topics on the fetal heart and how they manifest in the neonatal heart. The second part, **General Neonatal Issues**, includes epidemiology, transitional circulation, approach to history-taking and physical examination of the newborn suspected to have cardiac disease, and discussions on the common manifestations – cyanosis, tachypnea, hypoperfusion, and dysmorphism. The third part, **Diagnostic Procedures**, has seven chapters that discuss the various tools for an accurate and comprehensive diagnosis of neonatal heart disease. The fourth part, **Specific Morphologic Conditions**, comprises 41 chapters that provide comprehensive discussions on the various cardiac defects that are made easy to understand through generous use of figures and tables. The fifth part, **Rhythm Disturbances in the Newborn**, provides a four-chapter discussion of neonatal rhythm disturbances, their presentation, evaluation, and management. The sixth part, **Special Issues in the Newborn**, includes important topics presented generously with visual aids. These are balloon atrial septostomy, interventional therapeutic procedures, the Hybrid procedure, neonatal cardiac surgical procedures, extracorporeal membrane oxygenation, ventricular assist device, cardiac transplantation, and postoperative care. The seventh and last part, **Neonatal Formulary**, details the various cardiac medications used in the neonatal age group as well as provides guidance for nutritional care.

This book will hopefully be a major resource for pediatric cardiologists, neonatologists, residents, fellows, sonographers, nurses, and other allied professionals who take care of newborns with heart disease.

Ernerio T. Alboliras
Ziyad M. Hijazi
Leo Lopez
Donald J. Hagler

List of Contributors

Ra-Id Abdulla, MD
Professor
Department of Pediatrics
Chief, Section of Pediatric Cardiology
Rush University Medical Center
Chicago, IL, USA

Michael J. Ackerman, MD, PhD
Professor in Medicine, Pediatrics, and Pharmacology
Windland Smith Rice Sudden Death Genomics Laboratory
Mayo Clinic
Rochester MN, USA

Hitesh Agrawal, MD
Fellow in Pediatric Cardiology
Texas Children's Hospital
Houston, TX, USA

Ernerio T. Alboliras, MD
Medical Director
Genus Heart Center
Scottsdale, AZ, USA

Zahid Amin, MD
Professor and Chief
Division of Pediatric Cardiology
Children's Hospital of Georgia
Augusta University
Augusta, GA, USA

Robert H. Anderson, MD
Honorary Visiting Professor
Institute of Genetic Medicine
Newcastle University;
Division of Biomedical Sciences
St George's, University of London
London, UK

Enrique Oliver Aregullin, MD
Pediatric Cardiologist
Helen DeVos Children's Hospital (Congenital Heart Center CVTS)
Grand Rapids, MI, USA

Sawsan Awad, MD
Associate Professor
Section of Pediatric Cardiology
Rush University Medical Center
Chicago, IL, USA

Carl L. Backer, MD
Division of Cardiovascular-Thoracic Surgery
Ann & Robert H. Lurie Children's Hospital of Chicago;
Department of Surgery
Northwestern University Feinberg School of Medicine
Chicago, IL, USA

Sowmya Balasubramanian, MD, MSc
Clinical Assistant Professor
Division of Cardiology
Department of Pediatrics
Stanford Medical School
Stanford, CA, USA

Piers C.A. Barker, MD
Professor of Pediatrics and Obstetrics and Gynecology
Division of Pediatric Cardiology
Duke University Medical Center
Durham, NC, USA

Sergio Bartakian, MD
Assistant Professor of Pediatrics;
Director of Pediatric and Congenital Cardiac Catheterization Laboratory
Division of Pediatric Cardiology
University of Texas at San Antonio
San Antonio, TX, USA

Aaron Bell, MD
Department of Paediatric Cardiology
Evelina Children's Hospital
London, UK

Hannah Bellsham-Revell, MD
Department of Paediatric Cardiology
Evelina Children's Hospital
London, UK

Darren P. Berman, MD
Co-Director of Cardiac Catheterization and Interventional Therapy
Division of Cardiology
Nationwide Children's Hospital
Columbus, OH, USA

Rebecca S. Beroukhim, MD
Director of Pediatric Echocardiography and Fetal Cardiology
Massachusetts General Hospital for Children
Boston, MA, USA

Deepti Bhat, MD
Pediatric Cardiologist
Cardon Children's Hospital
Mesa, AZ, USA

John W. Bokowski, PhD
Instructor, Section of Pediatric Cardiology
Rush Center for Congenital and Structural Heart Disease
Chicago, IL, USA

William L. Border, MBChB
Director of Noninvasive Cardiac Imaging
Children's Healthcare of Atlanta Sibley Heart Center;
Associate Professor of Pediatrics
Emory University School of Medicine
Atlanta, GA, USA

J. Martijn Bos, MD, PhD
Assistant Professor in Pediatrics
Windland Smith Rice Sudden Death Genomics Laboratory
Mayo Clinic
Rochester, MN, USA

Jessica Bowman, MD
Pediatric Cardiologist
Nationwide Children's Hospital
Columbus, OH, USA

David W. Brown, MD
Pediatric Cardiologist, Director of Clinical Training Program
Department of Cardiology
Boston Children's Hospital;
Associate Professor of Pediatrics
Harvard Medical School
Boston, MA, USA

Nigel A. Brown, MD
Professor
Division of Biomedical Sciences
St George's, University of London
London, UK

Sujatha Budde, MD, MS
Pediatric Cardiologist
Seattle Children's Hospital;
Assistant Professor
Department of Pediatrics
University of Washington School of Medicine
Seattle, WA, USA

Harold M. Burkhart, MD
Professor of Surgery and Chief
Division of Cardiovascular and Thoracic Surgery
University Health Sciences Center
Oklahoma City, OK, USA

Allison K. Cabalka, MD
Professor of Pediatrics
Division of Pediatric Cardiology
Mayo Clinic
Rochester, MN, USA

Bryan Cannon, MD
Associate Professor of Pediatrics;
Director, Pediatric Arrhythmia and Pacing Service
Mayo Clinic
Rochester, MN, USA

Qi-Ling Cao, MD
Medical Director Echo and Research Laboratory
Sidra Cardiovascular Center of Excellence
Sidra Medical and Research Center
Doha, Qatar

Frank Cetta, MD
Professor of Medicine and Pediatrics
Division of Pediatric Cardiology
Mayo Clinic
Rochester, MN, USA

Sarah Chambers Gurson, MD
Pediatric Cardiology Associates PC
Fairfax, VA, USA

Grace Choi, MD
Ann & Robert H. Lurie Children's Hospital of Chicago
Northwestern University Feinberg School of Medicine
Chicago, IL, USA

Nadine Choueiter, MD
Assistant Professor in Pediatrics
Albert Einstein College of Medicine;
Director of Non-Invasive Imaging
Children's Hospital at Montefiore
Bronx, NY, USA

Meryl S. Cohen, MD
Attending Cardiologist, Professor of Pediatrics
Perelman School of Medicine at the University of Pennsylvania;
Director, Cardiology Fellowship Training Program
The Children's Hospital of Philadelphia
Philadelphia, PA, USA

Timothy M. Cordes, MD
Director of Pediatric Echocardiography Laboratory;
Associate Professor of Pediatrics
Riley Children's Hospital,
Indiana University School of Medicine
Indianapolis, IN, USA

Clifford L. Cua, MD
Pediatric Cardiologist
Nationwide Children's Hospital
Columbus, OH, USA

Barbara J. Deal, MD
Division Head, Cardiology
Ann & Robert H. Lurie Children's Hospital;
Getz Professor of Cardiology
Northwestern University Feinberg School of Medicine
Chicago, IL, USA

Joseph A. Dearani, MD
Professor of Surgery
Division of Cardiovascular Surgery
Mayo Clinic
Rochester, MN, USA

Karim A. Diab, MD
Associate Professor
Director of Echocardiography Laboratory
Rush Center for Congenital Heart Disease
Chicago, IL, USA

Adam L. Dorfman, MD
Professor of Pediatrics
Division of Pediatric Cardiology
University of Michigan Congenital Heart Center
C.S. Mott Children's Hospital
Ann Arbor, MI, USA

Howaida El-Said, MD, PhD
Director of the Cardiac Catheterization Laboratory
Rady Children's Hospital, San Diego;
Clinical Professor of Pediatrics at UC San Diego
San Diego, CA, USA

Osama Eltayeb, MD
Assistant Professor of Surgery
Department of Surgery, Northwestern University Feinberg School of Medicine;
Division of Cardiovascular-Thoracic Surgery
Ann & Robert H. Lurie Children's Hospital of Chicago
Chicago, IL, USA

Lowell Frank, MD
Attending Cardiologist and Director of Cardiology Fellowship Training Program
Children's National Medical Center;
Assistant Professor of Pediatrics
George Washington University School of Medicine
Washington, DC, USA

Mark K. Friedberg, MD
Assistant Professor, Department of Pediatrics
University of Toronto;
Co-Director Echo Research Laboratory
Division of Pediatric Cardiology
The Labatt Family Heart Center
Hospital for Sick Children
Toronto, Canada

Miwa K. Geiger, MD
Assistant Professor, Pediatrics
Division of Pediatric Cardiology;
Director, Fetal Heart Program
Mount Sinai Hospital
NY, USA

Salwa Gendi, MD
Assistant Professor of Pediatrics
University of Mississippi Medical Center
Jackson, MS, USA

Tal Geva, MD
Cardiologist-in-Chief
Department of Cardiology
Boston Children's Hospital;
Professor of Pediatrics
Harvard Medical School
Boston, MA, USA

Donald J. Hagler, MD
Professor of Pediatrics and Medicine
Division of Pediatric Cardiology
Mayo Clinic
Rochester, MN, USA

Denise A. Hayes, MD
Assistant Professor
Hofstra Northwell School of Medicine;
Pediatric Cardiologist
Cohen Children's Medical Center
Queens, NY, USA

Camden L. Hebson, MD
Assistant Professor of Medicine
Division of Cardiology
Department of Medicine
Emory University School of Medicine
Atlanta, GA, USA

Ziyad M. Hijazi, MD, MPH
Acting Chief Medical Officer - Chair of the Department of Pediatrics & Director
Sidra Cardiovascular Center of Excellence
Doha, Qatar

Ralf J. Holzer, MD
Chief, Division of Pediatric Cardiology
New York-Presbyterian/Weill Cornell Medical Center;
Director of Pediatric Cardiac Catheterization
The Komansky Children's Hospital
New York, NY, USA

Lisa Hornberger, MD
Professor of Pediatrics and Obstetrics and Gynecology
University of Alberta;
Director of Fetal and Neonatal Cardiology Program,
Section Head of Pediatric Echocardiography
Stollery Children's Hospital
Edmonton, Alberta, Canada

James C. Huhta, MD
Pediatric Cardiology Associates
St. Petersburg, FL, USA;
Professor of Pediatrics, Adjunct Professor
Institute of Clinical Medicine
University of Tromso, Norway

Darren Hutchinson, MBBS
Paediatric and Fetal Cardiologist
Department of Cardiology
Royal Children's Hospital Melbourne
Victoria, Australia

Amish Jain, MD
Division of Neonatology
Department of Pediatrics
Mount Sinai Hospital;
Department of Pediatrics
University of Toronto
Toronto, Canada

Jonathan N. Johnson, MD
Assistant Professor of Pediatrics
Division of Pediatric Cardiology
Mayo Clinic
Rochester, MN, USA

Supaluck Kanjanauthai, MD
Advocate Heart Institute for Children
Department of Pediatric Cardiology
Advocate Children's Hospital
Oak Lawn Campus
Oak Lawn, IL, USA

Deepak Kaura, MD
Executive Chair
Foundation Medical Services
Sidra Medical and Research Center
Doha, Qatar

Damien Kenny, MB, MD
Pediatric Cardiologist
Our Lady's Children's Hospital
Crumlin, Dublin, Ireland

H. Helen Ko, BS
Technical Director/Operations Manager of Pediatric Echocardiography
Division of Pediatric Cardiology
Mount Sinai Medical Center
New York, NY, USA

Peter Koenig, MD
Ann & Robert H. Lurie Children's Hospital of Chicago
Northwestern University Feinberg School of Medicine
Chicago, IL, USA

Wyman W. Lai, MD, MPH
Medical Director, Echocardiography and Co-Medical Director
Heart Institute, Children's Hospital of Orange County
Orange, CA, USA

Leo Lopez, MD
Director of Cardiac Non-Invasive Imaging
Nicklaus Children's Hospital;
Clinical Professor of Pediatrics
Herbert Wertheim College of Medicine
Florida International University
Miami, FL, USA

Irene D. Lytrivi, MD
Associate Professor of Pediatrics
Division of Pediatric Cardiology
Mount Sinai Medical Center
New York, NY, USA

Kiran K. Mallula, MD
Assistant Professor of Clinical Pediatrics
Division of Cardiology
Louisiana State University School of Medicine;
Interventional Cardiologist
Children's Hospital of New Orleans
New Orleans, LA, USA

Samer Masri, MD
Pediatric Cardiologist
American University of Beirut
Beirut, Lebanon

Marie McDonald, MD
Professor of Pediatrics
Division of Medical Genetics
Department of Pediatrics
Duke University Medical Center
Durham, NC, USA

Timothy J. Mohun, PhD
Developmental Biology Division
The Francis Crick Institute Mill Hill Laboratory
London, UK

Michael C. Mongé, MD
Division of Cardiovascular-Thoracic Surgery
Ann & Robert H. Lurie Children's Hospital of Chicago
Department of Surgery
Northwestern University Feinberg School of Medicine
Chicago, IL, USA

Anita J. Moon-Grady, MD
Professor, Clinical Pediatrics;
Director, Fetal Cardiovascular Program
University of California at San Francisco
San Francisco, CA, USA

Gareth J. Morgan, MD
Pediatric Cardiologist
Children's Hospital of Colorado;
Associate Professor of Pediatrics
University of Colorado School of Medicine
Aurora, CO, USA

Shaine A. Morris, MD, MPH
Pediatric Cardiology and Cardiac Non-Invasive Imaging
Texas Children's Hospital;
Assistant Professsor – Pediatrics-Cardiology
Baylor College of Medicine
Houston, TX, USA

Brieann Muller, MD
Assistant Professor of Pediatrics
Section of Pediatric Cardiology
Rush University Medical Center
Chicago, IL, USA

John J. Nigro, MD
Chief of Cardiac Surgery
Rady Children's Hospital;
Director, Rady Children's Heart Institute
Rady Children's Hospital-San Diego
San Diego, CA, USA

Patrick W. O'Leary, MD
Consultant, Division of Pediatric Cardiology;
Professor of Pediatrics, College of Medicine
Mayo Clinic
Rochester, MN, USA

Neil D. Patel, MD
Fellow in Pediatric Cardiology
Children's Hospital of Los Angeles
Los Angeles, CA, USA

Andrada R. Popescu, MD
Division of Cardiovascular-Thoracic Surgery
Ann & Robert H. Lurie Children's Hospital of Chicago;
Assistant Professor of Radiology
Department of Surgery
Northwestern University Feinberg School of Medicine
Chicago, IL, USA

Stephen Pophal, MD
Division of Cardiology
Phoenix Children's Hospital
Phoenix, AZ, USA

Rajesh Punn, MD
Clinical Assistant Professor
Division of Pediatric Cardiology
Department of Pediatrics
Stanford Medical School
Stanford, CA, USA

Robert Puntel, MD
Division of Cardiology
Phoenix Children's Hospital
Phoenix, AZ, USA

Michael D. Quartermain, MD
Division of Cardiology
The Children's Hospital of Philadelphia and Perelman School of Medicine
University of Pennsylvania
Philadelphia, PA, USA

Muhammad Yasir Qureshi, MBBS
Division of Pediatric Cardiology
Mayo Clinic
Rochester, MN, USA

Shakeel A. Qureshi, MD
Professor and Consultant Paediatric Cardiologist
Evelina London Children's Hospital
London, UK

Randy Richardson, MD
Department of Radiology
St. Joseph's Hospital and Medical Center
Creighton University School of Medicine
Phoenix, AZ, USA

Anthony F. Rossi, MD
Director of Cardiac Critical Care
The Heart Program
Nicklaus Children's Hospital
Miami, FL, USA

Hyde M. Russell, MD
Department of Surgery
Northwestern University Feinberg School of Medicine
Division of Cardiovascular-Thoracic Surgery
Ann & Robert H. Lurie Children's Hospital of Chicago
Chicago, IL, USA

Justin Ryan, PhD
Division of Cardiology
Phoenix Children's Hospital
Phoenix, AZ, USA

Sameh M. Said, MD
Instructor of Surgery
Division of Cardiovascular Surgery
Mayo Clinic
Rochester, MN, USA

Vikas Sharma, MBBS
Assistant Professor of Surgery, Thoracic and Cardiac Surgery
University of Utah Health Care-Hospital and Clinics
Salt Lake City, UT, USA

Gregory J. Schears, MD
Professor of Anesthesiology
Mayo Clinic
Rochester, MN, USA

Ira Shetty, MD
Department of Pediatric Cardiology
Advocate Heart Institute for Children
Advocate Children's Hospital
Oak Lawn Campus
Oak Lawn, IL, USA

Timothy C. Slesnick, MD
Director of Pediatric Cardiac Magnetic Resonance Imaging;
Pediatric Cardiologist, Sibley Heart Center
Children's Healthcare of Atlanta;
Associate Professor of Pediatrics
Emory University
Atlanta, GA, USA

Shubhika Srivastava, MBBS
Professor of Pediatrics;
Director of Echocardiography Laboratory
Division of Pediatric Cardiology
Mount Sinai Medical Center
New York, NY, USA

Nicole Sutton, MD
Assistant Professor of Pediatrics
Albert Einsein College of Medicine;
Pediatric Cardiologist
Children's Hospital at Montefiore
Bronx, NY, USA

Nathaniel W. Taggart, MD
Assistant Professor of Pediatrics
Division of Pediatric Cardiology
Mayo Clinic
Rochester, MN, USA

Gregory H. Tatum, MD
Associate Professor of Pediatrics
Division of Pediatric Cardiology
Duke University Medical Center
Durham, NC, USA

Darshit Thakrar, MD
Assistant Professor of Radiology
University of Pittsburgh
Pittsburgh, PA, USA

Sabrina Tsao, MBBS
Director, Electrophysiology
Division of Cardiology
Ann & Robert H. Lurie Children's Hospital;
Assistant Professor of Pediatrics (Cardiology)
Feinberg School of Medicine
Northwestern University Feinberg School of Medicine
Chicago, IL, USA

Gregory Webster, MD, MPH
Director, Electrocardiogram Laboratory, Cardiology
Ann & Robert H. Lurie Children's Hospital;
Assistant Professor of Pediatrics
Northwestern University Feinberg School of Medicine
Chicago, IL, USA

Stephanie Burns Wechsler, MD
Associate Professor of Pediatrics
Divisions of Pediatric Cardiology and Medical Genetics
Duke University Medical Center
Durham, NC, USA

Mark Wylam, MD
Associate Professor of Pediatrics and Medicine
Division of Pediatric Pulmonology and Critical Care Medicine
Department of Pediatric and Adolescent Medicine
Mayo Clinic
Rochester, MN, USA

Evan M. Zahn, MD
Director
Congenital Heart Program and Division of Pediatric Cardiology
Cedars-Sinai Medical Center
Los Angeles, CA, USA

Mark V. Zilberman, MD
Director, Pediatric Echocardiology and Fetal Cardiology;
Pediatric Cardiologist, Boston Floating Children's Hospital;
Associate Professor of Pediatrics
Tufts University School of Medicine
Boston, MA, USA

Part I

Prenatal and Perinatal Issues

1

Cardiac Embryology and Embryopathy

Robert H. Anderson [1,2], *Nigel A. Brown* [2], *and Timothy J. Mohun* [3]

[1] *Institute of Genetic Medicine, Newcastle University, UK*
[2] *Division of Biomedical Sciences, St. George's, University of London, UK*
[3] *Developmental Biology Division, The Francis Crick Institute Mill Hill Laboratory, London, UK*

As long ago as the beginning of the twentieth century, Abbott [1] argued that knowledge of embryology was essential for interpretation of congenital cardiac malformations. Only recently, however, have the necessary facts regarding the formation of the heart been sufficiently robust to underscore interpretations of the morphology of the lesions themselves. Our knowledge of cardiac development, based as it is on evidence rather than speculation, is now sufficient to help in understanding the morphology, not only of the normal heart, but also most significant congenital cardiac malformations. The advances have been made possible in no small part by the development of techniques that reveal the three-dimensional changes occurring during the processes of cardiac development [2].

Initial Stages of Development

When first recognized as having endodermal, ectodermal, and mesodermal germ layers, the developing human embryo is discoid, and the endodermal and ectodermal layers are continuous at the margins of the disc with the walls of the amnion and the yolk sac, respectively [3]. Already at this early stage, the presence of the primitive streak, with the node at its cranial end, permits recognition of the right and left sides of the developing embryo. During the subsequent stage of gastrulation, cells migrate into the mesodermal region on both sides through the primitive streak, fusing to produce the cardiac crescent. Concomitant with embryonic folding, there is folding of a trough derived from the heart-forming areas that produces the primary linear heart tube. It used to be thought that all the components of the definitive heart were present in the original tube. It is now known that, with ongoing development, new material is added to the tube at both its ends. The material of the initial tube eventually provides no more than the apex of the left ventricle (LV), and part of the muscular ventricular septum [4]. It remains moot as to whether the newly migrating cells are derived from a so-called second heart field, and whether this alleged field itself has cranial and caudal components. Suffice it to say that new cells, both myocardial and non-myocardial, continue to be added at both ends of the heart tube as it loops and separates into its right and left sides [5].

Looping of the Heart Tube

Development of the human heart is usually described using the Carnegie stages, which extend from 1 through 23, although the heart continues to show marked morphologic changes subsequent to stage 23, which is equivalent to about 8 weeks of development. The heart becomes recognizable at stage 9, equivalent to about 20 days of development. The myocardial part is then no more than a strip, anterior to paired vascular channels, with endocardial jelly interposed between the myocardial and endothelial layers [3]. By the next stage, the myocardial component has folded around the vascular elements, which are now fused to produce a tube with a solitary lumen. The connections of the lumen with the developing embryonic circulatory systems then permit recognition of the arterial and venous poles of the tube. At stage 11, representing about 25 days of development, it is possible to recognize the ventricular loop, with the atrioventricular (AV) canal positioned between the developing atrial component and the inlet of the loop. These features are seen in the developing mouse at embryonic day 9.5 (Figure 1.1). Looping is a key feature of development. The tube usually curves to the right, with the apical component of the LV then developing from the inlet part of the loop, and the apical part of the right ventricle (RV) from the outlet (Figure 1.2). The apical components of the ventricles, therefore, develop

Visual Guide to Neonatal Cardiology, First Edition. Edited by Ernerio T. Alboliras, Ziyad M. Hijazi, Leo Lopez, and Donald J. Hagler.

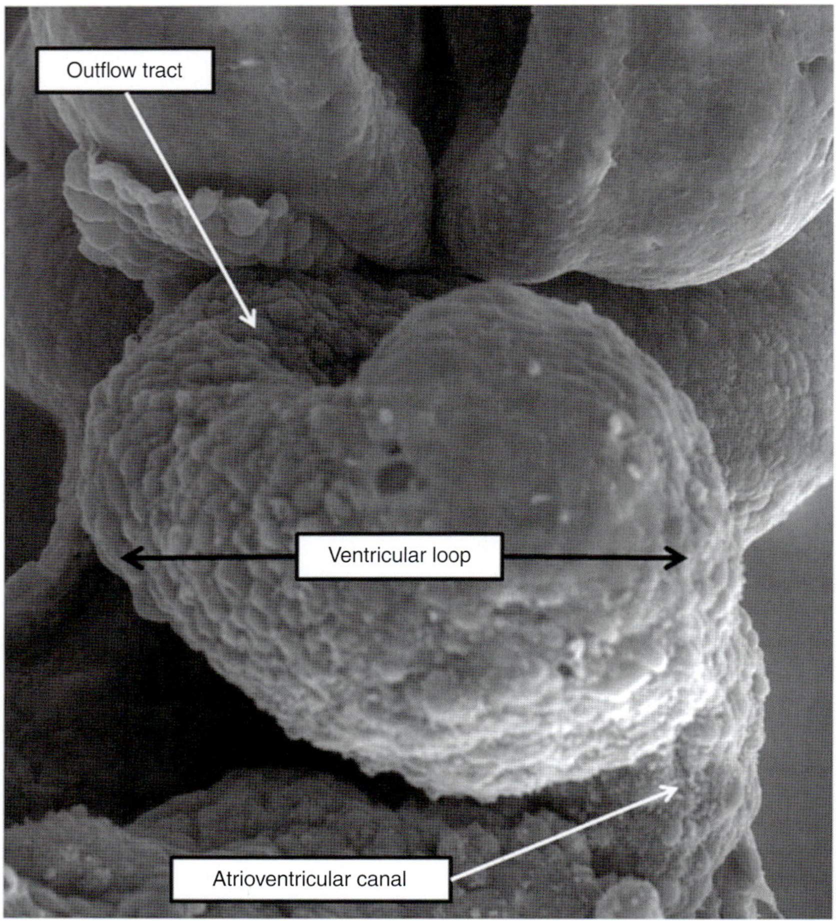

Figure 1.1 The scanning electron micrograph image shows the developing heart of the mouse at E9.5. The heart has been revealed by removing the ventral wall of the pericardial cavity. The ventricular loop extends from the atrioventricular (AV) canal, and supports the outflow tract.

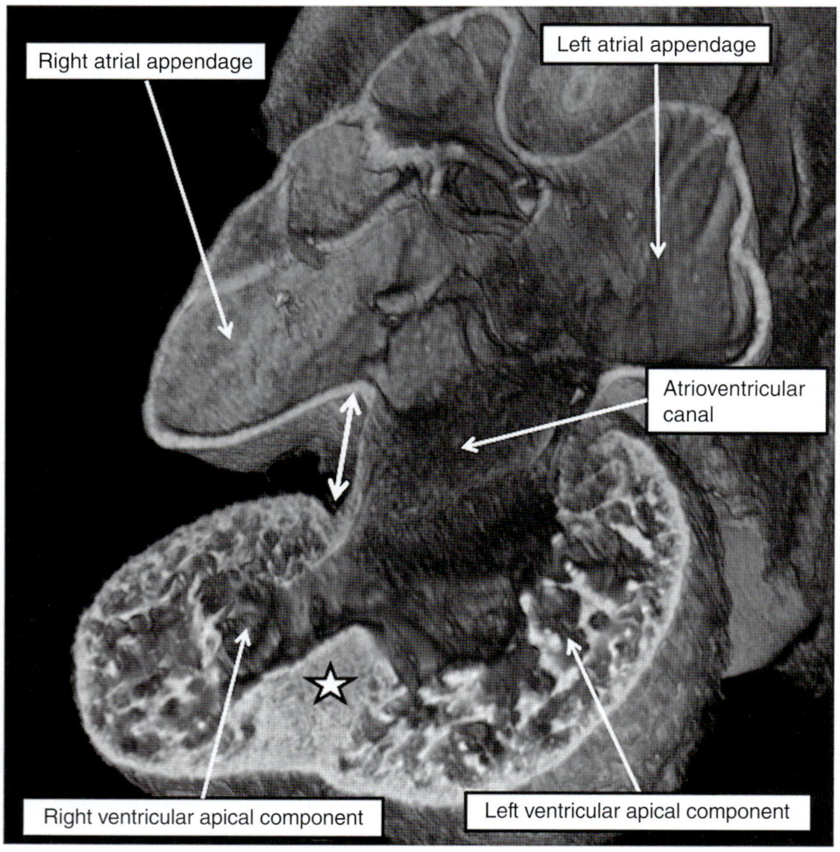

Figure 1.2 The image is prepared using an episcopic dataset from a developing mouse embryo early on embryonic day 11.5. The four-chamber section shows how the atrial appendages are beginning to balloon in parallel fashion from the common atrial chamber, while the apical components of the developing ventricles are ballooning in series from the ventricular loop. The process of ballooning of the apical ventricular components produces the muscular ventricular septum formed between them (star). The AV canal connects predominantly to the developing left ventricle (LV), but already its right wall has provided contiguity between the right atrium (RA) and the developing right ventricle (RV; double-headed white arrow).

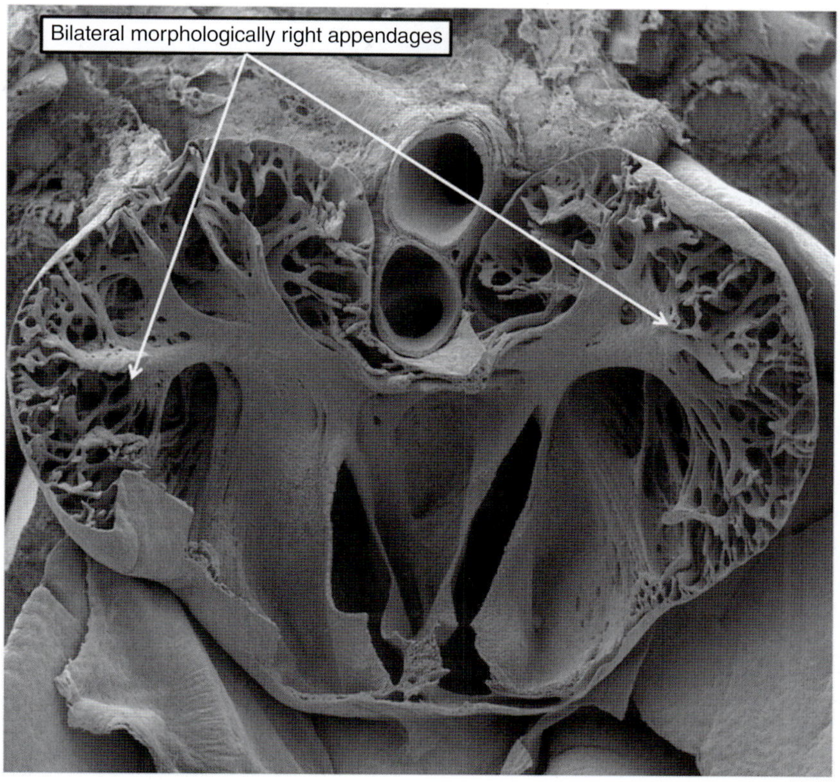

Figure 1.3 The scanning electron microscopic image prepared from a *Pitx2c* knock-out mouse shows the atrial chambers, viewed from the ventricular aspect, having cut the heart in its short axis. There is isomerism of the RA appendages.

in series, unlike the atrial appendages, which develop in parallel from the atrial component of the developing heart. In the setting of visceral heterotaxy, therefore, in which there is isomerism of those features that are usually lateralized, it is only the atrial appendages that show evidence of symmetry [6]. Indeed, isomeric right atrial appendages are the prime cardiac feature of mice genetically modified by knocking out *Pitx2c* [7], one of the genes responsible for producing morphologic leftness (Figure 1.3). For the ventricles, however, because the apical part of each ventricle develops from a part of the tube containing both the initial right and left sides, knocking out *Pitx2c* does not produce evidence of ventricular isomerism. The direction of ventricular looping is random in the syndromes of visceral heterotaxy [8].

The Process of Ballooning

Subsequent to looping, it is possible to recognize the morphologic features of the developing cardiac chambers. The relations of the atrial appendages to the developing AV canal permit distinction of the morphologically right and left atrial chambers, while it is the eventual structure of the apical components that distinguishes between the definitive RV and LV. These parts, the appendages and the apical components, are produced by the process now described as ballooning [9]. Remodeling of the initial cavity of the linear tube then permits the atrial cavities, subsequent to their separation, to become connected directly to their respective ventricles, and the arterial trunks to be brought into union with their appropriate ventricles. When the ventricular loop is first seen, however, the circumference of the AV canal is supported almost exclusively by the developing LV (Figure 1.4), while the developing outlet component, which has a solitary lumen, arises in its entirety from the developing RV. The default options for development therefore are double inlet to the LV, and double outlet from the RV. When first formed, furthermore, the RV possesses only apical trabecular and outlet components (Figure 1.5), although from the outset its wall is continuous through the right side of the AV canal with the developing right atrium (RA; Figure 1.2).

Formation of the Atrial Chambers

The systemic venous tributaries drain to the developing atrial component of the heart tube at the venous pole. This situation, established by Carnegie stage 11 in the human heart, is equivalent to embryonic day 9.5 in the mouse. At this early stage, the atrial part of the heart tube is also attached to the pharyngeal mesenchyme through the dorsal mesocardium. The systemic venous tributaries initially open in relatively symmetrical fashion to either side of this area of attachment. The reflections of the pharyngeal mesenchyme in the area of the attachment

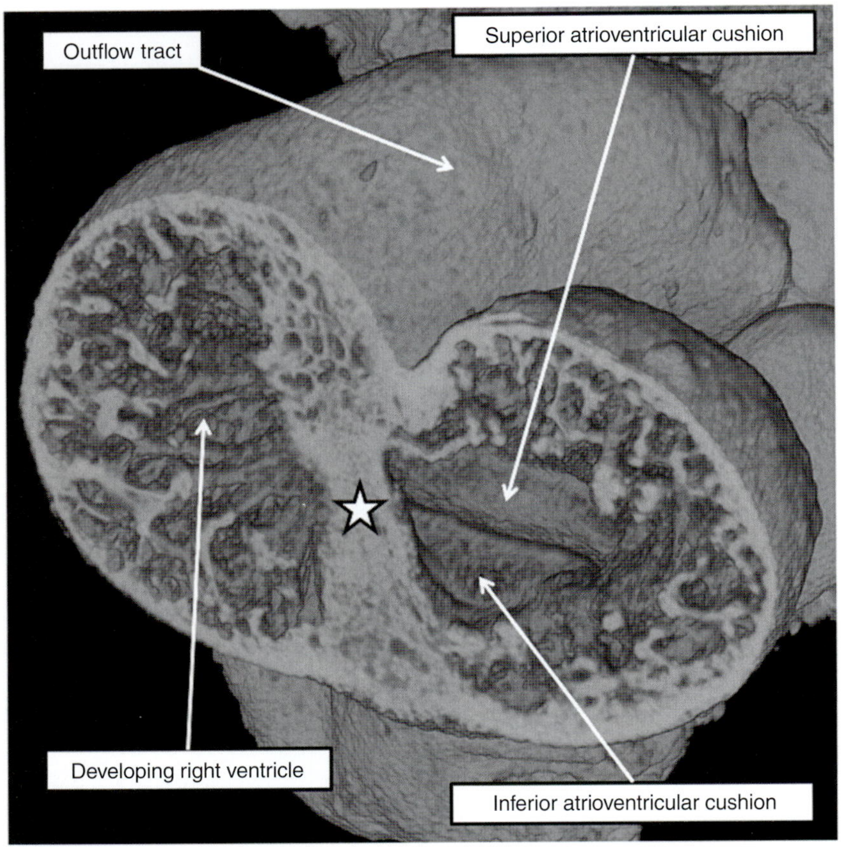

Figure 1.4 The image is from an episcopic dataset prepared from a mouse at early embryonic day 11.5. A short axis cut has been made through the ventricular loop, which is then viewed from the aspect of the transected apical components. The star shows the developing ventricular septum. The opening between the AV cushions opens exclusively into the cavity of the developing LV. The outflow tract is supported by the developing RV.

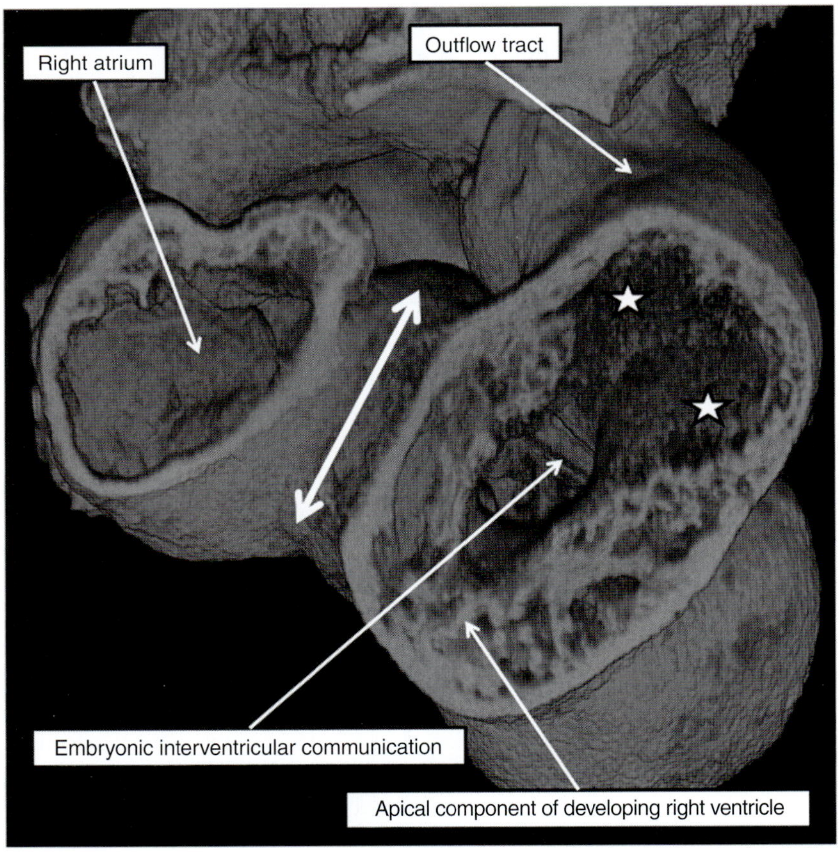

Figure 1.5 The image is from an episcopic dataset prepared from a mouse at early embryonic day 11.5. The apical trabecular component of the RV is beginning to balloon from the outlet component of the ventricular loop. As yet, there is no direct communication between the cavities of the RA and the RV, the blood flowing into the developing RV through the embryonic interventricular communication. Already, however, the right wall of the AV canal (double-headed arrow) provides continuity between the RA and RV walls. The outflow tract arises exclusively from the RV, with the proximal outflow cushions already visible within its lumen (stars).

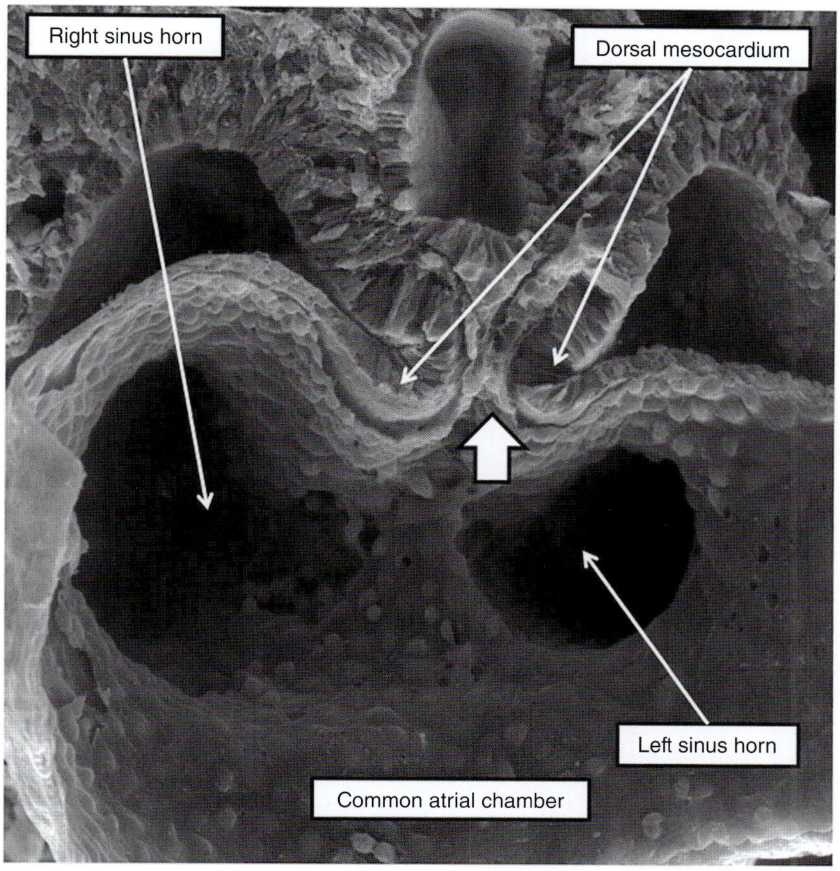

Figure 1.6 The scanning electron micrograph image shows evidence of the initial symmetry of the systemic venoatrial connections at embryonic day 9.5 in the mouse, albeit that the left horn is smaller than the right. The section is taken through the dorsal mesocardium, and shows the pulmonary pit (thick arrow). As yet, there is no formation of the lungs.

enclose a midline pit (Figure 1.6). With subsequent formation of the lungs, and canalization of a venous channel in the mediastinum, the blood from both developing lungs enters the atrial cavity through this pit. By the time the pulmonary vein has canalized and gained its cardiac connection, there has been realignment of the left-sided systemic venous channels. Thus, during E10.5 in the mouse, the left-sided systemic venous tributary becomes incorporated into the developing left AV groove. As it is incorporated within the groove, it retains its own walls (Figure 1.7). Folds then become evident within the developing RA. Known as the venous valves, they guard the entrances of the systemic venous tributaries, now recognizable in the human heart as the superior and inferior caval vein and the coronary sinus, the latter formed from the left sinus horn (Figure 1.8). Should the intrapericardial part of this left-sided channel persist postnatally, it is seen as the left superior caval vein, which is always present in the mouse heart. The pulmonary vein in humans initially has a solitary atrial orifice, which empties into the left atrium (LA) adjacent to the left AV junction (Figure 1.9). Only much later in humans does the pulmonary venous component enlarge in size, with the veins migrating onto the atrial roof so that, eventually, one vein connects at each corner of the definitive LA [10]. A similar expansion in mouse produces a fold dorsally between the connections of the pulmonary veins to the LA, and the wall of the RA (Figure 1.10). Remodeling of the pulmonary venous component is part and parcel of the processes of atrial septation.

Atrial Septation

Atrial septation is heralded by the appearance of the primary atrial septum, or septum primum, in the atrial roof (Figure 1.7). The primary septum grows towards the AV canal, interposing between the openings of the systemic channels, now committed to the RA, and the orifice of the newly formed pulmonary vein (Figure 1.11). Within the AV canal, the process known as endothelial-to-mesenchymal transformation has already converted the endocardial jelly into superior and inferior AV cushions (Figure 1.10). The space between the leading edge of the primary atrial septum and the atrial surfaces of the cushions is the primary atrial foramen, or "ostium primum." The cranial border of the foramen is formed by a mesenchymal cap carried on the leading edge of the developing primary atrial septum (Figure 1.11). Continuing growth of the primary septum

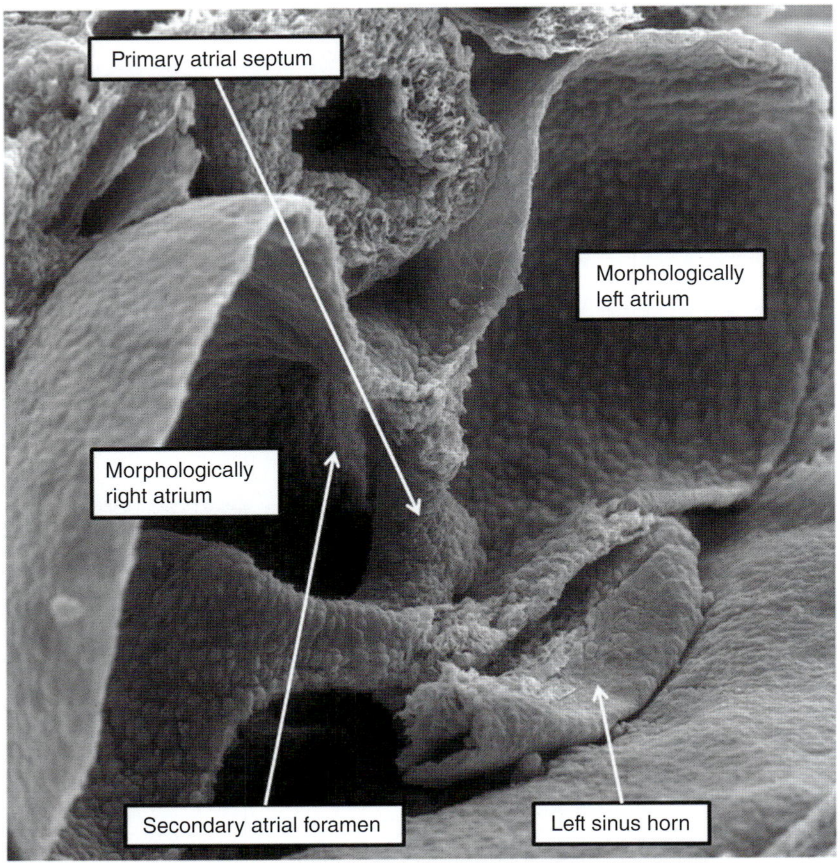

Figure 1.7 The scanning electron microscopic image shows the atrial chambers, viewed from the aspect of the removed ventricular chambers, from a developing mouse heart obtained late at E10.5. The dissection shows how the left sinus horn, with its own discrete walls, has become incorporated into the developing left AV junction. Note the secondary atrial foramen.

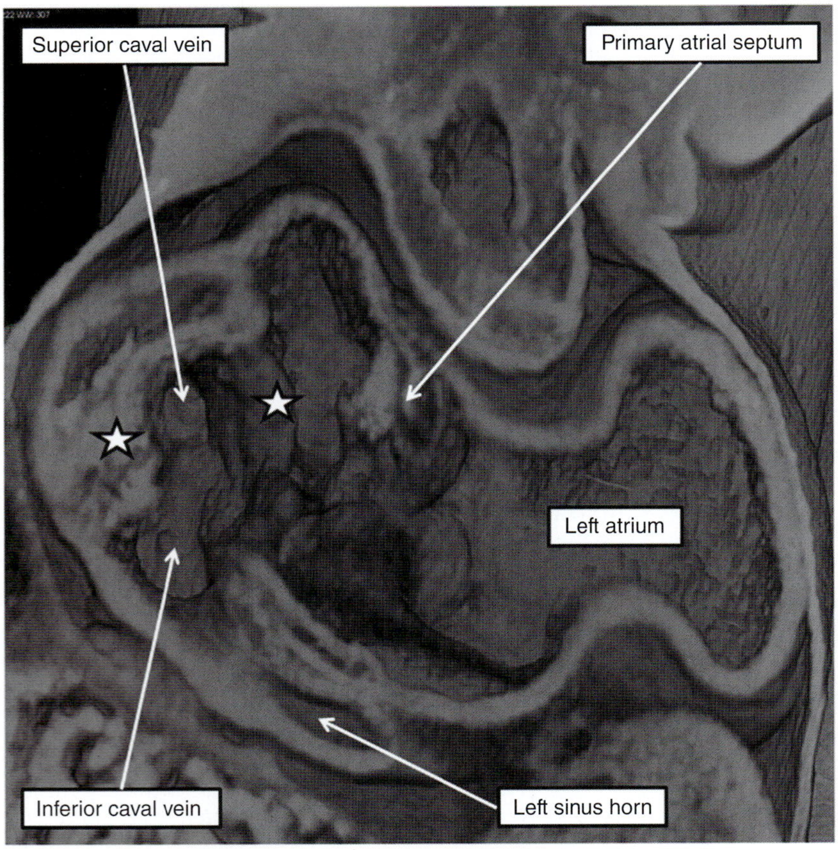

Figure 1.8 The image is from an episcopic dataset prepared from a human embryo at Carnegie stage 14. It shows the atrial cavities viewed from the ventricular aspect. The left sinus horn has been incorporated in the left AV groove, and the openings of the caval veins are seen within the confines of the venous valves (stars). Note the location of the primary atrial septum, which is growing from the atrial roof.

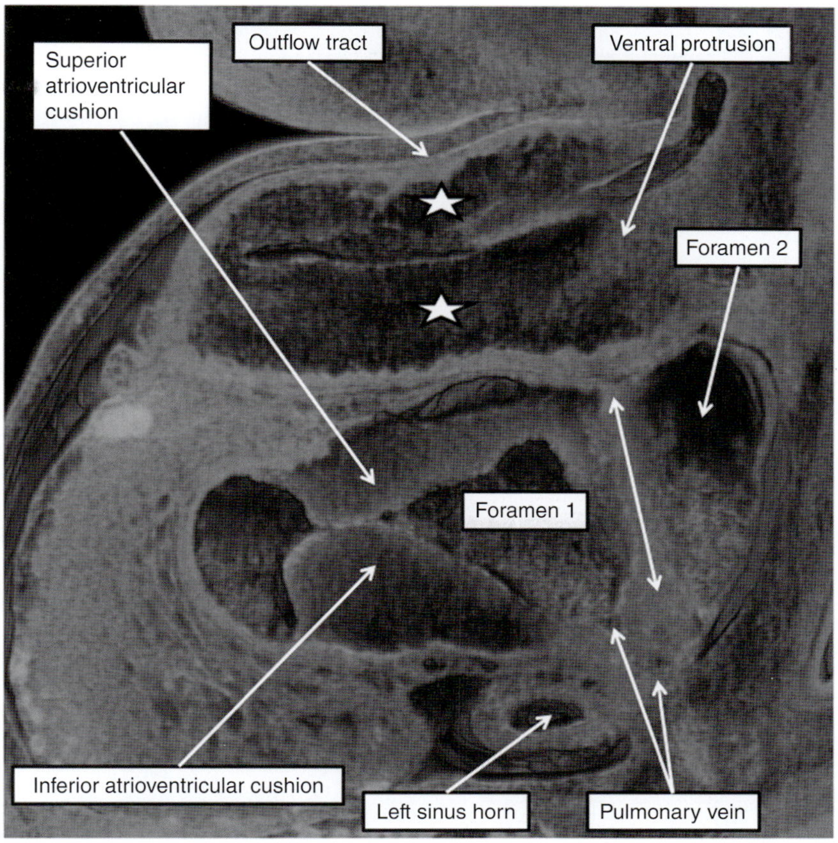

Figure 1.9 The image is from the same dataset as shown in Figure 1.8, but is cut in the sagittal plane, replicating the long axis parasternal echocardiographic plane. It shows the AV cushions facing one another in the AV canal, and the outflow cushions (stars) extending the full length of the outflow tract. Note also the ventral protrusion from the dorsal wall of the aortic sac. The section also cuts through the solitary pulmonary vein, and its entrance to the developing LA, which at this stage is adjacent to the developing AV junction. The double-headed white arrow shows the sectioned primary atrial septum, which separated the primary (Foramen 1) and secondary (Foramen 2) atrial foramens. Note the discrete walls of the left sinus horn, now incorporated within the left AV junction.

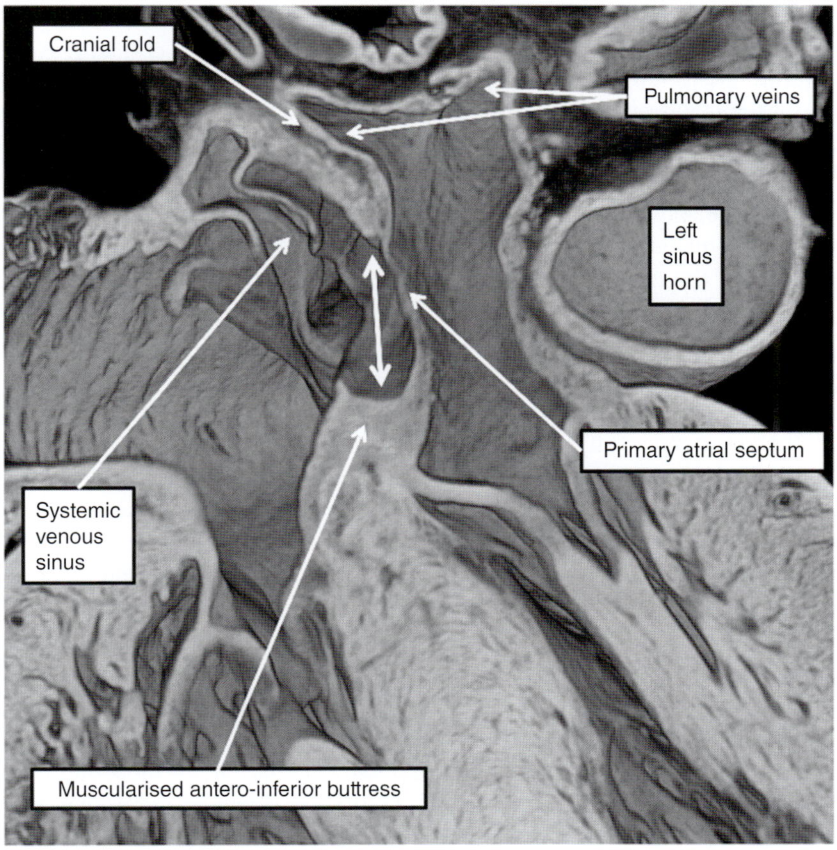

Figure 1.10 The four-chamber section is prepared from an episcopic dataset from a mouse heart at embryonic day 18.5. The mesenchymal cap and vestibular spine have muscularized to form the anteroinferior buttress of the oval fossa (double-headed white arrow). The cranial margin of the fossa, however, is a deep fold between the RA wall and the attachments of the pulmonary veins to the LA. The floor of the oval fossa is formed by the primary atrial septum. Note the discrete walls of the left sinus horn, which in the mouse persists as a left superior caval vein.

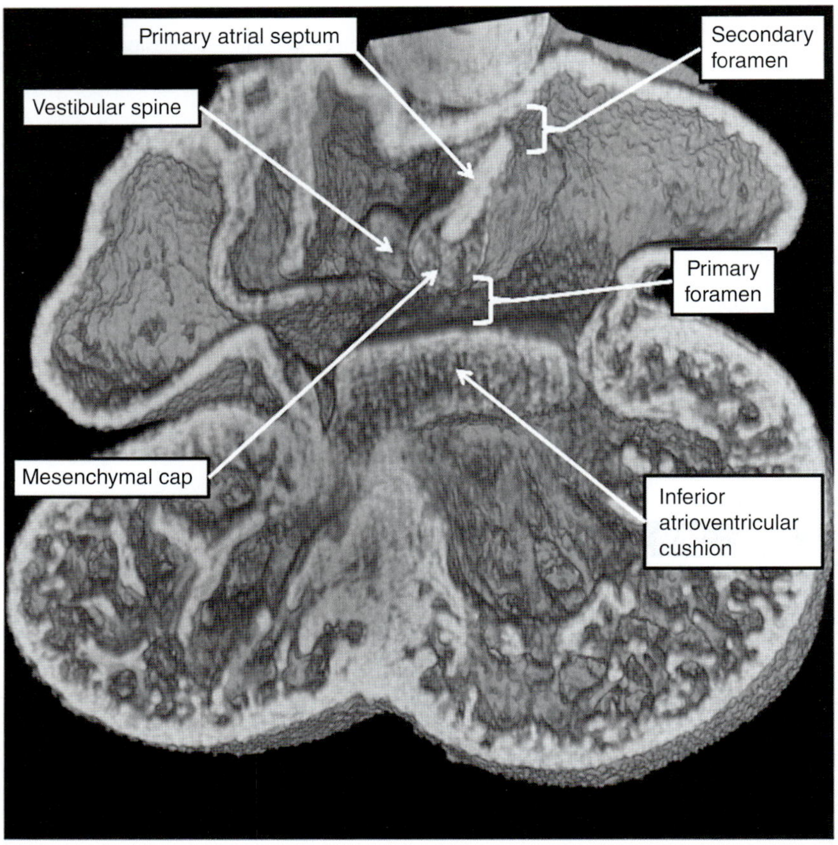

Figure 1.11 The four-chamber section is from an episcopic dataset prepared from a mouse heart at embryonic day 11.5. It shows the building blocks of the atrial septum. The primary septum has broken away from the atrial roof to form the secondary foramen. The space between the mesenchymal cap on its leading edge and the inferior AV cushion is the primary atrial foramen. Note the vestibular spine at the leading edge of the valves guarding the systemic venous sinus of the RA.

then reduces the size of the primary foramen. Before the primary foramen can close, the cranial origin of the septum breaks down, producing the secondary atrial foramen, or "foramen secundum." This second hole is an essential component of the developing fetal circulation, because the richly oxygenated blood derived from the placenta needs to reach the left side of the developing heart. It is fusion of the mesenchymal cap with the atrial surfaces of the AV endocardial cushions that obliterates the primary foramen, with the process reinforced by additional intracardiac migration of tissues from the pharyngeal mesenchyme.

The new cells enter the heart through the right margin of the pulmonary pit, which expands to become the vestibular spine (Figure 1.12). Expansion of the spine carries forward the inferior ends of the venous valves, anchoring them to the right side of the fused endocardial cushions. The mesenchymal tissues derived from the cap and the spine (Figure 1.13) subsequently muscularize to form the anteroinferior buttress of the definitive atrial septum, with the primary atrial septum forming the floor of the oval fossa (Figure 1.10). Although the cranial margin of the oval fossa is often depicted as growing from the atrial roof, this margin in the postnatal heart is a fold rather than a muscular ridge. It is not seen during development until after the right pulmonary veins have achieved their definitive position on the roof of the LA. In the mouse, the fold is produced dorsally rather than cranially. As in humans, it does not become apparent until after the pulmonary veins have remodeled towards the end of development (Figure 1.10).

Full anatomic fusion between the flap valve derived from the primary septum and the rims of the oval foramen occurs in only three-quarters to two-thirds of the overall population [11]. Lack of anatomic fusion results in persistent patency of the oval foramen. A short primary septum, or perforations within it, produces the "secundum" defects, which should properly be described as "foramen secundum" defects, or better considered as holes within the oval fossa. Inappropriate fusion and muscularization of the components of the anteroinferior buttress can also produce holes within the septum, which are well described as vestibular defects [12]. The "ostium primum" defect is an AV, rather than an atrial, septal defect. Its pathognomonic feature is the presence of a common AV junction, along with a trifoliate left AV valve. The feature underscoring this, and other AV septal defects with common AV junction, is failure of formation of the vestibular spine (compare Figures 1.13 and 1.14) [13]. The sinus venosus defect is the consequence of abnormal connection of one or more of the right pulmonary veins to the superior or inferior caval vein, with the anomalous pulmonary vein or veins retaining its or their LA connection [14]. The known spectrum of

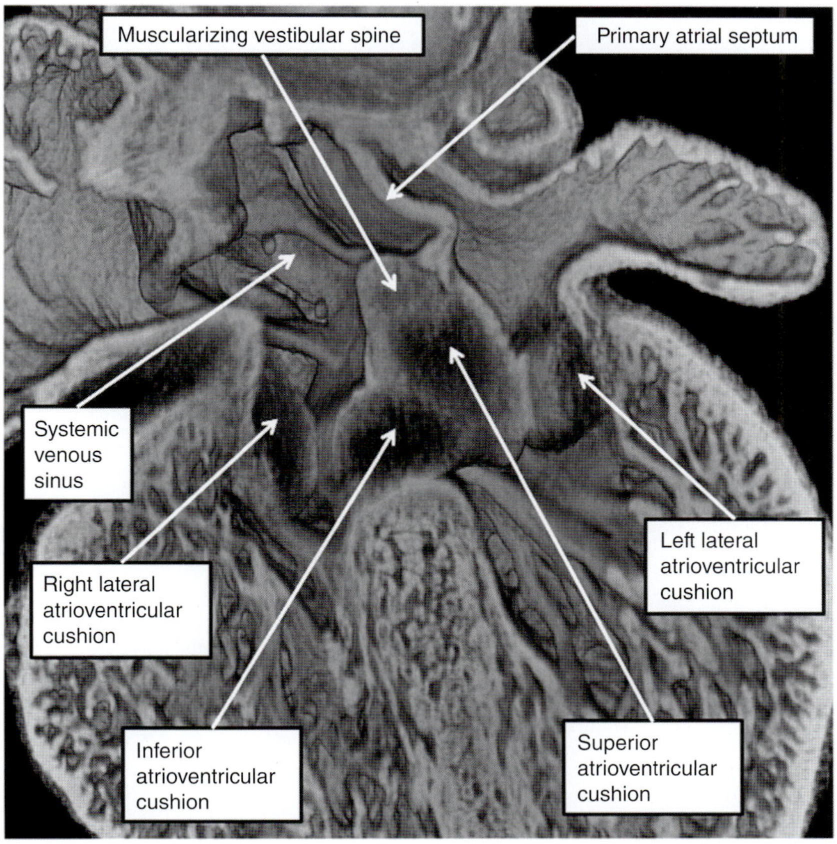

Figure 1.12 The four-chamber section is from an episcopic dataset prepared from a mouse heart at embryonic day 13.5. The mesenchymal cap on the atrial septum has fused with the AV cushions to close the primary atrial foramen. The section is cut more dorsally, and shows how the vestibular spine has reinforced the right side of the area of fusion. The spine is beginning to muscularize to form the anteroinferior buttress of the oval fossa (see Figure 1.10).

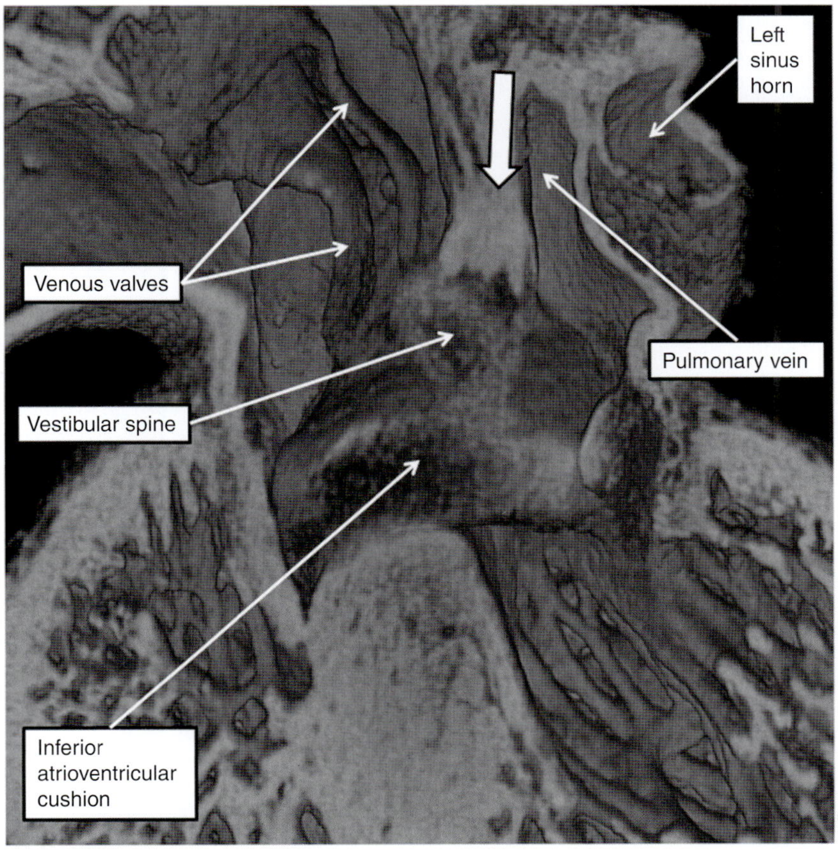

Figure 1.13 The four-chamber section is from an episcopic dataset prepared from a mouse heart at embryonic day 12.5. It shows the vestibular spine growing from the site of the right pulmonary ridge. The arrow shows the connection with the pharyngeal mesenchyme. The spine is carrying forward to inferior zone of apposition of the venous valves that guard the systemic venous sinus. Note the left superior caval vein, derived from the left sinus horn, entering the left AV junction.

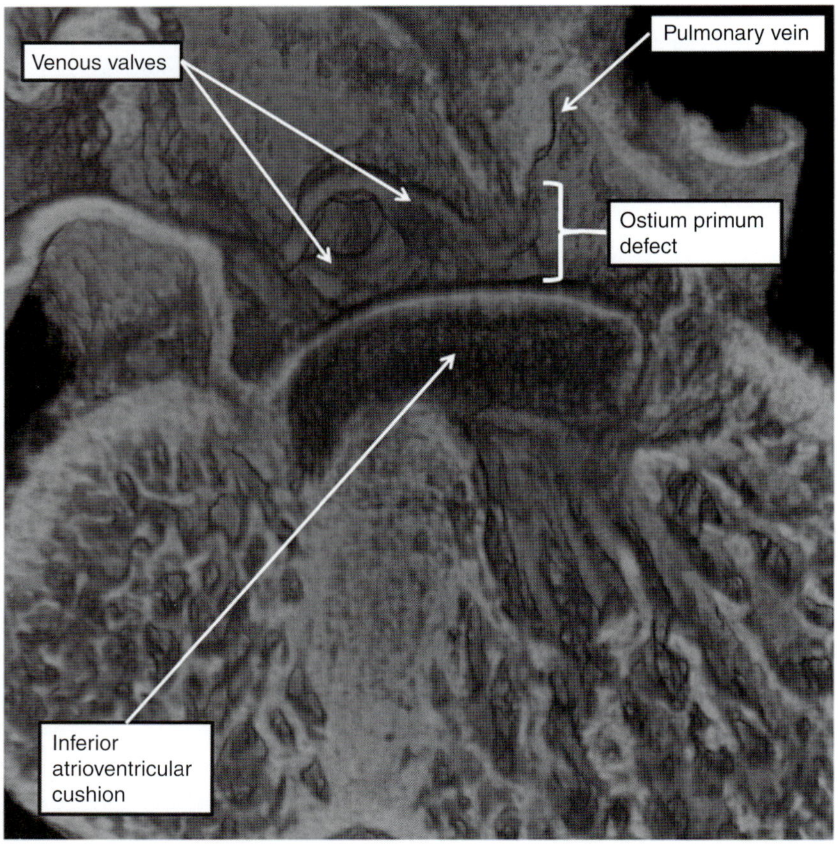

Figure 1.14 The four-chamber section is from an episcopic dataset prepared from a *Tbx1* null mouse at embryonic day 12.5. The mouse has an AV septal defect, with this section showing the ostium primum defect. There is total lack of formation of the vestibular spine. Note the hypoplastic nature of the right pulmonary ridge.

malformations, which extends from fenestration of the coronary sinus to its complete unroofing, shows that erosion of walls of both the coronary sinus and the LA are required to produce the coronary sinus defect [15].

Ventricular Development

Ballooning of the apical trabecular components from the ventricular loop heralds the appearance of the apical muscular ventricular septum. When first seen, the primary interventricular foramen is bounded by the crest of the muscular septum and the inner heart curvature (Figure 1.15). This foramen is never closed. Instead, it is remodeled so that the right half of the AV canal is placed in direct communication with the apical part of the RV, and the developing aortic outlet brought into communication with the apical part of the LV. Prior to remodeling of the foramen, the right AV groove interposes between the cavities of the developing RA and RV (Figure 1.5). Failure of expansion of this groove produces classic tricuspid atresia, which is a result of absence of the right AV connection [16]. With normal remodeling of the AV canal, the apical muscular interventricular septum is brought in line with the underside of the fused AV cushions, the RA then connecting directly with the cavity of the RV (Figure 1.16).

The formation of additional lateral cushions in the newly created ventricular inlets then sets the scene for development of the leaflets of the tricuspid valve (TV) and mitral valve (MV) (Figure 1.17). In the right-sided channel, the lateral cushion forms the primordiums of the anterosuperior and inferior, or mural, leaflets, with the conjoined AV cushions providing the substance for formation of the septal leaflet (Figure 1.18). On the left side, the developing MV initially has a trifoliate configuration [17]. It is only subsequent to transfer of the aorta to the LV that the fused superior and inferior cushions are moved away from the septum to form the aortic leaflet of the MV (Figure 1.19). Failure of complete fusion produces clefting of the aortic mitral leaflet. In both ventricles, the trabecular layers of the myocardium condense to form the papillary muscles, with delamination from the parietal ventricular walls producing the septal and inferior leaflets of the TV, and the mural leaflet of the MV [17]. Abnormal persistence of the myocardial components accounts well for the so-called arcade lesion, in which the leading edge of the valvar leaflets remains myocardial. It is failure of delamination of the inferior and septal leaflets from the myocardium of the RV inlet that produces Ebstein's malformation [17].

Completion of ventricular formation requires transfer of half of the outflow tract to the developing LV, again achieved by remodeling of the cavity of the initial linear

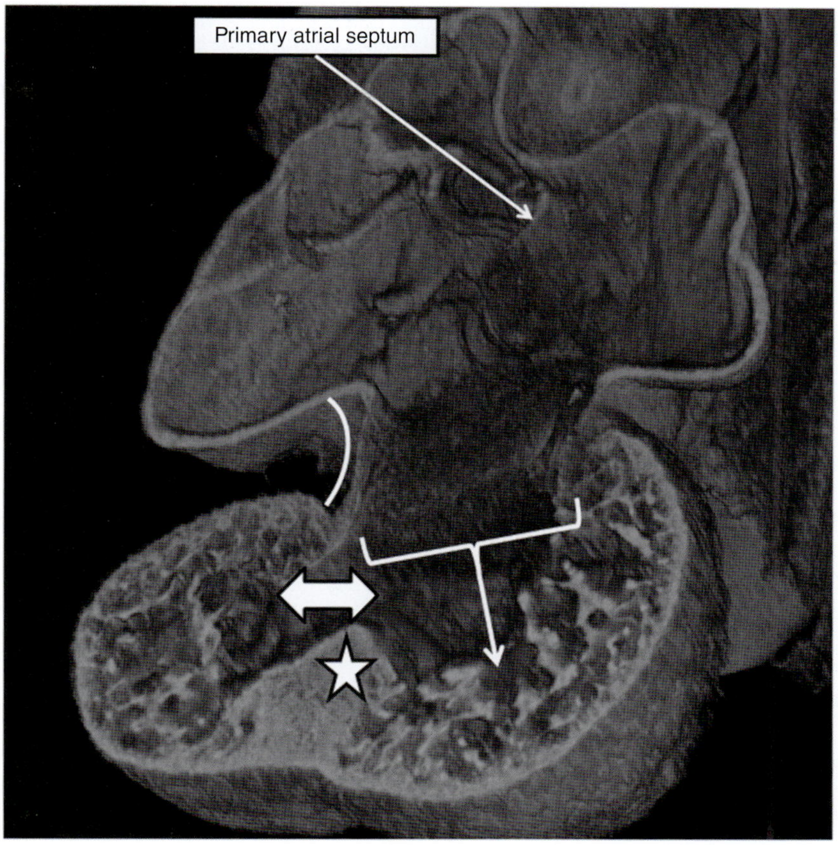

Figure 1.15 The image is the same as that used for Figure 1.2, and comes from a developing mouse embryo early on embryonic day 11.5. It is re-labeled to show how, at this early stage, the AV canal connects almost exclusively with the cavity of the developing LV (bracket). The blood then enters the developing RV through the embryonic interventricular communication (double-headed white arrow), which is bounded caudally by the developing muscular ventricular septum (star), and cranially by the right margin of the inner heart curvature (white curve).

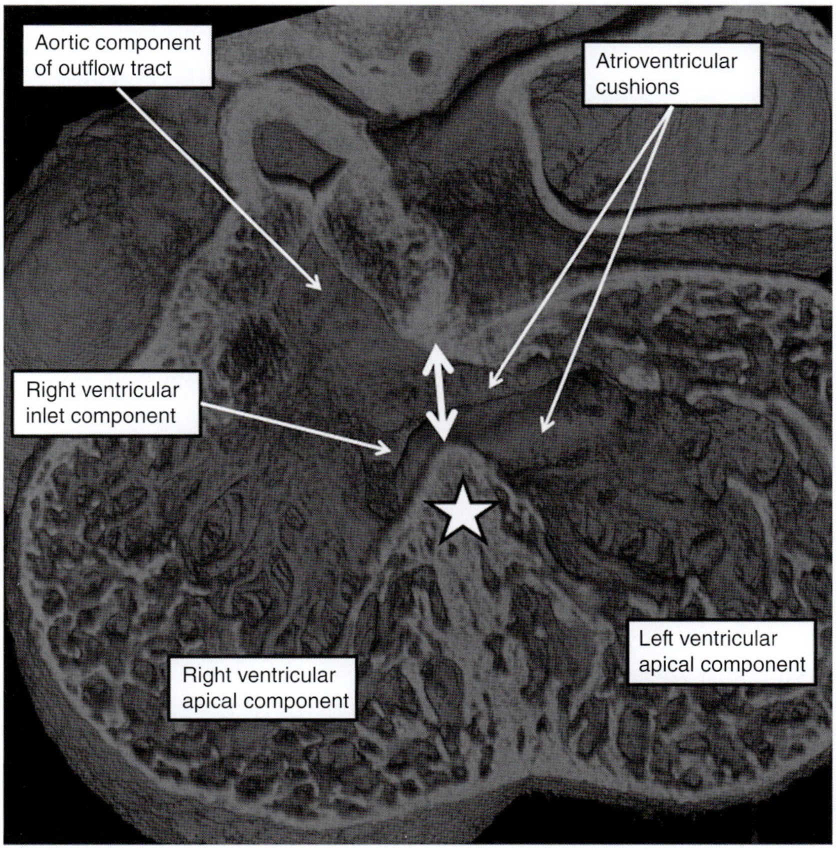

Figure 1.16 The image is a frontal section through an episcopic dataset prepared from a developing mouse early on E12.5. The AV canal has expanded so that the cavity of the developing RA is now in direct continuity with the cavity of the RV, thus producing the RV inlet. The larger parts of the AV cushions, however, remain committed to the LV. The aortic component of the developing outflow tract, in contrast, remains supported by the developing RV, so that the blood entering the aorta must still pass through the embryonic interventricular communication (white arrow). The star shows the crest of the muscular interventricular septum.

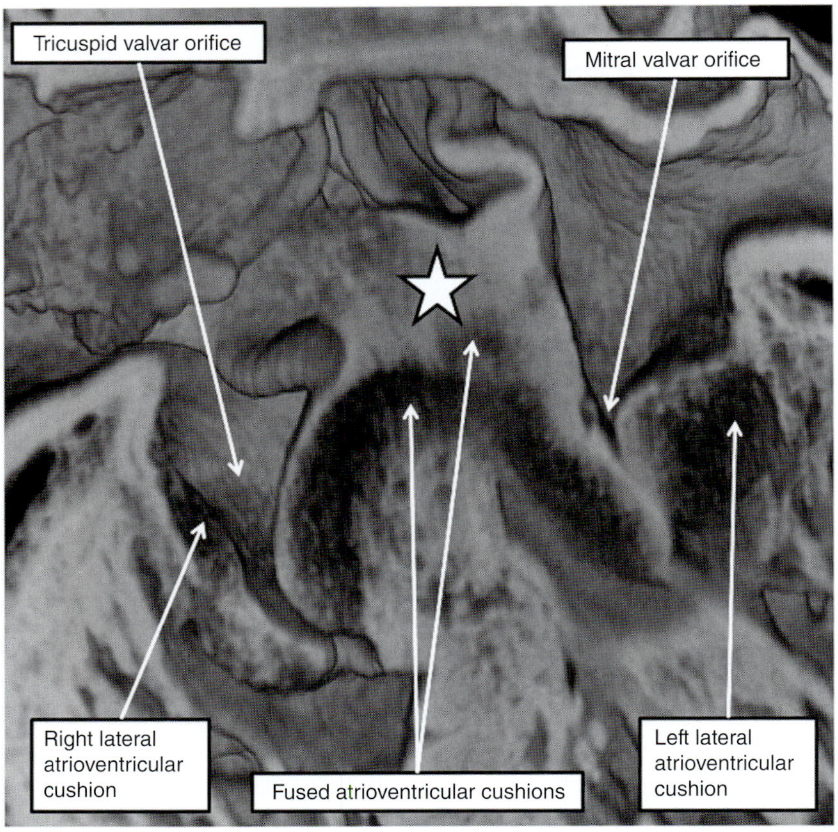

Figure 1.17 The image shows a four-chamber section through the AV junctions later on embryonic day 12.5 in the developing mouse heart. The major AV endocardial cushions have now fused to divide the junction into the tricuspid (TV) and mitral valve (MV) orifices. Lateral cushions have now developed in the newly formed right and left junctions, and will form the mural leaflet of the MV, and the anterosuperior and inferior leaflets of the TV (see Figure 1.18). The star shows the muscularizing vestibular spine and mesenchymal cap, which bind the atrial septum to the surface of the cushions.

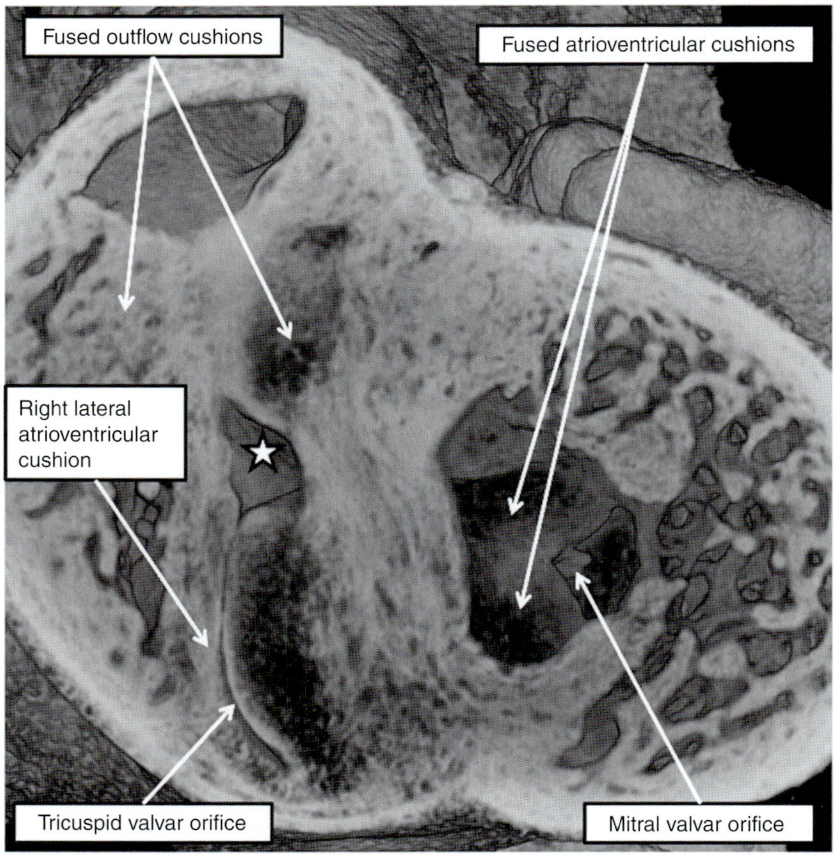

Figure 1.18 The image shows a short axis section from an episcopic dataset prepared from an embryonic mouse at day 13.5. The bulk of the fused AV cushions remains within the LV and have fused to form what will become the aortic leaflet of the MV. At this stage, however, the aortic outflow tract remains supported by the RV (star). The right lateral cushion and the rightward margins of the fused AV cushions guard the developing TV orifice.

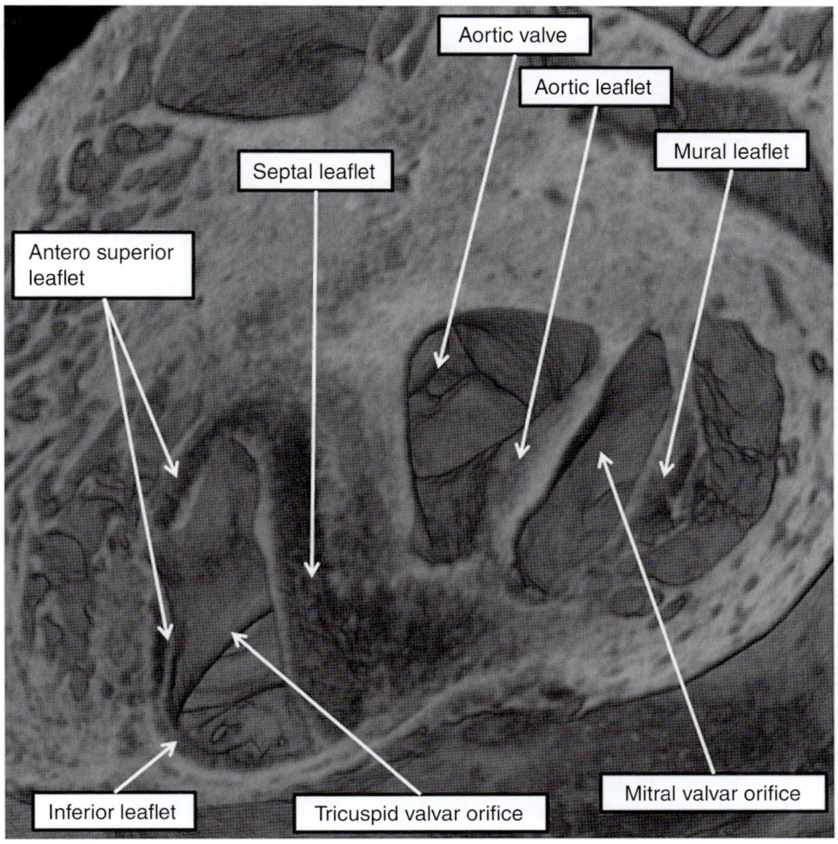

Figure 1.19 The image showing the short axis of the ventricular mass viewed from the apex is from an episcopic datasets prepared from a mouse at embryonic day 14.5. The aortic root has now been transferred into the LV, interposing between the septum and the MV so that the latter valve now possesses aortic and mural leaflets. The TV is developing its anterosuperior and inferior leaflets, but the septal leaflet has not yet delaminated from the muscular ventricular septum.

heart tube. Prior to the remodeling, the outflow tract itself is divided into pulmonary and aortic channels by the development of endocardial cushions that extend throughout its length (Figure 1.9) [18]. The distal parts of these cushions fuse each other, and with a protrusion from the dorsal wall of the aortic sac, to separate the intrapericardial arterial trunks. The intermediate components fuse and form the adjacent leaflets and sinuses of the arterial valves. Remodeling of the inner curve then brings the fused proximal cushions in line with the crest of the muscular ventricular septum (Figure 1.20). It is muscularization of their fused surface that produces the RV infundibulum (Figure 1.21). The persisting central part of the initial interventricular communication (Figure 1.20) can then be closed by apposition of the rightward edges of the superior and inferior AV cushions with each other, and with the muscularized outflow cushions (Figure 1.22). Failure of this process accounts well for the production of perimembranous ventricular septal defects, while failure of muscularization of the outflow cushions provides a good explanation for the doubly committed and juxta-arterial defects. Muscular defects are well explained on the basis of failure of compaction of the apical muscular septum.

Development and Maldevelopment of the Outflow Tract

When first seen, the outflow component of the linear heart tube extends from the RV to the margins of the pericardial cavity, and has exclusively myocardial walls [18]. Its lumen, at the margins of the pericardial cavity, becomes continuous with the lumens of the bilateral and initially symmetrical arteries that develop within the pharyngeal arches (Figures 1.23 and 1.24). The confluence within the pharyngeal mesenchyme that gives rise to the arteries is known as the aortic sac. The arteries percolating through the arches are never all seen at the same time. By the time the arteries of the fourth and sixth arches have appeared, the arteries of the first three arches have lost their original connection with the aortic sac. Eventually, the right-sided channels disappear, with the artery of the left fourth arch becoming the transverse aorta, and the left sixth arch artery persisting in the fetal circulation as the arterial duct (Figure 1.25).

The multiple variants of vascular rings are well explained on the basis of retention of the various components of the initially bilaterally symmetrical system [19]. As already discussed, the initially common lumen of the

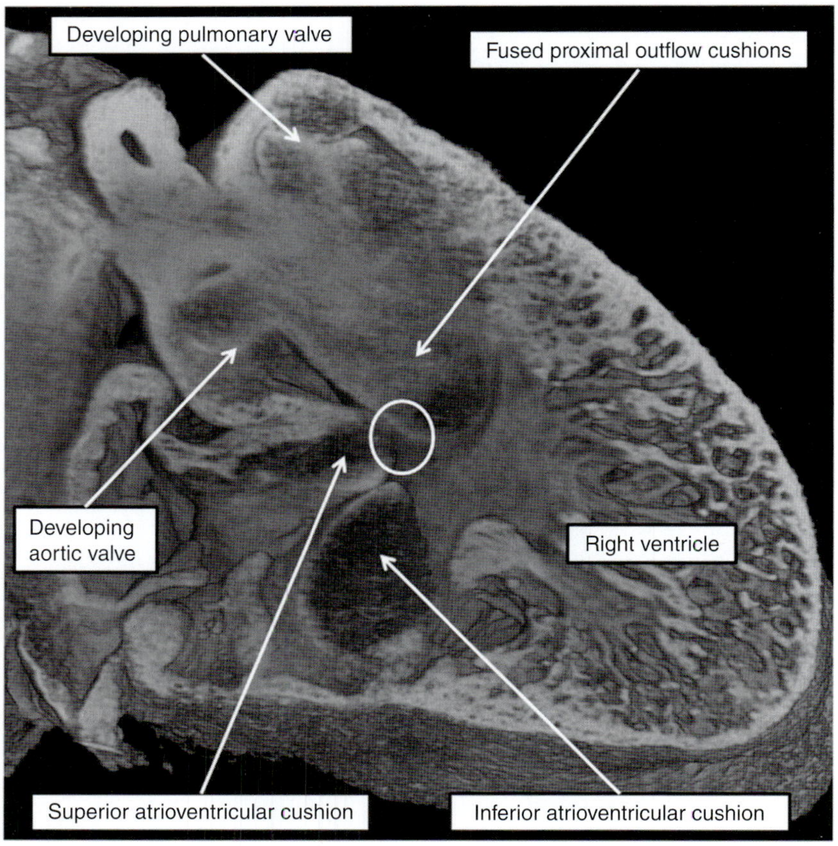

Figure 1.20 The episcopic section shows the right side of the developing mouse heart at embryonic day 13.5. The proximal outflow cushions have fused to form the cranial margin of the persisting embryonic interventricular communication (white circle).

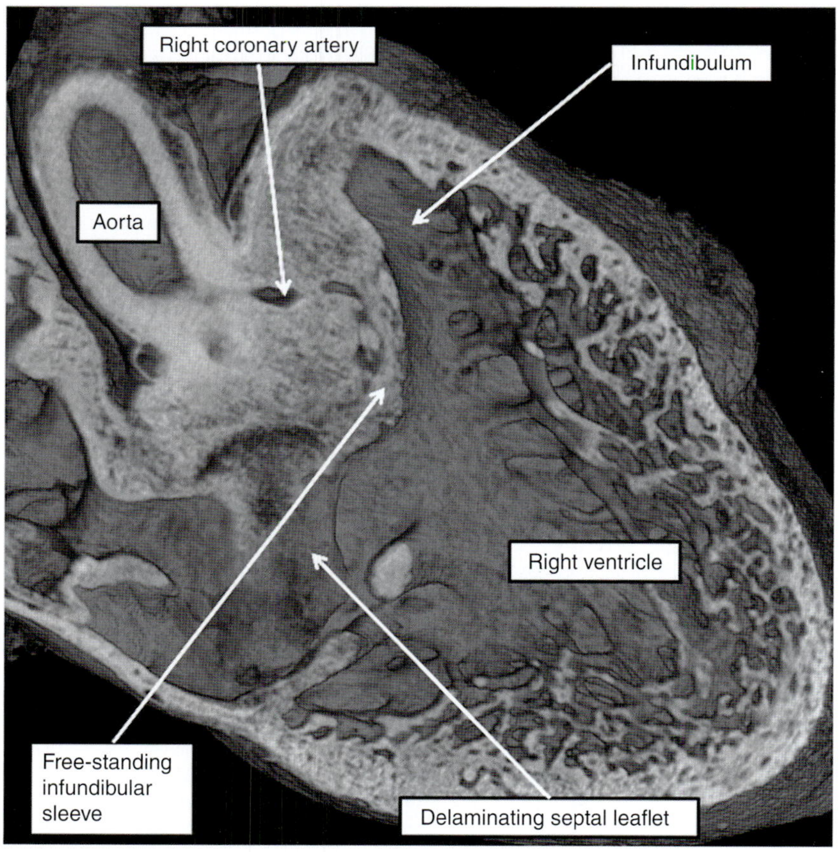

Figure 1.21 This episcopic section, in the same plane as Figure 1.20, is from a mouse at embryonic day 14.5. The surface of the fused proximal cushions has muscularized to form the margin of the free-standing infundibular sleeve adjacent to the aortic root.

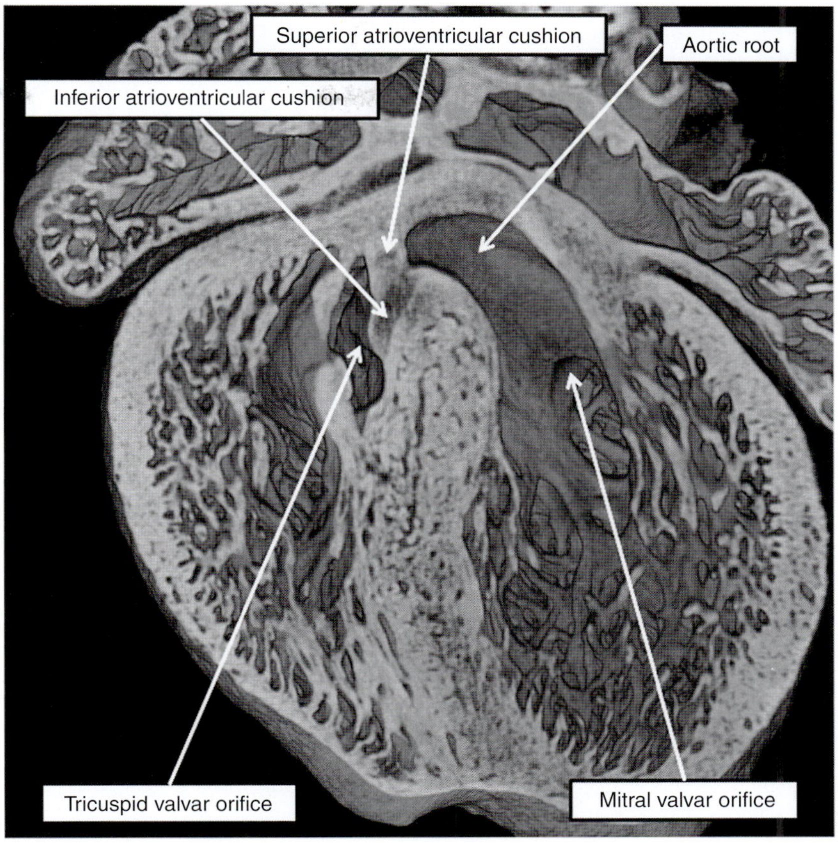

Figure 1.22 This episcopic section, again from a mouse at embryonic day 14.5, but now in four-chamber projection, shows how the rightward margins of the AV endocardial cushions have fused to close the RV entrance to the subaortic vestibule, thus forming the membranous septum, and completing the process of ventricular septation.

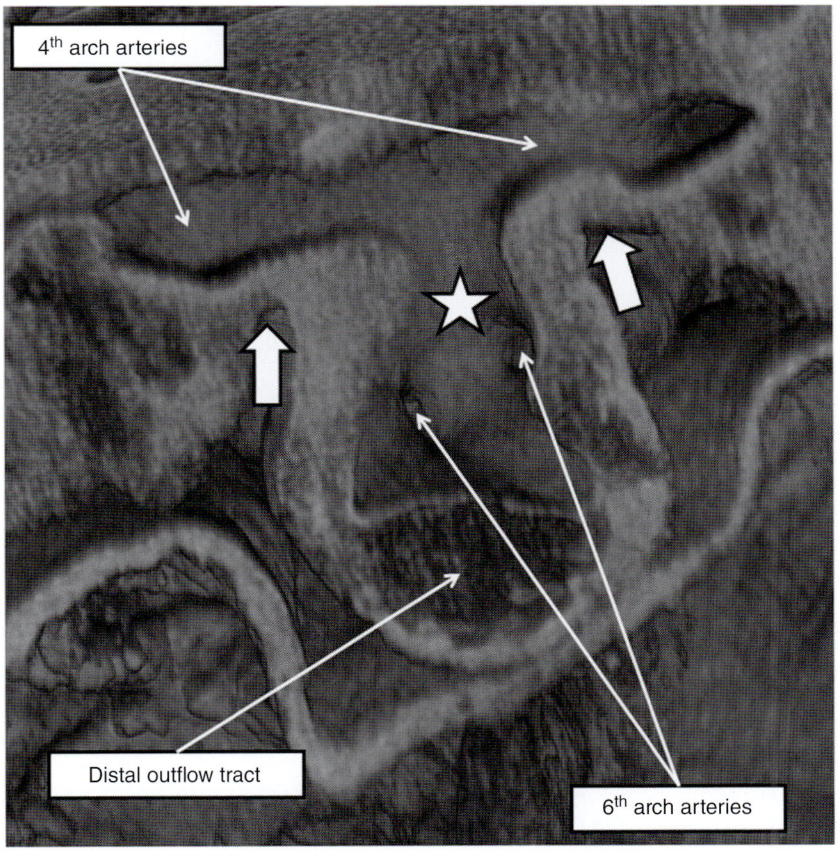

Figure 1.23 The image is from an episcopic dataset prepared from a human embryo at Carnegie stage 13. The cavity of the distal outflow tract becomes continuous with the lumen of the aortic sac at the level of the pericardial reflections (thick arrows). Arising from the aortic sac are the arteries running through the fourth and sixth pharyngeal arches. The fourth arch arteries will become the systemic channels, while the sixth arch arteries will supply the developing pulmonary arteries, so at this stage the dorsal wall of the sac (star) is the putative aortopulmonary septum.

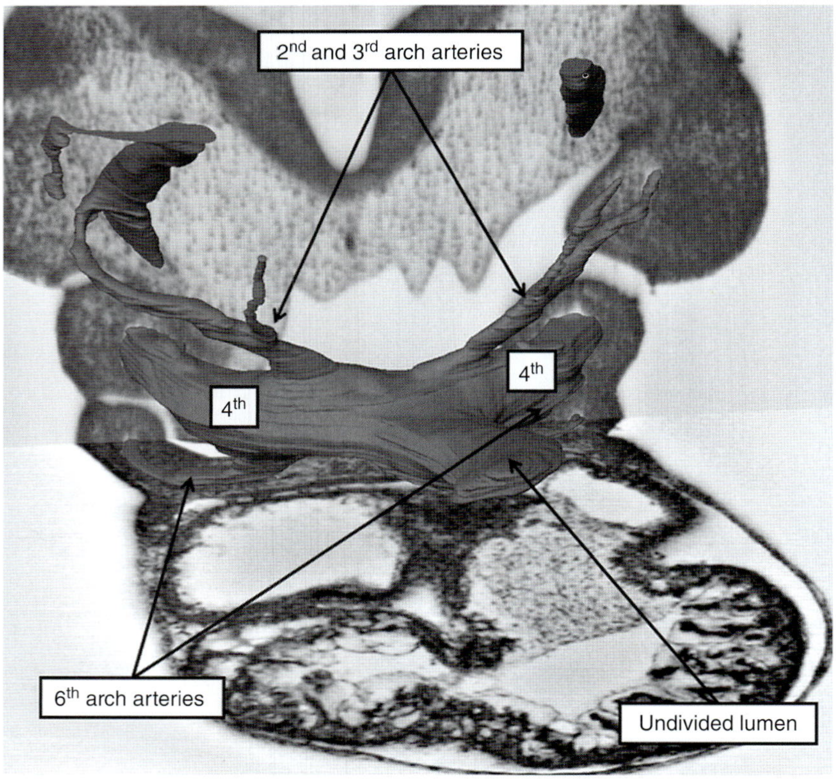

Figure 1.24 The image shows orthogonal sections from an episcopic dataset from a mouse at embryonic day 11.5, with reconstruction of the arteries running through the pharyngeal mesenchyme. At this stage, the arteries of the fourth arch are dominant, and bilaterally symmetrical, as are the arches of the first through third arches, which are diminishing in importance, and those of the sixth arches, which are still developing.

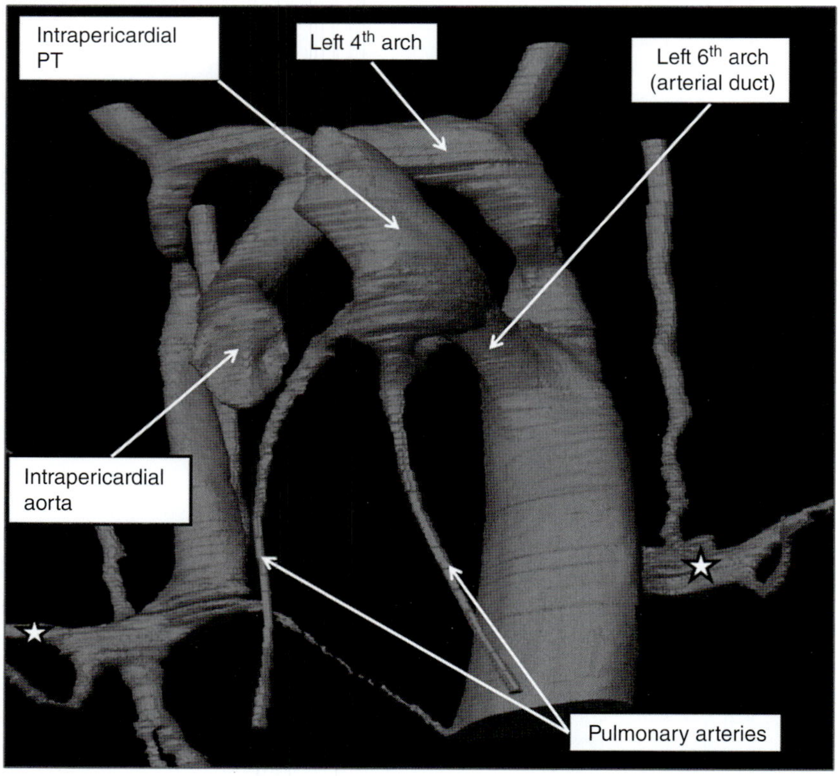

Figure 1.25 The image is a reconstruction made from an episcopic dataset prepared from a mouse at embryonic day 14.5. It shows how, because of regression of the right-sided components of the initially bilaterally symmetrical arteries coursing through the pharyngeal pouches, the system has been transformed into the arch of the aorta and the arterial duct. The seventh intersegmental arteries (stars), however, have still to migrate cranially to become the subclavian arteries. PT, pulmonary trunk.

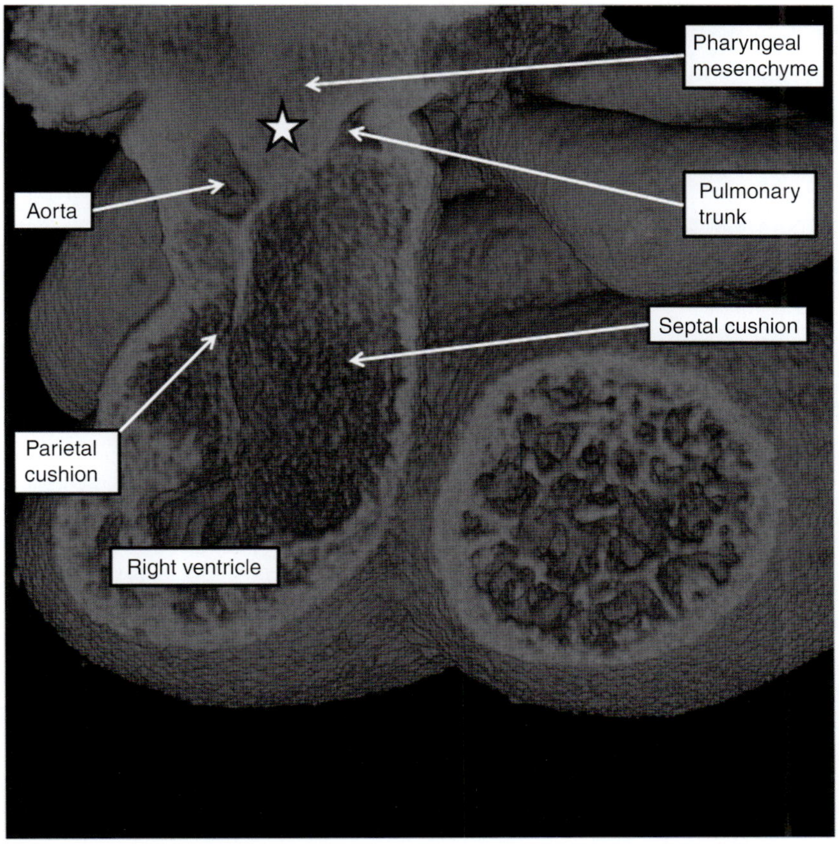

Figure 1.26 The image is from an episcopic dataset prepared from a developing mouse heart at embryonic day 11.5. It shows a long axis cut through the developing outflow tract. The parietal walls of the aorta and pulmonary trunk have grown into the heart from the second heart field. The distal outflow tract is now undergoing separation by fusion of a ventral intraluminal protrusion from the pharyngeal mesenchyme enclosing the aortic sac (star) with the distal ends of the cushions that extend through the outflow tract.

outflow tract is separated into pulmonary and systemic channels by fusion of a protrusion that grows ventrally from the dorsal wall of the aortic sac with the distal end of the spiraling cushions that have developed throughout the extent of the tract (Figure 1.26) [18]. Prior to fusion of these components, further non-myocardial tissues have grown into the heart from the second heart field to produce the walls of the intrapericardial aorta and pulmonary trunk. Fusion of the protrusion from dorsal wall of the aortic sac with the distal cushions obliterates a transient aortopulmonary foramen. The protrusion is covered by cells derived from the neural crest, and the cushions are filled with neural crest cells. Failure to close the foramen results in an aortopulmonary window [18]. Overall failure of the cushions to fuse results in common arterial trunk, with the different variants of common trunk depending on the contribution made by the ventral protrusion [18]. The outflow tract is initially supported exclusively by the RV, with a significant part of normal development being the transfer of the aorta to the LV. Incomplete transfer therefore explains well the various lesions with overriding of the aortic valve, such as tetralogy of Fallot, or the Eisenmenger variant of ventricular septal defect. Double outlet RV is the default option for maldevelopment of the outflow tract. Discordant ventriculo-arterial connections, or transposition, however, require straight as opposed to spiraling formation of the outflow cushions. Inappropriate transfer of the pulmonary trunk in this setting, as opposed to the aorta, then explains well the spectrum known as the Taussig–Bing malformation [20].

Development of the Coronary Circulation

The coronary arteries, which supply blood to the various tissues within the walls of the heart, and the coronary veins, which return the deoxygenated blood, are epicardially derived. Most of the cells are derived from the epicardial organ, which grows over the entire epicardial surface of the heart as far as the distal outflow tract [21]. An additional population of cells then forms around the distal outflow tract [22]. The proximal coronary arteries bud out from the aortic wall, with the openings initially seen distal to the junction between the developing sinuses and the intrapericardial component of the aorta (Figure 1.27). The buds growing from the aortic trunk make contact with the plexuses forming around the distal outflow tract, which in turn communicate with the overall epicardial plexus [22]. Subsequent to the separation of the aortic and pulmonary roots by fusion of the outflow cushions, the origins of the coronary arteries

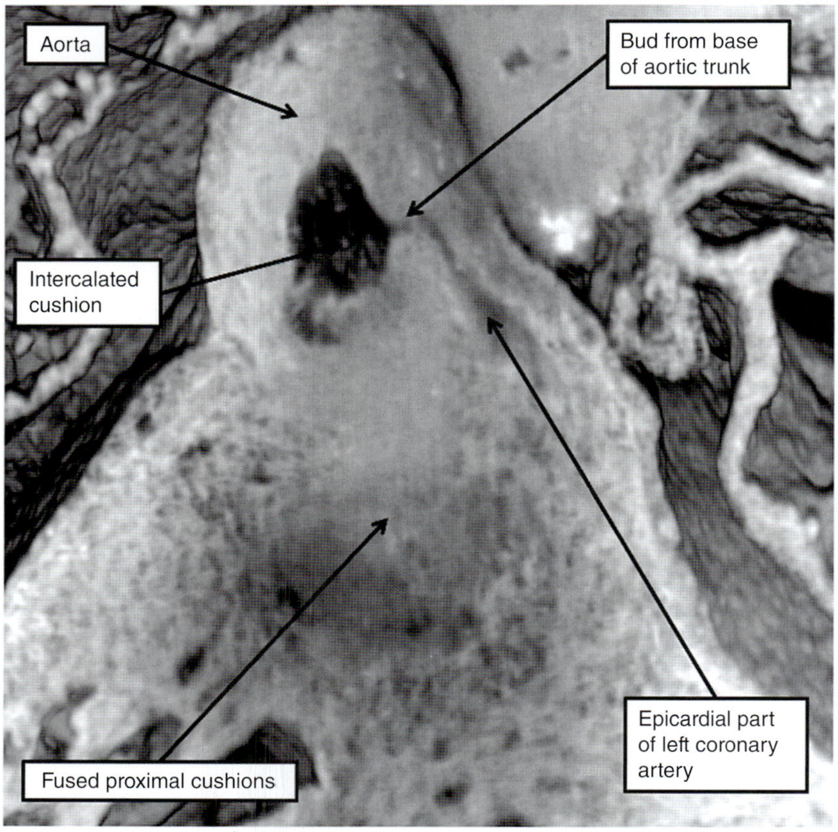

Figure 1.27 The image is from an episcopic dataset prepared from a developing mouse heart at embryonic day 13.5. It is a frontal section showing the part of the aortic root adjacent to the newly separated pulmonary root. Note the fused mass of the proximal outflow cushions that produced the separation. The bud of the left coronary artery, arising from the aortic trunk distal to the ends of the outflow cushions, which will cavitate to form the aortic valvar leaflets. The bud has joined with the epicardial component of the developing left coronary artery.

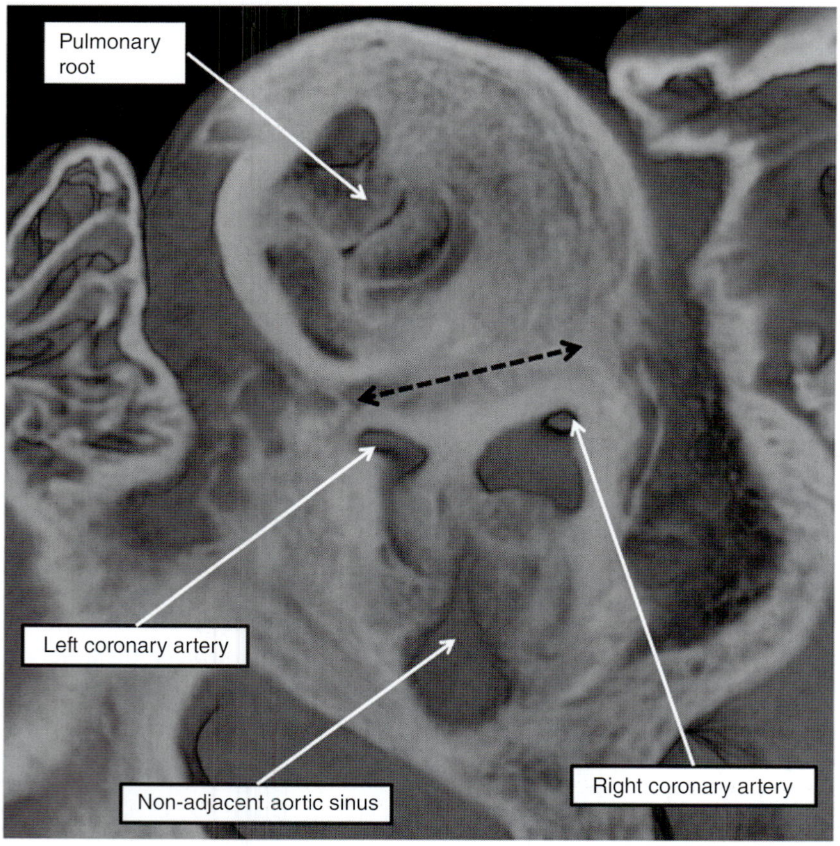

Figure 1.28 The image, this time in short axis, and viewed from above, is from an episcopic dataset prepared from a mouse heart at embryonic day 15.5. The origins of the coronary arteries, which were originally formed distal to the junction between the developing sinuses and the intrapericardial aorta (see Figure 1.27), have now been incorporated within the aortic valvar sinuses adjacent to the pulmonary root. Dashed line, transient aortopulmonary foramen.

are incorporated within the two aortic valvar sinuses formed adjacent to the pulmonary trunk (Figure 1.18). Inappropriate connection with a pulmonary valvar sinus provides the explanation for anomalous origin of a major coronary artery from the pulmonary trunk, while abnormal incorporation within the developing aortic sinuses explains well the various lesions seen in which the coronary arteries arise from inappropriate sinuses.

Acknowledgments

Our chapter is based heavily on the similar chapter we produced for the forthcoming textbook to be published by Springer, edited by the team working in Denver, Colorado (see reference [3]). We have also analyzed the material in preparation for submission of a review of ventricular septation to *Anatomical Record*, our figures for this chapter being prepared from the same datasets that will be used for the more formal publication. We retain our intellectual copyright in the images prepared from the episcopic datasets. We are indebted to Dr. Simon Bamforth, from Newcastle University, for permitting us to use the reconstructions he prepared to illustrate the concepts shown in Figures 1.24 and 1.25. We also thank Dr. Robert Kelly, from the University of Marseilles, for sharing with us his observations showing that the proximal coronary arterial stems grow out from the developing aortic root, and for making available mice lacking the vestibular spine.

References

1 Abbott ME. (1936) *Atlas of Congenital Cardiac Disease*, American Heart Association, New York, p. 2.

2 Mohun TJ, Weninger WJ. (2011) Imaging heart development using high-resolution episcopic microscopy. *Curr Opin Genet Dev*, **21**, 573–578.

3 Anderson RH, Moorman AFM, Brown NA, *et al.* (2014) Normal and abnormal development of the heart, in *Pediatric and Congenital Cardiology, Cardiac Surgery and Intensive Care* (eds E da Cruz, D Ivy, and J Jaggers), Springer, New York, pp. 151–177.

4 Aanhaanen WT, Brons JF, Dominguez JN, *et al.* (2009) The Tbx2+ primary myocardium of the atrioventricular canal forms the atrioventricular node and the base of the left ventricle. *Circ Res*, **104**, 1267–1274.

5 Moorman AFM, Christoffels VM, Anderson RH, van den Hoff MJB. (2007) The heart-forming fields: one or multiple? *Phil Trans Roy Soc Biol*, **362**, 1257–1265.

6 Uemura H, Ho SY, Devine WA, Kilpatrick LL, Anderson RH. (1995) Atrial appendages and venoatrial connections in hearts with patients with visceral heterotaxy. *Ann Thorac Surg*, **60**, 561–569.

7 Brown NA, Anderson RH. (1999) Symmetry and laterality in the human heart: developmental implications, in *Heart Development* (eds RP Harvey, N Rosenthal), Academic Press, San Diego, pp. 447–462.

8 Cohen MS, Anderson RH, Cohen MI, *et al.* (2007) Controversies, genetics, diagnostic assessment, and outcomes relating to the heterotaxy syndrome. *Cardiol Young*, **17** (Suppl 2), 29–43.

9 Moorman AFM, Christoffels VM. (2003) Cardiac chamber formation: development, genes, and evolution. *Physiol Rev*, **83**, 1223–1267.

10 Webb S, Kanani M, Anderson RH, Richardson MK, Brown NA. (2001) Development of the human pulmonary vein and its incorporation in the morphologically left atrium. *Cardiol Young*, **11**, 632–642.

11 Hagen PT, Scholz DG, Edwards WD. (1984) Incidence and size of patent foramen ovale during the first decades of life: an autopsy study of 965 normal hearts. *Mayo Clin Proc*, **59**, 17–20.

12 Sharratt GP, Webb S, Anderson RH. (2003) The vestibular defect: an interatrial communication due to a deficiency in the atrial septal component derived from the vestibular spine. *Cardiol Young*, **13**, 184–190.

13 Anderson RH, Wessels A, Vettukattil JJ. (2010) Morphology and morphogenesis of atrioventricular septal defect with common atrioventricular junction. *World J Ped Card Surg*, **1**, 59–67.

14 Butts RJ, Crean AM, Hlavacek AM, *et al.* (2011) Veno-venous bridges: the forerunners of the sinus venosus defect. *Cardiol Young*, **21**, 623–630.

15 Knauth A, McCarthy KP, Webb S, *et al.* (2002) Interatrial communication through the mouth of the coronary sinus. *Cardiol Young*, **12**, 364–372.

16 Scalia D, Russo P, Anderson RH, *et al.* (1984) The surgical anatomy of hearts with no direct communication between the right atrium and the ventricular mass: so-called tricuspid atresia. *J Thorac Cardiovasc Surg*, **87**, 743–755.

17 Kanani M, Moorman AFM, Cook AC, *et al.* (2005) Development of the atrioventricular valves: clinicomorphologic correlations. *Ann Thorac Surg*, **79**, 1797–1804.

18 Anderson RH, Brown NA, Chaudhry B, *et al.* (2012) Formation of the intrapericardial arterial trunks in the developing human and mouse heart. *Cardiovasc Res*, **95**, 108–115.

19 Edwards JE. (1948) Anomalies of the derivatives of the aortic arch system. *Med Clin N Am*, **32**, 925–948.

20 Stellin G, Zuberbuhler JR, Anderson RH, Siewers RD. (1987) The surgical anatomy of the Taussig–Bing malformation. *J Thorac Cardiovasc Surg*, **93**, 560–569.

21 Pérez-Pomares JM, Phelps A, Sedmerova M, *et al.* (2002) Experimental studies on the spatiotemporal expression of WT1 and RALDH2 in the embryonic avian heart: a model for the regulation of myocardial and valvuloseptal development by epicardially derived cells (EPDCs). *Dev Biol*, **247**, 307–326.

22 Parisot P, Théveniau-Ruissy M, Kelly R. (2011) Conotruncal and coronary artery development in two mouse models of congenital heart defects. *Arch Cardiovasc Dis Suppl*, **3**, 101.

2

Maternal, Familial, and Non-Cardiac Fetal Conditions Affecting the Fetal and Neonatal Heart

Miwa K. Geiger[1] and Anita J. Moon-Grady[2]

[1] Mount Sinai Hospital, New York, NY, USA
[2] University of California at San Francisco, San Francisco, CA, USA

Genetic, epigenetic, intrauterine, and extrauterine factors impact the embryogenesis, development, and function of the human cardiovascular system. Although many of these interactions are incompletely understood, a number of maternal, placental, and fetal conditions that disrupt normal fetal cardiac development and/or function have been identified.

Maternal Factors

Metabolic

Pregestational maternal diabetes is associated with up to a fivefold risk of structural cardiac malformations [1]. The most commonly reported defects are ventricular septal defects (VSD), conotruncal anomalies (particularly transposition of the great arteries), as well as single ventricle malformations [2] and pulmonary valve abnormalities. Poorly controlled diabetes later in gestation increases the risk for fetal hypertrophic cardiomyopathy (HCM), with a dose–response relationship between the degree of hyperglycemia and hypertrophy (negligible risk when HbA1C is maintained <6%) [3]. Infants with HCM tend to have asymmetric septal hypertrophy (Figure 2.1) and yet have a good prognosis as hypertrophy generally regresses with time. While most of these infants are asymptomatic, some with severe hypertrophy develop congestive heart failure because of reduced ventricular compliance and/or severe left ventricular outflow tract obstruction and may require supportive care.

Maternal phenylketonuria confers a 10- to 15-fold higher risk of structural heart defects when maternal phenylalanine levels are >15 mg/dL [4]. Cardiac defects more commonly seen are hypoplastic left heart syndrome, coarctation of the aorta, and tetralogy of Fallot.

Autoimmune

Anti-Ro and anti-La autoantibodies, often seen in women with lupus, other autoimmune conditions, as well as asymptomatic women, can cause fetal complete atrioventricular block (CAVB) and/or cardiomyopathy associated with endofibroelastosis (Figure 2.2). In known seropositive women, the prevalence of fetal heart block is reported to be 1–5%, increasing to 11–19% in pregnancies with a previously affected child [5]. Systemic inflammatory response to these antibodies is thought to lead to the fetal myocardial and conduction system injury and fibrosis. Fetuses with CAVB present with bradycardia (ventricular rates 50–70 bpm), leading to cardiomegaly and ventricular hypertrophy. Heart rates <55 bpm increase fetal risk for hydrops and poor outcome. Neonatal mortality is reported to be 19–31%. Pacemaker placement is indicated in infants with hydrops or other evidence of poor cardiac output. In utero treatment of acquired AV block (prior to the onset of third degree block) with maternal dexamethasone has been reported but remains controversial [6].

Infection

Maternal infections have been implicated in fetal structural heart defects and myocarditis. Rubella infection is associated with postnatal patent ductus arteriosus, pulmonary stenosis, branch pulmonary artery stenosis, and VSDs. It has been reported that any febrile illness in the first trimester can increase the risk for congenital heart defects [2]. Fetal myocarditis has also been attributed to coxsackievirus, adenovirus, cytomegalovirus, toxoplasma, and HIV infections during pregnancy. Maternal parvovirus B19 infection is a rare cause of fetal anemia (and non-immune hydrops) as well as myocarditis [7].

Visual Guide to Neonatal Cardiology, First Edition. Edited by Ernerio T. Alboliras, Ziyad M. Hijazi, Leo Lopez, and Donald J. Hagler.

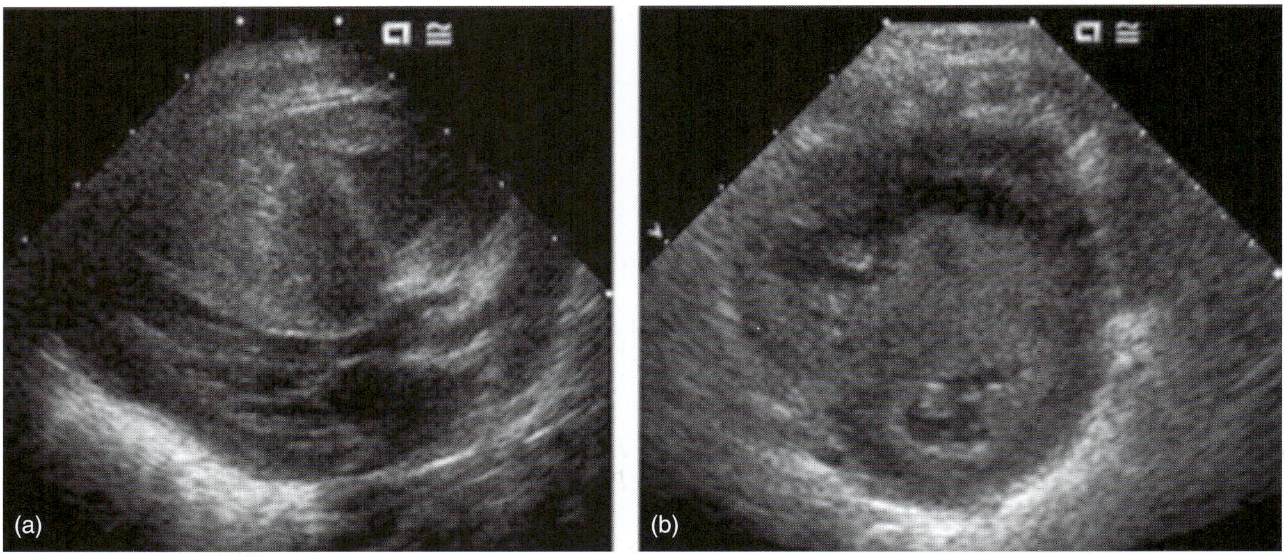

Figure 2.1 Neonatal hypertrophic cardiomyopathy associated with maternal diabetes. (a) Parasternal long axis and (b) short-axis images demonstrate asymmetric septal hypertrophy with near obliteration of the left ventricular cavity. The development of hypertrophy is associated with maternal hemoglobin A1C levels >6 g/dL in the latter part of gestation and generally resolves slowly after birth. *Source*: Jaeggi *et al.* [3]. Reproduced with permission of John Wiley & Sons Inc.

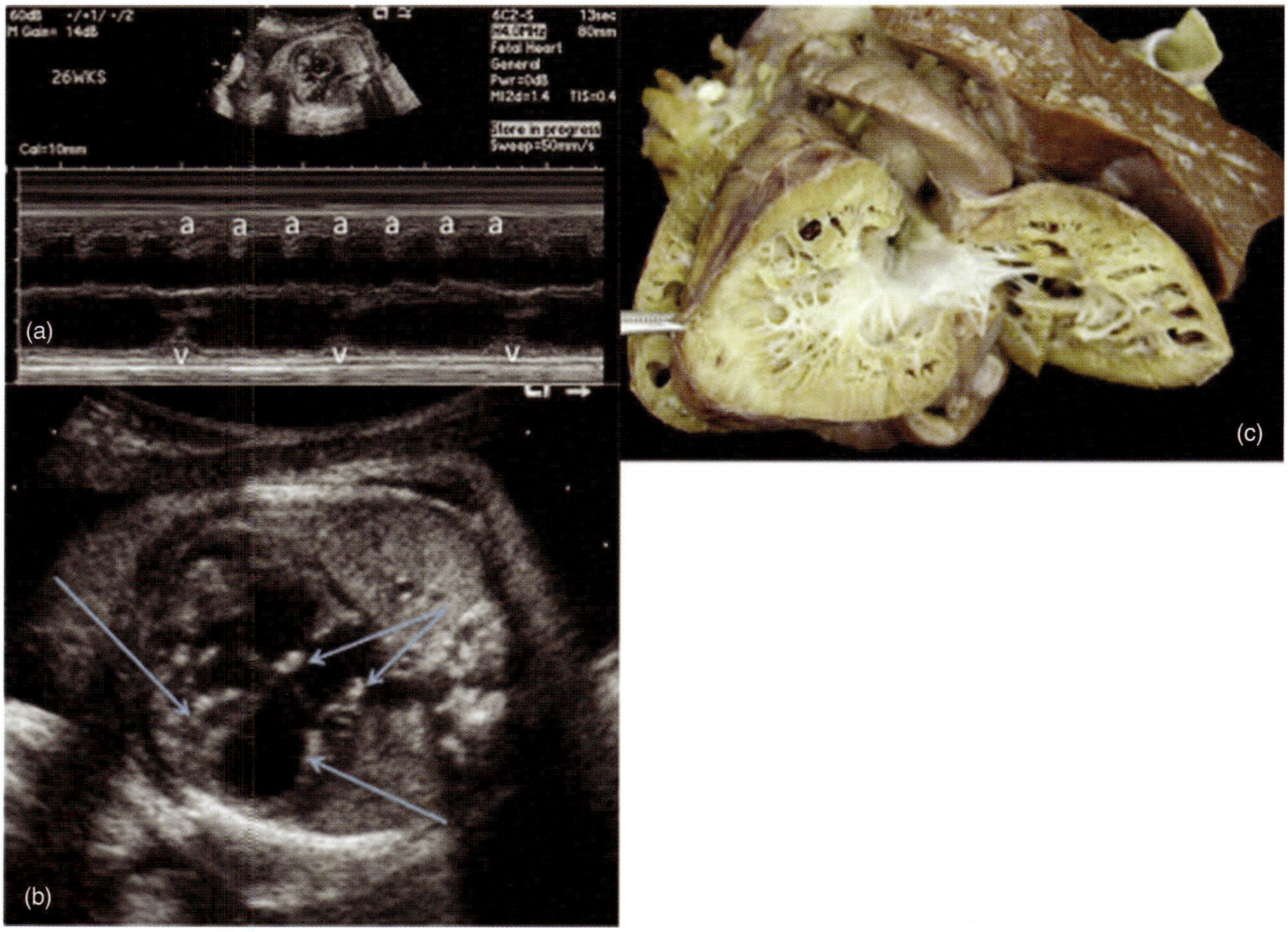

Figure 2.2 Maternal autoantibody-associated heart block and cardiomyopathy. (a) M-mode tracing in a 26 weeks' gestation fetus with AV dissociation consistent with third-degree AV block (a, atrial contraction; v, ventricular contraction) in the setting of SSA+ mother. Endocardial fibroelastosis involving the left ventricle is seen (b) by fetal echocardiography, as echo-bright areas of atrial and ventricular endocardium (arrows) and (c) autopsy specimen. Heart block is usually not reversible once it occurs; cardiomyopathy, associated with high rates of death or transplantation in the first year of life, may be treated in utero or in the neonatal period with dexamethasone and intravenous immunoglobulin with improvement in survival [18]. Photo (c) courtesy of Norman H. Silverman, MD, DSc (MED).

Cardiac Teratogens

Anticonvulsants, lithium, retinoic acid, selective serotonin reuptake inhibitors, and angiotensin converting enzyme inhibitors have been linked to structural cardiac defects if fetal exposure occurs during the first trimester.

Indomethacin (used to treat preterm labor and polyhydramnios) can cause premature constriction of the ductus arteriosus as can other non-steroidal medications (Figure 2.3). In general, this is reversible within a few days of discontinuation of the medication [8]. If ductal constriction continues, severe right ventricular dysfunction, tricuspid regurgitation, and hydrops can develop. Delivery may be indicated and these infants are at an increased risk for neonatal pulmonary hypertension.

Twins

Cardiac malformations are more common in twin than in singleton pregnancies, and monozygotic twins are at a higher risk than dizygotic twins. Monozygotic twins have up to a ninefold risk of congenital heart defect (CHD) even in the absence of twin–twin transfusion syndrome (TTTS) [9], the majority having one twin affected, despite identical genetic makeup [10].

Familial

In the absence chromosomal deletion syndromes, the risk of cardiac malformations in offspring of a parent with a CHD has been reported to be from 3% to 14%, depending on the lesion [11, 12]. Recurrence risk is 3% for a couple with one previous fetus with CHD and estimated to be 10% with more than one affected pregnancy.

A family history of single gene deletions with Mendelian autosomal dominance, such as Noonan, Williams, and Alagille syndromes, significantly increases the risk of CHD (Table 2.1) [13]. However, in some diseases such as Marfan syndrome, the cardiac phenotype may not manifest until childhood or later and therefore may not be detectable in fetal or neonatal life without genetic testing.

Fetal and neonatal familial cardiomyopathies represent more severe forms of these diseases and generally portend poor prognosis. X-linked cardiomyopathies can occur with fetal dilated or non-compaction cardiomyopathy (Figure 2.4). Rarely, fetuses with metabolic abnormalities, such as glycogen storage diseases and cytochrome oxidase deficiency, can exhibit hypertrophic cardiomyopathy in the prenatal or perinatal period. Other genetic diseases may have variable penetrance

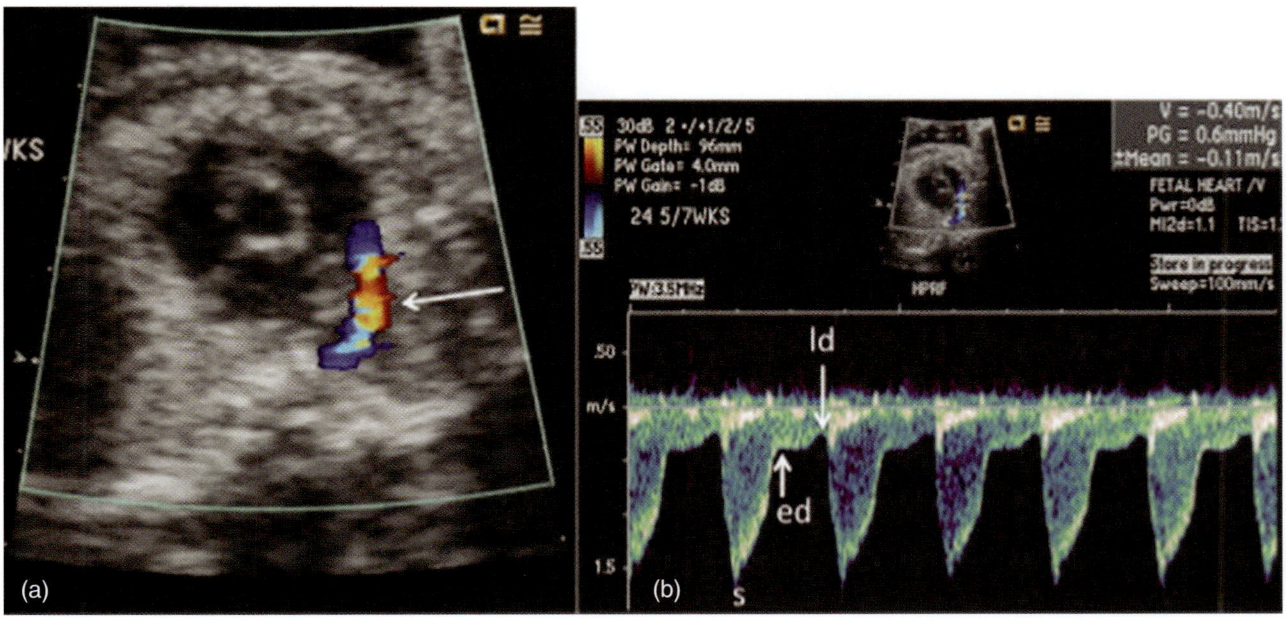

Figure 2.3 Constriction of the fetal ductus arteriosus resulting from maternal indomethacin exposure. (a) Short-axis image near the base of the fetal heart showing color Doppler aliasing (arrow) in the ductus with (b) corresponding spectral Doppler signal demonstrating increased velocities in systole (s), early diastole (ed), and late diastole (ld).

Table 2.1 Associated cardiac defects and frequency in various genetic disorders.

Genetic disorder	Common cardiac manifestations	Frequency of cardiac phenotype (%)
Alagille	PPS, PS, conotruncal defects	<90
Noonan	PS, HCM	<80
Williams–Beuren	Supravalvar AS, PS, PPS	<50
Holt–Oram	ASD, VSD, arrhythmia	<60
22q11 deletion (DiGeorge)	Conotruncal defects, arch anomalies, VSD	75
Ellis–van Creveld	ASD (common atrium)	50
Trisomy 9	PDA, VSD, TOF, DORV	<65
Trisomy 21	AVC, VSD, ASD, TOF	40–50
Trisomy 18	ASD, VSD, TOF, CoA, PDA, DORV	<90
Trisomy 13	PDA, ASD, VSD, HLHS, CoA	80
Klinefelter (XXY)	ASD, MVP, PDA, venous emboli	50
Turner (XO)	CoA, bicuspid aortic valve, AS	<25
Tuberous sclerosis	Cardiac rhabdomyomas	90
Marfan, Ehlers–Danlos	Aortic aneurysms, valve insufficiency	Rare in the fetus and neonate

AS, aortic stenosis; ASD, atrial septal defect; AVC, atrioventricular canal; CoA, coarctation of the aorta; DORV, double outlet right ventricle; HCM, hypertrophic cardiomyopathy; HLHS, hypoplastic left heart syndrome; MVP, mitral valve prolapse; PDA, patent ductus arteriosus; PPS, peripheral pulmonic stenosis; PS, pulmonary stenosis; TOF, tetralogy of Fallot; VSD, ventricular septal defect.
Source: Data from Pierpont *et al.* [13].

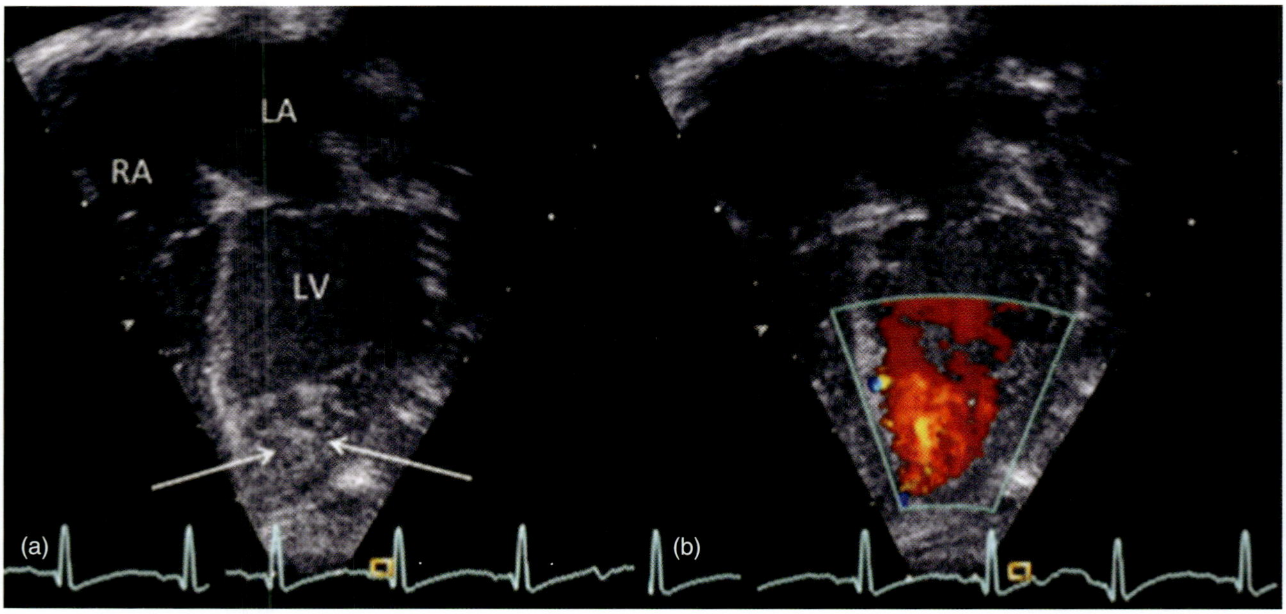

Figure 2.4 Left ventricular non-compaction cardiomyopathy. The left ventricular myocardium has a "spongy" appearance (a, arrows) with large non-compacted to compacted layer dimension, which can be demonstrated clearly by application of color Doppler over the area of interest (b). This neonate presented with poor cardiac output and the diagnosis was confirmed on gross and histologic examination of the explanted heart at the time of orthotopic heart transplantation soon after these images were obtained.

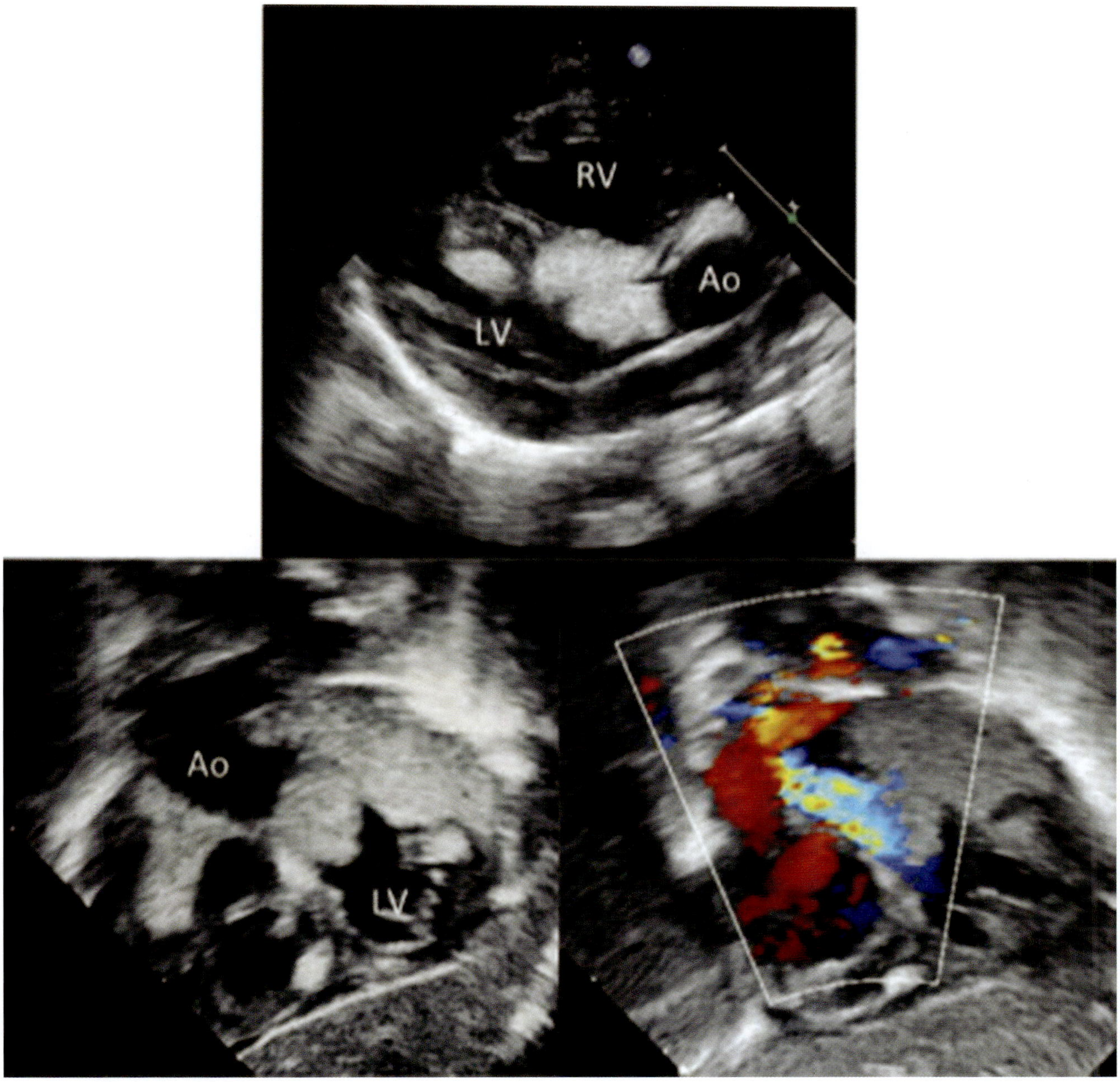

Figure 2.5 Multiple cardiac rhabdomyomas in a neonate with tuberous sclerosis. Though rarely obstructive, in this particular case there was moderate obstruction to the left ventricular outflow tract seen by color Doppler from the subcostal coronal image (lower right). These tumors can be detected in the mid-gestation fetus, and often enlarge at an alarming rate through the remainder of gestation, but will regress postnatally.

and/or expression in the heart including tuberous sclerosis (rhabdomyomas; Figure 2.5), idiopathic infantile arterial calcification, Noonan and other metabolic or storage disorders.

Hereditary anemias (homozygous alpha-thalassemia and Diamond–Blackfan) can lead to severe fetal anemia resulting in hydrops secondary to high output cardiac failure.

Non-cardiac Fetal Conditions

High Output Lesions

States of high cardiac output that can lead to fetal non-immune hydrops include severe fetal anemia, large arteriovenous malformations, hemangiomas, chorioangiomas, sacrococcygeal teratomas (Figure 2.6), TTTS,

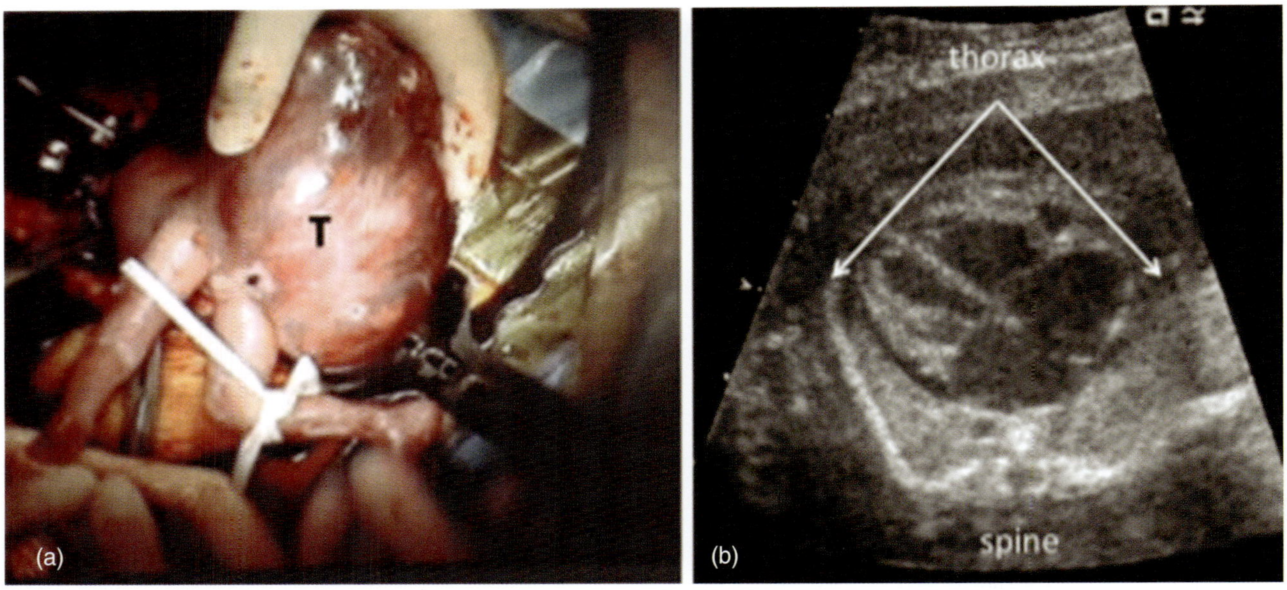

Figure 2.6 Fetus with large sacrococcygeal teratoma (SCT). (a) Intraoperative photo during fetal resection and debulking of the tumor (T); (b) Preoperative fetal echocardiography demonstrating cardiomegaly and pericardial effusion associated with impending hydrops because of high cardiac output. SCT is a germ cell tumor originating at the coccyx and growing outward and often occupying the fetal pelvis and abdomen that can grow to a substantial and highly vascular mass. SCT can cause high output cardiac failure because of increased preload which is exacerbated by its typically low vascular resistance which can compete with blood flow to placenta. With large SCT, the cardiac findings are ventricular hypertrophy and dilatation, with reduction in systolic function, atrioventricular valve regurgitation with development of hydrops and risk of fetal demise. Fetal surgical intervention or early delivery may be indicated for severe cases.

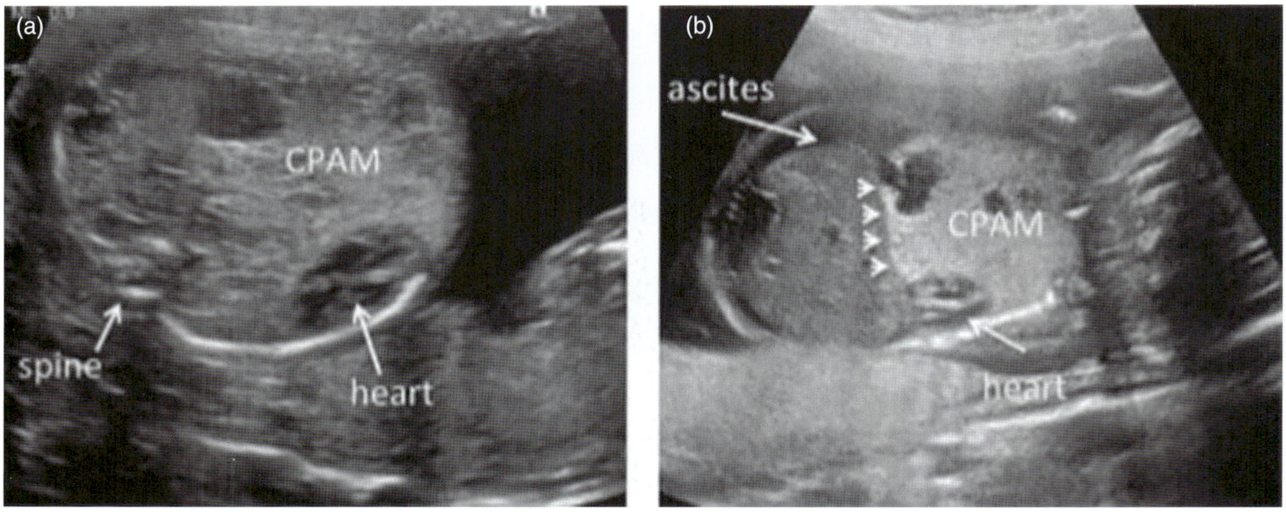

Figure 2.7 Congenital pulmonary airway malformation (CPAM, formerly congenital cystic adenomatoid malformations or CCAM). (a) Axial image of the thorax, note the extreme rightward shift and compression of the heart and the large mixed microcystic and macrocystic CPAM. (b) Sagittal image of the same fetus, demonstrating flattening of the left diaphragm (arrowheads) and a moderate accumulation of ascites. These lesions are complex histologically and may appear on ultrasound as homogeneous, cystic, or mixed type lesions. Compression of the heart and large veins can lead to impaired cardiac filling and hydrops. Myocardial function may appear preserved yet some studies have demonstrated reduced function over time. *Source*: Szwast *et al.* [19]. Reproduced with permission of John Wiley & Sons Inc.

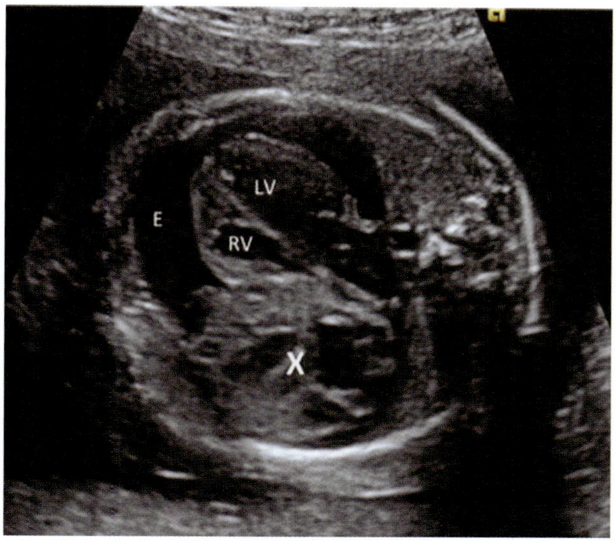

Figure 2.8 Fetal pericardial teratoma (X) with associated pericardial effusion at 26 weeks' gestation. The teratoma arises from the base of the heart near the aorta or right AV groove (here resulting in external compression of the right atrium) and usually receives blood supply from a vascular stalk from the ascending aorta. Though pericardial teratomas and their accompanying pericardial effusions are often well-tolerated, large teratomas can also have a compressive effect and lead to hydrops in the fetus or severe compromise in the newborn necessitating urgent surgery for decompression and/or removal of the tumor. E, effusion; LV, left ventricle; RV, right ventricle.

and twin reversal arterial and perfusion (TRAP) sequence. These diverse conditions result in increased cardiac workload (preload) for the fetal heart. Although the fetus may be able to generate several times a normal cardiac output before decompensation, the passive nature of the fetoplacental circulation is highly sensitive to small elevations in venous pressure. This, in combination with high capillary permeability and low fetal oncotic pressure, leads to extravasation of fluid into various compartments resulting in pericardial and pleural effusions, ascites, skin edema, polyhydramnios, and placental edema. Hydrops is diagnosed with accumulation of fluid into two or more of these spaces.

Space-Occupying Thoracic Lesions

Thoracic lesions can affect the position and occasionally the function and development of the heart. Congenital pulmonary airway malformations (formerly congenital cystic adenomatoid malformations) are benign tumors of the bronchioles that create cystic space occupying lesions, which, if large, can compress fetal lungs, esophagus, heart, and other vascular structures (Figure 2.7). Pericardial teratoma and its accompanying pericardial effusion may impact cardiac output (Figure 2.8). Congenital diaphragmatic hernia can lead to pulmonary hypoplasia and compression of the heart. Small left-sided cardiac structures and myocardial thinning have been described, though the left heart structures normalize in size after birth in the majority of cases [14]. Occasionally, hypoplastic left heart syndrome may be associated with a left-sided diaphragmatic hernia.

Placental Abnormalities

Monochorionic multiple gestation pregnancies are at risk for TTTS, a complex disease affecting approximately 15% of monochorionic pregnancies which, if untreated, results in demise of one or both fetuses in over 80% [15]. The disorder occurs most often in the second trimester and presents as polyhydramnios in the "recipient" twin and oligohydramnios in the other, the "donor." In severe cases, the recipient fetus can develop cardiomyopathy characterized by diastolic dysfunction, cardiac dilatation, and ventricular hypertrophy in response to the high preload and circulating vasoactive mediators. In addition to heart failure resulting in hydrops and fetal demise, the recipient is at increased risk for acquired structural heart defects, most commonly right ventricular outflow tract obstruction [9]. Fetal therapies for TTTS include amnioreduction and laser photocoagulation, the latter of which has been shown to reverse the majority of the cardiac manifestations in the recipient [16].

Placental "insufficiency" seen in association with intrauterine growth restriction is manifested by increased vascular resistance in the placenta and decreased oxygenated umbilical venous flow to the fetus. The fetal heart faces increased afterload and there is reduced oxygen delivery to fetal tissue resulting in preferential perfusion of the myocardium and brain (decreased cerebral vascular resistance and increased coronary flow are features [17]). As this condition progresses, diastolic and then systolic dysfunction can develop – flow reversal in the ductus venosus in atrial systole and umbilical venous pulsations are late findings associated with in utero fetal demise.

References

1 Ramos-Arroyo MA, Rodriguez-Pinilla E, Cordero JF. (1992) Maternal diabetes: the risk for specific birth defects. *Eur J Epidemiol*, **8** (4), 503–508. [Research Support, Non-US Govt]

2 Jenkins KJ, Correa A, Feinstein JA, *et al.* (2007) Noninherited risk factors and congenital cardiovascular defects: current knowledge: a scientific statement from the American Heart Association Council on

Cardiovascular Disease in the Young: endorsed by the American Academy of Pediatrics. *Circulation*, **115** (23), 2995–3014. [Review]
3 Jaeggi ET, Fouron JC, Proulx F. (2001) Fetal cardiac performance in uncomplicated and well-controlled maternal type I diabetes. *Ultrasound Obstet Gynecol*, **17** (4), 311–315.
4 Levy HL, Guldberg P, Guttler F, *et al.* (2001) Congenital heart disease in maternal phenylketonuria: report from the Maternal PKU Collaborative Study. *Pediatr Res*, **49** (5), 636–642. [Clinical Trial Research Support, Non-US Govt Research Support, US Govt, P.H.S.]
5 Buyon JP, Hiebert R, Copel J, *et al.* (1998) Autoimmune-associated congenital heart block: demographics, mortality, morbidity and recurrence rates obtained from a national neonatal lupus registry. *J Am Coll Cardiol*, **31** (7), 1658–1666. [Research Support, US Govt, P.H.S.]
6 Buyon JP, Clancy RM. (2003) Maternal autoantibodies and congenital heart block: mediators, markers, and therapeutic approach. *Semin Arthritis Rheum*, **33** (3), 140–154. [Research Support, Non-US Govt Research Support, US Govt, P.H.S. Review]
7 Ergaz Z, Ornoy A. (2006) Parvovirus B19 in pregnancy. *Reprod Toxicol*, **21** (4), 421–435. [Review]
8 Moise KJ Jr, Huhta JC, Sharif DS, *et al.* (1988) Indomethacin in the treatment of premature labor: effects on the fetal ductus arteriosus. *N Engl J Med*, **319** (6), 327–331.
9 Pettit KE, Merchant M, Machin GA, Tacy TA, Norton ME. (2013) Congenital heart defects in a large, unselected cohort of monochorionic twins. *J Perinatol*, **33** (6), 457–461.
10 Alrais F, Feldstein VA, Srivastava D, Gosnell K, Moon-Grady AJ. (2011) Monochorionic twins discordant for congenital heart disease: a referral center's experience and possible pathophysiologic mechanisms. *Prenat Diagn*, **31** (10), 978–984.
11 Fesslova V, Brankovic J, Lalatta F, *et al.* (2011) Recurrence of congenital heart disease in cases with familial risk screened prenatally by echocardiography. *J Pregnancy*, **2011**, 368067.
12 Nora JJ, Nora AH. (1976) Recurrence risks in children having one parent with a congenital heart disease. *Circulation*, **53** (4), 701–702. [Research Support, US Govt, P.H.S.]
13 Pierpont ME, Basson CT, Benson DW Jr, *et al.* (2007) Genetic basis for congenital heart defects: current knowledge: a scientific statement from the American Heart Association Congenital Cardiac Defects Committee, Council on Cardiovascular Disease in the Young: endorsed by the American Academy of Pediatrics. *Circulation*, **115** (23), 3015–3038. [Review]
14 Vogel M, McElhinney DB, Marcus E, *et al.* (2010) Significance and outcome of left heart hypoplasia in fetal congenital diaphragmatic hernia. *Ultrasound Obstet Gynecol*, **35** (3), 310–317. [Research Support, Non-US Govt]
15 Simpson LL. (2013) Twin–twin transfusion syndrome. *Am J Obstet Gynecol*, **208** (1), 3–18. [Practice Guideline]
16 Moon-Grady AJ, Rand L, Lemley B, *et al.* (2011) Effect of selective fetoscopic laser photocoagulation therapy for twin–twin transfusion syndrome on pulmonary valve pathology in recipient twins. *Ultrasound Obstet Gynecol*, **37** (1), 27–33. [Evaluation Studies Research Support, Non-US Govt]
17 Aburawi EH, Malcus P, Thuring A, Fellman V, Pesonen E. (2012) Coronary flow in neonates with impaired intrauterine growth. *J Am Soc Echocardiogr*, **25** (3), 313–318. [Research Support, Non-US Govt]
18 Trucco SM, Jaeggi E, Cuneo B, *et al.* (2011) Use of intravenous gamma globulin and corticosteroids in the treatment of maternal autoantibody-mediated cardiomyopathy. *J Am Coll Cardiol*, **57** (6), 715–723. [Multicenter Study]
19 Szwast A, Tian Z, McCann M, *et al.* (2007) Impact of altered loading conditions on ventricular performance in fetuses with congenital cystic adenomatoid malformation and twin–twin transfusion syndrome. *Ultrasound Obstet Gynecol*, **30** (1), 40–46. [Research Support, N.I.H., Extramural Twin Study]

3

The Natural and Unnatural History of Fetal Heart Disease

Karim A. Diab[1] *and Samer Masri*[2]

[1] *Rush Center for Congenital Heart Disease, Chicago, IL, USA*
[2] *American University of Beirut, Beirut, Lebanon*

The advent of fetal echocardiography has enhanced our understanding of how fetal cardiac disease progresses throughout gestation. Most major structural cardiovascular malformations develop during the first 6–7 weeks' gestation while other abnormalities develop or become apparent only later in gestation. These anomalies can continue to progress throughout gestation resulting in significant hemodynamic consequences. Recognition of the evolution of fetal heart disease is essential for proper prenatal counseling, adequate preparation for postnatal management, and for planning of any fetal cardiac intervention that could potentially alter the natural history of the disease.

Lesions that involve obstruction to blood flow at the level of the ventricular inflow or outflow are examples of lesions that can have critical sequelae on the growth of cardiac structures [1]. The algorithm in Figure 3.1 describes the progression of outflow obstructive lesions with advancing pregnancy. Following the progression of these lesions is important to better predict the postnatal management (Figures 3.2, 3.3, and 3.4). It can also be helpful in guiding the decision for intrauterine intervention, which can prevent the progression of disease severity. Fetuses with right-sided obstructive lesions, such as tetralogy of Fallot (TOF), may develop progressive pulmonary hypoplasia resulting in more severe obstruction or even pulmonary atresia.

Significant atrioventricular valve (AVV) regurgitation (i.e., AV canal, Ebstein anomaly) or semilunar valve regurgitation (i.e., truncus arteriosus, TOF with absent pulmonary valve syndrome) is usually poorly tolerated by the fetus [2]. The algorithm in Figure 3.5 describes the potential events in the progression of AVV regurgitation that can result in significant cardiovascular compromise in utero (Figures 3.6 and 3.7).

Other structural cardiac malformations can also progress in utero. In transposition of the great arteries, progressive hemodynamic changes can cause severe postnatal hypoxemia requiring urgent balloon atrial septostomy (Figures 3.8 and 3.9) [3]. Although many ventricular septal defects are not hemodynamically significant, it is important to know the natural history so as to counsel the family appropriately as some defects may evolve or even regress (Figure 3.10) [4].

Fetal arrhythmias occur in approximately 2% of pregnancies and can progress throughout gestation (Figure 3.11) [5]. Transplacental therapy may be necessary in order to modify the natural history of the disease.

Lastly, cardiac tumors can also change throughout fetal life and lead to secondary hemodynamic effects (Figure 3.12).

Visual Guide to Neonatal Cardiology, First Edition. Edited by Ernerio T. Alboliras, Ziyad M. Hijazi, Leo Lopez, and Donald J. Hagler.

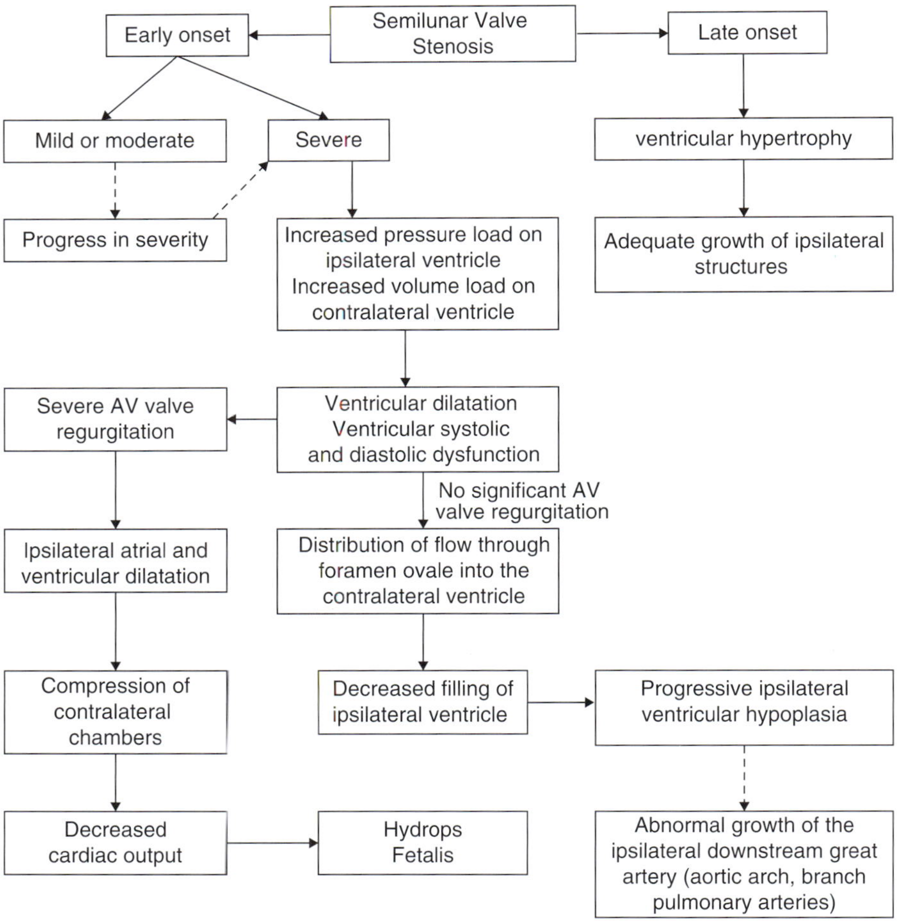

Figure 3.1 Natural progression of ventricular outflow obstruction (aortic/pulmonary stenosis).

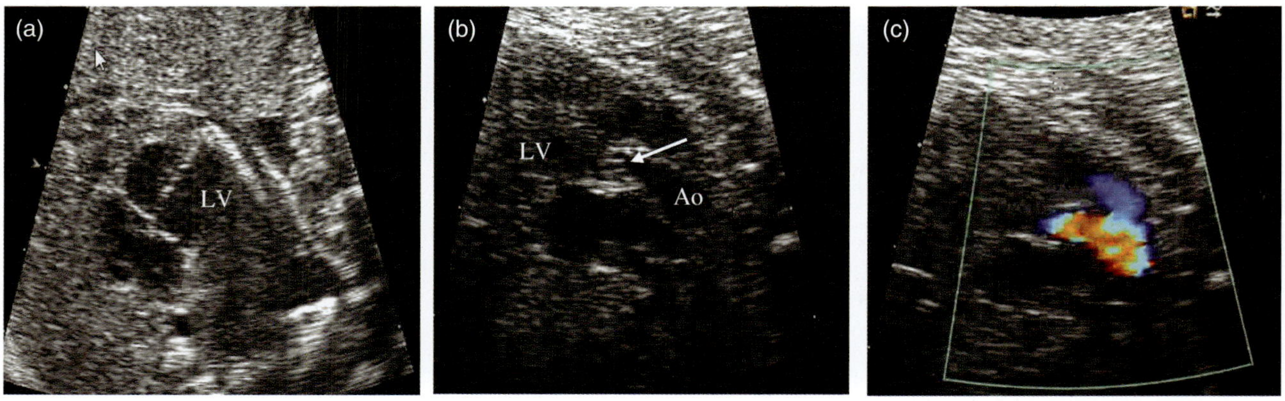

Figure 3.2 Progression of aortic stenosis in a fetus. The earlier the outflow obstruction develops in the fetus, the higher the likelihood of progression of left ventricle (LV) hypoplasia. (a) At 21 weeks, the LV has normal size and systolic function. (b) The aortic valve is thickened (arrow) causing LV outflow tract obstruction. (c) Color Doppler demonstrating turbulence across the LV outflow tract. (d) The peak gradient was 46 mmHg. (e) As the obstruction increases, the LV becomes progressively more dilated with reduced systolic function; there can be reversal of flow across the foramen ovale and aortic arch. To change the natural history of the disease and potential development of hypoplastic left heart syndrome, the patient underwent closed fetal cardiac intervention with balloon valvuloplasty of the aortic valve. (f) After the procedure, the LV is normal in size and function with normal right to left shunting across the patent foramen ovale. (g) Postnatally, the LV was normal in size and only aortic balloon valvuloplasty was needed. LV, left ventricle, Ao, ascending aorta.

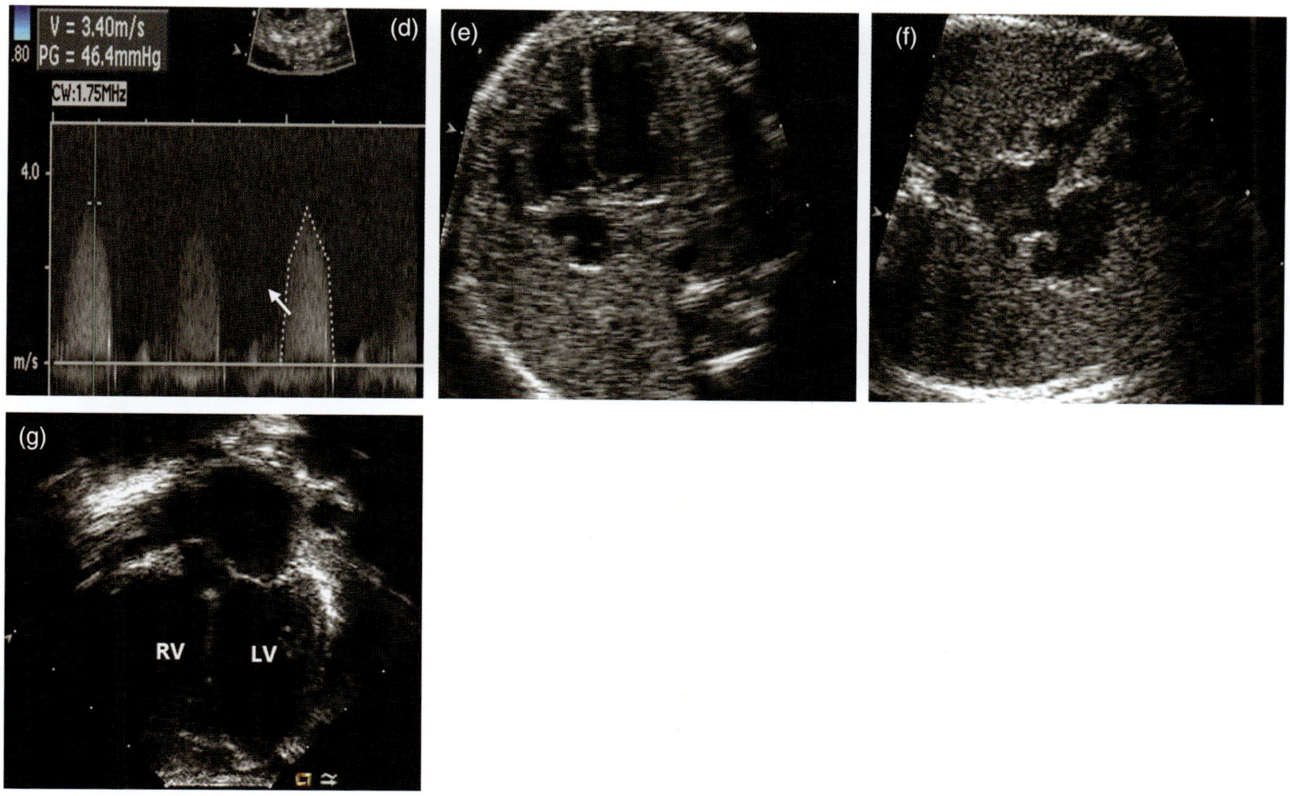

Figure 3.2 (*Continued*)

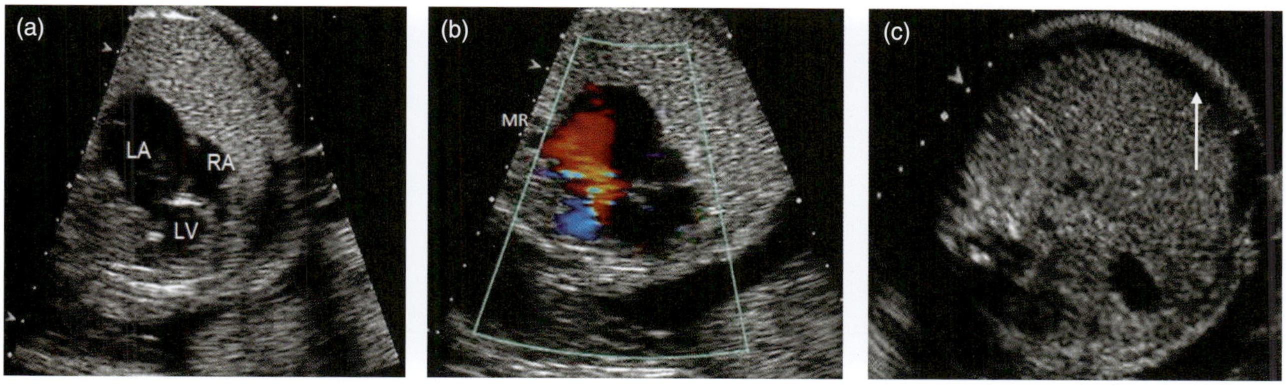

Figure 3.3 Echocardiographic imaging in a fetus with severe aortic valve stenosis resulting in hydrops fetalis. Unlike the previous case, at 30 weeks, severe mitral regurgitation (MR) was present. In the setting of outflow tract obstruction, the usual evolution is progressive ventricular hypoplasia. However, when significant atrioventricular valve insufficiency develops, the ventricle undergoes significant dilatation. (a) Four-chamber view shows severe left ventricle (LV) dilatation. There is severely decreased systolic function, and left atrium (LA) dilatation which compresses the right atrium (RA). (b) Severe mitral regurgitation. (c) Development of significant ascites and hydrops.

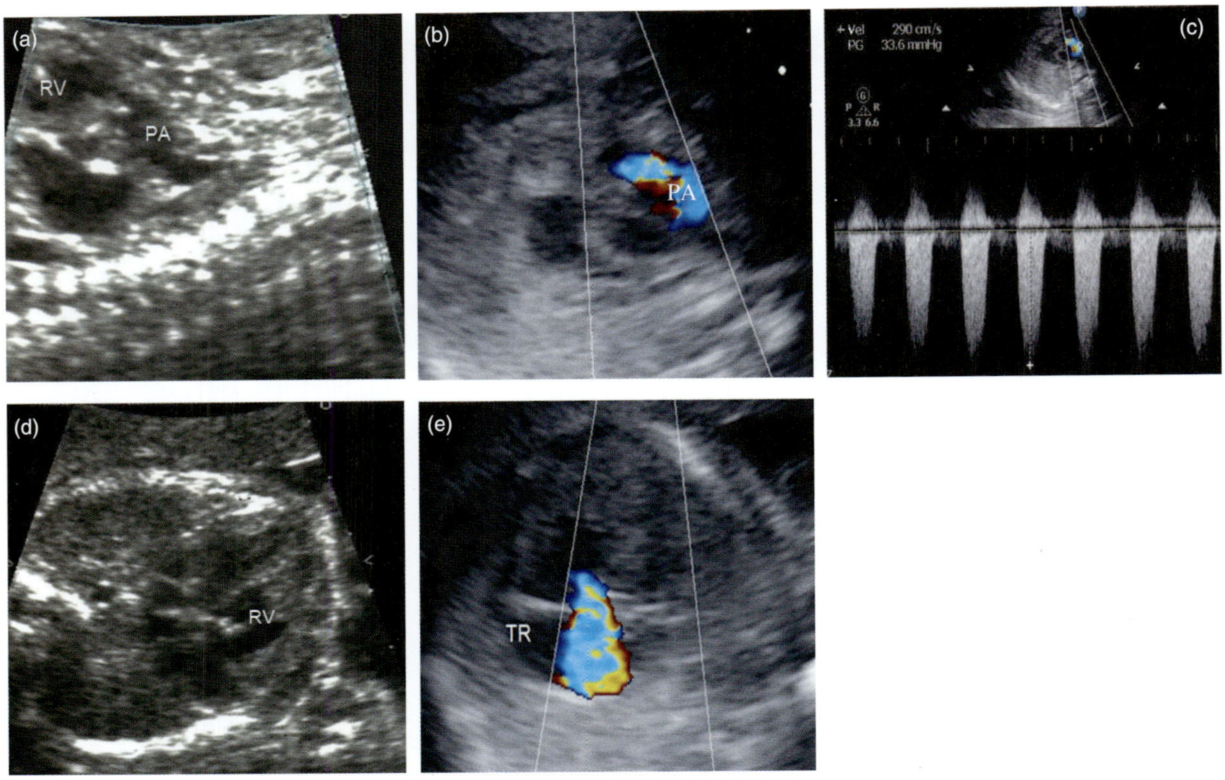

Figure 3.4 Progression of right ventricular outflow tract (RVOT) obstruction. (a) At 20 weeks, the pulmonary valve is doming and thickened. The right ventricle (RV) is mildly hypertrophied with normal systolic function. (b) Color flow mapping revealed turbulence at the level of the valve. (c) Peak gradient is 34 mmHg. (d) At 24 weeks, there is moderate RV hypertrophy and hypoplasia, with severe tricuspid regurgitation (TR) by color flow Doppler (e), predicting a suprasystemic right ventricular pressure (RVP). PA, pulmonary artery.

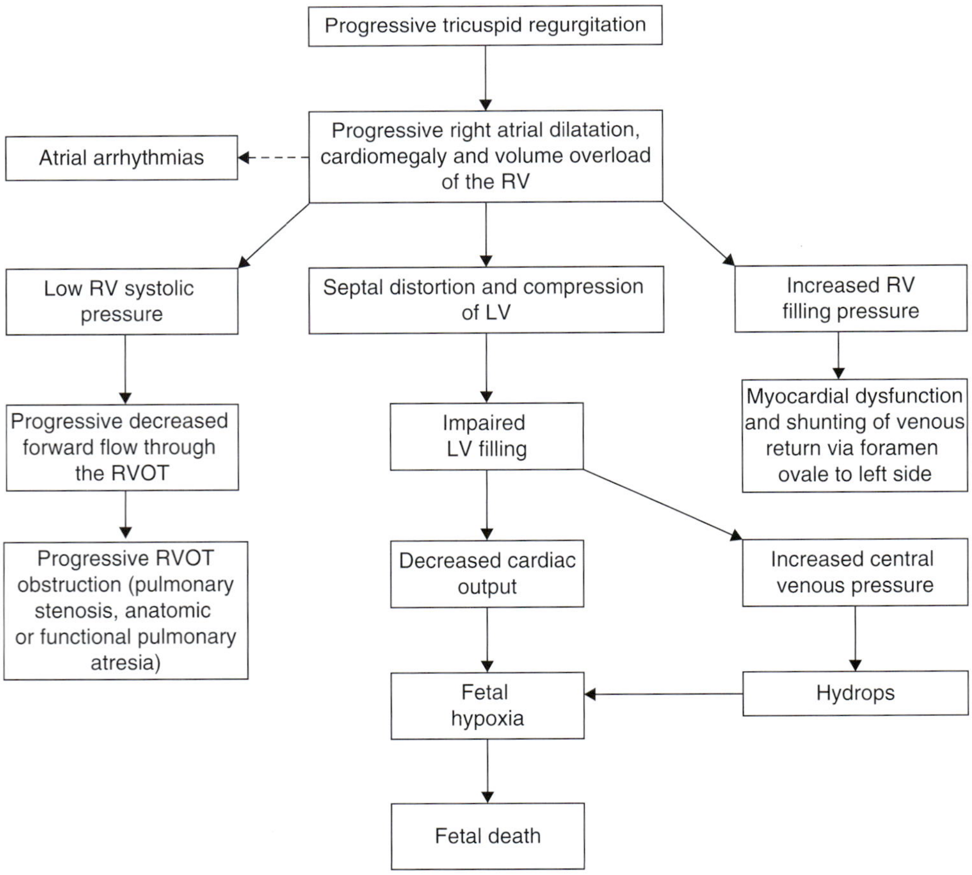

Figure 3.5 Natural history and progression in the fetus with significant atrioventricular valve regurgitation (e.g., Ebstein anomaly). LV, left ventricle; RV, right ventricle; RVOT, right ventricular outflow tract.

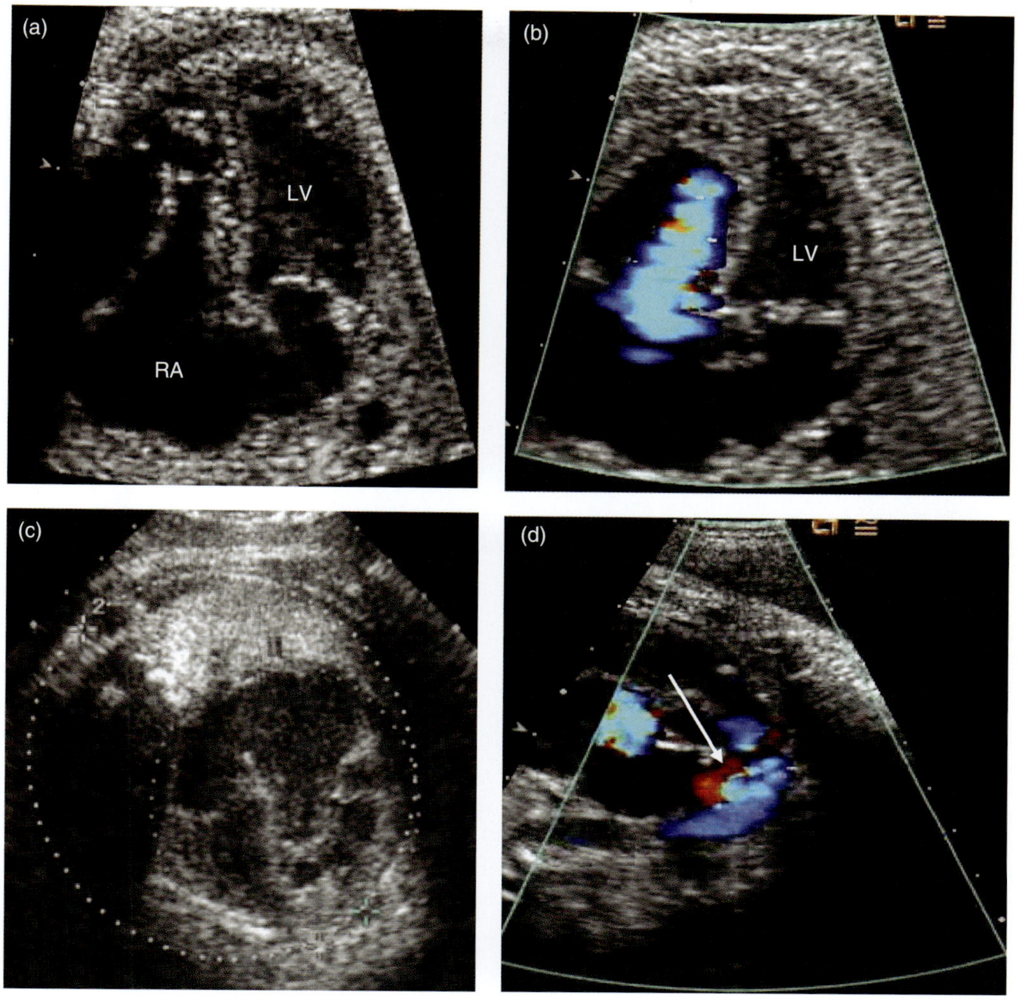

Figure 3.6 Severe Ebstein anomaly. (a,b) Severe tricuspid regurgitation with severe right atrial (RA) and right ventricular (RV) dilatation. This progressed in pregnancy and (c) resulted in significant increase in the cardiothoracic ratio and compression of the left ventricle (LV). (d) Decrease in forward flow through the RV outflow tract results in functional pulmonary atresia with reversal of flow in the ductus arteriosus (arrow).

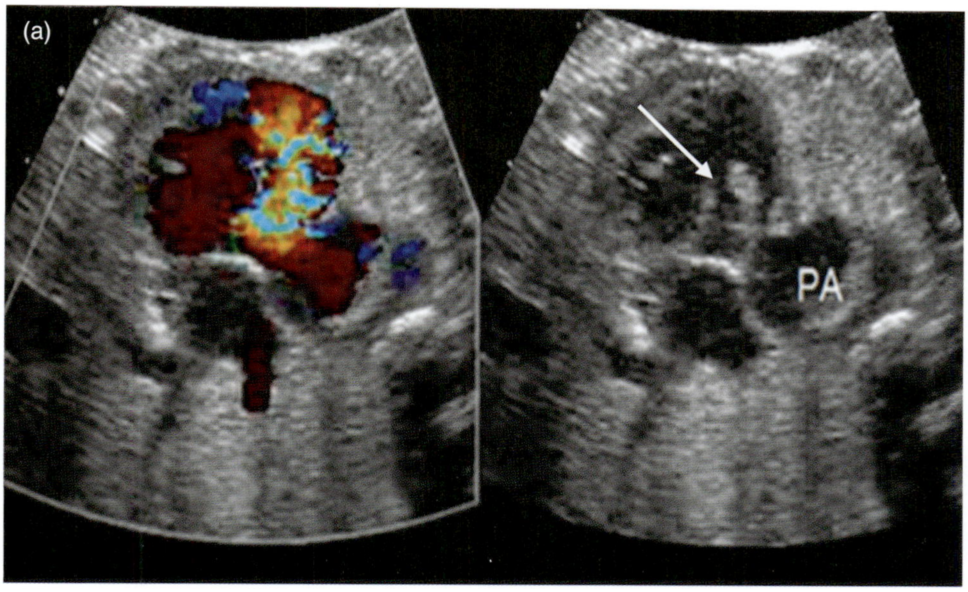

Figure 3.7 Tetralogy of Fallot with absent pulmonary valve syndrome. (a) Anterior malalignment ventricular septal defect (VSD; arrow) and free pulmonary regurgitation (color) cause progressive dilatation of the proximal pulmonary arteries (PA) which can result in significant compression on the tracheal–bronchial tree and esophagus. (b) Free pulmonary regurgitation shown by Doppler across the RV outflow tract.

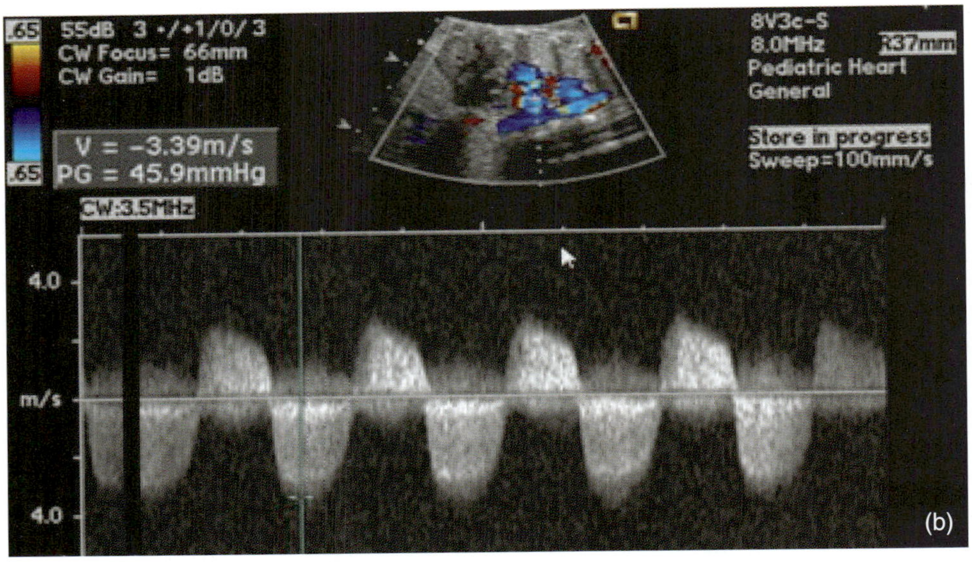

Figure 3.7 (*Continued*)

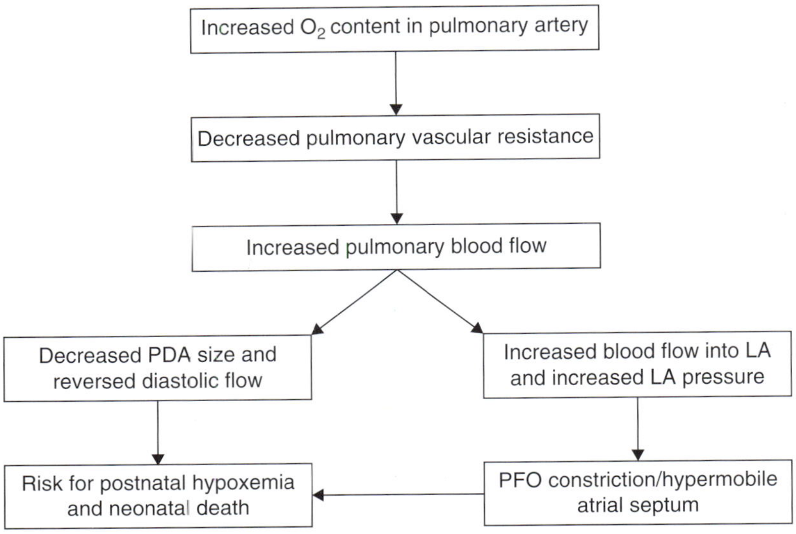

Figure 3.8 D-transposition of the great arteries. Progression of events leading to significant postnatal hypoxemia and need for urgent balloon atrial septostomy. LA, left atrium; PDA, patent ductus arteriosus; PFO, patent foramen ovale.

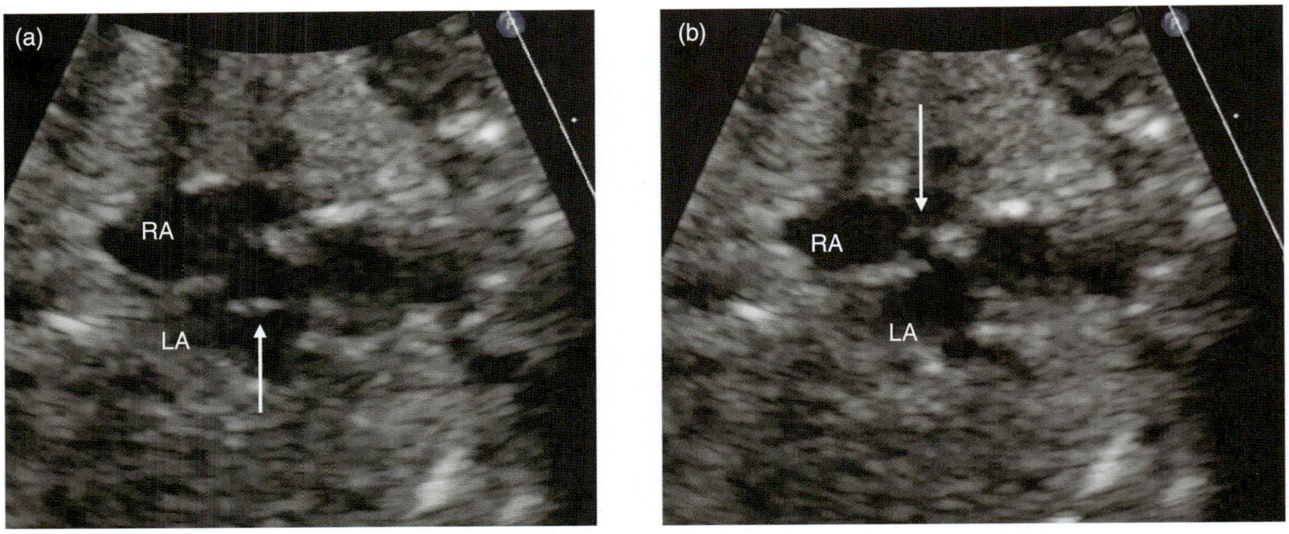

Figure 3.9 D-transposition of the great arteries. The progressive increase in the left atria blood flow results in increased pressure and causes the atrial septum to oscillate between (b) the right and (a) left atrium. This can be predictive of significant hypoxemia after birth requiring urgent balloon septostomy. LA, left atrium; RA, right atrium.

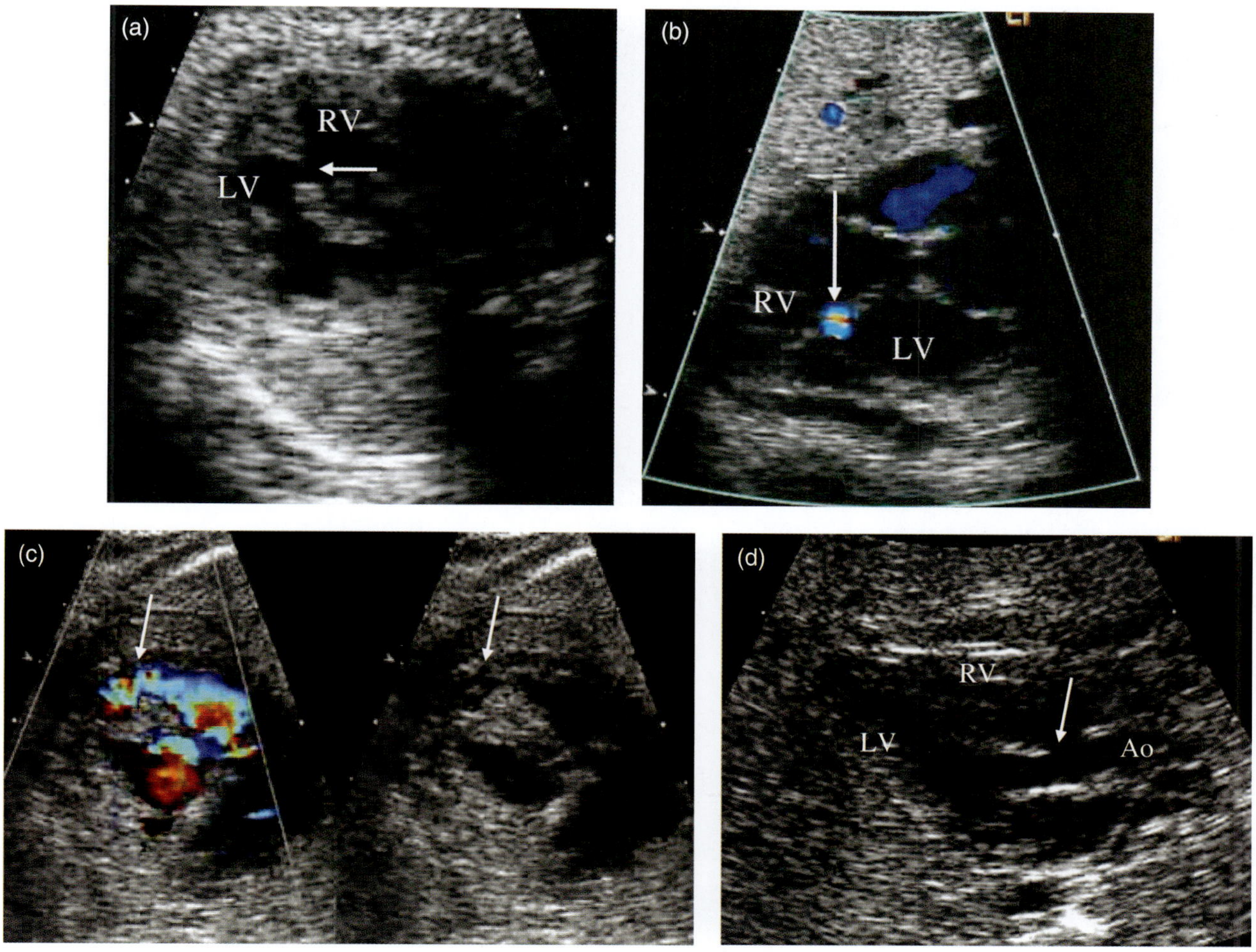

Figure 3.10 Ventricular septal defect (VSD). (a,b) Small mid-muscular VSD (arrow). Such defects often close spontaneously, up to one-third in utero. (c) Large muscular VSD in the apical muscular septum (arrow). This size of defect is less likely to close in utero and may require intervention postnatally. (d) Large posterior malalignment VSD with an overriding aorta (Ao). These defects do not close spontaneously and can be associated with chromosomal abnormalities.

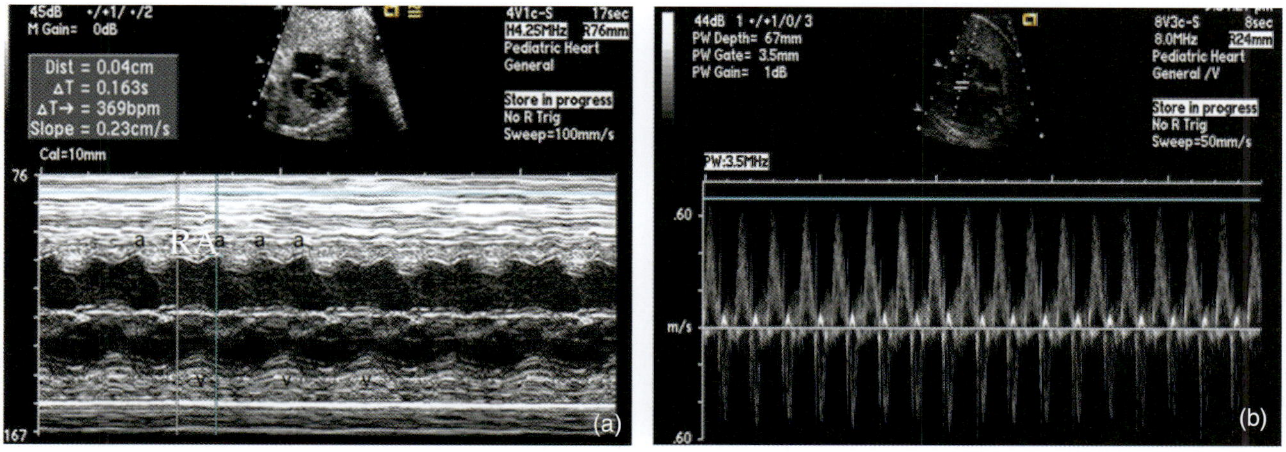

Figure 3.11 Fetal arrhythmias. (a) Atrial flutter; (b) supraventricular tachycardia. Fetal tachyarrhythmias, which usually develop in the late second or third trimesters, can progress and lead to significant fetal compromise necessitating early recognition and transplancental therapy. (c) Similarly, complete heart block, either associated with structural heart disease or more commonly with maternal autoantibodies, can lead to significant cardiovascular compromise.

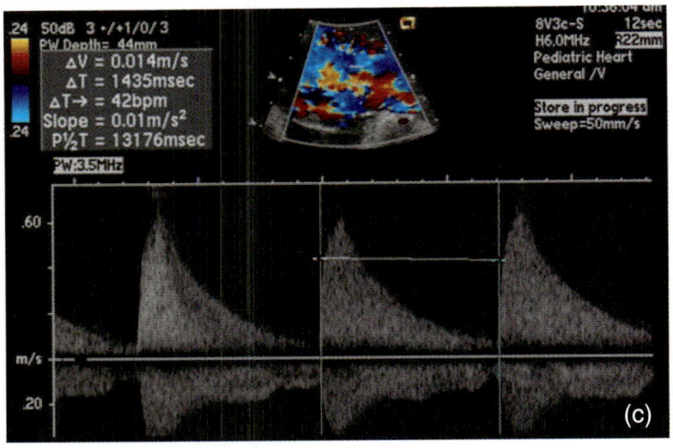

Figure 3.11 (*Continued*)

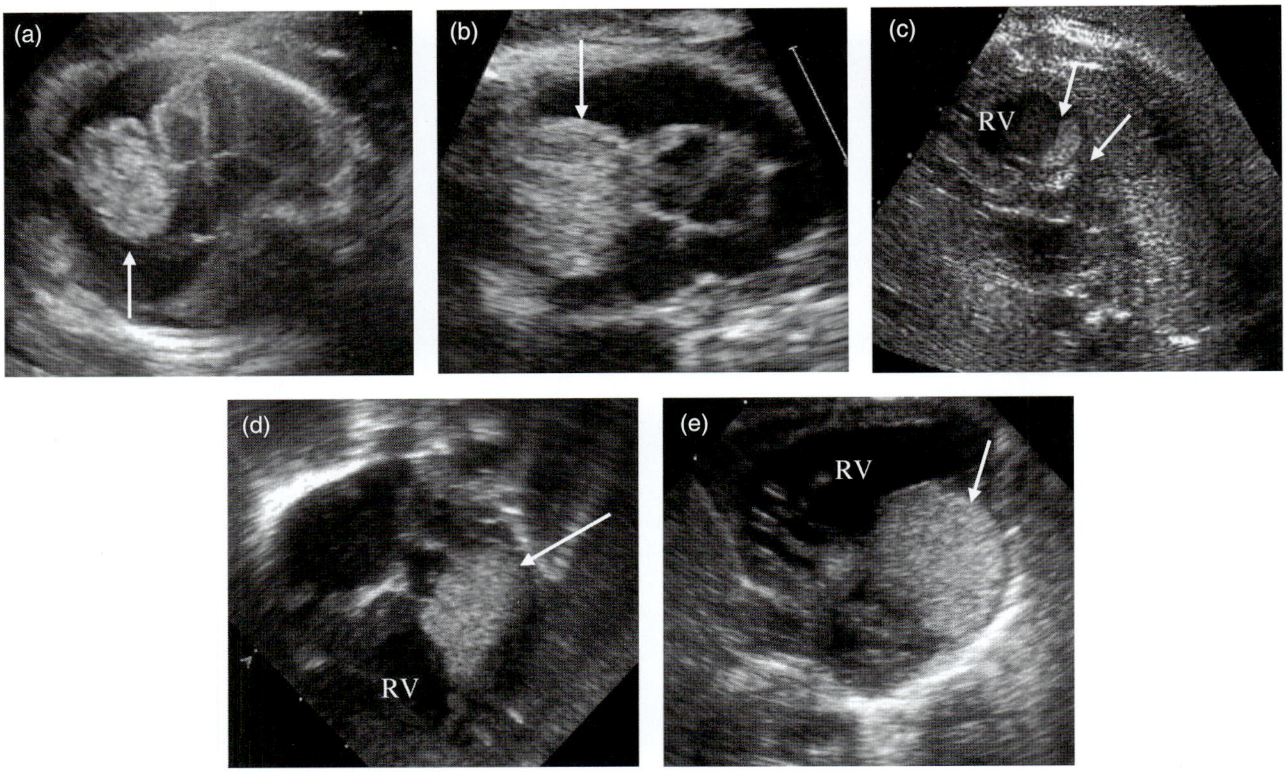

Figure 3.12 Cardiac tumors. (a,b) Pericardial teratoma (arrow) progresses in size and results in severe pericardial effusion and hydrops fetalis. (c) Rhabdomyomas tend to be multiple (arrows) and frequently increase in size potentially leading to inflow or outflow obstruction before regressing. (d,e) Large rhabdomyoma (arrows) occupying most of the LV and obstructing flow resulting across the LV outflow tract and resulting in near hypoplastic left heart syndrome.

References

1 Yamamoto Y, Hornberger LK. (2012) Progression of outflow tract obstruction in the fetus. *Early Hum Dev*, **88**, 279–285.

2 Acharya G, Archer N, Huhta JC. (2007) Functional assessment of the evolution of congenital heart disease in utero. *Curr Opin Pediatr*, **19**, 533–537.

3 Punn R, Silverman NH. (2011) Fetal predictors of urgent balloon atrial septostomy in neonates with complete transposition. *J Am Soc Echocardiogr*, **24**, 425–430.

4 Paladini D, Palmieri S, Lamberti A, *et al.* (2000) Characterization and natural history of ventricular septal defects in the fetus. *Ultrasound Obstet Gynecol*, **16**, 118–122.

5 Hornberger LK, Sahn DJ. (2007) Rhythm abnormalities of the fetus. *Heart*, **93**, 1294–1300.

Part II

General Neonatal Issues

4

Epidemiology of Heart Defects

Gregory H. Tatum and Piers C.A. Barker

Division of Pediatric Cardiology, Duke University Medical Center, Durham, NC, USA

Numerous epidemiology studies have demonstrated that congenital heart disease (CHD) is the most common type of birth defect noted in the USA (Table 4.1) [1] as well as other countries [2–4], accounting for 28% of major congenital anomalies [5]. Worldwide, approximately 1.35 million children are born with CHD every year [6]. CHD remains one of the leading causes of infant mortality [4, 7, 8]. Most mortality attributed to CHD occurs in the first year of life, but significant mortality persists into adulthood [9]. As a result of improvements in survival, it is now estimated that there are more adults living with CHD than children [10].

Prevalence of Individual Lesions

The prevalence of CHD is estimated to be around 8 per 1000 live births. Acyanotic CHD is more common than cyanotic heart disease, with ventricular septal defects being the most common lesion (Table 4.2). Tetralogy of Fallot and D-transposition of the great arteries are the most common cyanotic heart lesions (Table 4.3). Autopsy studies have demonstrated the presence of a patent foramen ovale in 27.3% [11] and bicuspid aortic valve in up to 2% of people [12]; however, asymptomatic cases of these two lesions are not included in most studies on prevalence of CHD.

Changes in Prevalence Over Time

The prevalence of CHD has increased in a non-linear fashion over time from 0.6 per 1000 live births in the 1930s to 9.1 per 1000 live births since 1995 [6]. The difference in prevalence rates may be multifactorial. In the 1930s–1950s, the expanding knowledge of CHD led to increased detection. Large prospective birth registries came into existence allowing for the study of the prevalence of CHD, but significant differences in methodology were used. Many studies only reported the most severe forms of CHD diagnosed by invasive methods leading to underestimation of the true prevalence rate. As echocardiography has become more common in clinical practice, some of the changes in the prevalence of CHD have been attributed to better detection [13]. Although a large part of the increase in prevalence of CHD is because of minor defects [14], which may not have been included in earlier studies, the rates of some more severe types of CHD have also increased [14], suggesting that the increasing prevalence of CHD is not because of better detection alone [6]. Childbirth is increasingly being delayed and advanced maternal age has been associated with CHD. There also has been improved survival of premature infants who are at increased risk for certain types of CHD such as a patent ductus arteriosus.

Regional and Racial Variation

Regional variations exist in the reported prevalence of CHD. The prevalence of CHD is highest in Asia (9.3 per 1000 live births) and lowest in Africa (1.9 per 1000 live births) [6]. The regional prevalence of CHD varies within as well between countries [5, 15]. In addition to variations in the overall prevalence, regional differences have been detected for individual lesions. Asia has reported a higher prevalence of right-sided obstructive lesions and lower prevalence of left-sided obstructive lesions [6, 16]. These regional differences suggest that genetic factors may affect the risk for CHD among different populations.

A correlation has been found between economic status of the countries and reported incidence of CHD, with a higher incidence in regions of more affluence [6]. The correlation between differences in socioeconomic status and birth prevalence of CHD suggest that lack of access to medical care may lead to underreporting of CHD in lower income populations.

Within the USA, several reports have shown racial differences in the prevalence of CHD [14, 17, 18] as well as among socioeconomic classes [18]. Tetralogy of

Visual Guide to Neonatal Cardiology, First Edition. Edited by Ernerio T. Alboliras, Ziyad M. Hijazi, Leo Lopez, and Donald J. Hagler.

Table 4.1 Prevalence of common birth defects in the United States [1], Canada [2], and Europe [3].

Type of birth defect	Rate per 10 000 live births		
	USA 2004–2006	Canada 1991–1993	Europe 2003–2007
Congenital heart disease	62–90[a]	79.1	73.2
Ventricular septal defect	–	30.4	30.4
Atrial septal defect	–	23.0	22.7
Atrioventricular septal defect	4.71	2.8	3.8
Tetralogy of Fallot	3.97	4.2	2.9
Transposition of the great arteries	3.0	4.2	3.2
Hypoplastic left heart syndrome	2.3	2.9	2.9
Truncus arteriosus	0.72	1.2	0.8
Trisomy 21	14.47	12.4	20.5
Cleft lip with or without cleft palate	10.63	10.7	9.4
Gastroschesis	4.49	–	2.5
Spina bifida without anencephaly	3.5	6.3	5.1
Congenital diaphragmatic hernia	2.61	–	2.8

a) Estimated rate derived from data published by Botto *et al.* [14].

Table 4.2 Acyanotic heart lesions prevalence per 1000 live births.

	Baltimore 1981–1982 [34]	Alberta 1981–1984 [35]	Qatar 1984–1994 [36]	Atlanta 1968–1997 [14]	Quebec 1985–2000 [10]
VSD	0.863	1.945	4.971	1.66	4.2
ASD	0.317	0.580	0.882	0.46	3.89
AVSD	0.362	0.242	0.341	0.12 (without trisomy 21 0.15 (with trisomy 21	0.57
Pulmonary stenosis	0.189		1.062	0.38	0.5
Patent ductus arteriosus	0.089	0.251	0.622	0.66	0.31
Aortic stenosis	0.111		0.3	0.1	0.27
Coarctation of the aorta	0.239		0.51	0.29	0.25

Table 4.3 Cyanotic heart disease prevalence per 1000 live births.

	Baltimore 1981–1982 [34]	Alberta 1981–1984 [35]	Qatar 1984–1994 [36]	Atlanta 1968–1997 [14]	Quebec 1985–2000 [10]
Tetralogy of Fallot	0.262	0.203	0.622	0.38	0.45
Transposition of the great arteries	0.211	0.28	0.381	0.25	0.27
Hypoplastic left heart syndrome	0.267		0.22	0.21	
Total anomalous pulmonary venous return	0.083	0.087	0.22	0.07	
Pulmonary atresia/intact septum	0.083		0.08	0.05	
Double outlet right ventricle	0.056	0.145	0.321	0.11	
Tricuspid atresia	0.039		0.1	0.3	
Ebstein anomaly			0.04	0.04	0.02
Truncus arteriosus	0.056			0.06	0.04

Box 4.1 Exposures associated with definite or possible risk of offspring with congenital cardiovascular defects

1) Maternal illness
   - Phenylketonuria – any defect
   - Pregestational diabetes – ventricular septal defect, d-TGA, aortic stenosis, pulmonary atresia, dextrocardia, PDA, and other conotruncal defects (tetralogy of Fallot, truncus arteriosus, and double outlet right ventricle)
   - Maternal rubella – VSD, PDA, pulmonary valve stenosis, peripheral pulmonary stenosis
   - Influenza – tricuspid atresia, coarctation of aorta, d-TGA, all right-sided or left-sided obstruction defect
   - Febrile illness – tricuspid atresia, coarctation of aorta, all right-sided or left-sided obstruction defect
   - Epilepsy – any defect
2) Maternal drug exposure
   - Anticonvulsants – any defect
   - Indomethacin for tocolysis – PDA constriction or intrauterine PDA closure
   - NSAID/Ibuprofen – d-TGA, AV canal, VSD
   - Thalidomide – any defect
   - Trimethoprim-sulfonamide – any defect
   - Retinoids – any defect
   - Marijuana – Ebstein anomaly, VSD
3) Environmental (maternal) – organic solvents
   - Organic solvents – AV canal defect, pulmonary stenosis, Ebstein anomaly, d-TGA, HLHS, conotruncal defects, TAPVR

AV canal, atrioventricular canal; d-TGA, dextro-transposition of great arteries; HLHS, hypoplastic left heart syndrome; PDA, patent ductus arteriosus; TAPVR, total anomalous pulmonary venous return; VSD, ventricular septal defect.

Fallot is seen more frequently in non-Hispanic black people than non-Hispanic white people and is seen least frequently in Hispanic people. Hispanic infants also had a lower incidence of hypoplastic left heart syndrome [17]. In studies comparing black with white populations, pulmonary stenosis has been found to occur more frequently in black people while D-transposition of the great vessels, coarctation of the aorta, and aortic stenosis were more frequent in white people [14, 18]. The discrepancy between races may have a genetic basis. However, access to healthcare also may have a significant role in the different prevalence rates. There are differences in infant mortality rates between the different races [8, 19], which would suggest that variable access to healthcare may be a factor in the reported racial differences.

Impact of Fetal Testing

The increased use of fetal testing has the potential to create differences between the fetal and postnatal prevalence of many lesions. While an in utero diagnosis permits better preparation of both the family and the medical team to optimize postnatal care, it also produces a decision whether to continue or terminate the pregnancy. Choices regarding termination vary greatly by country and are affected by gestational age at diagnosis and cardiac defect [20–24]. As an example, pregnancies complicated with pulmonary atresia with intact ventricular septum had a 61% termination rate in the UK 1991–1995 [25]. Overall, termination may decrease the prevalence of many types of CHD by 2–50%, with highest rates associated with single ventricle defects [26].

Non-Genetic Risk Factors

The understanding of the association between non-genetic factors and CHD continues to increase. Identified risk factors are presented in Box 4.1 [27]. Other risk factors remain more controversial. Several studies have reported an increased risk of CHD in pregnancies conceived with assisted reproductive technologies (ART), particularly septal defects [28, 29]. However, most studies examining the impact of ART are confounded by the increased fetal surveillance that typically occurs with a high-risk pregnancy, a lower likelihood of termination, and the inherent increased risks secondary to increased maternal age or causes of maternal infertility [30].

An association between maternal obesity and CHD has also been reported [31–33], with risk increasing with increased body mass index (BMI). Causal mechanisms for either ART or obesity producing an increased risk of CHD remain unclear beyond undiagnosed maternal diabetes or nutritional derangements. In contrast, maternal folic acid supplementation prior to conception and during early pregnancy may protect the fetus from the development of CHD, with further epidemiologic studies needed to confirm this effect [27].

References

1 Parker SE, Mai CT, Canfield MA, *et al.* (2010) Updated National Birth Prevalence estimates for selected birth defects in the United States, 2004–2006. *Birth Defects Res A Clin Mol Teratol*, **88** (12), 1008–1016. PubMed PMID: 20878909.

2 Johnson KC, Rouleau J. (1997) Temporal trends in Canadian birth defects birth prevalences, 1979–1993. *Can J Public Health*, **88** (3), 169–176. PubMed PMID: 9260357.

3 Dolk H, Loane M, Garne E. (2010) The prevalence of congenital anomalies in Europe. *Adv Exp Med Biol*, **686**, 349–364. PubMed PMID: WOS:000282382800020.

4 Billett J, Majeed A, Gatzoulis M, Cowie M. (2008) Trends in hospital admissions, in-hospital case fatality and population mortality from congenital heart disease in England, 1994 to 2004. *Heart*, **94** (3), 342–348. PubMed PMID: 17646196.

5 Dolk H, Loane M, Garne E; European Surveillance of Congenital Anomalies (EUROCAT) Working Group. (2011) Congenital heart defects in Europe prevalence and perinatal mortality, 2000 to 2005. *Circulation*, **123** (8), 841–849.

6 van der Linde D, Konings EE, Slager MA, *et al.* (2011) Birth prevalence of congenital heart disease worldwide: a systematic review and meta-analysis. *J Am Coll Cardiol*, **58** (21), 2241–2247. PubMed PMID: 22078432.

7 Heron M, Hoyert DL, Murphy SL, *et al.* (2009) Deaths: final data for 2006. *Natl Vital Stat Rep*, **57** (14), 1–134. PubMed PMID: 19788058.

8 Boneva RS, Botto LD, Moore CA, *et al.* (2001) Mortality associated with congenital heart defects in the United States: trends and racial disparities, 1979–1997. *Circulation*, **103** (19), 2376–2381. PubMed PMID: 11352887.

9 Gilboa SM, Salemi JL, Nembhard WN, Fixler DE, Correa A. (2010) Mortality resulting from congenital heart disease among children and adults in the United States, 1999 to 2006. *Circulation*, **122** (22), 2254–2263. PubMed PMID: 21098447.

10 Marelli AJ, Mackie AS, Ionescu-Ittu R, Rahme E, Pilote L. (2007) Congenital heart disease in the general population: changing prevalence and age distribution. *Circulation*, **115** (2), 163–172. PubMed PMID: 17210844.

11 Hagen PT, Scholz DG, Edwards WD. (1984) Incidence and size of patent foramen ovale during the first 10 decades of life: an autopsy study of 965 normal hearts. *Mayo Clinic Proc*, **59** (1), 17–20. PubMed PMID: 6694427.

12 Roberts WC. (1970) The congenitally bicuspid aortic valve: a study of 85 autopsy cases. *Am J Cardiol*, **26** (1), 72–83. PubMed PMID: 5427836.

13 Wilson PD, Correa-Villasenor A, Loffredo CA, Ferencz C. (1993) Temporal trends in prevalence of cardiovascular malformations in Maryland and the District of Columbia, 1981–1988. The Baltimore-Washington Infant Study Group. *Epidemiology*, **4** (3), 259–265. PubMed PMID: 8512990.

14 Botto LD, Correa A, Erickson JD. (2001) Racial and temporal variations in the prevalence of heart defects. *Pediatrics*, **107** (3), E32. PubMed PMID: 11230613.

15 Rankin J, Pattenden S, Abramsky L, *et al.* (2005) Prevalence of congenital anomalies in five British regions, 1991–99. *Arch Dis Child Fetal Neonatal Ed*, **90** (5), F374–379. PubMed PMID: 16113153. Pubmed Central PMCID: 1721948.

16 Jacobs EG, Leung MP, Karlberg J. (2000) Distribution of symptomatic congenital heart disease in Hong Kong. *Pediatr Cardiol*, **21** (2), 148–157. PubMed PMID: 10754087.

17 Canfield MA, Honein MA, Yuskiv N, *et al.* (2006) National estimates and race/ethnic-specific variation of selected birth defects in the United States, 1999–2001. *Birth Defects Res A*, **76** (11), 747–756.

18 Correa-Villasenor A, McCarter R, Downing J, Ferencz C. (1991) White–black differences in cardiovascular malformations in infancy and socioeconomic factors. The Baltimore-Washington Infant Study Group. *Am J Epidemiol*, **134** (4), 393–402. PubMed PMID: 1877600.

19 Yang Q, Chen H, Correa A, *et al.* (2006) Racial differences in infant mortality attributable to birth defects in the United States, 1989–2002. *Birth Defects Res A Clin Mol Teratol*, **76** (10), 706–713. PubMed PMID: 17022030.

20 Khoshnood B, De Vigan C, Vodovar V, *et al.* (2005) Trends in prenatal diagnosis, pregnancy termination, and perinatal mortality of newborns with congenital heart disease in France, 1983–2000: a population-based evaluation. *Pediatrics*, **115** (1), 95–101. PubMed PMID: 15629987.

21 Montana E, Khoury MJ, Cragan JD, *et al.* (1996) Trends and outcomes after prenatal diagnosis of congenital cardiac malformations by fetal echocardiography in a well defined birth population, Atlanta, Georgia, 1990–1994. *J Am Coll Cardiol*, **28** (7), 1805–1809. PubMed PMID: 8962570.

22 Nikkila A, Bjorkhem G, Kallen B. (2007) Prenatal diagnosis of congenital heart defects: a population based study. *Acta Paediatrica*, **96** (1), 49–52. PubMed PMID: 17187603.

23 Shevell T P-DA, Simpson L. (2001) Prenatal diagnosis of congenital heart disease and voluntary pregnancy termination: experience of a single tertiary care center. *Am J Obstet Gynecol*, **185** (6), S254.

24 Tegnander E, Williams W, Johansen OJ, Blaas HG, Eik-Nes SH. (2006) Prenatal detection of heart defects in a non-selected population of 30,149 fetuses: detection rates and outcome. *Ultrasound Obstet Gynecol*, **27** (3), 252–265. PubMed PMID: 16456842.

25 Daubeney PE, Sharland GK, Cook AC, *et al.* (1998) Pulmonary atresia with intact ventricular septum: impact of fetal echocardiography on incidence at birth and postnatal outcome. UK and Eire Collaborative Study of Pulmonary Atresia with Intact Ventricular Septum. *Circulation*, **98** (6), 562–566. PubMed PMID: 9714114.

26 Germanakis I, Sifakis S. (2006) The impact of fetal echocardiography on the prevalence of liveborn congenital heart disease. *Pediatr Cardiol*, **27** (4), 465–472. PubMed PMID: 16830077.

27 Jenkins KJ, Correa A, Feinstein JA, *et al.* (2007) Noninherited risk factors and congenital cardiovascular defects: current knowledge: a scientific statement from the American Heart Association Council on Cardiovascular Disease in the Young: endorsed by the American Academy of Pediatrics. *Circulation*, **115** (23), 2995–3014. PubMed PMID: 17519397.

28 Hansen M, Bower C, Milne E, de Klerk N, Kurinczuk JJ. (2005) Assisted reproductive technologies and the risk of birth defect: a systematic review. *Human Reprod*, **20** (2), 328–338. PubMed PMID: 15567881.

29 Reefhuis J, Honein MA, Schieve LA, *et al.* (2009) Assisted reproductive technology and major structural birth defects in the United States. *Human Reprod*, **24** (2), 360–366. PubMed PMID: 19010807.

30 Tandulwadkar S, Lodha P, Kharb V. (2012) Congenital malformations and assisted reproductive technique: where is assisted reproductive technique taking us? *J Hum Reprod Sci*, **5** (3), 244–247. PubMed PMID: 23533070. Pubmed Central PMCID: 3604829.

31 Madsen NL, Schwartz SM, Lewin MB, Mueller BA. (2013) Prepregnancy body mass index and congenital heart defects among offspring: a population-based study. *Congenit Heart Dis*, **8** (2), 131–141. PubMed PMID: 22967199.

32 Mills JL, Troendle J, Conley MR, Carter T, Druschel CM. (2010) Maternal obesity and congenital heart defects: a population-based study. *Am J Clin Nutr*, **91** (6), 1543–1549. PubMed PMID: 20375192. Pubmed Central PMCID: 2869507.

33 Stothard KJ, Tennant PW, Bell R, Rankin J. (2009) Maternal overweight and obesity and the risk of congenital anomalies: a systematic review and meta-analysis. *JAMA*, **301** (6), 636–650. PubMed PMID: 19211471.

34 Ferencz C, Rubin JD, McCarter RJ, *et al.* (1985) Congenital heart disease: prevalence at livebirth. The Baltimore-Washington Infant Study. *Am J Epidemiol*, **121** (1), 31–36. PubMed PMID: 3964990.

35 Grabitz RG, Joffres MR, Collins-Nakai RL. (1988) Congenital heart disease: incidence in the first year of life. The Alberta Heritage Pediatric Cardiology Program. *Am J Epidemiol*, **128** (2), 381–388. PubMed PMID: 3394704.

36 Robida A, Folger GM, Hajar HA. (1997) Incidence of congenital heart disease in Qatari children. *Int J Cardiol*, **60** (1), 19–22. PubMed PMID: 9209935.

5

The Transitional and Neonatal Heart and Cardiovascular System

Timothy M. Cordes

Riley Children's Hospital, Indiana University School of Medicine, Indianapolis, IN, USA

At the end of normal fetal gestation the fetus has several distinct cardiovascular structures and unique hemodynamic characteristics. These include venous return of blood to the right atrium from the ductus venosus, which contributes about 45% of the combined fetal cardiac output. A foramen ovale is present with right to left flow of about one-third of the combined cardiac output, and a ductus arteriosus with flow directed from the pulmonary artery to the descending aorta. The ductus arteriosus blood flow has been estimated to be about half of the combined cardiac output. In late gestation, only about 11% of the combined cardiac output is directed into the pulmonary circulation. The right ventricular dominance in utero is a unique hemodynamic characteristic. The right ventricle handles about 60% of the combined cardiac output, and the left ventricle handles about 40%. About 45% of the combined cardiac output circulates towards the low resistance placental vascular bed [1, 2].

Birth and Neonatal Period

Several significant cardiac vascular changes occur at delivery or shortly after. The ductus venosus functionally closes upon clamping of the umbilical cord. This becomes more permanently closed at 3–7 days after delivery. This reduction in venous preload to the right atrium effectively decreases right atrial pressure. At the same time, normal newborn respiration dramatically increases blood flow through the pulmonary circulation and return to the left atrium, thus increasing left atrial pressure to be slightly greater than that of the right atrium. This change in atrial pressure relationship forces the flap of the foramen ovale to close. This functional closure occurs very early but the foramen ovale does not permanently seal closed in most children for 2–5 years [3]. During this time it is not unusual to see a small amount of left to right shunting across the atrial septum (Figures 5.1 and 5.2).

The ductus arteriosus provides right to left flow in utero but several changes occur at the time of delivery that directly alter this. With the clamping of the umbilical vessels and removal of the placenta from the circulation, there is a rapid rise in systemic resistance. At the same time, there is a drop in pulmonary vascular resistance. Initially, the pulmonary vascular resistance may be slightly higher than systemic resistance and the ductus arteriosus will shunt either right to left or bi-directionally. In normal neonates, within a few hours pulmonary vascular resistance has decreased to be below systemic resistance, resulting in a small amount of left to right shunting across the ductus arteriosus. This left to right shunt increases the PO2 of the blood crossing the ductus arteriosus. The increased oxygen tension and the loss of placental prostaglandin E2 cause active constriction of the ductus arteriosus. There is functional closure of the ductus arteriosus in 93% of babies by 60 hours of age. Permanent closure occurs over the next 4–8 weeks by endothelial necrosis and subintimal proliferation (Figure 5.3).

Although there are dramatic changes in right and left ventricular volumes and outputs immediately after delivery, the size of the right ventricle is still relatively large compared to the left ventricle. Therefore, in neonatal echocardiograms the right ventricle will appear mildly dilated when compared to an infant or child [4, 5]. The right ventricle to left ventricle dimension ratio appears to return to normal at 2–4 weeks after delivery (Figure 5.4).

Flattening of the interventricular septum reflects elevated right ventricle and pulmonary artery pressures (Figures 5.5 and 5.6). At delivery, the pulmonary artery pressure and resistance are near systemic. This decreases in the first few hours to less than systemic, and to about 50% of systemic blood pressure in 24 hours. However two-dimensional and M-mode studies have shown that septal flattening can be seen for up to 5–7 days of age, and hyperdynamic septal wall motion, while still present at 1 week, has ceased by 1 month of age [6, 7].

Visual Guide to Neonatal Cardiology, First Edition. Edited by Ernerio T. Alboliras, Ziyad M. Hijazi, Leo Lopez, and Donald J. Hagler.

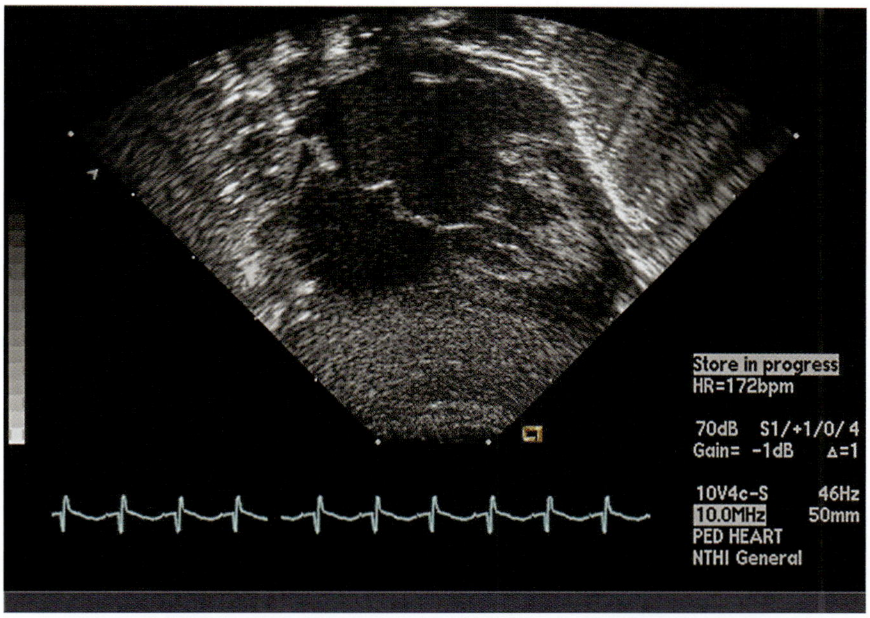

Figure 5.1 Two-dimensional subcostal view demonstrating small predominantly closed foramen ovale.

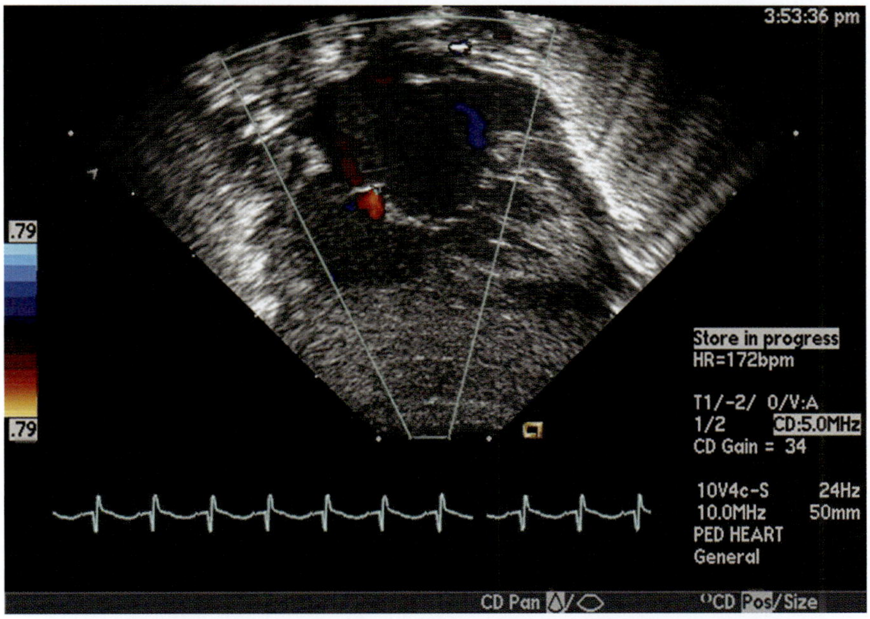

Figure 5.2 Color Doppler subcostal view demonstrating small amount of left to right shunting across a predominantly closed foramen ovale.

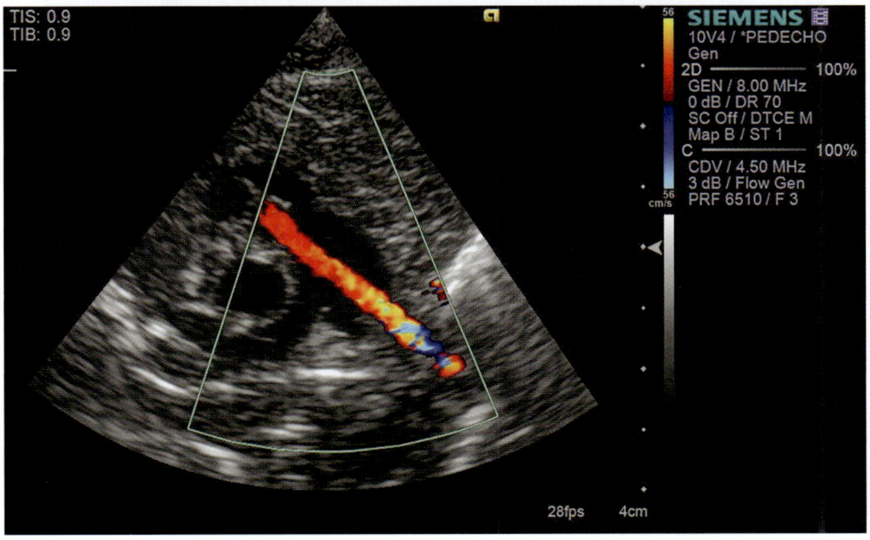

Figure 5.3 Color Doppler parasternal short axis view of a patent ductus arteriosus (PDA).

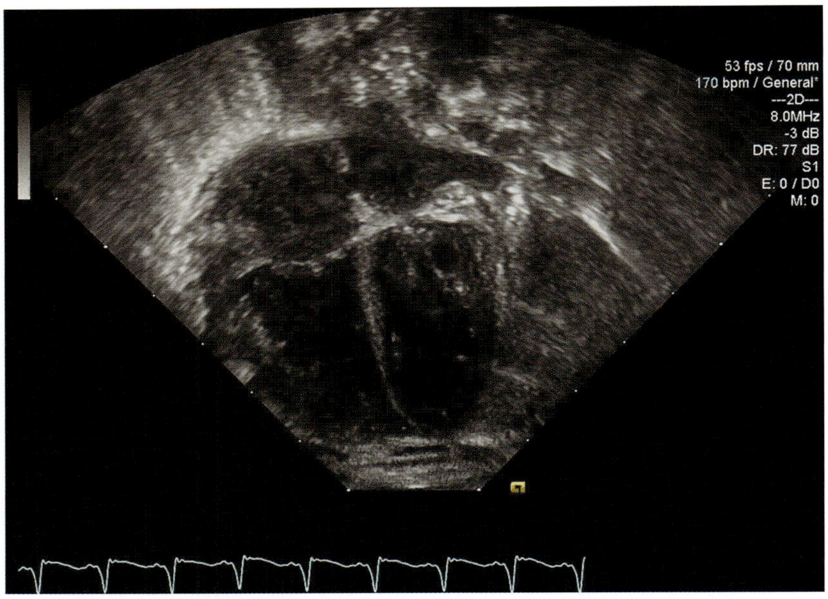

Figure 5.4 Four-chamber view showing dominance of right-sided chambers.

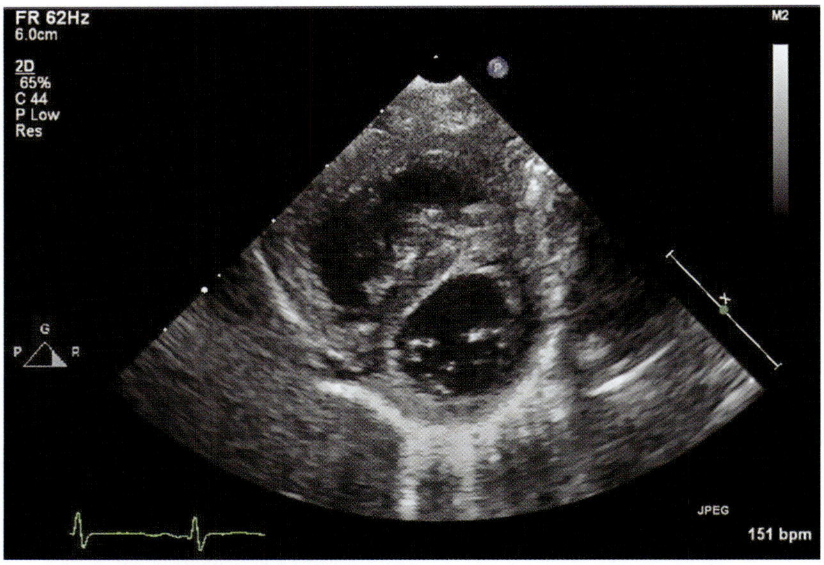

Figure 5.5 Parasternal short axis view showing both right ventricular (RV) volume and septal flattening in a normal newborn.

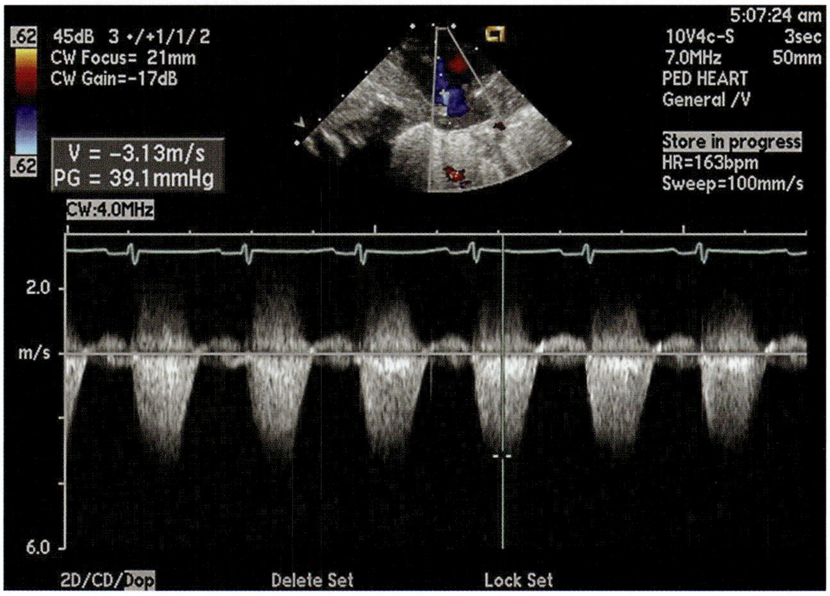

Figure 5.6 Parasternal long axis medially angulated tricuspid regurgitation Doppler pattern demonstrating elevated right ventricle and pulmonary artery systolic pressure.

As a result of the same volume and pressure physiology in utero, there is a difference in the pulmonary annulus and main pulmonary artery size compared to the aortic annulus and proximal ascending aorta of the neonate that changes over time (Figure 5.7) [8].

During the fetal period there is a size discrepancy between the main pulmonary artery which is carrying about 60% of the combined cardiac output, and the proximal branch pulmonary arteries which receive 8–11% of the combined cardiac output. This size discrepancy appears to create an acute angle of origin which contributes to physiologic peripheral branch pulmonary stenosis [9]. In addition, at birth, the branch pulmonary arteries resemble systemic arteries in that they have a thick media layer and relatively small lumen. This changes over time so that by approximately 6 months of age in babies with normal hearts the pulmonary arteries have the larger lumen and thinner media seen in older children and adults [10]. These anatomic findings in newborns and infants create a flow acceleration that is frequently seen on color and spectral Doppler echocardiographic imaging (Figures 5.8 and 5.9).

More recent studies are beginning to define the myocardial systolic and diastolic changes that occur in the neonate using tissue Doppler and strain methodologies [11, 12]. Further studies are needed to elucidate the transitional changes in myocardial function in the first days, weeks, and months after birth.

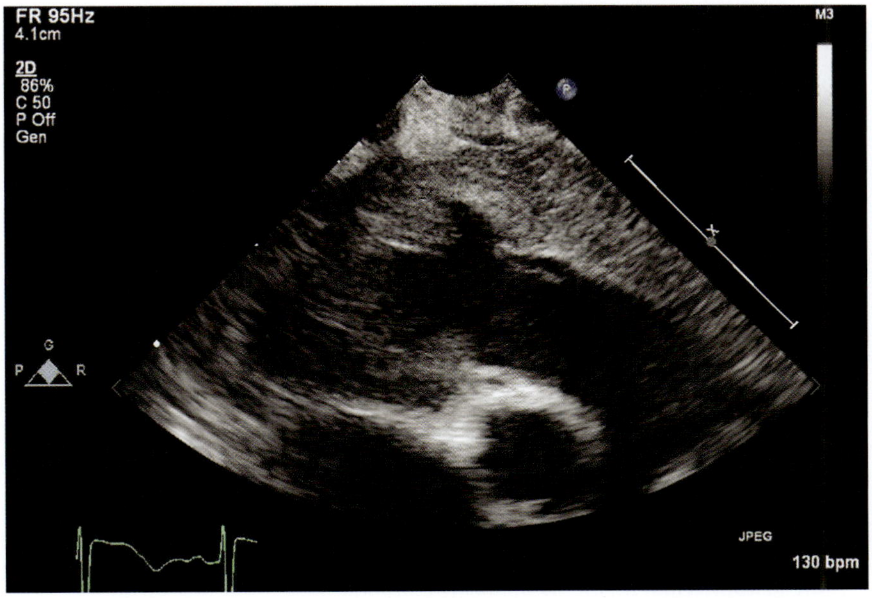

Figure 5.7 Cropped parasternal two-dimensional image of main pulmonary artery (MPA) and pulmonary annulus slightly larger than aorta.

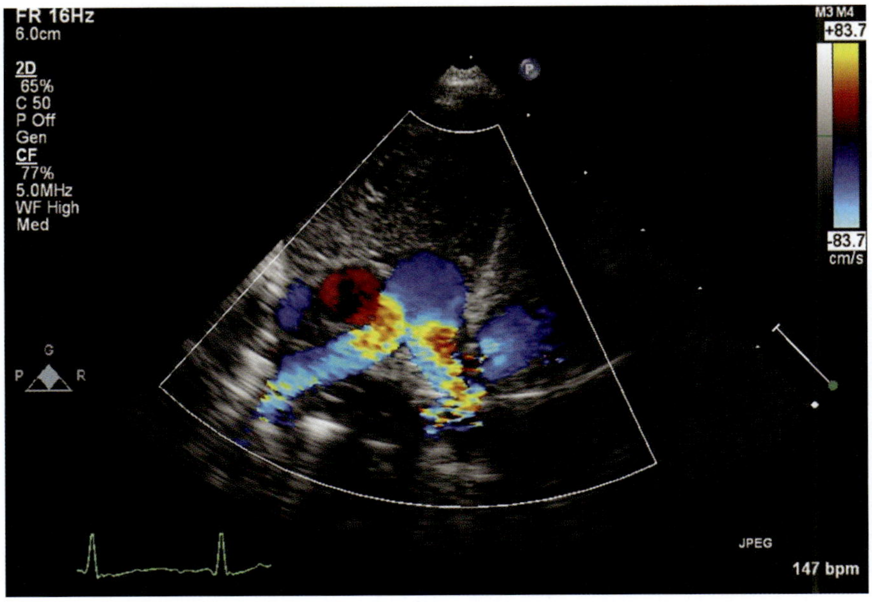

Figure 5.8 High parasternal short axis color Doppler image of flow acceleration at the origin of the branch pulmonary arteries.

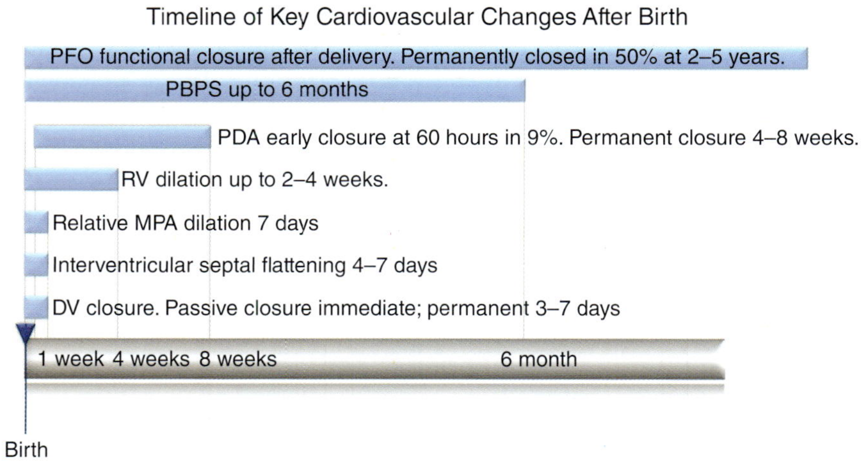

Figure 5.9 Summary timeline of key neonatal cardiovascular changes. DV, ductus venosus; MPA, main pulmonary artery; PBPS, peripheral branch pulmonary stenosis; PDA, patent ductus arteriosus; PFO, patent foramen ovale; RV, right ventricle.

Acknowledgment

The author would like to thank Elizabeth Brodell, RDCS, RDMS, RVT.

References

1 Mielke G, Benda N. (2001) Cardiac output and central distribution of blood flow in the human fetus. *Circulation*, **103** (12), 1662–1668.
2 Keane JF. (2006) Fetal and transitional circulation, in, *Nadas' Pediatric Cardiology*, 2nd edn (eds JF Keane, JE Lock, DC Fyler), Elsevier, USA, pp. 75–79.
3 Sharma A, Ford S, Calvert J. (2011) Adaptation for life: a review of neonatal physiology. *Anesthes Intensive Care Med*, **9**(3), 93–98.
4 Azancot A, Caudell TP, Allen HD, *et al.* (1983) Analysis of ventricular shape by echocardiography in normal fetuses, newborns, and infants. *Circulation*, **68** (6), 1201–1211.
5 Clark SJ, Yoxall CW, Subhedar NV. (2002) Measurement of right ventricular volume in healthy term and preterm neonates. *Arch Dis Child Fetal Neonatal Ed*, **87** (2), F89–93; discussion F93–94.
6 Rein AJ, Sanders SP, Colan SD, Parness IA, Epstein M. (1987) Left ventricular mechanics in the normal newborn. *Circulation*, **76** (5), 1029–1036.
7 Miyazaki A, Ichida F, Hashimoto I, Tsubata S, Okada T. (1992) Analysis of left ventricular regional wall motion in normal neonates. *Br Heart J*, **68** (6), 574–549.
8 Ichida F, Aubert A, Denef B, Dumoulin M, Van der Hauwaert LG. (1987) Cross sectional echocardiographic assessment of great artery diameters in infants and children. *Br Heart J*, **58** (6), 627–634.
9 Danilowicz DA, Rudolph AM, Hoffman JI, Heymann M. (1972) Physiologic pressure differences between main and branch pulmonary arteries in infants. *Circulation*, **45** (2), 410–419.
10 Dammann JF Jr., Muller WH Jr. (1953) The role of the pulmonary vascular bed in congenital heart disease. *Pediatrics*, **12** (3:1), 307–325.
11 Mori K, Nakagawa R, Nii M, *et al.* (2004) Pulsed wave Doppler tissue echocardiography assessment of the long axis function of the right and left ventricles during the early neonatal period. *Heart*, **90** (2), 175–180.

6

History and Physical Examination

Ernerio T. Alboliras

Genus Heart Center, Scottsdale, AZ, USA

The vast majority of serious cardiac diseases are detected at the neonatal stage although advances in maternal–fetal medicine and fetal cardiology allow for their antenatal detection. Although diagnostic tools, particularly echocardiography and electrocardiography, can provide accurate and prompt diagnosis of neonatal heart disease, even in the sick neonate a brief history and physical examination remain important and can be simultaneously carried out while diagnostic procedures are being performed.

In most situations where the neonate is stable, more comprehensive historical information can be gathered and a detailed physical examination can be performed. These procedures remain the hallmark for providing evidence for the presence of congenital heart disease and for justifying further diagnostic workup and therapy.

History

The most frequent reasons for referring a newborn for a cardiac evaluation include the following:

1) Prenatal diagnosis of fetal heart disease or fetal anomaly of other organ systems;
2) Heart murmur;
3) Abnormal heart rate and rhythm;
4) Cyanosis;
5) Signs of poor perfusion;
6) Non-palpable femoral pulses;
7) Respiratory distress of uncertain etiology;
8) Poor feeding;
9) Genetic or syndromic features; and
10) Abnormality of other organ systems with possible associated cardiac defect.

The comprehensiveness of history-taking upon first encounter with the neonate depends on the timing and severity of presentation. A brief but concise gathering of information should be satisfactory in the presence of life-threatening signs and symptoms in order to provide prompt diagnostic and therapeutic interventions. Detailed history-taking can be acquired later. Critical neonatal manifestations include severe bradycardia or tachycardia, respiratory distress, profound cyanosis, and diminished perfusion.

A quick review of the maternal record can provide information on the presence of maternal illness, medications, findings of a prior fetal echocardiogram, mode and difficulty of delivery, Apgar score, gestational age and size of the newborn, time of onset of symptoms, and results of any therapeutic modalities already performed prior to cardiology consultation. Obstetric records may reveal a history of a viral infection associated with cardiomyopathy, or presence of maternal lupus antibodies to account for a heart block. Prior medications given, such as indomethacin for premature labor, may cause constriction of the ductus arteriosus and consequent right heart failure. A fetal sonogram may have shown hallmarks of genetic anomalies associated with cardiac disease such as trisomy 21 and 18.

Extracardiac causes of respiratory distress such as transient tachypnea of the newborn, sepsis, diaphragmatic hernia, pneumothorax, and persistent fetal circulation should be ruled out. Perinatal asphyxia is associated with myocardial dysfunction and persistent pulmonary hypertension of the newborn. Neonatal distress may be seen in vascular obstruction of the airways. The earlier the onset of postnatal symptoms, the greater is the possibility of severe cardiac disease, typically seen in obstructed total anomalous pulmonary venous connection, hypoplastic left heart syndrome with intact atrial septum, and a closing ductus arteriosus in ductal-dependent lesions such as transposition of great arteries, tricuspid atresia with pulmonary stenosis, and tetralogy of Fallot with pulmonary atresia.

If the newborn being referred is not critically ill, there is more time to gather a more detailed history. Factors that increase the risk of having a cardiac disease should be identified: advanced maternal age, family history of cardiac or genetic defect, maternal diabetes, maternal

Visual Guide to Neonatal Cardiology, First Edition. Edited by Ernerio T. Alboliras, Ziyad M. Hijazi, Leo Lopez, and Donald J. Hagler.

drug intake, cigarette smoking, pregnancy screening test (quadruple and triple tests) positive for aneuploidy and birth defect, significant level of anti-Ro/SSA antibody, and increased fetal nuchal translucency. In utero detection of congenital heart disease or anomalies of other organ systems become more common as more women undergo fetal sonography and echocardiography.

The diagnosis being considered may depend on the timing of the onset of symptoms from birth. The baby may still be in the hospital as a result of premature birth or management of involvement of other organ systems such as diaphragmatic hernia, hydrocephalus, intestinal malrotation, or suboptimal feeding pattern, and a heart murmur is detected resulting in cardiology consultation. Many cardiac defects associated with significant left to right shunt, such as a large ventricular septal defect, patent ductus arteriosus, atrioventricular canal, truncus arteriosus, and aorticopulmonary window, develop symptoms after the postnatal drop in pulmonary resistance.

Physical Examination

If faced with a critically ill neonate, a concise sequence of physical examination can expedite placement of intravenous or umbilical vessel lines, possible intubation and mechanical ventilation, and performance of echocardiogram, electrocardiogram, and chest roentgenogram. This sequence of physical examination is directed towards confirmation of the suspected diagnosis and determining its severity and the presence of any associated problems. This sequence includes determining the weight and gestational age of the child, a cursory inspection of the face and limbs for major anomalies, inspecting the cardiac impulse, auscultating the heart for cardiac sounds, clicks, and murmurs, auscultating the lungs, palpating the abdomen for any organomegaly, palpating the femoral pulses, auscultating the head and liver for any bruit, and setting up the vital signs monitoring that can determine the heart rate and rhythm, oxygen saturation, respiratory rate, and blood pressure.

When the neonate is not critically ill, the temptation to immediately listen to the heart with a stethoscope should be avoided. The recorded weight, length, temperature, respiratory rates, heart rates, and oxygen saturation should be noted. Small and large for gestational age babies have increased risks for the presence of cardiac defects. A general survey is then performed that includes inspection of the head, torso, and limbs for any major anomaly, respiratory effort, color, skin perfusion, motor activity, and responsiveness to tactile stimuli. Mottling of the skin is normal in the newborn. Pressure on the skin should result in a quick refill. A sluggish refill may be normal soon after birth, but is also present in poor cardiac output. A vigorously crying baby should have a face that turns red. Acrocyanosis, a benign bluish or cyanotic discoloration of the hands, feet, and face, is common in the first 24 hours after birth. Cyanosis of the lips and oral mucosa, a sign of central cyanosis, is a sign of low oxygen saturation if persistent beyond the first few hours after birth. Plethora may be seen in the donor twin in twin–twin transfusion syndrome.

The head is examined for any facial dysmorphism seen in genetic or chromosomal anomalies with associated cardiac defect. The anterior fontanel is auscultated for any bruit of a cerebral arteriovenous malformation. The neck is examined for any redundancy of the skin. The chest should have symmetric movement. A newborn's respiratory rate is about 40–60 breaths per minute and not associated with alar flare or retractions. Auscultation should demonstrate equal breath sounds. Certain cardiovascular lesions can result in respiratory distress: pulmonary sling, vascular ring, and tetralogy of Fallot, with absent pulmonary valve syndrome where there maybe markedly dilated pulmonary arteries.

The heart is then examined. This should start with visual inspection and palpation of the cardiac impulse and for the presence of a thrill. Typically, the apex beat is higher than in older children. A prominent cardiac impulse at the right may suggest the presence of dextrocardia, left-sided pneumothorax, or left diaphragmatic hernia. Auscultation is then performed, which begins with identifying the first and second heart sounds. The first heart sound is more pronounced at the apex; the second heart sound more pronounced at the base. In spite of a fast heartbeat, the splitting of the second sound may be identified. A loud pulmonary component of the second sound may be present in pulmonary hypertension. A single second sound may be present in truncus arteriosus, tetralogy of Fallot with severe pulmonary stenosis or pulmonary atresia, aortic atresia, and in transposition of great arteries and double outlet right ventricle where the aortic and pulmonary valves have an anteroposterior relationship. A systolic ejection click is a high-pitched sound following the first sound heard in stenosis of the truncal valve and aortic or pulmonary valve.

Heart murmurs result from turbulence in blood flow across valves, chambers, septal defects, and vessels. They are described by their loudness (grades I–VI), timing based on the phase of the cardiac cycle, character, location, and radiation. Breath sounds should not be confused with murmurs. A closing ductus arteriosus is heard as transient soft systolic murmur at the left upper chest. A systolic murmur heard at birth may be a sign of a semilunar valve or truncal valve stenosis, or significant atrioventricular valve regurgitation. The absence of a heart murmur does not mean that a cardiac defect is not present. Ventricular septal defect usually manifests with a murmur only after the drop in pulmonary resistance.

Lesions such as transposition of great vessels, tetralogy of Fallot with pulmonary atresia, aortic atresia, and persistent pulmonary hypertension may not be associated with a murmur but manifest with overt cyanosis or poor perfusion. The continuous systolic–diastolic murmur typically described for patent ductus arteriosus is not observed at birth. A to-and-fro systolic–diastolic murmur may be heard at birth in coronary fistula, aorto-left ventricular tunnel, tetralogy of Fallot with absent pulmonary valve, and truncus arteriosus with valvar regurgitation.

The femoral and brachial pulses should be palpated. A generalized shallow pulse is seen in low cardiac output conditions such as severe dilated cardiomyopathy, supraventricular tachycardia, and complete heart block. The femoral pulse is diminished in coarctation of the aorta. If the right brachial artery and the femoral artery pulses are not palpable, an aberrant right subclavian artery below the coarctation may be present. A wide pulse pressure may be seen in an older premature baby with a patent ductus arteriosus and in high cardiac output failure such as neonatal thyrotoxicosis and arteriovenous malformation.

The abdomen should be palpated for hepatomegaly associated with right heart failure, and auscultated for bruit from an arteriovenous malformation. The presence of anasarca or hydrops may be signs of arteriovenous malformation, complete heart block, long-standing tachydysrhythmia, or severe cardiomyopathy.

A structured sequence of history-taking and physical examination can provide information needed for evaluation of the severity of neonatal cardiac illness and for selecting the appropriate diagnostic and treatment strategy.

Further Reading

Anderson RH, Macartney FJ, *et al.* (1987) History and physical examination, in, *Paediatric Cardiology*, vol. 1, Churchill Livingstone, Edinburgh, pp. 183–190.

Cassidy SC, Allen HD, Phillips JR. (2013) *Moss and Adams' Heart Disease in Infants, Children and Adolescents*, 5th edn (eds HD Allen, DJ Driscoll, RE Shaddy, TF Feltes), Wolters Kluwer, Lippincott Williams & Wilkins, Philadelphia, PA, pp. 82–92.

Fanaroff AA, Fanaroff JM. (2013) *Kalus and Fanaroff's Care of the High Risk Neonate*, 6th edn, Elsevier Saunders, Philadelphia, PA.

Keith JD. (1978) History and physical examination, in, *Heart Disease in Infancy and Childhood*, (eds JD Keith, RD Rowe, P Vlad), Macmillan, New York, NY, pp. 14–31.

7

The Cyanotic Newborn

Ernerio T. Alboliras

Genus Heart Center, Scottsdale, AZ, USA

Cyanosis is the bluish discoloration of the skin and mucous membranes caused by increased desaturated hemoglobin in the blood, but clinical assessment in the newborn can be difficult. Central cyanosis should be differentiated from acrocyanosis or peripheral cyanosis, which is a benign bluish discoloration of the hands, feet, or face. Extremity pulses and pulse oximetry are normal. This is thought to be from vasospasm of the cutaneous arterioles with sluggish capillary blood flow, oftentimes triggered by cold, and does not require treatment. Central cyanosis is clinically observable in the presence of >3 gm/dL of desaturated hemoglobin in the arterial blood and >5 gm/dL in capillary blood. The best method for clinical assessment is by looking at the tongue.

Non-cardiac causes of cyanosis should first be ruled out:

1) Primary lung disease (respiratory distress syndrome, pneumothorax and atelectasis);
2) CNS depression;
3) Diaphragmatic hernia;
4) Polycythemia; and
5) Methemoglobinemia.

Cyanotic heart diseases generally fall under two major groups:

1) Lesions with obstruction to pulmonary blood flow (PBF); and
2) Lesions with normal or increased PBF, but with parallel separation of the pulmonary venous return and systemic circulation.

In both, the effective PBF, or the amount of oxygenated blood that returns to the systemic circulation, is low. Right-to-left shunting across the foramen ovale and patent ductus arteriosus (PDA) can aggravate the severity of cyanosis.

The first group of cyanotic heart diseases presents radiographically with pulmonary oligemia: tetralogy of Fallot (TOF) with severe pulmonary stenosis or pulmonary atresia, tricuspid atresia with pulmonary stenosis, and severe persistent pulmonary hypertension in the newborn (PPHN). The second group presents with normal or increased pulmonary vascular markings: transposition of great arteries (TGA), total anomalous pulmonary venous return, and truncus arteriosus.

If cardiac disease is strongly suspected and echocardiography is not available, a hyperoxia test may be performed. The infant is given 100% FiO2 for 10 minutes and arterial blood gas is performed. In pulmonary disease, PaO2 usually increases to >100 mmHg, whereas infants with cyanotic heart disease show little change in PaO2. If the PaO2 does not increase beyond 100%, cyanotic heart disease may be present. The result may be misleading in certain conditions. In infants with severe PPHN, PaO2 may not elevate at 100% FiO2. Likewise, PaO2 >100 mmHg can be seen in certain forms of cyanotic heart disease with high pulmonary blood flow such as truncus arteriosus and tricuspid atresia with a large ventricular septal defect.

Simultaneous measurement of the oxygen saturations of the right hand and a foot is another method that provides a clue for the presence of critical congenital heart disease that warrant further diagnostic examination. This is based on the presence of a right-to-left shunt across the PDA in certain heart defects. Equal saturations between the right hand and a foot that is >95% is normal. A lower foot saturation (>3% on three occasions), called differential cyanosis, may mean right-to-left shunting across the PDA as seen in coarctation of aorta, interrupted aortic arch, and PPHN. A lower right hand saturation (>3% on three occasions), also called reverse differential cyanosis, is seen in TGA. Equal but low O2 saturations may still be seen in cardiac defects such as truncus arteriosus, TOF, or total anomalous pulmonary venous connection.

This screening method is advocated by the American Academy of Pediatrics and recommended for routine

Visual Guide to Neonatal Cardiology, First Edition. Edited by Ernerio T. Alboliras, Ziyad M. Hijazi, Leo Lopez, and Donald J. Hagler.

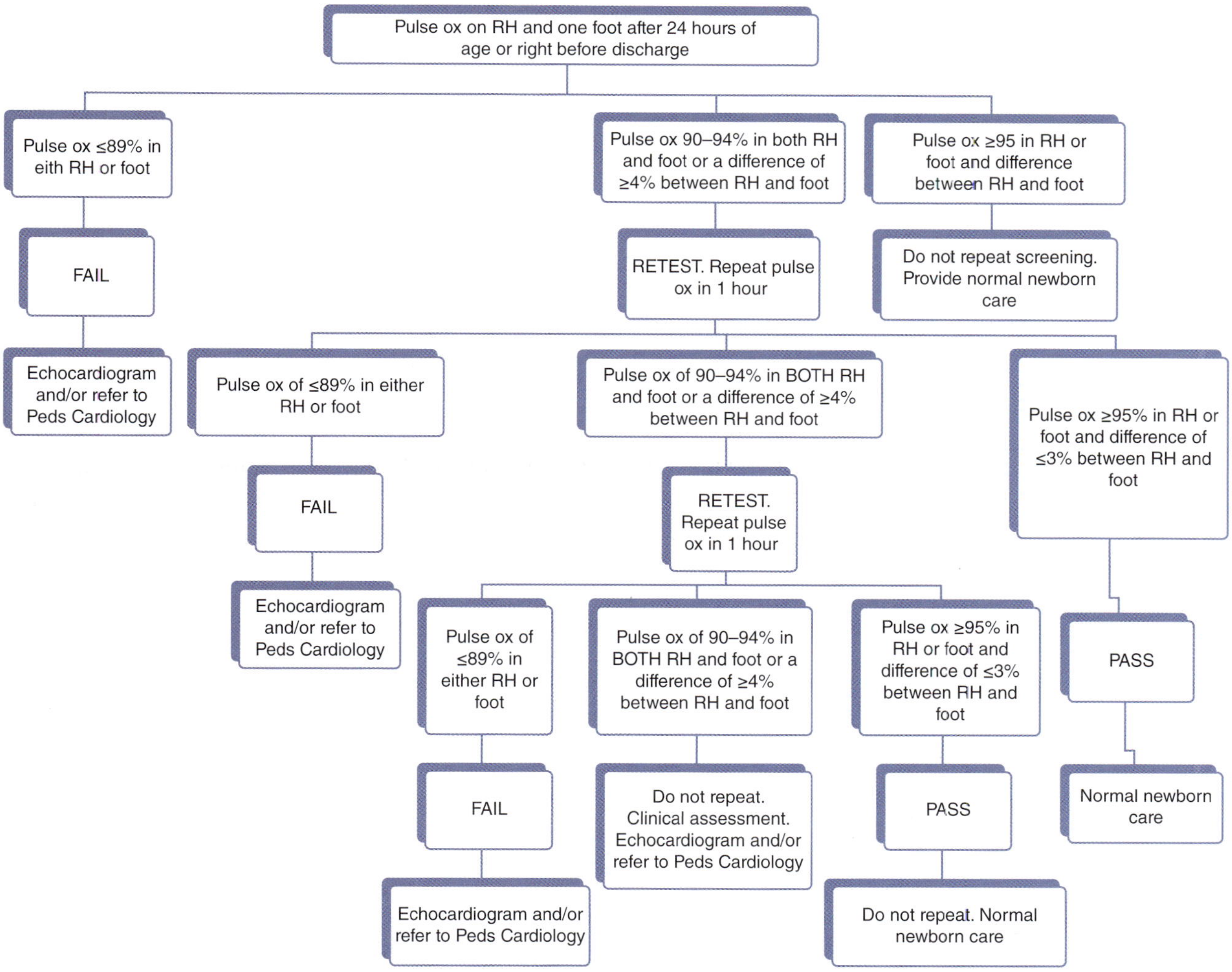

Figure 7.1 Recommended pulse oximetry screening for infants after 24 hours in the hospital and prior to hospital discharge. Any infant with a positive screen should have a diagnostic echocardiogram, which would involve an echocardiogram within the hospital or birthing center, transport to another institution for the procedure, or use of telemedicine for remote evaluation. The infant's pediatrician should be notified immediately and the infant might need to be seen by a cardiologist for follow-up. ox, oximetry; RH, right hand. *Source*: Adapted from Kemper *et al.* 2011 [1].

use by the Centers for Disease Control for asymptomatic newborns 24 hours from birth but before hospital discharge (Figure 7.1). Any infant with a positive screen should have a diagnostic echocardiogram, which would involve an echocardiogram within the hospital or birthing center, transport to another institution for the procedure, or use of telemedicine for remote evaluation. The infant's pediatrician should be notified immediately and the infant might need to be seen by a cardiologist for follow-up.

Stabilization is important if infant is not in a facility where echocardiography can be performed. Oxygen is given and prostaglandin started to keep the PDA patent even before evaluation is completed.

Reference

1 Kemper AR, Mahle WT, Martin GR, *et al.* (2011) Strategies for implementing screening for critical congenital heart disease. *Pediatrics*, **128**, e1259–1267.

Further Reading

Anderson RH, Macartney FJ, Shinebourne EA, *et al.* (1987) *Paediatric Cardiology*, vol. 1. Churchill Livingstone, Edinburgh.

Centers for Disease Control and Prevention (2017) Screening for critical congenital heart defects. http://www.cdc.gov/ncbddd/pediatricgenetics/pulse.html (accessed October 19, 2017).

Cloherty JP, Eichenwald EC, Stark AR. (2011) *Manual of Neonatal Care*, Wolters Kluwer, Lippincott Williams & Wilkins, Philadelphia, PA.

Keane JF, Lock JE, Fyler DC. (2006) *Nadas' Pediatric Cardiology*, Saunders Elsevier, Philadelphia, PA.

8

The Tachypneic Newborn

Ernerio T. Alboliras

Genus Heart Center, Scottsdale, AZ, USA

Problems in ventilation and oxygenation can be seen in conditions other than those principally affecting the respiratory system. The manifestations include rapid respirations, grunting, chest retractions, alar flaring, cyanosis, and even slow and shallow breathing or terminal apnea. A detailed history and physical examination, chest X-ray, complete blood count with hematocrit, blood sugar, arterial blood gas, and oxygen saturations should be determined. An electrocardiogram is valuable if there is persistent tachycardia or bradycardia. The timing of appearance of respiratory distress can provide clues to the kind of cardiac disease involved. The earlier the onset, the more severe the condition.

Pulmonary parenchymal disorders are the most common causes of respiratory distress in the neonate but other etiologies should also be considered (Box 8.1). A cardiovascular etiology may be seen with a heart murmur, abnormal cardiac silhouette and vascular markings on chest X-ray, difficult ventilation and oxygenation, and differential cyanosis on pulse oximetry of the right hand and a foot. In some pulmonary parenchymal or airway diseases, a separate associated cardiovascular disorder is seen. An echocardiogram should be performed if there is suspicion of cardiovascular disease.

In obstructive lesions of the left heart, there is significant impediment in blood flow to the systemic circulation, resulting in manifestations of pulmonary edema and respiratory distress. In total anomalous pulmonary venous connection (TAPVC), there could be obstruction to the egress of the pulmonary venous blood flow. Almost invariably, infradiaphragmatic TAPVC is associated with various areas of significant obstruction resulting in marked tachypnea with cyanosis. Tachypnea can be observed in coarctation of the aorta, critical aortic stenosis, and severe mitral stenosis in addition to systemic hypoperfusion.

A large communication between systemic and pulmonary circulations may result in overperfusion of the lungs. Fetal hydrops or early neonatal heart failure may be observed with large arteriovenous malformation and twin–twin transfusion. Except in premature infants with patent ductus arteriosus who may develop symptoms early, symptoms may occur late in other conditions of pulmonary overperfusion depending on the timing of the drop in pulmonary vascular resistance. These cardiac defects include ventricular septal defect, complete atrioventricular canal, truncus arteriosus, and aorticopulmonary window.

A distressed newborn may have cardiac conditions not associated with left-to-right shunts but with decreased output. These include supraventricular tachycardia, dilated cardiomyopathy, myocarditis, aortico-left ventricular tunnel, and severe congenital aortic or mitral regurgitation.

Mechanical obstruction of the airways and lung parenchyma with resultant respiratory distress may result from some cardiovascular disorders. There is only a fixed space within the thoracic cage such that marked enlargement of cardiac chambers can cause compression of the lungs and airways. In Ebstein anomaly, the severely regurgitant tricuspid valve may result in markedly dilated right ventricle and right atrium. Tetralogy of Fallot with absent pulmonary valve is associated with markedly dilated main pulmonary artery and proximal branches, resulting in mechanical obstruction of the bronchi and maldevelopment of the pulmonary arterial architecture. Congenital mitral regurgitation can create a giant atrium and dilated left ventricle with mass obstruction of the airway and compression of the lungs. A markedly dilated left ventricle can be seen in aortico-left ventricular tunnel, congenital aortic insufficiency, and dilated cardiomyopathy. Vascular anomalies such as double aortic arch, right aortic arch with an aberrant left subclavian artery and ligamentum arteriosum, and pulmonary sling cause direct airway compression. Pulmonary sling and complete tracheal rings can occur together resulting in a more difficult ventilation. Extrathoracic structures occupying the thorax in left-sided diaphragmatic hernia

Visual Guide to Neonatal Cardiology, First Edition. Edited by Ernerio T. Alboliras, Ziyad M. Hijazi, Leo Lopez, and Donald J. Hagler.

Box 8.1 Causes of neonatal respiratory distress

1) **Pulmonary disorders**
   - Respiratory distress syndrome
   - Transient tachypnea
   - Meconium aspiration syndrome
   - Pneumonia
   - Air leak syndrome
   - Pulmonary hypoplasia
2) **Systemic disorders**
   - Hypothermia
   - Metabolic acidosis
   - Anemia/polycythemia
   - Hypoglycemia
   - Pulmonary hypertension
   - Congenital heart disease
3) **Anatomic problems of the respiratory system**
   - Upper airway obstruction
   - Airway malformations
   - Space occupying lesions
   - Rib cage anomalies
   - Phrenic nerve injury
   - Neuromuscular diseases

Source: Martin and Crowley 2013 [1]. Reproduced with permission of Elsevier.

can be associated with hypoplastic left heart syndrome in addition to the pulmonary compression by the herniated viscera.

Details on the specific disorders can be seen in individual chapters.

Reference

1 Martin RJ, Crowley MA. (2013) Respiratory problems, in, *Klaus and Fanaroff's Care of the High-Risk Neonate*, 6th edn. (eds AA Fanaroff, JM Fanaroff), Elsevier Saunders, Philadelphia, PA, p. 248.

Further Reading

Anderson RH, Macartney FJ, Shinebourne EA, *et al.* (1987) *Paediatric Cardiology*, vol. 1. Churchill Livingstone, Edinburgh.

Fanaroff ASA, Fanaroff JM. (2013) *Klauss and Fanaroff's Care of the High Risk Neonate*, 6th edn. Elsevier-Saunders, Philadelphia, PA.

9

The Hypoperfused Newborn

Deepti Bhat

Cardon Children's Hospital, Mesa, AZ, USA

Among the most critically ill newborns are those that present with systemic hypoperfusion. While this clinical condition is usually non-cardiac in etiology, important cardiac lesions must be evaluated and excluded. The latter include conditions intrinsic to the cardiovascular system that prevent the systemic ventricle from generating adequate cardiac output to meet the metabolic demands of the body. Clinical signs may start insidiously but can progress rapidly, eventually leading to decompensated shock and death if there is delay in recognition and institution of appropriate treatment.

Etiology

The two major categories of cardiac conditions that lead to poor cardiac output are anatomic obstruction to the systemic ventricular outflow or from pump failure caused by diminished stroke volume.

Obstructive lesions of the heart may involve one or more components on the systemic side starting proximally from pulmonary veins and distally to the aorta (Box 9.1). These lesions may remain asymptomatic shortly after birth because of the presence of a patent ductus arteriosus (PDA) which provides perfusion antegradely into the descending aorta, and retrogradely into the ascending aorta and their branches, including the coronary arteries (ductal dependent systemic circulation). Once the PDA constricts, reduced systemic perfusion results and clinical signs become apparent. This may occur within a few days to weeks after birth. Timely administration of intravenous prostaglandin E (PGE) can be lifesaving.

The second category includes diseases of the cardiac muscle or cardiomyopathies where reduced contractility results in reduced stroke volume. Also, in persistent tachyarrhythmias or complete heart block, ventricular filling is interfered with leading to ineffective ventricular ejection by an otherwise healthy myocardium. These lesions are not dependent on a PDA and require treatment dependent on etiology, including inotropic support, antiarrhythmic agents, or even ventricular pacing.

History

A concise prenatal and postnatal history should be obtained. Fetal hydrops may indicate cardiomyopathy, tachyarrhythmia, or heart block. Maternal use of teratogens during pregnancy, diabetes, lupus, or abnormal genetic screening may point towards congenital heart lesions. A maternal history of a recent viral infection may suggest myocarditis. However, a history of fever, poor suck, vomiting, or diarrhea may indicate non-cardiac causes of hypoperfusion such as sepsis and hypovolemia.

Physical Examination

Physical examination findings include lethargy, pallor, cool extremities, absent or diminished peripheral pulses, and delayed capillary refill. Respiratory distress is common and results from pulmonary edema secondary to elevated pulmonary venous pressures and from progressive metabolic acidosis with lactic acidemia resulting from inadequate tissue perfusion. A gallop rhythm, single second heart sound, or a murmur may be helpful but difficult to appreciate because of tachycardia and poor heart function. Upper and lower extremity blood pressures may reveal a higher value in the arms by more than 10 mmHg in coarctation or an interrupted aortic arch. This difference may be small or absent if there is unrestricted PDA flow, aberrant right subclavian artery, or poor cardiac function. Pulse oximetry usually reveals

Visual Guide to Neonatal Cardiology, First Edition. Edited by Ernerio T. Alboliras, Ziyad M. Hijazi, Leo Lopez, and Donald J. Hagler.

Box 9.1 Causes of hypoperfusion in the neonate (see details in chapters on individual pathology)

Cardiac causes

1) Anatomic defects
   - Coarctation of the aorta
   - Hypoplastic transverse arch (usually associated with coarctation of aorta)
   - Interrupted aortic arch (all types)
   - Severe aortic valve, supravalvar, or subvalvar stenosis
   - Left ventricular atresia or severe hypoplasia (hypoplastic left heart syndrome)
   - Mitral valve atresia, severe hypoplasia, or severe stenosis
   - Supramitral ring, cor triatriatum with severe obstruction
   - Total anomalous pulmonary venous connection with severe obstruction
2) Functional defects
   - Dilated cardiomyopathy
   - Hypertrophic cardiomyopathy and storage disorders
   - Non-compaction of the left ventricle
   - Myocarditis
   - Myocardial dysfunction from perinatal asphyxia
   - Arrhythmias with fast ventricular rate: supraventricular tachycardia, atrial flutter
   - Complete (third degree) heart block

Non-cardiac causes

- Neonatal sepsis
- Hypovolemia
- Inborn errors of metabolism
- Adrenal insufficiency
- Severe anemia
- Neurologic instability

mild desaturation from right to left shunting across the foramen ovale or PDA. A higher value in the arm than the foot may indicate right to left shunting across the PDA in coarctation and interrupted aortic arch. Reversed differential cyanosis (higher saturation in the foot, lower in the arm) may be true in transposition of the great arteries (TGA) with PDA and pulmonary hypertension, or TGA with preductal aortic interruption or coarctation.

Diagnostic Tests

The arterial blood gas results may show metabolic acidosis with high lactate levels. A chest roentgenogram can determine the cardiac size and pulmonary vascular markings. A 12-lead electrocardiogram (ECG) should be obtained to identify tachyarrhythmias or heart block. ECG may also show inferolateral ischemia suggestive of anomalous left coronary artery, or prominent Q waves of endocardial fibroelastosis. As newborn sepsis can be lethal if untreated, a septic workup should be performed for all critically ill infants and antibiotics administered while awaiting definitive diagnosis. Urgent echocardiographic imaging is of paramount importance for accurate diagnosis.

Management

Irrespective of the etiology, initial treatment must consist of stabilization of the airway and correction of electrolyte abnormalities and metabolic acidosis. For suspected ductal dependent obstructive lesions, PGE should be immediately started. An initial dose of 0.01 μg/kg/min may maintain ductal patency, but, if the PDA is restrictive or closed, a much higher dose (0.05–0.1 μg/kg/min) may be required. Critically ill infants may become apneic with administration of PGE, especially at higher doses, and intubation of the newborn may be necessary. The receiving facility should be prepared for urgent interventions such as balloon atrial septostomy or aortic balloon dilatation. Patients with poor cardiac function require intravenous inotropes and continuous telemetry to monitor for arrhythmias. Mechanical ventilation may be required to reduce the work of breathing. Emergent treatment of arrhythmias may require medical or electrical cardioversion or ventricular pacing if the patient is hemodynamically unstable.

The prognosis of these lesions remains guarded even in the well-equipped tertiary facility. Prompt recognition, urgent evaluation with an echocardiogram, and communication between transferring and receiving facility are essential for better outcomes.

Further Reading

Fanaroff AA, Fanaroff JM. (2013) *Kalus and Fanaroff's Care of the High Risk Neonate*, 6th edn. Elsevier Saunders, Philadelphia, PA.

Meckler GD, Lowe C. (2009) To intubate or not to intubate? Transporting infants on prostaglandin E1. *Pediatrics*, **123** (1), e25–30.

Morris SA, Ethen MK, Penny DJ, *et al.* (2014) Prenatal diagnosis, birth location, surgical center, and neonatal mortality in infants with hypoplastic left heart syndrome. *Circulation*, **129** (3), 285–292.

Yap SH, Anania N, Alboliras, ET, Lilien LD. (2009) Reversed differential cyanosis in the newborn: a clinical finding in the supracardiac total anomalous venous connection. *Pediatr Cardiol*, **30** (3), 359–362.

10

The Dysmorphic Newborn

Stephanie Burns Wechsler and Marie McDonald

Duke University Medical Center, Durham, NC, USA

When a neonate is diagnosed with congenital heart disease (CHD), in the fetal period or after birth, the clinician should look for additional birth defects in other organ systems and in all other parts of the body, as in 25% of infants with CHD there will be additional findings in other areas. Sometimes there are obvious dysmorphic features from the time of birth such as cleft lip and/or palate or other organ system abnormalities such as omphalocele; these features are often diagnosed prenatally by fetal imaging. Other dysmorphic features are more subtle and can only be diagnosed postnatally by careful physical examination. Identifying a pattern of birth defects can indicate a specific genetic syndrome as a single unifying diagnosis. Diagnosing a syndrome early is important to the care of the baby and in counseling of the parents, though making a confirmed genetic diagnosis in the newborn period may not be possible because clues to a genetic diagnosis, such as developmental delay, will not yet be apparent. Nonetheless, it is important to look carefully for clues for a genetic diagnosis, to determine if genetic testing is needed, and to help plan the child's future care.

The approach to examining a newborn for dysmorphic features begins with a systematic, complete physical examination. There are specific anatomic regions that are "high yield" areas for finding dysmorphic features and delineating syndromes. It is beyond the scope of this chapter to include all details of a complete examination, so we concentrate on describing these "high yield" areas. In addition, we concentrate on features of genetic syndromes that are particularly associated with congenital heart disease.

First, size and growth are important, including birth weight, length, and head circumference. Small overall size, indicating poor growth in utero, is an important clue to a genetic diagnosis. Newborns with chromosomal anomalies such as trisomies 18 and 13 are small for gestational age at birth. Large size is less common and may be related to maternal diabetes (which can be associated with CHD). A few genetic syndromes are seen with large size in newborns, most commonly Beckwith–Weidemann syndrome (BWS). BWS is not commonly associated with CHD, but cardiomegaly can occur as well as other organomegaly. Significantly disproportionate size in a newborn is also unusual, and can indicate a specific diagnosis. Newborns with achondroplasia have macrocephaly with short proximal long bones (rhizomelia). Achondroplasia is not commonly associated with a higher incidence of CHD; however, these infants may be worked up for CHD because of cyanosis caused by respiratory problems from small chests and upper airway obstruction.

Examination of the head and face is a high yield area. Common head shape abnormalities seen in the newborn include brachycephaly (shortened anteroposterior dimension of the head), microcephaly, and macrocephaly. Brachycephaly is a common finding in trisomy 21/Down syndrome (Tri21/DS). Microcephaly can be present in many syndromes. Macrocephaly is less common but can be seen in BWS or hydrocephalus. Prominent forehead can be seen in infants with Noonan syndrome (Figure 10.1). A localized abnormality of the scalp in the parieto-occipital area, called cutis aplasia, is a hallmark feature of trisomy 13 (Figure 10.2a) and so is clouded cornea (Figure 10.2b).

Facial features like a low posterior hairline can suggest Turner or Noonan syndromes. The finding of a pupillary coloboma on eye examination can be a clue to CHARGE syndrome (**c**oloboma, **h**eart defects, choanal **a**tresia, **r**etarded growth and development, **g**enital abnormalities and **e**ar anomalies). Anomalies of eye spacing and placement of the palpebral fissures can be helpful. Upslanting palpebral fissures are a common feature in Tri 21/DS (Figure 10.3a) while downslanting palpebral fissures can occur in Noonan syndrome (Figure 10.1). Periorbital fullness with or without ptosis of the eyelids can be seen in 22q11 deletion syndrome (Figure 10.4), Noonan syndrome (Figure 10.1), and Williams syndrome

Visual Guide to Neonatal Cardiology, First Edition. Edited by Ernerio T. Alboliras, Ziyad M. Hijazi, Leo Lopez, and Donald J. Hagler.

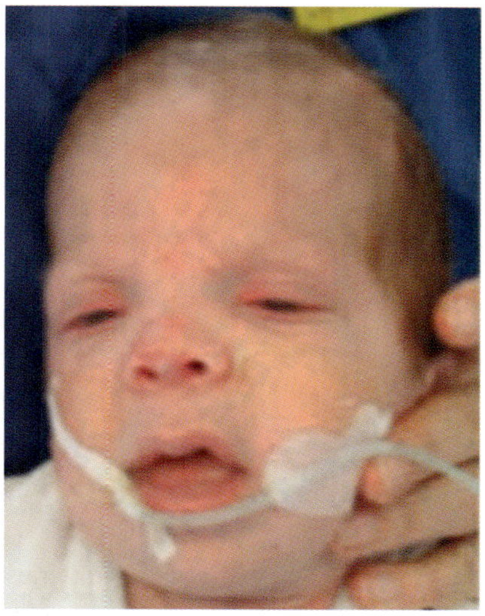

Figure 10.1 Noonan syndrome.

(Figure 10.5). Ear shape and placement is often noted as a minor dysmorphic feature with low set and posteriorly rotated ears being a common non-specific finding that does not give much clue to a specific genetic syndrome. There are other, more specific ear findings that can indicate a specific genetic syndrome such as the ear creases of BWS, the deficient lobe and "clipped-off" helix of the ear of CHARGE syndrome (Figure 10.6), and the small, cupped ear of Tri21/DS. A prominent nasal root, bulbous nasal tip with hypoplastic alae nasae, and bifid nasal tip of the nose are features of 22q11 syndrome (Figure 10.4c). Facial asymmetry can be an important clue to hemifacial microsomia, which can include CHD in the phenotype. Facial asymmetry with CHD is also seen in infants whose mothers took retinoic acid during pregnancy. Cleft lip and palate are not subtle physical findings; many cases of cleft lip and palate are apparently non-syndromic. Yet, the midline defects of cleft lip and palate can be a feature of trisomy 13.

Another high yield area for detection of dysmorphic features is the upper extremity, specifically the forearm, hand, and thumb. There are several "heart–hand" syndromes that include CHD as well as anomalies of the upper extremities. Holt–Oram syndrome (HOS) includes a spectrum of defects of the upper limb from minor changes in the bones of the wrist to hypoplastic, or even absent, thumbs or hypoplastic forearms because of radial defects along with cardiac septal defects (Figure 10.7a). Patients with HOS may also have progressive conduction defects but their electrophysiologic problems usually do not develop in the newborn period. Patients with Townes–Brock syndrome can have variable thumb anomalies along with ear anomalies, preauricular tags, and imperforate anus; these patients can also have CHD. Patients with thrombocytopenia with absent radius (TAR syndrome) have absence of the radius bilaterally though they do have thumbs; one-quarter to one-third of patients with TAR have CHD in addition to their limb anomalies. Patients with Fanconi anemia are often first noted to have limb anomalies and CHD as newborns, well before the characteristic anemia, because the hematologic findings do not develop for few years. The VACTERL association includes CHD in about 50% of patients along with limb anomalies with thumb (Figure 10.7b) and radial hypoplasia, and preaxial polydactyly as well as vertebral anomalies, anal atresia, tracheoesophageal fistula and renal anomalies. Polydactyly of the hands or the feet can be a clue to trisomies 13 and 18 (Figures 10.7c and 10.8a). Though not a skeletal anomaly per se, the puffy hands and/or feet with hyperconvex hypoplastic nails of a newborn girl with Turner syndrome are quite striking and should prompt evaluation for left-sided structural heart disease

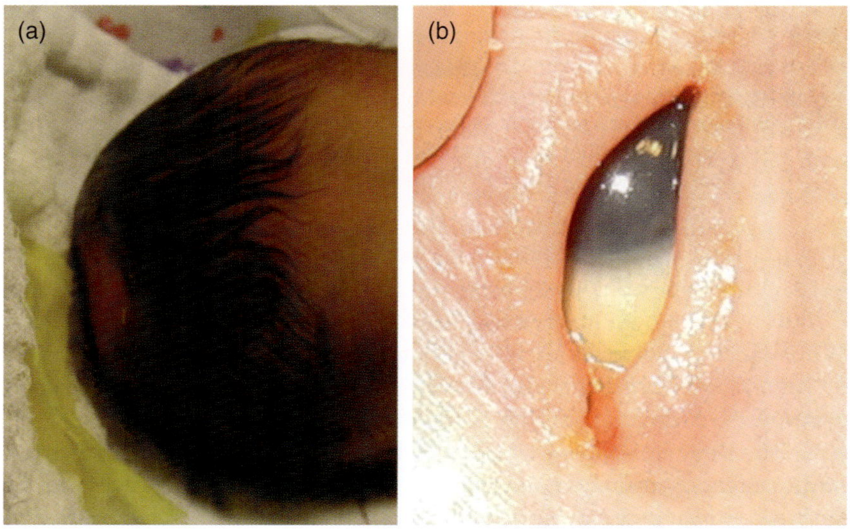

Figure 10.2 Trisomy 13: (a) cutis aplasia; (b) clouded cornea.

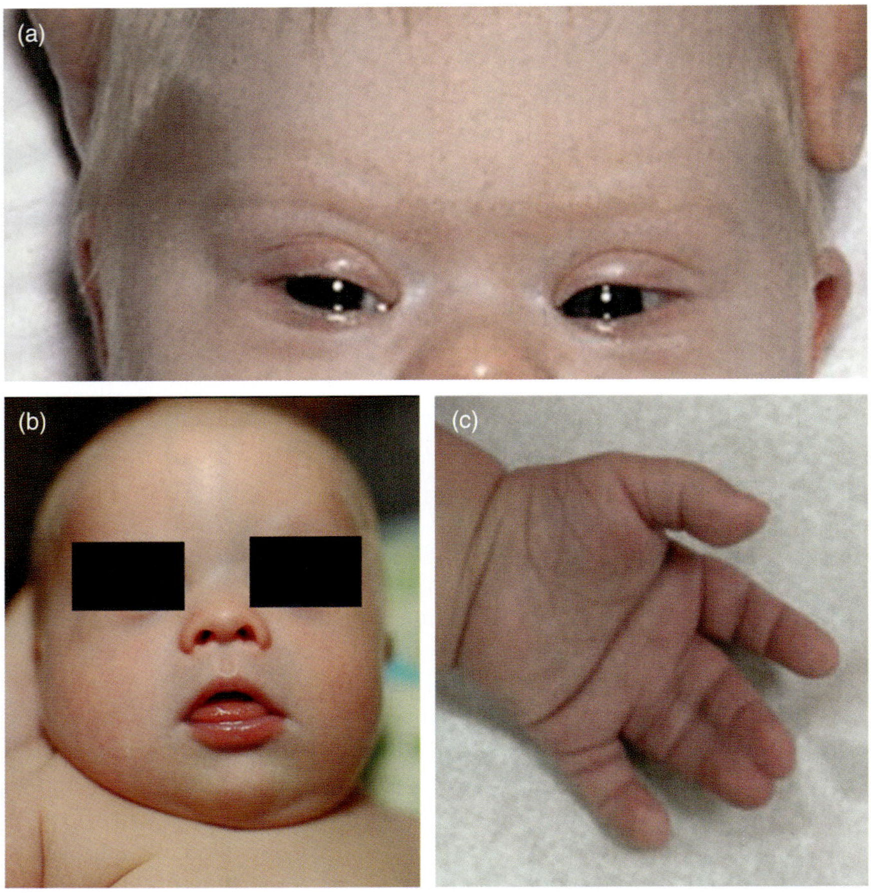

Figure 10.3 Trisomy 21/Down syndrome: (a) upslanting palpebral fissures and epicanthal folds; (b) low nasal bridge and prominent tongue; (c) single palmar crease.

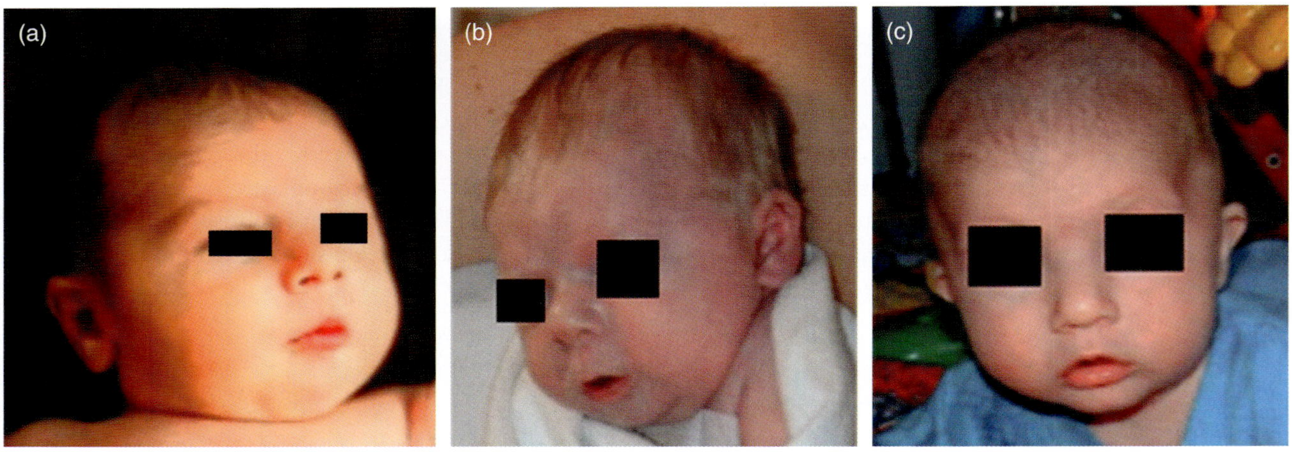

Figure 10.4 22q11 deletion syndrome: (a–c) periorbital fullness, prominent nasal root, bulbous nasal tip, and pinched alae.

(Figure 10.8b). Rocker-bottom feet are a common feature of trisomy 13 or 18 (Figure 10.8c).

Most neonates with suspected CHD have a chest X-ray. When skeletal anomalies are noted of the vertebral bodies and/or the ribs, this suggests a few specific genetic syndromes. Alagille syndrome is associated with butterfly vertebrae as well as CHD, particularly right-sided outflow tract abnormalities like pulmonary stenosis. The characteristic finding of hyperbilirubinemia and jaundice caused by a paucity of bile ducts in the patient with Alagille syndrome has not yet developed in newborns. Patients with Noonan syndrome may have vertebral segmentation defects. Vertebral defects are an important part of the VACTERL association. Thin posterior ribs are commonly noted in infants with trisomy 13.

There are some genetic syndromes, particularly some chromosomal conditions, that can and should be diagnosed in the newborn period. Tri21/DS is the most

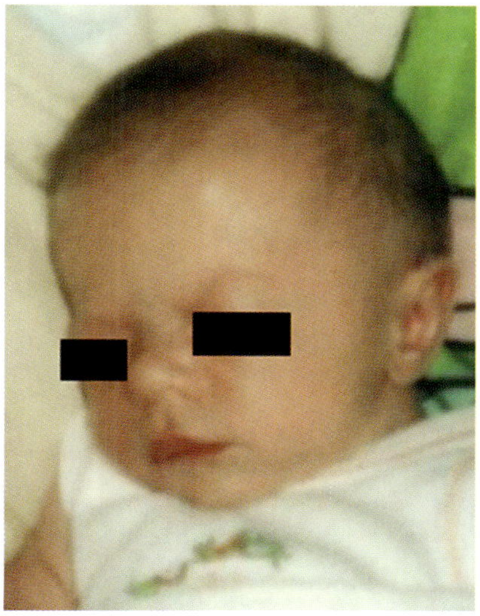

Figure 10.5 Williams syndrome.

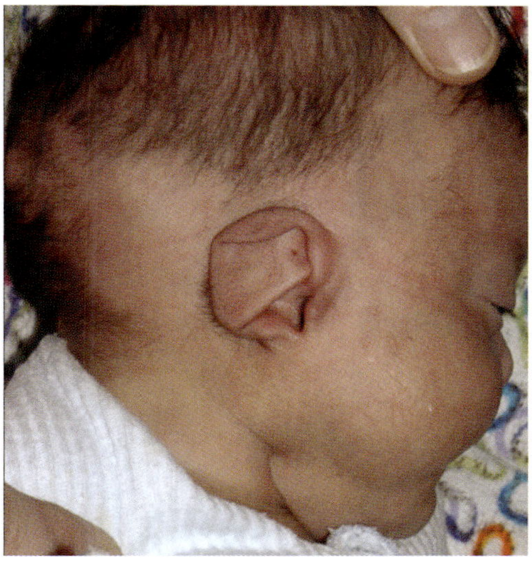

Figure 10.6 CHARGE syndrome ears. Deficient lobes and "clipped-off" helices.

common malformation syndrome and chromosomal defect occurring in live born infants. The classic facial features of epicanthal folds, low nasal bridge, upslanting palpebral fissures, small ears, prominent tongue, single palmar creases, and hypotonia usually make this diagnosis one that is made by clinical examination and confirmed by cytogenetic testing (Figure 10.3). CHD is quite common in Tri21/DS (40–50% of patients), so an infant suspected to have Tri21/DS should have an echocardiogram. If the scan in a newborn shows complete AV canal, careful examination for features of Tri21/DS is essential.

Timely diagnosis of trisomy 18 is important because there is a high mortality rate in these patients despite medical intervention. Many families and care teams decide against invasive options such as cardiac surgery for an infant with trisomy 18, so making the diagnosis is important for care decisions. The overall small size of infants with trisomy 18 along with small eyes, small mouth, short sternum, overlapping fingers, and fisted hands, rocker-bottom feet in association with CHD consisting of septal defects and redundant valvar tissue in virtually all of these infants alerts the clinician to likely trisomy 18 (Figures 10.7d and 10.8c). Similarly, patients with trisomy 13 have limited survival, so invasive cardiac procedures are often avoided. Infants with trisomy 13 may have midline defects such as cleft lip and palate (Figure 10.9) as well as holoprosencephaly along with thin ribs, rocker-bottom feet, clenched hands with overlapping fingers, polydactyly, and cutis aplasia (Figures 10.8c, 10.7d, and 10.7c). CHD in infants with trisomy 13 is common (up to 80% of those affected), but is mostly relatively simple septal defects and patent ductus arteriosus and rarely complex forms of CHD.

A female infant with CHD, especially in the spectrum of left-sided obstructive disease (from bicuspid aortic valve, aortic stenosis, coarctation of the aorta to full hypoplastic left heart syndrome) should be investigated for Turner syndrome, especially if there is also low posterior hairline and webbed neck, widely spaced nipples, some degree of pectus excavatum, lymphedema of the hands and feet, and hyperconvex nails (Figure 10.8b).

With the widespread use of microarray technology, chromosomal deletions are reported with increasing frequency. The 22q11 deletion is the most common deletion syndrome. These infants have a high incidence of conotruncal anomalies; truncus arteriosus and interrupted aortic arch especially should alert the clinician to consider 22q11 deletion. The facial features can be subtle and easy to overlook, though periorbital fullness, prominent nasal root with bulbous (even bifid tip), and "pinched" nasal alae with any degree of clefting of the hard and/or soft palate in the infant with CHD will strongly suggest this diagnosis, particularly if the metabolic finding of hypocalcemia is present as well (Figure 10.4). The infant with Williams syndrome, also a microdeletion syndrome, is small at birth and will have slow growth. Facial features of short palpebral fissures with epicanthal folds, periorbital fullness, depressed nasal bridge, anteverted nares, long philtrum, and wide mouth with prominent lips in conjunction with CHD that includes arterial stenoses of various arteries, especially supravalvar aortic stenosis, is strongly suggestive of Williams syndrome (Figure 10.5). Infants with Williams syndrome may have hypercalcemia as an important clinical clue to the diagnosis.

Several single gene disorders with CHD as an important part of the phenotype can be diagnosed in newborns. Noonan syndrome has head and neck features that can be seen from birth including a webbed neck and a

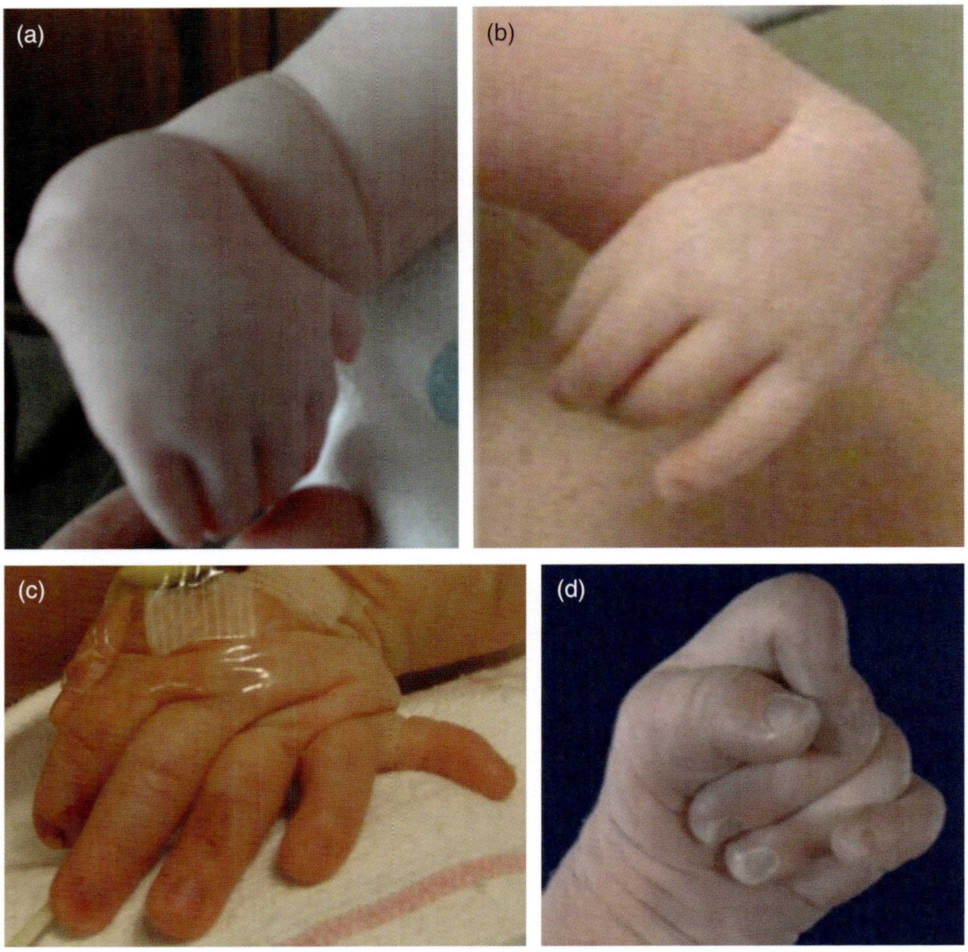

Figure 10.7 Upper extremity, hand, and finger anomalies: (a) hypoplastic thumb and wrist anomalies of Holt–Oram syndrome; (b) radial ray anomalies with absent radius and thumb in VACTERL syndrome; (c) polydactyly of the hand in trisomy 18; (d) overlapping fingers and clenched fists of trisomies 18 and 13.

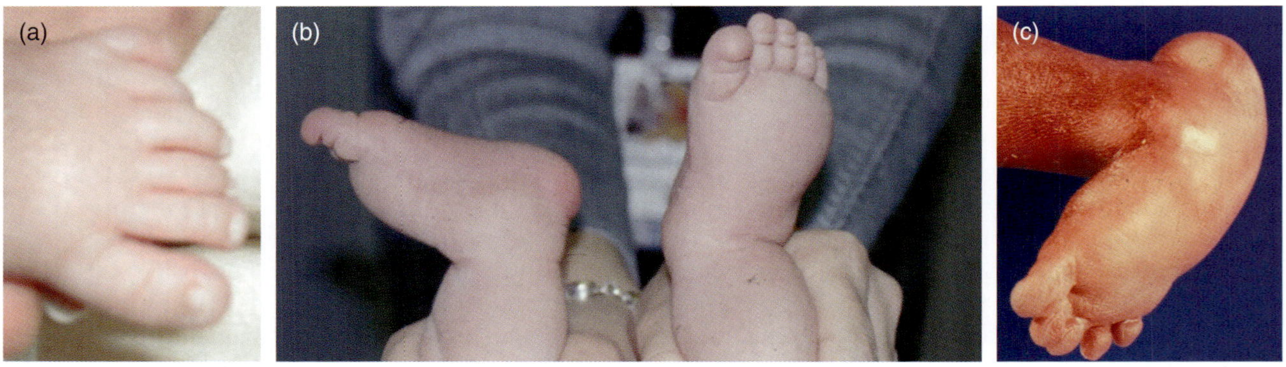

Figure 10.8 Foot and toe anomalies: (a) polydactyly of the foot; (b) dorsal lymphedema of the feet in Turner syndrome; (c) rocker-bottom feet of trisomies 18 and 13.

low posterior hairline along with ptosis, epicanthal folds, downslanting palpebral fissures, and low nasal bridge (Figure 10.1). These features, along with pulmonary valve stenosis, especially a dysplastic pulmonary valve, strongly suggest this disorder. Hypertrophic cardiomyopathy, sometimes of a striking degree, can also be present in the newborn with Noonan syndrome. CHARGE syndrome is now known to be caused by CHD7 mutations in most cases. These infants can be quite ill from birth given their potential respiratory, cardiac and gastrointestinal issues. The identification of several of the major criteria (from the mnemonic

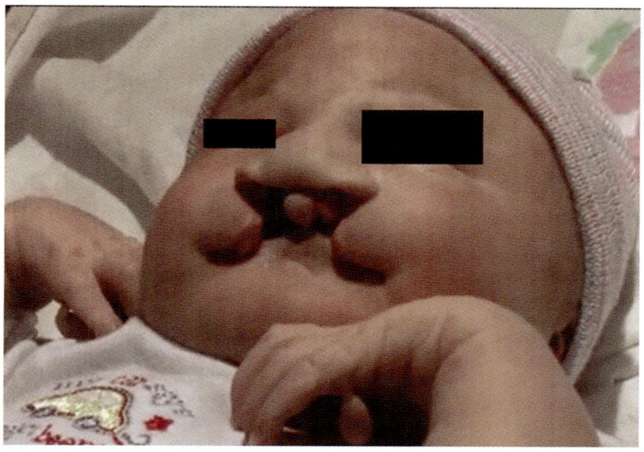

Figure 10.9 Cleft lip and palate in trisomy 13.

noted earlier), especially with the characteristic ear features (Figure 10.6), helps make the diagnosis in a newborn even though some of the features like hearing loss and developmental delay will not be apparent. Smith–Lemli–Opitz syndrome (SLO) is suggested by low cholesterol levels on chemistry panels in a newborn with overall small size, microcephaly, genital abnormalities, and CHD, especially endocardial cushion defects and septal defects. SLO is caused by a defect in cholesterol biosynthesis that causes abnormally low cholesterol levels; the diagnosis is made by finding elevated amounts of a cholesterol precursor, 7-dehydrocholesterol, in plasma.

CHD along with other birth defects can occur in infants who have been exposed to maternal medications or maternal metabolic diseases during pregnancy. Retinoic acid exposure is associated with CHD, specifically conotruncal malformations, and is also associated with facial asymmetry, sloping forehead with small abnormal ears. Fetal alcohol syndrome can include facial features such as long philtrum and thin upper lip as well as CHD. Maternal diabetes has long been associated with CHD in the infant along with large size at birth. Maternal phenylketonuria is associated with CHD, though the CHD is not of one type and can include septal defects as well as tetralogy of Fallot and coarctation of the aorta. These infants also have facial features of small eyes, epicanthal folds, long philtrum, and a thin upper lip along with other malformations such as cleft lip and palate.

While a specific diagnosis cannot be made in all neonates with dysmorphic features and CHD, genetic evaluation and follow-up, including different forms of genetic testing, can start in the newborn period and continue beyond. Making a specific genetic diagnosis is ultimately helpful to plan the best clinical care for the infant.

Further Reading

Jones KL. (2006) *Smith's Recognizable Patterns of Human Malformation*, 6th edn, Elsevier Saunders, Philadelphia, PA.

Pagon RA, Adam MP, Ardinger HH, *et al.* (eds) Gene Reviews® 1993–2014. University of Seattle, Seattle, WA. https://www.ncbi.nlm.nih.gov/books/NBK1116/ (accessed November 13, 2017).

Part III

Diagnostic Procedures

11

Chest Roentgenogram

Randy Richardson[1]*, Darshit Thakrar*[2]*, and Deepak Kaura*[3]

[1] St. Joseph's Hospital and Medical Center, Creighton University School of Medicine, Phoenix, AZ, USA
[2] University of Pittsburgh, Pittsburgh, PA, USA
[3] Sidra Medical and Research Center, Doha, Qatar

Several decades ago a chest X-ray had a key role in the diagnostic workup of a patient with congenital heart disease. Since then echocardiography, computed tomography, and magnetic resonance imaging have taken over as the non-invasive diagnostic modalities of choice for these patients. With a few exceptions, the radiograph does not typically have a significant role in making the diagnosis but it does have an important secondary role during the treatment and care of the neonate with congenital heart disease.

This chapter reviews the classic approach to radiographic interpretation in a neonate with congenital heart disease. It looks at some congenital heart lesions where the radiograph may have diagnostic value and reviews the secondary role of the radiograph in evaluating lines and tubes, looking for postoperative complications, and assessing fluid status.

Classic interpretation was based on evaluating the following: pulmonary vascularity, cardiomegaly, situs, great vessels, and extracardiac structures.

Pulmonary Vascularity

Pulmonary vascularity may be increased, decreased, or show evidence of pulmonary edema or heart failure. Increased pulmonary vascularity, which is also termed shunt vascularity, is suggested on radiographs where the pulmonary arteries appear enlarged but are still sharply demarcated from the lung parenchyma (Figure 11.1). Losing the distinctness or sharpness of the pulmonary vessels suggests that edema is infiltrating the parenchyma and silhouetting the vessels (Figure 11.2). Decreased pulmonary vascularity is seen when there is not adequate blood flow to the lungs. In this case the lungs appear more lucent and the vessels are smaller and less numerous than normal (Figure 11.3).

Differential diagnoses were traditionally based on these basic pulmonary vascularity findings in the patient with congenital heart disease. An acyanotic patient with increased pulmonary vascularity (shunt vascularity) would suggest one of the classic shunt lesions: atrial septal defect (ASD), ventricular septal defect (VSD), patent ductus arteriosus (PDA) or complete common atrioventricular canal (CCAVC) or endocardial cushion defect.

A cyanotic patient with increased pulmonary vascularity would suggest the differential diagnoses of transposition of the great arteries or vessels (TGA or TGV), total anomalous pulmonary venous return (TAPVR), truncus arteriosus, single ventricle and single atrium.

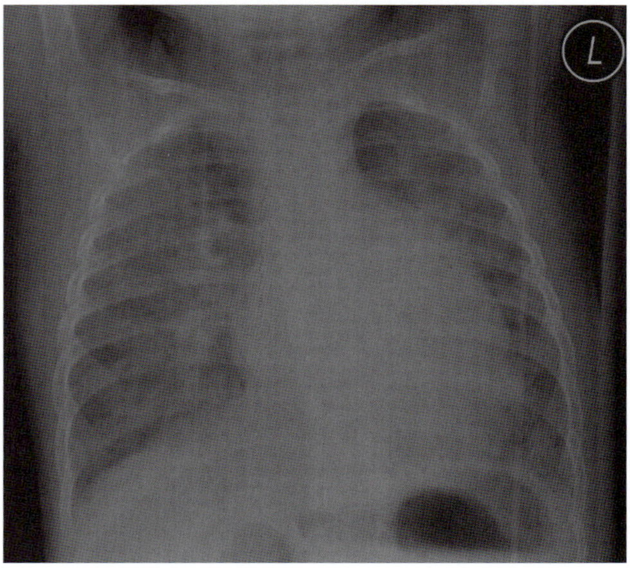

Figure 11.1 Frontal radiograph of the chest in a patient with a ventricular septal defect (VSD) shows increased pulmonary vascularity; prominent pulmonary vessels seen bilaterally.

Visual Guide to Neonatal Cardiology, First Edition. Edited by Ernerio T. Alboliras, Ziyad M. Hijazi, Leo Lopez, and Donald J. Hagler.

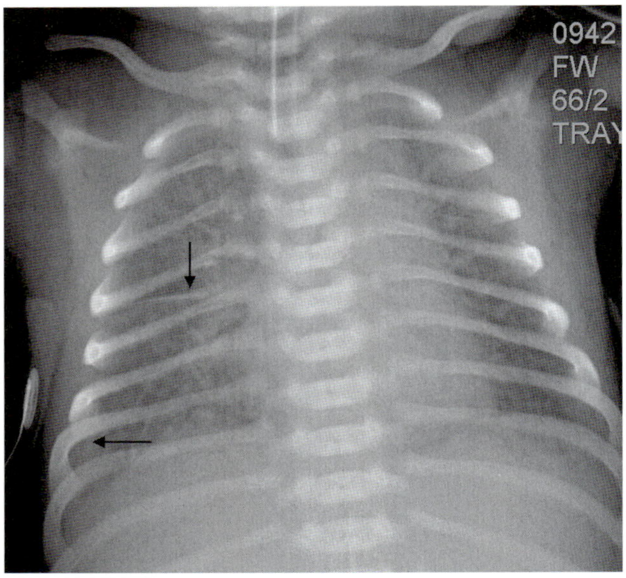

Figure 11.2 Frontal radiograph of the chest in a patient with obstructed total anomalous venous return shows increased indistinctness of the pulmonary vessels from diffuse pulmonary edema and fluid seen in the right costophrenic angle and horizontal fissure (black arrows).

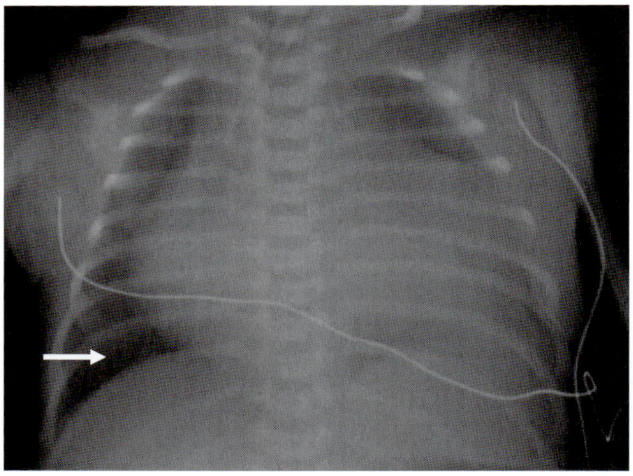

Figure 11.3 Frontal radiograph of the chest in a patient with Ebstein anomaly shows decreased pulmonary vascularity and marked cardiomegaly. Notice how clear the lungs are with very few vessels seen (arrow).

A cyanotic patient with decreased pulmonary vascularity would suggest differential diagnoses of tetralogy of Fallot, pulmonic atresia, tricuspid atresia, and Ebstein anomaly.

Finally, diffuse pulmonary edema in the perinatal period suggests heart failure with a wide number of possibilities in the differential diagnosis: obstructive left ventricular (LV) outflow lesions like severe coarctation, interruption of the aortic arch, aortic atresia, or severe aortic stenosis, hypoplastic left heart syndrome (HLHS) and mitral stenosis to name a few.

Cardiomegaly

In a neonate, the heart should not take up more than 50–55% of the chest width on frontal view. Contours of the heart should be assessed for specific chamber enlargement and other classic findings such as an upturned apex (boot shape) which suggests right ventricular hypertrophy (Figure 11.4). Cardiomegaly may be difficult to assess on a frontal neonatal radiograph. Thymic tissue is often prominent and may wrap around the heart and obscure the actual size of the heart on frontal view (Figure 11.5). The lateral radiograph will be normal in these patients.

Situs

Designation of situs should be attempted on all initial X-rays. Situs solitus is typically designated when the heart in normal position with the apex pointing to the left and the stomach on the left. Situs inversus typically shows the heart on the right with the apex pointing to the right and the stomach on the right side (Figure 11.6a). Situs ambiguous is anything that does not fit into the first two categories. The radiograph for situs ambiguous would typically show the apex of the heart on the left and the stomach on the right (Figure 11.6b). Situs

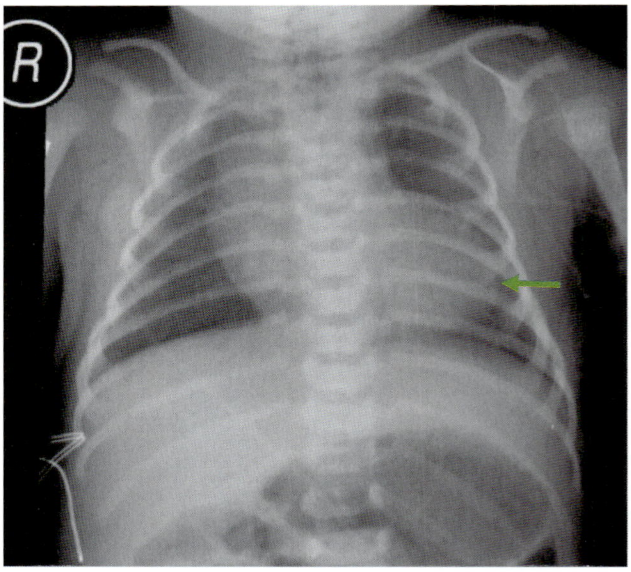

Figure 11.4 Frontal radiograph of the chest in a patient with tetralogy of Fallot shows decreased pulmonary vascularity and an upturned apex of the heart (arrow). This is often referred to as a "boot"-shaped heart.

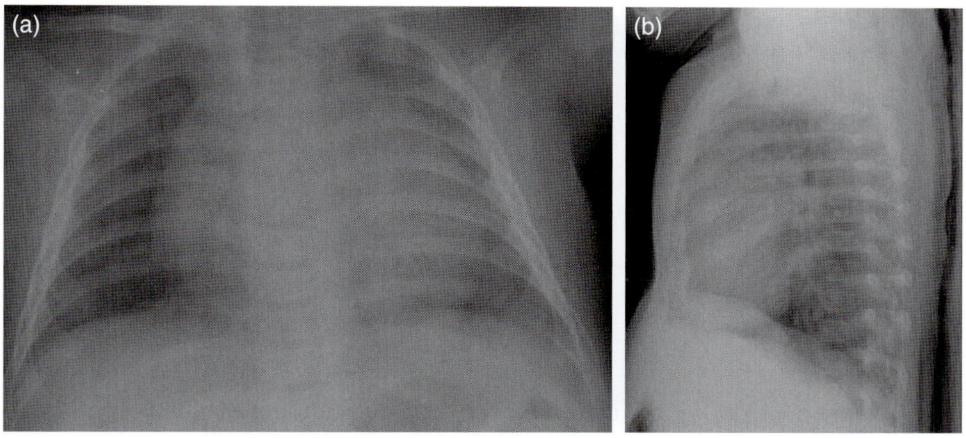

Figure 11.5 (a) Frontal and (b) lateral radiographs of the chest in an asymptomatic patient shows apparent cardiomegaly on the frontal view with a normal heart size on the lateral view. Thymic tissue in infants may make the cardiac silhouette appear enlarged.

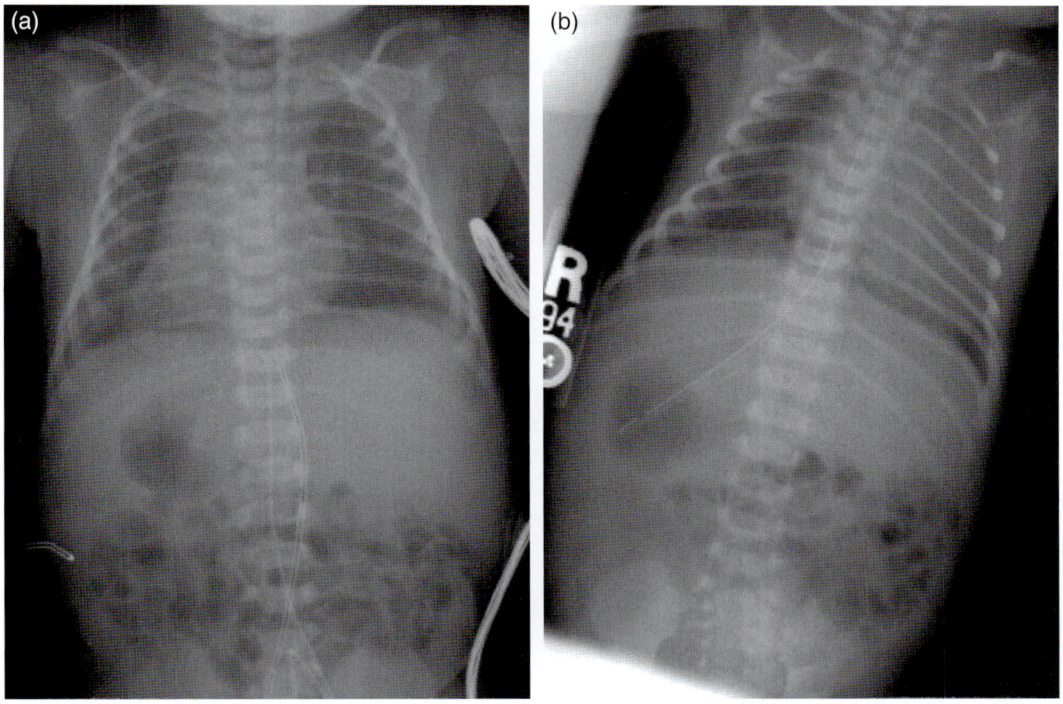

Figure 11.6 Both patients show the stomach to be on the right. (a) The patient has the cardiac apex on the right consistent with situs inversus; (b) the patient has the cardiac apex on the left consistent with situs ambiguous.

designation may not be possible on a radiograph of the chest if the stomach is not filled with air and/or if the heart is obscured by lung disease.

Great Vessels

Determining the side of the aortic arch may be difficult because of overlying thymic tissue. Three basic findings often help determine the side of the aortic arch. First, simply look for the arch in the upper mediastinum. It typically sits just above the main pulmonary artery and forms the first round prominence along the left upper mediastinum. Second, look for deviation of the trachea. Leftward deviation of the trachea suggests a right aortic arch (Figure 11.4). Finally, look for the descending aorta. It is often seen as a linear density paralleling the spine. A right aortic arch is often an important finding as it may be part of a vascular ring complex with an aberrant left subclavian and PDA completing the ring. A round density posterior to the intrathoracic trachea may be seen on lateral view and may cause some airway compression.

The main pulmonary artery typically forms the second round prominence along the left upper mediastinum. Look for enlargement of the pulmonary artery in patients with a left to right shunt and a diminutive pulmonary artery in patients with decreased pulmonary vascularity.

Extracardiac Evaluation

There are multiple associated findings seen in patients with congenital heart disease and a thorough evaluation of the extracardiac structures is warranted. VACTERL is a good mnemonic to remember as these represent associated findings seen in the neonate. V stands for vertebral. Vertebral anomalies are commonly with butterfly and hemivertebral bodies frequently seen. A is for atresias. On a chest X-ray, a dilated proximal pouch may be seen with esophageal atresia and a double bubble sign typically seen with duodenal atresia. C is for cardiac which is why we are following this mnemonic of associated findings. TE is for tracheo-esophageal fistula and may present as an isolated esophageal atresia. R is for renal and would be hard to evaluate by X-ray. L is for limb anomaly. The most common finding is an absent radius which may be inadvertently imaged on a neonatal chest X-ray (Figure 11.7).

Patients with Down syndrome commonly have congenital heart disease and some typical radiographic findings. On lateral view of the chest there may be a hypersegmented manubrium (Figure 11.8).

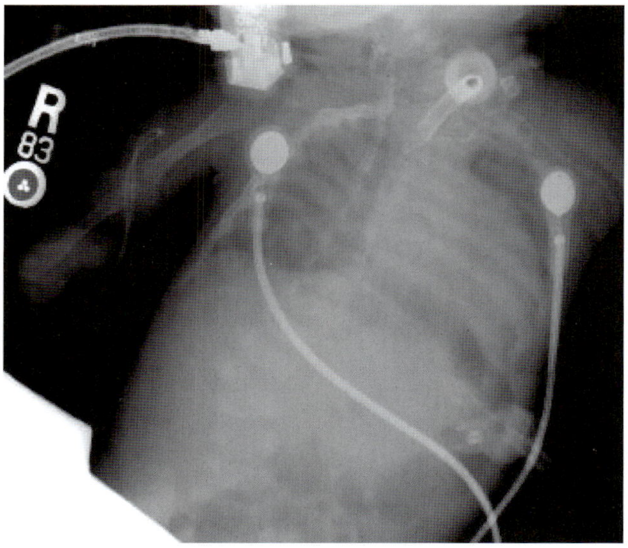

Figure 11.7 Frontal radiograph of the chest in a patient with repair of a prior tracheoesophageal fistula. Notice that there is cardiomegaly in this patient with a large atrial septal defect (ASD) and VSD. Also notice the hemivertebral body at L2 and the absent right radius. Patients with congenital disease heart often have associated anomalies that follow the VACTERL mnemonic.

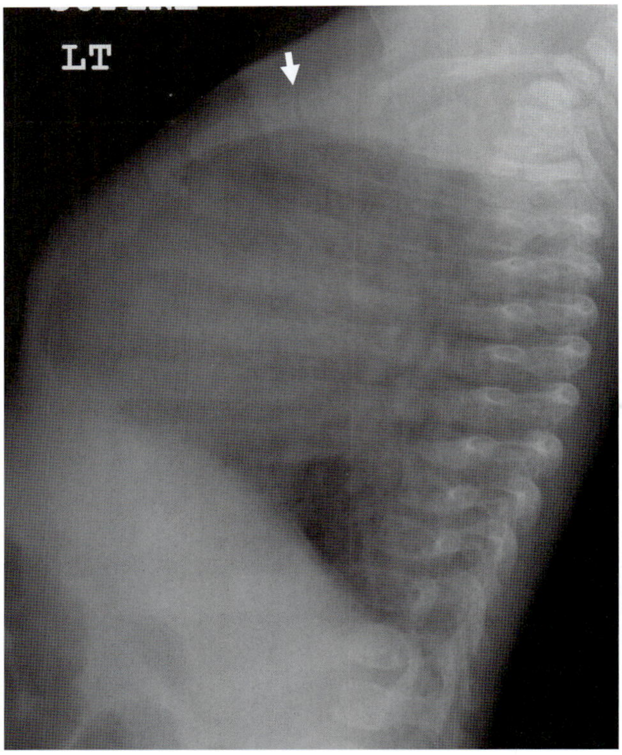

Figure 11.8 Lateral radiograph of the chest in a patient with known Down syndrome. Notice the hypersegmented manubrium (arrow) which is often seen in patients with Down syndrome on lateral view of the chest.

Patients with DiGeorge syndrome may not have thymic tissue although many of the patients with congenital heart disease may have decreased thymic tissue as there may be significant stress to their system from decreased blood oxygenation.

There are some cases in which the radiograph may be helpful in the diagnosis of some types of congenital heart disease. Scimitar syndrome is one where the radiograph may be diagnostic as the right lower lobe partial anomalous pulmonary venous return is visualized as a curvilinear vein coursing towards the inferior vena cava with associated hypoplasia of the right lung (Figure 11.9).

The "figure 3" sign is a classic finding on radiography in an older child with coarctation of the aorta with rib notching of the under surface of the 4–8th ribs (typically). Rib notching may be unilateral if the coarctation is proximal to the origin of the subclavian artery (Figure 11.10).

Ebstein anomaly has the so-called box-shaped heart with decreased pulmonary vascularity that is fairly characteristic (Figure 11.3). This heart shape is caused by the massive tricuspid regurgitation with enlargement of the right atrium and ventricle.

Diagnosis based on heart contour is not very reliable but there are some other classic findings that are often noted. The "snowman" sign seen with supracardiac type TAPVR (Figure 11.11) is caused by a prominent

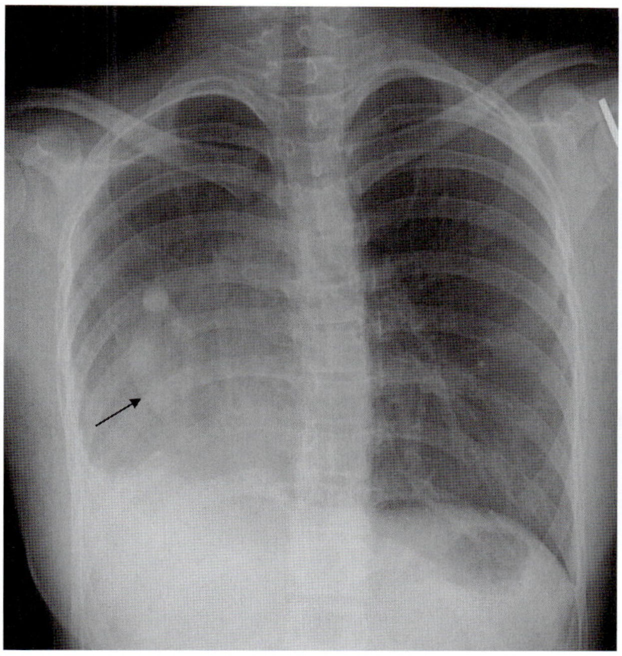

Figure 11.9 Frontal radiograph of the chest in an asymptomatic patient shows a curvilinear vein coursing anteromedically towards the inferior vena cava (black arrow). This was a partial anomalous venous return. Also notice the rightward mediastinal shift caused by hypoplasia of the right lung consistent with hypogenetic lung syndrome or scimitar syndrome.

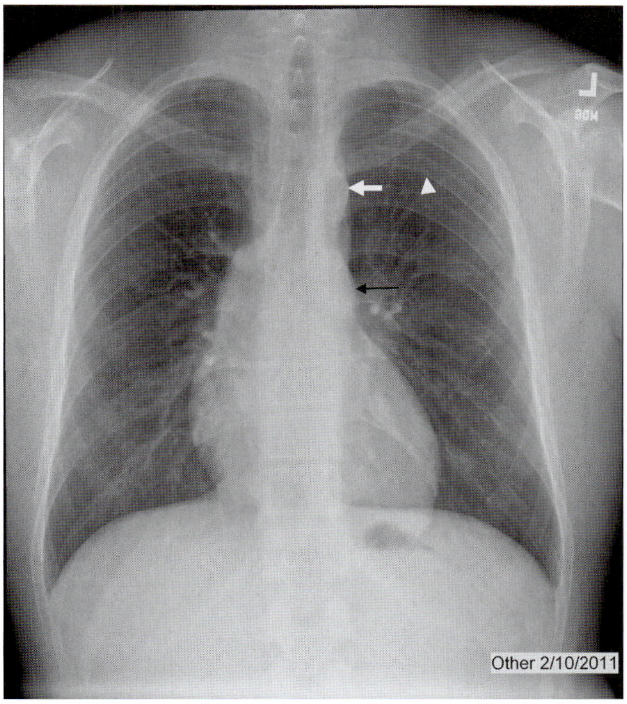

Figure 11.10 Frontal radiograph of the chest in a patient with high blood pressure in the upper extremity shows a classic "figure 3" sign from dilatation of the left subclavian artery (white arrow) and post-stenotic dilatation of the proximal descending thoracic aorta (black arrow) in a patient with coarctation. Subtle sclerosis and undulation of the inferior surface of the ribs is seen consistent with rib notching from prominent arterial collaterals (arrowhead).

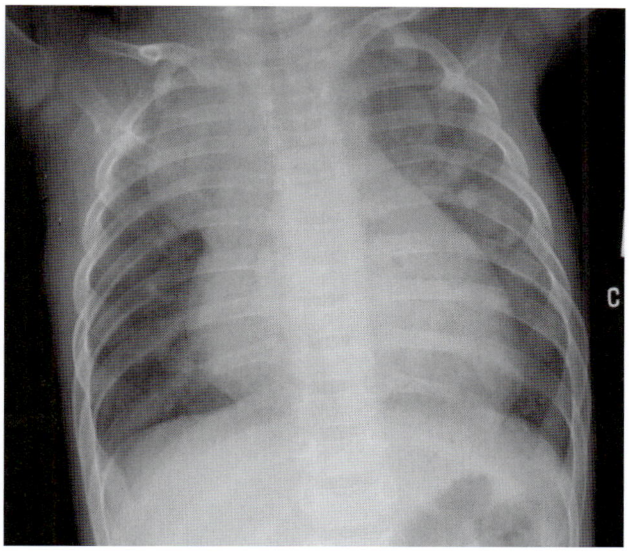

Figure 11.11 Frontal radiograph of the chest in a patient with supracardiac type total anomalous pulmonary venous return (TAPVR). Notice the prominent superior mediastinum from the anomalous venous drainage forming a snowman-like appearance of the mediastinum.

anomalous vertical vein typically ascending the left side of the superior mediastinum although a snowman sign is more commonly seen with a normal variant enlarged thymus.

The "egg on a string" sign seen with dextro-TGA (D-TGA) is caused by a characteristic globular shaped heart with a narrow superior mediastinum as the pulmonary artery is lined up posterior to the aorta causing the mediastinum to look narrowed (Figure 11.12).

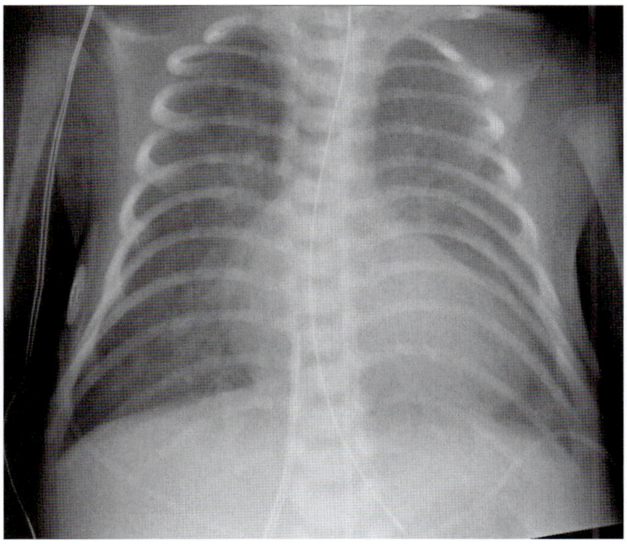

Figure 11.12 Frontal radiograph of the chest in a patient with dextro-transposition of the great arteries shows a globular or egg-shaped heart with a narrow mediastinum. The "egg on a string."

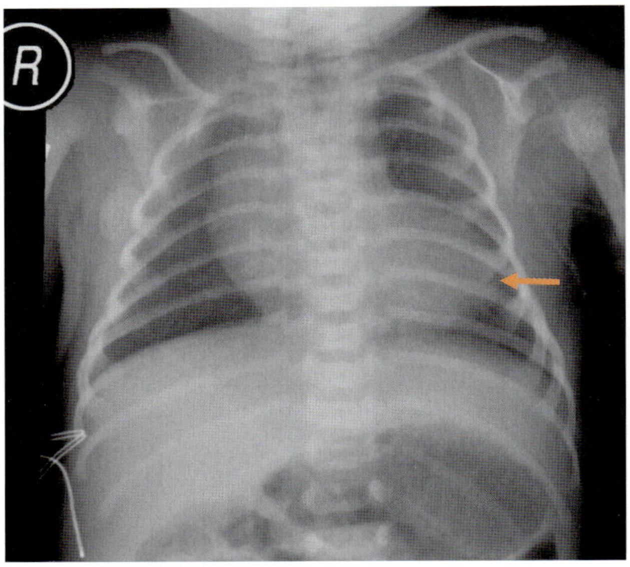

Figure 11.13 Frontal radiograph of the chest in a patient with tetralogy of Fallot shows decreased pulmonary vascularity and an upturned apex of the heart (arrow). This is often referred to as a "boot"-shaped heart.

The oft-quoted "boot-shaped" heart is classically seen in patients with tetralogy of Fallot but may be seen in other heart lesions where there is right ventricular hypertrophy (Figure 11.13). Finally, infracardiac type TAPVR with obstructed veins has a classic appearance with a normal heart size, pulmonary edema, and bilateral pleural effusion (Figure 11.2).

Lines and Tubes in Patients With Congenital Heart Disease

Although most lines and tubes are not unique to patients with congenital heart disease,there are some unique positions and types of lines for these patients.

A common difference seen with placement of a left subclavian line or PICC line may be that it courses down the left side of the mediastinum in patients with congenital heart disease. Although this could be an arterial stick with the tip coursing along the aorta, it is most often with a left-sided superior vena cava which is not uncommon in congenital heart patients (Figure 11.14).

Patients with situs anomalies are at an increased risk of malrotation of the midgut. Feeding tubes may be difficult to position in these patients and an urogenital examination may be helpful to elucidate the anatomy.

Temporary epicardial pacer wires are often placed after surgery and may not be completely removed. If coiled, these may be a contraindication to future MRI examinations.

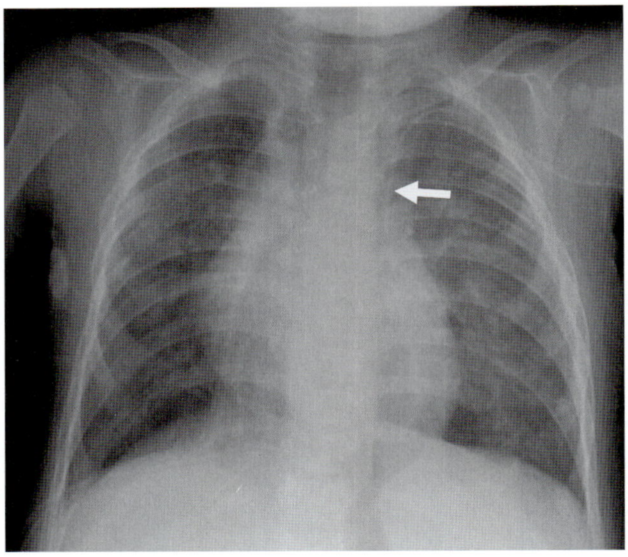

Figure 11.14 Frontal radiograph of the chest showing a left upper extremity PICC line descending along the left mediastinum in a left superior vena cava (arrow).

Epicardial biventricular pacer leads may be placed in patients. The round part of the lead should always face the heart.

Complications

Radiographic complications in the patient with congenital heart disease in the immediate postoperative period tend to be related to free air (pneumothorax,

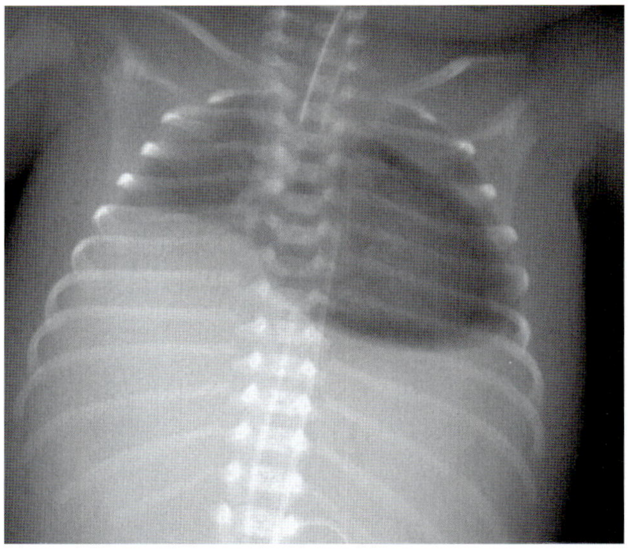

Figure 11.15 Frontal radiograph of the chest showing a large pneumopericardium in a patient after drainage of a large effusion.

pneumomediastinum, and pneumopericardium), as well as hemorrhage (Figure 11.15). Subsequent radiographic complications tend to be related to infectious etiologies such as pneumonia, and abscess formation.

In summary, radiographic evaluation of the patient with congenital heart disease does not typically have a key diagnostic role, with other non-invasive imaging modalities readily available with much higher sensitivity and specificity. Radiographs do have a secondary role in caring for the patient with congenital heart disease and knowing and understanding what to look for in these patients will contribute to their improved overall care.

12

Electrocardiogram

Bryan Cannon

Pediatric Arrhythmia and Pacing Service, Mayo Clinic, Rochester, MN, USA

One of the essential tools for evaluating the electrical activity of the heart is the electrocardiogram (ECG). This chapter focuses only on the basic principles of reading an ECG and does not discuss advanced concepts or arrhythmias. Before looking at the actual ECG tracing, it is important to understand some basic principles about how an ECG is performed.

ECG Leads

The limb leads consist of I, II, III, aVR, aVL, and aVF. These measure forces in a coronal plane. Each of these leads is assigned a vector (Figure 12.1). Forces directed towards these leads are represented on the ECG by upward (positive) deflections. Forces away from the lead are represented by downward (negative) deflections.

The precordial or chest leads consist of V1–V6 and measure cardiac forces in a transverse plane. Once again, forces toward these leads are represented by positive deflections, and forces away from the leads are represented by negative deflections. In this fashion, it is possible to tell the direction of electrical wavefronts in the heart.

Basic ECG Setup

The ECG is a measure of the electrical forces in the heart over time. The ECG is typically recorded on paper containing 1 × 1 mm squares. There are larger boxes that are 5 × 5 mm. As the ECG is printed out, the paper records the tracings over time. At a standard paper speed (25 mm/s), each small box is equal to 0.04 s (40 ms). Interval durations can be calculated by measuring along this axis. Vertical squares represent ECG voltages. These are important in determining atrial enlargement and ventricular hypertrophy. Each small box represents 0.1 mv, although deflections are typically recorded in millimeters rather than millivolts.

Wave Morphologies

The ECG contains several deflections which are named beginning with the letter P (Figure 12.2). The P wave represents depolarization of the atria. The QRS complex represents depolarization of the ventricles. The first initial downward deflection (if present) is called the Q wave. An upward deflection above the baseline following this Q wave is known as the R wave. The subsequent downward deflection below the baseline following the R wave is the S wave. The T wave represents repolarization of the ventricles. There may be an additional smaller deflection after the T wave which is called a U wave.

ECG Intervals

The PR interval is measured from the onset of the P wave to the onset of the QRS complex. This represents the time of the initial atrial depolarization and conduction through the atrioventricular node. The QT interval is measured from the *beginning* of the QRS complex to the *end* of the T wave. This represents the time from ventricular depolarization to ventricular repolarization. As the QT varies with heart rate, this interval must be corrected. This is most commonly by using Bazett's formula which involves dividing the QT interval (in seconds) by the square root of the previous RR interval (in seconds). The QT interval is best measured in leads II and V5 on the ECG. Measuring the QT interval in newborns can be difficult as they frequently have flattened T waves making determination of the exact end point of the T wave difficult. There may be transient prolongation of the QT interval seen immediately after

Visual Guide to Neonatal Cardiology, First Edition. Edited by Ernerio T. Alboliras, Ziyad M. Hijazi, Leo Lopez, and Donald J. Hagler.

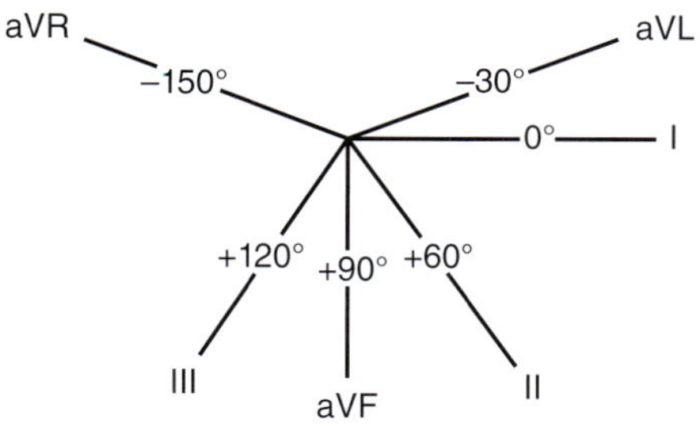

Figure 12.1 Orientation of leads of the electrocardiogram (ECG). Forces directed towards the leads are positive or upright deflections while forces moving away from the leads are negative or downward deflections.

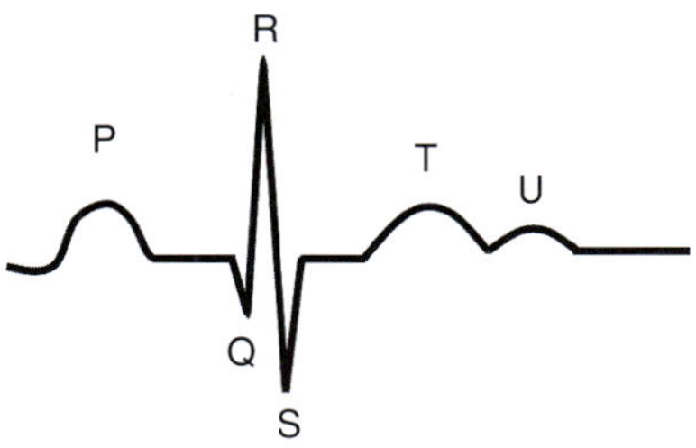

Figure 12.2 ECG tracing with P wave, QRS complex, T and U waves.

birth which may resolve in the first week of life. A QTc interval greater than 500 ms should always be considered abnormal and requires evaluation for either long QT syndrome (Figure 12.3) or a secondary cause of QT prolongation such as electrolyte disturbances, increased intracranial pressure, or medications.

Heart Rate

Heart rate can be estimated on the ECG and is typically measured in beats per minute. There are two methods of determining heart rate. The first method is to count the number of QRS complexes in a 10 s period (the typical length of the entire ECG) and then multiply this number by 6. If the heart rate is regular, a shortcut can be employed to quickly determine the heart rate. First, the amount of time (in milliseconds) between two consecutive QRS complexes is measured, remembering each small box is 40 ms. This number is then divided into 60 000 to determine the heart rate.

Cardiac Rhythm

In most neonates, atrial contractions are initiated by the sinus node located posteriorly at the junction of the superior vena cava and the right atrium. To call a rhythm sinus, it should meet three criteria. First, there must be a P wave before every QRS complex. Second, there must be a QRS complex after every P wave. Third, there must be a normal P wave axis (upright P wave in leads I and aVF). Most atrial impulses that do not have an upright P wave in leads I and aVF are not coming from the sinus node and may represent a cardiac arrhythmia.

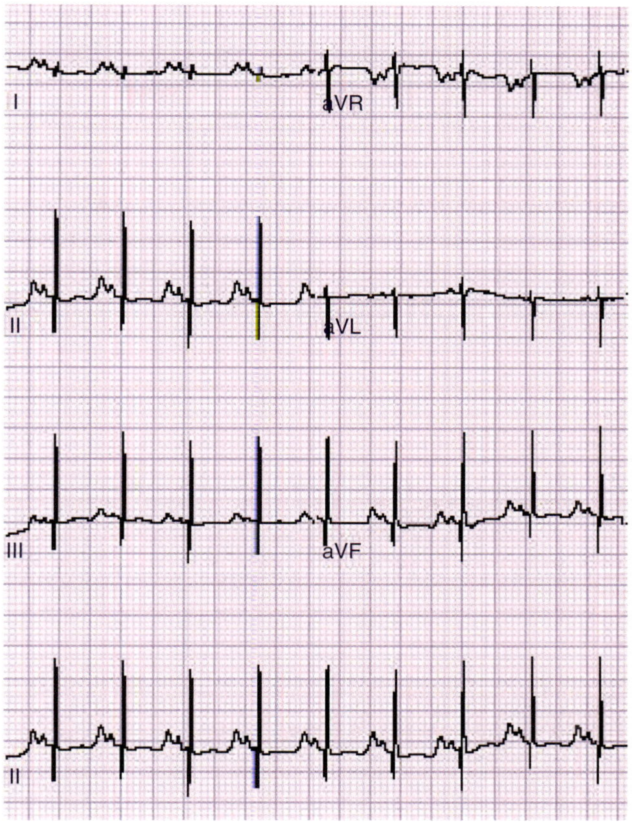

Figure 12.3 Long QT syndrome with corrected QT interval of 550 ms. Note that the T wave ends just before the onset of the next P wave.

Axis

The QRS axis gives information about the relationship of forces in the heart. The normal range for axis varies with age, with neonates having more dominance of the right-sided forces and a more rightward axis. The limb leads (I, II, III, aVR, aVL, and aVF) are used to calculate axis, but specifics about axis calculation are beyond the scope of this chapter. A normal axis in a neonate is between 60 and 190 degrees. Axis may be affected by ventricular hypertrophy, bundle branch block, or other conduction disturbances.

Right-sided Chest Leads

Many pediatric ECGs will include right-sided chest leads (V3R and V4R). These leads are placed in the same anatomic position as leads V3 and V4, but on the right side of the chest. These leads are helpful in determining right ventricular hypertrophy, right sided ischemia, and dextrocardia and are much more useful in the neonatal population than in older patients. If the combined voltages of the R and S waves are greater in leads V3R and V4R than in leads V3 and V4, the heart is positioned on the right side of the chest and the diagnosis of dextrocardia or dextroposition of the heart can be made. Some pediatric ECGs will also display lead V7, which has no well-defined use.

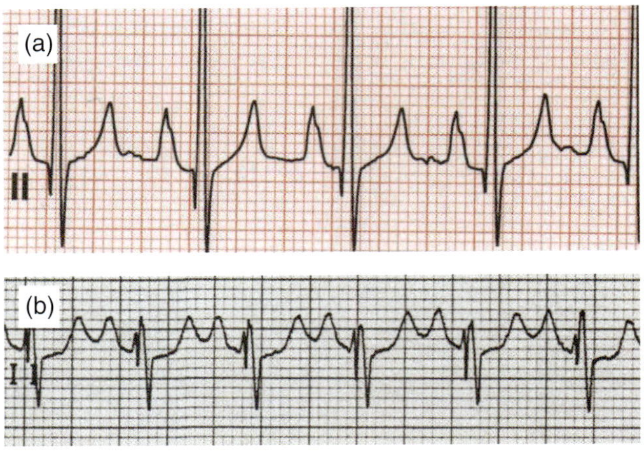

Figure 12.4 (a) Right atrial enlargement with P waves more than three boxes tall; (b) left atrial enlargement with P waves more than two boxes wide.

Abnormalities on the ECG

Atrial Enlargement

As the majority of the initial P wave deflection is caused by the right atrium, right atrial enlargement results in *tall* peaked P waves. P waves taller than 3 mm (three small boxes) in any lead are suggestive of right atrial enlargement. These changes are most commonly seen in leads II or V1, but may be seen in any lead.

As the left atrium is activated later in the P wave, left atrial enlargement results in *wide* P waves. P waves longer than 0.08 s (two small boxes) are suggestive of left atrial enlargement in a neonate. This is most commonly seen in leads II and V1, and lead V1 may have a broad notched or diphasic P wave with a negative terminal segment (Figure 12.4).

Ventricular Hypertrophy

Thickening of one or both of the ventricles may be suggested by findings on the ECG. The ECG is fairly good at predicting hypertrophy, particularly in neonates, although there is a relatively high incidence of false positive findings. Therefore, the presence of ventricular hypertrophy on ECG should be confirmed by echocardiography. ECG findings suggesting right and left ventricular hypertrophy are listed in Box 12.1. Extremely large voltages (so large it is difficult to contain them on the ECG paper) can be seen in patients with glycogen storage disease (most commonly Pompe disease, also known as acid maltase deficiency or glycogen storage disease type II) or in infants of diabetic mothers.

Low Voltage QRS

Low voltage QRS complexes are diagnosed if the R wave plus the S wave is less than 5 mm in the limb leads (I-aVF). Low voltage QRS complexes may be seen in normal newborns (especially premature neonates) as the myocardial mass is small in these small babies. This finding may also be present in patients with myocarditis, pericarditis, pneumothorax, or severe hypothyroidism.

QRS Duration

Similar to almost all other ECG intervals, the QRS duration is shorter in younger patients, particularly neonates.

Box 12.1 Criteria for right ventricular hypertrophy (RVH) and left ventricular hypertrophy (LVH)

Right ventricular hypertrophy

- R in V1 greater than upper limits for age
- Upright T in V1 after 7 days of age (normally may become upright again as early as 6 years old)
- Presence of Q wave >1 box in V1, V3R, or V4R
- rSR′ with R′ >15 mm in newborn
- Pure R wave in V1 in child older than 6 months

Possible RVH

- S in V6 greater than upper limits for age
- R/S ratio in V1 greater than upper limits for age

Left ventricular hypertrophy

- R in V6 greater than upper limits for age

Possible LVH

- S in V1 greater than upper limits for age
- Q wave in V5, V6, II, III, or aVF greater than upper limits for age
- R/S ratio in V1 less than lower limits for age

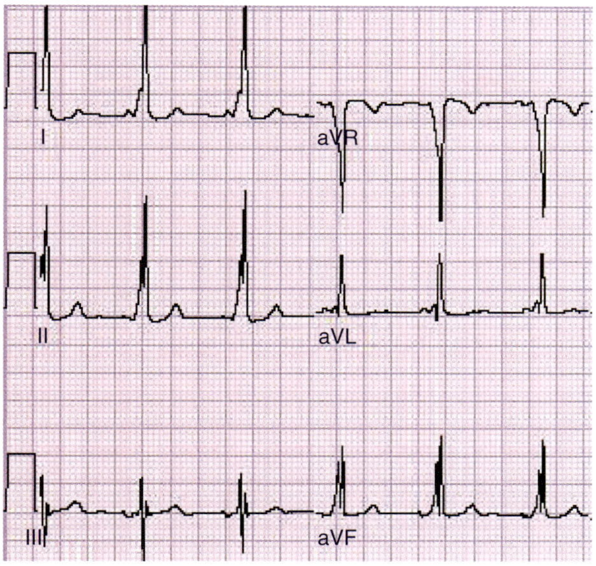

Figure 12.5 Wolff–Parkinson–White pattern with shortened PR interval and delta wave (slurring of the initial upstroke of the QRS complex).

The QRS duration in patients younger than 1 year is typically less than 0.08 s (two small boxes). A QRS duration of 0.08 s may appear narrow on a bedside monitor, so it is important to get a standard ECG to determine QRS duration. Prolonged QRS duration may be seen in patients with a bundle branch block or ventricular hypertrophy, and therefore should warrant further cardiac evaluation to determine any underlying defects or abnormalities.

Wolff–Parkinson–White

Wolff–Parkinson–White (WPW) syndrome is an accessory connection between the atrium and ventricle bypassing the AV node. This pattern is readily recognizable on the ECG as a shortened PR interval, slurring of the upstroke of the QRS (Figure 12.5). Patients with WPW are at increased risk for supraventricular tachycardia and this pattern has been associated with structural cardiac defects such as Ebstein anomaly in up to 20% of cases.

Abnormal Q Waves

The Q wave typically represents depolarization of the ventricular septum and may be present in almost any lead, but is commonly seen in leads II, III, and aVF. The normal duration of a Q wave is 0.01–0.015 s. In neonates, Q waves greater than 0.02 s (1/2 of a small box) are always abnormal. Wide Q waves may be seen in myocardial infarction, myocardial fibrosis, hypertrophic cardiomyopathy, WPW syndrome, and left ventricular non-compaction (a type of cardiomyopathy). The findings of deep and wide Q waves in leads I and aVL (infarction pattern) is a classic ECG finding in neonates with an anomalous left coronary artery and should prompt immediate referral to a pediatric cardiologist. In patients with anomalous left coronary artery, the left coronary originates from the pulmonary artery, causing an infarction of the myocardium supplied by the artery (resulting in the Q waves in leads I and aVL) (Figure 12.6).

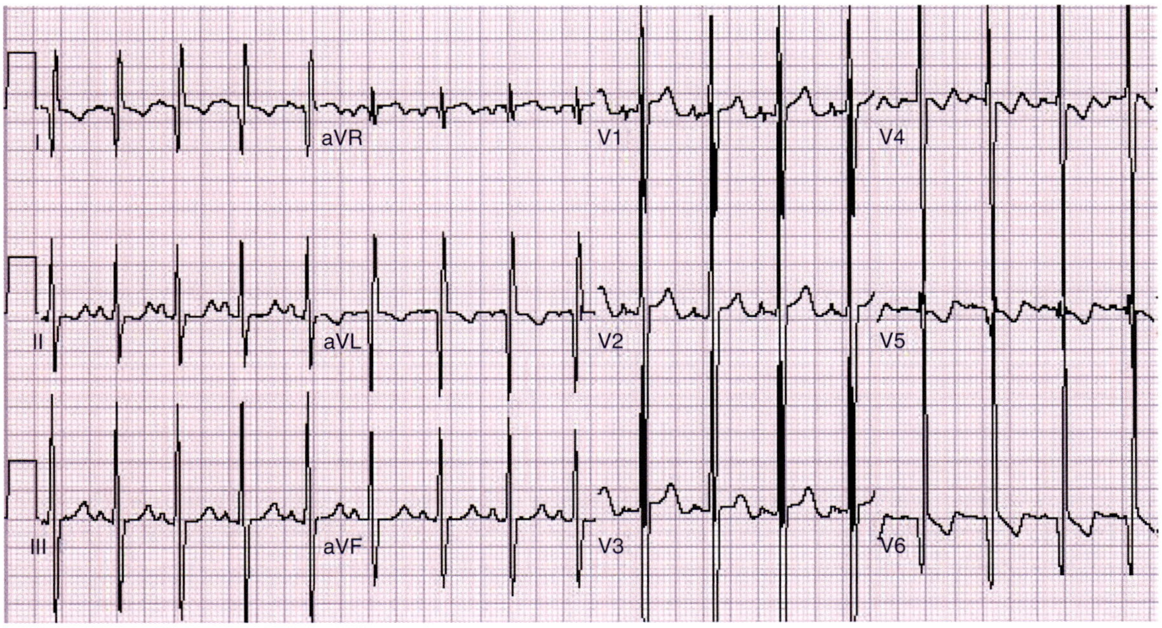

Figure 12.6 Anomalous left coronary artery with anterior infarction pattern (Q waves more than ½ box and ST segment changes in leads I and aVF. Note the abnormal Q waves and ST segment changes in lateral leads (V4–V6).

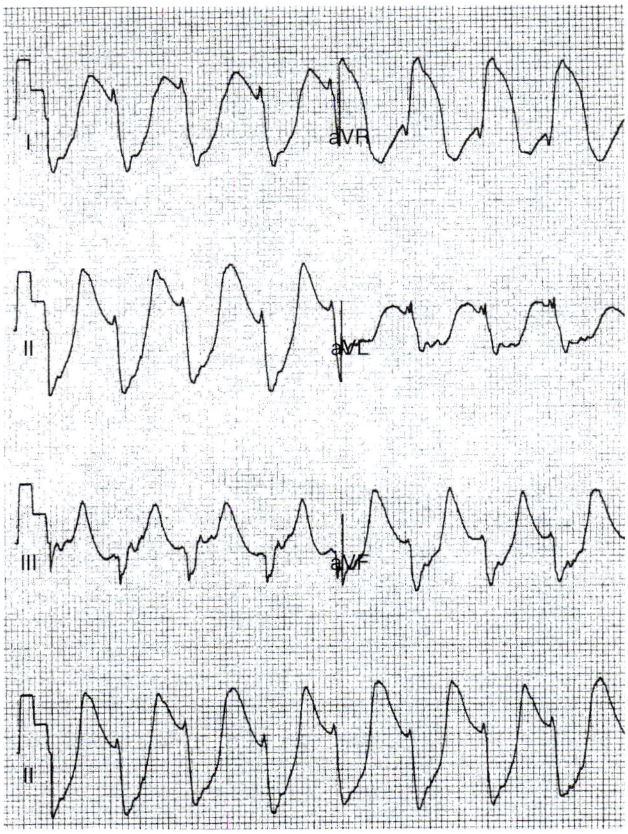

Figure 12.7 Loss of distinction between QRS complex and T wave (sine wave pattern) characteristic of hyperkalemia and severe acidosis or hypoxemia.

The infarction typically occurs around 2–4 months of age as the pulmonary pressures normally drop. Deep, but not wide, Q waves may indicate ventricular hypertrophy, but may also be normal variants.

T-wave Changes

Because ventricular repolarization is not as organized as ventricular depolarization, T-wave changes are non-specific. The T wave in lead V1 is upright at birth and then inverts during the first week of life. The T wave once again becomes upright around adolescence. An upright T wave between 1 week and 6 years of age is highly suggestive of right ventricular hypertrophy. Tall peaked T waves may be seen in hyperkalemia, left ventricular hypertrophy, and myocardial infarctions. In hyperkalemia, T waves begin to have a peaked appearance at a serum potassium around 6. As the potassium level increases, the QRS duration prolongs followed by prolongation of the PR interval then disappearance of the P wave. As the potassium level continues to rise, a wide-complex QRS with loss of distinction between the QRS and T wave results (often called a sine wave pattern; Figure 12.7). This is followed by ventricular fibrillation and cardiac arrest and should be treated by correcting the underlying abnormality rather than with antiarrhythmic medications. These ECG changes can also result with severe acidosis or hypoxemia. Even in neonates, T waves are almost always upright in leads V4–V6 and inversion of the T waves in these leads is highly suspicious for left ventricular pathology.

ST Segments

The ST segment is the segment between the QRS complex and the T wave. Abnormalities of the ST segment are defined based on the J point, the point at which the QRS complex terminates and the ST segment begins. An abnormal ST segment is indicated by elevation or depression of the J point greater than 1 mm in the limb leads (I–aVF) or greater than 2 mm in the precordial leads (V1–V6). ST segment changes may be seen in ventricular hypertrophy, myocarditis, ischemia or infarction, increased intracranial pressure, and electrolyte disturbances. Diffuse ST segment elevation is a classic finding in pericarditis, but may not be present in all cases and should not be used as the sole method for eliminating pericarditis from a differential diagnosis. Non-pathologic ST segment changes may be seen in a condition called early repolarization. In this condition, ST segments are elevated in leads with an upright T wave and depressed in leads with a negative T wave. In addition, the slope of the ST segment is in the same direction as the T wave.

Further Reading

Cannon B, Snyder C. (2012) Disorders of cardiac rhythm and conduction, in, *Moss and Adams' Heart Disease in Infants, Children, and Adolescents*, 8th edn (eds HD Allen, DJ Driscoll, RE Shaddy, TF Feltes). Lippincott Williams & Wilkins, Philadelphia, PA.

Park M, Guntheroth W. (2006) *How to Read Pediatric ECGs*, 4th edn. Mosby, St. Louis, MO.

Schwartz PJ, Garson A Jr, Paul T, *et al.* (2002) Guidelines for the interpretation of the neonatal electrocardiogram: a Task Force of the European Society of Cardiology. *Eur Heart J*, **23**, 1329–1344.

13

Echocardiogram

Michael D. Quartermain

Division of Cardiology, The Children's Hospital of Philadelphia and Perelman School of Medicine, University of Pennsylvania, Philadelphia, PA, USA

History

Ultrasound has been used to assess the cardiovascular system for over 50 years. Pediatric echocardiography and its application to congenital heart disease (CHD) has evolved rapidly since the 1970s. The development of high fidelity, pediatric-sized ultrasound probes has allowed for non-invasive assessment of the anatomy and physiology of complex CHD in even the smallest of neonates. From the bedside to the operating room, the field of echocardiography has revolutionized the way pediatric cardiology is practiced.

Physics

Knowledge of the physics behind ultrasound is necessary for understanding the functionality of the equipment as well as its applications and limitations. An echocardiography machine consists of three major parts: a transducer, central processing unit, and display screen with keyboard. The ultrasound waves are formed inside the transducer core by crystals with the ability to vibrate and produce sound waves of a particular frequency. Medical ultrasound waves represent a higher frequency than the human ear can hear and are referred to as "ultrasonic" [1]. As they travel through the body, the acoustic impedance of the tissue determines if the sound waves are reflected back to the transducer or emitted further into the imaging field. Resolution is the ability to separate two closely spaced structures, and an ultrasonic beam cannot resolve between two structures in space that are less than the wavelength of that beam. Given the formula $c = f \times w$, where c = speed of ultrasound in tissue (1540 m/s), f = frequency and w = wavelength, a higher frequency beam allows for better resolution of the small cardiac structures encountered in neonates.

Doppler echocardiography evaluates the direction and velocity of moving blood within the heart and blood vessels. The principle described by Christian Johann Doppler in 1843 states that the frequency of a sound wave will be altered if the source is in motion. An example is when the sound of a car horn increases in pitch as the car approaches a standing person and decreases as it drives away. The Doppler principle is utilized when the transducer emits "packets of energy" called pulse waves towards moving red blood cells. The cells reflect the beam with a shift in frequency based on their velocity, allowing for assessment of flow velocities throughout the heart and blood vessels. They can then be compared with published normal velocities in order to identify abnormal flow patterns [2]. In addition, velocity information for red blood cells crossing a stenotic valve can be used to calculate pressure gradients using the simplified Bernoulli equation $\Delta P = 4\ (V_2^2 - V_1^2)$, where V_1 is the velocity proximal to the valve and V_2 is distal to the valve. V_1 is normally much smaller than V_2 (<1 m/s), so it is usually ignored in the calculation resulting in an even simpler formula: $\Delta P = 4\,V^2$. For example, in a child with valvar aortic stenosis and a peak velocity across the valve of 3.5 m/s, the estimated peak aortic valve gradient is 48 mmHg using this equation. Echocardiographic Doppler gradients have become so reliable that the need for confirmation with invasive catheterization is uncommon even prior to complex heart surgery.

Performance of a Pediatric Echocardiogram

The average duration of a complete pediatric echocardiogram is 45–60 minutes for a standard patient and longer for patients with complex CHD [3]. Preparation and attention to patient safety are essential. Sedated

Visual Guide to Neonatal Cardiology, First Edition. Edited by Ernerio T. Alboliras, Ziyad M. Hijazi, Leo Lopez, and Donald J. Hagler.

studies are useful if patient agitation precludes obtaining complete images in patients for whom the clinical information is necessary at the time of the study [4]. However, most centers do not use conscious sedation in infants less than 50 weeks' gestation. Fetal imaging has also become commonplace and allows for diagnosis of complex CHD as early as 16–18 weeks' gestation [5]. Credentialing of pediatric echocardiography laboratories is necessary to ensure high quality and safe patient experiences. The accreditation process, established in 1998, has established standards and guidelines in terms of imaging and reporting as well as equipment and personnel. Within this context, the team is composed of a physician medical director, a technical director, sonographers certified in pediatric and/or congenital echocardiography, and attending physicians with specialized pediatric cardiology fellowship training. All members of the team must maintain continued medical education.

A comprehensive pediatric echocardiogram typically involves imaging of the heart from several orientations using multiple modalities (two-dimensional, spectral Doppler, and color flow echocardiography). Four primary views are recommended by the American Society of Echocardiography for pediatric imaging [6]: subcostal, apical, parasternal, and suprasternal notch (Figure 13.1). Echocardiography laboratories vary as to the order of the different views, but the subcostal view, when available, can document the abdominal situs and cardiac position.

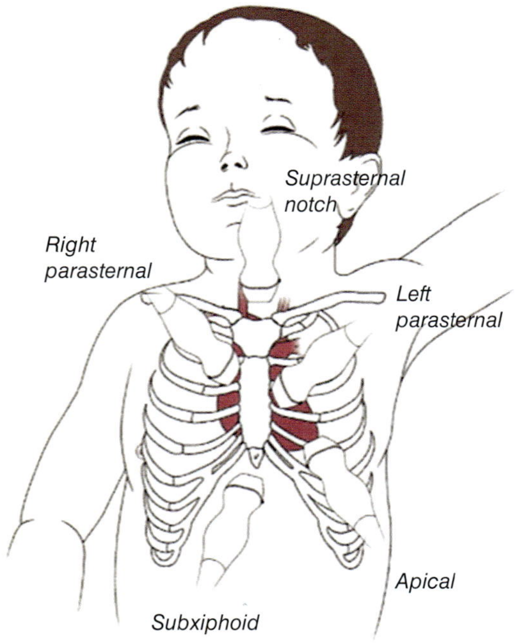

Figure 13.1 There are four main pediatric windows for optimal imaging: subcostal, apical, parasternal, and suprasternal views.

Table 13.1 Imaging views in pediatric patients with the cardiac features expected to be visualized.

View	Structure
Subcostal	Abdominal situs and cardiac position
	Atrial and ventricular septum
	Outflow tracts including aortic and pulmonary valves
Apical	Right and left ventricular size and function
	Mitral and tricuspid valves
	Right and left atrium
	Atrial and ventricular septum
Parasternal	Ventricular septum
	Mitral and tricuspid valves
	Aortic valve, aortic root, and ascending aorta
	Pulmonary valves, main and branch pulmonary arteries
	Coronary arteries
	Patent ductus arteriosus (high parasternal or "ductal" view)
Suprasternal notch	Pulmonary veins
	Superior vena cava
	Left innominate vein
	Ascending aorta
	Aortic arch (including arch sidedness)

Three imaging planes are utilized in most views: axial, sagittal, and coronal. Utilizing all views allows for assessment of valves, cardiac chambers, septum, arteries, veins, and outflow tracts in an orderly manner. Color flow Doppler is performed after two-dimensional imaging and provides information regarding blood flow in the heart, with red representing flow towards the transducer and blue representing flow away from the transducer. The color intensity is based on the magnitude of the blood flow velocity. Table 13.1 highlights the key structures for each imaging view in the pediatric patient.

Subcostal (Subxiphoid) View

Subcostal imaging is one of the most important views in pediatrics, particularly in neonates. This sweep begins with an axial cut through the abdomen to assess abdominal situs by identifying the positions of the stomach, liver, inferior vena cava, descending aorta, and heart. Patients with malposition of the heart (such as dextrocardia) or abnormalities of visceral situs (such as heterotaxy syndrome) are identified in this view (Figure 13.2). The

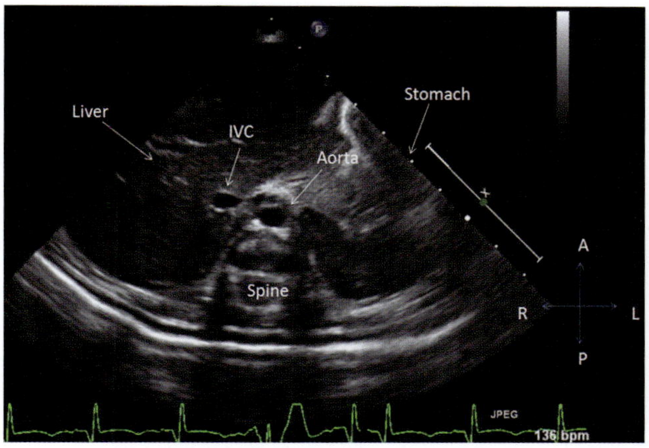

Figure 13.2 Subcostal transverse abdominal views in a patient showing the normal position of the liver on the right and the stomach on the left. The inferior vena cava (IVC) sits rightward and anterior to the aorta which is located just leftward of the spine.

transducer is then adjusted to sweep the heart from a postero-inferior to an antero-superior plane and from right to left. Early in the subcostal frontal (coronal) sweep, the pulmonary venous return into the left atrium is seen postero-inferiorly. The atrial septum is then well seen, followed by visualization of the ventricular septum. A more anterior sweep reveals the left and right ventricular outflow tracts, respectively. Sagittal sweeps and oblique imaging provide additional information. Figure 13.3 shows the normal structures identified in a subcostal frontal sweep. Doppler interrogation of the descending aorta at the level of the diaphragm will identify abnormal flow patterns, such as those seen with aortic coarctation and a patent ductus arteriosus.

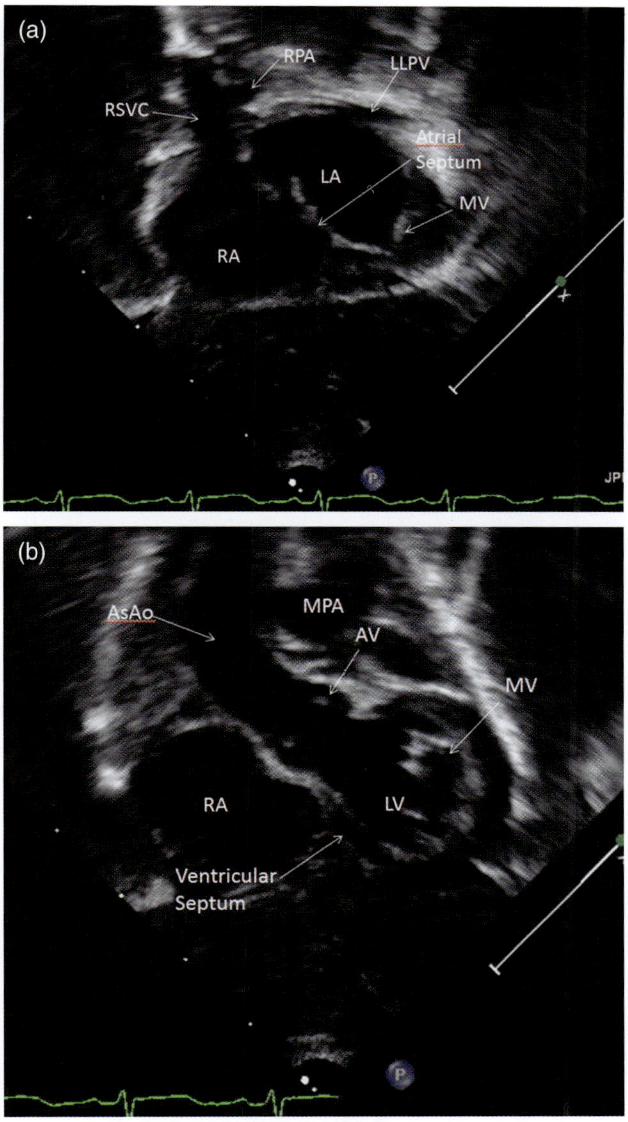

Figure 13.3 (a) Subcostal frontal views starting posteriorly allowing visualization of the atrial septum. In this case there is a small patent foramen ovale. Both the left atrium (LA) and right atrium (RA) are well seen as is the left lower pulmonary vein (LLPV) and right superior vena cava (RSVC). The right pulmonary artery (RPA) is identified posterior to the RSVC. (b) Subcostal frontal image sweeping anterior demonstrating the left ventricle (LV), mitral valve (MV), and outflow tract. The aortic valve (AV) and ascending aorta (AsAo) are well visualized. Just leftward of the aorta is the main pulmonary artery (MPA). The ventricular septum is also well seen in this image.

Apical View

Apical imaging allows for simultaneous visualization of all four chambers (Figure 13.4), with a sweep from posterior structures to more anterior ones (the atrioventricular valves, the septum, and the left and right ventricular outflow tracts). Two-dimensional and Doppler assessment of the mitral and tricuspid valves identifies valve pathology and provides information about diastolic function. Atrial and ventricular size and ventricular systolic function can also be evaluated. The ventricular septum is interrogated to exclude defects. Color flow mapping and Doppler interrogation are performed to identify valvar regurgitation or stenosis.

Parasternal View

Parasternal long-axis views allow for measurements of aortic annular and root diameters (Figure 13.5). Short-axis views identify abnormalities of the right ventricular outflow tract and pulmonary arteries (Figure 13.6). M-mode assessment of the left ventricle in a short-axis view allows for quantification of left ventricular dimensions and function. Although new measurements and techniques have become available, M-mode is still the basis of most clinical decisions in children with abnormal ventricular size and function.

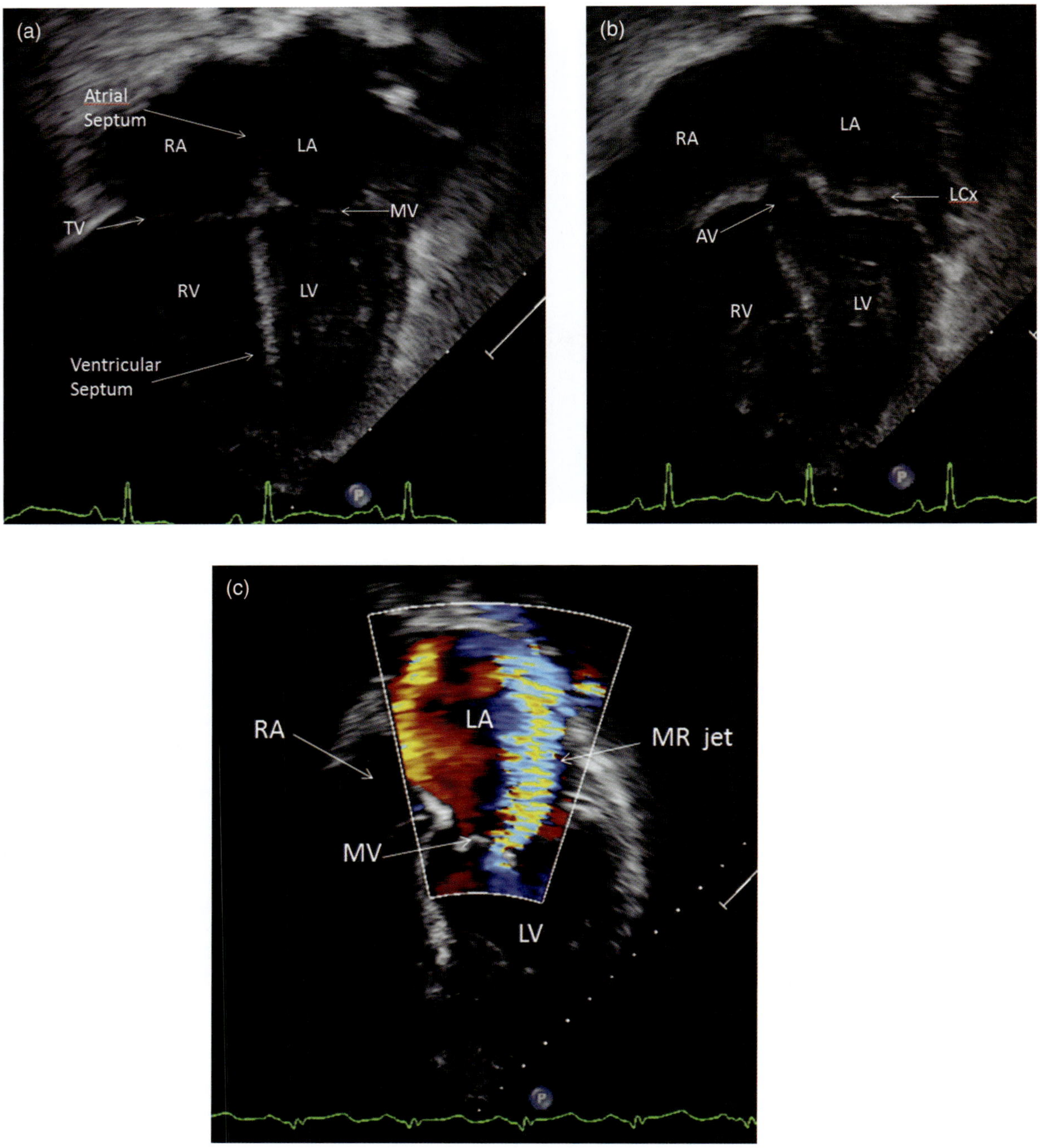

Figure 13.4 (a) Apical view demonstrating all four chambers: the left atrium (LA), right atrium (RA), left ventricle (LV), and right ventricle (RV). Both the mitral valve (MV) and tricuspid valve (TV) are well seen. (b) Tilting the probe anterior from the four-chamber view allows for visualization of left ventricular outflow tract and aortic valve (AV). The left circumflex coronary artery (LCx) is seen running adjacent to the mitral valve. (c) Apical four-chamber view with color flow placed over the mitral valve demonstrating a significant jet of mitral regurgitation (MR) directed back into the left atrium. The bright blue and yellow colors produced by the MR jet are related to the direction of flow and high velocity of the blood as it regurgitates back into left atrium (LA).

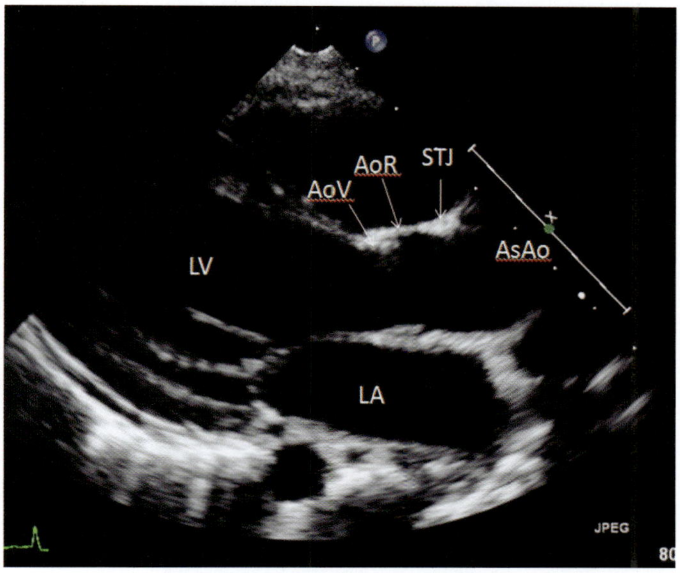

Figure 13.5 Parasternal long axis imaging of the left ventricular outflow tract allowing for visualization of the aortic valve (AV), aortic root (AoR), sinotubular junction (STJ), and ascending aorta (AsAo). Assessments of the mitral valve and left ventricle (LV) can also be made from this view.

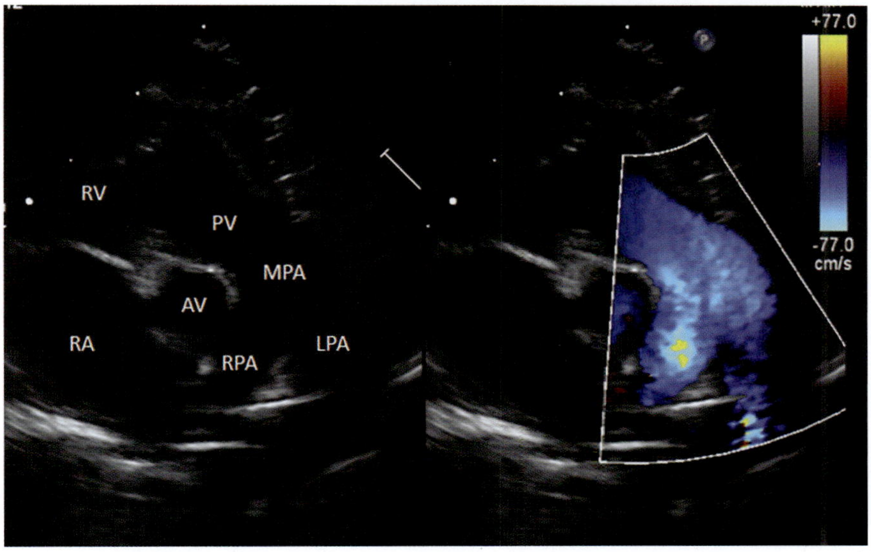

Figure 13.6 A color compare image taken in a parasternal short-axis view demonstrating the right ventricular outflow tract, main pulmonary artery (MPA), and both left (LPA) and right pulmonary arteries (RPA). Two-dimensional view on the left and color flow of the same image on the right. The right atrium (RA), right ventricle (RV), and aortic valve (AV) are also identified in this view.

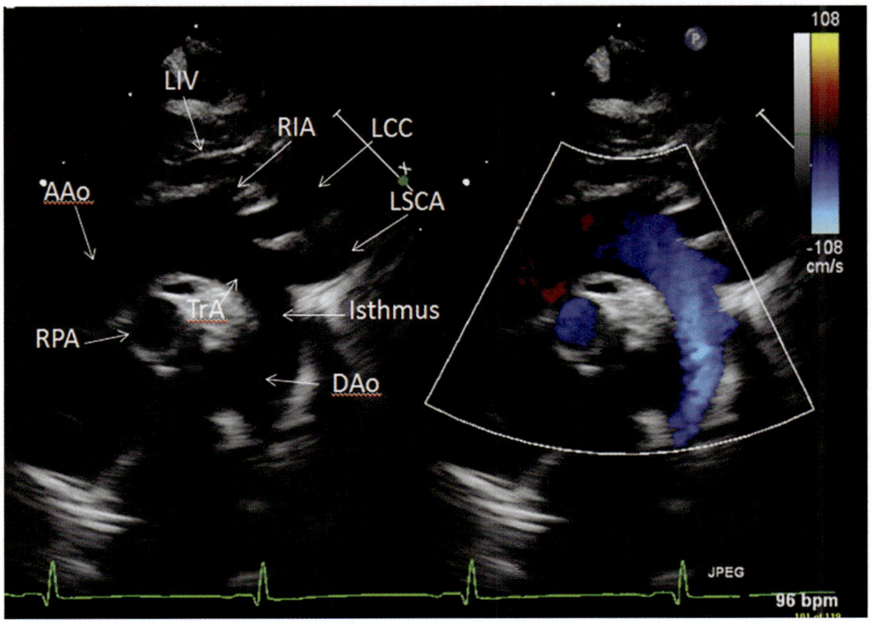

Figure 13.7 From suprasternal notch the "candy cane" view of the aortic arch demonstrates the ascending (AAo), transverse (TrA) and descending aorta (DAo) along with the head and next branches including the left innominate artery, left common carotid (LCC), and the left subclavian artery (LSCA). The aortic isthmus and descending aorta (DAo) are visualized. The left pulmonary artery is seen coursing underneath the aorta and the left innominate vein (LIV) runs superior and anterior to the aortic arch.

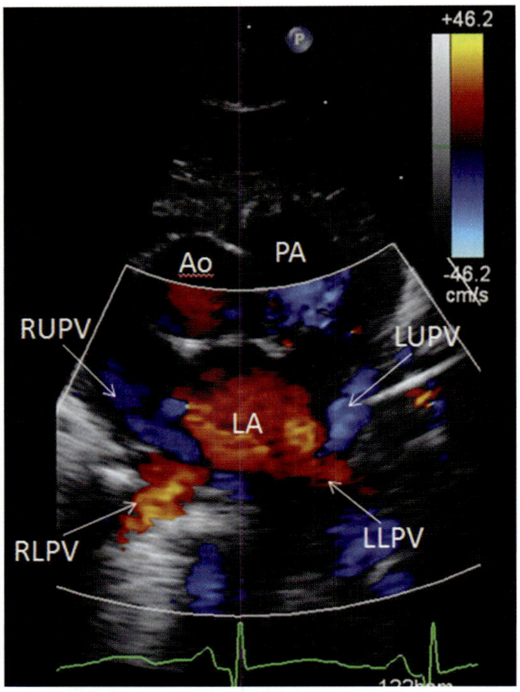

Figure 13.8 Parasternal imaging of the left atrium (LA) in the "crab view" provides identification of all four pulmonary veins. The left upper (LUPV), left lower (LLPV), right upper (RUPV) and right lower (RLPV) pulmonary vein are all identified by color flow assessment. The aorta (Ao) and pulmonary artery (PA) are visualized superior to the LA.

Other structures seen in this view include the coronary arteries, aortic valve, and patent ductus arteriosus if present.

Suprasternal View

The suprasternal notch view allows for assessment of the aortic arch with the "candy cane" view (Figure 13.7). Color mapping and Doppler interrogation delineates flow abnormalities in the aortic arch and descending aorta and identifies clinically important obstruction (aortic coarctation), aortic arch sidedness and the branching pattern are particularly important when symptoms suggest a vascular ring. A high parasternal transverse "crab" view identifies all the pulmonary veins draining into the left atrium (Figure 13.8). Superior systemic venous return can also be assessed with visualization of the superior vena cava and innominate vein.

Quantification in pediatric echocardiography is important, and guidelines have been published [7], including assessment of atrial and ventricular size as well as ventricular systolic and diastolic function. Pediatric guidelines regarding more advanced modalities such as three-dimensional echocardiography and strain analysis have not yet been published.

References

1 Suetens P. (2002) Ultrasonic imaging, in, *Fundamentals of Medical Imaging*. Cambridge University Press, Cambridge, pp. 145–183.
2 Grenadier E, Lima CO, Allen HD, *et al.* (1984) Normal intracardiac and great vessel flow velocities in infants and children. *J Am Coll Cardiol*, **4**, 343–350.
3 Kisslo J, Byrd BF, Geiser EA, *et al.* (1995) Recommendations for continuous quality improvement in echocardiography. *J Am Soc Echocardiogr*, **8**, S1–S28.
4 American Academy of Pediatrics: Committee on Drugs (1992) Guidelines for monitoring and management of pediatric patients during and after sedation for diagnosis and therapeutic procedures. *Pediatrics*, **89**, 1110–1115.
5 Rychik J, Ayres N, Cuneo B, *et al.* (2004) American Society of Echocardiography guidelines and standards for performance of the fetal echocardiogram. *J Am Soc Echocardiogr*, **17**, 803–810.
6 Lai WW, Geva T, Shirali GS, *et al.* (2006) Guidelines and standards for performance of a pediatric echocardiogram: a report from the Task Force of the Pediatric Council of the American Society of Echocardiography. *J Am Soc Echocardiogr*, **19**, 1413–1430.
7 Lopez L, Colan SD, Frommelt PC, *et al.* (2010) Recommendations for quantification methods during the performance of a pediatric echocardiogram: a report from the Pediatric Measurements Writing Group of the American Society of Echocardiography Pediatric and Congenital Heart Disease Council. *J Am Soc Echocardiogr*, **23**, 465–495.

14

Cardiac Catheterization and Angiocardiography

Howaida El-Said[1] *and Sergio Bartakian*[2]

[1] *Rady Children's Hospital, San Diego, CA, USA*
[2] *University of Texas at San Antonio, San Antonio, TX, USA*

Significant advances in non-invasive fetal imaging over the past decade have improved the ability to diagnose most congenital heart defects with a high level of accuracy. This has resulted in a lesser need for performing neonatal heart catheterizations for diagnostic purposes. Most pediatric catheterization laboratories are now equipped to perform interventional procedures on infants born with congenital heart disease. Despite this transformation, a solid understanding of the angiographic anatomy of the normal, as well as the abnormal, anatomy is vital. There are numerous textbooks for the purpose of discussing basic principles of angiography [1]. This chapter provides only a cursory view of cardiac catheterization and angiography in the neonate. A detailed review of all possible congenital heart defects is beyond the scope of this chapter.

Patent Ductus Arteriosus (Figures 14.1 and 14.2)

Among the most common of the congenital heart defects encountered in the neonatal setting, patent ductus arteriosus (PDA) can vary considerably from the benign silent ductus requiring no intervention, to a large shunting ductus causing rapid heart failure.

Pulmonary Valve Stenosis (Figure 14.3)

This lesion can range from very mild to critical (where a PDA is needed to maintain cardiac output), the latter of which requires urgent attention in the catheterization laboratory to perform a balloon valvuloplasty to relieve the obstruction and establish improved cardiac output.

Critical Aortic Valve Stenosis (Figure 14.4)

Somewhat similar to critical pulmonary valve stenosis already described, this lesion requires a significant amount of additional care to ensure the proper balance between relieving the obstruction and minimizing insufficiency is achieved. The goal is not to eliminate obstruction completely, but rather to reduce it to a tolerable amount. Ideally, no amount of aortic valve insufficiency results; however, a trivial to mild degree is often tolerated in exchange for relieving a severe obstruction sufficiently to postpone any surgery.

Coarctation of the Aorta (Figure 14.5)

Coarctation encountered in the neonatal period can include a simple discrete lesion (Figure 14.5a), complex (Figure 14.5b), a long segment coarctation or hypoplasia (Figure 14.5c), as well as a post-surgical re-coarctation (Figure 14.5d). The primary means of therapy for the former three is surgical repair, balloon angioplasty in the catheterization laboratory may be used for the latter.

Major Aorto-Pulmonary Collateral Arteries (Figure 14.6)

Major aorto-pulmonary collateral arteries (MAPCAs) form in utero as a result of pulmonary valve atresia and can vary from multiple to a single collateral providing the entirety of pulmonary blood flow. The native pulmonary arteries may be confluent and encouraged to grow further by addition of a surgical shunt or, as is often the case, may be extremely hypoplastic such that they cannot be relied upon as a source for future rehabilitation. In the latter case, the MAPCA vessels

Visual Guide to Neonatal Cardiology, First Edition. Edited by Ernerio T. Alboliras, Ziyad M. Hijazi, Leo Lopez, and Donald J. Hagler.

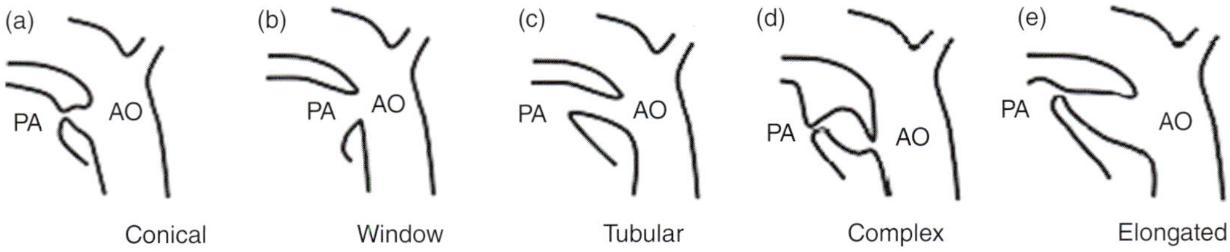

Figure 14.1 Various types of patent ductus arteriosus (PDA) using the classification of Krichenko *et al*. [2]. AO, aorta; PA, pulmonary artery.

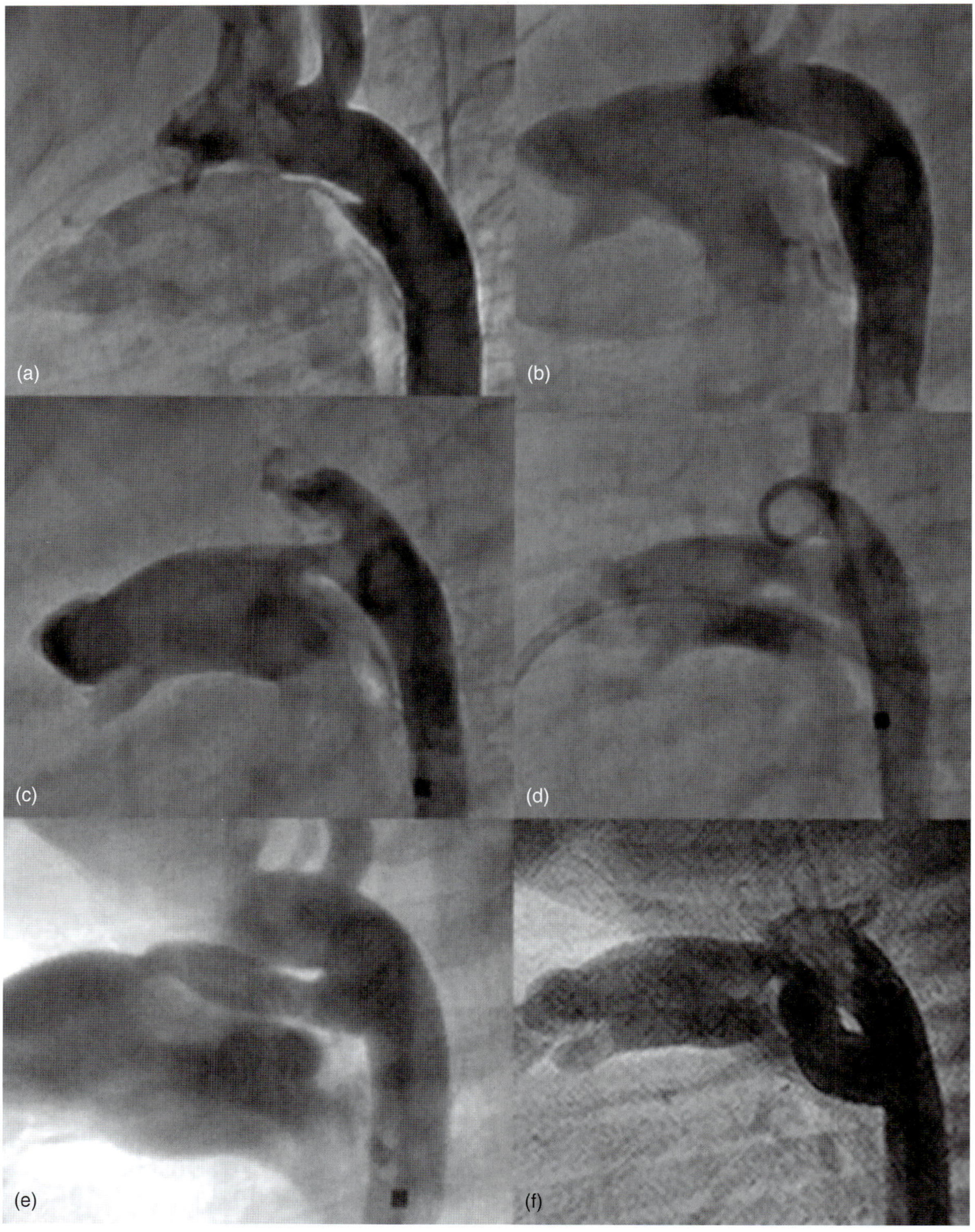

Figure 14.2 Various morphologies of PDA. (a) Silent ductus; (b–c) small to large type A ductus; (e) complex type D ductus; (f) serpiginous ductus often seen in tricuspid or pulmonary atresia.

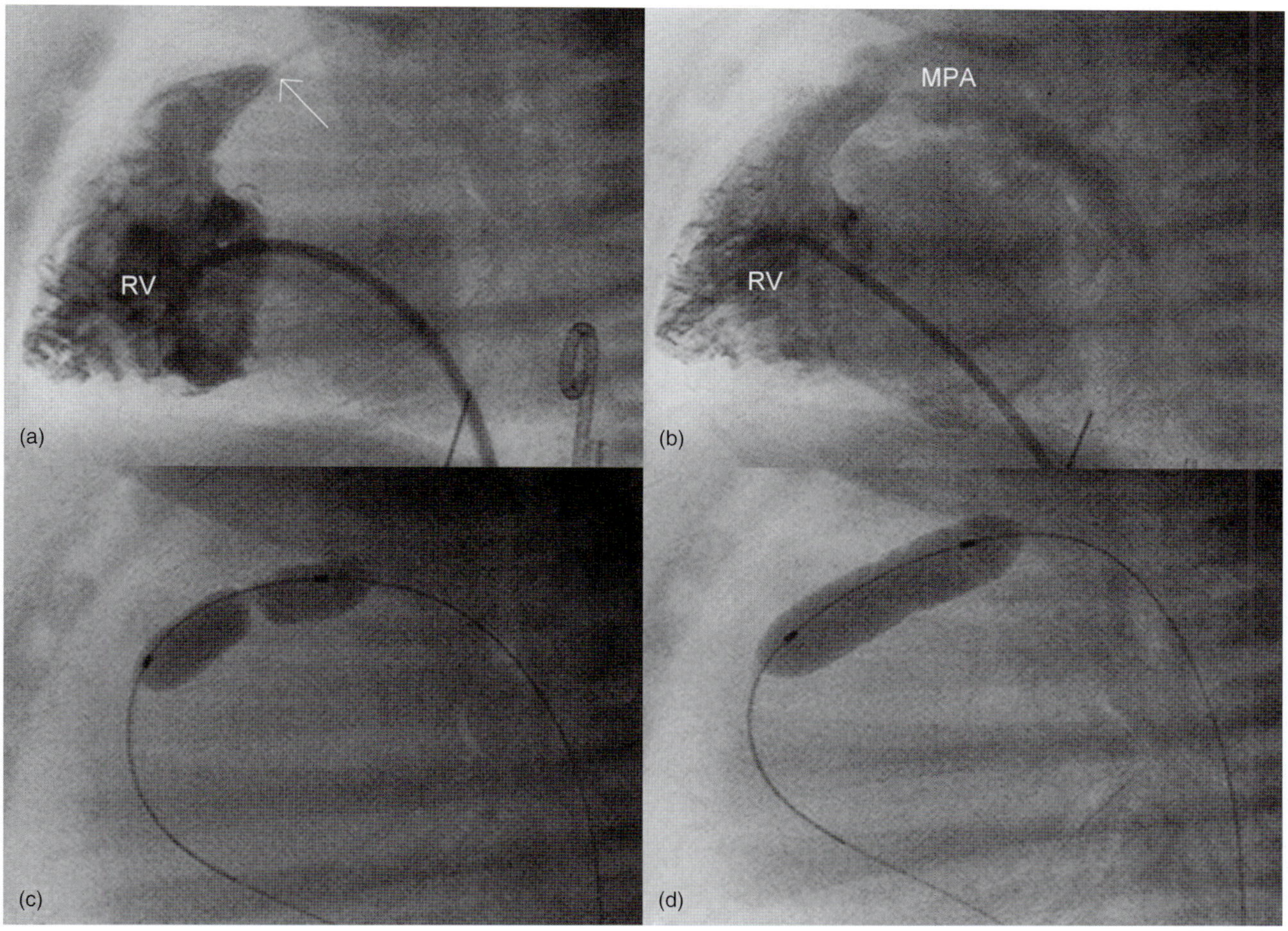

Figure 14.3 Patient with critical pulmonary valve stenosis. (a) Pulmonary valve jet (arrow) from right ventricle into main pulmonary artery before valvuloplasty; (b) improved flow across valve post valvuloplasty; (c) waist on balloon depicts the location of the valvar stenosis; (d) resolution of waist indicating successful valvuloplasty. MPA, main pulmonary artery; RV, right ventricle.

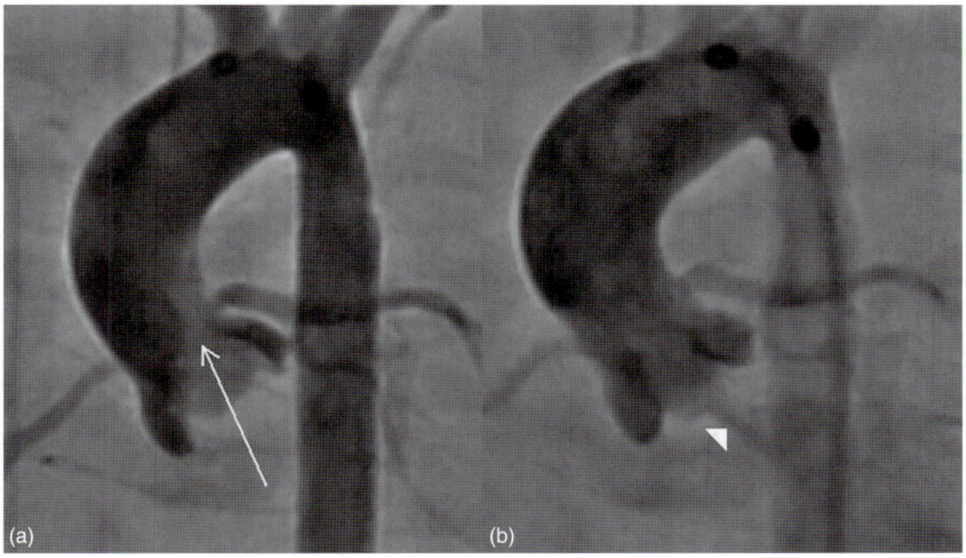

Figure 14.4 (a) Severe valvar aortic stenosis. The arrow depicts negative contrast (area of non-contrast opacified blood entering the contrast opacified aortic root) indicating the effective orifice of the valve. (b) Image performed post valvuloplasty reveals mild aortic valve insufficiency (arrowhead).

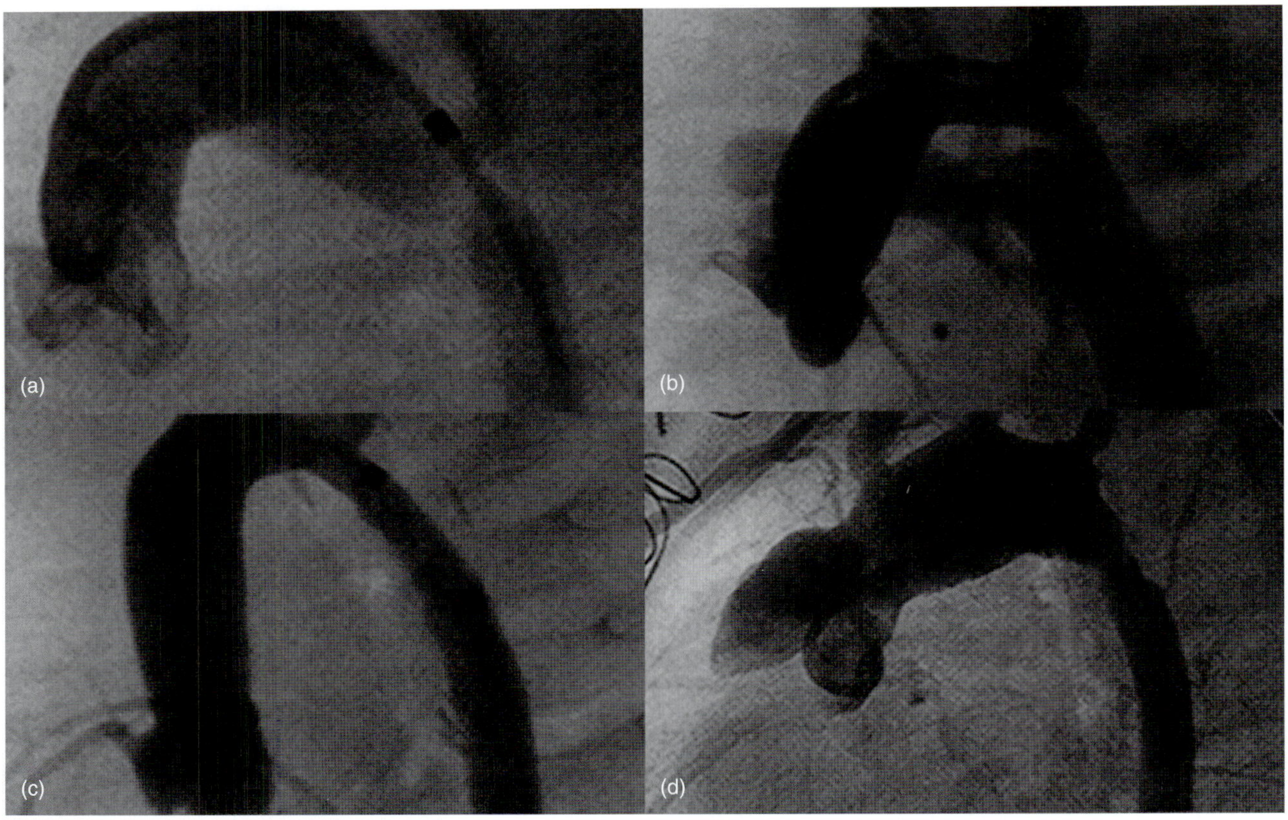

Figure 14.5 Various forms of coarctation of the aorta in the neonatal period.

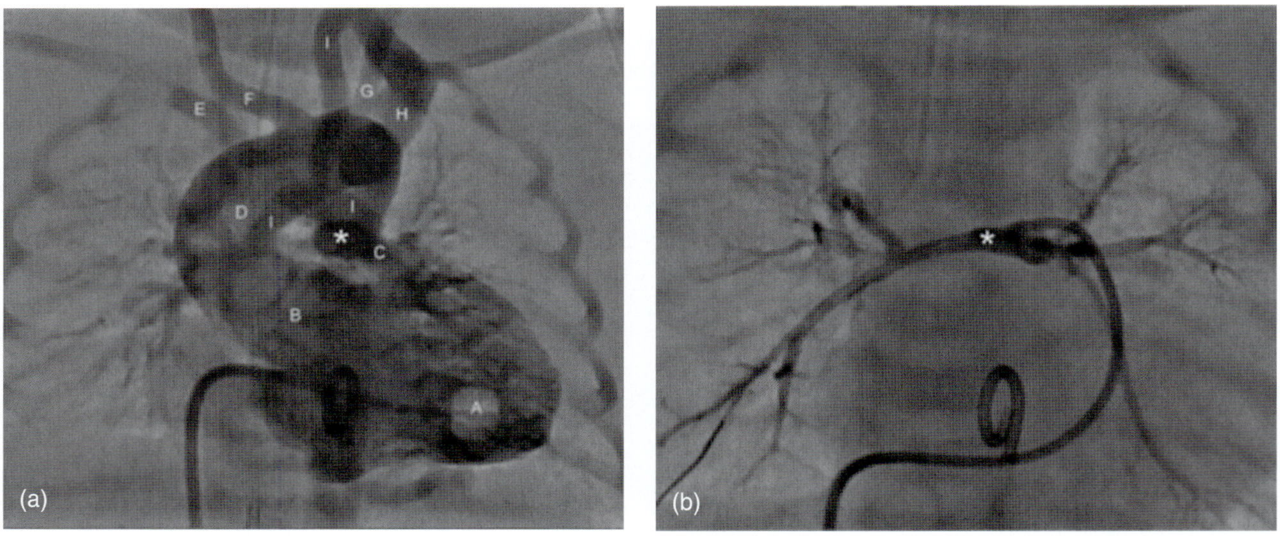

Figure 14.6 (a) A: Balloon angiographic catheter positioned in the right ventricle. B: level of aortic valve. C: right ventricular outflow tract. The asterisk marks the same spot in both panels (just past level of pulmonary valve annulus) and is where the tip of the catheter is in (b). D: ascending aorta. E: 4th aortic branch – anomalous right subclavian artery originating from descending aorta. F: 1st aortic branch – right common carotid artery. G: 2nd aortic branch – left common carotid artery. H: 3rd aortic branch – origin of left subclavian artery, which branches medially into: I: the single large MAPCA which descends caudally and branches to supply both right and left pulmonary circulations. (b) Having crossed the level of the atretic pulmonary valve, the severely hypoplastic native pulmonary arteries are shown to be confluent but measuring less than 2 mm in diameter.

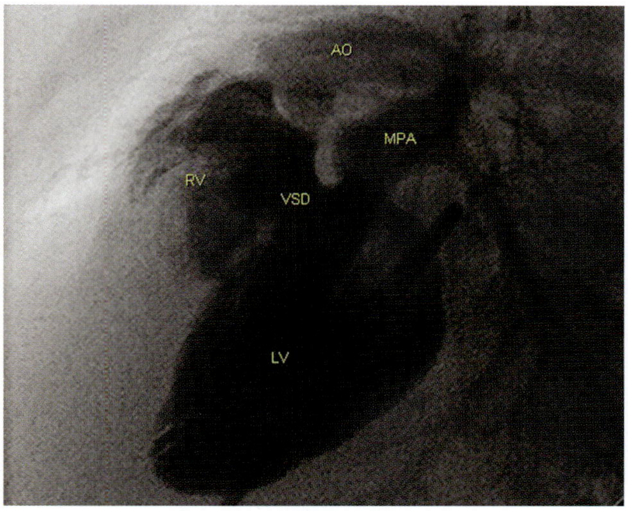

Figure 14.7 Lateral projection angiogram with 60° left anterior oblique (LAO) and 30° cranial angulation. Shows a smooth walled, posterior left ventricle (LV) communicating with the pulmonary arteries (MPA). The right ventricle (RV), which is not completely filled with contrast, communicates with the transposed and anterior aorta (AO). There is a ventricular septal defect (VSD) seen as well, which is sometimes present in this lesion.

can be unifocalized (if multiple) and anastomosed to the right ventricle by means of a right ventricle–pulmonary artery (RV–PA) conduit.

Transposition of the Great Arteries (Figure 14.7)

In the normal heart, the aortic valve lies posterior and rightward of the pulmonary valve. In the most common form of transposition of the great arteries (D-TGA), the aortic valve remains rightward but is now anterior to the pulmonary valve. This causes communication of the aorta with the anterior right ventricle. The resulting deoxygenated blood from the right ventricle is pumped through the aorta and circulated to the body, bypassing the lungs, while the left ventricle pumps oxygenated blood back into the lungs through the pulmonary artery. In effect, two separate parallel circulatory systems are created.

Hypoplastic Left Ventricle (Figure 14.8)

There is a wide spectrum of congenital heart disease that involves varying degrees of left-sided obstructive lesions,

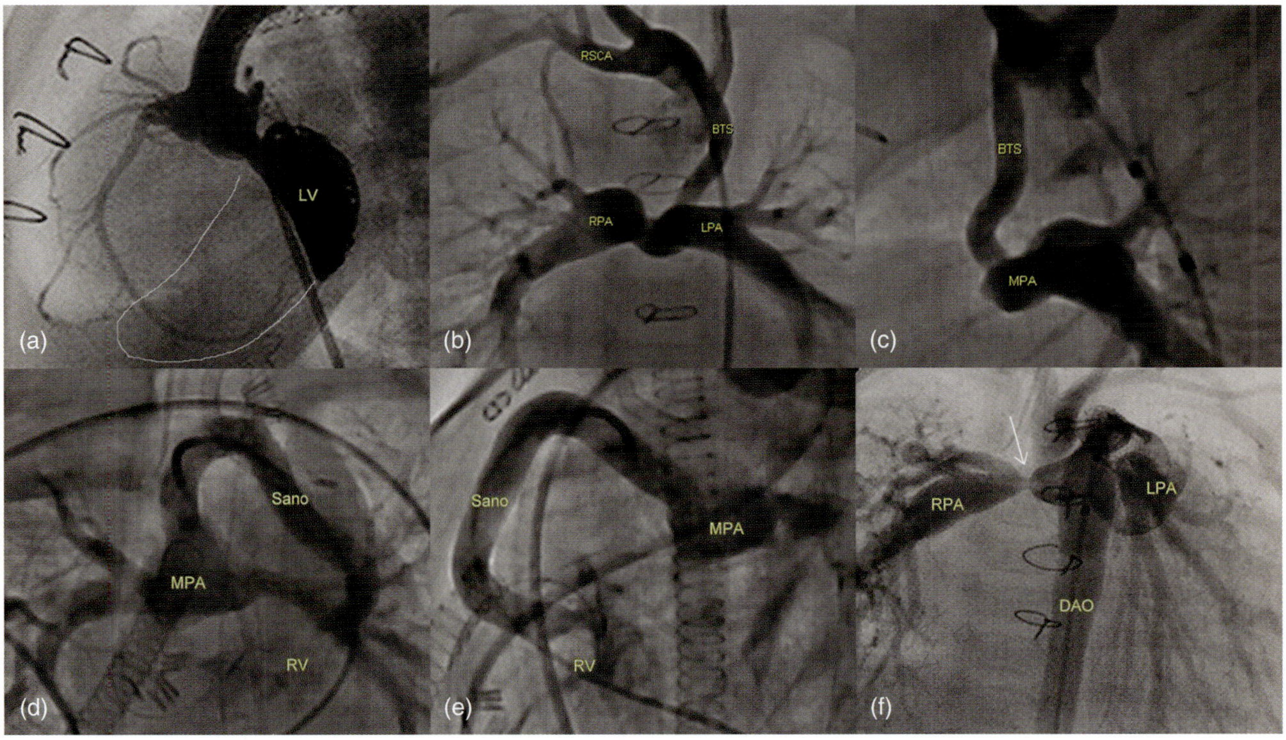

Figure 14.8 (a) A severely hypoplastic left ventricle following Norwood procedure. The area traced by the white line represents that which a normal-sized left ventricle might occupy in a normal heart. (b,c) A Blalock–Taussig shunt (BTS) originating from the region of the right common carotid artery and right subclavian artery (RSCA) and inserting into the region of the main pulmonary artery (MPA). LPA, left pulmonary artery; RPA, right pulmonary artery. (d,e) A comparable Sano shunt originating from the right ventricle (RV) and inserting into the MPA. (f) An alternative hybrid procedure with placement of bands on the pulmonary arteries to restrict pulmonary blood flow (arrow).

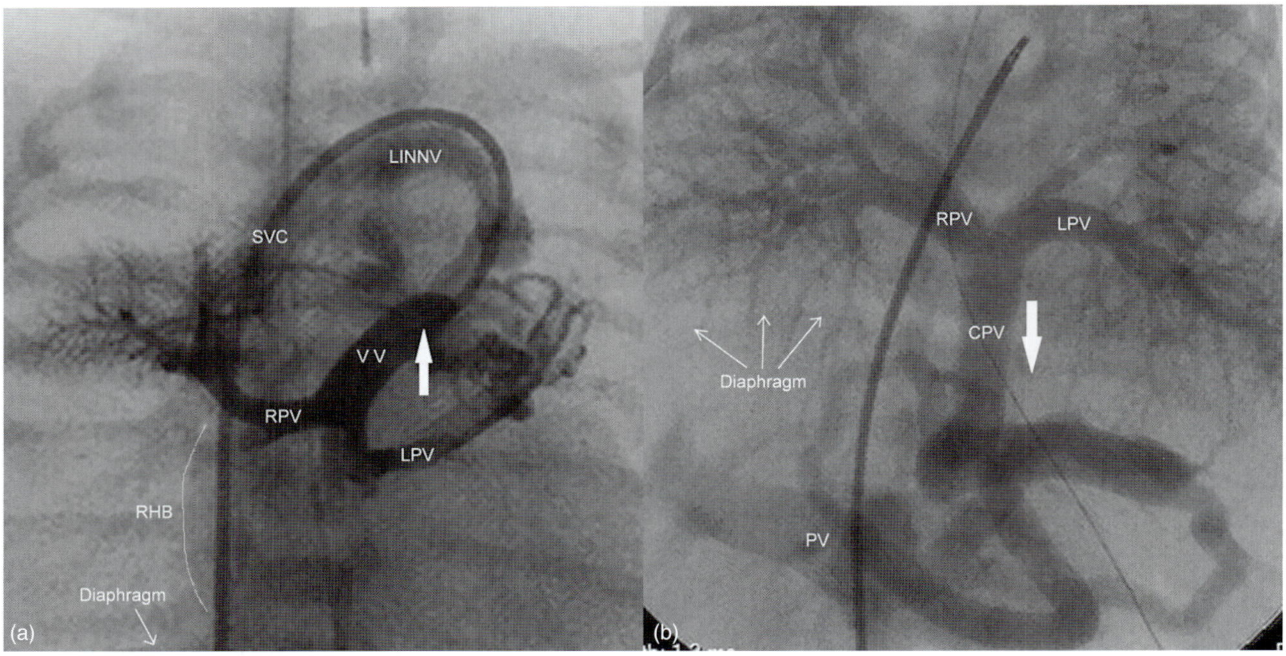

Figure 14.9 (a) A supracardiac total anomalous pulmonary venous connection (TAPVC). In this example, drainage of the pulmonary veins is to the vertical vein (VV), left innominate vein (LINNV), superior vena cava (SVC), and finally to the right atrium. (b) An infra-diaphragmatic TAPVC where drainage is via the common pulmonary vein (CPV), below the diaphragm, to the portal venous (PV) system, and finally to the right atrium via the inferior vena cava. Note the level of the diaphragm shown in the two examples. Solid arrows represent direction of flow through the connecting vein. LPV, left pulmonary vein; RHB, right heart border; RPV, right pulmonary vein.

which lead to the inability to sustain systemic cardiac output. Either the Blalock–Taussig shunt or the Sano shunt (combined with the Norwood procedure) are currently the two options for the first stage of a three-step palliative and reparative process. The hybrid procedure is an alternative which involves the surgeon placing bands on the pulmonary arteries followed by a stent being placed in the ductus arteriosus by the interventional cardiologist, to supply systemic output. An alternative to these is primary orthotopic cardiac transplantation, an option that is limited by the number of available organs.

Total Anomalous Pulmonary Venous Connection (Figure 14.9)

This is a result of an embryologic failure of the common pulmonary vein to connect with the pulmonary venous plexus. The consequence is a failure of the normal pulmonary venous return to the left atrium. The Darling classification is the most widely accepted nomenclature in referring to total anomalous pulmonary venous connection (TAPVC) [3]. In type I, the anomalous connection is typically either to a remnant of the left superior vena cava or to the right superior vena cava. In type II, the anomalous connection is to the heart, either to the right atrium directly or to the coronary sinus. In type III, the anomalous connection is at the infra-cardiac level (below the diaphragm), with the pulmonary venous return entering the right atrium ultimately via the inferior vena cava. Type IV TAPVC simply is some combination of the above [4].

Rotational Angiography (Figure 14.10)

With modern angiographic systems, many catheterization laboratories are now capable of performing three-dimensional rotational angiography, which can provide additional vital data. When combined with standard angiographic techniques, a more comprehensive evaluation of the anatomy is possible.

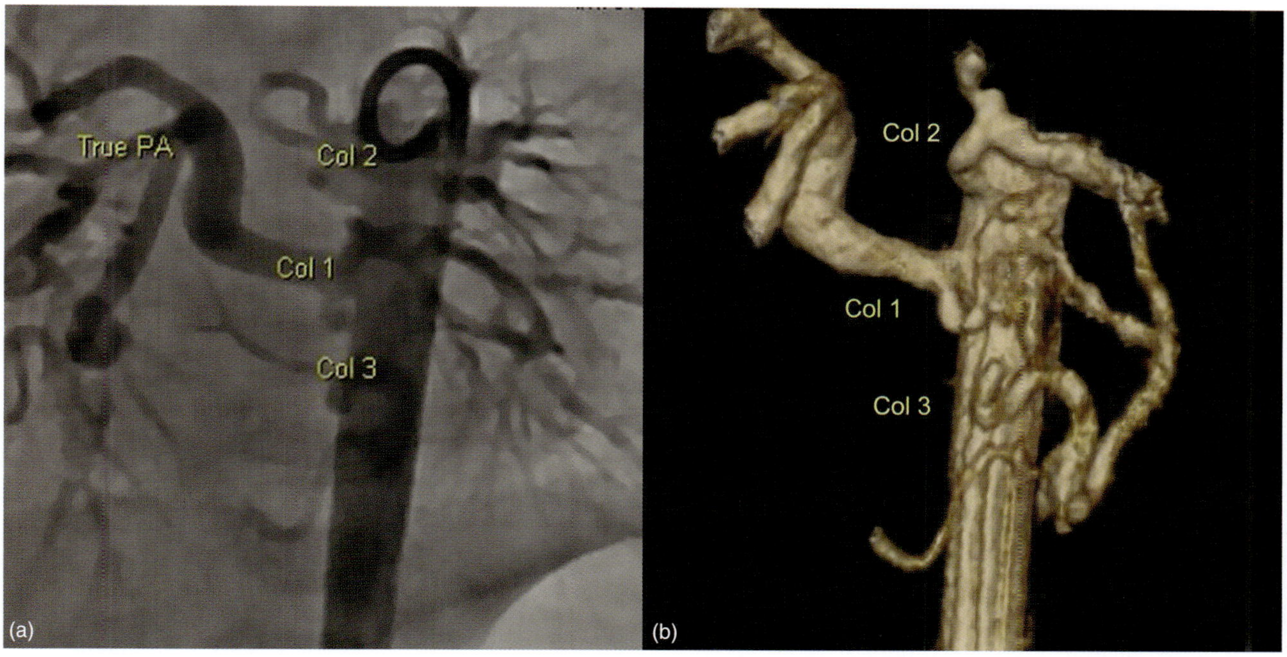

Figure 14.10 Three-dimensional rotational reconstruction allows the operator (and surgeon) to appreciate the interrelationship of the three collateral arteries (in this case, MAPCAs) which was not seen with the initial standard angiogram. Col, collateral; PA, pulmonary artery.

References

1 Freedom RM, Mawson JB, Yoo S, Benson LN. (2003) *Congenital Heart Disease: Textbook of Angiography*, Wiley-Blackwell, Oxford.

2 Krichenko A, Benson LN, Burrows P, *et al.* (1989) Angiographic classification of the isolated, persistently patent ductus arteriosus and implications for percutaneous catheter occlusion. *Am J Cardiol*, **63**, 877–879.

3 Darling RC, Rothney WB, Craig JM. (1957) Total pulmonary venous drainage into the right side of the heart. *Lab Invest*, **6**, 44–64.

4 Herlong JR, Jaggers JJ, Ungerleider RM. (2000) Congenital Heart Surgery Nomenclature and Database Project: pulmonary venous anomalies. *Ann Thorac Surg*, **69**, S56–S69.

15

Computed Tomography

Randy Richardson

St. Joseph's Hospital, Creighton University School of Medicine, Phoenix, AZ, USA

Multidetector cardiac computed tomography (CT) scanning with rapid rotational speeds and high spatial and temporal resolution has dramatically changed the possibilities for imaging the heart in the neonate. As with any imaging modality that requires ionizing radiation, careful adherence to proper technique is required with special attention paid to utilizing the latest technology to reduce the radiation dose to the infant while still obtaining the necessary information. In this chapter we review basic protocols for obtaining a high quality cardiac CT in a neonate while emphasizing radiation lowering techniques, discuss the advantages of cardiac CT over other cross-sectional modalities, and show the post-processing techniques available with cardiac CT.

Scanning Technique for Cardiac CTA in Neonates

To utilize the advantages of cardiac computed tomography angiography (CTA) safely, it is important to consider radiation exposure and optimize scanning techniques. Fast scanning times and high-quality evaluation of both complex cardiac and coronary anatomy have enabled CTA to aid in patient management and treatment planning. Currently, there are two accepted cardiac CTA scanning techniques for infants with congenital heart disease: retrospective and prospective ECG-gated scanning.

General anesthesia is routinely administered in neonates to optimize the scans and minimize motion artifacts. Iodinated contrast medium is used at 1 mL/lb body weight, with an injection rate of 0.5–0.7 mL/s. Although there are several intravenous sites for injection, the left upper extremity may be preferable in patients with congenital heart disease to visualize a possible left superior vena cava (SVC). For neonates, a weight-based protocol is used, with 80-kVp tube voltage and tube current adjusted according to body weight for prospective scanning. The gantry speed is set as fast as possible, often using half or quarter turn technology to keep up with the rapid heart rate of an infant. Slice thickness is typically 0.6 mm and detector coverage about 40 mm. Timing of the bolus is key to optimize scans and many autodetection programs exist. The patient is scanned in a craniocaudal direction starting at the level of the subclavian artery and ending at the level of the diaphragm. The anesthesiologist assists with a breath hold during the scan to minimize motion artifact. Beta-blockers are not usually used to decrease the heart rate in children with congenital heart disease.

During retrospective scanning, the X-ray beam is turned on during the entire cardiac cycle and spiral scanning continues during table motion (Figure 15.1). Retrospective gating uses a low pitch (0.2) to obtain attenuation measurements at all spatial locations in the heart and to scan during all phases of the cardiac cycle, including the entire R-R interval. CT scans using a retrospective technique will have a significantly higher radiation exposure.

The vast majority of scanning should be carried out using the prospective ECG-triggered scanning technique to minimize radiation dose. This technique uses a non-spiral step-and-shoot axial scanning process in which the X-ray beam is on for a short time and is turned off as the table moves. The imaging window can be at any point along the cardiac cycle. Because the infant's heart rate is high, short acquisition times with padding may be used to capture up to 50% of the cardiac cycle to evaluate function (Figure 15.2). When functional analysis is needed, 175 ms of padding is typically used. For adults, end systole is the optimal time for imaging the coronary arteries in between 65% and 80% of the cardiac cycle. In infants, the optimal time for imaging the coronary arteries is typically during systole, at 45–55% of the cardiac cycle.

Visual Guide to Neonatal Cardiology, First Edition. Edited by Ernerio T. Alboliras, Ziyad M. Hijazi, Leo Lopez, and Donald J. Hagler.

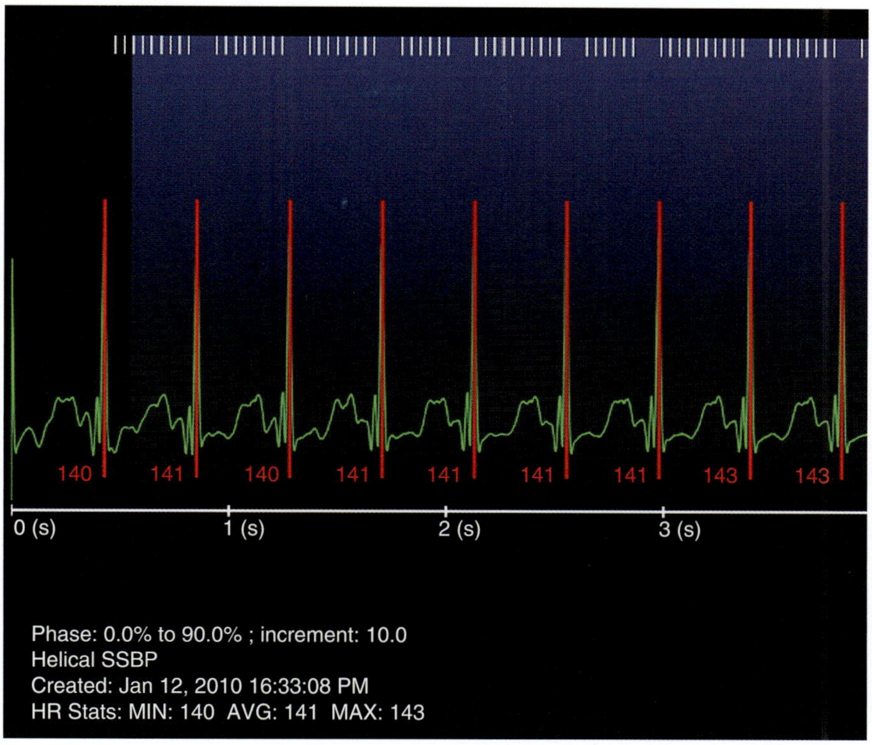

Figure 15.1 Retrospective ECG-gated scan. The X-ray beam (in blue) is on through multiple cardiac cycles.

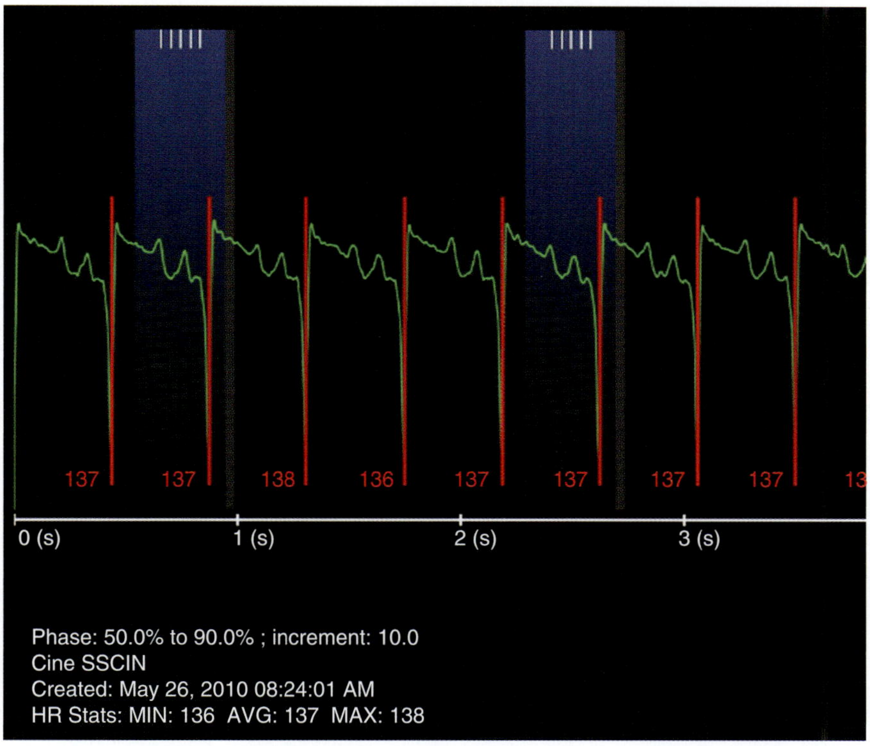

Figure 15.2 Prospective ECG-gated scan. The X-ray beam (in blue) is not on during the entire cardiac cycle. In this case enough padding was used to cover 50–90% of the cardiac cycle. Notice the rapid heart rate of 137 bpm. The X-ray beam is triggered by the timing of the cardiac cycle.

Performing CT scans using the lowest possible radiation dose should always be a priority. Using a prospective ECG-gated technique and a weight-based protocol for infants will significantly lower the radiation dose. Pre- and post-processing noise reduction techniques are now standard on most CT scanners and can be used for further radiation saving without significantly compromising image quality. Modulation techniques are also used to lower radiation dose but tend to be less successful with the rapid heart rate of a neonate.

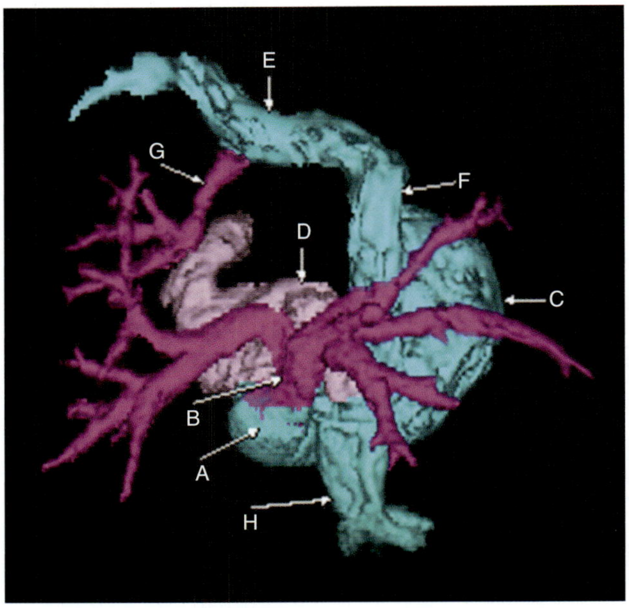

Figure 15.3 Posterior projection from a 3D color-coded cardiac CT in a patient with mixed type total anomalous pulmonary venous return. The entire right-sided pulmonary veins and left lower pulmonary vein (pink) drain through a common channel (B) to a dilated coronary sinus (A) to the right atrium (C). The left upper pulmonary vein (G) drains to the left brachiocephalic vein (E). The inferior vena cava (IVC) (H) and superior vena cava (SVC) (F) are shown.

Advantages of Cardiac CTA Over Other Imaging Modalities

Cardiac CTA produces the highest spatial resolution images of all cross-sectional imaging modalities. For this reason, CTA offers the best chance to visualize the coronary arteries, aortopulmonary collaterals, and pulmonary arteries, which may be as small as 1–2 mm in diameter in the neonate. With this high spatial resolution comes the ability to perform the best possible detail for three-dimensional (3D) reconstructions which can be important in patients with complex congenital heart disease to help with presurgical planning (Figure 15.3).

In addition to 3D reconstructions, the high spatial resolution also gives the most accurate volumetric analysis of the ventricles, giving the best information to determine the viability of a two ventricle repair in a patient with hypoplastic right or left ventricle.

Cardiac CTA, with its high special and fast temporal resolution, is the best imaging modality to image the coronary arteries. Coronary artery anomalies are associated with congenital heart disease and may be important for presurgical planning. Even with the very rapid heart rate of an infant, a cardiac CT scan can reliably demonstrate the coronary arteries.

Other cross-sectional modalities may allow identification of the origins of the coronary arteries; however, cardiac CTA affords a more reliable evaluation of the

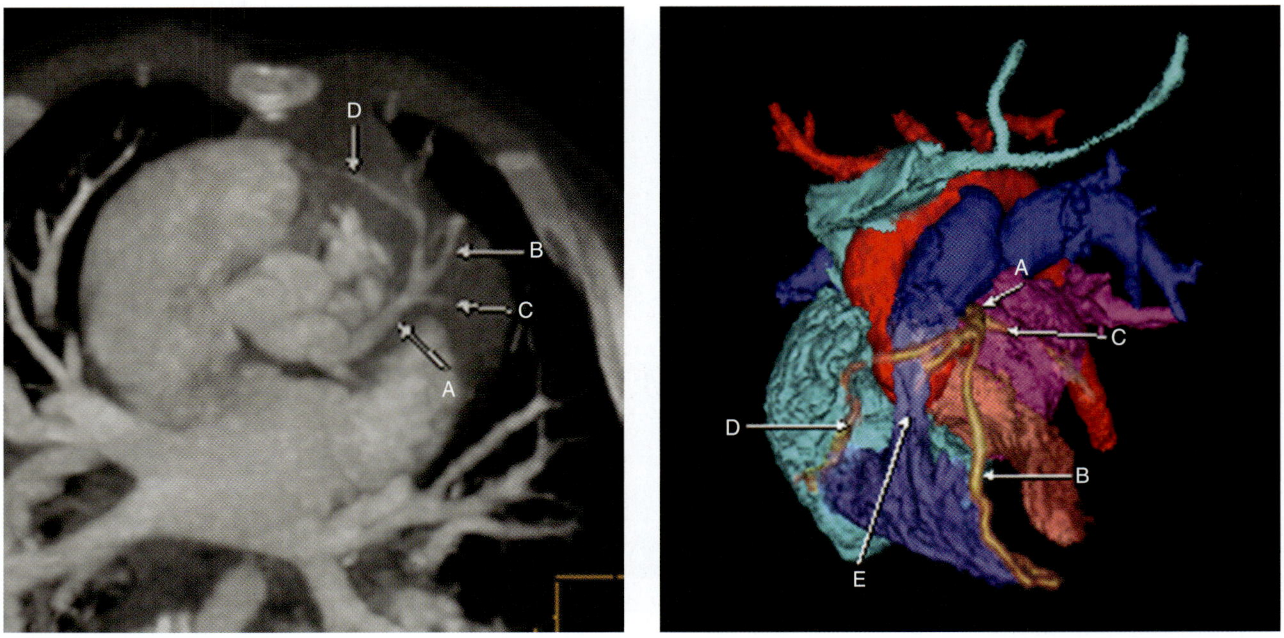

Figure 15.4 Axial maximum intensity projection (MIP) and frontal color-coded 3D images from a cardiac CT shows a single left coronary artery (A) arising from the left coronary sinus with the circumflex (C), left anterior descending (LAD) (B), and right coronary (D) arteries all arising from the left coronary artery. Notice that the right coronary crosses in front of the narrowed right ventricular outflow tract (E). The surgeon would need to be notified of this finding before surgery to plan the best approach.

course and termination of the coronary arteries. For example, visualizing the coronary artery as it passes in front of the pulmonary outflow tract in a patient with tetralogy of Fallot (Figure 15.4) or with coronary artery fistulas in patients with pulmonic atresia.

CT offers an excellent evaluation of the airway and lungs which is limited with magnetic resonance imaging (MRI) and echocardiography. Airway anomalies are common in patients with congenital heart disease and airway abnormalities can cause significant pre- and post-operative morbidity. Bronchomalacia is also common in patients with congenital heart disease and dynamic CT can show the findings of bronchomalacia without additional imaging or bronchoscopy.

Cardiac CT requires short anesthesia times, and a typical scan takes only seconds to perform. Short anesthesia

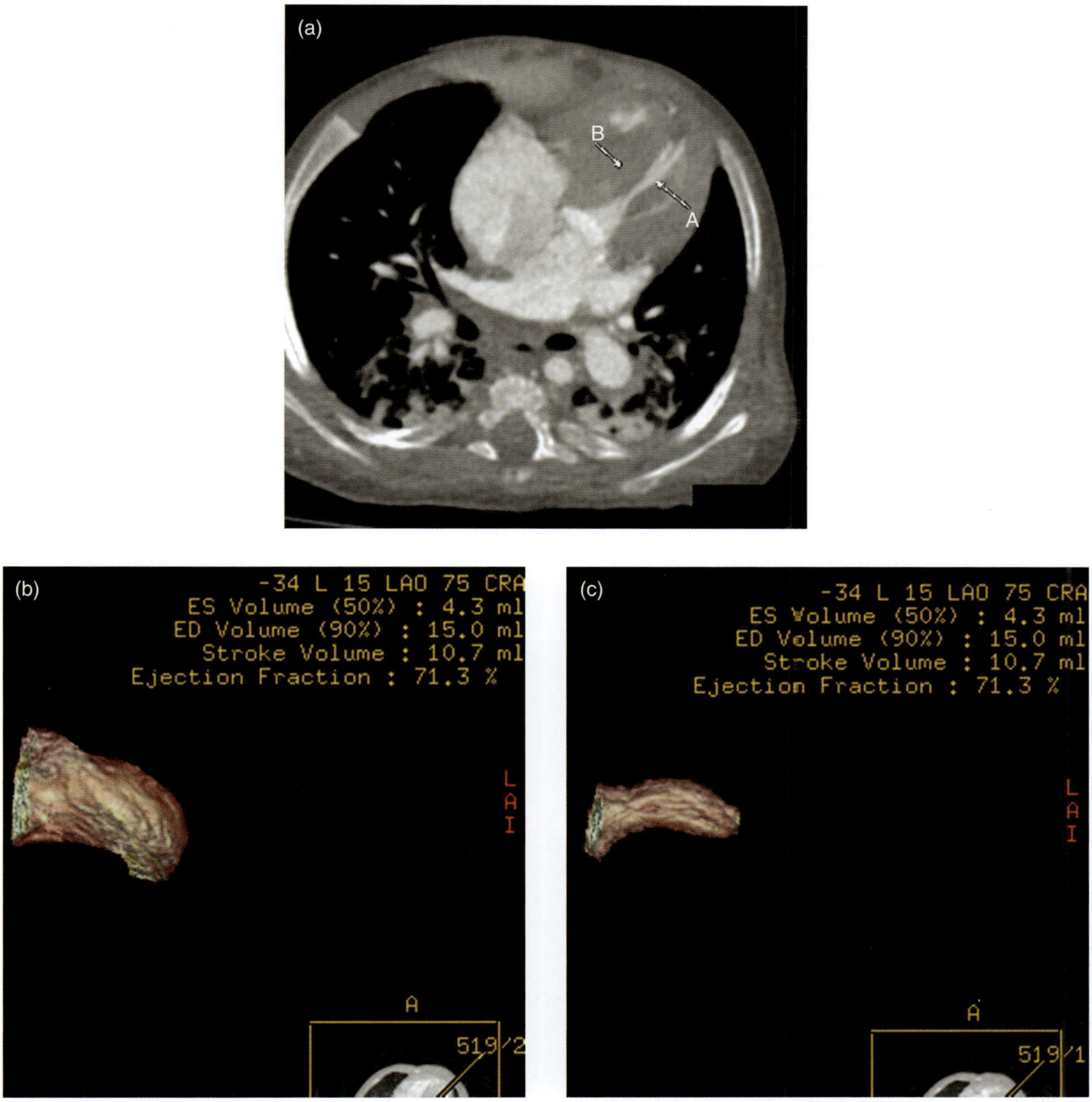

Figure 15.5 (a) An axial and (b,c) two volumetric images from a cardiac CT in an infant with an obstructive cardiomyopathy shows marked thickening of the muscular ventricular septum and left ventricle. The post-processed functional analysis shows a hyperdynamic ejection fraction measuring 71.3%. Notice the gross volume measurements: end systolic (ES) volume = 4.3 mL, end diastolic (ED) volume = 15 mL, and stroke volume = 10.7 mL. Indexed volumes may be obtained by dividing the gross volume by the body surface area.

times are an advantage in the patient with complex congenital heart disease. Anesthesia management may be very difficult for long periods of time outside the intensive care unit, making MRI difficult to perform. A typical cardiac CTA takes 4–5 s of scanning time.

Postprocessing of Cardiac CTA

Commercially available workstations have software packages to provide volumetric analysis for cardiac CTA. End-systolic and end-diastolic volumes are easily obtained for both right and left ventricles. Once volumes have been determined for end systole and end diastole, the ejection fraction and stroke volume can be calculated and provided as part of the report. It is helpful to divide the end-diastolic and end-systolic volumes by body surface area to provide indexed volumes. Indexed volumes are obtained by dividing the gross end-diastolic and end-systolic volume of the right and left ventricles by the body surface area (Figure 15.5).

Volumetric CT post-processing of pulmonary vasculature may be performed using a commercially available 3D workstation. The pulmonary vasculature (pulmonary arteries and veins) is grown out with the aid of an automated vessel selection tool. The right pulmonary blood volume percentage is obtained by dividing the pulmonary blood volume from the right side by the total pulmonary blood volume from both the right and left sides. The same calculation is performed to determine the percentage of pulmonary blood volume on the left (Figure 15.6). This

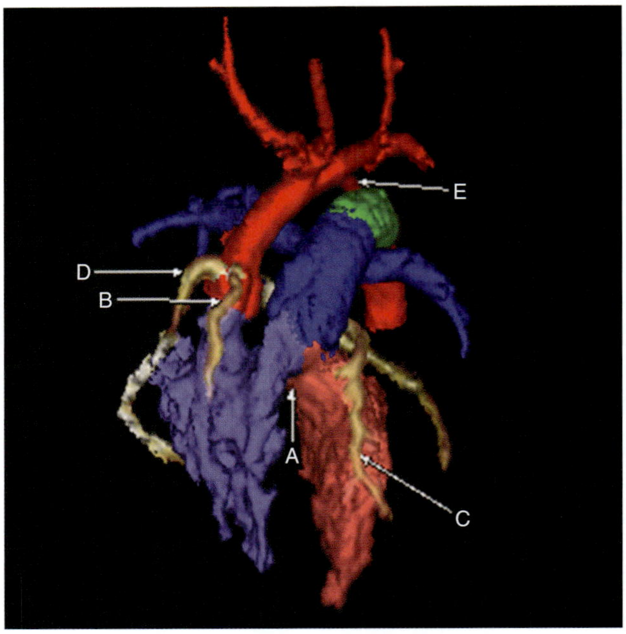

Figure 15.7 A frontal and posterior projection from a 3D color-coded cardiac CT in a patient with transposed double outlet right ventricle. Notice that the right ventricle (purple) gives rise to the aorta (red) and contributes to the main pulmonary artery (blue). A subpulmonic ventral septal defect (VSD) (A) is shown. The descending aortic arch is hypoplastic (E). A PDA (green) is widely patent and needed to get enough blood to the descending aorta. An accessory LAD (B) originates from the right coronary sinus adjacent to the origin of the right coronary artery (D). The LAD (C) originates from the left coronary artery.

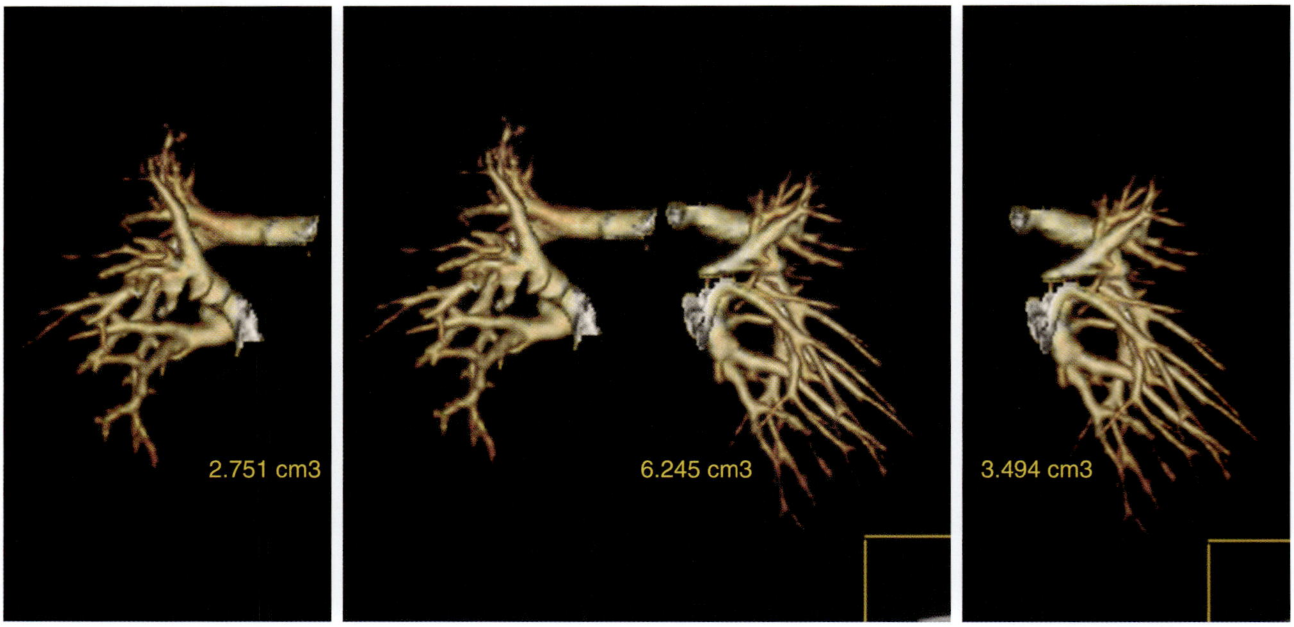

Figure 15.6 Volume rendered images of the pulmonary vasculature showing the gross volumes for the right and left pulmonary arteries in an infant where the patent ductus arteriosus (PDA) is inserted into the left pulmonary artery. The volume percentage on the right = 2.751/6.245 = 44/%. The volume percentage on the left = 3.494/6.245 = 56%.

technique can be used, in some cases, instead of performing a nuclear medicine lung perfusion scan.

3D models of cardiac anatomy are commonly used in patients with complex congenital heart disease and can be produced on standard post-processing workstations. After segmenting the pieces of anatomy out individually, the pieces are reassembled and colored. A standardized 3D color-coding scheme can also be utilized to help communicate findings and to improve the understanding of complex anatomy (Figure 15.7).

Using the images in conferences and consultations allows viewers to understand the anatomy quickly and efficiently. The color scheme is derived from a palette of commonly used colors currently associated with the arterial and venous structures, such as red for the aorta, blue for the pulmonary arteries, purple for the right ventricle, salmon for the left ventricle, light blue for the right atrium and systemic veins, pink for the left atrium and pulmonary veins, and so forth.

Once the segmentation and coloring of the models is complete, the data exist to create a 3D resin model of the anatomy. A 3D rapid prototyping machine may be used to create models of the heart (Figure 15.8). These models are to scale and may be sterilized and used in the operating room.

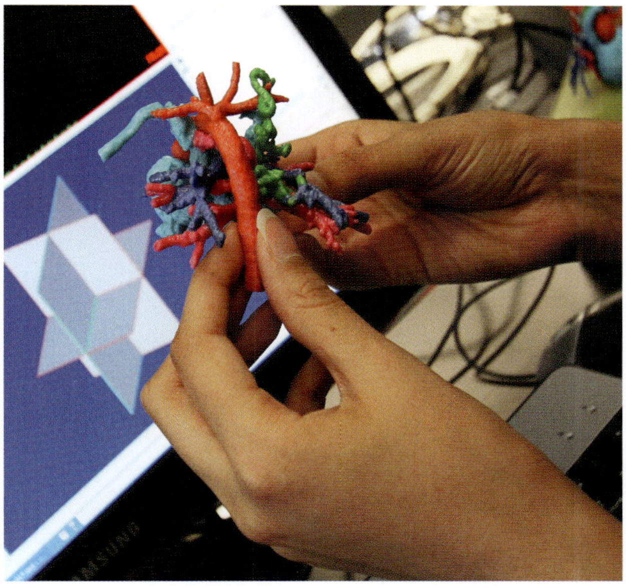

Figure 15.8 Posterior view of a resin 3D color-coded model in a patient with tetralogy of Fallot. Notice the green aortopulmonary collaterals arising from the descending aorta and right brachiocephalic artery (red).

Further Reading

Goo HW. (2011) Cardiac MDCT in children: CT technology overview and interpretation. *Radiol Clin North Am*, **49** (5), 997–1010. doi: 10.1016/j.rcl.2011.06.001 [Review]

Huang MP, Liang CH, Zhao ZJ, *et al.* (2011) Evaluation of image quality and radiation dose at prospectiveECG-triggered axial 256-slice multi-detector CT in infants with congenital heart disease. *Pediatr Radiol*, **41** (7), 858–866. doi: 10.1007/s00247-011-2079-2.

Kim YM, Yoo SJ, Kim TH, *et al.* (2002) Three-dimensional computed tomography in children with compression of the central airways complicating congenital heart disease. *Cardiol Young*, **12** (1), 44–50.

Krishnamurthy R. (2010) Neonatal cardiac imaging. *Pediatr Radiol*, **40** (4), 518–527.

Lapierre C, Déry J, Guérin R, *et al.* (2010) Segmental approach to imaging of congenital heart disease. *Radiographics*, **30** (2), 397–411.

Lee YW, Yang CC, Mok GS, Wu TH. (2012) Infant cardiac CT angiography with 64-slice and 256-slice CT: comparison of radiation dose and image quality using a pediatric phantom. *PLoS One*, **7** (11), e49609. doi:10.1371/journal.pone.0049609.

Long YG, Yang YY, Huang IL, *et al.* (2010) Role of multi-slice and three-dimensional computed tomography in delineating extracardiac vascular abnormalities in neonates. *Pediatr Neonatol*, **51** (4), 227–234.

Watanabe N, Hayabuchi Y, Inoue M, *et al.* (2009) Tracheal compression due to an elongated aortic arch in patients with congenital heart disease: evaluation using multidetector-row CT. *Pediatr Radiol*, **39** (10), 1048–1053.

Young C, Taylor AM, Owens CM. (2011) Paediatric cardiac computed tomography: a review of imaging techniques and radiation dose consideration. *Eur Radiol*, **21** (3), 518–529. doi: 10.1007/s00330-010-2036-8. Review.PubMed PMID: 21188593.

16

Magnetic Resonance Imaging

Shaine A. Morris[1] *and Timothy C. Slesnick*[2]

[1] *Texas Children's Hospital and Baylor College of Medicine, Houston, TX, USA*
[2] *Sibley Heart Center Children's Healthcare of Atlanta; Emory University, Atlanta, GA, USA*

Echocardiography remains the mainstay for diagnosis and surgical planning of children with congenital heart disease (CHD). With advancements in technology, both pre- and postnatal echocardiography accurately and efficiently delineates cardiovascular anatomy, function, and hemodynamics. Even with careful and skilled examination, however, for selected patients additional diagnostic information may be needed. In the past, cardiac catheterization was required for these patients, but over the last 30 years, cardiovascular magnetic resonance imaging (CMR) has become an option that allows complete assessment of the cardiovascular anatomy while avoiding the inherent risks of catheterization. CMR offers excellent spatial and temporal resolution, is not limited by acoustic windows that may impair echocardiography, is non-invasive, and does not involve ionizing radiation. Neonatal imaging requires modifications to standard pulse sequences to adjust for the children's small sizes and increased heart rates. These limitations notwithstanding, CMR is used in neonates to evaluate cardiac and vascular anatomy, ventricular function, hemodynamic flow quantification, and tissue characterization in cases of cardiac tumors.

Modern magnetic resonance magnets have strong, homogeneous gradients, allowing comprehensive anatomic and functional assessment. Minimal patient motion is essential to high image quality, and this can be achieved with either deep sedation or general anesthesia. All CMR studies are performed using vectorcardiographic gating to freeze cardiac motion. Eliminating respiratory motion is also advantageous in some patients, in which case either respiratory triggering or general anesthesia with breath holding for brief periods of time are utilized (Figure 16.1).

In addition to modifications to account for respiratory motion, performance of CMR in neonates requires attention to the scanning environment. Neonates are at risk of hypothermia, even in short periods of time, so warm blankets or heating packs are needed to ensure maintenance of euthermia throughout the study. The examination should be tailored to the specific clinical question to minimize the total scan time. Neonatal CMR imaging can be performed in as little as 5–10 minutes depending on the specific scenario, though the typical study lasts 45–60 minutes.

Neonatal CMR studies typically begin with bright blood, steady state free precession (SSFP), static images in the axial, coronal, and sagittal planes that are used to prescribe the remaining image planes. Cine SSFP imaging is the primary pulse sequence for neonatal CMR, providing bright blood, dynamic images with multiple phases throughout the cardiac cycle. Bright blood cine imaging is performed in multiple cardiac geometries, including the two-chamber, four-chamber, short axis, and outflow tract planes, in addition to supplemental planes such as straight axial or coronal to fully define the cardiac and vascular anatomy.

Static black blood imaging is utilized to a lesser extent, but can aid in vascular assessment, airway evaluation, and in the case of cardiac tumors tissue characterization. Typically, fast spin-echo with double inversion recovery technique or spin-echo echoplanar imaging sequence is performed (Figure 16.2). Velocity encoded cine phase contrast imaging allows quantification of blood flow direction and volumes. This technique allows calculation of shunts, differential pulmonary blood flow, and assessment of valvar and vascular pathology via analysis of stenotic jets and regurgitation.

Contrast enhanced magnetic resonance angiography (CEMRA) using gadolinium injection followed by a T1-weighted gradient echo pulse sequence provides high spatial resolution three-dimensional (3D) datasets which can then be reformatted in any plane. By using parallel imaging and advanced k-space filling techniques, multiple dynamics can be obtained with relatively high temporal resolution (1–4 s) to allow contrast tracking, lung perfusion data, and separation of pulmonary arterial, systemic arterial, and systemic venous phases. These

Visual Guide to Neonatal Cardiology, First Edition. Edited by Ernerio T. Alboliras, Ziyad M. Hijazi, Leo Lopez, and Donald J. Hagler.

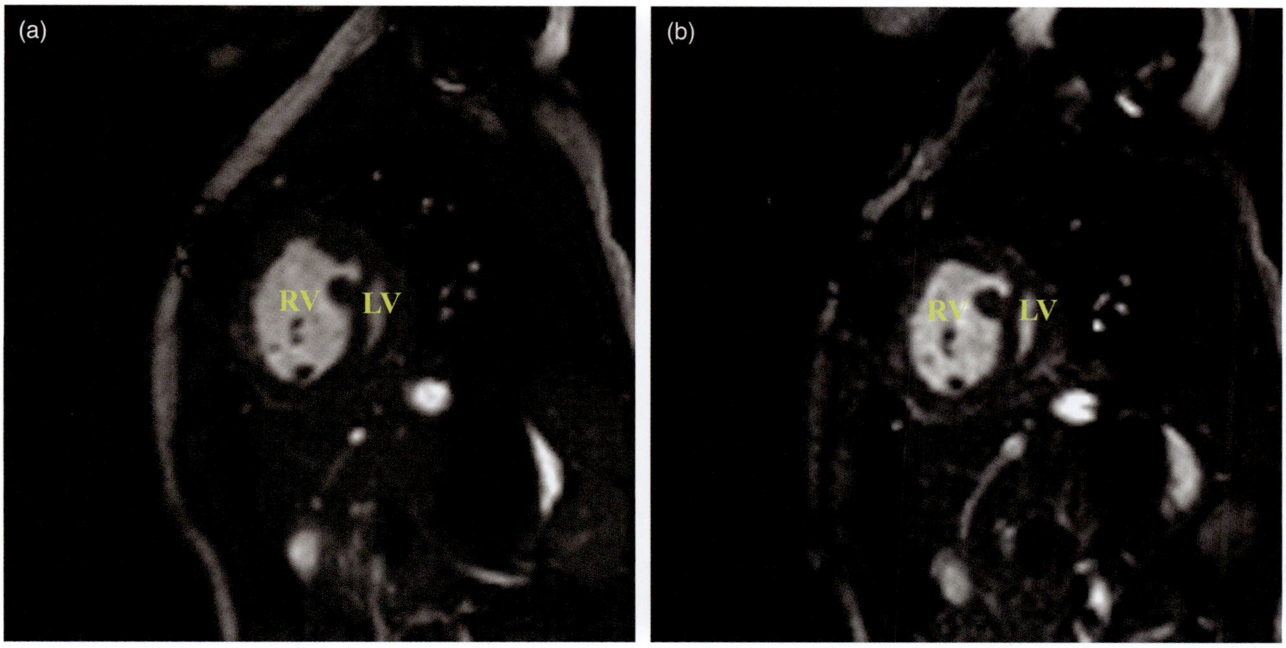

Figure 16.1 Short axis cine steady state free precession (SSFP) images in a child with an unbalanced atrioventricular septal defect using (a) multiple signal averages and (b) respiratory triggering; both images display similar image quality. LV, left ventricle; RV, right ventricle.

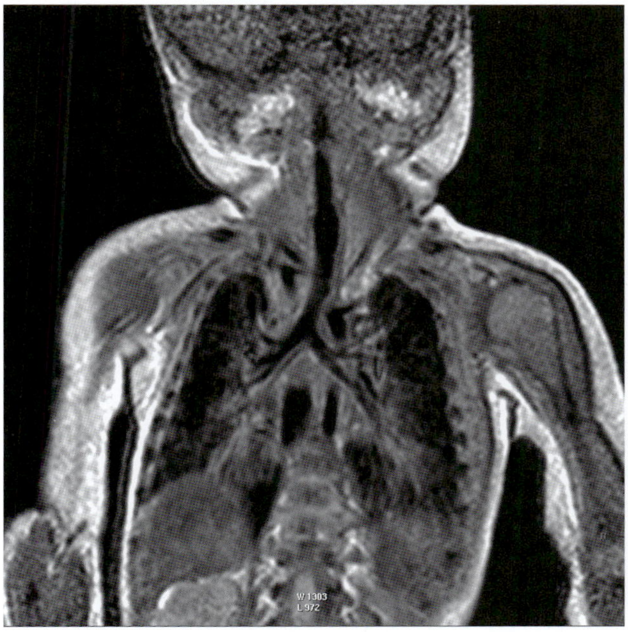

Figure 16.2 Respiratory triggered, spin-echo echoplanar imaging in the paracoronal plane in a child with heterotaxy syndrome. Note the symmetric trachea-bronchial pattern showing bilateral right-sided (eparterial) bronchi.

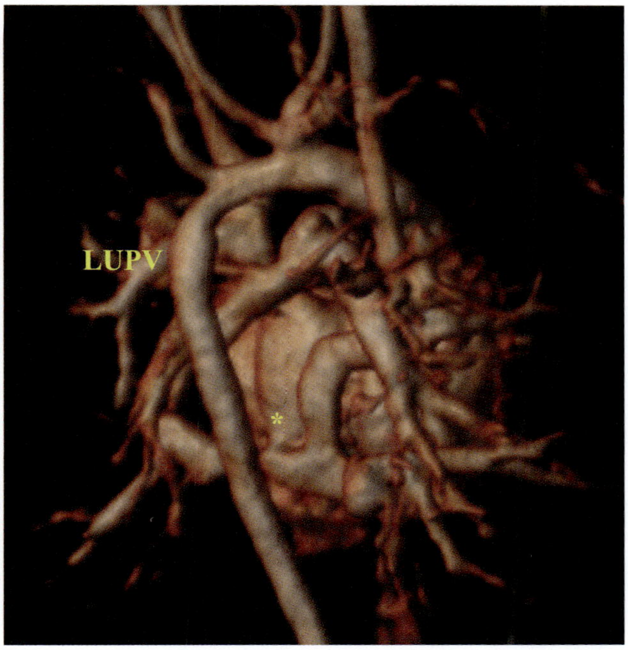

Figure 16.3 Three-dimensional (3D) volume rendered image from a postoperative contrast enhanced MRA of the chest demonstrating a child with heterotaxy syndrome and history of obstructed supracardiac total anomalous pulmonary venous return. The right and left lower and the right upper pulmonary veins now return to a posterior confluence whose anastomosis to the atrium is now severely stenotic (*) while the left upper pulmonary vein drains to the left superior vena cava. LUPV, left upper pulmonary vein.

data permit double oblique reconstructions to accurately measure cross-sectional areas of any thoracic vascular structure and assess for distal stenosis. Finally, 3D volume-rendered images provide an excellent overview of complex anatomy (Figure 16.3). Post-contrast imaging using inversion recovery gradient echo sequence to assess for late gadolinium enhancement (LGE) allows for detection and quantification of myocardial fibrosis.

Indications for Neonatal CMR

Intrathoracic Vascular Evaluation

Echocardiography provides excellent intracardiac evaluation, but assessment of extracardiac vasculature can sometimes be limited by aeration of the lungs as well as the small size and tortuous courses of arterial and venous vessels. Using a combination of high spatial resolution, thin slice images, and phase contrast velocity mapping, aortic arch abnormalities can be assessed (as in complex coarctation or interruption of the aortic arch; Figure 16.4). For neonates with known or suspected vascular rings, both vascular and airway anatomy can be assessed using thin slice black blood imaging (Figure 16.5). Pulmonary blood flow and distal pulmonary artery architecture, whether supplied via the main pulmonary artery, patent ductus arteriosus, or aorto-pulmonary collateral arteries, can be demonstrated using thin slice cine LGE images combined with contrast-enhanced magnetic resonance imaging (CEMRA). Anomalies of systemic venous return can be difficult to fully visualize by echocardiography, particularly in the setting of complex malformations such as heterotaxy syndrome, and CMR can define anomalous venous return (Figure 16.6) and any evidence of obstruction (extrinsic compression or from intravascular thrombus). Finally, pulmonary venous anomalies can be demonstrated, particularly in cases of partial or total anomalous pulmonary venous return where

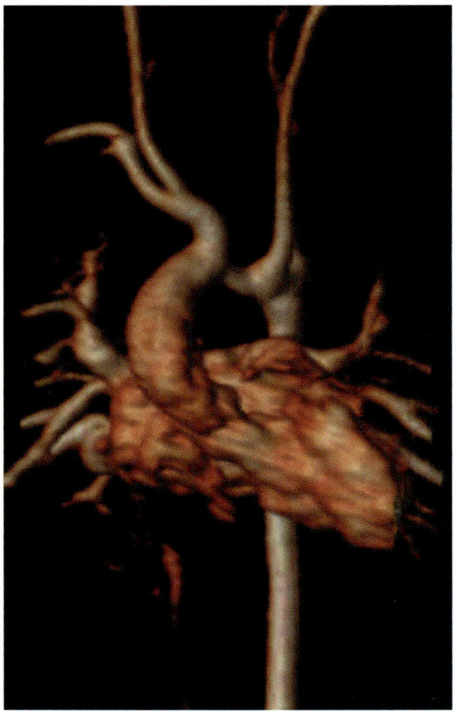

Figure 16.4 3D volume rendered image of a child with complex coarctation of the aorta with transverse arch hypoplasia.

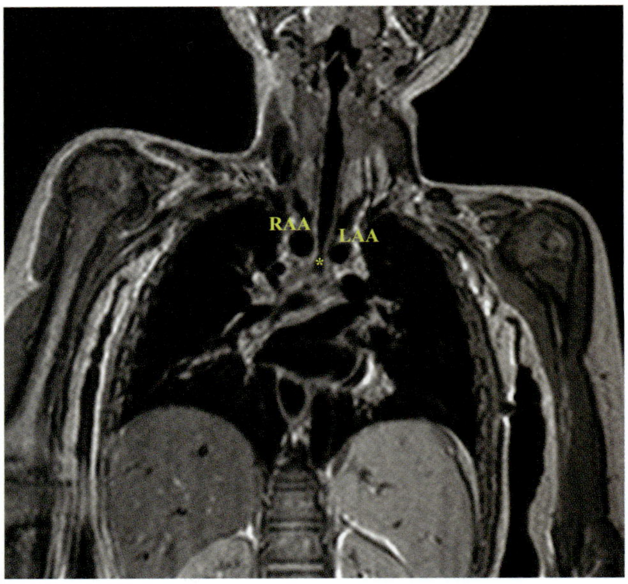

Figure 16.5 Spin-echo echoplanar imaging in the paracoronal oblique plane in a child with a double aortic arch showing airway narrowing (*) at the level of the double arch. LAA, left aortic arch; RAA, right aortic arch.

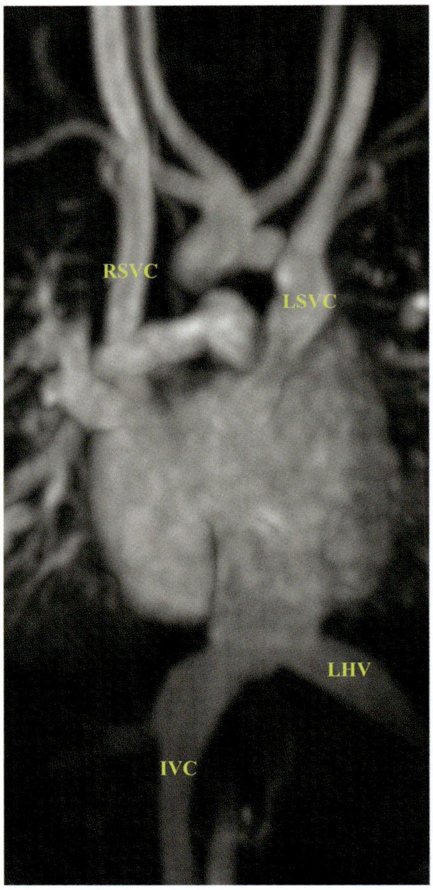

Figure 16.6 Maximum intensity projection image from a contrast enhanced MRA of the chest in a child with heterotaxy syndrome demonstrating systemic venous anomalies including an inferior vena cava that ascends on the right and then enters into the left-sided atrium with the hepatic veins and bilateral superior vena cava to the ipsilateral atria. IVC, inferior vena cava; LHV, left hepatic vein; LSVC, left superior vena cava; RSVC, right superior vena cava.

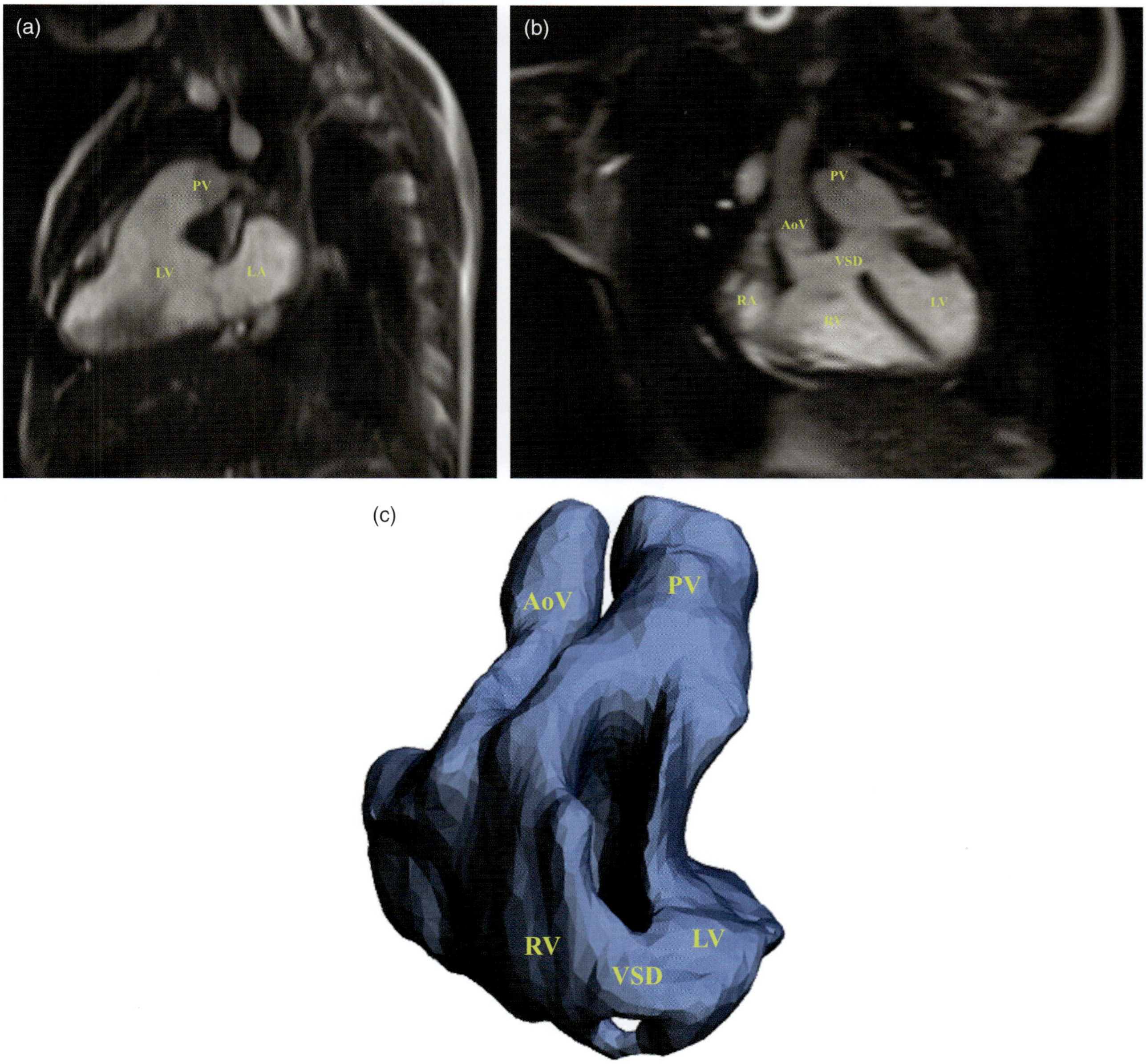

Figure 16.7 Steady state free precession image demonstrating (a) the left ventricular pulmonary outflow tract, (b) the right ventricular systemic outflow tract, and (c) a computational model of the blood pool demonstrating the complex ventricular septal defects and relationship to the semilunar valves in a child with d-transposition of the great arteries and VSD. AoV, aortic valve; LA, left atrium; LV, left ventricle; PV, pulmonary valve; RA, right atrium; RV, right ventricle; VSD, ventricular septal defect.

echocardiography is unable to delineate the anatomy (Figure 16.3).

Native Intracardiac Anatomy and Surgical Planning

For select cases, echocardiography may be insufficient for pre-operative planning, and CMR can often replace cardiac catheterization without the risks inherent to invasive procedures and ionizing radiation. For neonates with borderline hypoplastic ventricular chambers where the decision to proceed with a biventricular repair or a staged single ventricle palliation is unclear, CMR provides accurate ventricular volumes to assess the balance between the left and right ventricles, as well as demonstrating the size and commitment of AV valves to the ventricles [1]. When endocardial fibroelastosis is suspected, CMR can assess myocardial viability using LGE imaging. In cases of double outlet right ventricle or transposition of the great arteries with ventricular septal defect, double oblique planes allow unique insight into the relationship of these structures, assisting the surgeon's decision whether an arterial switch procedure or interventricular tunnel is possible to achieve a biventricular repair (Figure 16.7).

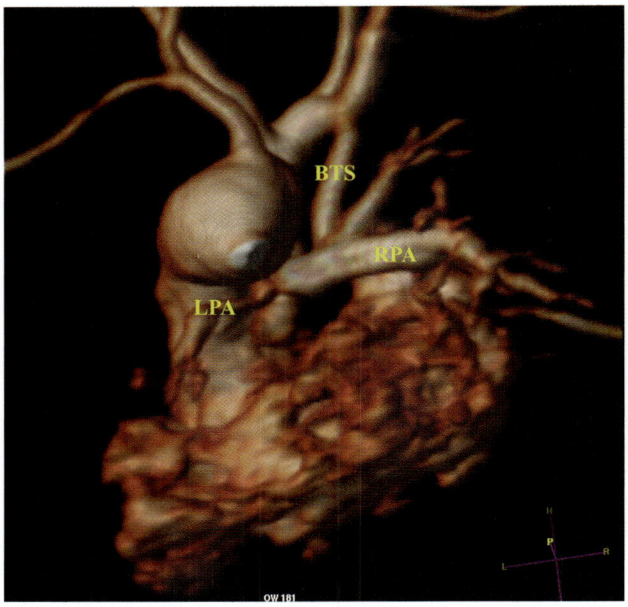

Figure 16.8 3D volume rendered image of a child with hypoplastic left heart syndrome, status post Norwood procedure using a Blalock–Taussig shunt, now with severe stenosis of the proximal left pulmonary artery just leftward of the insertion of the shunt. BTS, Blalock–Taussig shunt; LPA, left pulmonary artery; RPA, right pulmonary artery.

Postoperative Assessment

With improvements in congenital heart surgery, many children undergo either complete anatomic repair or staged palliation during the neonatal period. For the majority of these children, echocardiography is well equipped to follow their postoperative anatomy and hemodynamics, but at times further information is needed. CMR can provide information regarding residual lesions or complications, including intracardiac shunts, intracardiac and vascular obstruction (Figures 16.3 and 16.8), aneurysms, and presence and extent of intravascular thrombus.

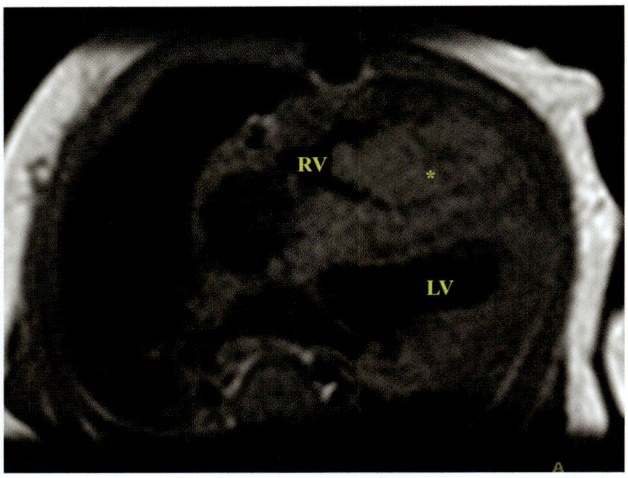

Figure 16.9 T1-weighted imaging in the four-chamber geometry of a child with a large rhabdomyoma (*) of the interventricular septum. LV, left ventricle; RV, right ventricle.

Neonatal Tumor Evaluation

Neonatal primary myocardial tumors are rare, and the vast majority are benign. Most cases represent rhabdomyomas in association with tuberous sclerosis or fibromas. The echocardiographic characteristics of these types of masses are well described, and for many children echocardiography alone is sufficient. For occasional cases, the findings may be atypical, such that further imaging is required. CMR provides tissue characterization, mass location and extension, and resultant hemodynamic effects from impingement on adjacent cardiovascular structures (Figure 16.9) [2].

References

1 Grosse-Wortmann L, Yun TJ, Al-Radi O, *et al.* (2008) Borderline hypoplasia of the left ventricle in neonates: insights for decision-making from functional assessment with magnetic resonance imaging. *J Thorac Cardiovasc Surg*, **136** (6), 1429–1436. PubMed PMID: 19114185.

2 Beroukhim RS, Prakash A, Buechel ER, *et al.* (2011) Characterization of cardiac tumors in children by cardiovascular magnetic resonance imaging: a multicenter experience. *J Am Coll Cardiol*, **58** (10), 1044–1054. PubMed PMID: 2186784.

17

Electrophysiologic Testing, Transesophageal Pacing and Pacemakers

Bryan Cannon

Pediatric Arrhythmia and Pacing Service, Mayo Clinic, Rochester, MN, USA

Pacemakers

Neonates with very slow heart rates as a result of conduction disturbances, such as complete AV block, may occasionally require implantation of a permanent pacing system in order to maintain an adequate heart rate and subsequent systemic perfusion.

The most common indication for placement of a permanent pacing system in the neonatal population is complete AV block. Not all patients with complete AV block require a pacemaker immediately, as many patients with complete AV block are completely asymptomatic for long periods of time. Indications for immediate placement of a pacemaker in patients with complete AV block are:

1) Presence of symptoms (e.g., lethargy, poor feeding, and poor weight gain);
2) Wide-complex escape rhythm;
3) Significant pauses (more than 3 s or more than 2–3× the underlying basic cycle length) on Holter monitor or ECG monitoring;
4) Mean ventricular rate below 55 bpm (70 bpm in patients with coexisting significant congenital heart disease);
5) Ventricular dysfunction;
6) Complex ventricular ectopy.

In addition, neonates with AV block (complete or 2 : 1) caused by long QT syndrome are at a particularly high risk of life-threatening ventricular arrhythmias and sudden death (up to 50% incidence). Rapid atrial or ventricular pacing may be effective in preventing ventricular arrhythmias in this population and placement of a permanent pacemaker is indicated in these patients prior to discharge. Other indications for pacemaker placement are listed in Box 17.1.

If there is an indication, pacemakers can be placed using a transvenous (insertion through the subclavian vein, across the tricuspid valve into the right ventricle) or epicardial approach where leads are directly sewn onto the epicardial surface of the heart after a sternotomy. In general, because of the small size of the veins and heart, an epicardial approach is almost always used in neonates (Figure 17.1). Using a programming computer (each device company has a specific programmer) it is possible to change the pacing rate as well as other settings by simply placing the programming wand over the pacemaker non-invasively. Many devices also incorporate home monitoring so that settings and problems can be evaluated from the patient's home.

Implantable Cardioverter-Defibrillators

Implantable cardioverter-defibrillator (ICD) implantation is indicated in the survivor of cardiac arrest after evaluation to define the cause of the event and to exclude any reversible causes. ICD placement is usually not possible in neonates and small infants because of the large size of the ICD, ICD lead, and coil necessary for the system to function properly. It can be considered in children less than 1 year who are at high risk for recurrent life-threatening ventricular arrhythmias (such as long QT syndrome with multiple ventricular tachycardia/fibrillation episodes). Placing an ICD in young children is typically via an epicardial approach requiring a median sternotomy to position (Figure 17.2). This was previously performed with epicardial patches, but there were many complications with fibrosis and system failure, so this approach has largely been abandoned.

Electrophysiology Studies

An electrophysiology study involves placing specialized catheters that are able to pace the atria and ventricles as well as record, characterize, and track the electrical wavefronts in the heart. Catheters are typically placed at strategic positions in the heart: typically, the atria, ventricles, and bundle of His. By observing the intrinsic electrical activity of the heart as well as pacing from

Visual Guide to Neonatal Cardiology, First Edition. Edited by Ernerio T. Alboliras, Ziyad M. Hijazi, Leo Lopez, and Donald J. Hagler.

Box 17.1 Recommendations for permanent pacing in neonates and children.

Permanent pacemaker implantation is indicated for:

1) Advanced second- or third-degree AV block associated with symptomatic bradycardia, ventricular dysfunction, or low cardiac output
2) Marked sinus node dysfunction with correlation of symptoms during age-inappropriate bradycardia
3) Postoperative or catheter-induced advanced second- or third-degree AV block that is not expected to resolve
4) Sustained pause dependent VT, with or without QT prolongation.

Permanent pacemaker implantation is reasonable for:

1) Sinus bradycardia with complex congenital heart disease with a resting heart rate of less than 40 bpm or pauses in ventricular rate longer than 3 s
2) Patients with congenital heart disease and impaired hemodynamics caused by sinus bradycardia or loss of AV synchrony

Permanent pacemaker implantation is *not* indicated for:

1) Transient postoperative AV block with return of normal AV conduction in the otherwise asymptomatic patient
2) Asymptomatic type I second-degree AV block
3) Symptomatic sinus bradycardia with the longest relative risk interval less than 3 s and a minimum heart rate of more than 40 bpm.

Adapted from Epstein *et al.* 2008 [1].

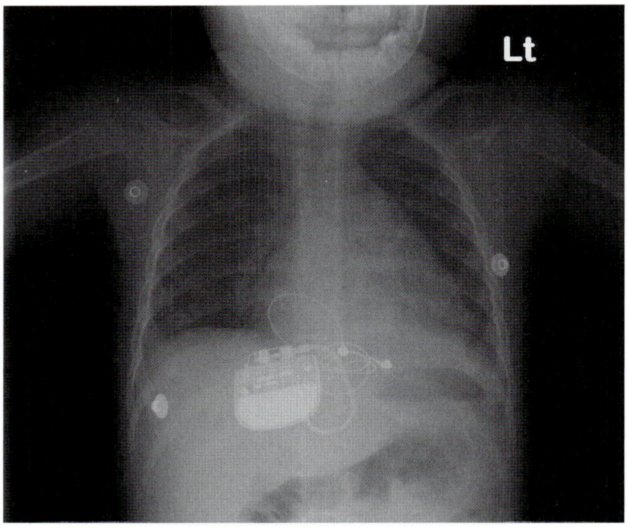

Figure 17.1 Epicardial pacing system. A bipolar lead delivers energy to pace heart between two electrodes that is sewn directly onto the epicardial surface of the heart. The leads are then tunneled to the generator (also known as the "can") in the abdomen which contains the computer and battery for the pacemaker.

the atria and ventricles, it is possible to determine the cardiac conduction properties as well as delineate the mechanism of many arrhythmias. The catheters are inserted through the veins into the heart. The femoral, internal jugular, and umbilical veins can be used to insert these catheters into the heart, in a similar way to procedures using hemodynamic catheters. The catheters used vary from 4 French (Fr) to 8 Fr and can have between two and twenty poles to measure the pinpoint electrical wavefronts passing through the myocardium. It is also possible to pace the heart from any of these poles. Some catheters have the potential for delivering radiofrequency energy or cryo-energy from the tip of the catheter to destroy abnormal areas of the heart responsible for arrhythmias in the process of ablation.

The role of electrophysiology studies in the neonate is limited. The small size of the vessels limits access to the heart and only allows for placement of a small number of catheters. The catheters used are relatively stiff and are at risk for perforating the relatively thin neonatal myocardium. In addition, almost all of the important information about arrhythmias can be obtained non-invasively. Ablation procedures in neonates are only typically performed in multidrug-refractory arrhythmias that are severely affecting ventricular function. They are not performed routinely as most neonatal tachycardias will resolve spontaneously, and the risk of performing an ablation is significantly higher in children less than 4–5 years of age and 15 kg (significant complication in around 10%) compared with children above this age and weight range (significant complication in less than 2%). However, in the neonate with severely depressed function resulting from arrhythmias that are not able to be controlled with high doses of three or more medications, there may be no other option than attempting to eliminate the source of the arrhythmia by ablation. A pediatric cardiovascular surgeon and capability for extracorporeal membrane oxygenation (ECMO) or mechanical support should be readily available if there is a major complication during the procedure or if there is hemodynamic collapse from the arrhythmia.

Transesophageal and Temporary Pacing

In patients with normal anatomy, the left atrium sits anteriorly and immediately adjacent to the esophagus. For this reason, an electrophysiology catheter placed

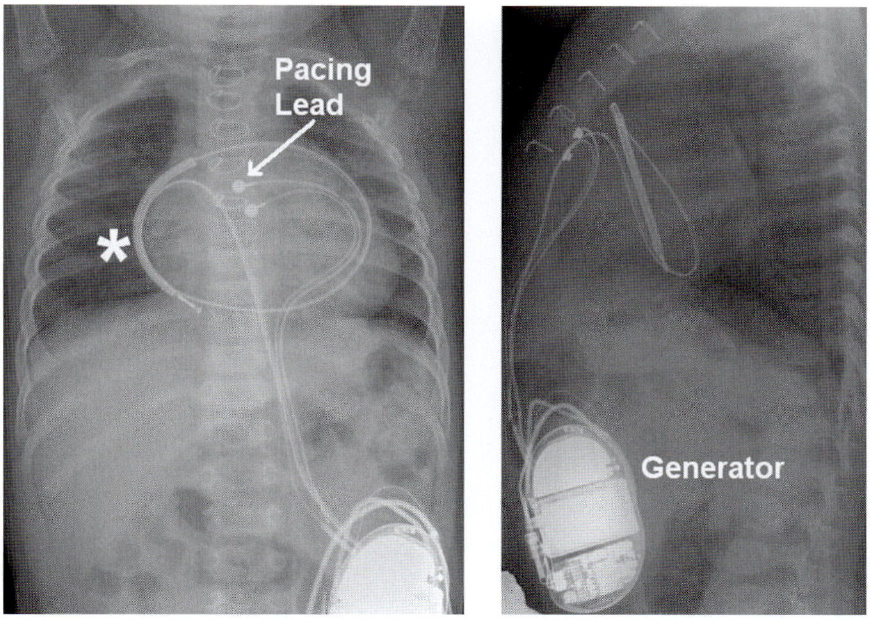

Figure 17.2 Epicardial implantable cardioverter-defibrillator (ICD) system. A standard bipolar pace sense lead is placed on the epicardial surface. A shocking coil (*) is then placed in the pericardial sac and the leads are tunneled to an ICD generator placed in the abdomen. The pacing lead is able to recognize arrhythmia and the generator can deliver a defibrillation shock to the coil to convert potentially fatal ventricular arrhythmias. (Note: The use of a coil in the pericardial sac is an off-label use.)

through the mouth or nose into the esophagus is an excellent way to both pace the left atrium and record the atrial activity of the heart. A *soft* electrophysiology catheter (either a small transvenous catheter or a specialized catheter made for transesophageal placement) can be placed in the esophagus and positioned behind the left atrium. This can either be accomplished fluoroscopically (ideally) or by placing the catheter and observing for cardiac electrical signals. The lead can be connected to the ECG machine or electrophysiology recording system to obtain a recording of the left atrial signal.

It can also be connected to a temporary pacing device or stimulator to pace the atrium. This may be uncomfortable for the patient and should not be used to pace for more than 24–48 hours as there is a risk of esophageal erosion. In general, the ventricle cannot be paced transesophageally, and if ventricular pacing is needed this is best achieved by placing a transvenous temporary pacing lead. The femoral vessels are the best route for placement, but the internal jugular or umbilical veins can also be used, but these approaches typically require a sheath that is left in place through which the pacing lead is placed. There are several types of temporary pacing leads that can be used. The first is a balloon tipped catheter that can be directed into the ventricle by using the blood flowing through the heart. In patients with no underlying ventricular rate, it is not possible to pass this catheter as is depends on blood flow to carry the catheter to the ventricle. The second type of catheter is a fixed curve catheter that can be directed into the ventricle by manipulating the catheter typically under fluoroscopic guidance. The third type is a temporary catheter with a small screw at the tip that can be placed in the ventricle fluroscopically and then screwed into the myocardium. A fourth possibility is to use a permanent pacing lead that has an active fixation screw that can be deployed through the tip. Transcutaneous pacing that can be performed using an external defibrillator is technically challenging because of the large size of the two pads that must be placed on the chest in order to pace. The external pads can be cut to fit small neonates, but this goes against the manufacturer's recommendations for most devices. In general, ventricular pacing is only useful when there is a primary electrical problem with the heart such as AV block. In situations like hypoxia or acidosis where there is a secondary bradycardia, temporary pacing will not be effective as it is frequently difficult to electrically capture the heart. Treatment of the primary etiology of the bradycardia should be undertaken rather than attempting temporary pacing.

Reference

1 Epstein AE, DiMarco J, Ellenbogen K, *et al.* (2008) ACC/AHA/HRS 2008 Guidelines for device-based therapy of cardiac rhythm abnormalities. *J Am Coll Cardiol*, **51** (21), e1–62.

Part IV

Specific Morphologic Conditions

18

Total Anomalous Pulmonary Venous Connection

David W. Brown and Tal Geva

Department of Cardiology, Boston Children's Hospital;, Department of Pediatrics, Harvard Medical School, Boston, MA, USA

Definition

Total anomalous pulmonary venous connection (TAPVC) occurs when all pulmonary veins connect to the systemic venous circulation. TAPVC is a rare congenital anomaly, reported in 9 in 100 000 live births [1, 2]. The most commonly used classification of TAPVC is based on the site of connection(s) between the pulmonary and systemic veins (Figure 18.1) [3]:

1) *Supracardiac* – connections to the innominate vein, azygous vein, or to the superior vena cava;
2) *Cardiac* – anomalous connections to the coronary sinus;
3) *Infradiaphragmatic* – connections below the diaphragm; and
4) *Mixed* – connections to more than one location.

With all types, an interatrial communication to allow blood to enter the systemic circulation is necessary to sustain life, so that a patent foramen ovale or atrial septal defect is considered part of the malformation.

Etiology

Most cases of pulmonary venous anomalies are sporadic. However, there are known syndromic associations for TAPVC including cat-eye, Holt–Oram, and the asplenia syndromes. Numerous case reports of non-syndromic familial cases suggest a heritable genetic cause, with heterogenous genetic loci reported; one gene for familial total anomalous pulmonary venous return in a large Utah kindred was mapped to chromosome 4p13-q12 [4].

Embryologic Basis

An understanding of the embryologic development of the pulmonary veins helps to explain the various patterns of pulmonary to systemic venous connections seen with TAPVC. The lungs and tracheobronchial tree derive from the foregut, and the pulmonary vascular bed from a portion of the splanchnic plexus. Thus, early in gestation, the primitive lung drains by the splanchnic venous plexus into the systemic circulation via the umbilicovitelline and cardinal venous systems. At 32–33 days' gestation, the pulmonary veins subsequently establish a communication with the common pulmonary vein, which becomes incorporated into the posterior aspect of the developing left atrium, between the left and right horns of the sinus venosus, superior to the coronary sinus, and leftward of septum primum. Once this has occurred, the primitive connections of pulmonary venous to systemic venous systems typically regress [5].

TAPVC occurs because of failure to establish a normal connection between the pulmonary venous plexus and the common pulmonary vein before the connections with the splanchnic venous system have regressed. Thus, the anomalous left-sided connections observed are often to derivatives of the left cardinal vein (such as the left innominate vein and coronary sinus), right-sided connections to derivatives of the right cardinal system (superior and inferior vena cavae), and drainage that crosses the midline is possible because the splanchnic venous plexus is a midline structure. The persistent embryologic connection between the pulmonary and systemic veins is often named a vertical vein because of its orientation.

Anatomy

Supracardiac TAPVC is the most common type (47% in the largest published series [3]), most commonly to the leftward aspect of the innominate vein (Figures 18.1a, 18.2, and 18.3). A pulmonary venous confluence is typically present posterior to the left atrium that drains via a left-sided ascending vertical vein to the innominate vein. This vertical vein usually passes anterior to the left pulmonary artery and mainstem bronchus, although

Visual Guide to Neonatal Cardiology, First Edition. Edited by Ernerio T. Alboliras, Ziyad M. Hijazi, Leo Lopez, and Donald J. Hagler.

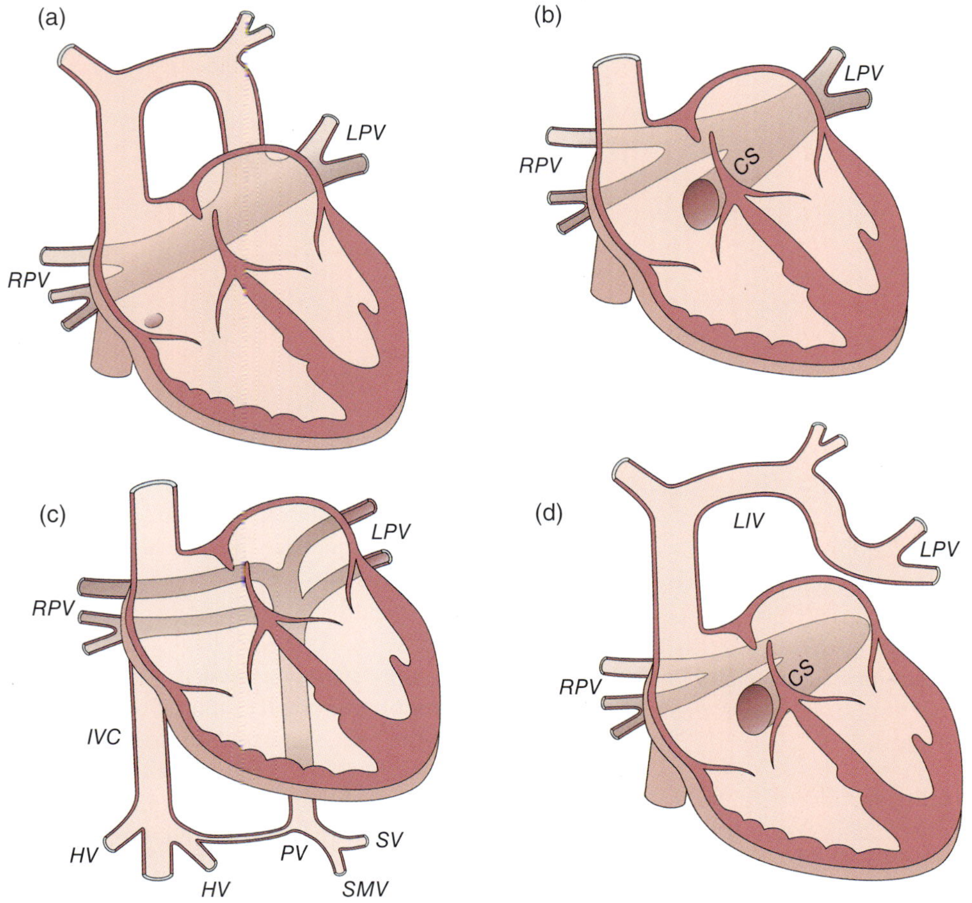

Figure 18.1 Variants of total anomalous pulmonary venous connection (TAPVC). (a) Supracardiac: both right (RPV) and left (LPV) pulmonary veins join a common pulmonary venous confluence behind the heart, which drains via a vertical vein to the undersurface of the left innominate vein, and thence to the right atrium. (b) Cardiac: the pulmonary venous confluence connects to the coronary sinus (CS), and thence to the right atrium via the coronary sinus ostium. (c) Infradiaphragmatic: the pulmonary venous confluence drains inferiorly via a vertical vein to the portal vein (PV) or hepatic veins (HV) and thence to the right atrium. IVC, inferior vena cava; SMV, superior mesenteric vein; SV, splenic vein. (d) Mixed connections: left pulmonary veins drain to the left innominate vein (LIV), and right pulmonary veins to the coronary sinus in this example. *Source*: Brown 2009 [9]. Reproduced with permission of John Wiley & Sons.

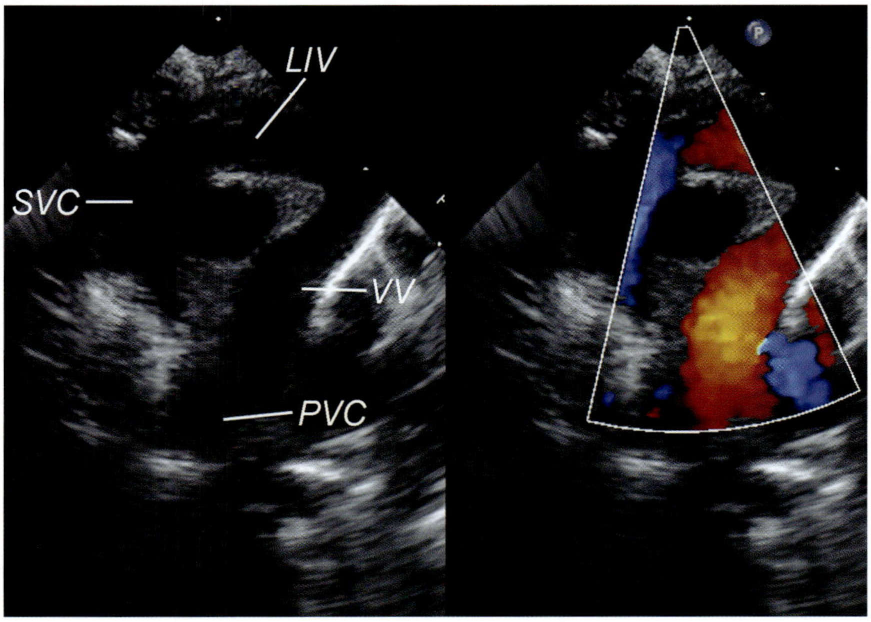

Figure 18.2 Parasternal short axis echocardiogram view with color Doppler flow mapping in this patient with supracardiac TAPVC to the left innominate vein (LIV) shows the pulmonary venous confluence (PVC) which drains via the vertical vein (VV) toward the leftward aspect of the innominate vein. SVC, superior vena cava.

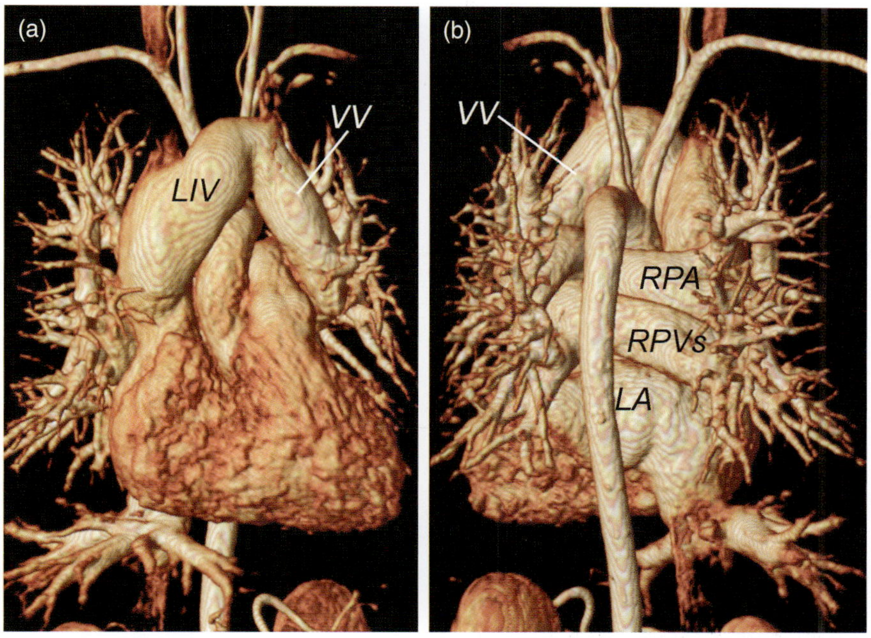

Figure 18.3 Anterior and posterior views of volume-rendered cardiac magnetic resonance angiogram in a 50-year-old man with uncorrected supracardiac TAPVC to the left innominate vein.The right ventricle was severely dilated (end-diastolic volume index 216 mL/m^2) and the pulmonary-to-systemic flow ratio measured 3.9. Succesful surgical repair was performed after cardiac catheterization confirmed mildly elevated pulmonary artery pressure and resistance (2.1 Wood units).

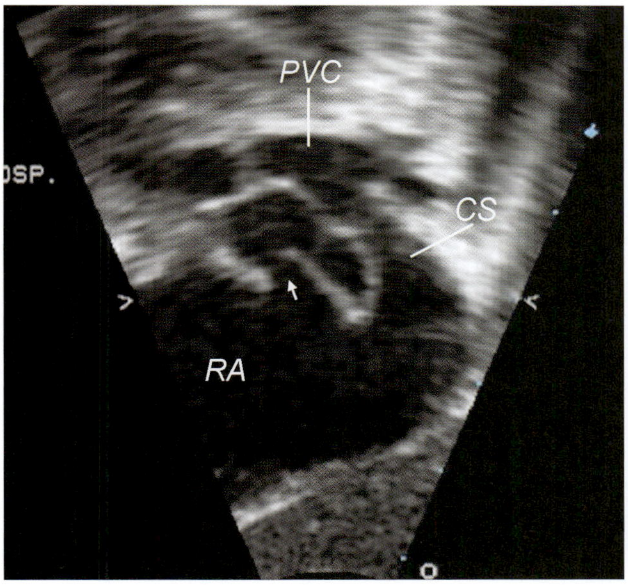

Figure 18.4 Cardiac TAPVC. Subxiphoid short axis two-dimensional echocardiogram view in a patient with TAPVC to the coronary sinus shows the pulmonary venous confluence (PVC) draining via a communicating vein to the severely dilated coronary sinus (CS). Note the relative hypoplasia of the left atrium and the obligate open position of the patent foramen ovale (arrow) which allows filling of the left heart. RA, right atrium.

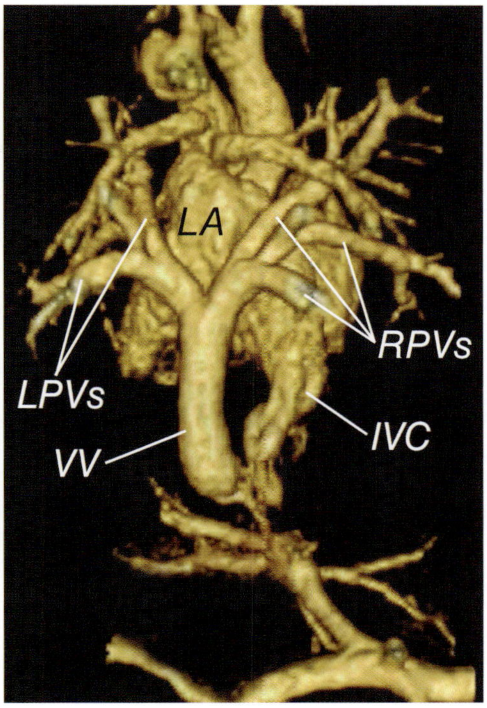

Figure 18.5 Posterior view of volume-rendered cardiac magnetic resonance angiogram in a 2-day-old infant girl with infradiaphragmatic TAPVC to the portal vein. The individual left and right pulmonary veins (LPVs and RPVs, respectively) join a vertical confluence (VV) that courses posterior and inferior to the left atrium (LA) before joining the portal vein. Pulmonary venous blood then returns to the right atrium through the inferior vena cava (IVC).

occasionally it passes *between* these structures, which usually results in obstruction to pulmonary venous flow.

Cardiac TAPVC occurs in 16% of cases [3], and involves anomalous connection between the pulmonary venous confluence and the coronary sinus, with a venous vessel connecting typically in the region of the left atrioventricular groove (Figures 18.1b and 18.4). The coronary veins drain normally into the proximal end of the coronary sinus, and the typically severely dilated coronary sinus drains normally into the right atrium; the coronary sinus septum is usually intact.

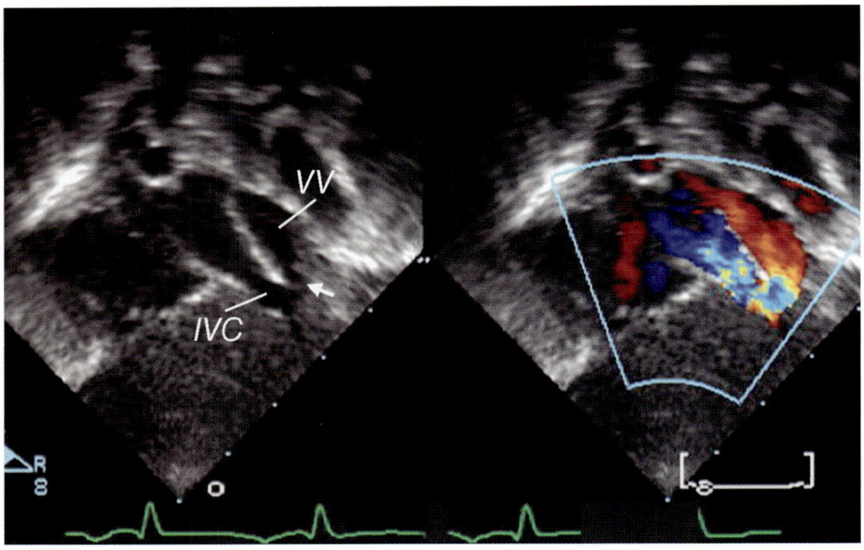

Figure 18.6 Infradiaphragmatic TAPVC. The subxiphoid short axis echocardiogram view in this patient with infradiaphragmatic TAPVC with two-dimensional and color Doppler flow mapping shows the vertical vein (VV) descending just below the level of the diaphragm, and then coursing anteriorly to drain directly into the inferior vena cava (IVC). Note the narrowing of the venous connection to the IVC (arrow), with color Doppler flow acceleration at the connection to the IVC.

Infradiaphragmatic TAPVC occurs in 13–23% [3], usually connecting to the umbilicovitelline system below the diaphragm (Figures 18.1c, 18.5, and 18.6). A descending vertical vein typically originates from the confluence of pulmonary veins to course below the diaphragm to form connections with the portal venous system (most common), the ductus venosus, hepatic vein, or inferior vena cava. Obstruction is frequently present with infradiaphragmatic forms of TAPVC for a number of reasons, most commonly caused by intrinsic narrowing of the connecting vessel, the interposition of the hepatic sinusoids between the pulmonary venous drainage and the heart for those that drain via the portal vein, and constriction of the ductus venosus.

Mixed TAPVC is the least common type occurring in 7–10% [3, 6], often with complex variations of the above forms of venous connections represented (Figures 18.1d and 18.7).

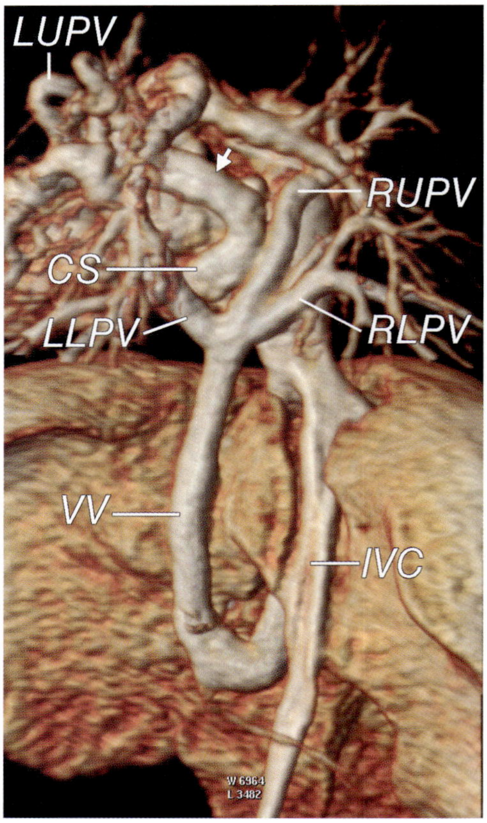

Figure 18.7 Mixed TAPVC. Posterior view of volume-rendered cardiac magnetic resonance angiogram in a 3-day-old infant girl with mixed-type TAPVC. The left upper (LUPV) and lingular pulmonary veins join a semihorizontal vein (arrow) that drains into the coronary sinus (CS). The left lower (LLPV) and both right upper and lower (RUPV and RLPV, respectively) join a vertical vein (VV) that courses infradiaphragmatically and drains into the inferior vena cava (IVC) through the portal vein.

Pathophysiology

The pathophysiology of TAPVC depends greatly upon the presence or absence of pulmonary venous obstruction, as well as the adequacy of the interatrial defect to allow flow to the systemic circulation. In the absence of pulmonary venous obstruction, there is complete mixing of systemic and pulmonary venous blood in the right atrium. As the resistance to pulmonary blood flow is significantly lower than that of the systemic circulation, there is significant pulmonary overcirculation (often 3–5 times normal) and the systemic saturation may be 90% or higher, often resulting in clinically inapparent

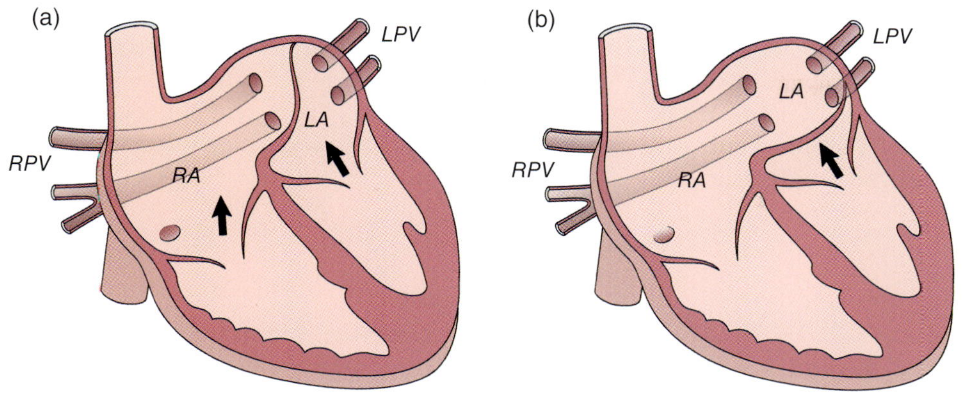

Figure 18.8 Anomalous pulmonary venous drainage with malposition of septum primum. (a) Mild leftward malposition with normal pulmonary venous connections results in anomalous drainage of the right upper and lower pulmonary veins to the right atrium. (b) With more severe malposition of septum primum, drainage of all four pulmonary veins is directed anomalously into the right atrium. Note the absence of a well-developed septum secundum; this is common in patients with the polysplenia forms of heterotaxy syndrome. LA, left atrium; LPV, left pulmonary veins; RA, right atrium; RPV, right pulmonary veins. *Source*: Brown 2009 [9]. Reproduced with permission of John Wiley & Sons.

cyanosis. Right ventricular dilation and hypertrophy frequently occur, along with varying degrees of pulmonary hypertension. The size of the interatrial communication with TAPVC has a critical role. With worsening restriction to flow across the atrial septum, there is not only a dramatic increase in pulmonary overcirculation and worsening pulmonary hypertension, but also diminished systemic output. Infants with obstructed TAPVC typically present in the first days of life, with a rapid and fulminant progression of dyspnea to cardiorespiratory failure. In patients with TAPVC without obstruction, clinical detection can be delayed.

Total Anomalous Pulmonary Venous Drainage

TAPVC must be distinguished from total anomalous pulmonary venous drainage, which results when despite normal pulmonary vein connections to the left atrium, abnormal anatomy of the atrial septum directs pulmonary venous drainage into the right atrium (Figures 18.8 and 18.9). This is often caused by anatomically leftward malposition or malattachment of septum primum (commonly encountered in polysplenia syndrome [6]), which results in partial or total anomalous pulmonary venous drainage, depending upon the degree of malposition and number of veins affected.

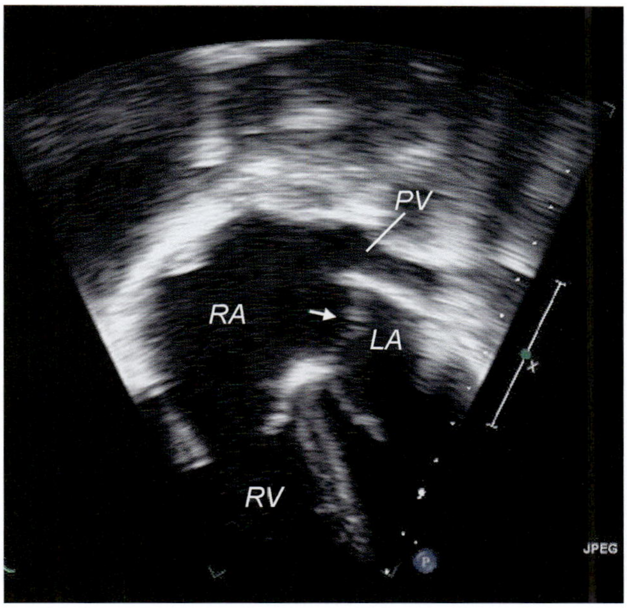

Figure 18.9 Anomalous pulmonary venous drainage. Apical two-dimensional echocardiogram image in a patient with severe leftward malposition of septum primum shows the lack of septum secundum superiorly, normal pulmonary venous connections to the posterior aspect of the left atrium (LA), and leftward malposition of septum primum (arrow), resulting in drainage of all pulmonary veins into the right atrium (RA). PV, pulmonary veins; RV, right ventricle.

Treatment

The treatment of TAPVC is surgical correction. It usually consists of creation of an anastomosis between the pulmonary venous confluence and the back wall of the left atrium. Given the natural history of the disease, surgery is typically undertaken upon diagnosis, and is frequently emergent because of the presence of pulmonary venous obstruction in the neonatal period. While 3-year survival for patients with a two-ventricle circulation is good, approaching 90% in one large series [7], similar term survival for those with single-ventricle anatomy is considerably worse (47% in the same series). Recurrent pulmonary venous obstruction is a major cause of late mortality after repair of TAPVC, occurring in 10–15% of patients and typically becoming manifest in the first 6 months after repair [7, 8]. This can occur both at the level of the anastomosis of the confluence to the left atrium, as well as the individual pulmonary veins. Outcomes of treatment of recurrent pulmonary venous obstructive disease in this population remain poor.

References

1 Ferencz C, Rubin JD, McCarter RJ, *et al.* (1985) Congenital heart disease: prevalence at livebirth. The Baltimore-Washington Infant Study. *AmJ Epidemiol*, **121** (1), 31–36.
2 Hoffman JI, Kaplan S. (2002) The incidence of congenital heart disease. *J Am Coll Cardiol*, **39** (12), 1890–1900.
3 Burroughs JT, Edwards JE. (1960) Total anomalous pulmonary venous connection. *Am Heart J*, **59**, 913–931.
4 Bleyl S, Nelson L, Odelberg SJ, *et al.* (1995) A gene for familial total anomalous pulmonary venous return maps to chromosome 4p13-q12. *Am J Hum Genet*, **56** (2), 408–415.
5 Rammos S, Gittenberger-de Groot AC, Oppenheimer-Dekker A. (1990) The abnormal pulmonary venous connexion: a developmental approach. *Int J Cardiol*, **29** (3), 285–295. PubMed PMID: 2283187. Epub 1990/12/01. eng.
6 Lucas RV Jr, Adams P Jr, Anderson RC, *et al.* (1961) Total anomalous pulmonary venous connection to the portal venous system: a cause of pulmonary venous obstruction. *Am J Roentgenol Radium Ther Nucl Med*, **86**, 561–575.
7 Hancock Friesen CL, Zurakowski D, *et al.* (2005) Total anomalous pulmonary venous connection: an analysis of current management strategies in a single institution. *Ann Thorac Surg*, **79** (2), 596–606.
8 Seale AN, Uemura H, Webber SA, *et al.* (2013) Total anomalous pulmonary venous connection: outcome of postoperative pulmonary venous obstruction. *J Thorac Cardiovasc Surg*, **145** (5), 1255–1262. PubMed PMID: 22892140.
9 Brown DW. (2009) Pulmonary venous anomalies, in, *Echocardiography in Pediatric and Congenital Heart Disease: From Fetus to Adult* (eds WW Lai, LL Mertens, MS Cohen, T Geva) Wiley-Blackwell, Oxford, pp. 119–142.

19

Other Anomalies of Pulmonary and Systemic Venous Connections

Mark V. Zilberman[1] *and Clifford L. Cua*[2]

[1] *Pediatric Echocardiology and Fetal Cardiology; Pediatric Cardiologist, Boston Floating Children's Hospital; Associate Professor of Pediatrics, Tufts University School of Medicine, Boston, MA, USA*
[2] *Nationwide Children's Hospital, Columbus, OH, USA*

Partial abnormal pulmonary venous return (PAPVR) is a condition in which at least one of the pulmonary veins drains into the left atrium while the rest are connected to the systemic venous circuit. There are multiple variations of this condition; from one to three pulmonary veins can drain into the superior vena cava (SVC), coronary sinus, and/or inferior vena cava (IVC). However, the most common forms are left pulmonary vein drainage into the superior vena cava via the left innominate vein, and the anomalous connections of the right pulmonary veins to the inferior vena cava, known as scimitar syndrome. A partition deficiency between the right superior vena cava and right upper pulmonary vein is always associated with superior sinus venosus atrial septal defect and is described elsewhere. Atrial septal defect is commonly present in PAPVR [1]. When PAPVR is an isolated lesion, its physiology is that of pulmonary volume overload of variable significance. The clinical picture is similar to that of an atrial septal defect with comparable left-to-right shunt. Like an isolated atrial septal defect, it rarely causes symptoms during the neonatal period. Contrary to this, infants with scimitar syndrome are often symptomatic during the first few months of life [2]. PAPVR is usually diagnosed by echocardiography and can be definitively confirmed by either computer tomography (CT) or magnetic resonance angiography (MRA). Cardiac catheterization is rarely needed and is considered only when pulmonary venous stenosis is suspected.

The left pulmonary veins drain into the left innominate vein via the vertical vein. This venous arrangement (vertical to the left innominate, to the right SVC) might create a typical X-ray figure of "snowman" on the chest X-ray. However, this classic feature is almost never seen in neonates because of the presence of a thymus shadow. The diagnosis is made when the Doppler echocardiography demonstrates a venous flow directed cephalad – away from the heart (Figure 19.1). A single abnormally draining pulmonary vein as an isolated lesion requires no intervention. Multiple abnormally draining veins require surgery later in childhood.

Scimitar syndrome has been reported in 3–6% of patients with PAPVR [3]. In scimitar syndrome, all the right pulmonary veins, or occasionally the veins draining the right middle and right lower lobes, enter the IVC either just above or below the diaphragm. This malformation frequently is associated with other anomalies, including hypoplasia of the right lung, anomalies of the bronchial system, horseshoe lung, secondary dextrocardia, hypoplasia of the right pulmonary artery, anomalous arterial connection to the right lung from the aorta, and pulmonary sequestration. Although patients with scimitar syndrome might have minimal symptoms, many of them present in infancy with signs of congestive heart failure and pulmonary hypertension. These patients usually have additional congenital cardiac abnormalities, most commonly atrial and/or ventricular septal defects [2]. Scimitar syndrome is suspected when an infant presents with symptoms of congestive heart failure and dextroposition of the heart on the chest radiology imaging. The diagnosis is confirmed by echocardiography and CT/MRA (Figure 19.2). Symptomatic infants require intervention with occlusion of the arterial collaterals and repair of venous return, or even pulmonectomy [2]. Persistence of pulmonary hypertension after surgery is a rare but ominous sign that lung transplantation may be necessary [3].

Congenital anomalies of the systemic venous connection to the heart represent a wide and heterogeneous group of malformations. Often systemic venous anomalies are part of complex congenital heart defects discussed elsewhere; however, they may present as isolated lesions. Some of them, such as persistent left SVC to the coronary sinus (Figure 19.3), or retro-aortic innominate vein (Figure 19.4) [4], have no clinical significance. Others become clinically evident during the newborn period either because of systemic arterial

Visual Guide to Neonatal Cardiology, First Edition. Edited by Ernerio T. Alboliras, Ziyad M. Hijazi, Leo Lopez, and Donald J. Hagler.

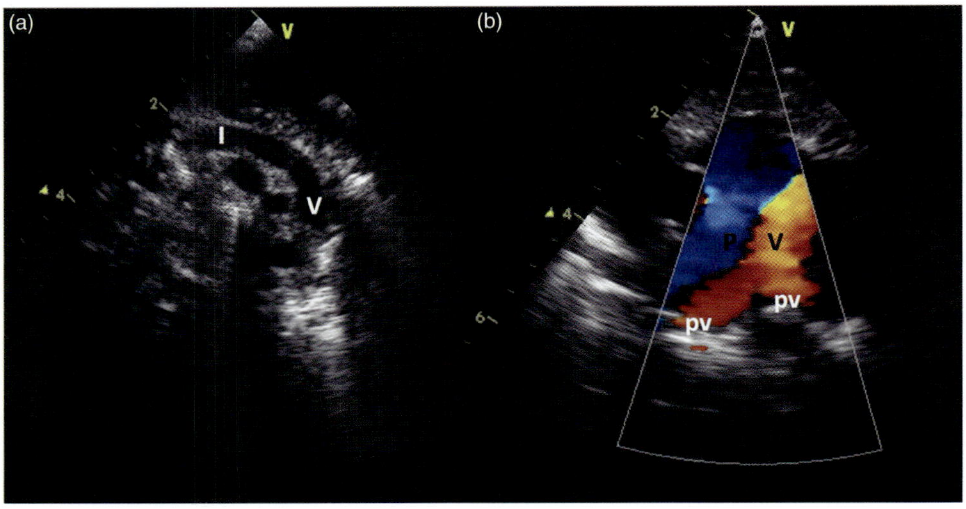

Figure 19.1 Supracardiac abnormal pulmonary drainage. Echocardiographic suprasternal views: (a) connection of the vertical vein (V) to the left innominate vein (I) forming the top part of a "snowman" figure; (b) two pulmonary veins (pv) connected to the vertical vein (V). The flow is away from the heart. The left pulmonary artery (P) is to the right.

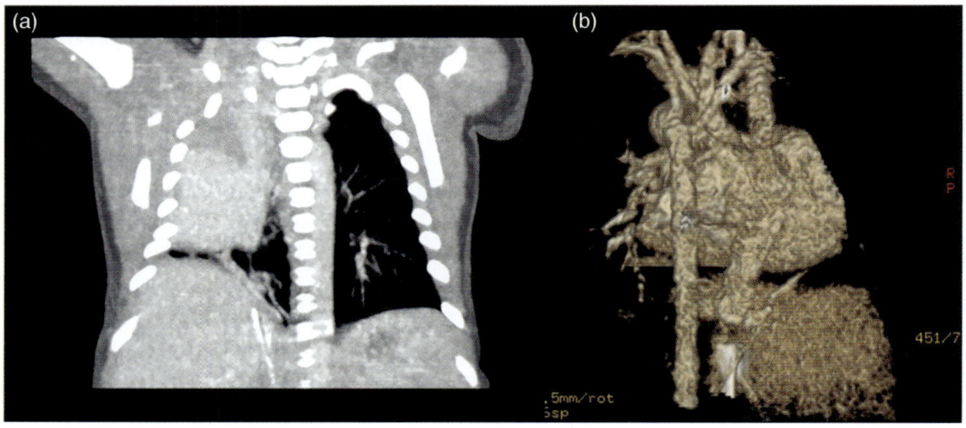

Figure 19.2 Scimitar syndrome. CT images: (a) hypoplastic right lung and dextroposition of the heart; (b) a volume-rendered angiogram. A small right pulmonary vein connects to the IVC–right atrial junction.

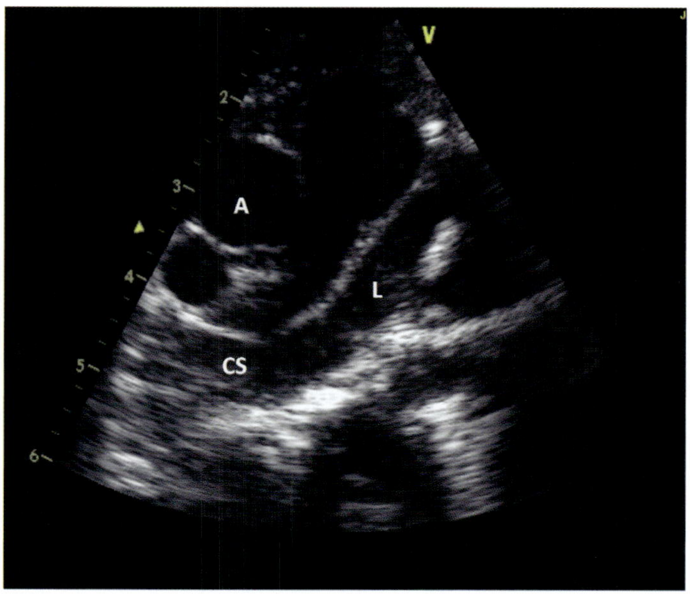

Figure 19.3 Echocardiographic image of the left superior vena cava (SVC) in a patient with L-transposition and a ventricular septal defect (VSD). The left SVC (L) connects to the dilated coronary sinus (CS).

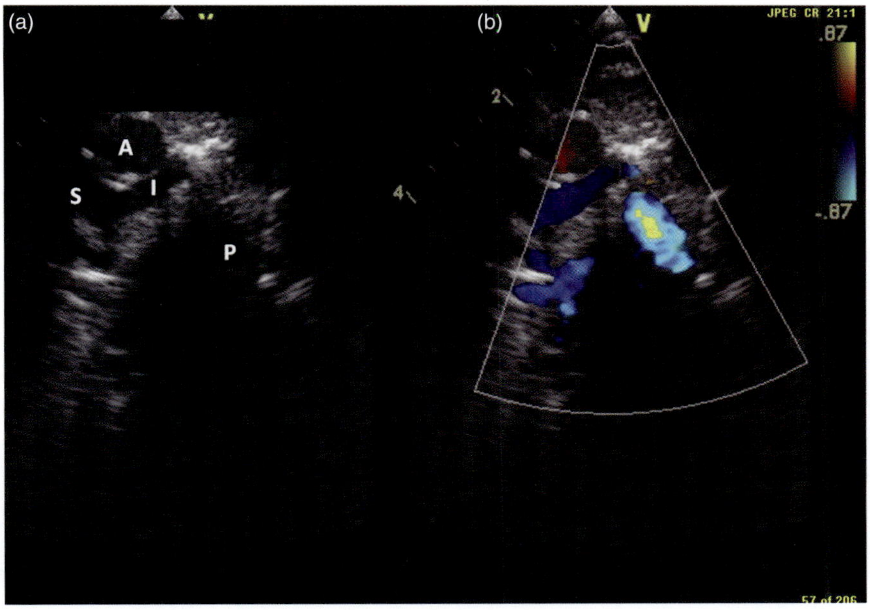

Figure 19.4 (a) Suprasternal echocardiographic image of the left innominate vein (I) coursing inferior to the aorta (A) and connecting to the right superior vena cava (S). (b) Right-sided color Doppler panel shows blob flow in the abovementioned vessels as well as some turbulence in the left pulmonary artery (P).

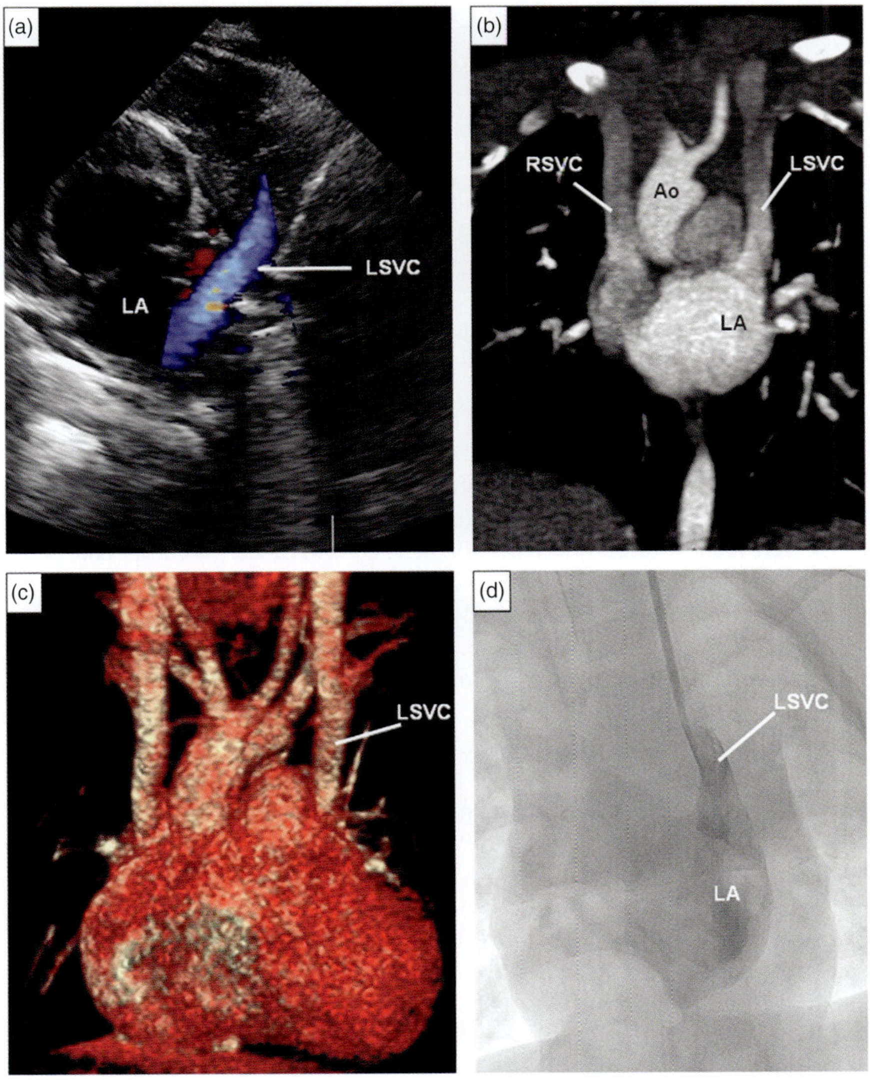

Figure 19.5 (a) Two-dimensional echocardiography showing the persistent left SVC draining into the left atrium. (b) Computed tomography scan showing bilateral superior venae cavae without the left innominate vein. (c) Three-dimensional CT scan reconstruction showing the absence of communication between the bilateral SVCs. (d) Angiography confirming direct connection of the left SVC to the roof of the left atrium. Ao: aorta; LA: left atrium; LSVC, left superior vena cava; RSVC: right superior vena cava. Source: Tampere *et al.* 2012 [19]. Copyright (C) 2012 Elsevier Masson SAS. All rights reserved. Reprinted with permission.

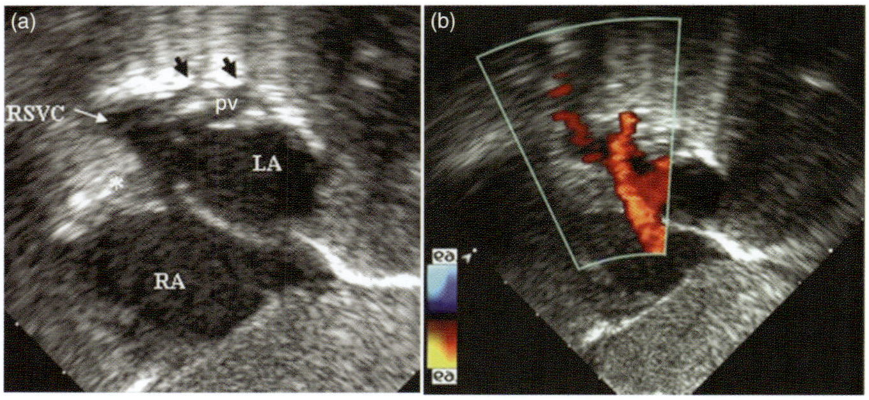

Figure 19.6 Two-dimensional echocardiography. (a) Right superior vena cava (RSVC) connected to the left atrium (LA). (b) Left-to-right shunting across the non-restrictive secundum atrial septal defect and flow from the right pulmonary veins (pv) into the RSVC. Source: Vassallo *et al.* 2006 [13]. Reproduced with permission of John Wiley & Sons.

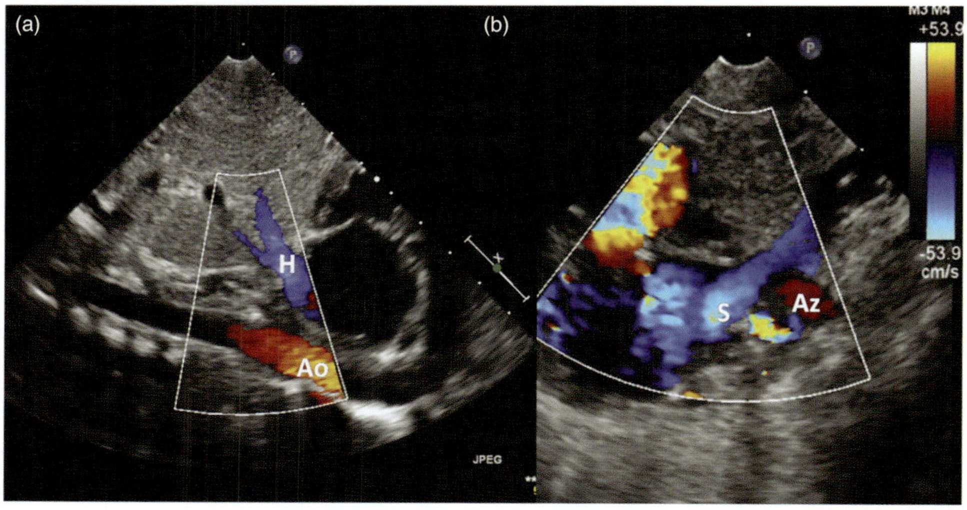

Figure 19.7 Two-dimensional echocardiography of interrupted IVC with azygos continuation in a patient with heterotaxy. (a) The hepatic vein (H) entering the right atrium directly. (b) The azygos vein (Az) entering the right SVC.

desaturation, or an unusual course of central or umbilical venous catheters. Arterial desaturation develops when systemic venous flow reaches the left atrium. There are few possible arrangements: the left SVC could drain to the left atrium directly (Figure 19.5), it could reach the left atrium through the unroofed coronary sinus, or the right SVC could drain directly to the left atrium (Figure 19.6). Unusual catheter course is seen in cases of interrupted IVC with azygos continuation (Figure 19.7), umbilical vein anomalies (Figure 19.8), or abnormalities of the ductus venosus.

Persistence of the left SVC is a relatively common anatomic variant. In the vast majority of patients, it drains via the intact coronary sinus to the right atrium, resulting in normal systemic venous return and has no clinical sequelae. In combination with a normal right SVC, the incidence is 0.3% in autopsy studies [5]. Presence of the left SVC in the absence of the right SVC is much less common. Nearly half of these patients have additional cardiac abnormalities [6]. These patients have a significantly higher incidence of atrial arrhythmias than those with bilateral SVCs [7]. Patients with persistent left SVC in combination with other cardiac defects show high incidence of extracardiac anomalies [8]. The diagnosis of a persistent LSVC is suspected when dilated coronary sinus is seen by echocardiography (Figure 19.4), or a specific course of a central venous catheter from the left subclavian or jugular vein.

In about 8% of patients with persistent left SVC, the vein drains to the left atrium through an unroofed coronary sinus [5]. Left SVC draining directly into the left atrium is almost always a part of a complex congenital heart defect of left atrial isomerism. As an isolated lesion, it is unlikely to cause clinically detectable cyanosis, but it does place patients at risk for paradoxical embolus, cerebrovascular accident, and intracranial abscess [9, 10].

Isolated drainage of the right SVC into the left atrium is exceedingly rare [11]. The anomaly presents with cyanosis. The diagnosis is usually confirmed by contrast echocardiography or angiography. The condition requires surgical repair [12, 13].

Persistent azygos vein in association with interrupted IVC is observed in 0.6% of all congenital heart disease

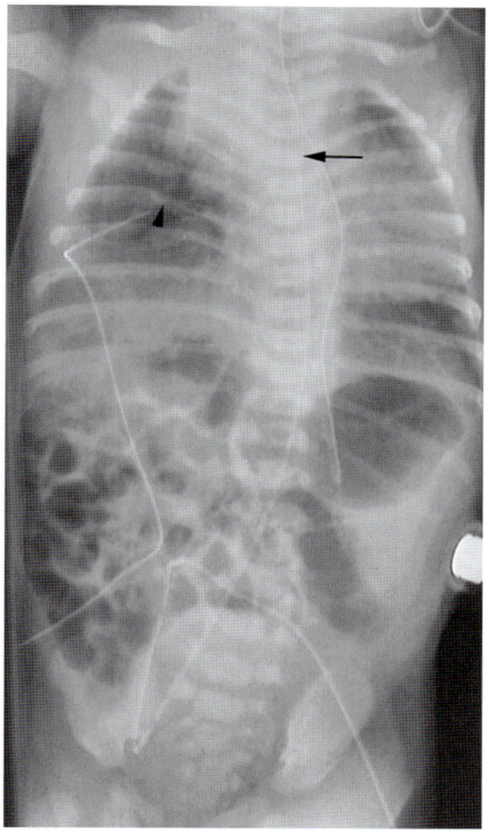

Figure 19.8 X-ray of a newborn with persistent right umbilical vein. The catheter in the umbilical artery courses in a normal fashion via the right iliac artery up into the descending aorta with the tip at the level of Th3 (arrow). Catheter inserted in the umbilical vein goes towards the right costophrenic angle ad turns with the tip in a medial direction (arrowhead). Source: Nikstad and Smevik 2004 [22]. Copyright @ 2004 Nakstad and Smevik. Reprinted with permission.

[11] and is usually associated with left atrial isomerism. Persistent azygos vein with an uninterrupted IVC is not associated with heterotaxy but has a significant incidence of abnormal drainage of the right pulmonary veins into the azygos or the SVC. Interestingly, these patients have a normal size IVC when compared with matched controls [14].

Absent ductus venosus has a reported prevalence of 6/1000 fetal examinations [15]. It can be an isolated anomaly leading to fetal cardiomegaly and dilated IVC, although it may present as a dilatation of the umbilical vein, or portal sinuses. Fetuses develop either intrahepatic or extrahepatic drainage of the umbilical vein, in the latter case it drains into either the right atrium or into different parts of the IVC. Fetuses with absent ductus venosus must be followed for signs of congestive heart failure requiring premature delivery. However, those with isolated absence of ductus venosus and no fetal hydrops had an excellent short-term postnatal survival rate [16]. Postnatal development of diaphragmatic hernia was described in those with umbilical vein draining above the diaphragm [17].

Normally, functional ductus venosus closure occurs within 14–18 days of life. Primary failure of spontaneous ductus venosus closure is a rare abnormality that can cause cholestasis and hepatic dysfunction. Patent ductus venosus can be addressed either surgically [18] or with a coil occlusion [19].

Incomplete regression of the right sinus horn (sinus venosus) structures can lead to the presence of a fenestrated membranous structure within the right atrium known as a Chiari network. A Chiari network has no clinical significance per se but has a known association with hypoplasia of the right-sided cardiac structures [20].

Achnowledgment

The authors are grateful to Ms. Joyce Cordier, RDCS for her help in preparing the figures.

References

1 Hlavacek AM, Shirali GS, Anderson RH. (2010) Pulmonary venous abnormalities, in, *Paediatric Cardiology*, 3rd edn. (ed. RH Anderson), Churchill Livingstone, Philadelphia, pp. 497–521.
2 Huddleston CB, Exil V, Canter CE, Mendeloff EN. (1999) Scimitar syndrome presenting in infancy. *Ann Thorac Surg*, **67**, 154–160.
3 Vida VL, Padalino MA, Boccuzzo C, *et al.* (2010) Scimitar syndrome: a European Congenital Heart Surgeons Association (ECHSA) Multicentric Study. *Circulation*, **122**, 1159–1166.
4 Gerlis L, Ho SJ. (1989) Anomalous subaortic position of the brachiocephalic (innominate) vein: a review of published reports and report of three new cases. *Br Heart J*, **61**, 540–545.
5 Geva T, Van Praagh S. (2008) Abnormal systemic venous connections, in, *Moss And Adams' Heart Disease in Infants, Children, and Adolescents: Including the Fetus and Young Adult*, 7th edn. (eds AJ Moss and HD Allen), Wolters Kluwer Health/Lippincott Williams & Wilkins, Philadelphia, pp. 792–803.
6 Bartram U, Van Praagh S, Levine JC, *et al.* (1997) Absent right superior vena cava in visceroatrial situs solitus. *Am J Cardiol*, **80**, 175–183.
7 Ratnasamy C, Idris SF, Carboni MP, Kanter RJ. (2009) Arrhythmias in children having a single left superior

vena cava and minimal structural heart disease. *J Cardiovasc Electrophysiol*, **20**, 182–186.
8 Postema PG, Rammeloo LAJ, van Litsenburg R, Rothuis EGM, Hruda J. (2008) Left superior vena cava in pediatric cardiology associated with extra-cardiac anomalies. *Int J Cardiol*, **123**, 302–306.
9 Butera G, Salvia J, Carminati M. (2012) When side matters: contrast echocardiography with injection from the left antecubital vein to detect a persistent left superior vena cava draining to the left atrium in a patient with cerebral stroke. *Circulation*, **125** (1), e1.
10 Vizzardi E, Fracassi F, Farina D, *et al.* (2008) Persistence of left superior vena cava, absence of coronary sinus and cerebral ictus. *Int J Cardiol*, **126** (2), e39–41.
11 Smallhorn JF, Anderson RH. (2010) Anomalous systemic venous return, in, *Paediatric Cardiology*, 3rd edn. (ed. RH Anderson), Churchill Livingstone, Philadelphia, pp. 485–496.
12 Gorenflo M, Sebening C, Ulmer HE. (2006) Anomalous connection of the right superior caval vein to the morphologically left atrium. *Cardiol Young*, **16**, 184–186.
13 Vassallo M, Pascotto M, Pisacane C, *et al.* (2006) Right superior vena cava draining into the left atrium: prenatal diagnosis and postnatal management *Ultrasound Obstet Gynecol*, **27**, 445–448.
14 Punn R,Olson I. (2010) Anomalies associated with a prominent azygos vein on echocardiography in the pediatric population. *J Am Soc Echocardiogr*, **23**, 282–285.
15 Acherman, RJ, Evans WN, Galindo A, *et al.* (2007) Diagnosis of absent ductus venosus in a population referred for fetal echocardiography. *J Ultrasound Med*, **26**, 1077–1082.
16 Thomas JT, Petersen S, Cincotta R, Lee-Tannock A, Gardener G. (2012) Absent ductus venosus: outcomes and implications from a tertiary centre. *Prenat Diagn*, **32**, 686–691.
17 Jowett V, Paramasivam G, Seale A, *et al.* (2013) Diaphragmatic hernia: a postnatal complication of anomalous drainage of the umbilical vein. *Ultrasound Obstet Gynecol*, **41** (5), 589–591.
18 Yoshimoto Y, Shimizu R, Saeki T, *et al.* (2004) Patent ductus venosus in children: a case report and review of the literature. *J Pediatr Surg*, **39**, E1.
19 Schwartz YM, Berkowitz D, Lorber A. (1999) Transvenous coil embolization of a patent ductus venosus in a 2-month-old child. *Pediatrics*, **103**, 1045.
20 Loukas M, Sullivan A, Tubbs RS, *et al.* (2010) Chiari's network: review of the literature. *Surg Radiol Anat*, **32**, 895–901.
21 Tampere L, Paranon S, Seguela PE. (2012) Percutaneous closure of a left superior vena cava draining directly into the left atrium in a child. *Arch Cardiovasc Dis*, **1051**, 53–55.
22 Nikstad B, Smevik B. (2004) Abnormal systemic venous connection possibly associated with a persistent right umbilical vein; a case report. *BMC Pediatrics*, **4**, 7.

20

Anomalies of Atrial Septation

Darren Hutchinson[1] *and Lisa Hornberger*[2]

[1] *Department of Cardiology, Royal Children's Hospital Melbourne, Victoria, Australia*
[2] *University of Alberta; Section Head of Pediatric Echocardiography, Stollery Children's Hospital, Edmonton, Alberta, Canada*

A communication between the left and right atrium, an atrial septal defect (ASD), is the third most common form of congenital heart disease [1]. While isolated ASDs are common, ASDs are even more commonly seen in conjunction with other structural heart defects. This chapter reviews isolated ASDs.

Background and Anatomy

The actual reported incidence of ASDs varies significantly depending on what definition is used, especially if you include patent foramen ovale.

In fetal life, the foramen ovale has an essential role in distributing blood from the right atrium to the left heart. The Eustachian valve preferentially streams the most highly oxygenated blood entering the right atrium to the left atrium via the foramen ovale. In studies using transesophageal echocardiogram and agitated saline, a patent foramen ovale is seen in up to 10% of adults [2]. Fetal diagnosis of pathological ASDs are possible, especially in primum defects, but is limited because of the uniform presence of the patent foramen ovale.

ASDs can be divided into four main groups: ostium secundum, ostium primum, sinus venosus, and coronary sinus defects (Figure 20.1). Ostium secundum defects are the most common form of ASD and account for at least two-thirds of all ASDs with a prevalence of 10.3 per 10 000 births [1]. Secundum ASDs form as a consequence of a defect in the ovale fossa and may be single or represent multiple fenestrations in the septum primum (Figure 20.2). Sinus venosus defects occur most commonly near the superior vena cava (SVC) entry to the right atrium, but can also be seen associated with the inferior vena cava (Figure 20.3). Superior sinus venosus defects are usually associated with abnormal drainage of the right upper pulmonary vein to either the SVC or the right atrium itself, and inferior sinus venosus defects are often associated with anomalous drainage of the right low pulmonary vein. Coronary sinus defects are rare and occur as a consequence of a defect in the roof of the coronary sinus. Finally, ostium primum defects are related to partial or complete atrioventricular septal defects (Figure 20.4) and although mentioned briefly here are discussed in detail in Chapter 22.

Secundum ASD appears to be more frequent with lower gestational age, lower birth weight, and intrauterine growth restriction [3]. Associated chromosomal anomalies, including trisomy 21, are seen in 6–14% [3]. Other syndromes also seen in association with isolated secundum ASD including VACTERL, Holt–Oram syndrome, and 22Q deletion.

Neonatal Presentation

Diagnosis of an isolated ASD in the neonatal period is exceedingly rare unless it is an incidental finding on echocardiogram performed for another indication. Even in the presence of moderate to large ASDs, the majority of affected patients remain asymptomatic for many years or even decades. The compliant right atrium, along with the normally elevated right ventricular and pulmonary artery pressures in the neonatal period, mean the left to right shunt at atrial level is often hemodynamically insignificant in the newborn. Even if present, volume loading of the right ventricle is generally well tolerated. In the setting of severe pulmonary hypertension such as persistent pulmonary hypertension of the newborn (PPHN), an ASD may shunt right to left causing the newborn to be cyanosed. Rarely, some children may become symptomatic in the first few years of life but generally not until 3–4 years of age at the earliest. Possible symptoms include poor weight gain, mild shortness of breath on exertion, and predisposition to respiratory infections.

Clinical examination in the neonatal period from an isolated ASD would almost always be normal. In later

Visual Guide to Neonatal Cardiology, First Edition. Edited by Ernerio T. Alboliras, Ziyad M. Hijazi, Leo Lopez, and Donald J. Hagler.

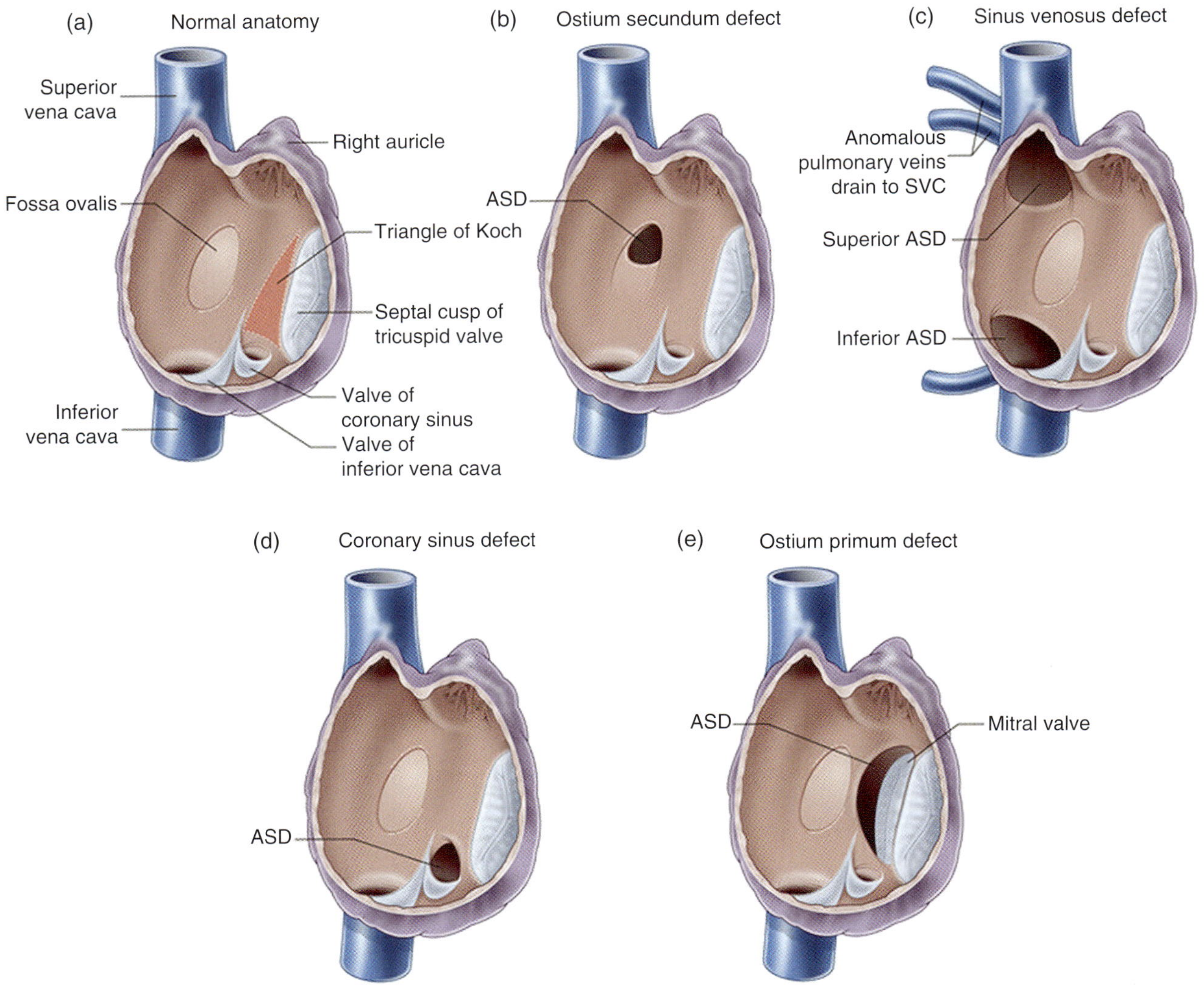

Figure 20.1 (a) Normal atrial septal anatomy looking from the right atrial aspect. The fossa ovalis, a normal structure, is seen covered by the flap valve that is held open in fetal life. (b) Secundum atrial septal defect (ASD) forms as a consequence of a defect in the fossa ovalis. Note the ovale shape of the defect, which means measurement of the defect should be performed in multiple planes when imaging. (c) Sinus venosus ASDs occur related to the superior vena cava (superior ASD) or inferior vena cava (inferior ASD). Anomalous drainage of right-sided pulmonary veins is common with anomalous veins draining to the SVC shown in this image. (d) Coronary sinus ASD seen intimately related to the mouth of the coronary sinus. The left atrium (not shown) is where there will be varying degrees of unroofing of the coronary sinus also. (e) Ostium primum ASD occurs immediately above the atrioventricular valves and may be part of the partial or complete atrioventricular septal defect.

childhood, clinical findings may reveal a wide and fixed splitting of the second heart sound. An ejection systolic murmur may be heard from increased flow across a normal pulmonary valve and a soft mid-diastolic murmur may be heard from increased flow across a normal tricuspid valve.

Chest X-ray can show mild cardiomegaly with right atrial enlargement, prominence of the main pulmonary artery, and, rarely, increased pulmonary vascular markings. Features on electrocardiogram include first degree heart block, a 'pseudo' right bundle branch block (secondary to prolonged repolarization of the dilated RV), abnormal P wave access (especially in sinus venous defects), rightward axis, and right ventricular hypertrophy.

Two-dimensional echocardiography combined with color Doppler aims to define the position, including the length of the septal rims, size, and hemodynamic effect of an ASD. Assessment of all parts of intracardiac anatomy is essential at first diagnosis to exclude associated congenital heart disease. As ASDs are seldom anatomically round defects, ASDs need to be assessed in multiple imaging planes to assess their size correctly. The same rule is true when assessing the rims of the ASD which needs to include views of the inferior, anterior (aortic), IVC and SVC rims. Hemodynamic significance

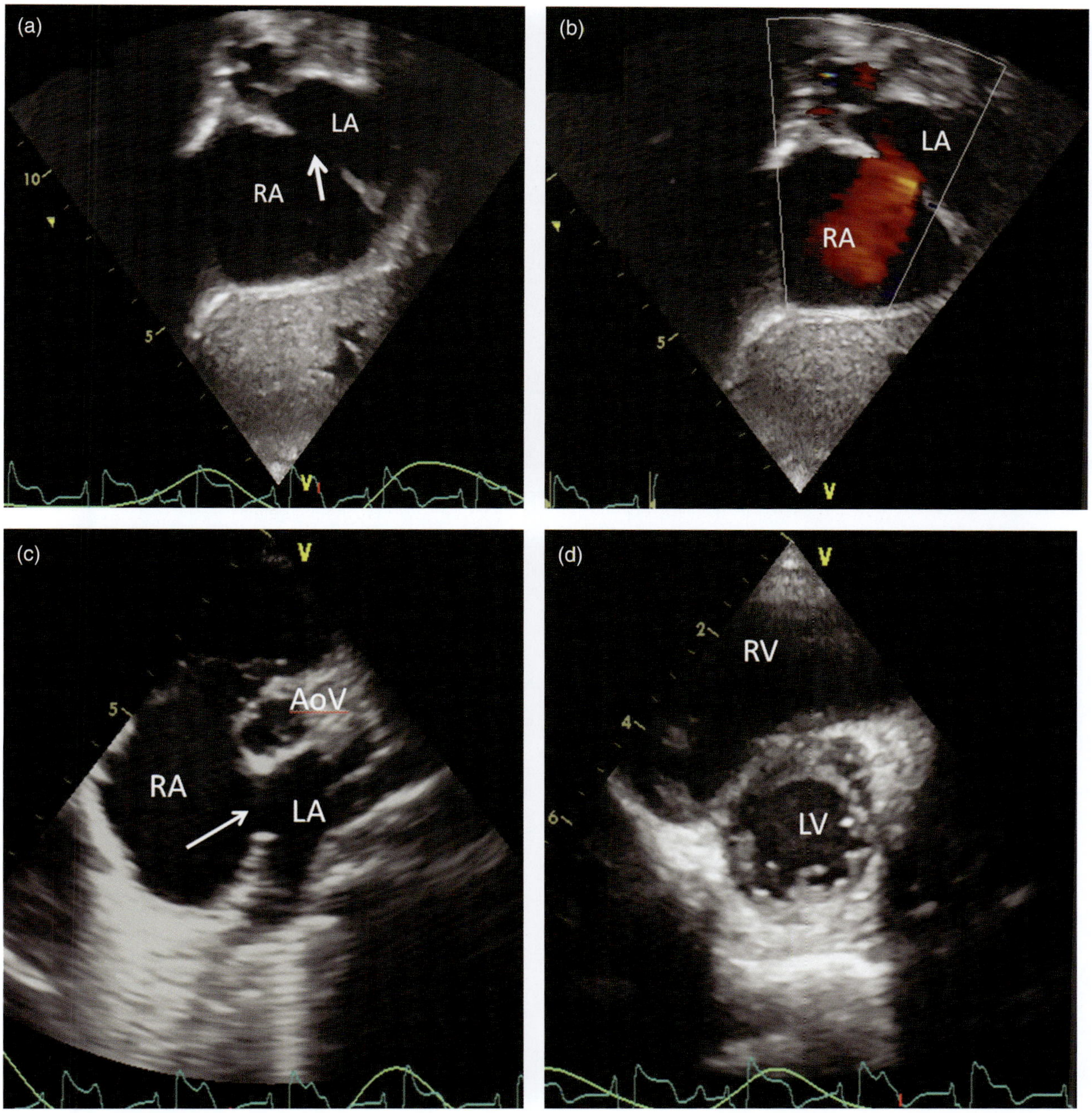

Figure 20.2 Secundum ASD. (a) Subcostal image demonstrating a central appearing large secundum ASD (arrow). (b) By color flow mapping, the patency of the ASD and the left to right shunt (arrow) can be seen. (c) In a parasternal short axis view of the same patient, the secundum ASD (arrow) can be clearly seen positioned immediately behind the aorta, thus suggesting little anterior rim and a fairly good-sized posterior rim. (d) Right ventricular (RV) dilation and diastolic septal flattening in the parasternal short axis image confirm the hemodynamic importance of the ASD with RV volume overload. AoV; aortic valve; LA, left atrium; LV, left ventricle; RA, right atrium; RV, right ventricle.

may be indicated by right atrial and right ventricular enlargement, increased pulmonary valve flow velocity, and dilation of the main pulmonary artery. Assessment for leak of the AV valves is important in primum ASDs.

In some cases, additional imaging with either cardiac magnetic resonance imaging (MRI) or computed tomography (CT) may be required to fully define the ASD anatomy and pulmonary venous drainage; this is most frequently true of sinus venosus ASD.

Management and Treatment Options

It is important to recognize that most secundum ASDs found in neonates will close spontaneously. A study of

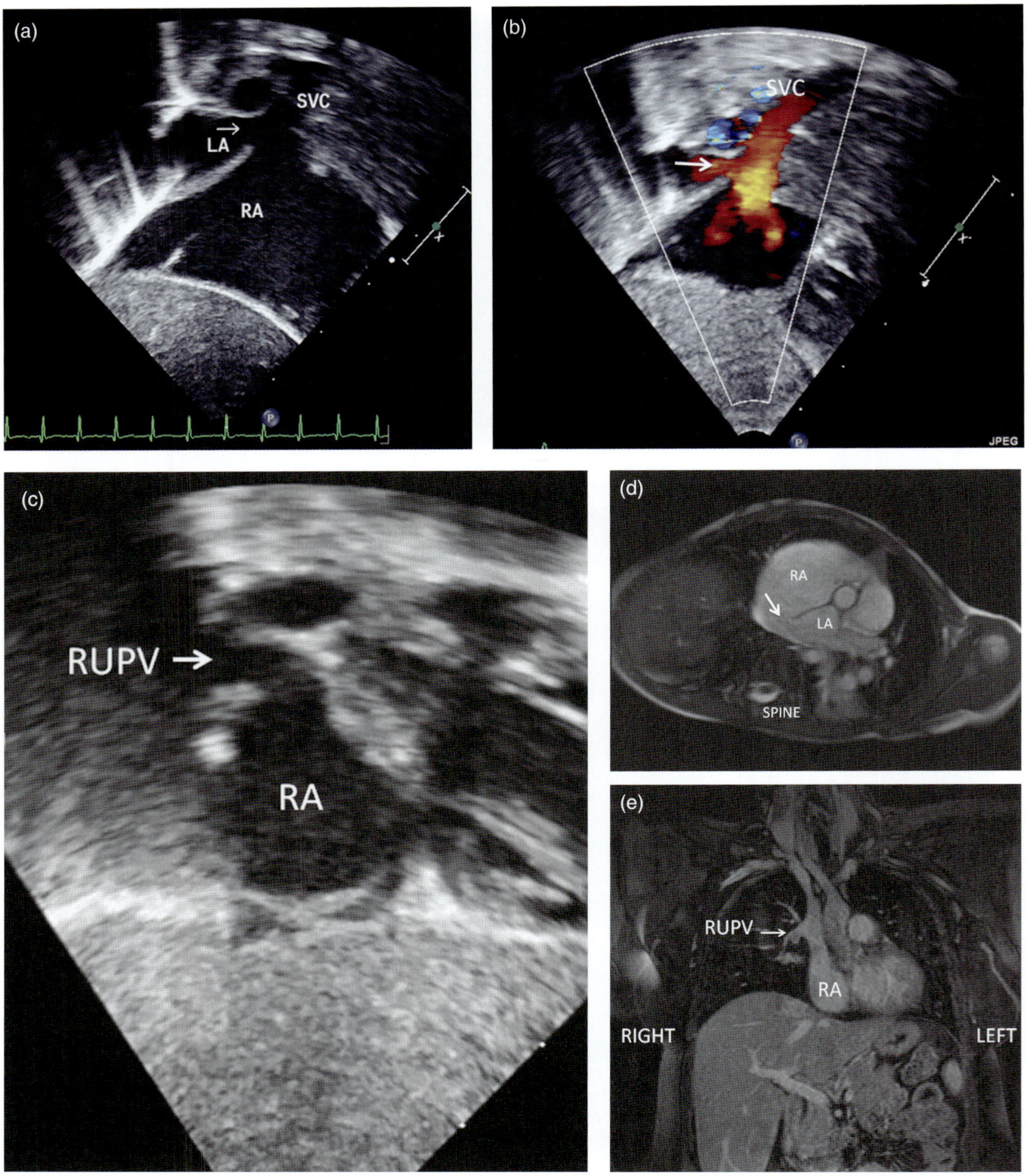

Figure 20.3 Sinus venosus ASD. (a) Subcostal echo image demonstrating a superior sinus venosus ASD (arrow) just beneath the superior vena cava (SVC). (b) Color flow mapping confirms the presence of the atrial level shunt (arrow) which courses from right atrium (RA) to left atrium (LA). (c) Further two-dimensional image, sweeping from the SVC inferiorly, the anomalous connection of the right upper pulmonary vein (RUPV) into the SVC at the RA–SVC junction. (d) Magnetic resonance angiography in an axial view through the chest confirms the presence of a superior and posterior sinus venosus ASD (arrow). (e) Anomalous RUPV can be quite difficult to see consistently by echocardiography but their connection with the SVC can be confirmed by MRI as shown in this coronal view through the chest.

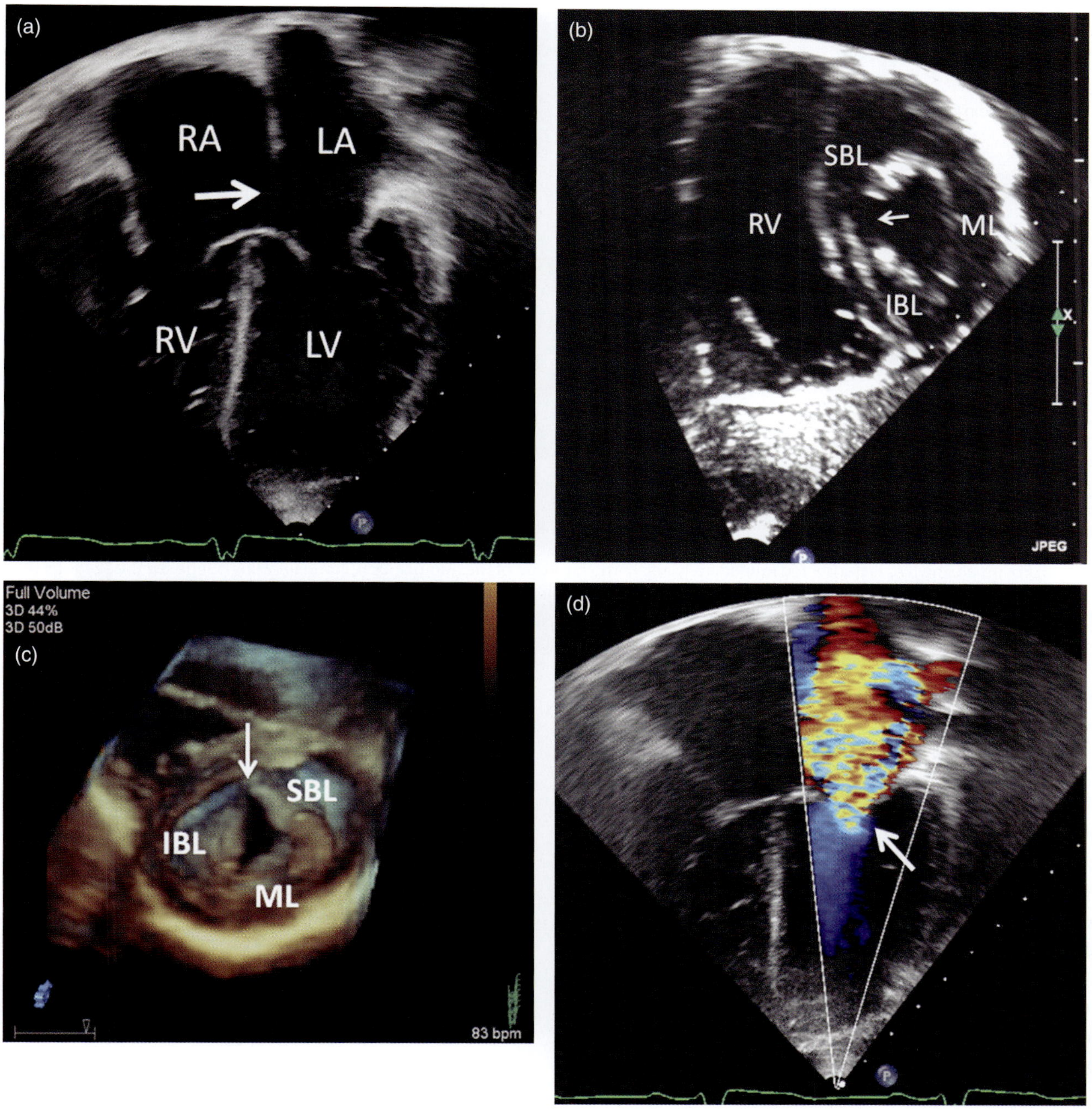

Figure 20.4 Primum ASD. (a) An echocardiographic four chamber view that demonstrates the atrioventricular (AV) valves hinging at the same level with a defect in the atrial septum just above the AV valves. This defect is a primum ASD. (b) The presence of a cleft in the left AV valve (arrow) as shown in this subcostal short-axis image is a critical component for the diagnosis of a primum ASD. The three left AV valve leaflets include the superior bridging leaflet (SBL), the inferior bridging leaflet (IBL), and the mural leaflet (ML), with a cleft between the SBL and IBL. (c) The anatomy of the left AV valve is even better demonstrated by three-dimensional echocardiography as shown in this image demonstrated as if one were looking up from the left ventricular apex. (d) As is true for many affected patients, there is often left AV valve insufficiency (arrow), which usually stems from the cleft between the SBL and IBL.

101 infants diagnosed with secundum ASD prior to 3 months showed spontaneous closure in 87%, with all defects <3 mm closing at follow-up [4]. Only defects with a diameter of >8 mm were shown not to close on their own.

Although it is extremely rare for an ASD to need treatment in the neonatal period, it is important to be aware of treatment strategies in later childhood and beyond. Routine follow-up for neonates found to have a moderate or large secundum ASD, ≥3 mm, should be offered annually, and include clinical assessment and echocardiography. All patients with ASDs other than secundum type should also be followed.

If a patient were found to be symptomatic with a small ASD, <8 mm, first line medical therapy with diuretics could be considered. The aim would be to reduce

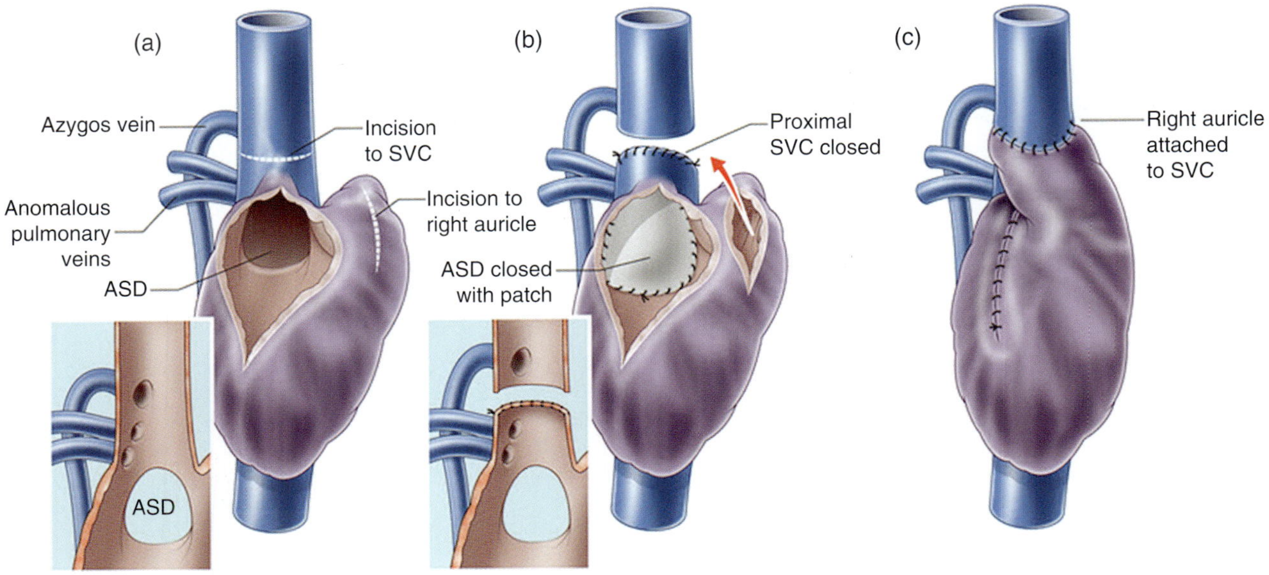

Figure 20.5 Sinus venosus ASD repair. (a) Superior sinus venosus ASD intimately related to the SVC entrance into the right atrium. Anomalous drainage of right-sided pulmonary veins to the SVC (inset). The azygous vein is seen entering the SVC above the anomalous veins. (b) For repair, the SVC is transected immediately above the insertion of the anomalous pulmonary veins but below the azygous vein. The auricle of the right atrium is opened and the ASD is patched, baffling the anomalous right-sided pulmonary veins from the right to the left atrium. (c) The SVC is anastomosed to the right atrial auricle.

symptoms to allow either spontaneous closure of the defect or dilation of the defect to facilitate device closure. Endocarditis prophylaxis is not indicated for an isolated ASD.

The aim of closure of an ASD is first to ameloriate symptoms and secondly to avoid the potential risk of causing irreversible pulmonary hypertension. The aim is generally to offer closure to patients whose Qp : Qs is thought clinically to be above 1.5 : 1, generally those with right atrium and/or right ventricle dilation.

For hemodynamically significant secundum ASDs, the current treatment of choice is device closure via cardiac catheterization just before school age (2–5 years). Success rates, compared with surgical repair, are equal, with a lower complication rate and a shorter duration of hospitalization [5]. In certain cases where the secundum ASD is particularly large, the patient is particularly small, or the rims on which to anchor the device are deficient, surgical repair will be chosen.

Surgical repair is the treatment of choice for ostium primum, sinus venosus, and coronary sinus ASDs. Closure of sinus venosus ASDs is a challenge as a consequence of the presence of anomalous pulmonary veins. Use of the "Warden procedure," with transection of the distal SVC (above the anomalous veins), baffling of the anomalous veins to the left atrium, and then attachment of the SVC to the right atrial appendage is currently the treatment of choice (Figure 20.5).

References

1 Reller MD, Strickland MJ, Riehle-Colarusso T, *et al.* (2008) Prevalence of congenital heart defects in metropolitan Atlanta, 1998–2005. *J Pediatr*, **153**, 807–813.

2 Fisher D, Fisher E, Budd J, Rosen S, Goldman M. (1995) The incidence of patent foramen ovale in 1,000 consecutive patients: a contrast transesophageal echocardiogram study. *Chest*, **107** (6), 1504–1509.

3 Ferencz C, Loffredo CA, Correa-Villasenor A, Wilson PD, eds. (1997) Atrial septal defect, in, *Genetic and Environmental Risk Factors of Major Cardiovascular Malformations: The Baltimore-Washington Infant Study 1981–1989*, Futura, Armonk, NY, pp. 267–283.

4 Radzik D, Davignon A, van Doesburg N, *et al.* (1993) Predictive factors for spontaneous closure of atrial septal defects diagnosed in the first 3 months of life. *J Am Coll Cardiol*, **22** (3), 851–853.

5 Du Z, Hijazi Z, Kleinman C, Silverman N, Larntz K. (2002) Comparison between transcatheter and surgical closure of secundum atrial septal defect in children and adults: results of a multicenter nonrandomized trial. *J Am Coll Cardiol*, **39** (11), 1836–1844. doi: 10.1016/S0735-1097(02)01862-4.

21

Atrial Chamber Obstruction

Lisa Hornberger

University of Alberta; Section Head of Pediatric Echocardiography, Stollery Children's Hospital, Edmonton, Alberta, Canada

Obstruction within the atrial chambers is a rare form of congenital heart disease. When present, intra-atrial obstruction has the potential to produce significant symptoms and even collapse in the neonatal period. Here we discuss left intra-atrial obstruction in the form of cor triatriatum sinister, and briefly mention the even more rare right-sided intra-atrial obstruction, cor triatriatum dexter.

Cor Triatriatum Sinister

Background and Anatomy

Cor triatriatum sinister accounts for only 0.1% of all congenital heart defects [1]. The embryologic basis of cor triatriatum is still not fully understood, with multiple theories being proposed but none agreed upon.

In all cases, there is a fibromuscular division within the left atrium resulting in two distinct chambers. There is a distal chamber, which usually receives blood from the pulmonary veins, and a proximal chamber, which delivers blood to the mitral valve and left ventricle. There is generally a communication between the two chambers via a defect in the fibromuscular division (Figure 21.1a and 21.2a,b). The size of the communication between the two chambers is directly related to symptoms and presentation.

In approximately 60% of cases, there is communication between the left and right atrium, usually between the right atrium and proximal left atrial chamber [2]. In approximately 50% of patients, additional cardiac anomalies are present. Commonly associated heart lesions include persistent left superior vena cava, total or partial anomalous pulmonary venous drainage (TAPVD or PAPVD), and ventricular septal defects.

Neonatal Presentation

In two large review studies, the mean age at diagnosis was 7 months of age [2, 3]. Importantly, 25% of patients with cor triatriatum presented in the neonatal period [2]. In this same study, a further 28% presented within the first year of life.

Presentation is directly related to the size of the communication between the proximal and distal chambers in the left atrium. Other cardiac defects, when present, also affect the timing and severity of presentation. The presenting features stem mostly from left atrial hypertension with pulmonary edema of varying severity. Typical presenting features in the neonatal period include tachypnea, tachycardia, poor feeding with failure to thrive, and possible cyanosis [1–3]. Reduced cardiac output from left ventricular inflow obstruction is also possible [3].

Physical examination may reveal a right ventricular heave and on auscultation a loud P2 may be heard. Infants will usually be normally saturated with this condition and should respond, to some degree, to oxygen therapy if required (in contrast to TAPVD). Many of the presenting features share common ground with TAPVD.

Investigations to Make the Diagnosis

Chest X-ray will show cardiomegaly with features of left atrial hypertension and pulmonary venous obstruction in most patients who present in the neonatal period. Electrocardiography may show an exaggerated rightward cardiac axis, more than is usual for the newborn.

Neonatal echocardiography is now the gold standard for diagnosis of cor triatriatum. The aim of echocardiography is to both make the diagnosis of cor triatriatum and to assess for other associated congenital heart lesions. B-mode, color Doppler, and pulsed wave Doppler are essential in the assessment of cor triatriatum. More recently, three-dimensional echocardiography has been used to more clearly define the anatomy and spacial relationships. Particular attention is paid to assessing pulmonary venous connections, the presence of an atrial septal defect as well as the size of and flow across the connection between the proximal and distal chambers.

Visual Guide to Neonatal Cardiology, First Edition. Edited by Ernerio T. Alboliras, Ziyad M. Hijazi, Leo Lopez, and Donald J. Hagler.

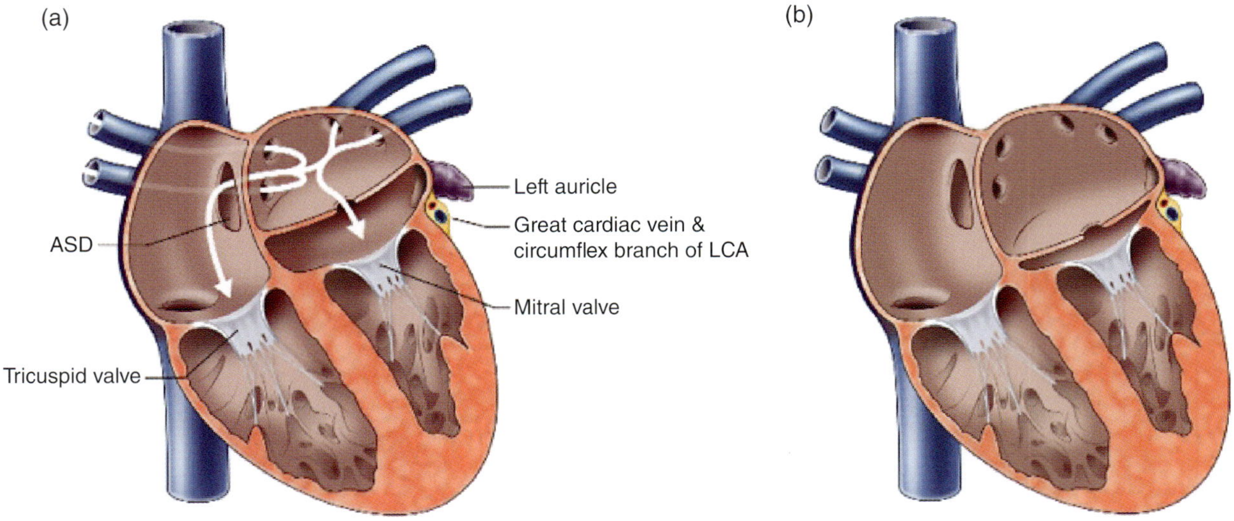

Figure 21.1 Diagrams demonstrating cor triatriatum sinister and supramitral ring. (a) Cor triatriatum sinister with fibromuscular division within the left atrium which is above the left auricle. An atrial septal defect (ASD) is seen between the left atrial distal chamber receiving the pulmonary venous return and the right atrium. A defect is seen within the fibromuscular ridge allows some blood to pass from the distal to proximal left atrial chamber and then through the mitral valve. LCA, left coronary artery. (b) Supramitral ring (SMR) is a fibromuscular membrane closely adherent to the mitral valve on the atrial side. This rarely presents in the neonatal period but is a differential diagnosis to cor triatriatum sinister.

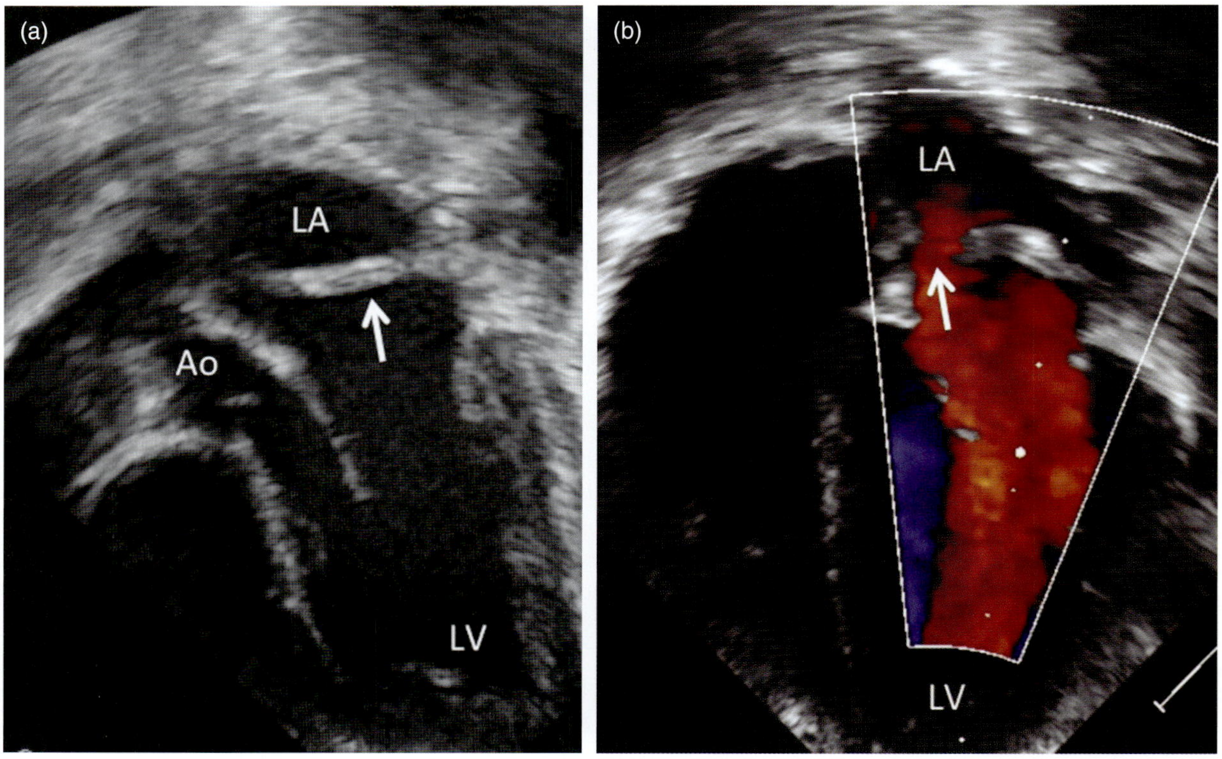

Figure 21.2 Echocardiography images demonstrating cor triatriatum sinister. (a) Anatomic features of cor triatriatum as seen from a "five chamber" view. The thick fibromuscular membrane within the left atrium is seen (arrow) dividing the left atrium into two chambers. (b) Using color flow mapping, the defect within the fibromuscular membrane is seen with flow between the distal and proximal chamber seen (arrow). Ao, aorta; LA, left atrium; LV, left ventricle.

Echocardiography should also be able to distinguish cor triatriatum sinister from a supramitral ring (Figure 21.1b). In supramitral ring there is a fibromuscular membrane adherent to the atrial side of the mitral valve. The obstruction is below the level of the atrial appendage which differs from cor triatriatum sinister where the obstruction is above the atrial appendage. Supramitral ring is typically a progressive lesion associated with other left heart obstructive lesions including other forms of mitral stenosis and coarctation, and is not a cardiac lesion seen in the newborn period.

In the current era the need for cardiac catheterization with angiography in cor triatriatum is unusual, especially for patients diagnosed in the neonatal period.

The presence of extracardiac anomalies in cor triatriatum is seen in up to one-third of patients [3], with chromosomal abnormalities seen in 12% [3].

Other diagnoses to consider in the differential include TAPVD, isolated pulmonary vein stenosis, and congenital mitral stenosis. All of these conditions should be distinguishable on echocardiography.

Management

Symptomatic medical management, such as diuretic therapy, may be used until surgical repair is performed. Definitive surgical correction of the defect is the treatment of choice and carries very low morbidity and mortality in experienced centers [2, 3]. Surgery should be performed soon after the diagnosis is made and may need to be performed as an emergency if there is significant decompensation. Surgical repair is via median sternotomy and is usually performed through a right atrial approach [2]. The obstructive membrane is resected and the procedure is curative.

Cor Triatriatum Dexter

Cor triatriatum dexter involves division within the right atrium and is an even rarer form of congenital heart disease than cor triatriatum sinister [1]. The basis of cor triatriatum dexter is from persistence of embryonic venous valve tissue that usually regresses during late fetal life (Figure 21.3a,b) [5]. In postnatal life, remnants of these valves can be seen as the Eustachian valve, Thebesian valve, and crista terminalis [5].

Persistence of right atrial venous valve tissue can cause varying degrees of obstruction to right ventricular inflow (Figure 21.4). The venous valve tissue may be significantly fenestrated, such as with a Chiari network of the right atrium, or may be nearly intact causing significant obstruction to right ventricular inflow. Interestingly, an intact membrane is usually seen when associated with pulmonary or tricuspid atresia and as such the obstruction is of little hemodynamic significance in these cases. If there is patent right ventricular inflow and outflow, then the obstruction to right ventricular inflow and shunting of deoxygenated from the right to left atrium can cause neonatal cyanosis. Surgical repair is warranted in the newborn period and the type of

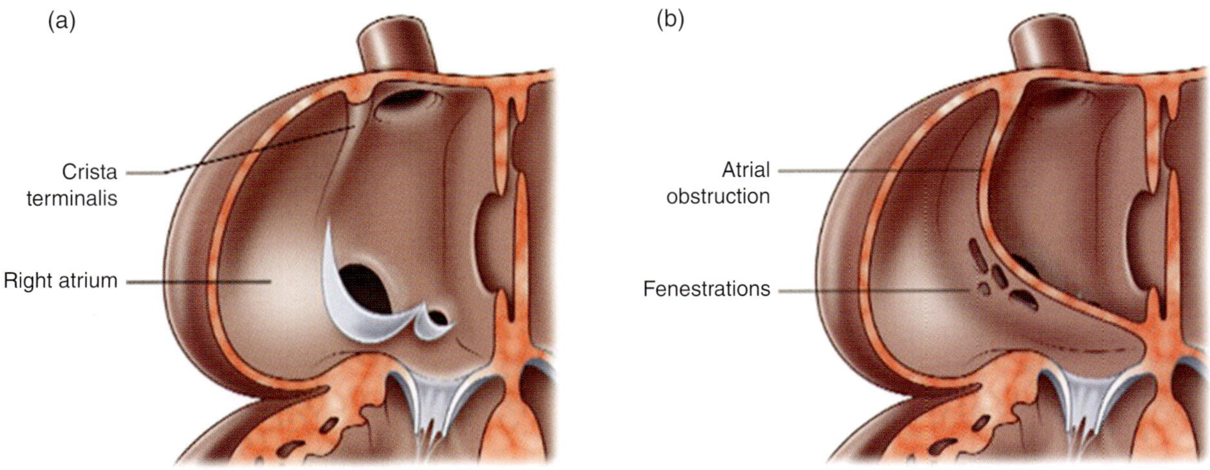

Figure 21.3 Diagram demonstrating the features of cor triatriatum dexter. (a) Normal embryonic venous valve tissue in the right atrium. The persistence of embryonic venous valve tissue in postnatal life can lead to development of right atrial chamber obstruction. (b) Obstructive tissue within the right atrium occurring between the systemic venous inflows (inferior and superior vena cava) and the tricuspid valve. Fenestration within this tissue allows varying degrees of flow from the systemic venous return to the tricuspid valve.

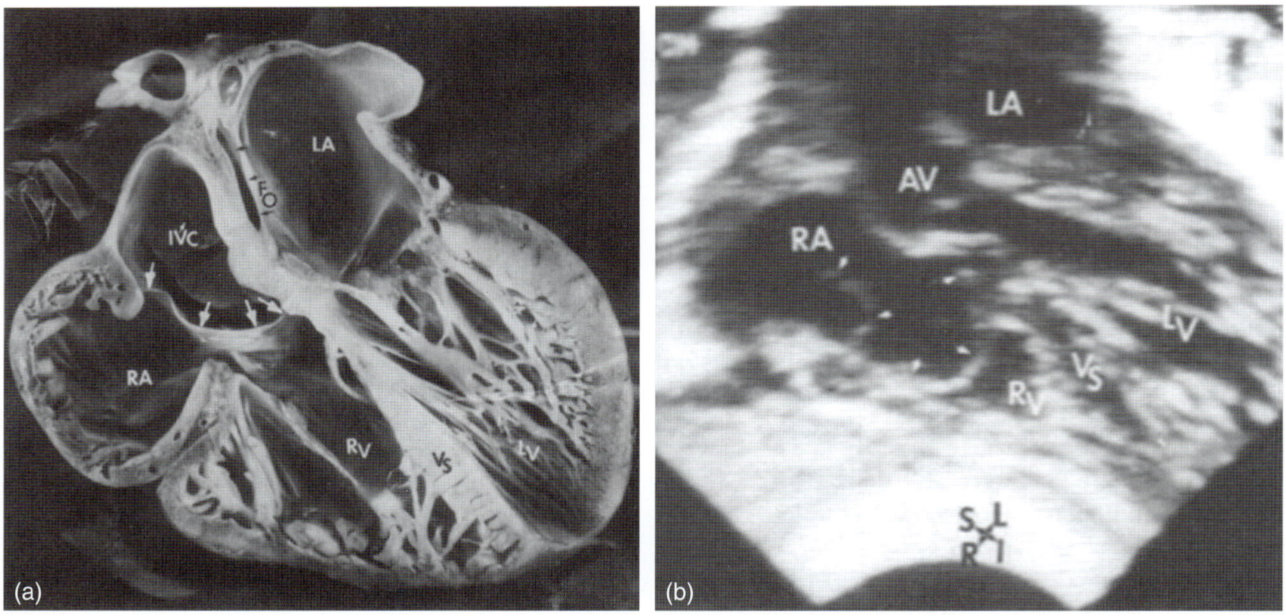

Figure 21.4 (a) Postmortem specimen bisected to simulate the subcostal four-chamber view (compare with Figure 20.5). The membrane (white arrows) divides the right atrial cavity in two. The smooth-walled portion of the right atrium. which receives the venae cavae is medial to the membrane whereas the pectinate muscles, atrial appendage (not seen) and tricuspid valve orifice are lateral. The lower portion of the membrane is shaped like a windsock and overlies the tricuspid valve orifice. Both ventricles have trabecular (spongy) apices. (b) Subcostal four-chamber echocardiographic view during systole. The echo-dense membrane (bordered by arrowheads) is within the right atrium, septating the atrium into two chambers. The inferior portion of the membrane is shaped like a windsock with its convexity facing the tricuspid valve. The right atrial portion medial to the membrane is distended with systemic venous blood entering the right atrium.

References

1 Anderson R, Redington RN. (2009) Division of atrial chambers, in, *Paediatric Cardiology*, 3rd edn (eds RH Anderson, EJ Baker, D Penny, *et al.*). Churchill Livingstone, Philadelphia, PA, pp. 547–552.

2 Alphonso N, Norgaard M, Newcomb A, *et al.* (2005) Cor triatriatum: presentation, diagnosis and long-term surgical results. *Ann Thorac Surg*, **80**, 1666–1671.

3 Humpl T, Reineker K, Manlhiot C, *et al.* (2010) Cor triatriatum sinistrum in childhood: a single institution's experience. *Can J Cardiol*, **26** (7), 371–376.

4 Konstantinov I, Yun TJ, Calderone C, Coles JG. (2004) Supramitral obstruction of left ventricular inflow tract by supramitral ring. *Oper Tech Thorac Cardiovasc Surg*, **9** (3), 247–251.

5 Trento A, Zuberbuhler JR, Anderson RH, Park SC, Siewers RD. (1988) Divided right atrium (prominence of the Eustachian and Thebesian valves). *J Thorac Cardiovasc Surg*, **96**, 457–463.

22

Common Atrioventricular Canal Defects

Meryl S. Cohen, MD

Division of Cardiology, The Children's Hospital of Philadelphia; Perelman School of Medicine, University of Pennsylvania, Philadelphia, PA, USA

Pathophysiology

Common atrioventricular canal (CAVC) describes a cluster of cardiac defects with an atrioventricular (AV) septal defect and abnormal development of the AV valves typically resulting in a common inlet into both ventricles [1]. In embryologic development, CAVC results from failed fusion of the endocardial cushions that form the canal portion of the atrial and ventricular septum along with the AV valves [2]. CAVC defects, also known as AV septal defects, are associated with trisomy 21 (Down syndrome) [3] and heterotaxy syndrome.

CAVC presents an anatomic and physiologic continuum from a primary atrial to a primary ventricular communication. Though absent AV septum occurs in all forms of the defect, the AV valve position dictates the size of the atrial and ventricular communications [4, 5]. Complete CAVC includes a large atrial septal defect (ASD) adjacent to the AV valves, a large posterior (inlet) ventricular septal defect (VSD) (Figure 22.1), and a common AV valve (Figure 22.2). The common AV valve has two leaflets crossing the defect superiorly (superior bridging leaflet) and inferiorly (inferior bridging leaflet). Incomplete (or partial) CAVC, also known as ostium primum ASD, is characterized by an atrial communication without a VSD component because the AV valve is adherent to the ventricular septum (Figures 22.3 and 22.4). In incomplete CAVC, there are two AV valve openings with a common annulus. There is never a normal tricuspid and mitral valve, and it is more appropriate to use the terms right and left AV valves here. The left AV valve has a "cleft" which is the commissure between the superior and inferior bridging leaflets where they meet at the ventricular septum (Figures 22.5 and 22.6) [4, 5]. Some cases (called transitional CAVC) have a large ASD with a small restrictive VSD through chordal attachments that are adherent to the crest of the ventricular septum. AV valve regurgitation in the setting of all forms of CAVC is common (Figure 22.7).

The relationship of the atrial and ventricular septum to the common AV valve may be evenly distributed or malaligned to one chamber or the other. Atrial septal malalignment results in a double outlet atrium (Figure 22.8). Ventricular septal malalignment occurs more frequently with the common AV valve opening more into one ventricle. Here, the contralateral ventricle is often hypoplastic (Figure 22.9), causing problems when considering biventricular repair [6, 7].

Associated lesions include tetralogy of Fallot, patent ductus arteriosus, coarctation of the aorta, and left ventricular (LV) outflow tract obstruction.

Clinical Manifestation

CAVC can be diagnosed in fetal life (Figure 22.10). Unless there is significant AV valve regurgitation, most fetuses with these defects have an uneventful gestation. Severe common AV valve regurgitation increases the risk for hydrops fetalis. If CAVC is suspected in utero, genetic testing should be performed to exclude Down syndrome.

CAVC and its variants are typically quiescent in newborns. The clinical course depends on the amount of atrial and ventricular shunting, AV valve regurgitation, the degree of malalignment if present, and other associated lesions. In complete CAVC, the VSD is large and unrestrictive with systemic right ventricular (RV) and pulmonary artery pressures; left-to-right shunting is almost exclusively determined by the pulmonary vascular resistance with the shunt increasing over the first 6–8 weeks of life. Symptoms of congestive heart failure including growth failure, respiratory symptoms, difficulty eating, and tachycardia are common.

When the ASD is the primary lesion (incomplete CAVC), the amount of left-to-right shunt is determined by the relative compliance of the RV and LV. The consequence of atrial shunting is dilation of the right atrium,

Visual Guide to Neonatal Cardiology, First Edition. Edited by Ernerio T. Alboliras, Ziyad M. Hijazi, Leo Lopez, and Donald J. Hagler.

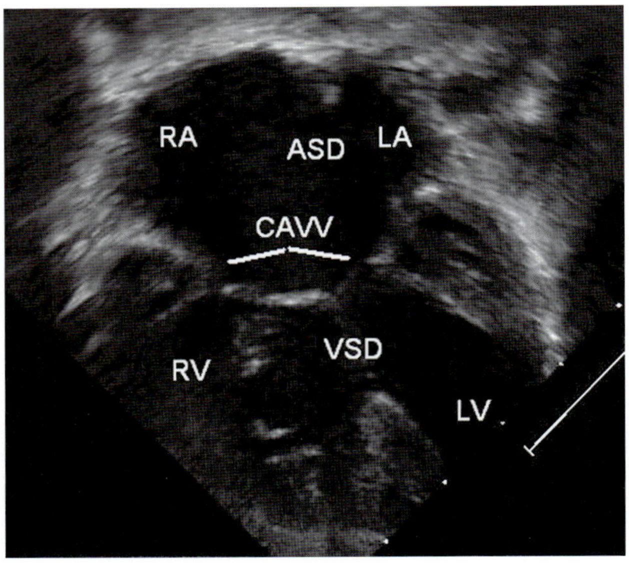

Figure 22.1 Apical four-chamber view of a complete common atrioventricular canal with a large atrial septal defect (ASD) and large ventricular septal defect (VSD) and a common atrioventricular valve (in the closed position). CAVV, common atrioventricular valve; LA, left atrium; LV, left ventricle; RA, right atrium; RV, right ventricle.

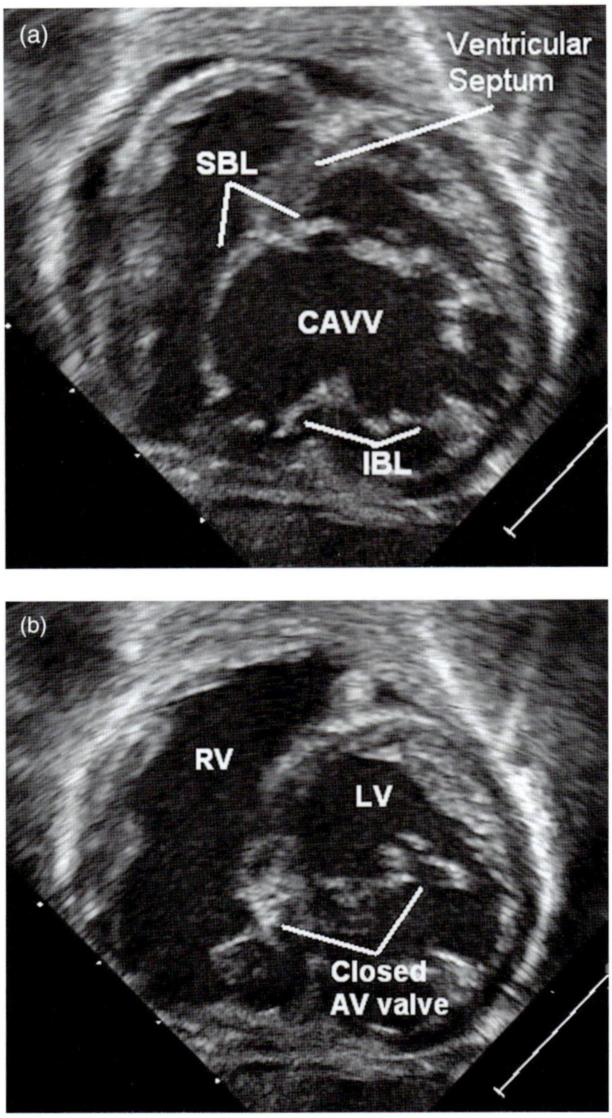

Figure 22.2 (a) Subxiphoid left anterior oblique view of a patient with complete common atrioventricular canal with a common atrioventricular valve (CAVV) seen straddling the ventricular septum in the open position. Note the superior bridging leaflet (SBL) and inferior bridging leaflet (IBL) crossing the ventricular septum. (b) Same view of the complete common atrioventricular canal with the CAVV in the closed position demonstrating the leaflets crossing the ventricular septum. LV, left ventricle; RV, right ventricle.

RV, and pulmonary arteries. Most children are initially asymptomatic, but failure to thrive and respiratory symptoms can occur. AV valve regurgitation, if significant, can cause chamber dilation and symptoms of heart failure.

CAVC requires surgery. If unrepaired, early death is likely. In complete CAVC, pulmonary vascular disease can occur within the first year of life. The restrictive VSD in transitional CAVC can close spontaneously with AV valve tissue; however, the ostium primum ASD and the large inlet VSD do not typically close without surgery. Children with Down syndrome and CAVC are at higher risk for pulmonary vascular disease [8].

Investigations

Echocardiography is the primary imaging modality used to diagnose CAVC. Fetal diagnosis is readily made at 18–20 weeks' gestation (Figure 22.10). After birth, two-dimensional imaging provides anatomic detail of all components of CAVC, and color and spectral Doppler techniques highlight flow across the ASD and VSD, severity of AV valve regurgitation, and presence of a patent ductus arteriosus. Three-dimensional echocardiography can augment standard imaging by highlighting details of AV valve anatomy and function (Figure 22.11) [9]. Transesophageal echocardiography is often used for patients undergoing surgical repair and those with suboptimal transthoracic windows and/or inconclusive diagnosis. Cardiac magnetic resonance (CMR) imaging can delineate anatomic features difficult to visualize by echocardiography such as pulmonary venous connections and coronary artery anatomy, but it is rarely required for diagnosis, particularly in neonates with good echocardiographic windows. CMR can also measure shunts and AV valve regurgitant fractions. Rarely, preoperative cardiac catheterization is performed to measure pulmonary vascular resistance if there is concern.

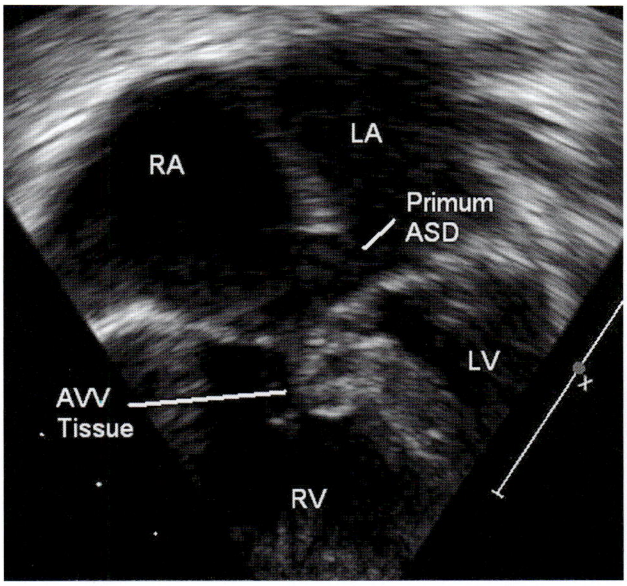

Figure 22.3 Apical four-chamber view of an incomplete common atrioventricular canal. The ostium primum atrial septal defect is seen. There is atrioventricular (AVV) tissue adherent to the ventricular septum closing off the ventricular septal defect component such that shunting only occurs at the atrial level. ASD, atrial septal defect; AVV, atrioventricular; LA, left atrium; LV, left ventricle; RA, right atrium; RV, right ventricle.

Management

CAVC requires surgery to repair the defect(s). In complete CAVC, surgery is performed when heart failure symptoms occur (generally at 2–6 months of age). Surgery for complete CAVC entails closure of the ASD and VSD along with division and resuspension of the AV valve [10]. The left-sided cleft is often surgically closed to prevent regurgitation (Figure 22.12). Those with transitional or incomplete (partial) CAVC do not require surgery until early childhood (1–4 years of age). Patch closure of the ASD is performed along with cleft closure of the left AV valve. Some children require re-operation, typically because of severe left AV valve regurgitation (Figure 22.13), residual ASD or VSD, or LV outflow tract obstruction (Figure 22.14) [11–13]. Complete heart block may occur, and pacemaker implantation may be necessary [14].

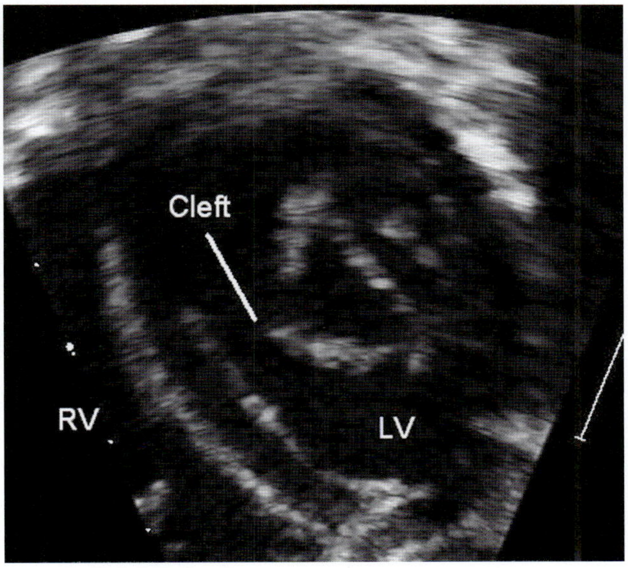

Figure 22.5 Subxiphoid view of an incomplete common atrioventricular canal with a "cleft" in the left atrioventricular valve. Note the vale is trifoliate rather than the normal mitral valve which is bifoliate. The so-called cleft is where the superior and inferior bridging leaflets meet at the ventricular septum. LV, left ventricle; RV, right ventricle.

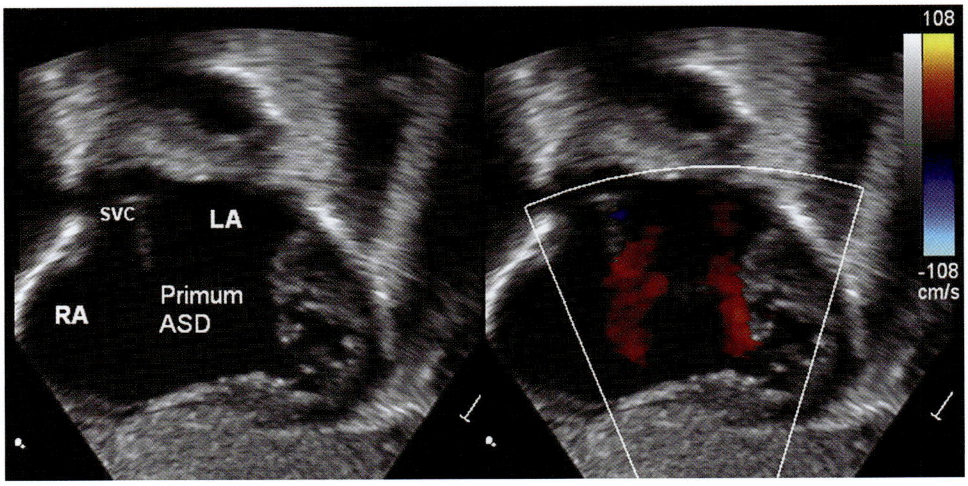

Figure 22.4 Subxiphoid view in color compare mode of a large ostium primum atrial septal defect in a patient with incomplete common atrioventricular canal. Left to right flow across the defect can ben seen (red flow seen on right side of panel). ASD, atrial septal defect; LA; left atrium; RA, right atrium; SVC, superior vena cava.

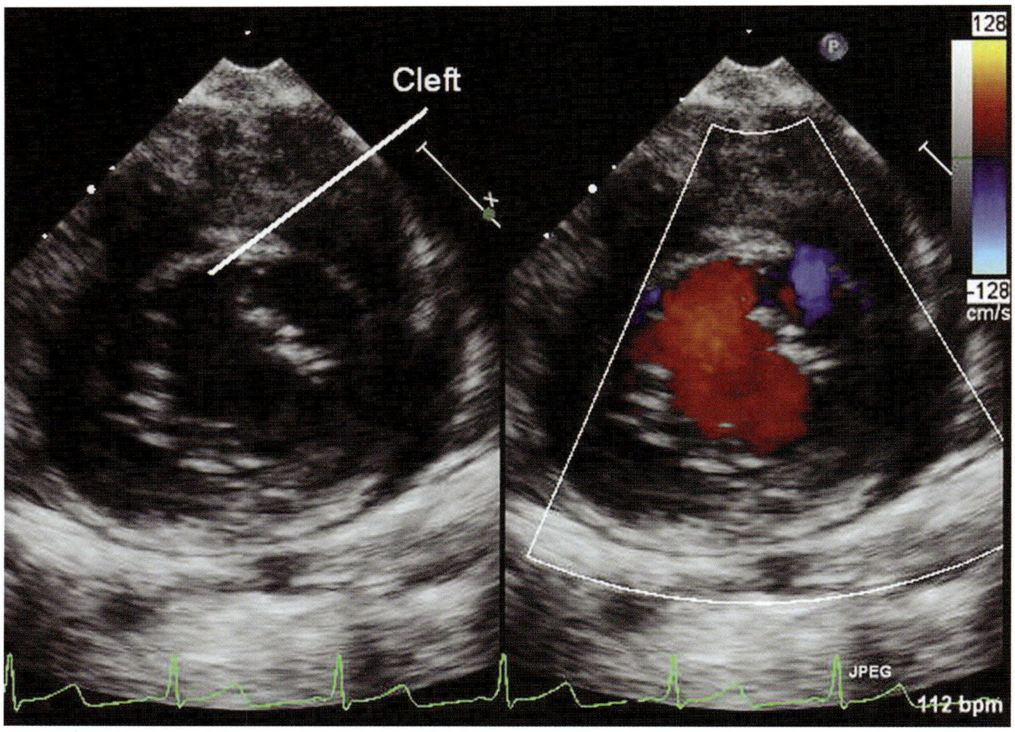

Figure 22.6 Parasternal short-axis view in color compare mode demonstrating the cleft in the left atrioventricular valve in a patient with incomplete common atrioventricular canal.

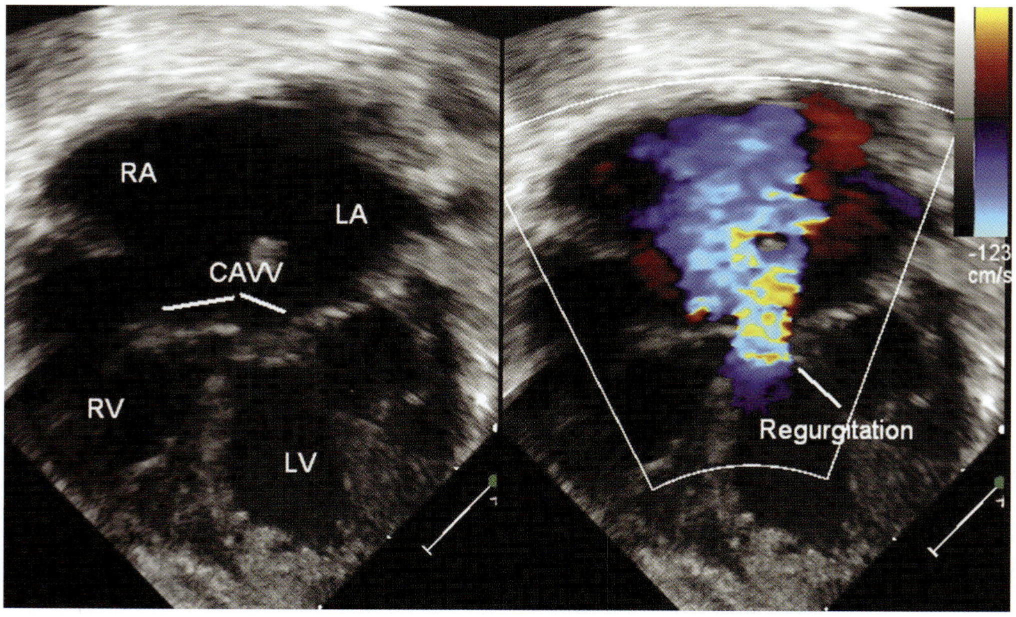

Figure 22.7 Apical four-chamber view of a complete common atrioventricular canal in color compare mode with the common atrioventricular valve in the closed position. Significant common atrioventricular valve regurgitation is seen into both atria. CAVV, common atrioventricular valve; LA, left atrium; LV, left ventricle; RA, right atrium; RV, right ventricle.

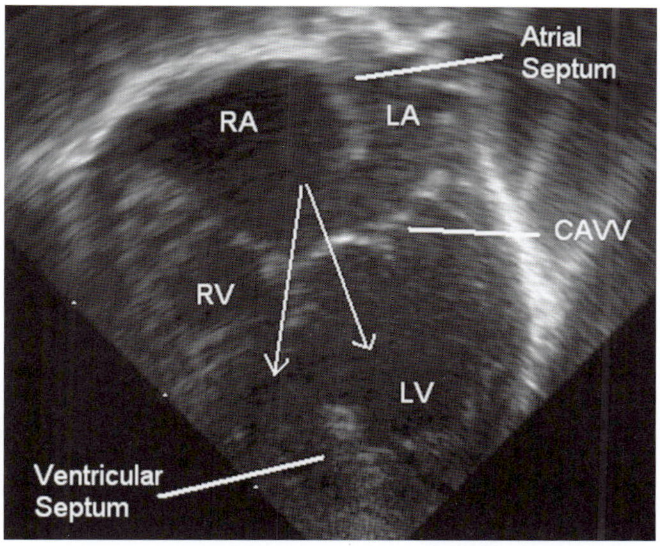

Figure 22.8 Apical four-chamber view of a patient with a malaligned atrial septum in the setting of complete common atrioventricular canal resulting in double outlet right atrium. Note the atrial septum is misaligned with the ventricular septum such that the right atrium (RA) can empty into both ventricles (white arrows). CAVV, common atrioventricular valve; LA, left atrium; LV, left ventricle; RA, right atrium; RV, right ventricle.

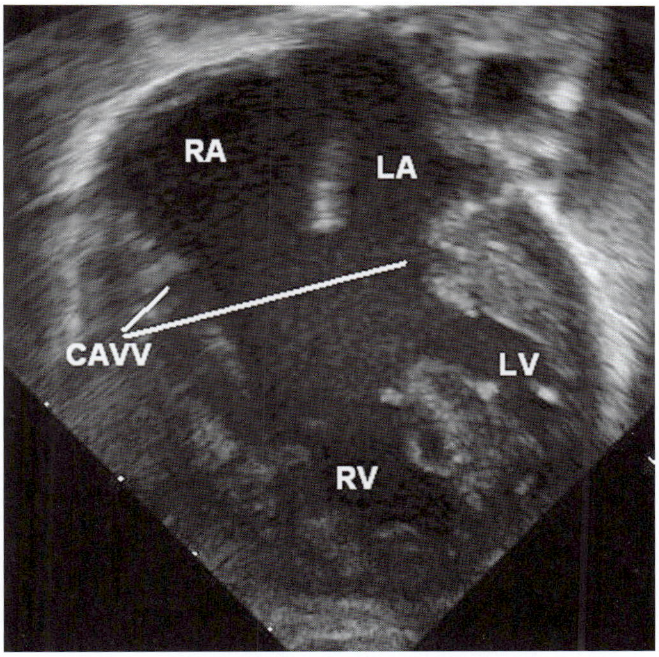

Figure 22.9 Apical four-chamber view of a patient with complete common atrioventricular canal unbalanced to the right. The common atrioventricular valve (CAVV) is in the open position. There is more valve over the right ventricle than the left ventricle and the left ventricle is small compared to the right. CAVV, common atrioventricular valve; LA, left atrium; LV, left ventricle; RA, right atrium; RV, right ventricle.

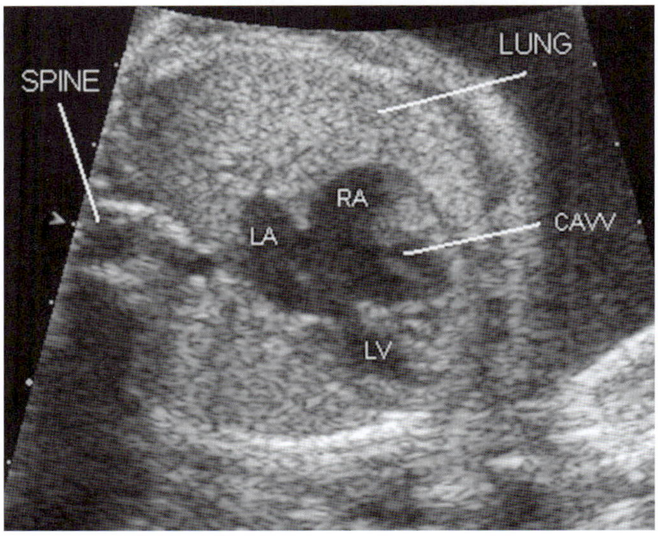

Figure 22.10 Fetal echocardiogram in the four-chamber view demonstrating a complete common atrioventricular canal with the common atrioventricular valve (CAVV) in the open position. Note the large atrioventricular septal defect at the center of the heart. CAVV, common atrioventricular valve; LA, left atrium; LV, left ventricle; RA, right atrium; RV, right ventricle.

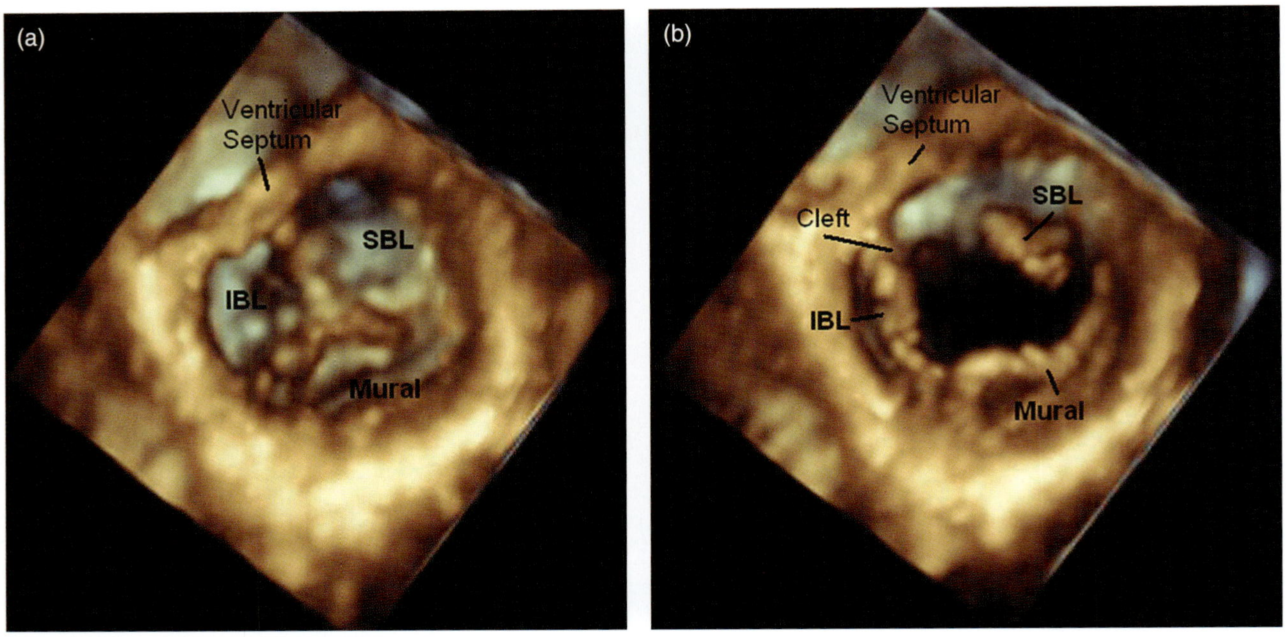

Figure 22.11 (a) Three-dimensional (3D) echocardiographic image cut from the left ventricle looking up toward the left atrioventricular valve in a patient with incomplete common atrioventricular valve. In the closed position, the trifoliate appearance of the valve is highlighted well. (b) Same image with the left atrioventricular valve in the open position shows the leaflets well with the "cleft" seen directed toward the ventricular septum. IBL, inferior bridging leaflet; SBL, superior bridging leaflet.

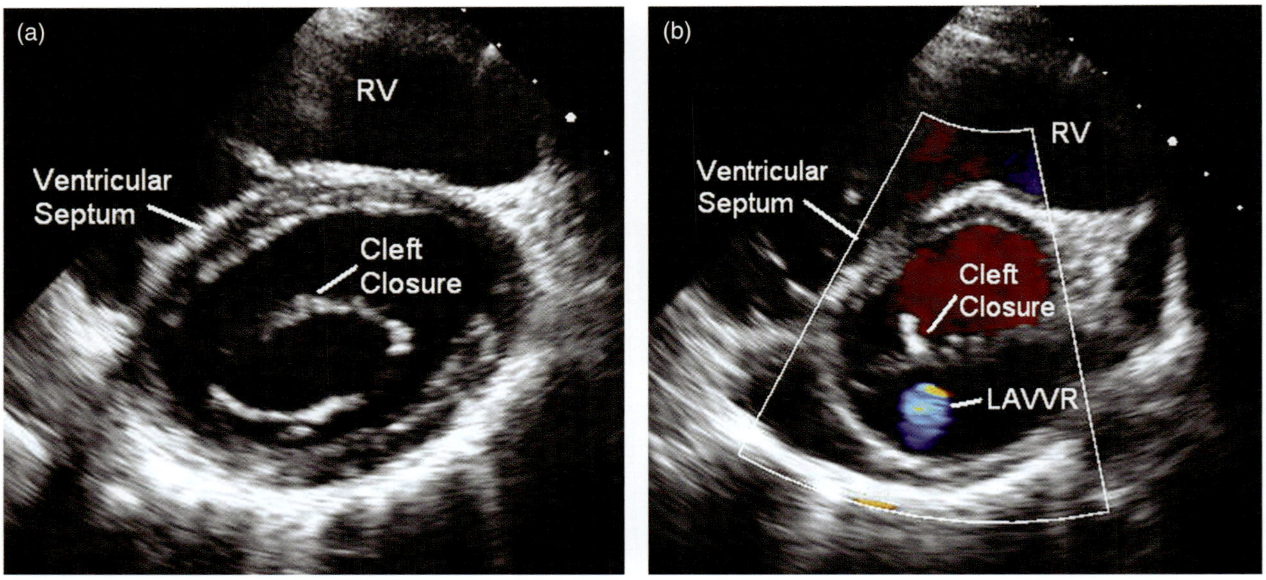

Figure 22.12 (a) Parasternal short-axis view of a patient with complete common atrioventricular canal who has undergone repair including closure of the cleft in the left atrioventricular portion of the valve. The region where the superior and inferior bridging leaflets are sewn together is highlighted. (b) Image using color Doppler in the same patient. There is a trivial jet of residual atrioventricular valve regurgitation seen at the edge of the cleft closure. LAVVR, left atrioventricular valve regurgitation; RV, right ventricle.

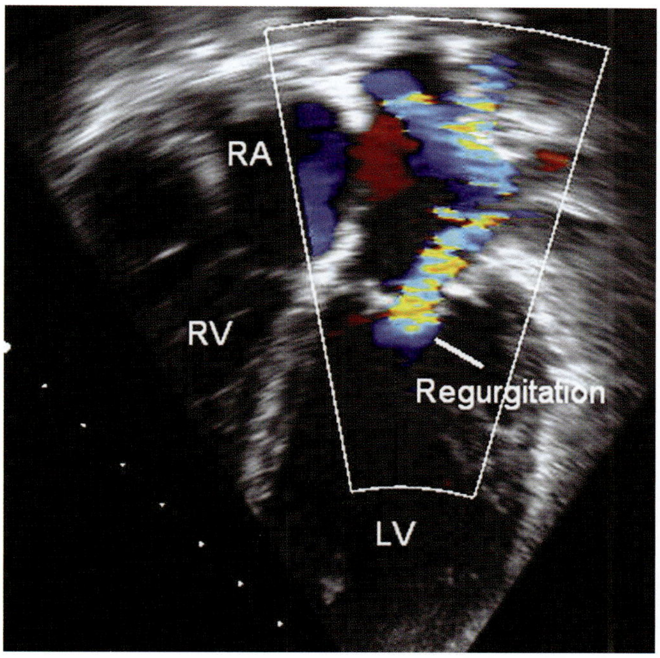

Figure 22.13 Apical four-chamber view with color Doppler in a patient who has undergone repair of complete common atrioventricular canal. There is a jet of residual left atrioventricular valve regurgitation seen. LV, left ventricle; RA, right atrium; RV, right ventricle.

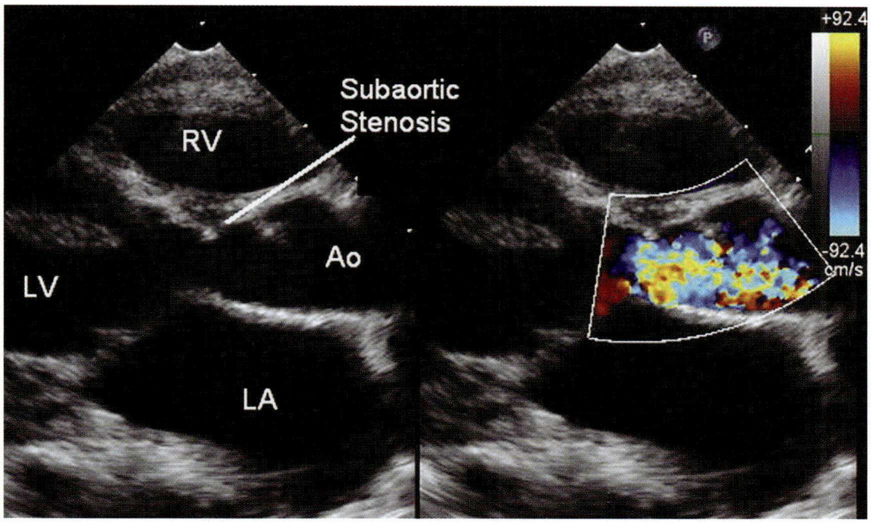

Figure 22.14 Parasternal long-axis view in color compare mode of a patient who has undergone repair of incomplete common atrioventricular valve. Within 1 year of surgery, the patient developed significant subaortic stenosis. Note the narrowing under the aorta and the color Doppler on the right panel which shows turbulent flow. The subaortic obstruction is from abnormal attachments of the left atrioventricular valve to the ventricular septum. Ao, aorta; LA, left atrium; LV, left ventricle; RV, right ventricle.

References

1 Bharati S, Lev M. (1973) The specturm of common atrioventricular orifice (canal). *Am Heart J*, **86**, 553–561.

2 Loewy Kirby M. (2007) *Endocardium, Cardiac Cushions, and Valve Development in Cardiac Development*, Oxford University Press, New York, NY, pp. 119–131.

3 Marx GR, Fyler DC. (2006) Endocardial cushion defects, in, *Nadas' Pediatric Cardiology*, (eds JF Keane, JE Lock, DC Fyler), Saunders Elsevier, Philadelphia, PA, pp. 663–674.

4 Anderson RH, Ho SY, Falcao S, *et al.* (1998) The diagnostic features of atrioventricular septal defect with common atrioventricular junction. *Cardiol Young*, **8**, 33–49.

5 Cohen MS. (2009) Atrioventricular canal defects, in, *Echocardiography in Pediatric and Congenital Heart Disease: From Fetus to Adult* (eds WW Lai, L Mertens, MS Cohen, T Geva), Blackwell Publishers, Oxford, pp. 230–248.

6 Szwast AL, Marino BS, Rychik J, *et al.* (2011) Usefulness of left ventricular inflow index to predict successful biventricular repair in right-dominant unbalanced atrioventricular canal. *Am J Cardiol*, **107**, 103–109.

7 Cohen MS, Jegatheeswaran A, Baffa JM, *et al.* (2013) Echocardiographic features defining right dominant unbalanced atrioventricular septal defect: a multi-institutional study of the Congenital Heart Surgeon's Society. *Circ Cardiovasc Imag*, **6**, 508–513.

8 Clapp S, Perry BL, Farooki ZQ, *et al.* (1990) Down syndrome, complete atrioventricular canal and pulmonary vascular obstructive disease. *J Thorac Cardiovasc Surg*, **100**, 115–121.

9 Barrea C, Levasseur S, Roman K, *et al.* (2005) Three-dimensional echocardiography improves the understanding of left atrioventricular valve morphology and function in atrioventricular septal defects undergoing patch augmentation. *J Thorac Cardiovasc Surg*, **129**, 746–753.

10 Rastelli GC, Ongley PA, Kirklin JW, McGoon DC. (1968) Surgical repair of complete form of persistent common atrioventricular canal. *J Thorac Cardiovasc Surg*, **55**, 299–308.

11 Michielon G, Stellin G, Rizzoli G, *et al.* (1995) Left atrioventricular valve incompetence after repair of common atrioventricular canal defects. *Ann Thorac Surg*, **60** (6 Suppl), S604–609.

12 Draulans-Noe H, Weinink ACG. (1991) Anterolateral muscle bundle of the left ventricle in atrioventricular septal defect: left ventricular outflow tract and subaortic stenosis. *Pediatr Cardiol*, **12**, 83–88.

13 Ten Harkel AD, Cromme-Dijkhuis AH, Heinerman BC, *et al.* (2005) Development of left atrioventricular valve regurgitation after correction of atrioventricular septal defect. *Ann Thorac Surg*, **79**, 607–612.

14 Jacobs JP,Jacobs ML, Mavroudis C, *et al.* (2010) Atrioventricular septal defects: lessons learned about patterns of practice and outcomes from the congenital heart surgery database of the society of thoracic surgeons. *World J Pediatr Congenit Heart Surg*, **1**, 68–77.

23

Ventricular Septal Defect

Lowell Frank

Children's National Medical Center; George Washington University School of Medicine, Washington, DC, USA

Ventricular septal defects (VSDs) are the most common form of congenital heart disease, often representing an obligate component of complex lesions such as tetralogy of Fallot, double outlet right ventricle, truncus arteriosus, and atrioventricular septal defects.

Pathophysiology

VSDs shunt oxygenated blood from the left ventricle to the right ventricle and pulmonary circulation. The total left-to-right shunt is quantified as the pulmonary-to-systemic flow ratio (Qp : Qs), which is influenced by the size of the defect and the difference between the systemic and pulmonary vascular resistance (PVR). This is especially important in neonates with large defects who may be asymptomatic early in life while the PVR remains relatively elevated. Small restrictive defects typically remain asymptomatic because pulmonary blood flow is only trivially increased.

Clinical Presentation and Diagnosis

As the PVR declines, the degree of left-to-right shunting increases, resulting in increased pulmonary blood flow and symptoms of congestive heart failure. Patients may present with tachypnea during feeding, but the tachypnea may persist if the shunt is large enough. Tachycardia and diaphoresis often develop because of the upregulated neurohormonal cascade associated with congestive heart failure [1]. Poor weight gain can result from decreased caloric intake and increased cardiac metabolic demand.

Immediately after birth, the physical examination may be normal if the high PVR restricts flow across the VSD. A harsh holosystolic murmur along the left sternal border may be present, though it is often absent with large defects. Occasionally, there is an audible systolic ejection murmur at the base representing "relative pulmonic stenosis" because of the large volume of pulmonary blood flow crossing an otherwise normal pulmonary annulus.

Echocardiography is the primary imaging modality for the diagnosis of VSD. While electrocardiography can reveal left atrial enlargement and/or left ventricular hypertrophy and chest X-rays can show cardiomegaly and pulmonary edema (Figure 23.1), these findings have a low specificity. Echocardiography accurately assesses the morphology of the VSD, including its location and size as well as the direction and amount of shunting. Cardiac catheterization is rarely needed to obtain additional anatomic or physiologic data, and echocardiography is typically the sole pre-intervention imaging modality for patients undergoing surgical or percutaneous closure. Magnetic resonance imaging can also be useful to obtain diagnostic information if needed.

Nomenclature and Anatomy

VSDs can have complex, widely varying anatomy. Large defects of various types may have similar symptoms, but the options for surgical or transcatheter intervention can be quite different. Furthermore, the long-term sequelae and potential impact on surrounding structures depend on the precise location of the defect(s). Precise communication about the nature and details of the VSD between cardiologists and congenital cardiac surgeons is essential for successful repair.

There are many nomenclatures to describe the anatomic and (in some cases) embryologic substrate of VSDs, including those by Van Praagh [2], Anderson [3], and the Society for Thoracic Surgeons (Figure 23.2) [4]. Familiarity with the similarities and variations in each system is necessary for accurate communication.

Visual Guide to Neonatal Cardiology, First Edition. Edited by Ernerio T. Alboliras, Ziyad M. Hijazi, Leo Lopez, and Donald J. Hagler.

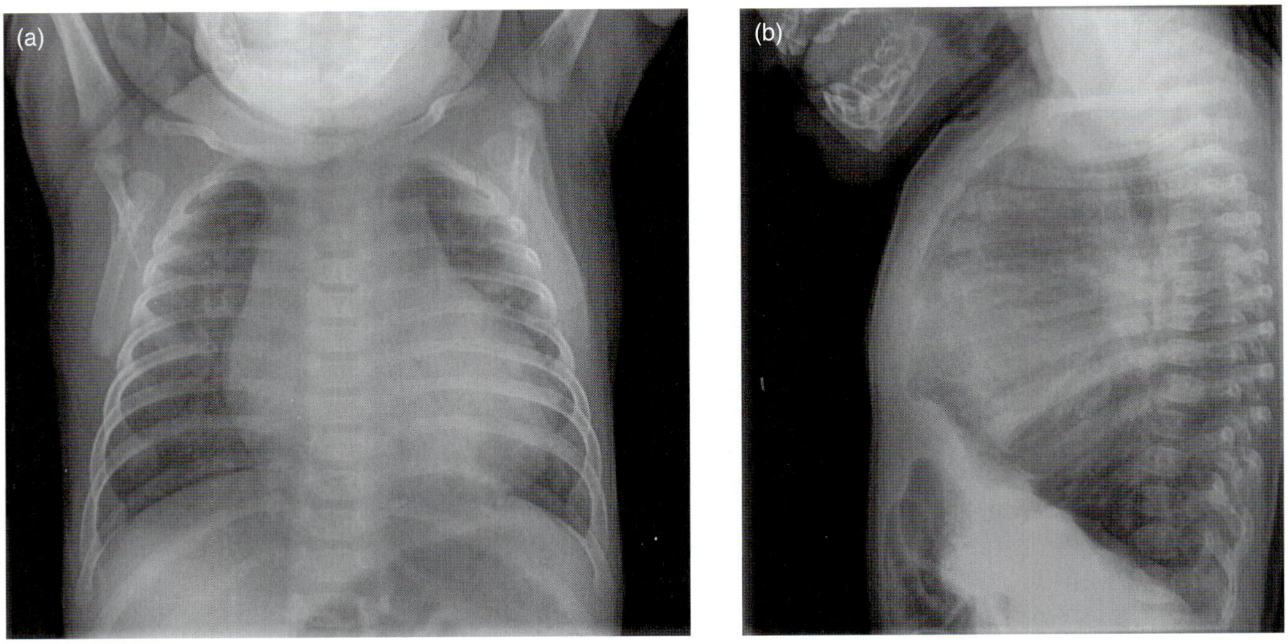

Figure 23.1 Chest X-ray of a patient with a large ventricular septal defect (VSD) in (a) anteroposterior and (b) lateral projections. Note the cardiomegaly with left atrial and left ventricular enlargement, increased pulmonary blood flow, and inferiorly directed cardiac apex.

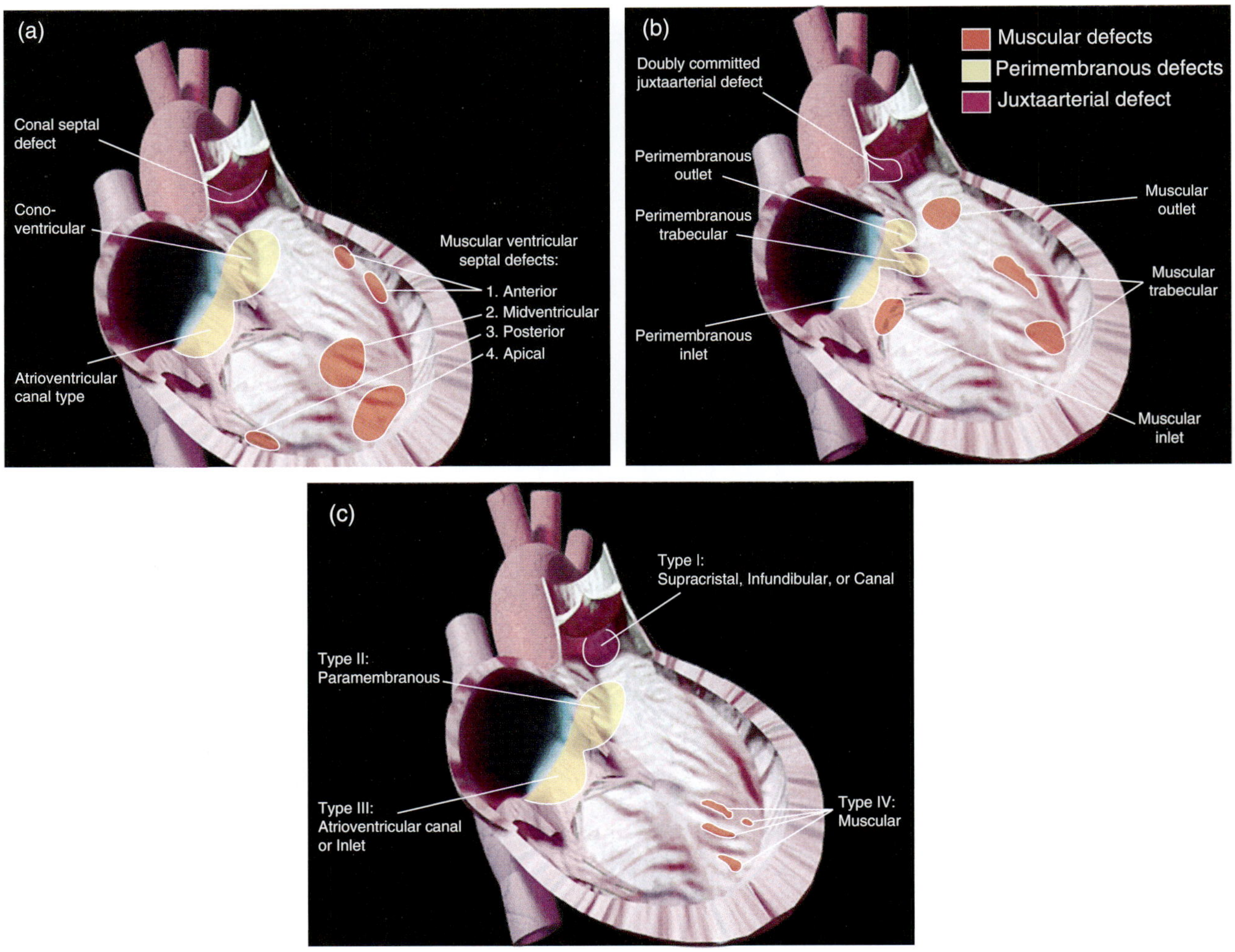

Figure 23.2 The nomenclature schemas to describe VSDs used by (a) Van Praagh, (b) Anderson, and (c) the Society for Thoracic Surgeons. *Source*: Jacobs *et al.* 2000 [4]. Reproduced with permission of Elsevier.

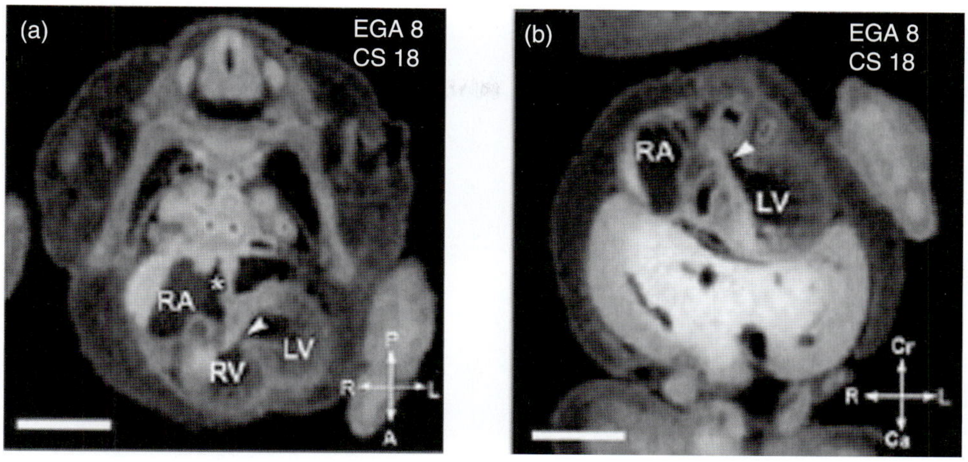

Figure 23.3 Magnetic resonance imaging of a human embryo at 8 weeks' gestation showing the growth of the muscular ventricular septum into the ventricular cavity with (a) an incomplete inlet ventricular septum (arrowhead) above the crest of the muscular septum, and (b) a formed outlet ventricular septum (arrowhead). *Source*: Dhanantwari *et al.* 2009 [5]. Reproduced with permission of Wolters Kluwer Health, Inc.

Ventricular septal development occurs between gestational age 7.8 and 9.4 weeks, with septation of the distal outflow segment occurring before the atrioventricular canal and membranous segment (Figure 23.3) [5]. The Van Praagh approach focuses on the four major components of the interventricular septum (Figure 23.4): (i) atrioventricular canal septum; (ii) muscular septum; (iii) septal band; and (iv) parietal band (also called conal septum or crista supraventricularis) [2]. In this system, VSDs are classified as conoventricular (with or without anterior or posterior malalignment), conal septal, atrioventricular canal-type, or muscular.

Conoventricular defects constitute the vast majority of VSDs (Figure 23.5) and are located at or around the junction of the conal and muscular portions of the interventricular septum, often associated with conal septal malalignment, such as the anterior malalignment present in tetralogy of Fallot contributing to the large VSD (Figure 23.5c,d). Similarly, posterior malalignment results in the complex of VSD, subvalvar aortic stenosis, and aortic coarctation. Conoventricular defects involve the "true" membranous septum, which is small and has both an interventricular and an atrioventricular component. Membranous VSDs are also known as "paramembranous" defects because they involve the membranous septum and surrounding areas. Others use the less accurate term "perimembranous" which implies complete surrounding of the membranous septum to describe defects bordered by the tricuspid and aortic valves without malalignment (Figure 23.5a,b). Small or moderate defects of this type may spontaneously close with accessory tricuspid valve apparatus. Occasionally, a prolapsing aortic valve leaflet closes the defect, but aortic insufficiency can develop secondary to continued valvar damage, usually necessitating surgical closure.

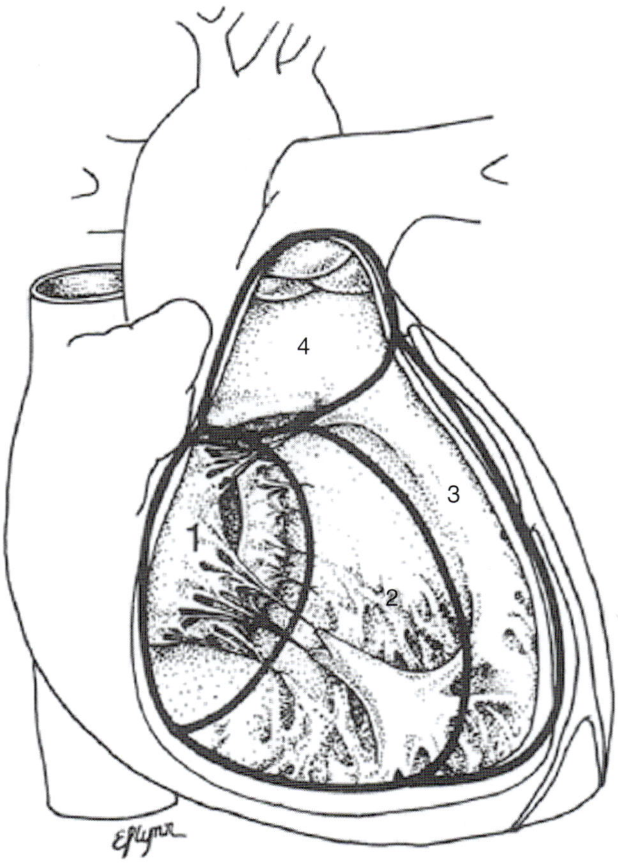

Figure 23.4 The four main components of the interventricular septum according to Van Praagh as viewed from the right left ventricle. 1 = atrioventricular canal septum; 2 = muscular ventricular septum; 3 = septal band; 4 = parietal band (also called the conal septum or crista supraventricularis). *Source*: Van Praagh *et al.* 1989 [2]. Reproduced with permission of Elsevier.

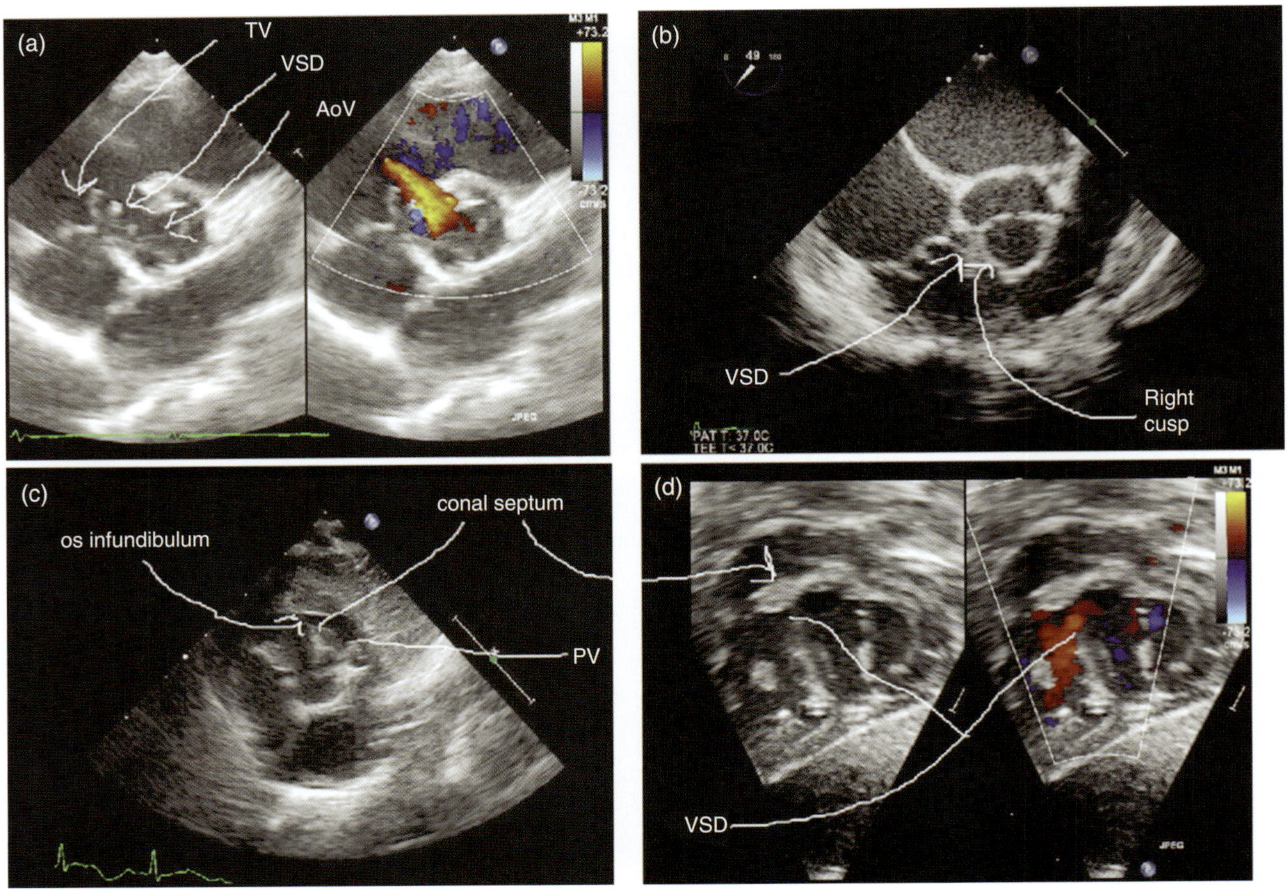

Figure 23.5 Conoventricular defects: (a) parasternal short-axis image without and with color showing the defect location between the aortic (AoV) and tricuspid valves (TV) without conal septal malalignment; (b) transesophageal view showing the right aortic cusp in the defect; (c) parasternal short-axis image showing anterior malalignment of the conal septum, narrowed os infundibulum, and small pulmonary annulus (PV) as seen in tetralogy of Fallot; and (d) subcostal sagittal image without and with color showing anterior malalignment of the conal septum.

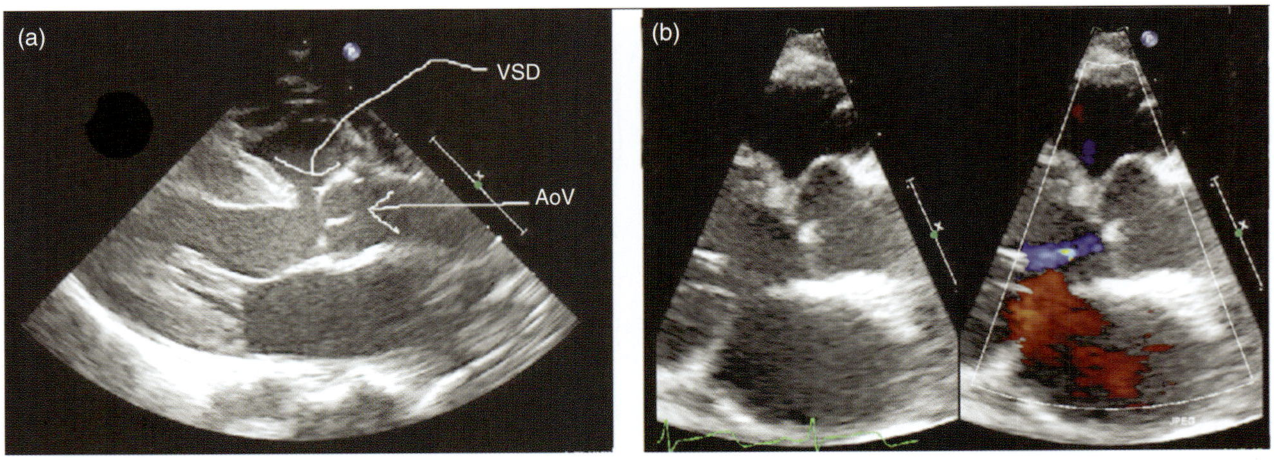

Figure 23.6 Conal septal defects: (a) parasternal long-axis image showing the relation to the aortic valve (AoV); (b) parasternal image without and with color showing closure of the defect by prolapsing AoV tissue and subsequent aortic insufficiency; (c) partial closure of the defect and small shunt; (d) parasternal short-axis image showing deficiency of the conal septum and aortic and pulmonary valvar continuity.

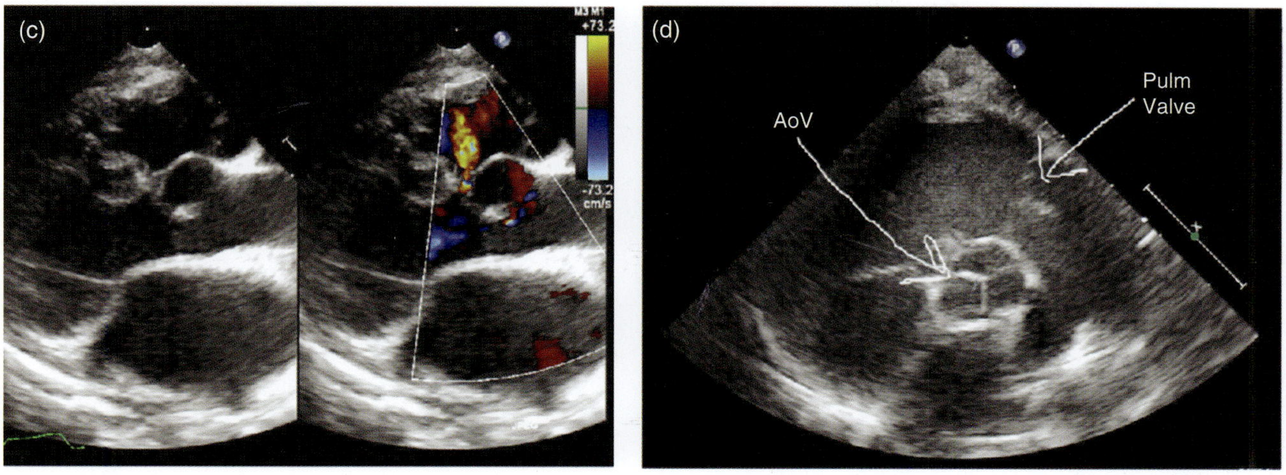

Figure 23.6 (*Continued*)

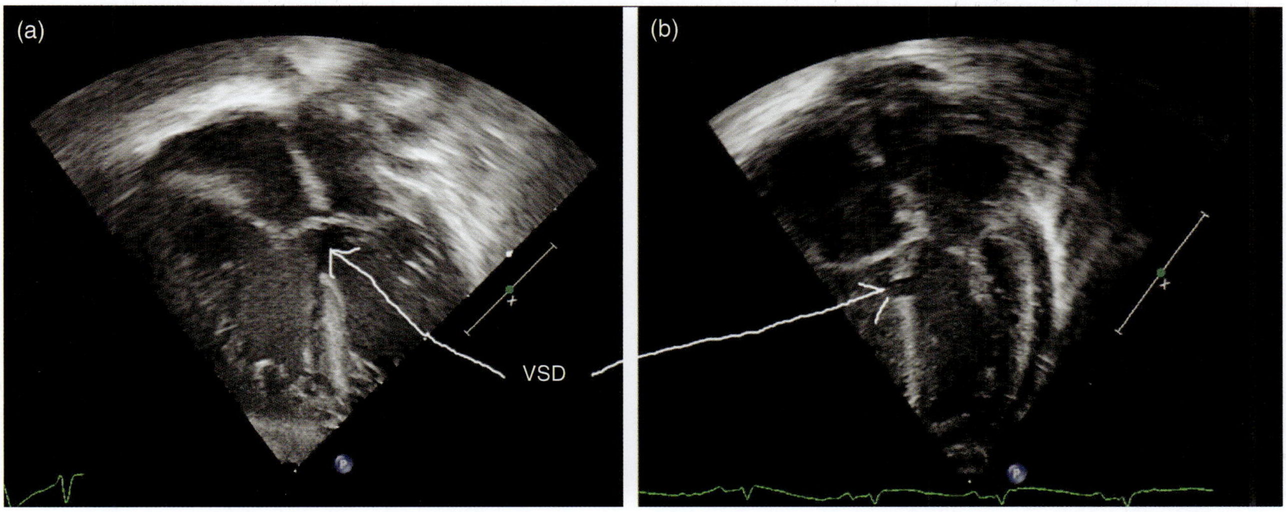

Figure 23.7 Comparison of (a) an atrioventricular canal-type defect with (b) a posterior muscular defect, in which there is a rim of muscular tissue in the more basilar aspect as well as offset of the tricuspid and mitral valves, which is not present in an atrioventricular canal defect.

Conal septal defects are located in the right ventricular outflow tract (or infundibulum) (Figure 23.6) and often known as "subpulmonary," "subarterial," "supracristal," and "doubly-committed juxtarterial" defects. The conal septum separating the subarterial outflow tracts is deficient, resulting in fibrous continuity between the semilunar valves. These defects are more common in Asian patients and are frequently associated with aortic valve prolapse (typically the right coronary cusp), necessitating close monitoring for aortic insufficiency.

Atrioventricular canal-type VSDs are bordered by the tricuspid and mitral valves and usually are associated with atrioventricular valve abnormalities ranging from a cleft mitral valve to a common atrioventricular valve. They are often referred to as "inlet" defects because of their relation to the atrioventricular valves; however, because posterior muscular VSDs also occur in the inlet portion of the septum with different embryologic origin and prognosis, the term "atrioventricular canal-type" is preferred by some (Figure 23.7).

Muscular VSDs are heterogeneous and imply that the defect is circumferentially surrounded by the trabecular septum. They have widely varied locations and are referred to as posterior, apical, mid-, and anterior muscular VSDs (Figure 23.8). A "Swiss cheese" septum occurs with multiple muscular defects. Muscular VSDs have a high rate of spontaneous closure, especially if anatomically small.

Management

Criteria for treatment have included elevated pulmonary artery pressure from large unrestrictive defects, left

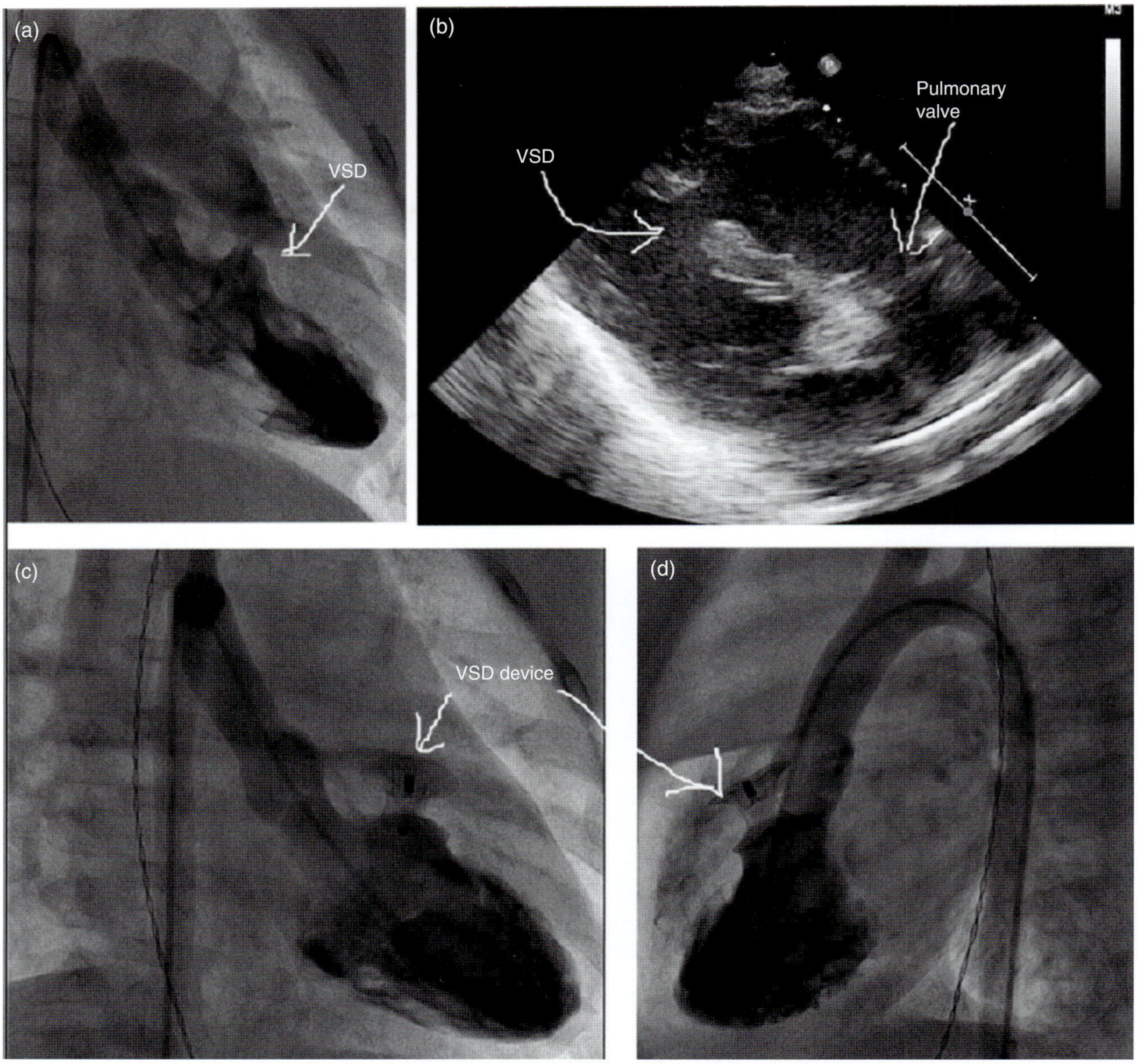

Figure 23.8 Anterior muscular defect: (a) long axial oblique angiography prior to intervention; (b) parasternal long-axis image showing the spatial relationship of the defect to the pulmonary valve; (c) long axial oblique; and (d) lateral view after device closure showing no residual shunt.

ventricular dilatation with normal pulmonary artery pressure, small defects with aortic valve prolapse and aortic insufficiency, pulmonary vascular disease, and endocarditis [6]. Conventional medical therapy for clinical symptoms have included diuretics, digoxin, and afterload reducing agents such as angiotensin converting enzyme inhibitors, all with varying degrees of success [7].

Unless spontaneous closure is possible, surgical closure for large defects is typically performed within the first few months of life, typically via a right atrial approach with visualization through the tricuspid valve. Exceptions include conal septal defects, which are best approached through the pulmonary valve, and muscular defects, which can be treated with catheter-based device closure (Figure 23.9) [8]. These latter defects can be difficult to visualize intraoperatively because of the coarse, irregular right ventricular trabeculations and their distance from the tricuspid valve. However, percutaneous closure requires a sizable venous sheath as well as a complex guidewire course and may not be practical in small infants.

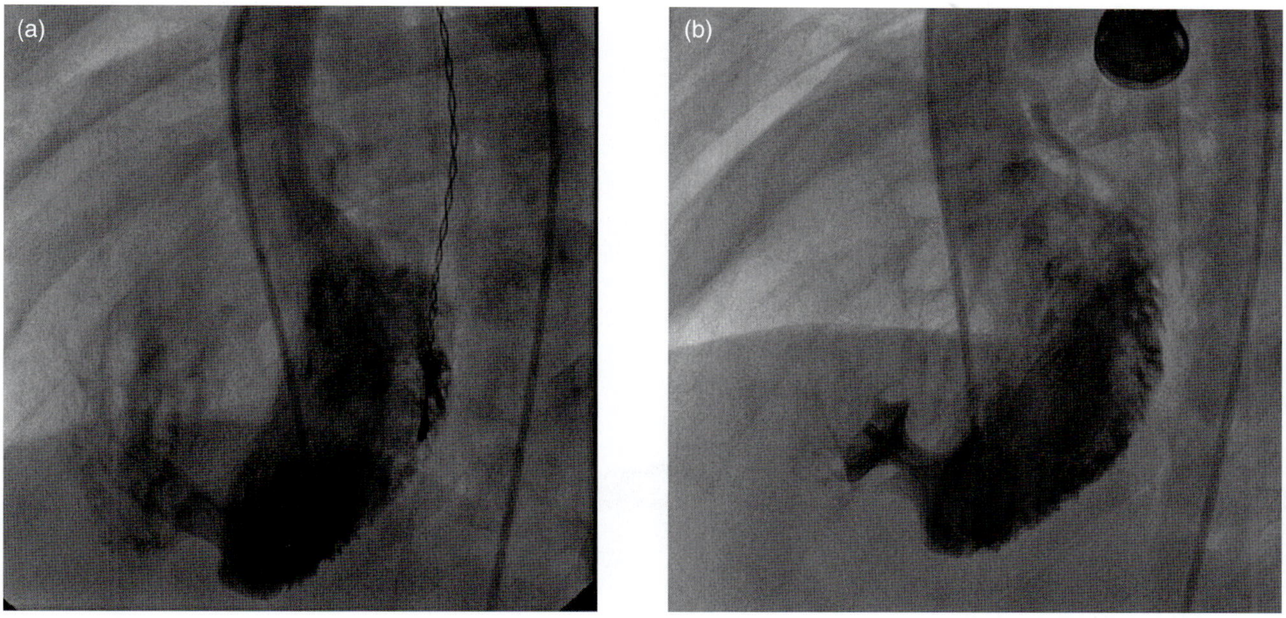

Figure 23.9 Left ventricular angiogram of an apical muscular VSD: (a) prior to intervention; and (b) after device closure with only trivial residual left-to-right shunting; the catheter courses retrograde from the aorta.

References

1 Hsu DT, Pearson GD. (2009) Heart failure in children: part I: history, etiology, and pathophysiology. *Circ Heart Fail*, **2**, 63–70.

2 Van Praagh R, Geva T, Kreutzer J. (1989) Ventricular septal defects: How shall we describe, name and classify them? *J Am Coll Cardiol*, **14**, 1298–1299.

3 Soto B, Becker AE, Moulaert AJ, Lie JT, Anderson RH. (1980) Classification of ventricular septal defects. *Br Heart J*, **43**, 332–343.

4 Jacobs JP, Burke RP, Quintessenza JA, Mavroudis C. (2000) Congenital Heart Surgery Nomenclature and Database Project: ventricular septal defect. *Ann Thorac Surg*, **69**, S25–35.

5 Dhanantwari P, Lee E, Krishnan A, *et al.* (2009) Human cardiac development in the first trimester: a high-resolution magnetic resonance imaging and episcopic fluorescence image capture atlas. *Circulation*, **120**, 343–351.

6 Penny DJ, Vick GW. (2011) Ventricular septal defect. *Lancet*, **377**, 1103–1112.

7 Hsu DT, Pearson GD. (2009) Heart failure in children: part II: diagnosis, treatment, and future directions. *Circ Heart Fail*, **2**, 490–498.

8 McCarthy KP, Ching Leung PK, Ho SY. (2005) Perimembranous and muscular ventricular septal defects: morphology revisited in the era of device closure. *J Interv Cardiol*, **18**, 507–513.

24

Tricuspid Atresia

Nathaniel W. Taggart

Division of Pediatric Cardiology, Mayo Clinic, Rochester, MN, USA

Tricuspid atresia (TA) is a rare form of cyanotic congenital heart disease, occurring in approximately 1 in 15 000 live births. Some reports suggest a slight male predominance, but this is not proven. There are no known genetic or teratogenic causes, although the incidence may be slightly higher among first-degree family members of affected individuals [1].

Anatomy

In place of a functional tricuspid valve, there may be a thin, imperforate membrane or a thick, muscular wall. The right ventricle (RV) is almost always hypoplastic (Figure 24.1). A patent foramen ovale (PFO) or atrial septal defect (ASD) allows for complete mixing of pulmonary and systemic venous return. A ventricular septal defect (VSD) allows blood to flow into the great artery which arises from the hypoplastic RV.

A number of different classifications schemes have been proposed for TA [2], but those most widely accepted categorize based upon two anatomic variables. Primary categorization (Type I, II, or III) describes the relationship of the great arteries – normally related, D-transposed (ventriculoarterial discordance), or L-transposed (atrioventricular and ventriculoarterial discordance). Type III is very rare and will not be discussed further. Subclassification (A, B, or C) describes the degree of pulmonary outflow obstruction (atresia, stenosis, or unobstructed, respectively). These anatomic variables effectively determine physiology. Therefore, this system provides a simple framework for understanding the physiology of TA and how best to manage neonates with this disease.

Physiology

With normal atrioventricular connections (Type I or II), desaturated systemic venous blood flow enters the right atrium and passes through a PFO or ASD into the left atrium. There, it mixes with saturated pulmonary venous blood and enters the left ventricle (LV). From there it is ejected out of the aorta and pulmonary artery (PA). Blood enters the PA either through the VSD and pulmonary valve or from the aorta via a patent ductus arteriosus (PDA). As a result, oxygen saturations measured in the aorta and PA are the same. The degree of cyanosis depends upon the ratio of pulmonary blood flow (Q_p) and systemic blood flow (Q_s). This ratio (Q_p/Q_s) is determined by the relative resistances of the pulmonary and systemic circulatory pathways. There are several potential resistors along the systemic and pulmonary pathways that affect Q_p/Q_s: the VSD, subvalvar infundibulum, the semilunar valves, the large vessels, and arteriolar beds.

Type I: Normally Related Great Arteries

Type I comprises approximately 70% of all TA. The aorta arises from the LV and the PA from the right; thus, "normally-related." Aortic stenosis (AS) and coarctation are rare. Therefore, in the absence of a PDA, Q_p is primarily dependent upon the VSD size and severity of PS (Figure 24.2).

Type I-A: Pulmonary Atresia

Type I-A comprises 10% of all TA. There is no direct communication between RV and PA. Neonates with Type I-A TA require a PDA for pulmonary blood flow. In

Visual Guide to Neonatal Cardiology, First Edition. Edited by Ernerio T. Alboliras, Ziyad M. Hijazi, Leo Lopez, and Donald J. Hagler.

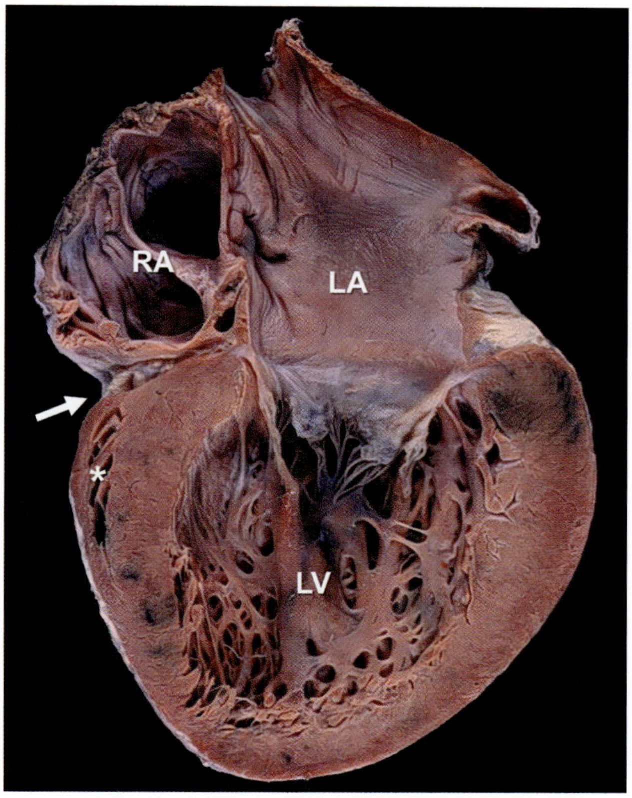

Figure 24.1 Gross pathologic specimen showing no communication between the right atrium (RA) and severely hypoplastic right ventricle (RV) (asterisk). LA, left atrium; LV, left ventricle.

the presence of a large, unrestrictive PDA, Q_p and SaO_2 are determined by the ratio of PVR to systemic vascular resistance (SVR). A restrictive PDA will cause a decrease in Q_p/Q_s and worsening cyanosis.

Type I-B: Pulmonary Stenosis and Restrictive VSD

Type I-B is the most common type of TA, accounting for 50% of all cases (Figure 24.3). There is flow across the VSD and pulmonary valve, but Q_p restricted either by the size of the VSD and resultant pulmonary stenosis (PS). With a PDA, these neonates may be reasonably well-saturated, but with ductal closure, Q_p decreases and SaO_2 drops. The degree of cyanosis then directly reflects the size of the VSD and degree of PS.

Type I-C: Large VSD and No PS

Type I-C comprises 10% of all TA (Figure 24.4). With a large VSD and no PS, Q_p depends solely upon PVR. As PVR drops, SaO_2 in these neonates may be normal or near-normal, reflecting high Q_p/Q_s. A PDA is not needed to maintain Q_p and may actually lead to pulmonary overcirculation or inadequate systemic perfusion.

Type II: D-Transposition of the Great Arteries

D-transposition of the great arteries (D-TGA) occurs in about 25–30% of TA. The aorta arises from the RV, typically anterior and rightward of the PA, which arises from a well-developed LV. As a result, PS or pulmonary atresia is much less common in Type II than in Type I TA. However, systemic output is dependent upon the size of the VSD. A small VSD frequently results in AS, arch hypoplasia, or coarctation and may manifest as poor perfusion or shock. Coarctation, in particular, is seen in nearly half of all Type II TA (usually Type II-C).

Type II-A: D-TGA with Pulmonary Atresia

Type II-A is very rare, comprising only 2% of TA. The entire cardiac output passes through the VSD into the aorta. As with Type I-A, Q_p at birth is entirely dependent upon a PDA. In the presence of a large PDA, PVR relative to SVR will determine Q_p/Q_s and SaO_2. Ductal constriction results in significant desaturation and cyanosis. Systemic obstruction (e.g., restrictive VSD, AS, coarctation) is very rare and would be catastrophic.

Type II-B: D-TGA with PS

Type II-B makes up 8% of TA. As with Type I-B, Q_p and SaO_2 are primarily determined by the severity of PS. While neonates with mild stenosis may be well-balanced or overcirculated, those with severe stenosis may require a PDA or surgical shunt to maintain adequate Q_p.

Type II-C: D-TGA with no PS

Type II-C accounts for 18% of all TA (Figure 24.5). In the absence of PS, Q_p/Q_s is determined by the relationship between PVR and any restriction to systemic circulation. This restriction can occur at the VSD, subvalvular outflow tract, aortic valve (i.e., AS), aorta (e.g., coarctation), or distal vasculature (e.g., elevated SVR). For example, in the presence of normal PVR, a severely restrictive VSD will force a greater proportion of the total cardiac output into the PA, resulting in a very high Q_p/Q_s and potentially normal SaO_2. However, systemic perfusion may be adversely affected because of low Q_s. If the obstruction is caused by coarctation, upper extremity perfusion may be adequate but lower body perfusion will suffer.

Physical Examination

Pulse oximetry generally reflects the severity of pulmonary outflow obstruction. $SaO_2 > 80–85\%$ suggests excessive Q_p. A large PDA may produce a widened pulse pressure.

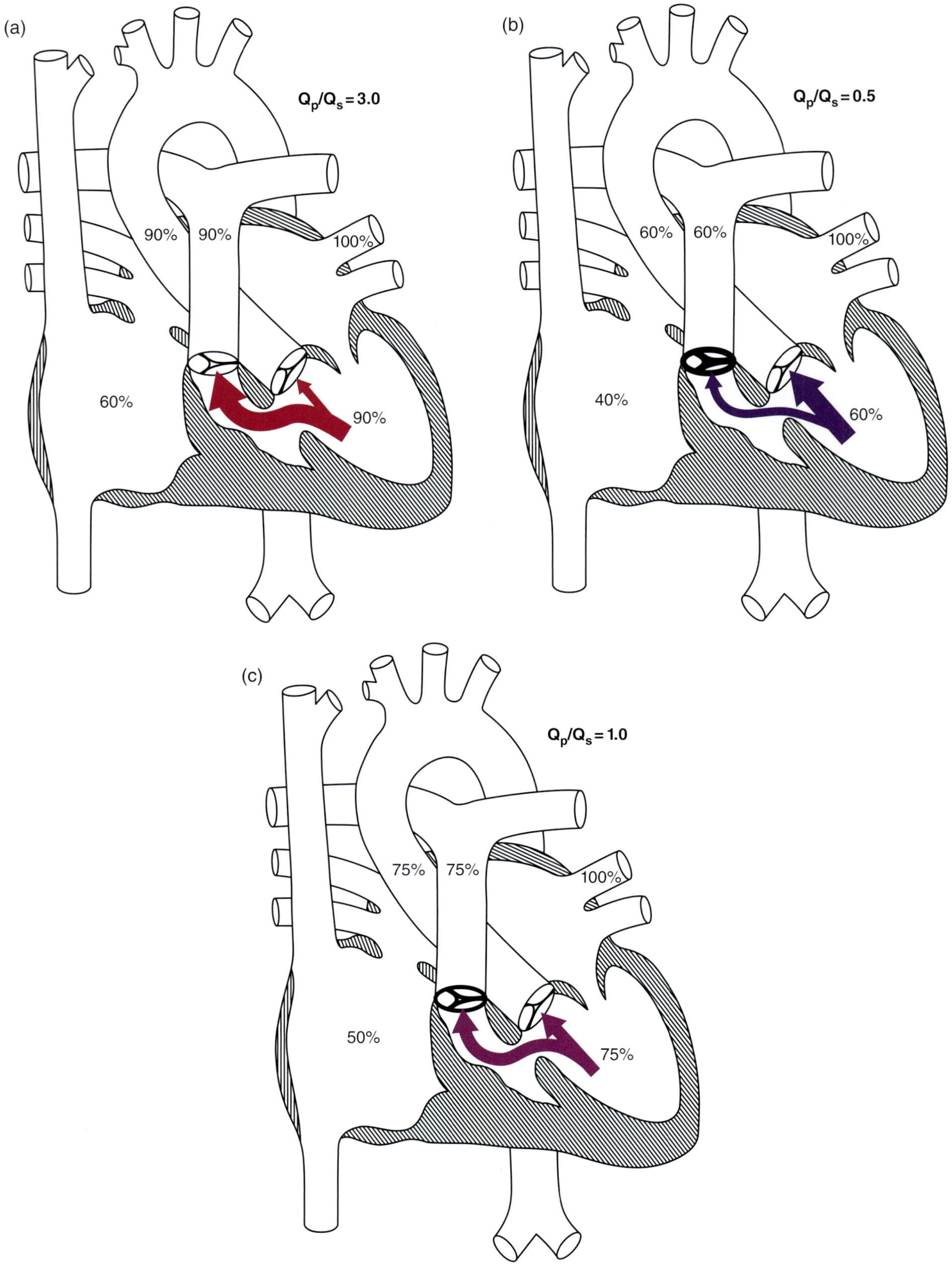

Figure 24.2 Hemodynamics of Type I tricuspid atresia with: (a) no pulmonary stenosis (PS); (b) severe PS; and (c) "well-balanced" PS.

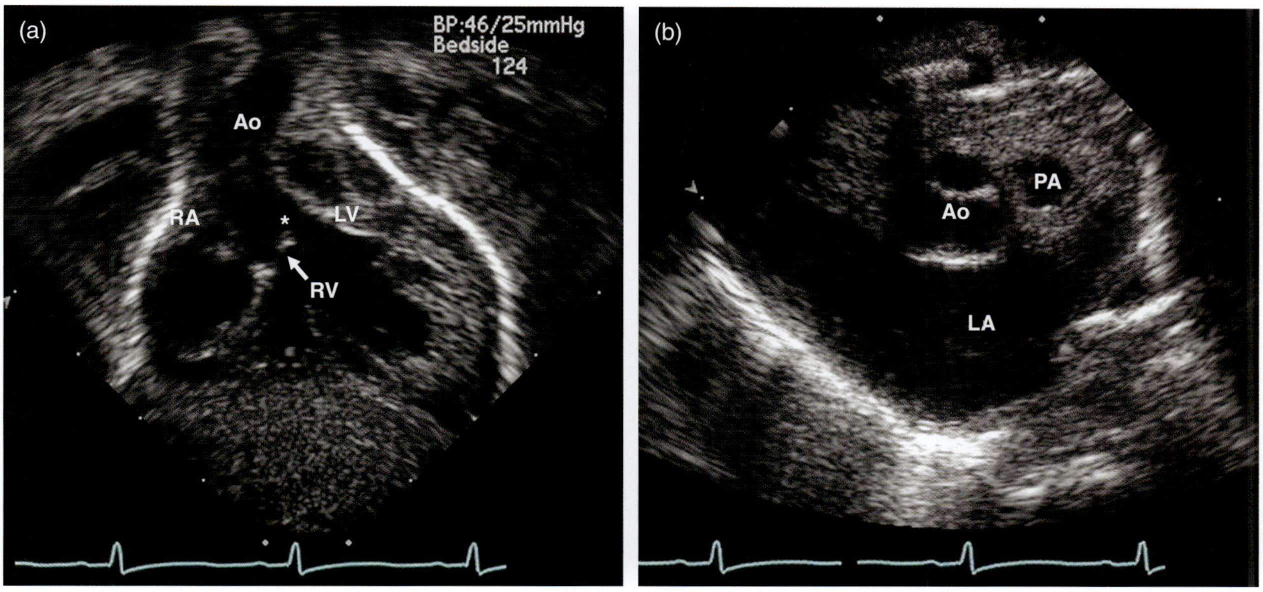

Figure 24.3 Type I-B tricuspid atresia. (a) Aorta (Ao) arises from the left ventricle (LV) with a restrictive ventricular septal defect (VSD) (asterisk). (b) The hypoplastic pulmonary artery (PA) is normally arranged anterior and leftward of the aorta (Ao). LA, left atrium.

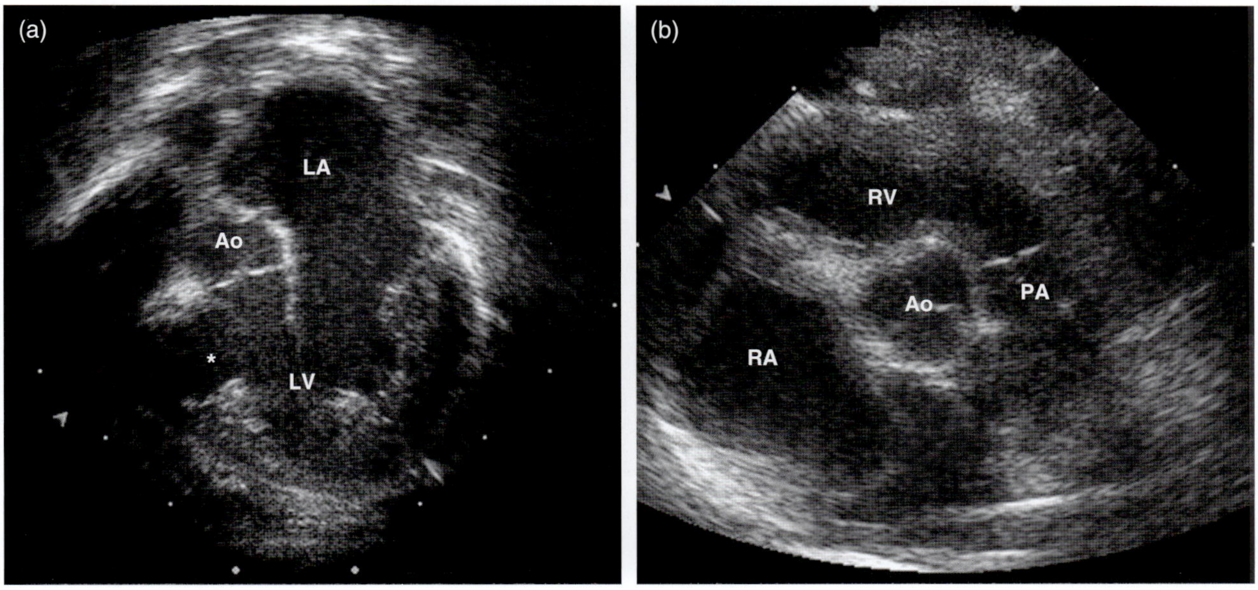

Figure 24.4 Type I-C tricuspid atresia. (a) Aorta arises from the LV. There is a large, unrestrictive VSD (asterisk). (b) The great arteries are normally related with a normally formed pulmonary valve.

When present, cyanosis is equal in the upper and lower extremities. Gradually increasing cyanosis suggests a closing PDA or Type I TA with a shrinking VSD. Pallor or mottling should raise concern for inadequate systemic perfusion caused by a Type II TA with a restrictive VSD, AS, or coarctation of the aorta.

Intercostal retractions, nasal flaring, and tachypnea are signs of pulmonary congestion and overcirculation, which would be seen in Type I-C or II-C TA.

Precordial impulse is displaced leftward because of RV hypoplasia and LV enlargement. S1 is single; S2 may be single (with pulmonary atresia) or narrowly split. A harsh, holosystolic murmur directed anteriorly and rightward represents flow across a restrictive VSD. A crescendo–decrescendo murmur over the precordium suggests PS or, less commonly, AS. Ductal constriction will be heard as a continuous murmur in the upper left precordium. A late systolic murmur heard over the back can indicate aortic coarctation. Absence of a murmur can be seen in either Type I-C or Type II-C with a large VSD and no obstructive lesions.

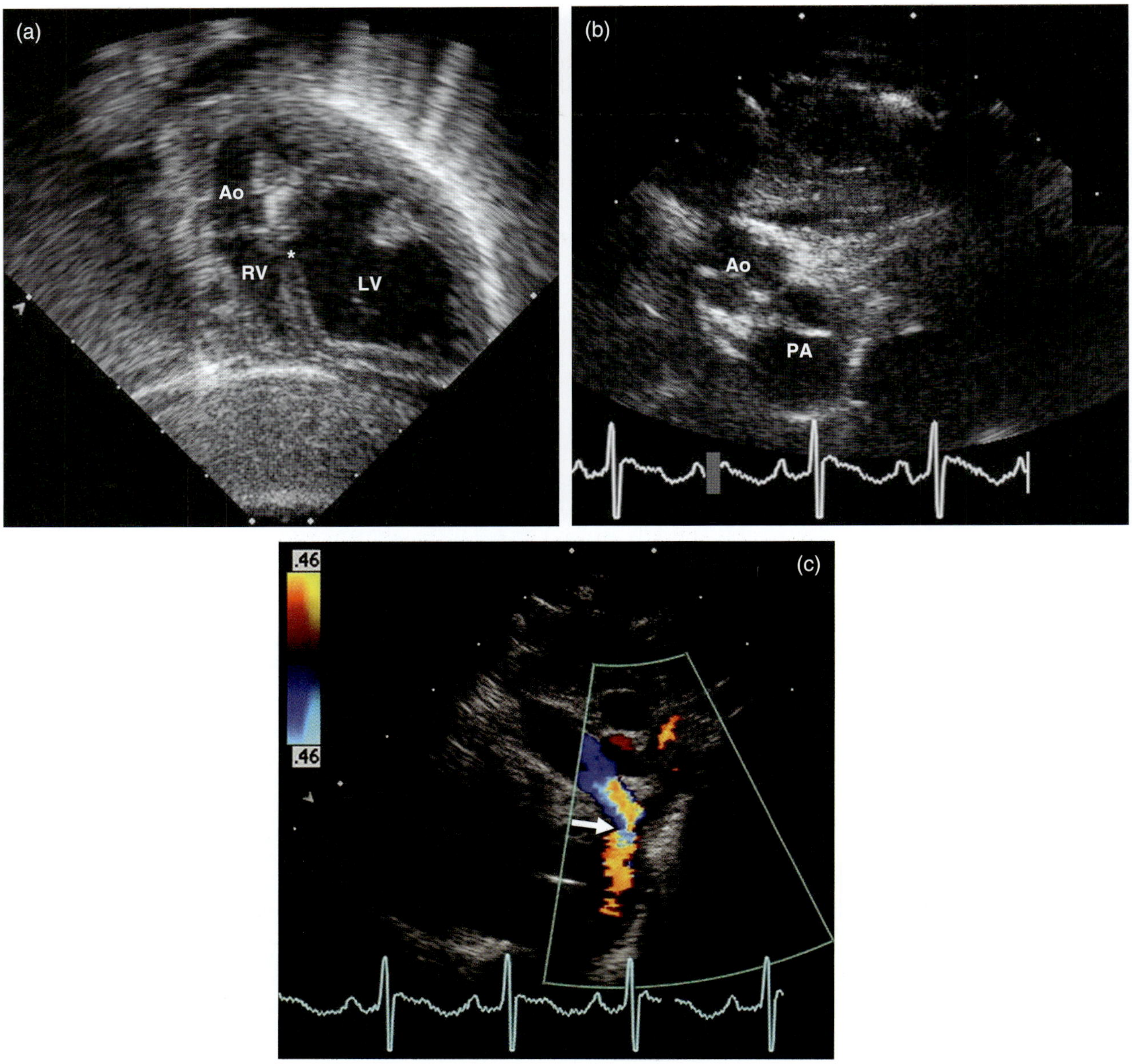

Figure 24.5 Type II-C tricuspid atresia. (a) The VSD is very restrictive (asterisk); the aorta arises from a hypoplastic RV. (b) The great arteries are transposed, with an anterior and rightward aorta. (c) Color flow Doppler of the aortic arch shows a discrete coarctation (arrow).

Electrocardiogram

Electrocardiogram typically shows peaked P-waves that may be widened or bifid, suggesting atrial enlargement. QRS axis is displaced leftward. RV voltages are diminished and precordial voltages can suggest LV hypertrophy.

Chest X-Ray

In the presence of significant PS or atresia, heart size may be normal or only mildly enlarged. Pulmonary vascular markings are usually diminished. The mediastinum may be narrow, particularly with pulmonary atresia. In the absence of PS or subvalvular obstruction, heart size is often moderately or severely enlarged and the lung fields are congested. The main PA trunk is usually prominent, except in D-TGA.

Echocardiography

Echocardiography almost always provides definitive diagnosis of TA. In addition to describing the anatomy, echocardiography allows for detailed physiologic assessment. Color flow and spectral Doppler can determine whether the atrial communication (PFO or ASD) is adequate or restrictive. Doppler techniques can also accurately define the severity of VSD restriction, AS, PS, and coarctation.

Cardiac Catheterization

In the modern era catheterization is rarely needed in the neonatal period. It can be necessary when echocardiography is inconclusive or incomplete, or to open a restrictive ASD or PFO.

Preoperative Management

The primary objective of medical management of the neonate with TA is to ensure adequate Q_p and Q_s and to relieve pulmonary overcirculation. Inadequate pulmonary or systemic perfusion caused by anatomic obstruction should be managed with intravenous prostaglandin E1 (PGE-1) to maintain ductal patency. PGE-1 administration should not be postponed until after echocardiography. It can later be discontinued if the echocardiogram demonstrates nonductal-dependent anatomy. Pulmonary congestion caused by overcirculation can be relieved with diuretics, such as furosemide.

A PDA is necessary in Types I-A and II-A TA, unnecessary in Type I-C and may be needed in Types I-B and II-B, depending upon the severity of PS. Type II-C does not require PGE-1 to improve Q_p, but may need it to support systemic circulation in the presence of significant systemic obstruction, such as coarctation.

It is important to know that the VSD in TA can become smaller over time, adversely affecting Q_p and SaO_2 (Type I) or Q_s (Type II). Early recognition of a newly restrictive VSD is vital and may require urgent surgical intervention if PGE-1 is unhelpful.

Surgical Management

The goal for neonates with TA is to provide a stable source of pulmonary blood flow, while preventing irreversible pulmonary vascular obstructive disease (Eisenmenger syndrome) as a result of excessive, high-pressure pulmonary blood flow. Neonates with TA and PDA-dependent pulmonary circulation will require a surgical shunt, either from the subclavian artery (modified Blalock–Taussig shunt) or ascending aorta/brachiocephalic artery (central shunt) to the PAs. The shunt replaces the PDA, which is ligated, and PGE-1 is discontinued.

Neonates with mild (Type I-B/II-B) or no PS (Type I-C/II-C) often manifest with $SaO_2 > 80–85\%$ (Figure 24.2a) resulting from pulmonary overcirculation and may require PA banding to reduce Q_p. In this surgical procedure, the main PA is constricted, lowering Q_p/Q_s closer to 1.0.

While severe PS results in inadequate Q_p (Figure 24.2b), in some cases of Type I-B and II-B, the degree of PS is such that $SaO_2 = 75–80\%$, representing a Q_p/Q_s near 1.0 (Figure 24.2c). These neonates are often referred to as being "well-balanced" and may not require shunt placement.

Additional surgical interventions may be needed in the neonatal period. Coarctation repair can be incorporated into or precede shunt placement. If AS, aortic arch hypoplasia, or a restrictive VSD is present, a Damus–Kaye–Stanzel end-to-side anastomosis of the main PA to the ascending aorta – with or without arch repair – may be necessary.

Postoperative Management

Neonates with a palliative surgical shunt are at risk for shunt thrombosis and occlusion and are prophylactically treated with antiplatelet therapy, usually aspirin 3–5 mg/kg/day. Desaturation or diminished perfusion with diminution of the continuous shunt murmur should raise concern for shunt occlusion. Urgent echocardiography should be performed. Intravenous heparin may be administered. Cardiac catheterization may be necessary to dilate or stent the shunt. Rarely, localized thrombolysis may be considered during catheterization. In some centers, surgical revision is the primary option for managing shunt occlusion.

References

1 Lok JM, Spevak PJ, Nichols DG. (2006) Tricuspid atresia, in, *Critical Heart Disease in Infants and Children*, 2nd edn. (eds DG Nichols, RM Ungerleider, PJ Spevak, *et al.*) Mosby Elsevier, Philadelphia, pp. 799–822.

2 Rao PS. (1980) A unified classification for tricuspid atresia. *Am Heart J*, **99** (6), 799–804.

25

Ebstein Malformation and Tricuspid Valve Dysplasias

Sameh M. Said, Donald J. Hagler, and Joseph A. Dearani

Division of Cardiovascular Surgery, Mayo Clinic, Rochester, MN, USA

Ebstein Malformation

Ebstein malformation (EM) accounts for 1% of all congenital heart disease [1]. The malformation is a right ventricular (RV) myopathy with highly variable tricuspid valve (TV) morphology (Figure 25.1). The main pathologic findings in EM include:

1) Failure of TV leaflet delamination;
2) Apical and posterior (downward) displacement of the functional annulus (septal > inferior > anterior);
3) Dilatation of the "atrialized" portion of the RV;
4) Fenestrations, redundancy, and tethering of the leaflets and chordae; and
5) Dilatation of the right atrioventricular junction (true tricuspid annulus).

Clinical Presentation

Newborn

EM in the neonatal period is characterized by cyanosis and severe right-sided heart failure. This occurs as a result of elevated right atrial pressures secondary to severe tricuspid regurgitation and low cardiac output. Cyanosis results from right-to-left shunting at the atrial level. Massive cardiomegaly is present and can compromise pulmonary function [2].

Children and Adults

In older children and adults the presentation is usually less dramatic with symptoms that range from being asymptomatic or fatigue, to decreased exercise intolerance, dyspnea, and cyanosis. With increasing age, atrial arrhythmias are common. Accessory conduction pathway(s) (Wolff–Parkinson–White syndrome) is present in approximately 15% of patients.

Preoperative Evaluation

Echocardiography is the diagnostic modality of choice in EM (Figure 25.2) and the following factors are considered favorable for "cone" valve repair: large, mobile anterior leaflet with the presence of some septal leaflet. Valve repair in the absence of septal leaflet generally consists of a monocusp approach. The Great Ormond Street Ebstein Score (GOSE score) is helpful preoperatively in evaluation in the neonate [3]. MRI allows accurate assessment of size and function of both the right and left ventricles. Electrophysiologic testing is performed when there is pre-excitation on preoperative electrocardiogram, recurrent supraventricular tachycardia, undefined wide-complex tachycardia, or syncope.

Indications for Surgery

Neonates

Surgery should be advised when there is:

1) Congestive heart failure and severe tricuspid regurgitation, or profound cyanosis with appropriate medical therapy;
2) Asymptomatic neonates who have a GOSE score of 3 or 4;
3) Symptomatic neonates with a GOSE score of 3 or 4 and mild cyanosis; and
4) A cardiothoracic ratio of >0.80.

There are two treatment pathways: the biventricular repair (Knott-Craig approach) (Figure 25.3) [4, 5], or the

Visual Guide to Neonatal Cardiology, First Edition. Edited by Ernerio T. Alboliras, Ziyad M. Hijazi, Leo Lopez, and Donald J. Hagler.

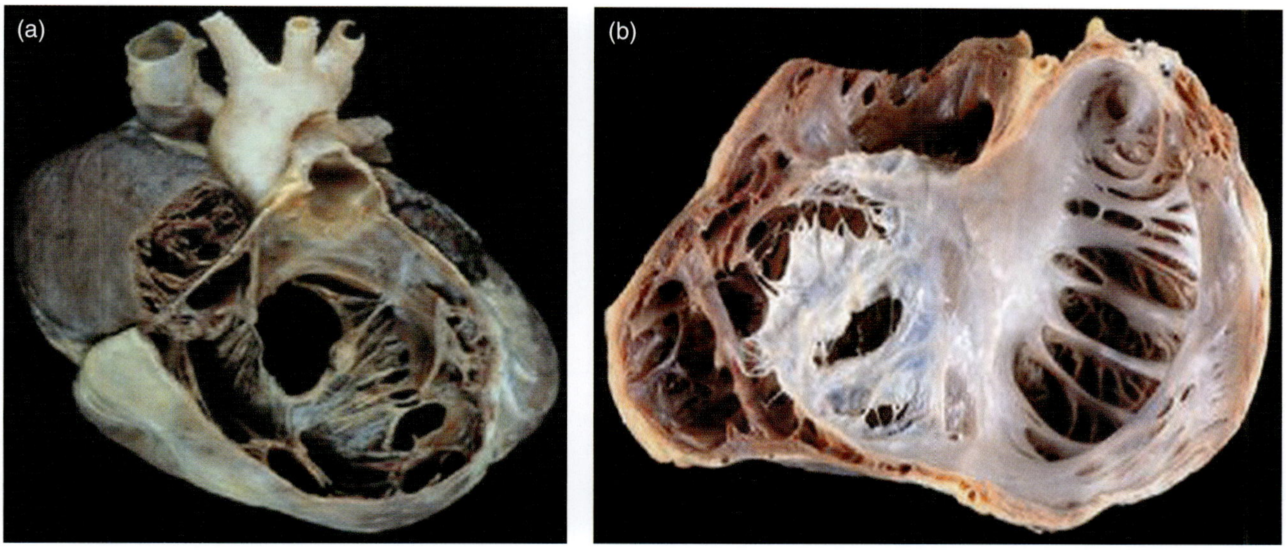

Figure 25.1 Ebstein heart: marked failure of delamination with fenestrations, and tethering of the anterior leaflet.

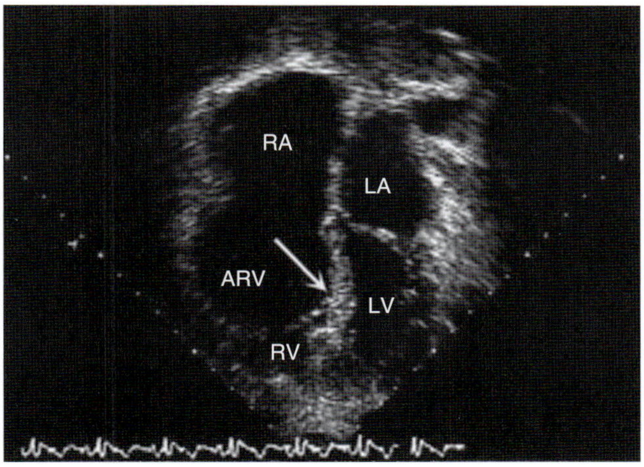

Figure 25.2 Example of an echocardiogram (four-chamber view, apex down): of a patient with severe Ebstein anomaly showing a grossly displaced septal leaflet (arrow). The anterior leaflet is severely tethered and nearly immobile from extensive failure of delamination. The functional right ventricle (RV) is small and the atrialized RV (ARV) is large. aRV, atrialized right ventricle; LA, left atrium; LV, left ventricle; RA, right atrium; RV, right ventricle.

single ventricle repair (i.e., right ventricular exclusion technique; Starnes approach) (Figure 24.4) [6].

Children and Adults

The indications for surgery in older children and adults:

1) The presence of symptoms – cyanosis, fatigue, shortness of breath;
2) Decreased exercise tolerance;
3) Progressive RV dilatation or progressive reduction of RV systolic function by echocardiography or MRI; and
4) Onset/progression of atrial or ventricular arrhythmias.

Surgical Techniques

Neonate

Biventricular repair is most often performed using a monocusp repair technique; application of the cone technique can be applied selectively depending on surgeon experience and stability of the child. In addition to TV repair, there is subtotal closure of the atrial septal defect, and selective plication of the atrialized RV. Sebening stitch (fixation of the major anterior papillary muscle to the ventricular septum) may be added to facilitate anterior leaflet–ventricular septal coaptation with the monocusp technique. Generous reduction right atrioplasty is performed routinely to make space for the lungs.

Univentricular strategy (RV exclusion) is chosen in the presence of less developed anterior leaflet, concomitant anatomic pulmonary atresia, or in the unstable neonate. This involves fenestrated TV patch closure, atrial septal defect enlargement, and a systemic-to-pulmonary artery shunt. If an incompetent pulmonary valve is present, the main pulmonary artery should be ligated or oversewn. Right atrial reduction is also routinely performed.

Children and Adults

Cone Repair

Despite good intermediate [7, 8] and long-term results of numerous repair techniques [9, 10], the need for re-operation persists for many (Figures 25.5 and 25.6). Cone repair (CR) is the most anatomic repair technique and includes 360 degrees of mobilized, surgically delaminated leaflet tissue which is then re-anchored at the true TV annular level [11]. The most difficult aspect of CR is *complete* surgical delamination which involves incision/excision of all muscular/fibrous attachments

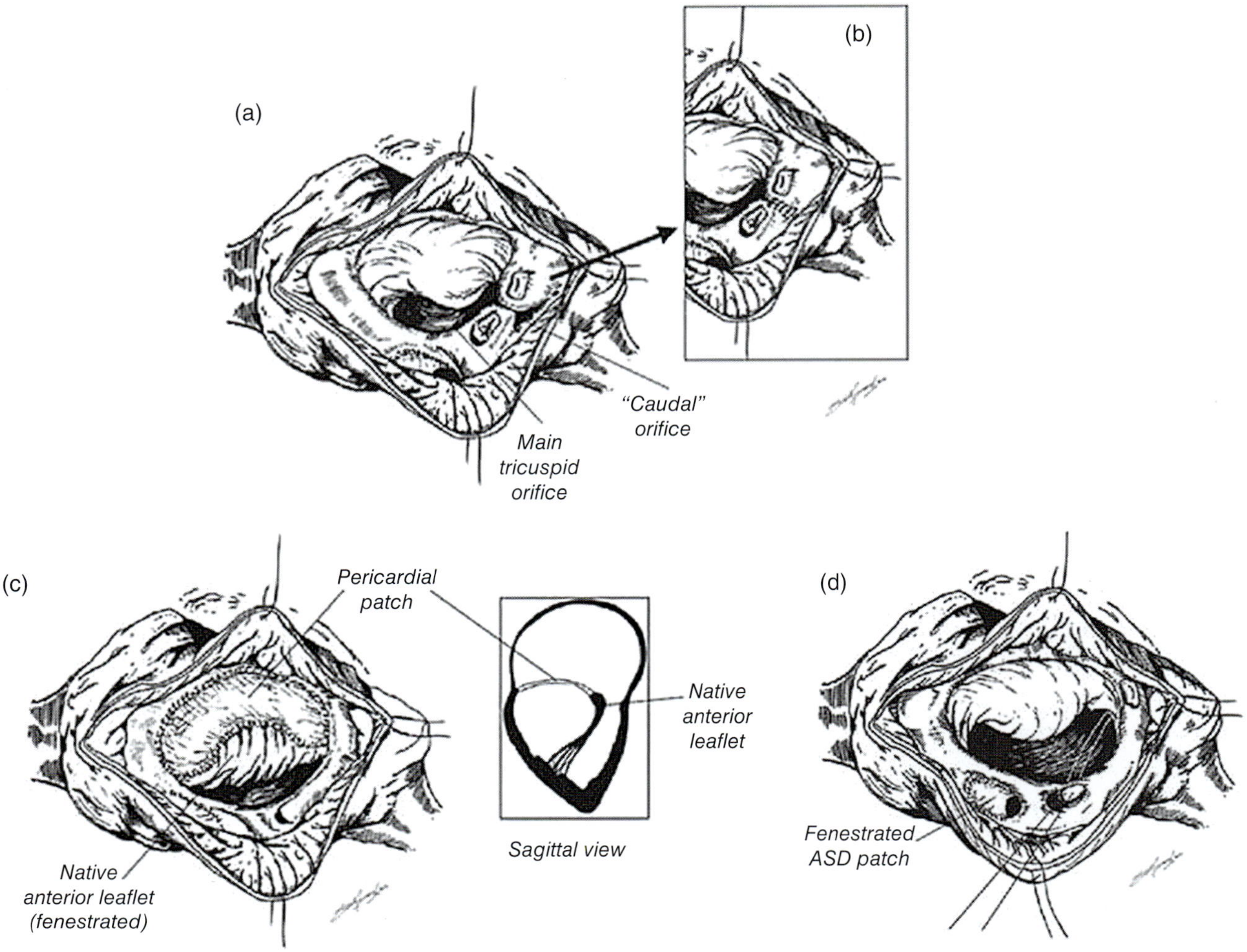

Figure 25.3 Biventricular repair of neonatal Ebstein (Knott-Craig). (a) Partition of the tricuspid valve (TV) orifice into two openings by approximation of the annuloplasty stitch. (b) Once the valve is judged to be competent, the "caudal" orifice is closed, thereby plicating the atrialized portion of the RV. (c) Creation of a competent monocuspid valve by taking down the anterior leaflet from the annulus, fenestrating it, and augmenting it with a pericardial patch. (d) The atrial septal defect (ASD) is closed with a fenestrated patch, and an annuloplasty stitch is placed with one pledgetted end in the coronary sinus and the other pledgetted end at the location of the commissure between anterior and posterior leaflets.

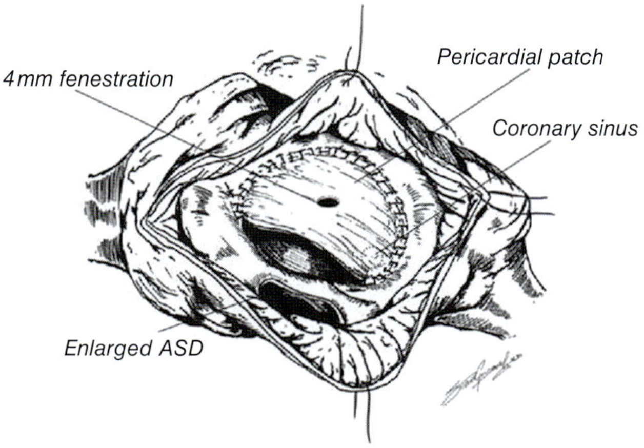

Figure 25.4 Starnes repair of neonatal Ebstein malformation.

between the body of the leaflet(s) and the RV free wall and ventricular septum. Second, recruitment of the septal leaflet (even when very diminutive) is critical in establishing 360 degrees of leaflet tissue to surround the TV orifice. In selected situations, the addition of supplemental tissue (autologous pericardium or cor-matrix membrane) to augment leaflet height can be helpful and increases leaflet-to-leaflet surface area and leaflet size. As an alternative to leaflet augmentation, the height of the native anterior leaflet can be increased by performing multiple plications along the detached edge (close to the annulus) of the mobilized anterior leaflet, thereby increasing the height of the leaflet in an effort to avoid the use of prosthetic material.

RV plication is performed of the inferior wall when it is smooth, thinned, and non-trabeculated. The inferior annulus plication is the site of greatest tension and the

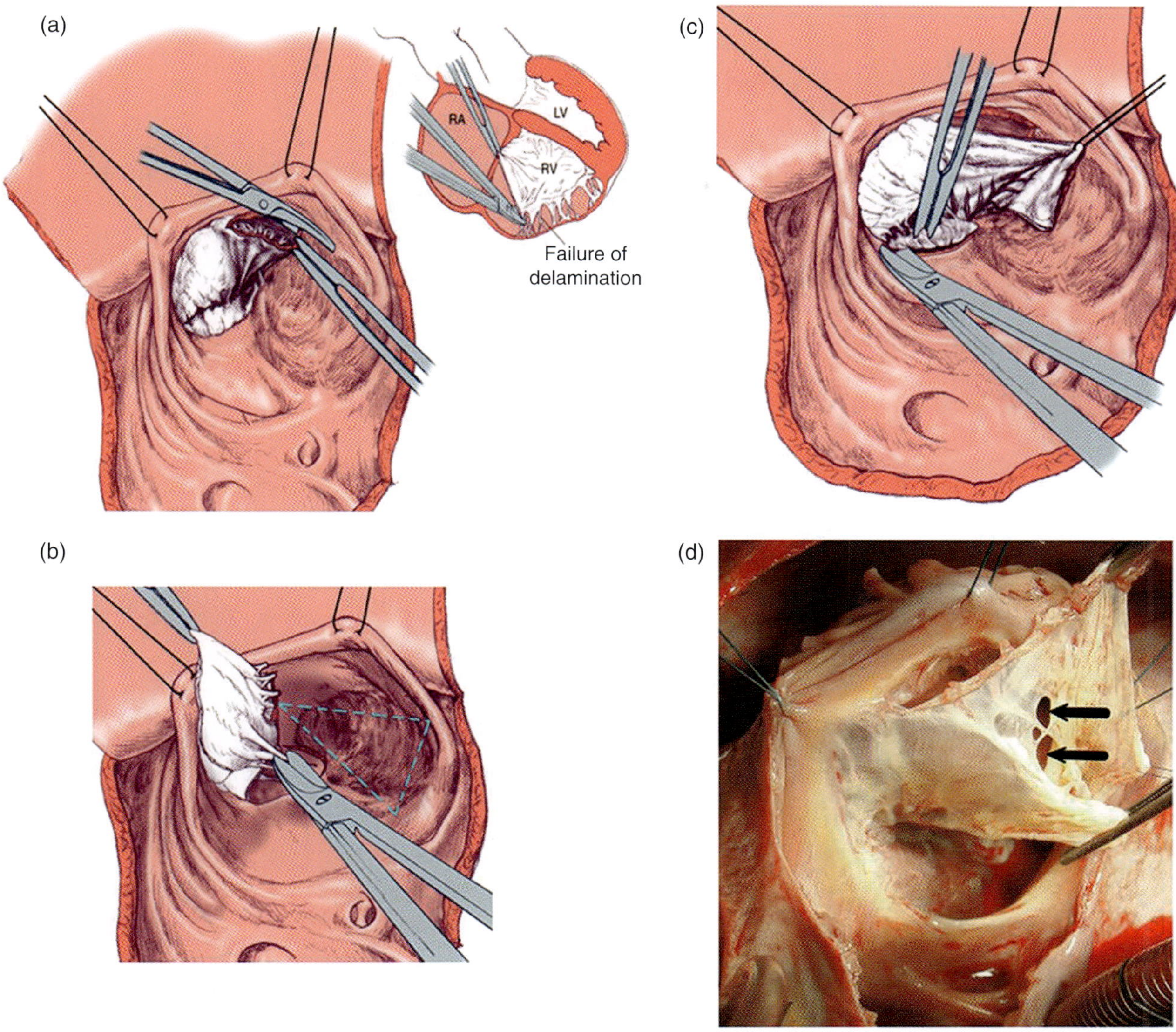

Figure 25.5 Operative steps for "cone repair." (a) The first incision is made in the anterior leaflet at 10:00 a few millimeters away from the true annulus. The incision is then extended in a clockwise fashion using a scissors. The delamination consists of incising/excising all fibrous and muscular attachments between the body of the leaflet and the right ventricular myocardium (moving apically toward the apex), but maintaining all chordal and (and occasionally muscular) attachments of the leaflet's leading edge to the underlying myocardium. LV, left ventricle; RA, right atrium; RV, right ventricle. (b) As the anterior and surgically delaminated inferior leaflet is reflected away from the RV myocardium, all fibrous and muscular attachments into the body of the underside of the leaflet are incised as shown with the scissors. The dotted triangle represents the atrialized RV, which is typically smooth, thinned and non-trabeculated. (c) The dissection should proceed medially all the way to the anteroseptal commissure. The leaflet tissue is typically very fragile and thin in this area. There can be marked variability in the status of the leading edge of the septal leaflet as was described for the anterior and inferior leaflets. (d) Intraoperative photo demonstrating the mobilized anterior and inferior (posterior) leaflets. Natural fenestrations are shown at the junction of the anterior and inferior leaflets (arrows).

most vulnerable to right coronary compromise. Evenly placed annular plication sutures around the entire anterior and inferior annulus may be preferable to an exaggerated plication in the inferior location. Septal re-attachment to the ventricular septum is performed caudal to the membranous septum and conduction tissue. Finally, the addition of an annuloplasty band stabilizes the repair (Figure 25.7a). An eccentric ring from antero-inferior commissure to coronary sinus is used when somatic growth is incomplete (Figure 25.7b) if there is concern of creating tricuspid stenosis. When RV dysfunction is severe, a bidirectional cavopulmonary anastomosis is performed. When RV dysfunction is moderately depressed, subtotal closure of the atrial septal defect is performed as an alternative to a bidirectional cavopulmonary anastomosis (BDCPA).

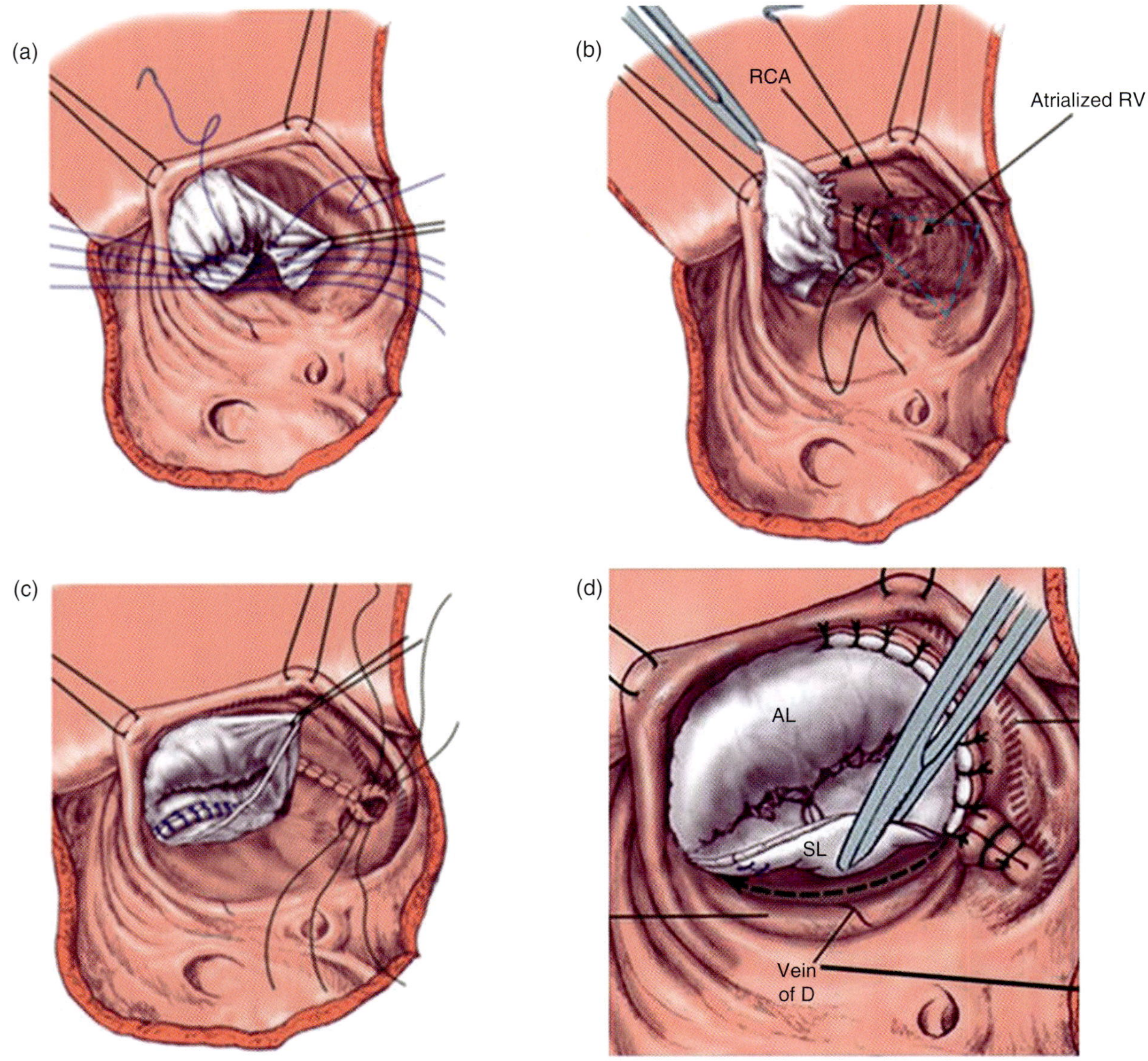

Figure 25.6 (a) After the anterior, inferior, and septal leaflets have been completely mobilized, the cut edge of the inferior leaflet is rotated clockwise to meet the proximal edge that has been prepared of the mobilized septal leaflet. The two are approximated with interrupted fine monofilament sutures completing the cone reconstruction. This results in 360° of leaflet tissue that will make up the new tricuspid valve orifice. (b) After the cone reconstruction is completed, the atrialized right ventricle (RV) is examined to determine if plication is necessary. Note the position of the right coronary artery (RCA) in the true tricuspid valve annulus and keep in mind that the main RCA or the posterior descending coronary artery can be compromised. This figure demonstrates the technique for internal plication of the atrialized RV from apex to base. Monofilament suture is utilized; the suture is begun distally toward the apex of the RV. It is important to frequently examine the outside of the inferior wall of the RV to insure that inadvertent compromise of the RCA is avoided. (c) The suture line is advanced toward the base of the heart (i.e., toward the atrioventricular groove). As the dotted lines of the triangle are effectively approximated, the atrialized RV is excluded. The suture line sometimes crosses the atrioventricular groove to reduce the size of the dilated annulus. After the sides of the triangle are approximated, the entrance into the excluded atrialized segment of the RV is then closed to eliminate the "blind pouch." (d) After the plication is completed, the newly constructed tricuspid valve is then re-attached at the level of the true tricuspid annulus. Because the neotricuspid valve will have an orifice that is smaller than the original dilated atrioventricular junction, a plication of the inferior annulus is usually necessary to meet the size of the smaller neotricuspid valve. Re-attachment of the septal leaflet should be performed to the ventricular septum and to the ventricular side of the conduction tissue which is usually marked by a small vein.

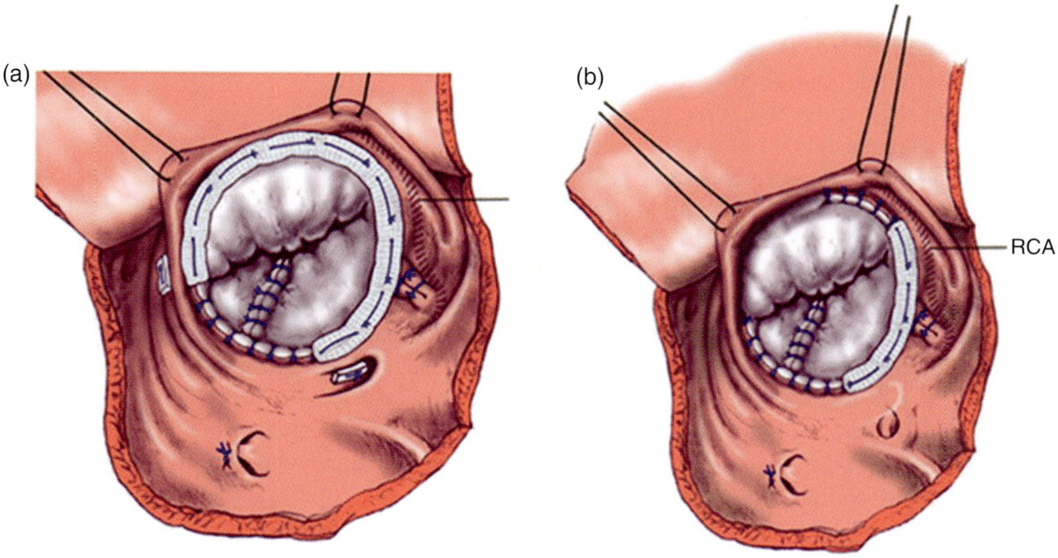

Figure 25.7 The tricuspid annulus is usually dilated and a flexible annuloplasty ring is typically used when somatic growth is complete (a); however, in younger patients when somatic growth is not complete, an eccentric ring confined to the inferior annulus (anteroinferior to inferoseptal commissures) can be used (b). RCA, right coronary artery.

Bidirectional Cavopulmonary Anastomosis

BDCPA reduces RV size and helps minimize compression of the left ventricle (LV), and provides preload to the LV. Importantly, low cardiac output syndrome is avoided [12]. The BDCPA is permissible when the mean pulmonary artery pressures are <18 mmHg and the LV end diastolic pressure is <10 mmHg. Indications for BDCPA include:

1) Severe right ventricular dilatation and/or dysfunction;
2) Leftward shift of the interventricular septum (D-shaped LV);
3) Preoperative cyanosis at rest or with exercise;
4) Post-bypass right atrium : left atrium pressure ratio of >1.5 : 1; and
5) Resultant TV repair with a small effective orifice (mean gradient >7–8 mmHg) [13].

TV Replacement

TV replacement is reserved for unsuccessful TV repair and for older patients (>55–60 years) with severe valve deformities, severe RV dilatation, or severe tricuspid annular dilatation. We prefer porcine bioprostheses to mechanical valves because of the relatively good durability in the tricuspid position and the lack of need for life-long anticoagulation [14]. However, mechanical valves in the tricuspid position are associated with higher frequency of thromboembolic complications especially in the presence of RV dysfunction [15]. The prosthetic valve suture line is deviated cephalad to the atrioventricular node, bundle of His, and membranous septum. This results in an intra-atrial position of the prosthesis. In order to avoid injury to the right coronary artery anteriorly, the suture line is deviated cephalad to the tricuspid annulus. The coronary sinus can be left to drain into the right atrium or into the RV. The bioprosthesis is oriented so that the recess between the struts of the prosthesis, straddle the area of the membranous septum and conduction tissue. It is important to downsize the prosthesis when a BDCPA has been performed because the amount of blood flow through the valve is reduced and leaflet opening or closing may be compromised.

Arrhythmia Surgery

A biatrial maze is performed when there is persistent atrial fibrillation. When atrial fibrillation is paroxysmal, the maze is usually confined to the right atrium. When atrial flutter is present, the cavotricuspid isthmus is cryoablated. A prophylactic right-sided maze is considered when there is significant atrial dilatation [16].

Postoperative Management

In children and adults, the postoperative period is generally straightforward when LV function is normal and RV dysfunction is not severe. Routinely, separation from bypass is accomplished with low dose epinephrine and milrinone infusions. Occasionally, low dose vasopressin is utilized when low systemic vascular resistance is present. This is not uncommon when right-sided heart failure is present. Volume administration is performed cautiously; a right atrial pressure of <12 mmHg is targeted and blood transfusions are avoided. In order to avoid RV dilatation, faster heart rates (100–120 bpm) with the use of temporary atrial pacing, if needed, is performed. A mild metabolic acidosis (base deficit of minus 5) is common early after operation; this usually resolves with careful volume administration and is not concerning provided urine output is satisfactory. Extubation is performed after metabolic parameters have normalized. Inotropic support is weaned over 24–48 hours and is determined by the degree of RV dysfunction, which can be severe after correction of tricuspid regurgitation.

When there is evidence of low cardiac output in the ICU following operation after optimization of inotropic support (e.g., low urine output, increasing creatinine, metabolic acidosis), consideration should be given to early re-operation for bidirectional cavopulmonary shunt. Delayed sternal closure, especially in patients with severe RV dilatation and dysfunction, can be life-saving.

To decrease RV afterload (i.e., decrease pulmonary arterial pressures), nitric oxide may be helpful in selected circumstances. Although RV and pulmonary artery pressures are usually normal or low in EM, temporary use of nitric oxide can be helpful to offset the pulmonary vasoconstrictive effects of inotropic support that is required in the early postoperative period. Atrial and ventricular arrhythmias should be treated aggressively through the optimization of metabolic parameters and the use of amiodarone, lidocaine, or beta-blocker therapy. In some patients, RV dysfunction is aggravated by atrial or ventricular arrhythmias, resulting in very low cardiac output. Also, some patients with postoperative severe RV dysfunction may respond to volume challenge with RV distention and progress to profound cardiogenic shock, rapidly. These situations can require immediate mechanical circulatory assistance.

Medical therapy after hospital discharge includes afterload reducing agents and beta blockade. This is generally accomplished with ACE-inhibitors; specific pulmonary vasodilators (e.g., sildenafil) are used selectively in the first 1–3 months after operation. When TV replacement has been performed, warfarin is utilized for 3 months postoperatively (target INR 2–3), in combination with lifelong aspirin (81 or 325 mg). If patients have any postoperative arrhythmias (particularly ventricular), amiodarone is used for a minimum of 3 months and then re-assessed. Atrial and/or ventricular arrhythmias are common late events after EM surgery, so a protocol for arrhythmia surveillance should be established for each institution with participation of the electrophysiology team. An exercise test and/or Holter monitoring should be performed between 6 and 12 months postoperatively to exclude the presence of any arrhythmias and prior to cessation of beta-blockers or other antiarrhythmic medications.

Mayo Clinic Experience

Our institutional experience with surgical treatment now exceeds 1000 patients. Results from the initial 539 patients were reported previously. More recently, we have adopted the cone repair; more than 150 have been performed. Our initial report of the first 89 patients (47 females; 53%) that underwent cone reconstruction (median age 19 years; range 19 days–68 years) were operated on between June 2007 and December 2011. Severe tricuspid regurgitation was present in 75 patients (84%). All patients underwent cone reconstruction (360 degrees leaflet tissue repair anchored at true annulus). Modifications included ringed annuloplasty in 57 (64%), leaflet augmentation in 28 patients (31%), and autologous chordae in 17 patients (19%). BDCPA was performed in 21 patients (24%). Early mortality occurred in 1 patient (1%). Early re-operation for recurrent tricuspid regurgitation occurred in 12 patients (13%); re-repair was performed in 6 patients (50%) and 6 (50%) required replacement. Mean follow-up was 19.7 ± 24.7 months. There was no late mortality or re-operation. At follow-up, 72 patients (87%) had no or mild tricuspid regurgitation, nine (11%) had moderate, and two patients (2%) had severe tricuspid regurgitation. Ringed annuloplasty was associated with less than moderate tricuspid regurgitation at dismissal ($p = 0.01$) [17].

We also reviewed our experience with re-repair of TV applying the principles of CR in 20 patients (median age 15 years) between June 2007 and October 2012 [18]. Four patients had prior BDCPA, and recurrent tricuspid regurgitation was mainly caused by incomplete leaflet coaptation with tethered anterior leaflet in all patients. Prior repair techniques consisted of annuloplasty maneuvers in all patients with no or incomplete surgical delamination. TV re-repair was possible in all patients with no mortality or re-operations during a mean follow-up period of 7.7 ± 10.7 months and at final echocardiography 18 patients had no or mild tricuspid regurgitation and 2 had moderate regurgitation.

Tricuspid Valve Dysplasia

In general, there are two categories of congenital TV dysplasia: those with and those without downward displacement. Cases with downward displacement, which is caused by failure of delamination of valve leaflets from the underlying myocardium, are, by definition, EM. When downward displacement is absent and dysplastic leaflets are fully delaminated, then the anatomic entity is referred to as "tricuspid valve dysplasia." Patients with pulmonary atresia and intact ventricular septum (PA/IVS) tend to have a higher incidence of a regurgitant TV secondary to TV dysplasia.

Uhl Anomaly

Uhl anomaly is extremely rare and can be associated with PA/IVS. In Uhl anomaly, there is complete or partial absence of the myocardial layer of the RV and the endocardium and the epicardium become opposed, but the septal component, septomarginal trabeculation, and the papillary muscles of the TV are normally muscularized [19]. The absence of myocardium may be the result of primary non-development of myocytes or a form of selective apoptosis. Most cases are sporadic and Feucht *et al.* [20] suggested the role of vascular endothelial growth factor in the induction of this cardiovascular malformation.

Congestive heart failure with associated peripheral edema and pleural effusion is the most frequent symptom. Arrhythmias and conduction disturbances are not common in Uhl anomaly as in arrhythmogenic RV dysplasia because of the absence of foci that transmit abnormal electrical activity [21].

Medical management of congestive heart failure and drainage of pleural effusions is often required. Surgical options include RV exclusion with atrial septectomy, BDCPA, and closure of the TV orifice [22]. One-and-half ventricle repair has been reported [23] and cardiac transplantation represents the therapy of last resort [24].

References

1 Mann RJ, Lie JT. (1979) The life story of Wilhelm Ebstein (1836–1912) and his almost overlooked description of a congenital heart disease. *Mayo Clin Proc*, **54**, 197–204.

2 Said SM, Dearani JA. (2013) Ebstein's anomaly, congenital tricuspid valve regurgitation, and dysplasia, in, *Moss and Adams' Heart Disease in Infants, Children, and Adolescents: Including the Fetus and Young Adult*, 8th edn (eds HD Allen, DJ Driscoll, RE Shaddy, TF Feltes), Lippincott Williams and Wilkins, Wolters Kluwer, pp. 889–912.

3 Celermajer DS, Cullen S, Sullivan ID, *et al.* (1992) Outcome in neonates with Ebstein's anomaly. *J Am Coll Cardiol*, **19**, 1041–1046.

4 Knott-Craig CJ. (2008) Management of neonatal Ebstein's anomaly. *Oper Tech*, **13**, 101–108.

5 Knott-Craig CJ, Goldberg SP, Overholt ED, *et al.* (2007) Repair of neonates and young infants with Ebstein's anomaly and related disorders. *Ann Thorac Surg*, **84**, 587–593.

6 Starnes VA, Pitlick PT, Bernstein D, *et al.* (1991) Ebstein's anomaly appearing in the neonate: a new surgical approach. *J Thorac Cardiovasc Surg*, **101**, 1082–1087.

7 Chen JM, Mosca RS, Altmann K, *et al.* (2004) Early and medium term results for repair of Ebstein anomaly. *J Thorac Cardiovasc Surg*, **127**, 990–998.

8 Wu Q, Huang Z, Pan G, *et al.* (2007) Early and midterm results in anatomic repair of Ebstein anomaly. *J Thorac Cardiovasc Surg*, **134**, 1438–1440.

9 Chauvaud S. (2000) Ebstein's malformation: surgical treatment and results. *Thorac Cardiovasc Surg*, **48**, 220–223.

10 Brown ML, Dearani JA, Danielson GK, *et al.* (2008) The outcomes of operations for 539 patients with Ebstein anomaly. *J Thorac Cardiovasc Surg*, **135**, 1120–1136.

11 da Silva JP, Baumgratz JF, Fonseca L, *et al.* (2004) Anomalia de Ebstein: resultados com a reconstrução cônica da valva tricúspide [in Spanish]. *Arq Bras Cardiol*, **82**, 212–216.

12 Chauvaud S, Fuzellier JF, Berrebi A, *et al.* (1998) Bi-directional cavopulmonary shunt associated with ventriculo and valvuloplasty in Ebstein's anomaly: benefits in high risk patients. *Eur J Cardiothorac Surg*, **13**, 514–519.

13 Quiñonez LG, Dearani JA, Puga FJ, *et al.* (2007) Results of the 1.5-ventricle repair for Ebstein anomaly and the failing right ventricle. *J Thorac Cardiovasc Surg*, **133**, 1303–1310.

14 Kiziltan HT, Theodoro DA, Warnes CA, *et al.* (1998) Late results of bioprosthetic tricuspid valve replacement in Ebstein's anomaly. *Ann Thorac Surg*, **66**, 1539–1545.

15 Sanfelippo PM, Giuliani ER, Danielson GK, *et al.* (1976) Tricuspid valve prosthetic replacement: early and late results with the Starr–Edwards prosthesis. *J Thorac Cardiovasc Surg*, **71**, 441–445.

16 Mavroudis C, Deal BJ, Back CL, *et al.* (2008) Arrhythmia surgery in patients with and without congenital heart disease. *Ann Thorac Surg*, **86**, 857–868.

17 Dearani JA, Said SM, O'Leary PW, *et al.* (2013) Anatomic repair of Ebstein's malformation: lessons learned with cone reconstruction. *Ann Thorac Surg*, **95** (1), 220–226; discussion 226–228.

18 Dearani JA, Said SM, Burkhart HM, *et al.* (2013) Strategies for tricuspid re-repair in Ebstein malformation using the cone technique. *Ann Thorac Surg*, **96** (1), 202–210.

19 Gould L, Guttman B, Carrasco J, *et al.* (1967) Partial absence of the right ventricular musculature: a congenital lesion. *Am J Med*, **42**, 636–641.

20 Feucht M, Christ B, Wilting J. (1997) VEGF induces cardiovascular malformation and embryonic lethality. *Am J Pathol*, **151**, 1407–1416.

21 Gerlis LM, Schmidt-Ott SC, HO SY, *et al.* (1993) Dysplastic conditions of the right ventricular myocardium: Uhl's anomaly versus arrhythmogenic right ventricular dysplasia. *Br Heart J*, **69**, 142–150.

22 Azhari N, Assaqqat M, Bulbul Z. (2002) Successful surgical repair of Uhl's anomaly. *Cardiol Young*, **12**, 192–195.

23 Yoshii S, Suzuki S, Hosaka S, *et al.* (2001) A case of Uhl's anomaly treated with a one and a half ventricle repair combined with partial right ventriculectomy in infancy. *J Thorac Cardiovasc Surg*, **122**, 1026–1028.

24 Ikari NM, Azeka E, Aiello VD, *et al.* (2001) Uhl's anomaly: differential diagnosis and indications for cardiac transplantation in an infant. *Arq Bras Cardiol*, **77**, 69–76.

26

Pulmonary Valve and Pulmonary Arterial Stenosis

Evan M. Zahn[1] *and Darren P. Berman*[2]

[1] *Congenital Heart Program and Division of Pediatric Cardiology, Cedars-Sinai Medical Center, Los Angeles, CA, USA*
[2] *Division of Cardiology, Nationwide Children's Hospital, Columbus, OH, USA*

Pulmonary Valve Stenosis

Pulmonary valve stenosis is one of the most common congenital heart lesions, accounting for 10% of all cardiac malformations; however, neonatal presentation is less common, representing 3–4% of infants referred for congenital heart disease. The most typical valve morphology is fusion of the individual valve leaflets at the commissures with the most severely obstructive valves presenting in the neonatal period as critical pulmonic stenosis. More rarely, patients can present with dysplastic pulmonary valve in which there is a trileaflet valve and the leaflets are thickened with limited mobility and often associated with some degree of annular hypoplasia.

It is important to distinguish between these two anatomic forms of pulmonic valve stenosis as therapeutic options vary depending on anatomic form. This differentiation is complicated by the fact that in the newborn period (and beyond) there is considerable overlap between simple pulmonic stenosis resulting form fusion of thin pliable valve leaflets and dysplastic thickened pulmonary valve, with most neonates having some qualities of both. Pulmonic valve stenosis typically presents as an isolated anatomic lesion but, if at all significant, is nearly always associated with significant right ventricular hypertrophy in the neonatal period as well as a patent foramen ovale with a bidirectional, mainly right to left, shunt pattern and a patent ductus arteriosus. Severe right ventricular systolic dysfunction is the norm in cases of critical pulmonic stenosis. With significant pulmonary valve obstruction in this age group there is nearly always tricuspid valve regurgitation, which may be associated with thickening of the tricuspid valve apparatus and leaflets. Occasionally, severe right ventricular hypoplasia can be seen similar to that observed in patients with pulmonary atresia and intact ventricular septum.

Most typically, neonates with pulmonary stenosis are full term, of normal birth weight, and normal appearing. Patients with mild to moderate obstruction usually present with the serendipitous auscultation of a systolic ejection murmur and no clinical symptomatology. Patients with severe stenosis typically exhibit severe symptomatology shortly after birth including cyanosis secondary to right to left shunting at atrial level, hepatic congestion, and low cardiac output. While with mild to moderate stenosis the neonatal ECG typically shows modest right ventricular hypertrophy, when the obstruction is critical, two distinct abnormal ECG patterns can be seen:

1) Severe right ventricular hypertrophy with right axis deviation (Figure 26.1); or
2) Left ventricular dominance and a lack of right heart forces.

The chest X-ray in moderate to severe stenosis will typically show some degree of cardiomegaly, often secondary to right atrial dilation, and diminished pulmonary vascular markings related to the right to left shunting at atrial level. The definitive diagnostic tool for this heart defect is echocardiography with color flow Doppler which provides all key anatomic and physiologic information including right ventricular size and function (Figure 26.2), pulmonary valve morphology, annular dimension (Figure 26.3), and pulmonary valve gradient, as well as status of the patent foramen ovale and patent ductus arteriosus and degree of tricuspid regurgitation. Not unusually, it can be difficult to discern whether in severe cases there is actually any antegrade flow across the pulmonic valve as retrograde flow from a large patent ductus arteriosus into the main pulmonary artery can obscure a small antegrade jet exiting the right ventricle via a critically stenotic pulmonary valve (Figure 26.4).

The timing and method of treatment is based primarily upon the severity of the obstruction as well as specific anatomic substrate. Infants with mild to moderate obstruction can be discharged home and followed as an outpatient once it has been determined that they are not

Visual Guide to Neonatal Cardiology, First Edition. Edited by Ernerio T. Alboliras, Ziyad M. Hijazi, Leo Lopez, and Donald J. Hagler.

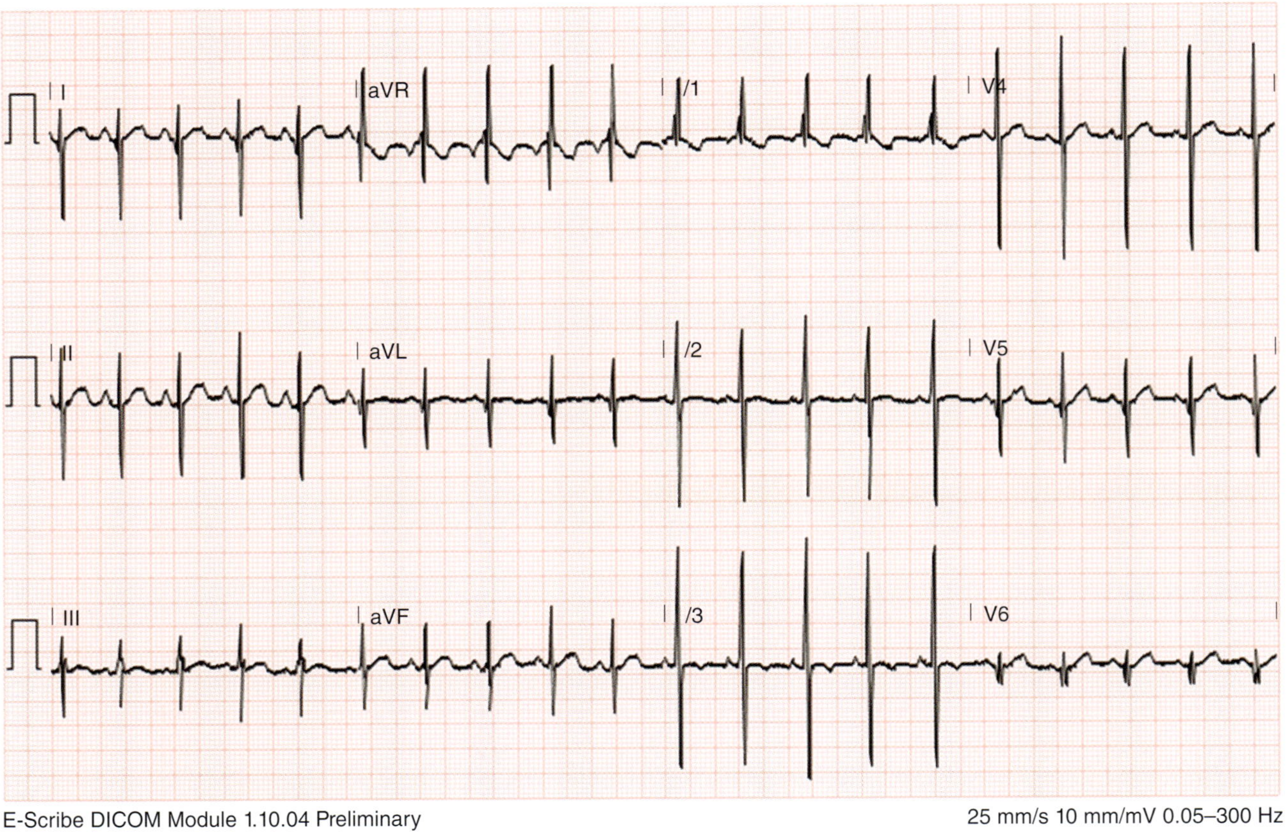

Figure 26.1 Twelve-lead electrocardiogram in a newborn with critical pulmonary valve stenosis. Note the right axis deviation and right ventricular hypertrophy.

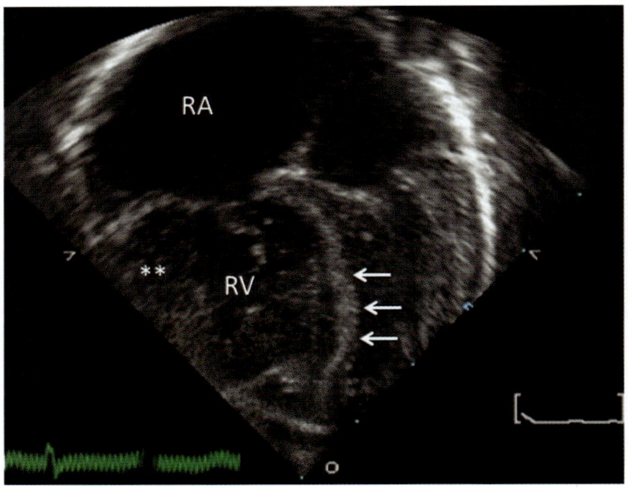

Figure 26.2 Transthoracic echocardiogram in a newborn with critical pulmonary valve stenosis. Note the dilated right atrium (RA) and the severely hypertrophied right ventricle (asterisks, RV). The bowing of the interventricular septum towards the left ventricle (white arrows) suggests a right ventricular pressure higher than the left ventricular pressure.

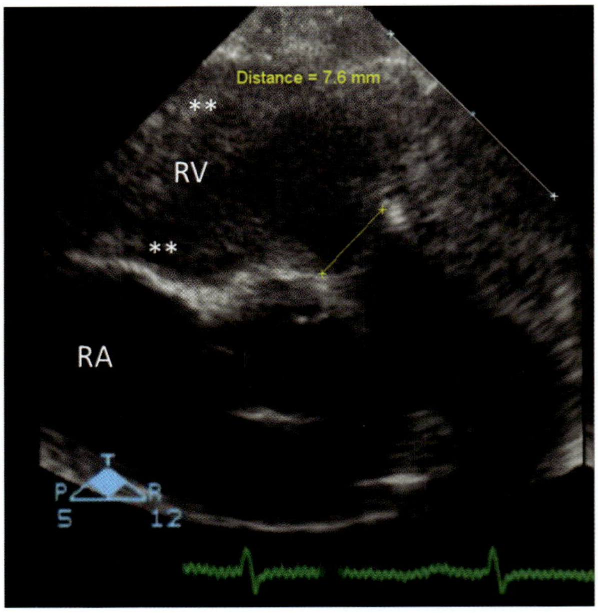

Figure 26.3 Parasternal short-axis transthoracic echocardiographic image taken in end-systole profiles the relationship of the right atrium (RA), right ventricle (RV), and measured pulmonary valve annulus. The measurement is taken at the hinge point of the leaflets and has a crucial role in the treatment algorithm for this disease. Note the lack of complete opening of the valve leaflets in systole and the severe right ventricular hypertrophy (asterisks).

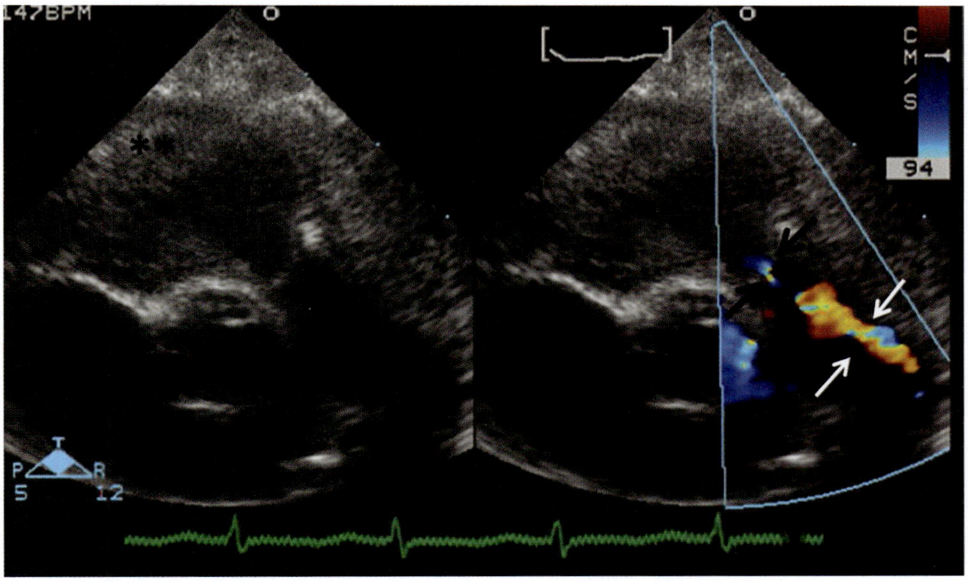

Figure 26.4 Parasternal short-axis transthoracic echocardiographic image taken in end-systole with and without color Doppler. Two-dimensional and color Doppler imaging across the right ventricular outflow tract demonstrate a patent infundibular region with poorly mobile pulmonary valve leaflets and a narrow jet of flow exiting through this critically stenotic valve (black arrows). Also seen is the left to right shunt via a patent ductus arteriosus which serves as this neonates primary source of pulmonary blood flow at this point in time (white arrows).

reliant on flow through a patent ductus arteriosus and patent foramen ovale to maintain adequate pulmonary blood flow and cardiac output, respectively.

Neonates who present with severe obstruction and clinical symptoms should be placed on prostaglandin E1 to maintain ductal patency and a therapeutic procedure performed prior to discharge. The procedure of choice is typically cardiac catheterization with balloon valvuloplasty [1, 2]. Usually performed from a femoral venous approach, an abbreviated hemodynamic evaluation should be performed focusing on the right ventricular pressure in relationship to either the directly measured aortic pressure or non-invasive cuff pressure. Following these measurements, a right ventricular angiogram should be performed in the frontal, or with slight right anterior oblique (RAO) and cranial angulation, and straight lateral 90 degrees left anterior oblique ILAO projections (Figure 26.5). These images are used to evaluate the degree of right ventricular dysfunction, hypertrophy, tricuspid regurgitation and, most importantly, obtain quantitative measurements of the pulmonary valve annulus, which will be used to determine the diameter of the valvuloplasty balloon (typically selected to be 1.1–1.3 times the annular diameter). The valve is then crossed with a soft-tipped guidewire which is positioned within a distal pulmonary artery branch or preferably across the ductus arteriosus and down into the descending aorta. An appropriate sized low-pressure balloon valvuloplasty catheter is selected based on the annular dimension and advanced over the guidewire to cross the valve (Figure 26.6). In severe cases, serial dilation using increasingly larger balloon diameters may be necessary. Typically, a tight "waist" is seen at the initiation of the balloon inflation, which disappears with an effective valvuloplasty. Repeat pressure measurements should focus upon any residual gradient across the pulmonary valve as the right ventricular pressure will typically remain elevated in the setting of a large patent ductus arteriosus. Additionally, because of a combination of immediate improvement in right ventricular contractility and severe hypertrophy of the infundibular portion of the right ventricle, these neonates can occasionally develop important dynamic subvalve pulmonic stenosis which in our experience is nearly always transient but can require the maintenance of PGE1 infusion or institution of beta-blocker therapy for a short period of time. Careful pullback pressure measurements along the right ventricular outflow tract as well as repeat right ventricular angiography are useful in determining the contribution of dynamic subpulmonic stenosis from residual valve stenosis which might require further therapy (e.g., valvuloplasty using a larger balloon diameter; Figure 26.7). In most cases following the procedure, PGE1 can be immediately discontinued. Hospital length of stay following the procedure is variable and depends on a number of factors including the effectiveness of the valvuloplasty and resolution of subvalvar obstruction, which can be followed by echocardiography (Figure 26.8). Rarely, a neonate may require a temporary additional source of pulmonary blood flow in the

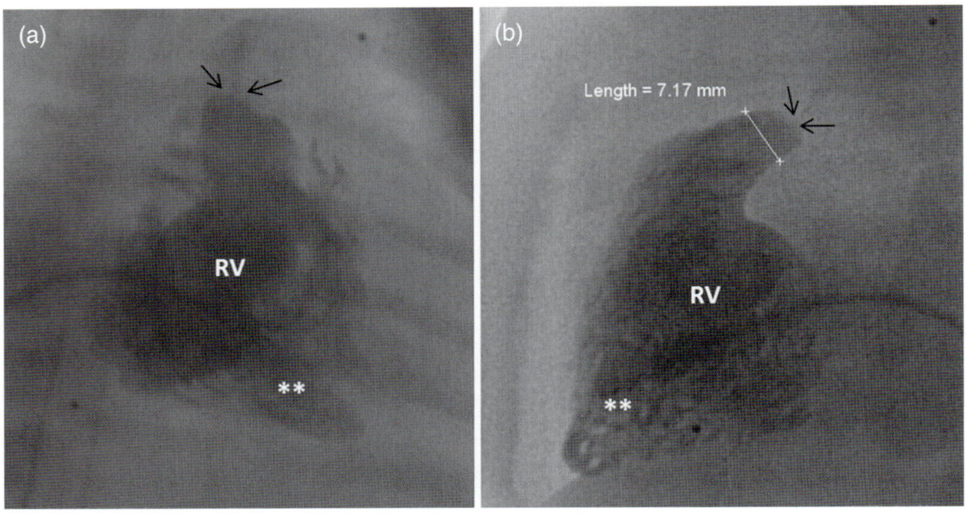

Figure 26.5 Right ventriculogram in a newborn with critical pulmonary valve stenosis performed in (a) frontal and (b) lateral projections. Right anterior oblique (RAO)/cranial angulation of the frontal camera helps profile the right ventricular outflow tract, doming pulmonary valve, and narrow jet of contrast exiting into the pulmonary artery (black arrows). Although hypertrophic (asterisks) and poorly functioning, the right ventricle can be seen to be normally formed (tripartite) in both projections. Although both projections are helpful, the lateral view provides an excellent angle for accurate measurement of the pulmonary valve annulus, which will determine the valvuloplasty balloon diameter and serve as an excellent roadmap for crossing the narrowed valve with a guidewire and positioning the balloon valvuloplasty catheter.

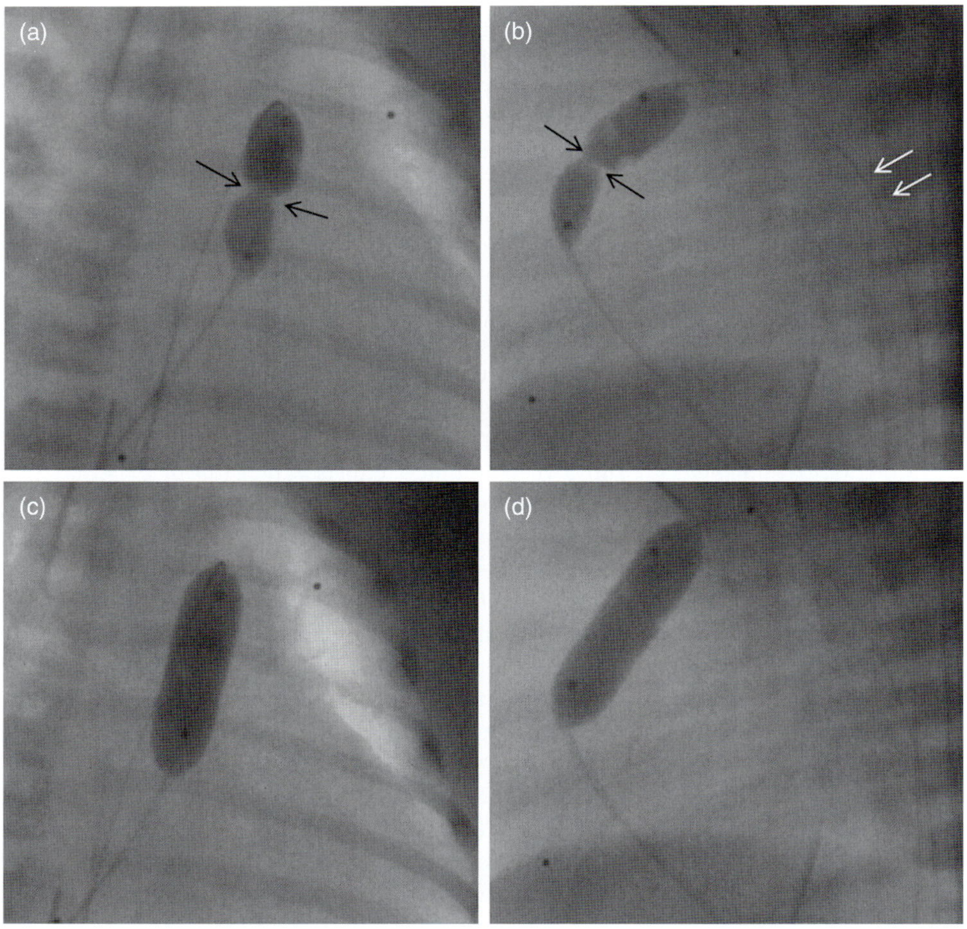

Figure 26.6 Balloon pulmonary valvuloplasty. An appropriate-sized balloon catheter (1.1–1.3 times the annular diameter) has been advanced across a stenotic pulmonary valve and inflated in the frontal (a,c) and lateral (b,d) projections. Early in the inflation (a,b), a tight "waist" in the mid-portion of the balloon (black arrows) confirms that the balloon is appropriately centered across the stenotic valve. At full inflation (c,d), the waist disappears, corresponding with relief of the stenosis. Note the distal guidewire position across the patent arterial duct and into the descending aorta (white arrows).

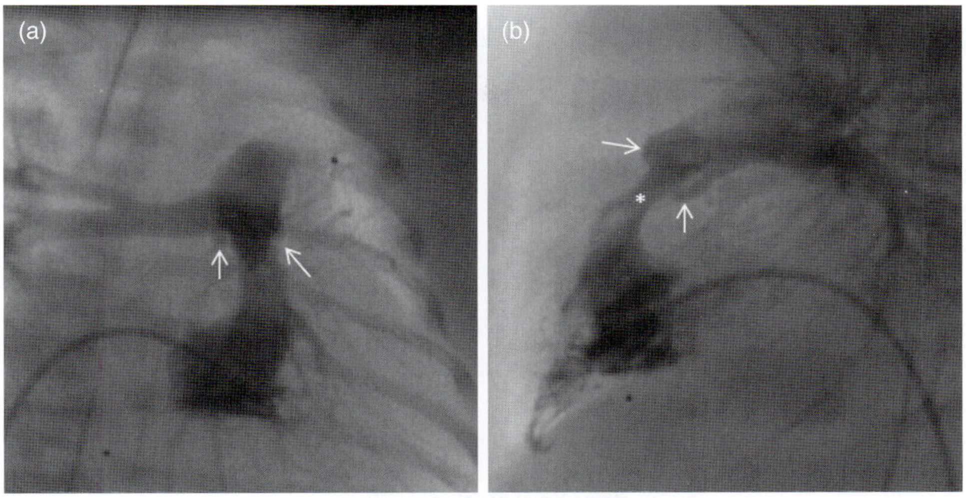

Figure 26.7 (a) Frontal and (b) lateral right ventriculogram following balloon pulmonary valvuloplasty. Valve leaflet mobility has dramatically improved, evidenced by the wider jet of contrast existing the RV and improved antegrade filling of the branch pulmonary arteries. The valve annulus is well profiled (white arrows) and the valve leaflets exhibit improved mobility. However, the improved contractility of the hypertrophied right ventricular infundibulum has resulted in significant subpulmonic obstruction seen best on the lateral projection (b) (asterisk). This phenomenon can be dramatic, effectively limiting antegrade flow from the RV leaving some neonates ductal dependent until there is further regression of right ventricular hypertrophy.

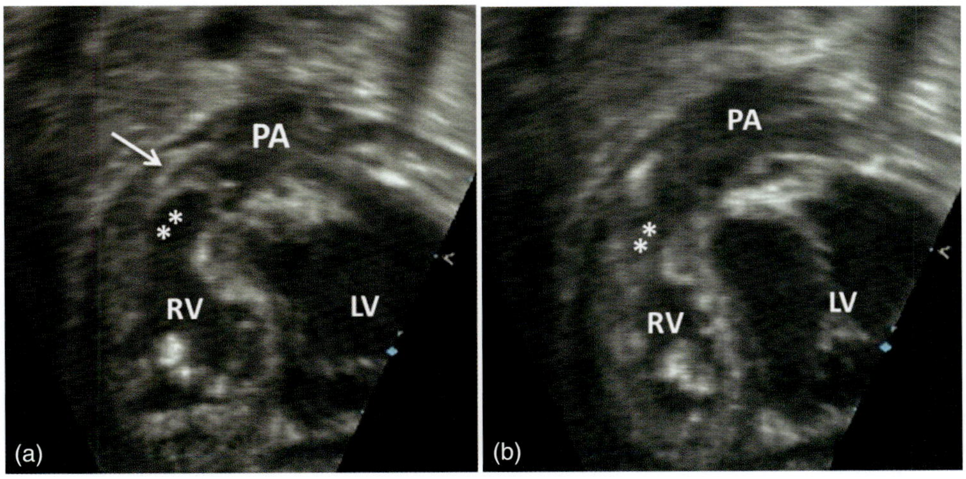

Figure 26.8 Transthoracic echocardiogram following successful balloon pulmonary valvuloplasty. (a) In ventricular diastole, note the significant degree of right ventricular hypertrophy, particularly in the region of the conal septum (infundibular region), which appears thickened but unobstructed (asterisks) at this point in the cardiac cycle. (b) During ventricular systole, the appearance of severe dynamic subvalve (infundibular) obstruction becomes evident (asterisks) as the hypertrophic infundibular muscle causes near obliteration of the outflow tract despite good systolic opening of the pulmonary valve leaflets.

form of stent implantation within the ductus arteriosis or a surgically placed modified Blalock–Taussig shunt [3]. Balloon valvuloplasty for pulmonary stenosis has a very high initial success rate; however, neonates with critical valvar stenosis have a higher reported need for re-intervention (as high as 30%). For the most part, prognosis is quite good; however, patients require lifelong follow-up for the both recurrence of stenosis as well as the development and/or progression of pulmonary valve regurgitation which can require treatment later in life.

Pulmonary Arterial Stenosis

Pulmonary arterial stenosis as an isolated defect is rare. When present as an isolated finding, an underlying congenital syndrome should be suspected including (but not limited to) Alagille, congenital rubella, Noonan, or Williams syndromes. Pulmonary arterial stenosis is more commonly found in association with other congenital heart defects occurring in 2–3% of all patients with other

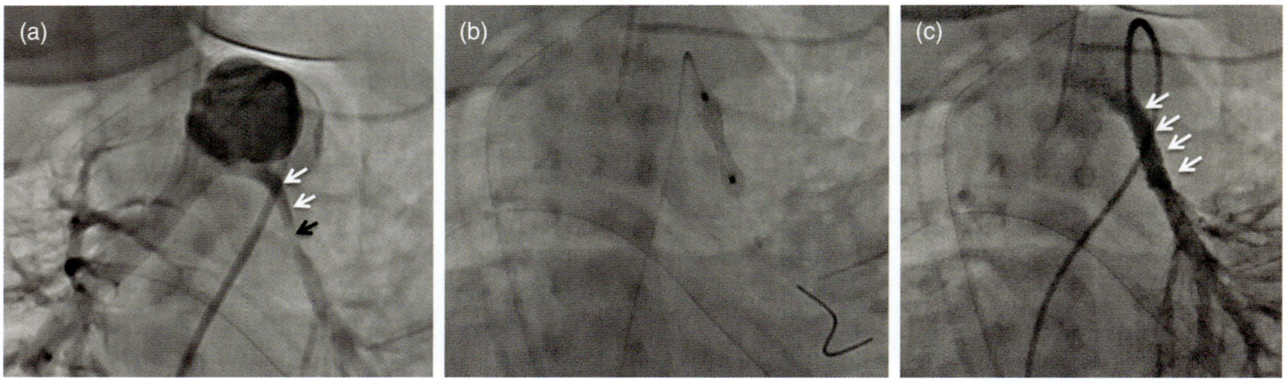

Figure 26.9 Branch pulmonary artery (BPA) stenosis in a newborn less than 24 hours after surgical correction of complex congenital cyanotic heart disease. (a) Angiography in the right ventricular outflow tract with extreme caudal angulation profiles the proximal BPAs well and reveals a severe long segment stenosis of the left pulmonary artery (PA; white arrows) as well as thrombus formation (black arrow). (b) Stent deployment across the narrowing led to an acute and dramatic rise in oxygenation because of successful reperfusion of the left lung. (c) Post-stent angiography shows the improvement in flow through the left PA. White arrows identify the stented portion of the PA. This stent will require further dilation and/or surgical enlargement as this infant grows.

underlying congenital heart disease, most commonly tetralogy of Fallot (particularly with pulmonary atresia) or truncus arteriosis; or following complex neonatal heart surgery that involves manipulating the pulmonary arteries.

Neonatal repair of complex conotruncal defects appears to be associated with the development of branch pulmonary artery stenosis [4]. Detection of pulmonary arterial stenosis may be difficult by echocardiography when the stenoses are in the periphery. Angiography, cardiac MRI, and CT are useful diagnostic tools in this setting. Treatment algorithms are variable and depend on the degree of the stenosis, location, and precise anatomic morphology. Mild to moderate isolated stenosis does not require treatment in a newborn and may spontaneously improve over time. Severe stenosis, either as an isolated finding, in association with other congenital heart disease, or following complex cardiac surgery often warrants treatment, particularly if right ventricular systolic pressure exceeds systemic blood pressure and/or signs or symptoms of right heart failure are present. Treatment options include percutaneous transcatheter balloon angioplasty with or without high pressure or cutting balloons, surgical angioplasty and, rarely, stent implantation in selected cases (Figure 26.9).

References

1 Radtke W, Keane JF, Fellows KE, Lang P, Lock JE. (1986) Percutaneous balloon valvotomy of congenital pulmonary artery stenosis using oversized balloons. *J Am Coll Cardiol*, **8**, 909–915.

2 Colli AM, Perry SB, Lock JE. (1995) Balloon dilation of critical valvar pulmonary artery stenosis in the first month of life. *Catheter Cardiovasc Interv*, **34**, 23–28.

3 Gudausky TM, Beekman RH. (2006) Current options, and long-term results for interventional treatment of pulmonary valvar stenosis. *Cardiol Young*, **16**, 418–427.

4 Lund AM, Vogel M, Marshall AC, *et al.* (2011) Early reintervention on the pulmonary arteries and right ventricular outflow tract after neonatal or early infant repair of truncus arteriosus using homograft conduits. *Am J Cardiol*, **108** (1), 106–113.

27

Pulmonary Atresia with Intact Ventricular Septum

Kiran K. Mallula[1] *and Zahid Amin*[2]

[1] *Division of Cardiology, Louisiana State University School of Medicine; Children's Hospital of New Orleans, New Orleans, LA, USA*
[2] *Children's Hospital of Georgia, Augusta University, Augusta, GA, USA*

Pulmonary atresia is a cyanotic congenital heart disease characterized by imperforate right ventricular outflow tract (RVOT) caused by a membrane or long segment muscular atresia with an intact ventricular septum. A patent ductus arteriosus (PDA) is the usual source of pulmonary blood flow. Other sources include direct aortopulmonary collaterals from the descending aorta or separate arterial ducts supplying non-confluent pulmonary arteries. In general, aorto-pulmonary collaterals are not as common as in pulmonary atresia with ventricular septal defect (VSD).

Incidence of the condition is 4.1 per 100 000 live births and prevalence is 0.083 per 1000 live births.

Embryology

It is usually agreed that the defect occurs after ventricular septation is complete. An abnormal intracardiac antegrade blood flow can cause atresia of the valve and affected ventricular growth. Blood entering the right ventricle (RV) has no egress and has to regurgitate through the tricuspid valve (TV). This may lead to hypoplasia of the annulus, formation of abnormal leaflets, and damage to the chords supporting the valve. Once the valve begins to leak, it is further structurally altered by turbulent flow.

High RV pressure can lead to development of ventriculo-coronary connections (VCCs) that partially decompress the RV during fetal life. The resulting shear forces can cause progressive stenosis and interruption of the coronary arteries and render major portions of heart muscle dependent on flow from the RV. This is known as right ventricular-dependent coronary circulation (RVDCC).

Pathology

The heart is mildly or severely enlarged with a huge right atrium occupying much of the right hemithorax. The RV may be profoundly thinned. Rarely, when the heart is significantly dilated, there are varying degrees of lung hypoplasia. On gross inspection, the coronary arteries are thickened and nodular with epicardial aneurysmal dilation. Rarely, they can be seen connecting with the pulmonary trunk. Dimples may be observed on the epicardial surface of the heart in association with the subepicardial coronary arteries and can represent the sites of VCCs. In patients with a well-formed infundibulum, the imperforate pulmonary valve exhibits three semilunar cusps with complete fusion of the commissure. The pulmonary valve is primitive in patients with a small RV and a severely atretic infundibulum. Because of the obligatory right-to-left shunt at atrial level, there is either a patent foramen ovale or true secundum atrial septal defect. The TV demonstrates a continuum of abnormalities ranging from severe stenosis to profound regurgitation. The z score of the TV correlates well with RV volume. Smaller TV size may serve as a surrogate for early RV inadequacy [1]. In some patients with small and extremely hypertensive RV, the convexity of the outlet portion of the interventricular septum, rarely results in severe left ventricular outflow tract obstruction leading to death after surgical creation of a cavopulmonary connection [2]. The myocardium can demonstrate ischemia, fibrosis, infarction, myocardial rupture, spongy myocardium, or endocardial fibroelastosis (EFE) [3]. There is an inverse relationship between ventricular EFE and extensive VCCs.

The RV can be divided into three portions: an inlet; a trabecular (apical) portion; and an infundibular portion. Bull *et al.* [4] distinguished three types of ventricles:

Visual Guide to Neonatal Cardiology, First Edition. Edited by Ernerio T. Alboliras, Ziyad M. Hijazi, Leo Lopez, and Donald J. Hagler.

those with generalized cavitary hypoplasia but with inlet, trabecular, and outlet portions (tripartite); those without a trabecular portion to the cavity (bipartite); and those in which both the trabecular and infundibular portions are entirely overgrown by hypertrophied myocardium (unipartite). The hypertensive RV supplies retrograde blood flow during systole via the VCCs for adequate myocardial perfusion. Unfortunately, this process can lead to further coronary arterial distortion. A negative z score for the TV annulus correlates with the presence of VCCs, which are more likely to be observed in patients whose ventricles have been categorized as unipartite or bipartite.

Physical Examination

After birth, functional and anatomic closure of the PDA leads to hypoxemia and cyanosis. Rarely, patients have restrictive interatrial communication, and the cardiac output is affected because of restrictive obligatory right-to-left shunt. The second heart sound is single. A holosystolic murmur is audible at the left lower sternal border, consistent with tricuspid regurgitation (TR). If the TR is severe, it can sometimes be associated with a thrill, and a mid-diastolic rumble may be audible. A systolic or continuous PDA murmur may be audible in the second and third left intercostal space. The arterial pulses are usually normal. If there is severe TR or restrictive atrial level communication, hepatomegaly can ensue.

Chest X-ray

The chest radiograph demonstrates mild to severe cardiomegaly. The pulmonary vascular markings are reduced. With massive cardiomegaly, the pulmonary markings may be difficult to evaluate.

Electrocardiography

The ECG demonstrates normal sinus rhythm, QRS axis of +30 to +90, left ventricular dominance or left ventricular hypertrophy, and right atrial enlargement. ST-T wave changes can be seen frequently, consistent with some degree of subendocardial ischemia.

Echocardiography

Although echocardiography is extremely important in primary identification of the lesion, it has several limitations. Identification of the extent of VCCs can be difficult (Figure 27.1). Reliable identification of coronary arterial stenosis or interruption may not be possible in neonates [5]. As a result of these limitations, angiography can be crucial in infants with severe RV hypoplasia, in whom a high incidence of VCCs is anticipated. The subcostal view can demonstrate the interatrial communication (Figure 27.2). The atrial septum is rarely aneurysmal. The size and morphology of the TV and TR should be assessed. It is sometimes difficult to detect forward flow

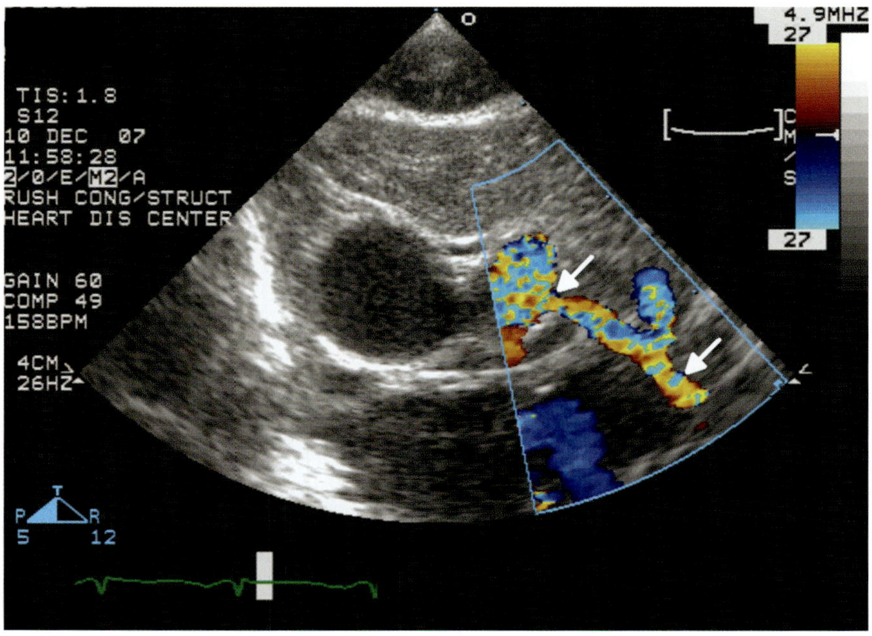

Figure 27.1 Parasternal short axis view with color Doppler demonstrating reversal of flow in the dilated coronary sinusoids with areas of multiple constrictions (white arrows).

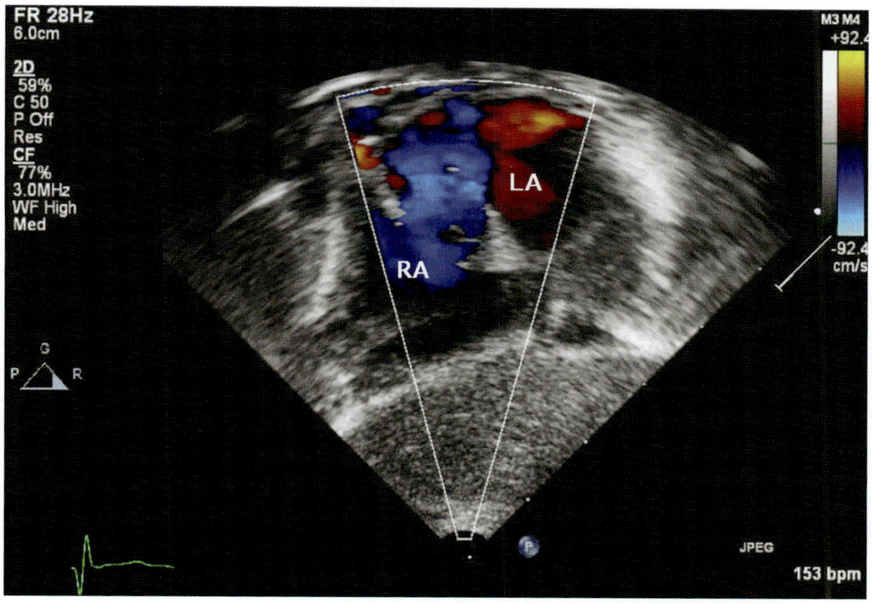

Figure 27.2 Subcostal view demonstrating obligatory right-to-left shunt from the right atrium (RA) to the left atrium (LA) across a non-restrictive foramen ovale.

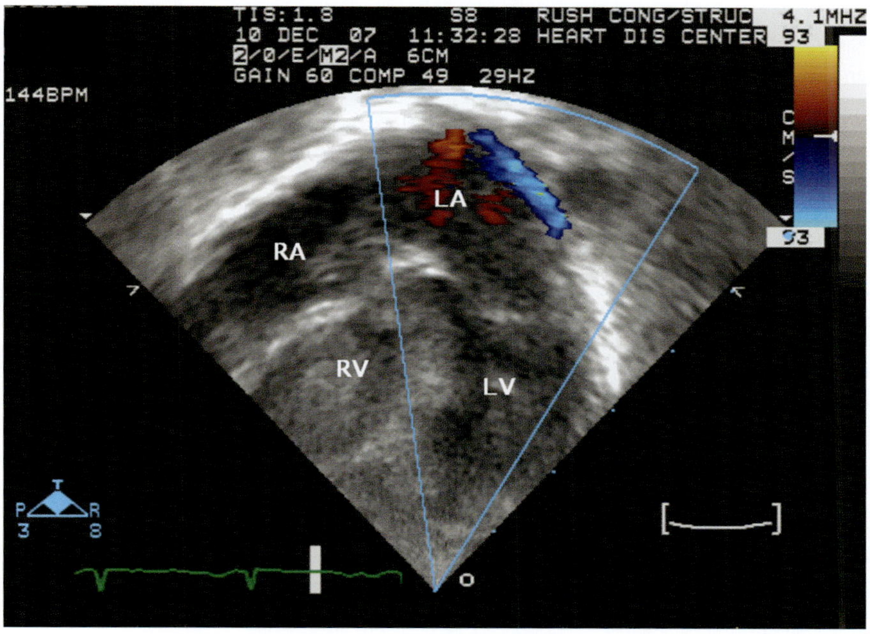

Figure 27.3 Apical four-chamber view demonstrating a small tricuspid valve with hypertensive thickened right ventricle (RV) and bowing of the interventricular septum into the left ventricle (LV). LA, left atrium; RA, right atrium.

across an extremely stenotic, obstructive TV and, in the absence of TR, the question of patency cannot always be resolved. The RV size, which usually corresponds to the dimension of the tricuspid annulus, can be imaged by a combination of subcostal and apical four-chamber views (Figure 27.3). It can be difficult to differentiate isolated pulmonary valve atresia from extremely severe stenosis. Even with Doppler echocardiography, this issue remains a problem because ductal flow can potentially mask a small forward flow jet. It is important to distinguish anatomic from a functional pulmonary atresia seen in elevated pulmonary resistance. Systolic regurgitation of the pulmonary valve caused by a jetting effect of the PDA against the valve and Doppler echocardiography during positive pressure ventilation, which transiently results in opening of the pulmonary valve and forward Doppler flow, can be evidence for functional rather than anatomic atresia [6].

Cardiac Catheterization

Hemodynamic assessment can demonstrate systemic or suprasystemic RV pressure in patients with hypertensive RV. The RV pressure may be subsystemic in those patients with massive cardiac enlargement, reflecting that the pulmonary valve is functionally atretic. The atrial mean pressures are equal in the presence

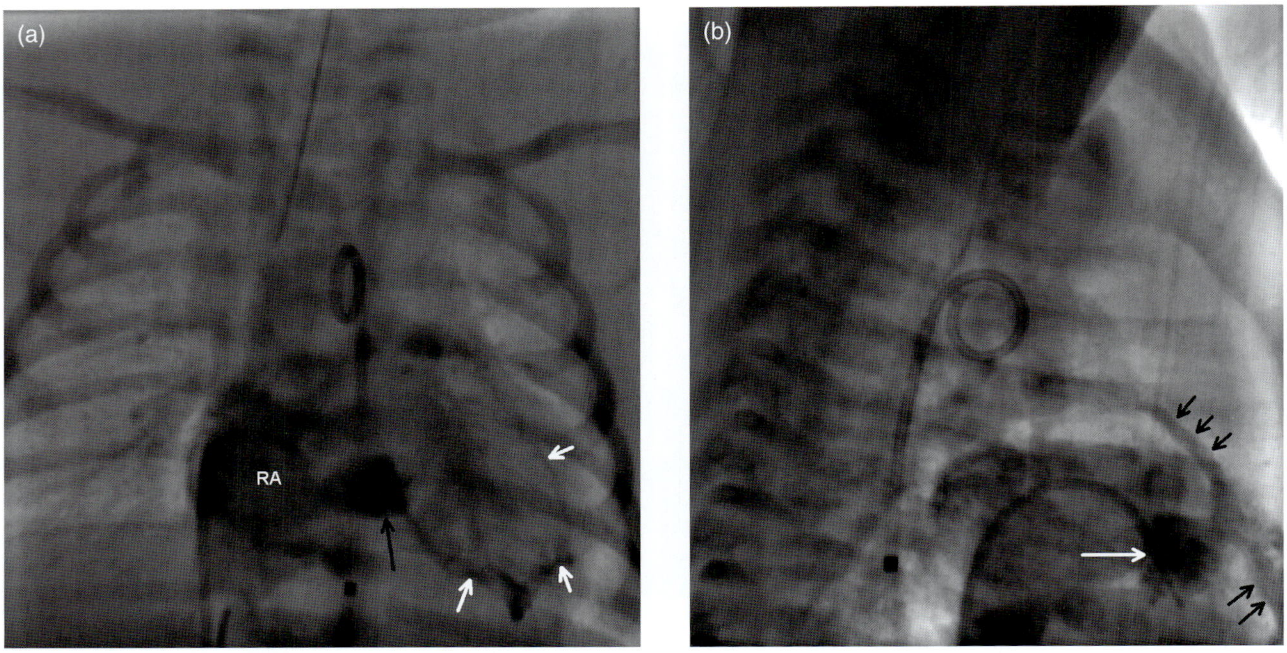

Figure 27.4 Cine angiographic image of right ventriculogram. (a) Frontal view demonstrates a small and diminutive unipartite RV (black arrow) with severe tricuspid valve regurgitation of the contrast in the right atrium (RA). A ventriculo-coronary connection (VCC) is seen with constrictions in the coronary artery (white arrows) supplying the inferior and lateral wall of the left ventricle. (b) Lateral view shows a hypoplastic RV (white arrow) with VCC (black arrows) arising from the RV and supplying the anterior and inferior walls of the left ventricle.

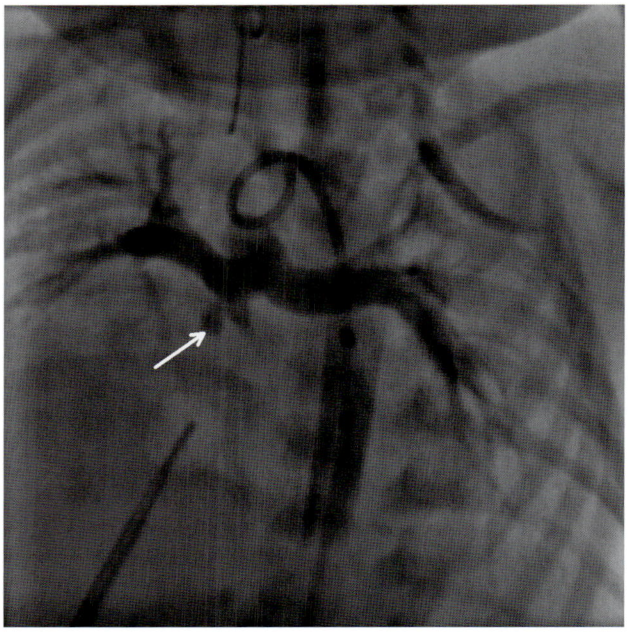

Figure 27.5 Cine angiographic image demonstrating confluent branch pulmonary arteries with no retrograde flow through the pulmonary valve (arrow). Injection is performed retrograde via a pigtail catheter in the aortic arch close to the origin of the ductus arteriosus.

of non-restrictive interatrial communication. If the interatrial communication is restrictive, a balloon atrial septostomy to avoid a low cardiac output syndrome is indicated.

Biplane angiography provides extensive information in the setting of pulmonary atresia with intact ventricular septum (PA/IVS). RV angiogram (Figure 27.4) demonstrates TR competence and structure, size of RV, extent of the apical trabecular zone, dimensions of the infundibulum, and establishes the presence or absence of VCCs. A selective RVOT injection can differentiate severe pulmonary valve stenosis from membranous atresia. An aortogram (Figure 27.5) defines the laterality of the aortic arch, the caliber of the subclavian arteries, the site of insertion of the PDA, the caliber of the pulmonary arteries, and coarctation of the pulmonary artery at the insertion of the arterial duct which may preclude treatment with a stent. In some patients with VCCs, a balloon catheter inflated in the RV or catheter-induced tricuspid insufficiency with simultaneous observation of electrocardiographic tracing may unmask a RVDCC. Additional information can be obtained with angulated views of the RV angiography in the setting of VCCs.

Medical Therapy

After birth, ductal patency should be maintained urgently by systemic administration of prostaglandin. Once pulmonary blood flow is established, it is important to recognize that systemic oxygen saturation is related to the amount of flow into the pulmonary circulation. A very low pulmonary vascular resistance and conversely high systemic vascular resistance can result in low cardiac output despite a high saturation.

Surgery

A single approach is impractical because of the wide spectrum of right heart morphology. Initial surgical considerations should include:

1) Evaluation for candidacy for a complete biventricular or a one-and-a half ventricular repair or a univentricular palliation;
2) Presence of VCCs and, if so, RVDCC;
3) Presence of an infundibulum;
4) Continuity of main pulmonary trunk with the imperforate pulmonary valve; and
5) Assessment of left ventricular function.

Palliative repairs aim at relief of cyanosis and ductal dependence by providing a reliable source of pulmonary blood flow. Relief of the RVOT obstruction establishes antegrade blood flow, which promotes growth of RV. Adequate decompression of RV allows regression of RV hypertrophy and promotes RV growth to an extent that definitive biventricular repair may be successfully achieved. A variety of methods including transpulmonary valvotomy, RVOT patch reconstruction, and balloon valvuloplasty are used to decompress the RV. If the RVOT remains atretic, growth of the RV is unlikely to occur, and thus a two-ventricle heart is unlikely to be achieved [7]. The exclusion of patients from the long-term aim of a biventricular repair is still unclear because the potential for RV growth after decompression of the RV is difficult to predict [8].

The most important problem when planning for definitive repair is the fact that RV growth and the contribution to pulmonary blood flow are difficult to predict. TV z value is an index of RV growth. Some patients are likely to require a so-called one-and-a-half ventricle repair, with the bidirectional superior cavopulmonary shunt effectively unloading the small right ventricle and potentially obstructive TV. Decompression of the hypertensive RV can be accomplished by removing the TV or performing a pulmonary valvotomy. Patients with markedly hypoplastic TV and RV or with RV-dependent coronary circulation should be candidates for a Fontan-type procedure. Complete anatomic repair of PA/IVS consists of relief of the residual RV outflow tract obstruction, closure of the atrial septal defect, and obliteration of a systemic to pulmonary (S-P) shunt if one has been performed.

In patients with RVDCC, a ductal stent or a S-P shunt (Figure 27.6) is the initial procedure of choice with a consideration for balloon atrial septostomy. The definitive repair in this situation should be a Fontan palliation. In some centers, these patients are considered for primary cardiac transplantation, especially if the coronary anomalies are particularly severe. In those patients with extreme Ebsteinoid or dysplastic TV and pulmonary atresia, contemporary approaches include cardiac transplantation and conversion to tricuspid atresia and construction of a S-P shunt with a later cavopulmonary palliation [9].

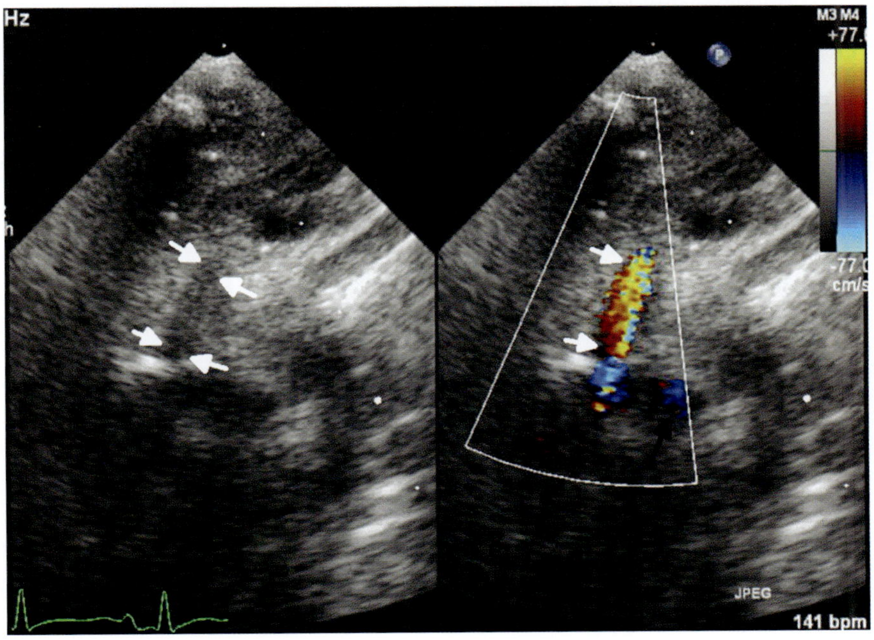

Figure 27.6 Modified suprasternal echocardiographic view demonstrating a right modified Blalock–Taussig shunt (white arrows) connecting the innominate and the right pulmonary artery (black arrow) on 2D and color Doppler.

Transcatheter Therapy

Transcatheter perforation of the atretic pulmonary valve with laser energy or radiofrequency energy followed by subsequent balloon dilation can be employed as an alternative to surgical valvotomy in selected patients. Radiofrequency energy has the advantages of being considerably less expensive, more portable, and less hazardous to staff. Other means of attaining perforation have been used, including mechanical wire perforation and standard electrode catheters.

Outcomes

Late patient-perceived physical functional health status and measured exercise status are reduced, regardless of PA/IVS repair pathway. For those with smaller initial TV z score, achievement of survival with biventricular repair may be at a cost of late deficits in exercise capacity, emphasizing that better outcomes may be achieved for borderline patients with a one-and-a-half ventricle (Glenn with RV to PA flow) or univentricular or Fontan repair strategy [10].

Conclusions

PA/IVS is one of the most complex cardiac lesions. Hence, managementdepends upon the morphology and the severity of the defect. In addition, management protocol is dictated based upon institutional results and protocols. The outcomes vary from a near-normal biventricular flow establishment to Fontan type repair. VCC remains the most complex part of management with high risk of sudden death resulting from associated coronary artery anomalies.

References

1. Hasan BS, Bautista-Hernandez V, McElhinney DB, *et al.* (2013) Outcomes of transcatheter approach for initial treatment of pulmonary atresia with intact ventricular septum. *Catheter Cardiovasc Interv*, **81** (1), 111–118.
2. Amin P, Levi DS, Likes M, Laks H. (2009) Pulmonary atresia with intact ventricular septum causing severe left ventricular outflow tract obstruction. *Pediatr Cardiol*, **30** (6), 851–854.
3. Hausdorf G, Gravinghoff L, Keck EW. (1987) Effects of persisting myocardial sinusoids on left ventricular performance in pulmonary atresia with intact ventricular septum. *Eur Heart J*, **8** (3), 291–296.
4. Bull C, de Leval MR, Mercanti C, Macartney FJ, Anderson RH. (1982) Pulmonary atresia and intact ventricular septum: a revised classification. *Circulation*, **66** (2), 266–272.
5. Selamet SE, Hsu DT, Thaker HM, Gersony WM. (2004) Complete atresia of coronary ostia in pulmonary atresia and intact ventricular septum. *Pediatr Cardiol*, **25** (1), 67–69.
6. Garcia JA, Zellers TM, Weinstein EM, Mahony L. (1998) Usefulness of Doppler echocardiography in diagnosing right ventricular coronary arterial communications in patients with pulmonary atresia and intact ventricular septum and comparison with angiography. *Am J Cardiol*, **81** (1), 103–104.
7. Shaddy RE, Sturtevant JE, Judd VE, McGough EC. (1990) Right ventricular growth after transventricular pulmonary valvotomy and central aortopulmonary shunt for pulmonary atresia and intact ventricular septum. *Circulation*, **82** (5 Suppl), 157–163.
8. Yoshimura N, Yamaguchi M. (2009) Surgical strategy for pulmonary atresia with intact ventricular septum: initial management and definitive surgery. *Gen Thorac Cardiovasc Surg*, **57** (7), 338–346.
9. Hanley FL, Sade RM, Blackstone EH, *et al.* (1993) Outcomes in neonatal pulmonary atresia with intact ventricular septum: a multiinstitutional study. *J Thorac Cardiovasc Surg*, **105** (3), 406–423, 424–427; discussion 423–424.
10. Karamlou T, Poynter JA, Walters HL 3rd, *et al.* (2013) Long-term functional health status and exercise test variables for patients with pulmonary atresia with intact ventricular septum: a Congenital Heart Surgeons Society study. *J Thorac Cardiovasc Surg*, **145** (4), 1018–1025; discussion 1025–1027.

28

Tetralogy of Fallot with Pulmonary Stenosis or Atresia

Muhammad Yasir Qureshi and Frank Cetta

Division of Pediatric Cardiology, Mayo Clinic, Rochester, MN, USA

Tetralogy of Fallot (TOF) is the most common cyanotic congenital heart disease. It occurs in 1 in 3500 live births and accounts for 7–10% of all congenital heart disease. The etiology of TOF is multifactorial, with 25% having chromosomal abnormalities. The familial recurrence risk is 3% (Table 28.1). It is a morphologic diagnosis, features of which include ventricular septal defect (VSD), right ventricular outflow tract (RVOT) obstruction, overriding aorta and right ventricular hypertrophy – all resulting from anterior deviation of the conal septum (Figure 28.1). Pulmonary valve atresia with ventricular septal defect (PAVSD) is sometimes considered the most extreme form of TOF and is also referred to as TOF with pulmonary atresia (Figure 28.2). PAVSD is commonly associated with complex pulmonary arterial architecture requiring more complex surgical management.

Table 28.1 Genetic mutations associated with tetralogy of Fallot.

Syndromes	Common mutations
Trisomies (21, 18, 13)	
DiGeorge	*22q11.2* deletion
Velocardiofacial	*TBX1*
Holt–Oram	*TBX5*
Alagille	*NOTCH2*
Cat eye	*22pter22q11* duplication
	NKX2.5
	GATA4
	NOTCH1
	FOXH1
	GDF1
	TDGF1
	ZFPM2
	GATA6
	CFC1
	TBX20
	JAG1
	TBX1
	CNVs

Tetralogy of Fallot with Pulmonary Stenosis

Morphologic and Anatomic Features

The key morphologic component of TOF is the anterior and superior deviation of conal septum (Figure 28.3). This deviation causes the conal septum to fail to meet the membranous and muscular septa and results in a large non-restrictive VSD. This malalignment also results in an overriding aorta and infundibular stenosis leading to hypoplasia of the pulmonary valve and pulmonary arteries. Right ventricular hypertrophy, the fourth component of TOF, results from the RVOT obstruction. The VSD is usually large with extension into the membranous and outlet septa. For this reason, the VSD in TOF is also referred to as conotruncal VSD. The aortic arch is right-sided in 25% of cases with TOF, but presence of a vascular ring is rare. Significant coronary arteries abnormalities can be present in up to 5% of cases. The most common abnormality is the anterior descending artery arising from the right coronary artery and traveling anterior to the RVOT, precluding the possibility of surgical incision in this region. About 2% of patients with TOF also have concomitant complete atrioventricular canal defect. In these patients, the VSD extends from the inlet septum to outlet septum in association with the atrioventricular canal defect. This entity is more common in patients with Down syndrome.

Clinical Manifestations

Many patients with TOF are diagnosed in utero as a result of advances in fetal echocardiography (Figure 28.4). Those who are not detected in fetal life may present in the neonatal period with a heart murmur and/or cyanosis. The auscultatory findings usually include a

Visual Guide to Neonatal Cardiology, First Edition. Edited by Ernerio T. Alboliras, Ziyad M. Hijazi, Leo Lopez, and Donald J. Hagler.

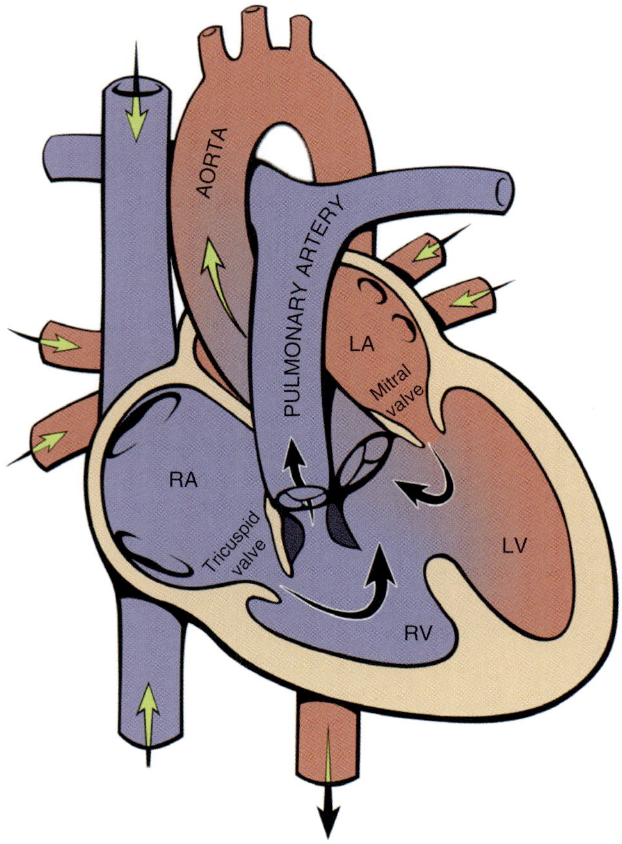

Figure 28.1 Anatomy and blood flow pattern in tetralogy of Fallot with pulmonary stenosis. LA, left artery; LV, left ventricle; right artery; RV, right ventricle.

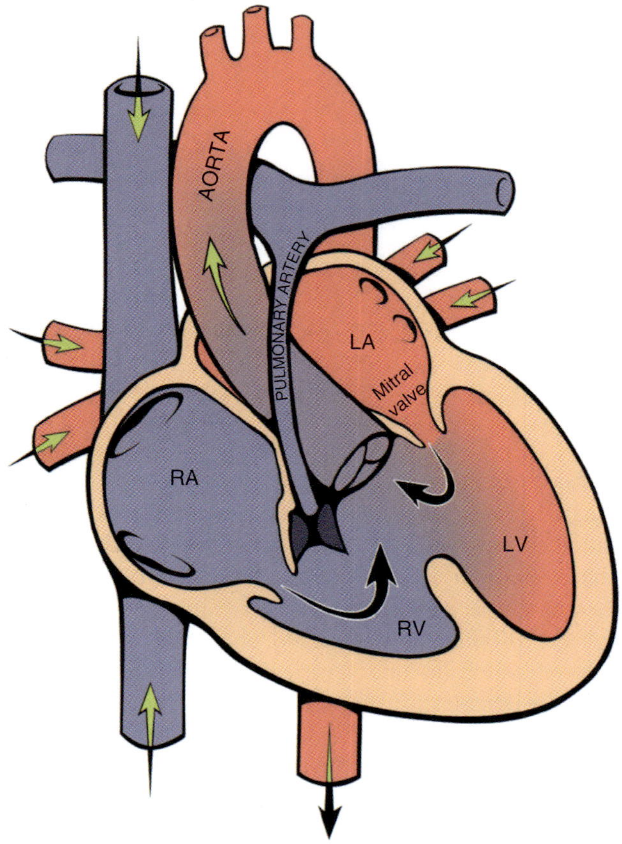

Figure 28.2 Anatomy and blood flow pattern in pulmonary atresia with ventricular septal defect.

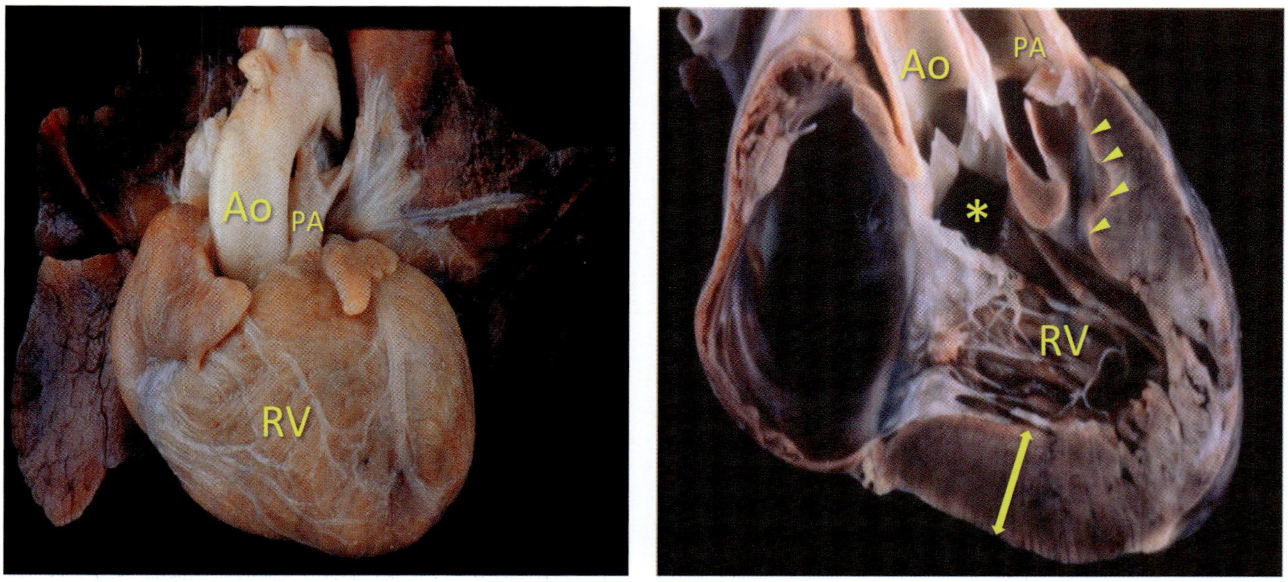

Figure 28.3 Pathology specimens of tetralogy of Fallot. The ventricular septal defect (*), infundibular stenosis (arrow heads) and right ventricular hypertrophy (arrow) can be noted. Ao, aorta; PA, pulmonary artery; RV, right ventricle.

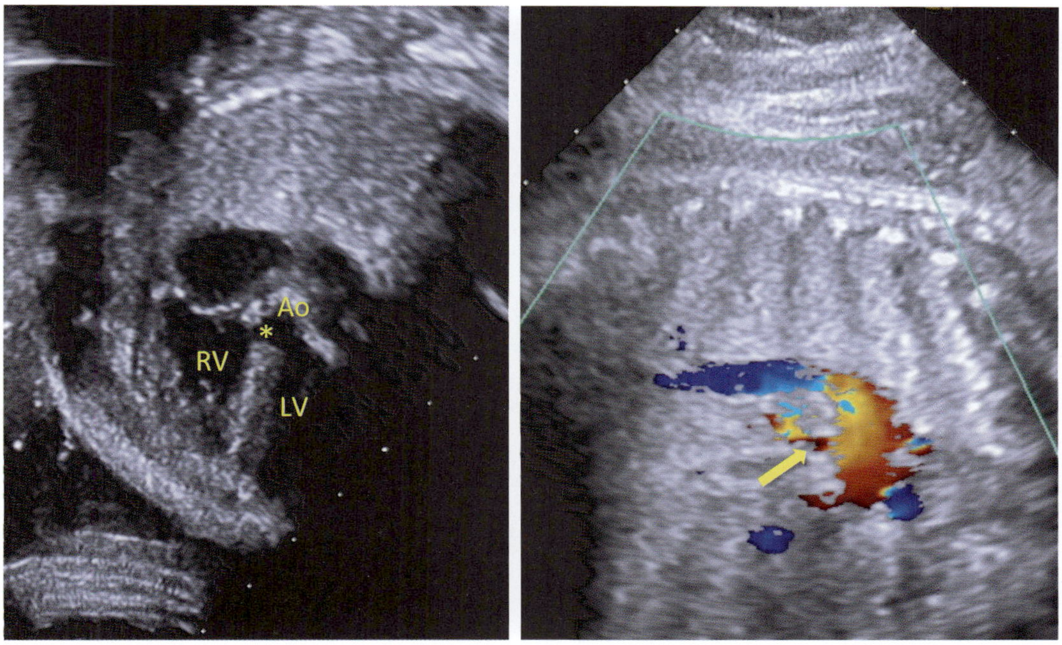

Figure 28.4 Four-chamber view (left panel) in a fetus with tetralogy of Fallot showing ventricular septal defect (*) and overriding aorta (Ao). Aortic arch with vertical ductus (arrow) is seen in the right panel. LV, left ventricle; RV, right ventricle.

normal S1 with a soft P2 component of the S2, or a single S2. An ejection click may be audible. A loud systolic ejection murmur is usually heard at the mid and upper left sternal border originating from RVOT stenosis. As the obstruction of the RVOT becomes more severe, the murmur becomes shorter and softer. The degree of cyanosis is dependent on the severity of RVOT obstruction. Severe RVOT stenosis results in increased right to left shunt across the VSD, leading to worse cyanosis. However, mild RVOT obstruction (the "pink tet") may result in a clinical picture of a large VSD with non-restrictive pulmonary blood flow. These patients may not have cyanosis and present with tachypnea, tachycardia, or diaphoresis as the pulmonary vascular resistance falls. In most of these patients, the degree of RVOT obstruction worsens with time and cyanosis eventually is manifest.

Laboratory and Imaging Investigations

The ECG usually shows right axis deviation and right ventricular (or biventricular) hypertrophy. The classic chest radiograph finding of a "boot-shaped" heart is actually rare (<25% of patients) (Figure 28.5). More common findings include "black lungs" caused by reduced pulmonary vascular markings, but in acyanotic TOF pulmonary vascular markings may be prominent.

Echocardiography is the mainstay of diagnosis in TOF (Figures 28.6–28.11). In most cases, transthoracic echocardiography is the only imaging study needed prior to surgical intervention. The parasternal long-axis view can show the anatomy of the VSD and overriding aorta. The parasternal short-axis, subcostal coronal, and subcostal sagittal views show the RVOT and pulmonary valve anatomy. Doppler interrogation in these views allows quantification of RVOT obstruction. The parasternal short axis and high parasternal windows allow optimal imaging of the branch pulmonary arteries. In neonates, echocardiography alone is sufficient to demonstrate coronary artery anomalies. It is important to exclude coronary artery branches crossing anteriorly over the RVOT. This alerts the surgeon to avoid inadvertent transection of that branch during augmentation of the RVOT. Associated anomalies such as a persistent left superior vena cava or secundum atrial septal defect should also be sought. In cases where the branch pulmonary arteries or coronary artery anatomy are not clearly defined by echocardiography, other imaging modalities such as computed topography angiography (CTA), magnetic resonance imaging (MRI), or cardiac catheterization can be used.

Management

Medical management is limited in TOF. Hypercyanotic "tet spells" usually do not occur in the neonatal period (Figure 28.12). The peak incidence for these spells is at 2–4 months of age. Therefore, parents should

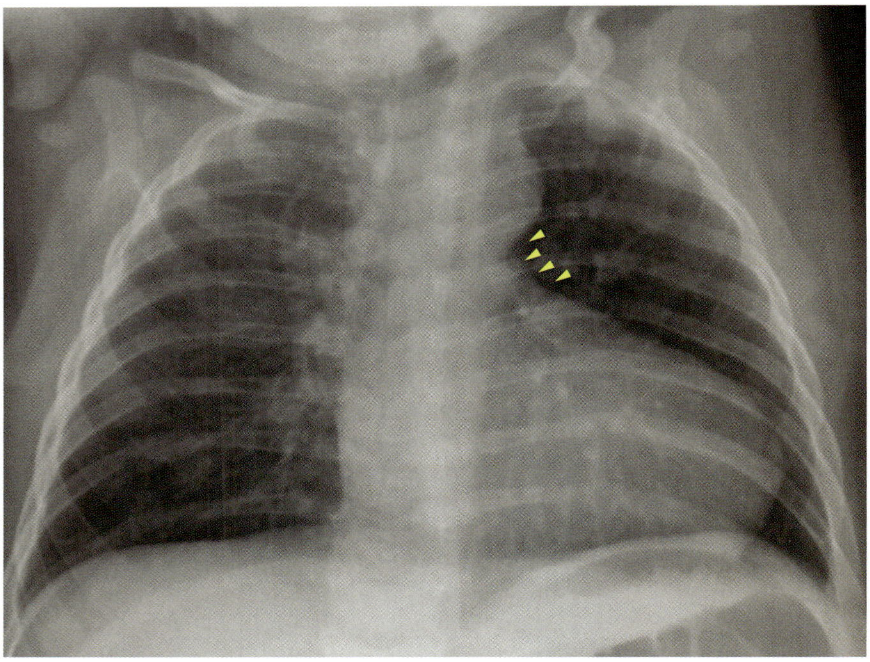

Figure 28.5 Chest radiograph of a neonate with pulmonary atresia with ventricular septal defect showing a classic "boot-shaped heart." Concavity (yellow arrow heads) in left border of cardiac silhouette is due to the absence of the central pulmonary artery. The cardiac apex is lifted off the diaphragm because of right ventricular hypertrophy. Note the absence of a thymic shadow raising suspicion of *22q11* deletion.

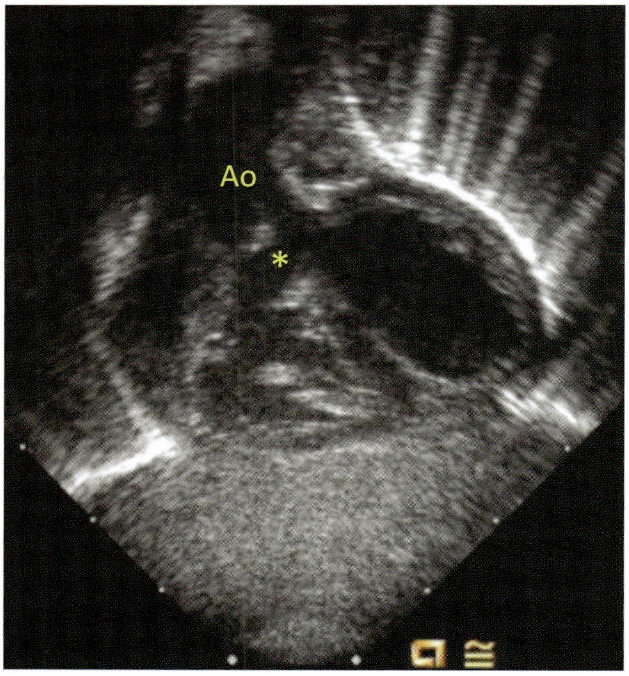

Figure 28.6 Subcostal coronal view showing ventricular septal defect (*) and overriding aorta (Ao).

be educated from the neonatal period about identification and initial management of these spells. Oral beta-blockers are sometimes used to prevent hypercyanotic spells. In acyanotic TOF, heart failure symptoms from pulmonary overcirculation can be managed by using diuretic therapy and high calorie formula. In cyanotic TOF, initial surgical management includes creation of a systemic to pulmonary shunt to augment pulmonary blood flow. A complete repair then follows this by 1 year of age (Figure 28.13). Some institutions prefer neonatal complete repair instead of a palliative shunt procedure. However, initial palliation with a shunt procedure is preferred in patients with severely hypoplastic pulmonary arteries and in those with coronary anomalies (Figure 28.14). The shunt procedure usually includes insertion of a Gore-Tex tube connecting the innominate artery (modified Blalock–Taussig shunt) or ascending aorta (central shunt) to the pulmonary artery. The complete repair includes patch closure of VSD via transatrial or transpulmonary approach, and resection of muscle bundles in RVOT. If the pulmonary valve and infundibulum are severely hypoplastic, augmentation with a transannular patch may be necessary. This leaves the infant with significant pulmonary valve regurgitation, causing long-term complications of right ventricular dilation and dysfunction. In the current era, efforts are made to preserve the native pulmonary valve, even accepting moderate residual pulmonary stenosis, in order to avoid the long-term sequelae of free regurgitation. Presence of an anomalous coronary artery anterior to RVOT may require institution of an RV to PA conduit, which is usually performed after 1 year of age.

Outcome

Long-term complications include pulmonary valve regurgitation requiring re-operation and valve replacement.

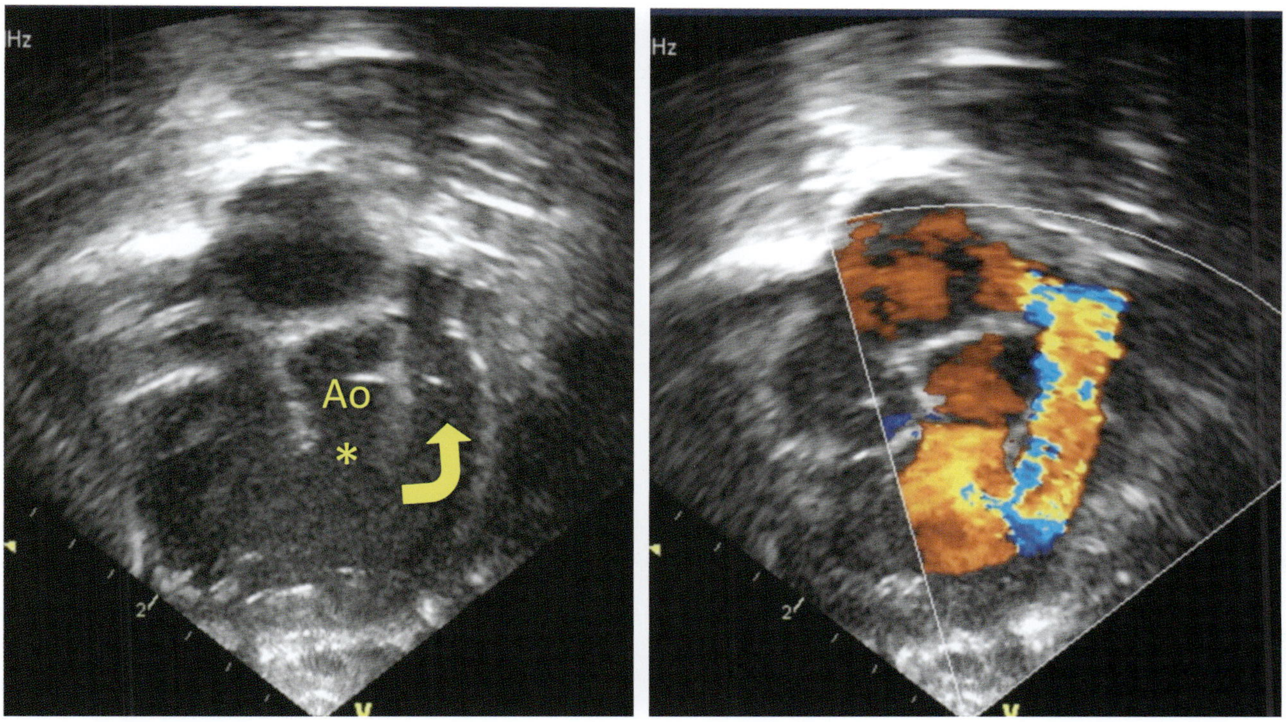

Figure 28.7 Subcostal right anterior oblique (right ventricular inflow–outflow) view showing ventricular septal defect (*) and infundibular stenosis (arrow) with aliasing of flow with color Doppler interrogation.

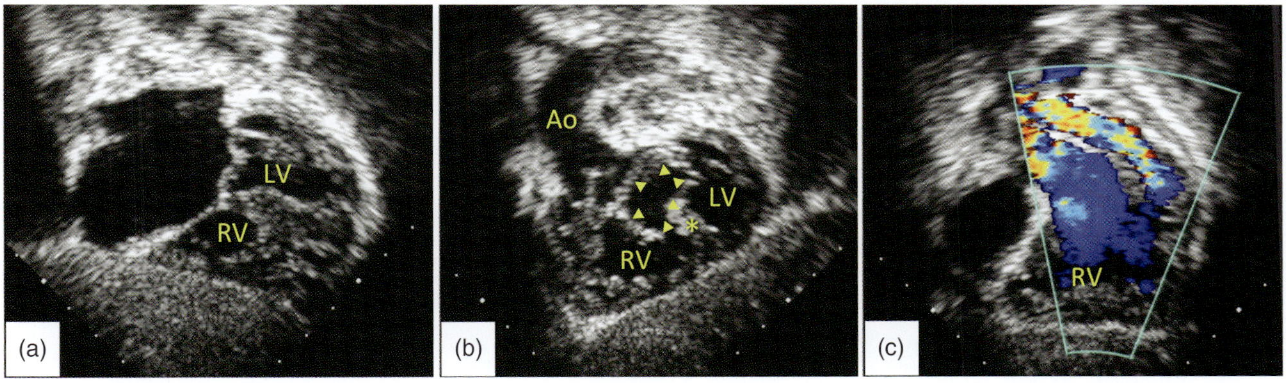

Figure 28.8 Echocardiography of a patient with tetralogy of Fallot with complete atrioventricular canal defect ("tet canal"). (a) Subcostal coronal (four-chamber) view showing a common atrioventricular valve with a large primum atrial septal defect. (b) Subcostal view in the plane of the atrioventricular valve (arrow heads). Interventricular septum is marked by asterisk (*). (c) Color Doppler image with slightly anterior tilt of transducer from (b). The laminar outflow from the right ventricle (RV) is through ventricular septal defect into the aorta (Ao). The turbulent flow is through the stenotic infundibulum into the main pulmonary artery. LV, left ventricle.

Rarely, complete heart block can be seen in immediate postoperative period. The survival rate in TOF with surgical intervention is >96% in the first 2 years of life and >90% for 30 years. However, long-term survival is less than the general population. Atrial re-entrant tachycardia occurs in more than 30% of patients and important ventricular arrhythmias occur in up to 10%. The overall incidence of sudden death is 0.2% per year. These are important issues as this patient population ages.

Pulmonary Valve Atresia with Ventricular Septal Defect (Tetralogy of Fallot with Pulmonary Atresia)

Morphologic and Anatomic Features

Similar to TOF with pulmonary stenosis, PAVSD has a non-restrictive malalignment VSD with overriding aorta (Figure 28.2). In contrast to TOF, the RVOT in PAVSD

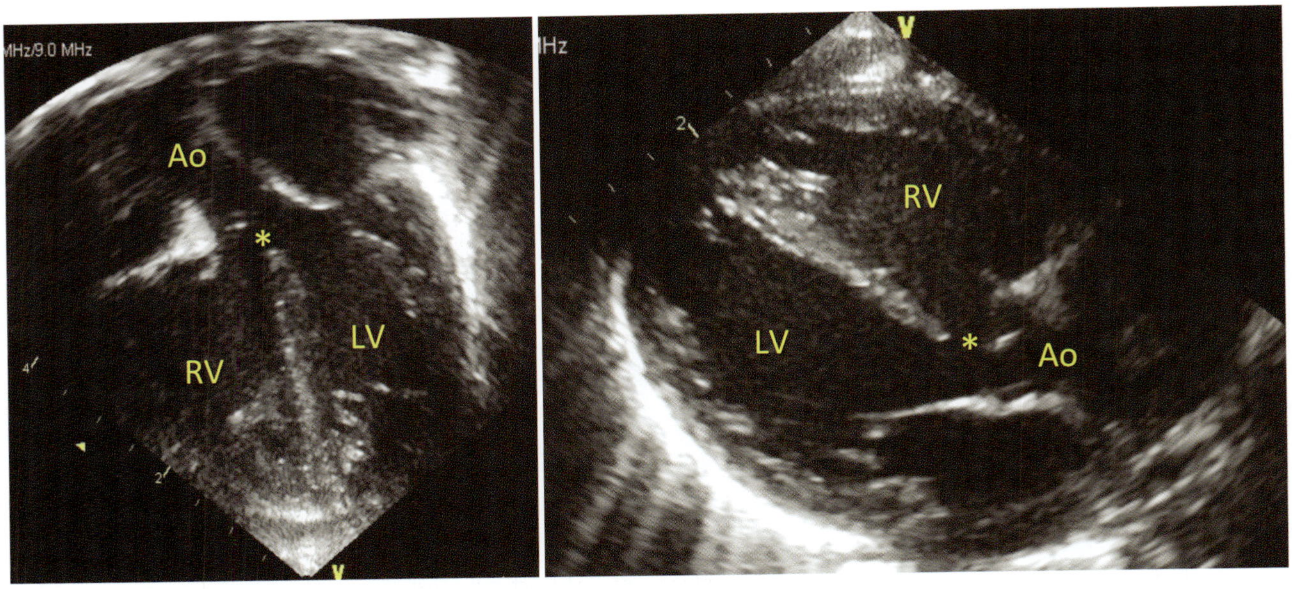

Figure 28.9 Ventricular septal defect (*) and overriding of aorta (Ao) can be seen on apical (left panel) and parasternal long-axis views (right panel). LV, left ventricle; RV, right ventricle.

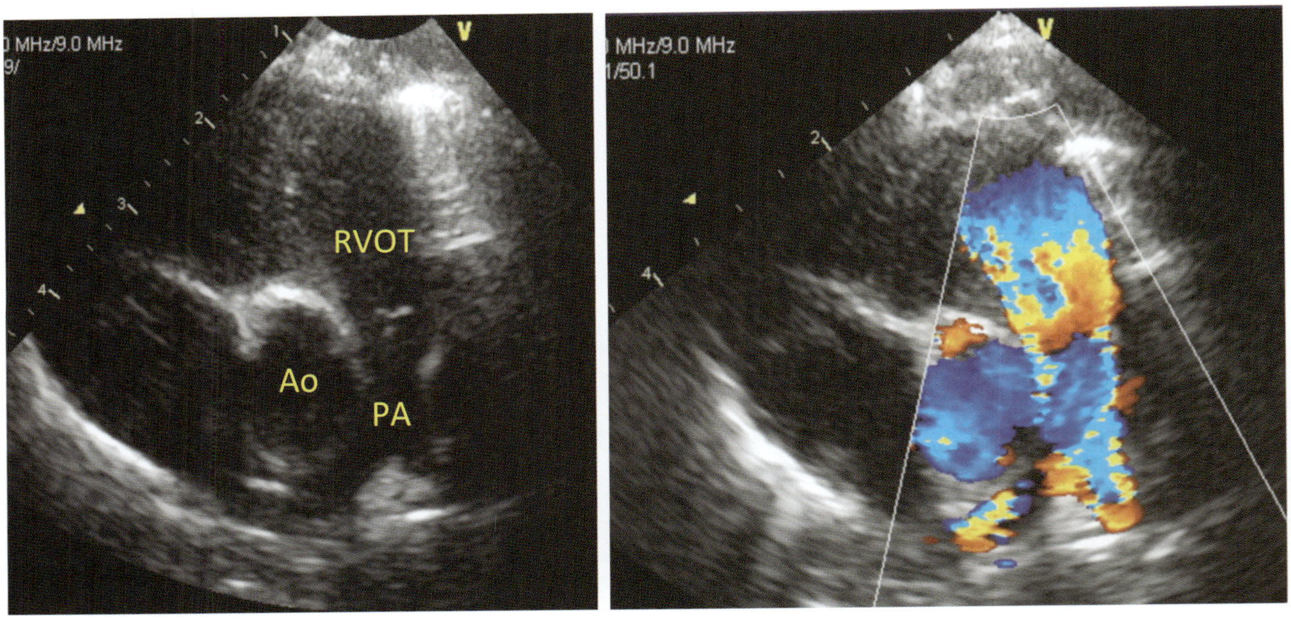

Figure 28.10 Parasternal short-axis view in two-dimensional and color Doppler imaging showing aliased flow in the right ventricular outflow tract (RVOT) and pulmonary arteries (PA).

ends in a blind pouch. A diminutive main pulmonary artery segment is usually present, which connects to the branch pulmonary arterial confluence. The pulmonary blood flow is supplied from the aorta either through a ductus arteriosus (70% of cases) (Figure 28.15) or through multiple major aortopulmonary collateral arteries (30%). In most cases, both ductal and collateral vessels coexist but the degree of collateral supply is directly related to the severity of central pulmonary artery hypoplasia. The ductus arteriosus in PAVSD has a unique morphology and is sometimes described as a "vertical ductus" (Figure 28.16). This is brought about by the reversed direction of its blood flow in utero: from aortic arch to pulmonary artery. This orients the ductus more in line with the curve of aortic arch. In severe cases, the central pulmonary arteries may be discontinuous and independent collateral arteries supply most of the pulmonary blood flow (Figure 28.17). In PAVSD, the pulmonary arteries are frequently hypoplastic. Even with confluent central pulmonary arteries, the distribution of one or both pulmonary arteries may be incomplete (arborization abnormalities), with the

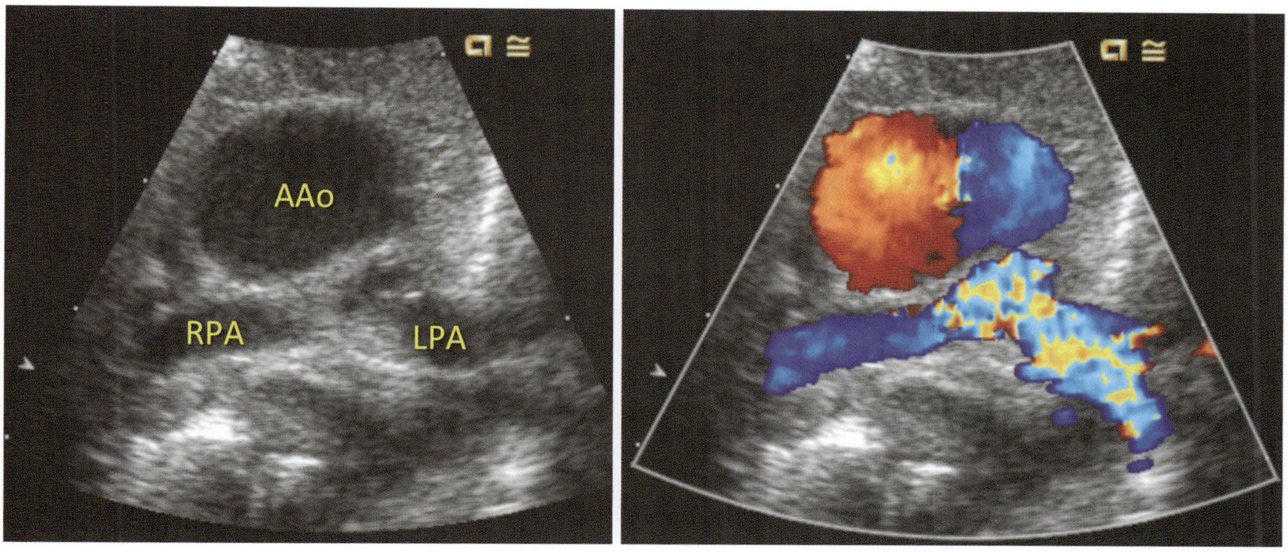

Figure 28.11 High parasternal short-axis view showing the confluence of the branch pulmonary arteries. AAo, ascending aorta; LPA, left pulmonary artery; RPA, right pulmonary artery.

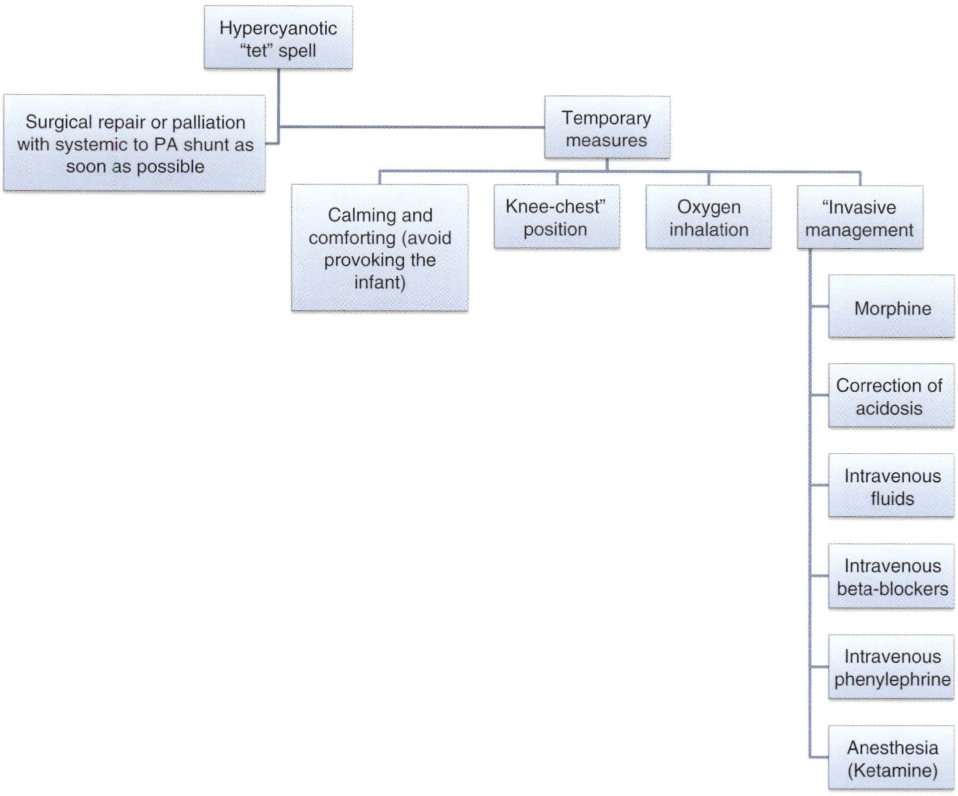

Figure 28.12 Management of a hypercyanotic "tet spell" in patients with tetralogy of Fallot.

remainder of lung segments being supplied solely by collateral arteries. Collateral arteries arise predominantly from the descending aorta or subclavian arteries. The major collaterals can vary from 1 to 6 in number and measure from 1 to 20 mm in diameter. Collateral arteries can anastomose with central pulmonary arteries (*communicating collaterals*) and become stenotic at their origins or at the site of connection with pulmonary arteries. Other collateral arteries tend to travel parallel to the bronchi as bronchial arteries and may be the only blood source of various bronchopulmonary segments (*non-communicating collaterals*).

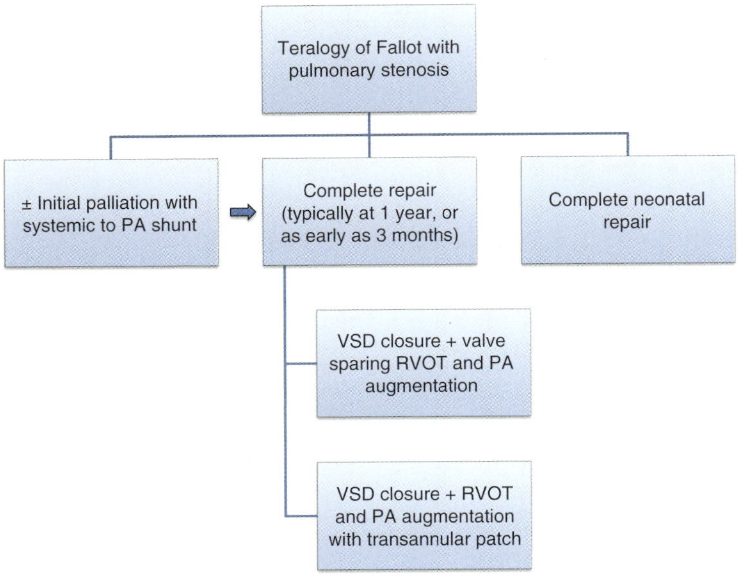

Figure 28.13 Surgical management options for patients with tetralogy of Fallot.

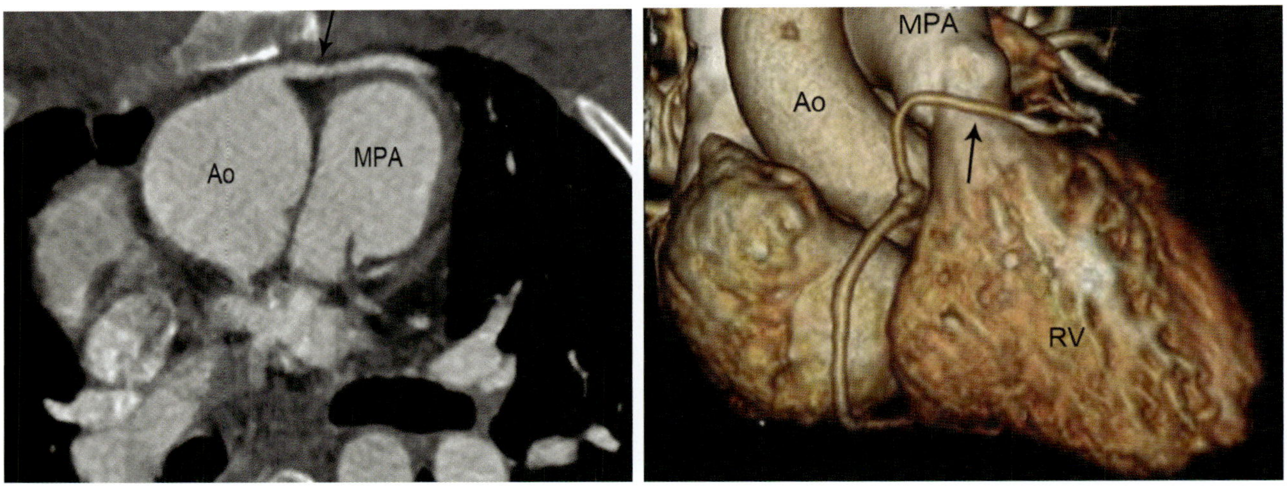

Figure 28.14 Anomalous origin of the left anterior descending (LAD) coronary artery from the right coronary artery as it travels anterior to the right ventricular outflow tract (RVOT). This anomaly is important to recognize in patients with tetralogy of Fallot where a transannular incision in the RVOT may result in transection of the LAD. Ao, aorta; LV, left ventricle; MPA, main pulmonary artery; RV, right ventricle.

Clinical Manifestations

Fetal echocardiography can identify most of these patients in utero. Otherwise, they will present with cyanosis or murmur as a newborn. The murmur is usually faint and continuous, originating either from the ductus or the collateral arteries. S1 is normal and S2 is single and loud. The degree of cyanosis is dependent on the amount of blood flow from patent ductus arteriosus or collateral arteries. Therefore, this is a ductal-dependent lesion that requires administration of prostaglandin E1 infusion to maintain ductal patency until surgery. Some neonates with PAVSD may not be cyanotic because of extensive collateral arterial blood supply. However, the natural tendency of these collateral vessels is to become stenotic which then results in cyanosis. Some infants may even present with heart failure symptoms caused by excessive pulmonary blood flow from collateral arteries. This usually occurs after the pulmonary vascular resistance has fallen (4–6 weeks of age).

Laboratory and Imaging Investigations

ECG and chest radiograph findings are usually similar to TOF. The intracardiac anatomy can be well evaluated by echocardiography, similar to TOF. The VSD and overriding aorta can be seen in similar imaging planes. The more critical evaluation is that of the central and branch pulmonary arteries. High parasternal and suprasternal windows allow superior evaluation of the central pulmonary arteries and vertical ductus in neonates.

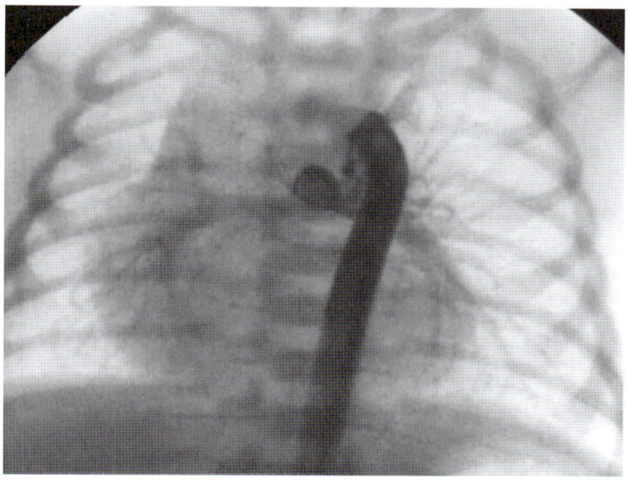

Figure 28.15 Descending aorta angiogram filling the confluent central pulmonary arteries with good distribution to both lungs.

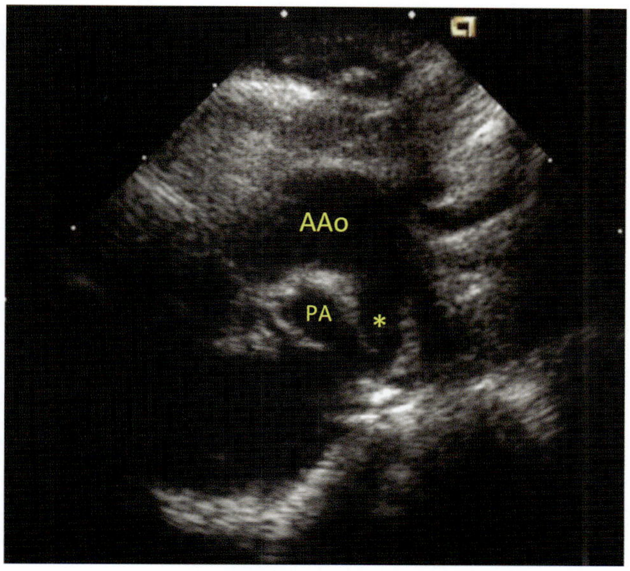

Figure 28.16 Vertical ductus (*) in pulmonary atresia with ventricular septal defect. The contour of ductus is in line with ascending aorta (AAo) and aortic arch.

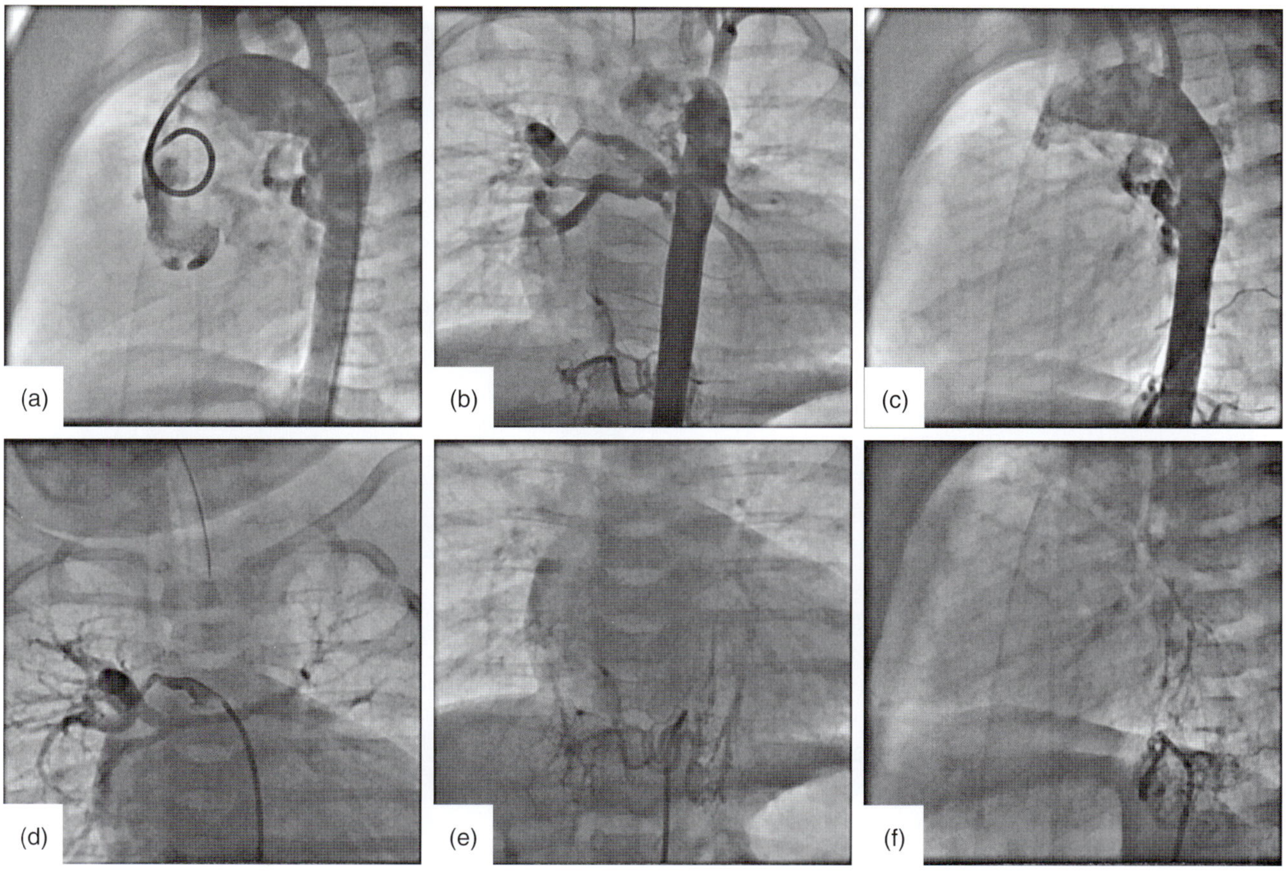

Figure 28.17 Cardiac catheterization in a patient with pulmonary atresia with ventricular septal defect. (a) Lateral projection of ascending aorta angiogram. (b,c) AP and lateral projections of descending aorta angiogram showing multiple collateral arteries, with some that communicate with the central pulmonary arteries. (d–f) Selective angiograms of collateral arteries with only one (d) communicating with the central pulmonary arteries.

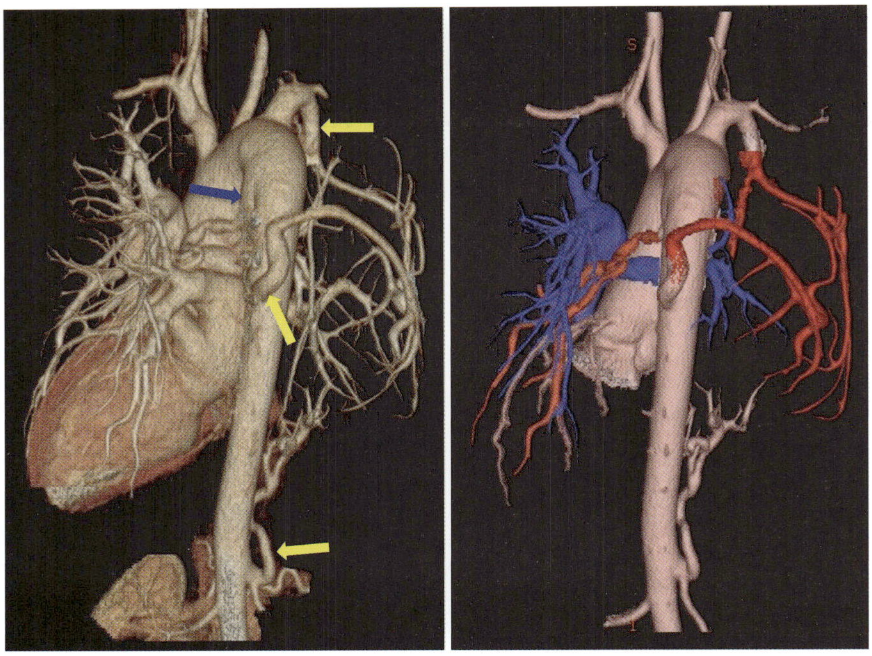

Figure 28.18 Computed tomography angiography of a patient with pulmonary atresia with ventricular septal defect. Multiple major aortopulmonary collateral arteries (yellow arrows) can be seen. Blue arrow points at the patent ductus arteriosus perfusing the central pulmonary arteries. The color coded image (right panel) highlights native pulmonary arteries (blue), collateral arteries (red), and aorta (pink). One major collateral is arising from the right renal artery.

The origin of collateral arteries from the descending aorta can sometimes be seen by echocardiography, but their distribution is better assessed with other imaging modalities.

Further non-invasive imaging of pulmonary and collateral arteries can be performed with CTA (Figure 28.18) or MRI (Figure 28.19). Pulmonary and collateral arteries can be seen well with either of these modalities. However, distinction between communicating and non-communicating collateral arteries can be challenging. Time resolved imaging in MRI or CTA perfusion may allow this distinction, but the gold standard for evaluation of collateral arteries is selective angiograms with invasive cardiac catheterization.

Neonates with larger central pulmonary arteries and no major collateral arteries seen by echocardiography may not need cardiac catheterization prior to initial surgical palliation. Patients with small central pulmonary arteries and those with complex collateral supply must undergo diagnostic cardiac catheterization to define the collaterals prior to surgery. During this diagnostic catheterization, size and distribution of the pulmonary and collateral arteries is assessed. The central pulmonary arteries are accessed through the ductus arteriosus for angiographic imaging. If the procedure is being performed after the ductus has closed, retrograde wedge injection of pulmonary veins or selective angiogram of communicating collateral artery can help in imaging the pulmonary arteries. Selective angiograms of collateral arteries help in surgical planning and allow the identification of the vessels that should be included during unifocalization surgery.

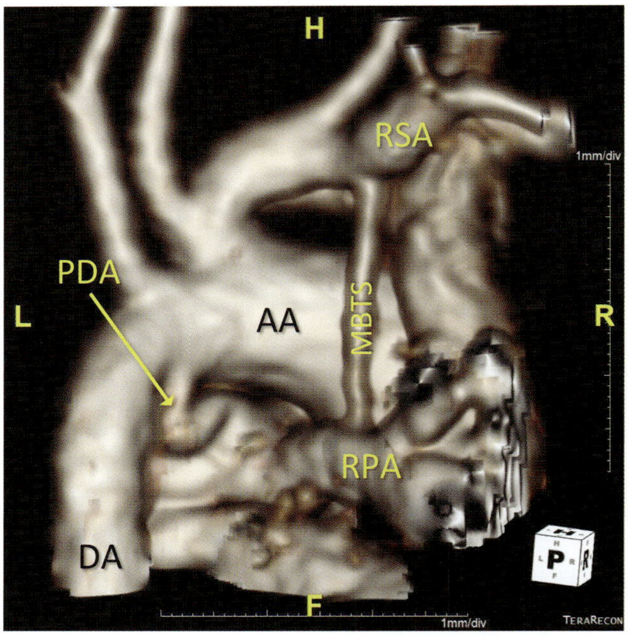

Figure 28.19 Three-dimensional volume rendering of magnetic resonance angiogram performed on an infant with pulmonary atresia and ventricular septal defect, viewed from posterior aspect. Confluent central pulmonary arteries receive blood from patent ductus arteriosus (PDA) and modified Blalock–Taussig shunt (MBTS). AA, aortic arch; DA, descending aorta; RPA, right pulmonary artery; RSA, right subclavian artery.

Management

Initial medical management for PAVSD involves stabilization of the neonate with prostaglandin E1 infusion, which must be initiated as soon as the diagnosis is suspected. Imaging of collateral arteries with cardiac

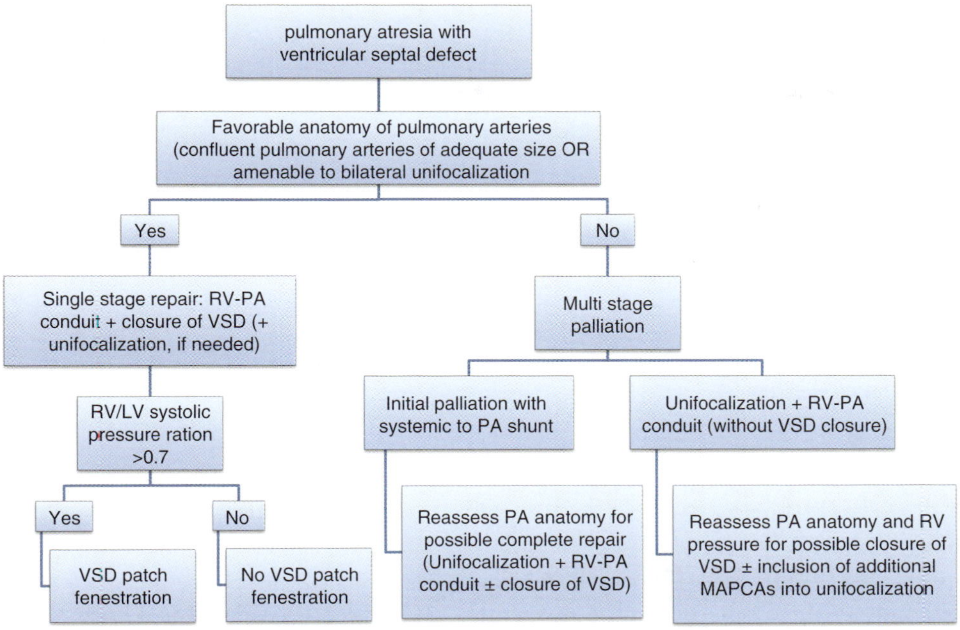

Figure 28.20 Surgical management options for pulmonary atresia with ventral septal defect (VSD).

catheterization, MRI, or CTA should be performed as soon as feasible. The goal of surgery is palliative in those who do not possess favorable pulmonary arterial architecture (Figure 28.20). This includes an initial systemic to pulmonary artery shunt, modified Blalock–Taussig shunt, or Mee procedure, or a limited unifocalization surgery with a conduit from the right ventricle to the pulmonary arteries. The goal of surgical management in infants whose pulmonary arteries are amenable to reconstruction includes establishment of connection between the right ventricle and the pulmonary arteries, as soon as possible, to allow continued growth of the central pulmonary arteries. In the ideal situation, a single stage repair involves insertion of a conduit connecting the right ventricle to adequate sized pulmonary arteries and closure of the VSD. If major collateral vessels exist, these need to be incorporated into pulmonary circulation with unifocalization procedures. Unifocalization involves disconnection of major collateral arteries from their aortic origin and anastomosing these to the central pulmonary arterial confluence. Connection of the lung segments that are not communicating with pulmonary arteries is established with incorporation of their collateral arteries into central pulmonary circulation. The goal is to incorporate the maximum number of pulmonary segments (at least 14) into the eventual RVOT reconstruction. At the end of surgery, if the right ventricular systolic pressure is >70% of systemic, the VSD is fenestrated.

Outcome

Surgical mortality is <5%, with timing of complete surgical repair reportedly ranging from 1 day to >50 years of age. Presence of major aortopulmonary collateral arteries and the need to reopen the VSD are factors associated with late mortality. Children in whom repair is not carried out and without adequate collateral supply have a poor prognosis.

Further Reading

O'Leary PW, Edwards WD, Julsrud PR, Burkhart HM. (2013) Pulmonary atresia and ventricular septal defect, in, *Moss and Adams' Heart Disease in Infants, Children, and Adolescents*, 8th edn (eds HD Allen, DJ Driscoll, RE Shaddy, TF Feltes), Lippincott Williams & Wilkins, Philadelphia. [Kindle Location 43410.]

Roche SL, Greenway SC, Redington AN. (2013) Tetralogy of Fallot with pulmonary stenosis and tetralogy of Fallot with absent pulmonary valve, in, *Moss and Adams' Heart Disease in Infants, Children, and Adolescents*, 8th edn (eds HD Allen, DJ Driscoll, RE Shaddy, TF Feltes), Lippincott Williams & Wilkins, Philadelphia, PA. [Kindle Location 43909.]

Villafane J, Feinstein JA, Jenkins KJ, et al. (2013) Hot topics in tetralogy of Fallot. *J Am Coll Cardiol*, **62**, 2155–2166.

Vyas H, Johnson J, Eidem BW. (2015) Tetralogy of Fallot, in, *Echocardiography in Pediatric and Adult Congenital Heart Disease*, 2nd edn (eds BW Eidem, PW O'Leary, F Cetta), Wolters Kluwer, Philadelphia, PA, pp. 305–319.

29

Absent Pulmonary Valve

Brieann Muller and Sawsan Awad

Section of Pediatric Cardiology, Rush University Medical Center, Chicago, IL, USA

Absent pulmonary valve (APV) is a rare congenital cardiac malformation, the exact incidence of which is not certain because it is often reported with other cardiac malformations, such as tetralogy of Fallot (TOF). The key anatomic feature of APV is a rudimentary and dysplastic non-coaptating pulmonary valve (Figure 29.1 and 29.2). This abnormal valve can be seen in isolation (Figures 29.3 and 29.4), which is extremely rare, or associated with other cardiac lesions. Often, it is referred to as absent pulmonary valve syndrome when the dysplastic valve is associated with a malalignment-type ventricular septal defect (VSD) and dilated pulmonary arteries. The most commonly associated cardiac lesions that have been described with APV include VSD, absent arterial duct, and TOF. The incidence of APV in patients with TOF is 2–6%; whereas about 80% of patients with APV will also have TOF. Rarely, APV can be seen with tricuspid atresia.

The morbidity of APV is related to the degree of pulmonary artery dilation. The severe pulmonary stenosis and regurgitation that occur because of the dysplastic valve non-coaptating ultimately lead to significant dilation of the main and branch pulmonary arteries (Figures 29.1b and 29.2a). These dilated arteries cause bronchial compression leading to bronchomalacia and even severe respiratory distress at birth. Complete airway occlusion leading to pulmonary fluid retention and heart displacement has been described [1]. Chronic obstructive pulmonary disease is seen in those patients that survive beyond the neonatal period.

Over the last 20 years, three large case series have reported fetal and postnatal survival rates for APV below 20% [1]. Cardiac failure is the main reason for death related to APV, but pregnancy termination and intrauterine death (Figure 29.1) also contribute to its high mortality rate [2]. APV is suspected prenatally when fetal echocardiography reveals dilation of the right side of the heart and isolated pulmonary regurgitation (Figures 29.1c and 29.3b). Aneurysmal branch pulmonary arteries can also be seen in fetal life (Figure 29.1b). Confirmatory diagnosis is made by neonatal transthoracic echocardiogram.

Management of patients with APV involves careful surgical planning. Surgical repair includes pulmonary valve replacement and plication of redundant aneurysmal pulmonary arterial walls.

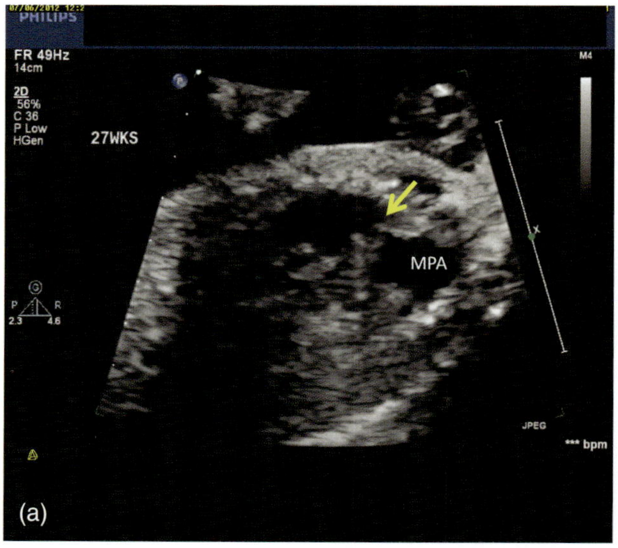

Figure 29.1 Fetal echocardiogram of a fetus at 27 weeks' gestation with tetralogy of Fallot and absent pulmonary valve. This fetus developed hydrops as evidenced by increased skin thickness, abnormal ductus venosus, and increased cardiothoracic ratio (not shown) and ultimately had intrauterine demise. (a) The dysplastic pulmonary valve (yellow arrow) and dilated main pulmonary artery (MPA) can be seen in this two-dimensional (2D) view. (b) 2D and color view showing dilated right (RPA) and left (LPA) pulmonary artery branches characteristic of absent pulmonary valve syndrome. (c) Doppler evaluation of the pulmonary valve demonstrating significant pulmonary valve regurgitation (blue arrow; positive wave, above the baseline) and pulmonary valve stenosis (yellow arrow; negative wave, below the baseline).

Visual Guide to Neonatal Cardiology, First Edition. Edited by Ernerio T. Alboliras, Ziyad M. Hijazi, Leo Lopez, and Donald J. Hagler.

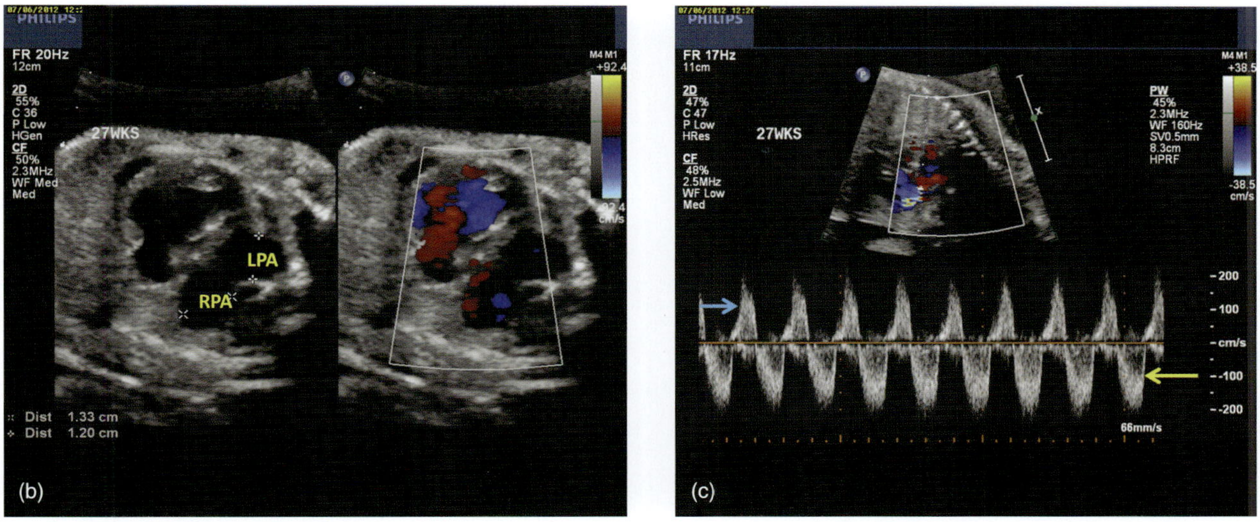

Figure 29.1 (*Continued*)

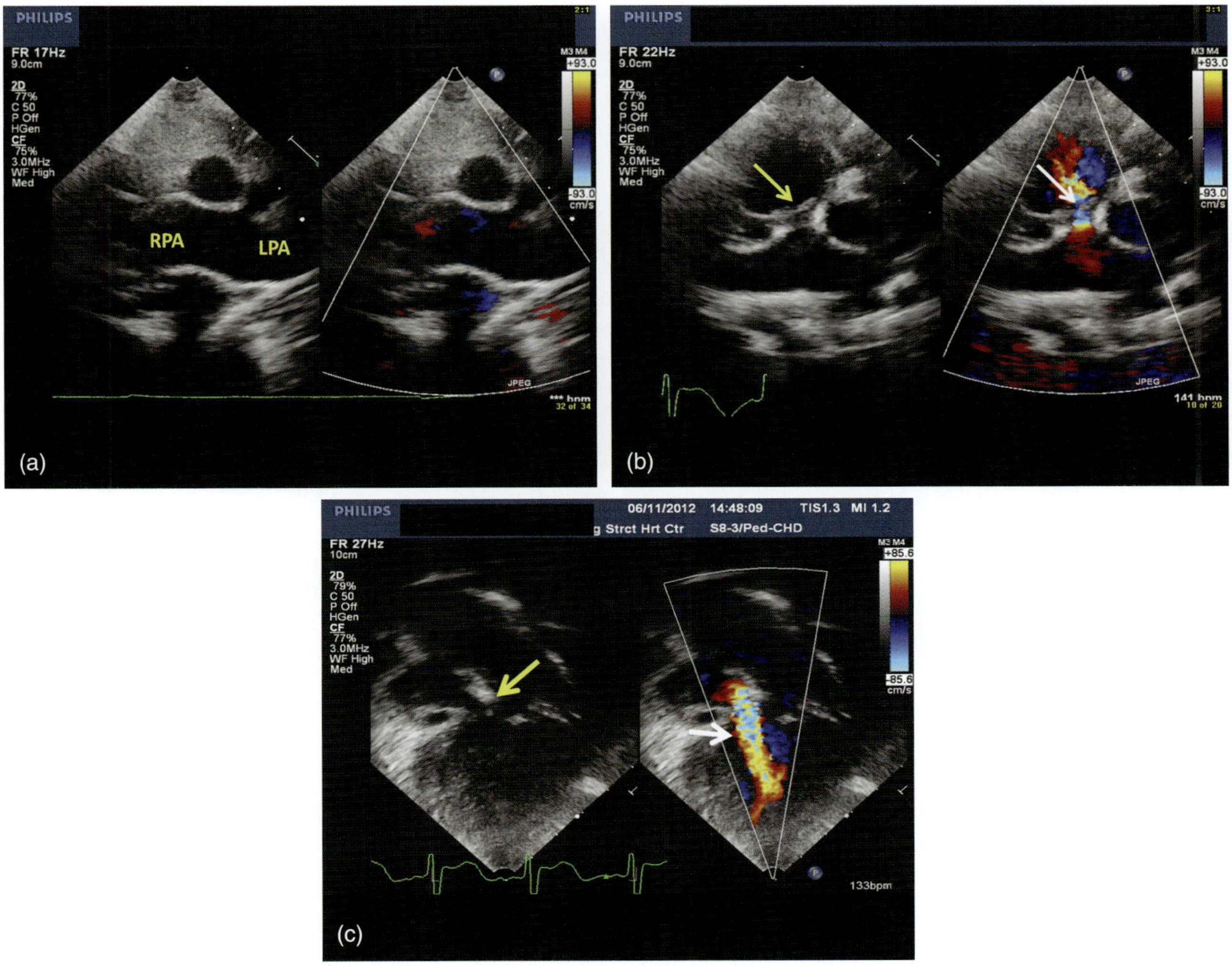

Figure 29.2 Postnatal transthoracic echocardiogram of a patient with visceral situ inversus, dextrocardia, and tetralogy of Fallot/absent pulmonary valve. (a) 2D and color image from high short parasternal view showing severely dilated branch pulmonary arteries. LPA, left pulmonary artery; RPA, right pulmonary artery. (b) 2D and color image from short parasternal view showing dysplastic pulmonary valve (yellow arrow) with turbulence of flow through the valve (white arrow). (c) Subcostal 2D and color image showing dysplastic pulmonary valve (yellow arrow) and significant pulmonary valve regurgitation (red color jet; white arrow).

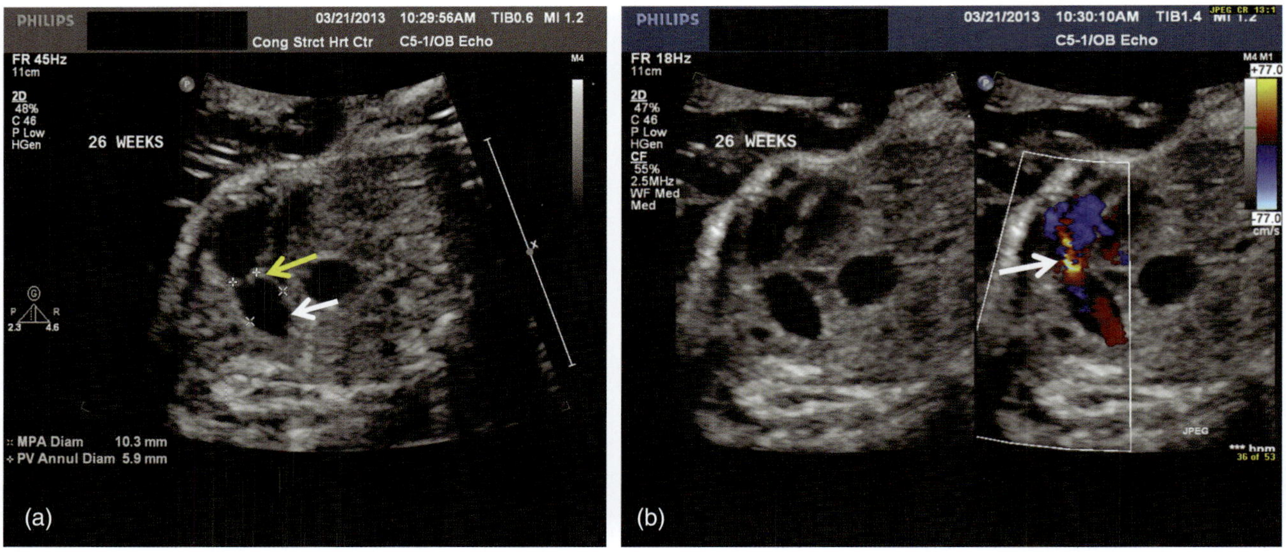

Figure 29.3 Fetal echocardiogram images of a fetus at 26 weeks' gestation with absent pulmonary valve and muscular ventricular septal defect (VSD; not associated with TOF). This patient also had cardiac dextroposition secondary to left-sided diaphragmatic hernia. Patient was placed on extracorporeal membrane oxygenation (ECMO) at birth and diaphragmatic hernia was subsequently repaired. Patient expired after 11 days on ECMO support secondary to poorly developed lung parenchyma bilaterally. (a) 2D image showing the dysplastic pulmonary valve (yellow arrow) and dilated main pulmonary artery (white arrow). (b) This 2D and color image shows pulmonary regurgitation (white arrow).

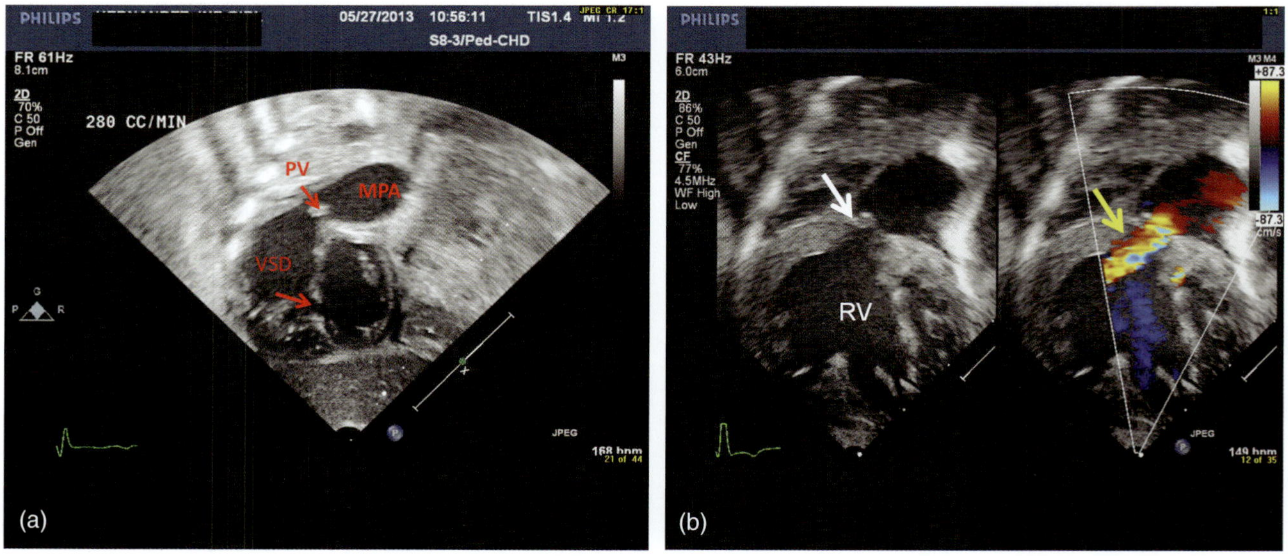

Figure 29.4 Postnatal transthoracic echocardiogram images of the same patient as in Figure 29.3. (a) The dysplastic pulmonary valve (PV) and dilated main pulmonary artery (MPA) can be seen as well as a muscular ventricular septal defect (VSD). Notice that transthoracic echocardiogram is performed while patient is on 280 mL/min ECMO flow (full support). (b) 2D and color images of a subcostal view showing significant pulmonary valve regurgitation (yellow arrow). Thickened, dysplastic pulmonary valve (white arrow) is well demonstrated. Notice also dilated, hypertrophied right ventricle (RV). (c) Subcostal 2D and color images demonstrate the dysplastic valve (PV) with poor coaptation (yellow asterisk) as well as a severely dilated main pulmonary artery (MPA).

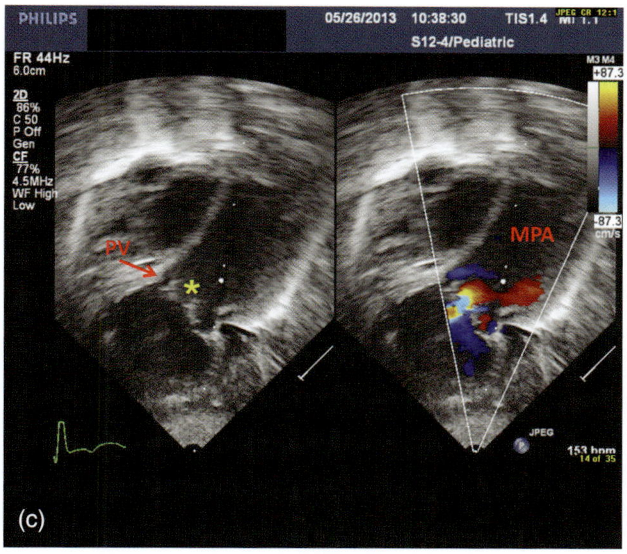

Figure 29.4 (*Continued*)

References

1 Wertaschnigg D, Jaeggi M, Chitayat D, *et al.* (2013) Prenatal diagnosis and outcome of absent pulmonary valve syndrome: contemporary single-center experience and review of the literature. *Ultrasound Obstet Gynecol*, **41**, 162–167.

2 Volpe P, Paladini D, Marasini M, *et al.* (2004) Characteristics, associations and outcome of absent pulmonary valve syndrome in the fetus. *Ultrasound Obstet Gynecol*, **24**, 623–628.

30

Transposition of the Great Arteries

Adam L. Dorfman

Division of Pediatric Cardiology, University of Michigan Congenital Heart Center, C.S. Mott Children's Hospital, Ann Arbor, MI, USA

Transposition of the great arteries (TGA) is defined as ventriculo-arterial discordance, a reversal of the usual relationship of the great arteries with the ventricles. In this scenario, the left ventricle is related to the pulmonary artery, while the right ventricle is related to the aorta. There is typically reversal of the topologic position of the great arteries too, such that the aorta is located anterior and variably rightward of the pulmonary artery, with conus supporting the aorta and causing fibrous discontinuity between the aortic and tricuspid valves. However, these anatomic details can vary. This chapter is dedicated to discussion of {S,D,D} TGA, with situs solitus of the atria, D-looping of the ventricles, and D-positioning of the aorta. This lesion is commonly referred to as "D-looped TGA" or as "complete TGA" or TGV (transposition of great vessels), signifying that the systemic and pulmonary circulations are in parallel. Congenitally corrected TGA is covered separately in Chapter 31.

The typical anatomy of this lesion is delineated in Figure 30.1. Note the rightward and superior positioning of the aorta from the anterior, normally positioned right ventricle, with the pulmonary artery to the left and slightly inferior from the posteriorly positioned left ventricle, with fibrous continuity between the pulmonary and mitral valves. A patent foramen ovale (PFO) and a patent ductus arteriosus (PDA) are also present.

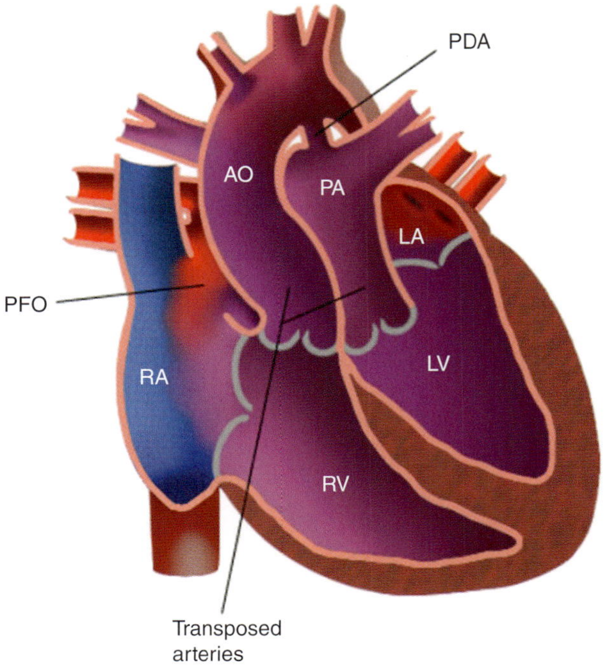

Figure 30.1 Diagram of {S,D,D} transposition of the great arteries. Note the ventriculo-arterial discordance, with mitral–pulmonary valve fibrous continuity and separation of the tricuspid and aortic valves by conal muscle. There is a small atrial septal defect with left atrial to right atrial shunting and a patent ductus arteriosus with aortic to pulmonary artery shunting. Ao, aorta; LA, left atrium; LV, left ventricle; PA, main pulmonary artery; PDA, patent ductus arteriosus; PFO, patent foramen ovale; RV, right ventricle.

The pathophysiology of TGA stems from the parallel circulations. Oxygen depleted blood from the systemic veins is recirculated to the aorta, while oxygen rich pulmonary venous blood is recirculated to the pulmonary arteries. Survival as a neonate is dependent on mixing of these two circulations, usually from a PFO and a PDA (Figure 30.1), and in approximately half of cases, via a ventricular septal defect (VSD). Adequate mixing of circulations is critical for allowing systemic oxygen delivery.

The incidence of associated cardiac lesions is high, requiring careful diagnostic attention. A VSD is the most commonly associated lesion; this includes VSDs of any type; frequently these are moderate to large defects beneath the pulmonary valve (paramembranous), but can include atrioventricular canal defects, infundibular (sub-aortic) defects, or muscular defects which can sometimes be small and not require surgical intervention. The presence of a VSD does not guarantee adequate mixing of venous and arterial. Additional lesions are more common in TGA with an associated VSD than in those with intact ventricular septum. While either semilunar valve can be stenotic, more common is left ventricular outflow tract obstruction and valvar

Visual Guide to Neonatal Cardiology, First Edition. Edited by Ernerio T. Alboliras, Ziyad M. Hijazi, Leo Lopez, and Donald J. Hagler.

pulmonary stenosis. Pulmonary atresia is also seen. When valvar aortic stenosis is present, it can also be associated with aortic coarctation or interrupted aortic arch. There can also be abnormalities of the atrioventricular valves, including straddling or overriding valves that can sometimes lead to ventricular hypoplasia. Abnormalities of the coronary artery origins are also relatively common, more so when the aorta and pulmonary artery have more of a right–left side-to-side orientation, as opposed to anterior–posterior. There are many possible orientations of the coronary artery origins, with "usual" origins defined as the left main coronary artery arising from the left-facing aortic sinus and bifurcating, and the right coronary artery arising from the right-facing sinus (Figure 30.2); when the vessels are oriented anterior–posterior, the facing sinuses are the posterior sinuses of the aorta [1]. The most common abnormality is the circumflex coronary artery arising from the right, and passing posterior to the pulmonary root as it courses to the left atrioventricular groove. Either coronary artery can have an intramural course (within the adventitia of the aorta), which can pose surgical difficulties.

Clinical presentation is typically with cyanosis and hypoxia. In situations in which circulatory mixing is not adequate, neonates can quickly develop life-threatening levels of hypoxia and acidosis requiring emergent intervention. Conversely, if the PFO and PDA are non-restrictive, the cyanosis can be clinically subtle, and it may be less pronounced as well in the presence of a

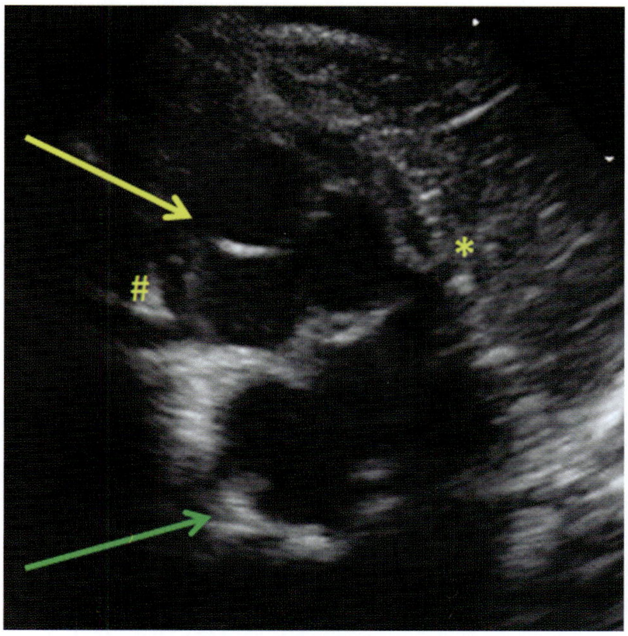

Figure 30.2 Echocardiogram: parasternal short-axis image displaying the anterior and slightly rightward aortic valve (yellow arrow) and posterior pulmonary valve (green arrow). The origins of the right (#) and left (*) coronary arteries can be seen arising from the facing sinuses of the aorta.

large VSD. Anecdotally, some of these infants have been discharged home undiagnosed when the cyanosis is not recognized. If discharged without diagnosis, infants with intact ventricular septum will exhibit progressive cyanosis, or may present *in extremis* if the PDA closes. Infants with an associated large VSD will present in the first few weeks of life with signs and symptoms of congestive heart failure. An associated severe coarctation or interrupted aortic arch will result in circulatory failure if the PDA closes after the infant is discharged.

Diagnosis typically begins with recognition of cyanosis. While cyanosis in the neonate can occasionally go undetected, uniform pulse oximetry in neonates prior to hospital discharge has been recommended by the US Secretary of Health and Human Services, and endorsed by the American Academy of Pediatrics [2]. This screening can be life-saving in cases in which the infant would have otherwise been discharged home. Perinatal findings on cardiac examination may be subtle. In the absence of associated lesions, there may be no murmur present. The second heart sound will typically sound single because of the prominence of the anterior aortic valve. Palpation of the precordium is often unremarkable. Associated non-cardiac lesions are rare. Electrocardiogram in the perinatal period is usually normal. Chest X-ray can also be normal, but can include findings such as a narrow mediastinum because of the anterior–posterior arrangement of the great arteries, and potentially increased pulmonary vascular markings, particularly in the context of an associated VSD.

Diagnosis of TGA can be made by fetal echocardiography. However, this diagnosis can be easily missed on a screening fetal ultrasound, so TGA should be considered in the differential diagnosis of neonatal cyanosis even with a history of a normal level II ultrasound. The mainstay of detailed anatomic diagnosis postnatally is echocardiography. In an urgent situation, the presence of TGA can be quickly recognized by the appearance of outflow tracts in parallel from the parasternal long-axis view (Figure 30.3) or an anatomic sweep from the subcostal coronal view. With this sweep, the pulmonary artery is seen arising from the left ventricle (Figure 30.4a), followed by the anterior aorta arising from the right ventricle (Figure 30.4b). After recognition of this diagnosis in the acutely ill neonate, the atrial septum should be assessed for the size of any defect, which is usually a PFO. The aortic arch and presence of a PDA should also be evaluated. In the more common scenario in which the neonate is hemodynamically stable, a complete echocardiogram is performed to assess the anatomy of the great arteries, as well as to perform a detailed evaluation of the remainder of the anatomy, with particular attention to assessing for the associated cardiac lesions discussed earlier. The echocardiogram should be performed with the detail necessary for planning

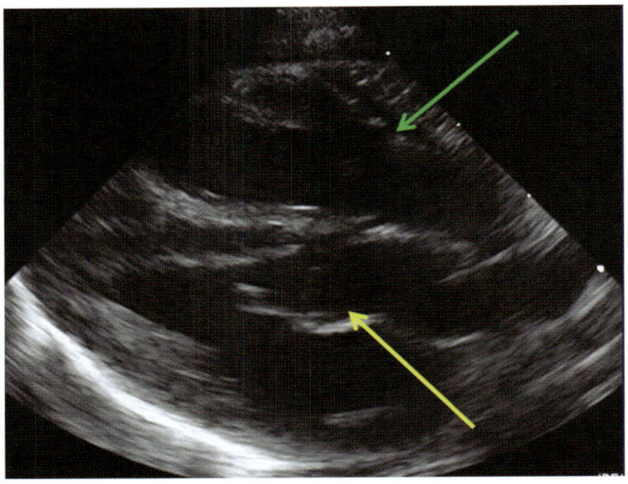

Figure 30.3 Echocardiogram: parasternal long-axis view displaying parallel outflow tracts, with the pulmonary artery arising posteriorly from the left ventricle (yellow arrow), and the aorta arising anteriorly from the right ventricle (green arrow). Note the fibrous continuity between the open mitral valve and the closed pulmonary valve.

surgery. If immediate medical attention or intervention is required, the remainder of the echocardiogram can be completed subsequent to stabilization of the patient. In unusual scenarios such as particularly complex aortic arch anatomy, cross-sectional imaging (CT or MR) may be useful for further delineation of anatomy. Rarely, invasive angiography is helpful to diagnose coronary artery abnormalities. However, echocardiography can provide the complete diagnosis in the vast majority of cases.

The first line of medical therapy for the neonate with TGA with intact ventricular septum is prostaglandin E1 infusion to maintain ductal patency. This is essential when there is an associated ductal-dependent lesion such as interrupted aortic arch or pulmonary atresia. In some cases of TGA without associated lesions and with a large atrial level shunt, there can be adequate mixing of the circulations without a PDA. Prostaglandin infusion can be complicated by apnea and/or systemic hypotension, so close monitoring is essential, and endotracheal intubation may become necessary. Fluid bolus can be helpful for hypotension and to increase circulatory mixing.

TGA has been associated with pulmonary vascular disease, particularly in the presence of a VSD with systemic pulmonary arterial pressure. Pulmonary vascular disease in these patients by age 1 year is nearly ubiquitous. However, pulmonary hypertension is seen sporadically in neonates with TGA, either before or after corrective surgery. Inhaled nitric oxide is sometimes required in the critical care setting for management of this problem.

If the neonate is cyanotic in the presence of inadequate mixing at the atrial septal level, a balloon atrial septostomy (BAS) can be considered. This procedure is covered in depth in Chapter 63. It can be performed in the catheterization laboratory under fluoroscopic guidance, or at the bedside with guidance by echocardiography (Figure 30.5). The result of the BAS is fracturing of the atrial septum (Figure 30.6), enabling greater mixing of the circulations and allowing for improved oxygenation. This is a temporizing procedure, performed to provide clinical stability prior to ultimate surgical correction. Following BAS, oxygenation will sometimes

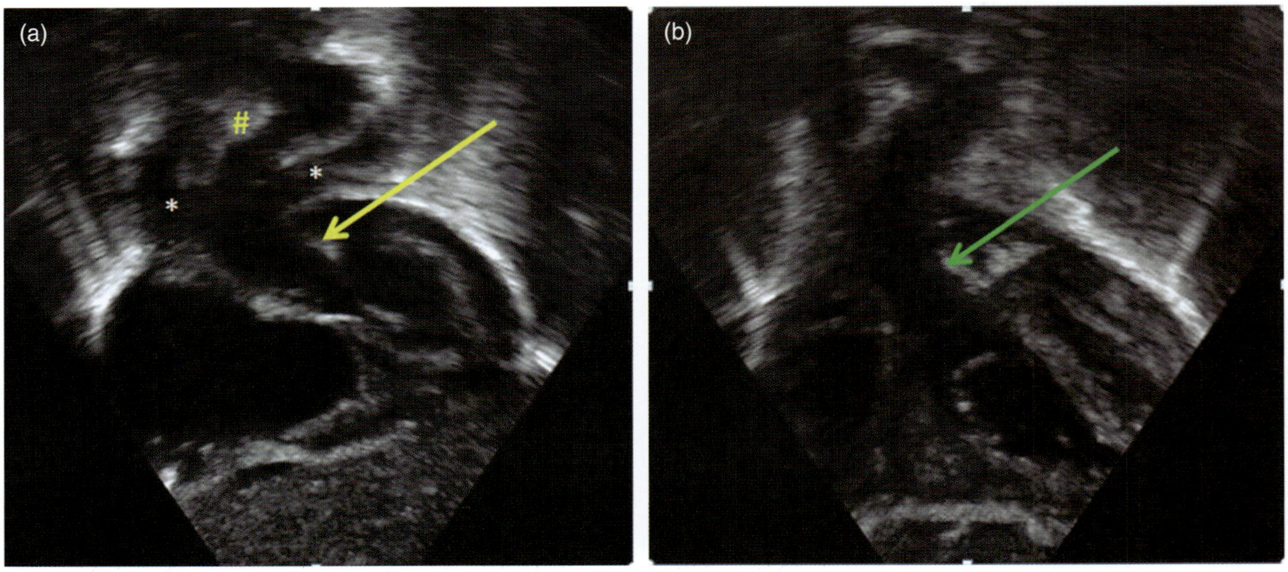

Figure 30.4 (a) Echocardiogram: subcostal coronal view showing the pulmonary artery arising from the left ventricle (yellow arrow). The early branching of the main pulmonary artery into the branches is seen (*), as well as the presence of a large patent ductus arteriosus (#). (b) Subcostal coronal view in more anterior plane, showing the aorta arising from the right ventricle (green arrow). Note the lack of fibrous continuity between the open tricuspid valve and the closed aortic valve.

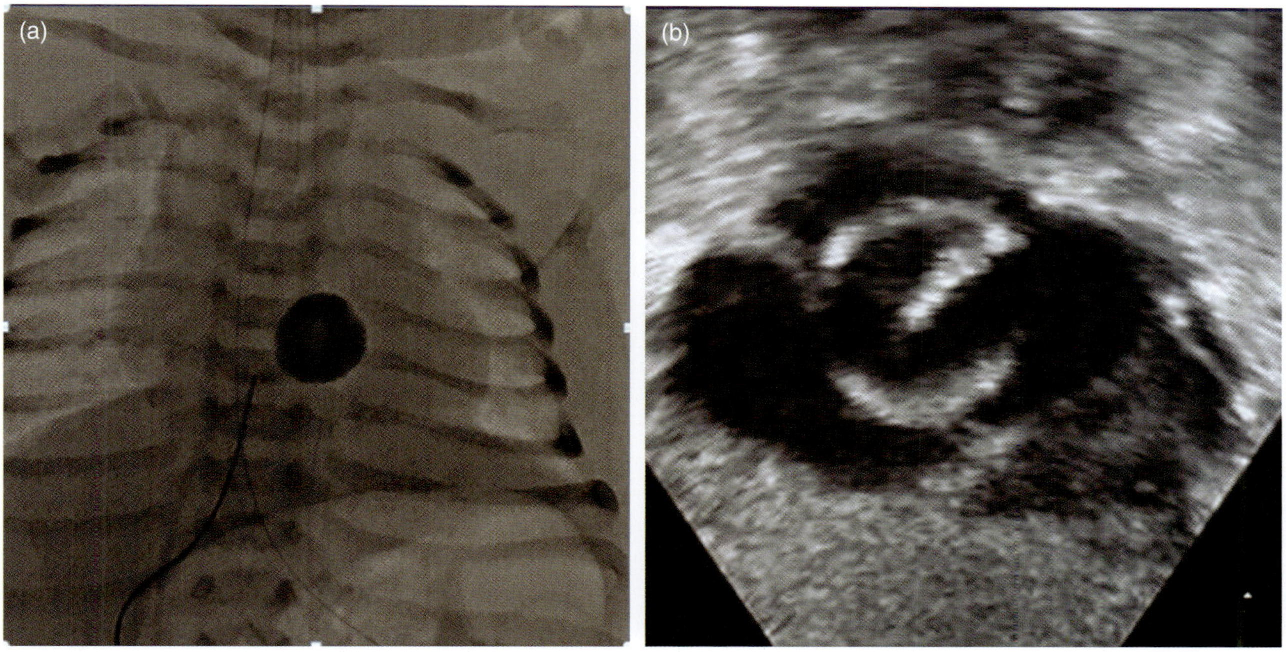

Figure 30.5 (a) Fluoroscopic image of a balloon inflated in the left atrium, ready to be pulled across the atrial septum for a balloon atrial septostomy. (b) Echocardiographic image of a balloon filling most of the left atrium prior to balloon atrial septostomy. Note the tenting of the atrial septum towards the right atrium, with tension placed on the balloon catheter.

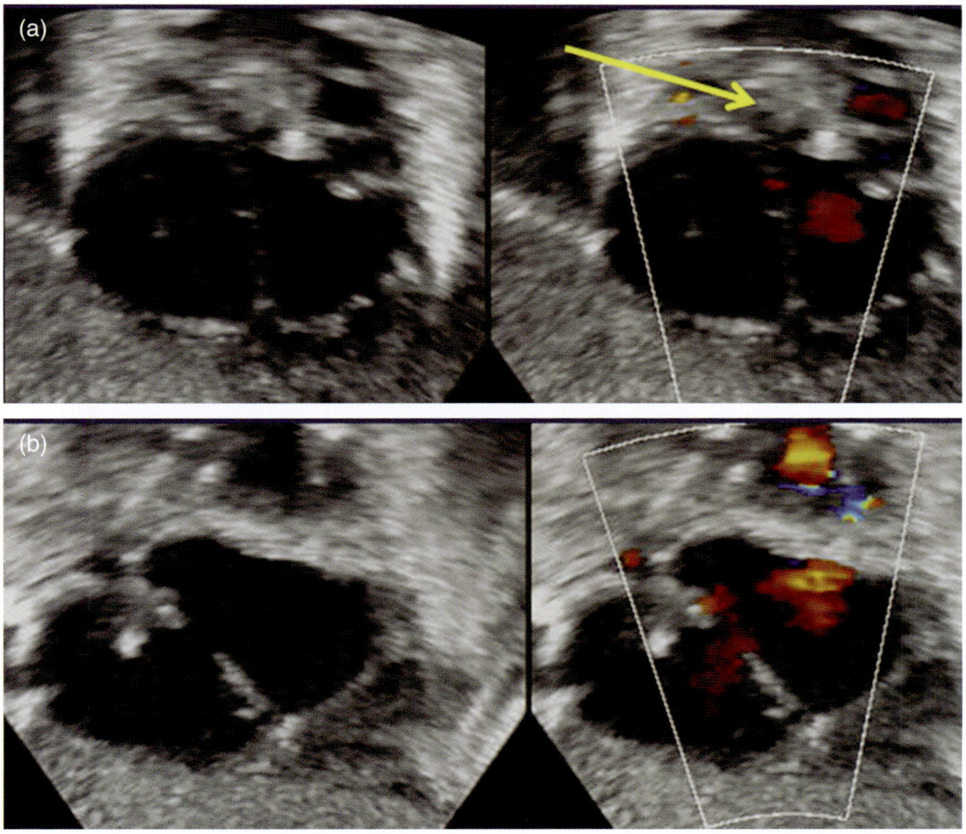

Figure 30.6 (a) Echocardiogram: subcostal coronal view showing the atrial septum prior to balloon atrial septostomy, with a tiny patent foramen ovale seen on the color image, with red color showing flow from the left atrium to the right atrium. (b) Atrial septum of the same patient following balloon atrial septostomy. Note the much larger hole in the atrial septum, with red color depicting a wide jet of left atrial to right atrial flow.

be adequate to allow discontinuation of prostaglandin infusion while awaiting surgery.

Preferred surgery for TGA is the arterial switch operation (ASO), which was first reported by Jatene in 1976 [3] and came into widespread use by the late 1980s. A detailed description of this operation is found in Chapter 66. In brief, the coronary arteries are excised with a button of tissue from the native aorta. The aorta and pulmonary artery are transected, and the pulmonary artery pulled anterior to the aorta (known as the Lecompte maneuver). The coronary buttons are then re-attached to the neo-aorta. Associated lesions are addressed at the same time. The ASO is typically performed within the first 2 weeks of life. In some situations, most commonly involving a congenitally abnormal pulmonary valve, the ASO cannot be performed. In the situation of TGA with pulmonary stenosis or atresia and a large VSD, preferably of the paramembranous or infundibular type, the preferred alternative operation is the Rastelli procedure, in which the left ventricular outflow is directed through the VSD with a patch to the native aortic valve, and a conduit is placed from the right ventricle to the pulmonary artery.

Current short and mid-term prognosis for TGA with an arterial switch operation is excellent. At experienced centers, survival to discharge as a neonate is widely reported to be well over 95%. Mortality rates are somewhat lower for TGA with intact ventricular septum compared to those with VSDs and other associated lesions. Longer term outcomes are also good [4]. Potential hemodynamic lesions that could require re-intervention include:

- Coronary artery insufficiency;
- Right ventricular outflow tract obstruction (usually valvar or supravalvar pulmonary stenosis);
- Branch pulmonary artery stenosis;
- Neo-aortic root dilatation; and
- Neo-aortic regurgitation.

References

1 Pasquini L, Sanders SP, Parness IA, *et al.* (1994) Coronary echocardiography in 406 patients with d-loop transposition of the great arteries. *J Am Coll Cardiol*, **24**, 763–768.

2 Mahle WT, Martin GR, Beekman RH III,, *et al.* (2012) Endorsement of health and human services recommendation for pulse oximetry screening for critical congenital heart disease. *Pediatrics*, **129**, 190–192.

3 Jatene AD, Fontes VF, Paulista PP, *et al.* (1976) Anatomic correction of transposition of the great vessels. *J Thorac Cardiovasc Surg*, **72**, 364–370.

4 Khairy P, Clair M, Fernandes SM, *et al.* (2013) Cardiovascular outcomes after the arterial switch operation for D-transposition of the great arteries. *Circulation*, **127**, 331–339.

31

Congenitally Corrected Transposition of the Great Arteries

Camden L. Hebson[1] *and William L. Border*[2]

[1] *Division of Cardiology, Department of Medicine, Emory University School of Medicine, Atlanta, GA, USA*
[2] *Children's Healthcare of Atlanta Sibley Heart Center; Emory University School of Medicine, Atlanta, GA, USA*

Congenitally corrected transposition of the great arteries (CCTGA) refers to the cardiac morphologic abnormality consisting of discordant atrioventricular and ventriculo-arterial connections. In other words, the morphologically right atrium is connected to a morphologically left ventricle across a mitral valve, with the left ventricle then connected to the pulmonary trunk. The morphologically left atrium is then connected to the morphologically right ventricle across the tricuspid valve, with the morphologically right ventricle connected to the aorta. Usually, the morphologic left ventricle is situated on the right side, and the morphologically right ventricle is on the left side (Figures 31.1 and 31.2). The physiology is described as "congenitally corrected" because the flow of blood is essentially normal, with the deoxygenated systemic venous blood being pumped to the lungs and the oxygenated pulmonary venous blood being pumped to the body. CCTGA is one of the more rare cardiac lesions, with a reported incidence of approximately 0.05% of congenital cardiac malformations [1, 2].

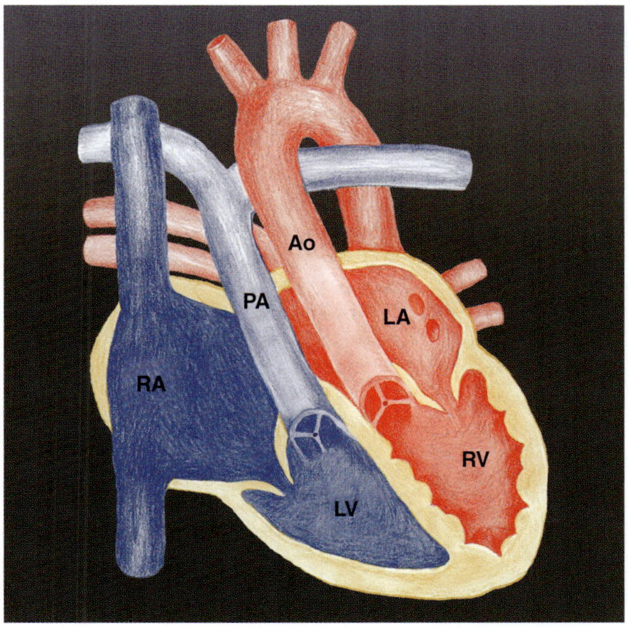

Figure 31.1 Diagram of an apical four-chamber view. There is atrioventricular discordance and ventriculo-arterial discordance. Note the smooth-walled morphology of the right-sided morphologically left ventricle, indicative of ventricular inversion. Ao, aorta; LA, left atrium; LV, left ventricle; PA, pulmonary artery; RA, right atrium; RV, right ventricle.

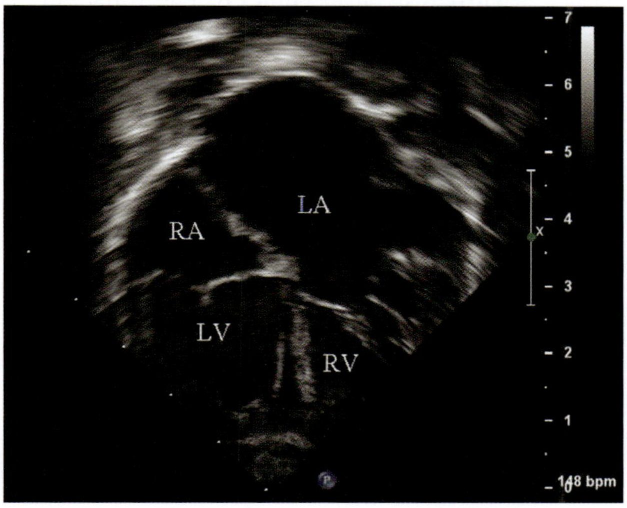

Figure 31.2 A two-dimensional (2D) echocardiography apical four-chamber view at the level of the atrioventricular valves. Note the malalignment of the atrial septum compared to the ventricular septum. The apical displacement of the tricuspid valve compared to the mitral valve, along with the smooth-walled morphology of the left ventricle, are clues to the presence of ventricular inversion. LA, left atrium; LV, left ventricle; RA, right atrium; RV, right ventricle.

Morphology and Associated Lesions

Typically, the atrial chambers are in their known positions with the right atrium on the right, the left atrium on the left, and there is L-looping (otherwise known as left-hand ventricular topology) of the ventricles. Usually, when the ventricular septum is intact, there is a

Visual Guide to Neonatal Cardiology, First Edition. Edited by Ernerio T. Alboliras, Ziyad M. Hijazi, Leo Lopez, and Donald J. Hagler.

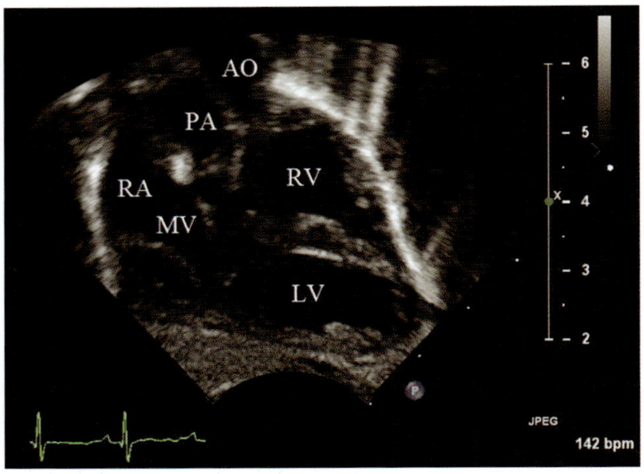

Figure 31.3 A 2D echocardiography subcostal coronal view. Pertinent visible anatomy includes mitral–pulmonic fibrous continuity (no subpulmonary conus), the smooth-walled right-sided morphologic LV, and the parallel relationship of the great vessels with the aorta leftward of the proximal pulmonary artery. AO, aorta; LV, left ventricle; MV, mitral valve; PA, pulmonary artery; RA, right atrium; RV, right ventricle.

reverse-offsetting of the attachments of the leaflets of the atrioventricular (AV) valve to the septum, with the mitral valve on the right side attached appreciably higher than the tricuspid valve on the left side at the crux of the heart (Figure 31.2). There is fibrous continuity between the leaflets of the pulmonary and mitral valves (Figure 31.3). In addition, the pulmonary valve is wedged between the atrial septum and the mitral valve, resulting in a deviation of the atrial septum away from the ventricular septum (Figure 31.2). The epicardial distribution of the coronary arteries usually follows their respective ventricles. Thus, the right-sided coronary artery will exhibit the path of a morphologically left coronary artery, with its short main stem dividing into ventricular and circumflex branches. The left-sided coronary artery is arranged as a morphologic right coronary artery, giving origin to the infundibular and marginal branches. The anterior interventricular artery is a good guide to the location of the muscular ventricular septum. The atrioventricular conduction system is abnormally positioned in CCTGA because of the malalignment of the atrial septum and ventricular septum. The AV node is located beneath the opening of the right atrial appendage, at the lateral margin of the area of pulmonary–mitral fibrous continuity. This abnormal course of the conduction system can be problematic when closing ventricular septal defects (VSDs) during surgical repair.

There are a number of associated lesions that can occur with CCTGA, and these usually occur in over 90% of patients. The most common are VSDs, followed by obstruction of the pulmonary outflow tract and abnormalities of the tricuspid valve [3]. The majority of the VSDs are paramembranous, located below the pulmonary valve with extension into the inlet of the morphologically left ventricle (Figure 31.4). Muscular defects can also be found as well as subarterial or conal defects. Obstruction to pulmonary outflow can occur at both the valvar and subvalvar level. When subvalvar, it can be muscular or fibrous (Figure 31.5). Finally, the tricuspid valve, which is the morphologic right AV valve on the left side, can have various abnormalities. Most commonly, it is apically displaced, earning it the description of Ebstein malformation. The tricuspid valve could be thickened

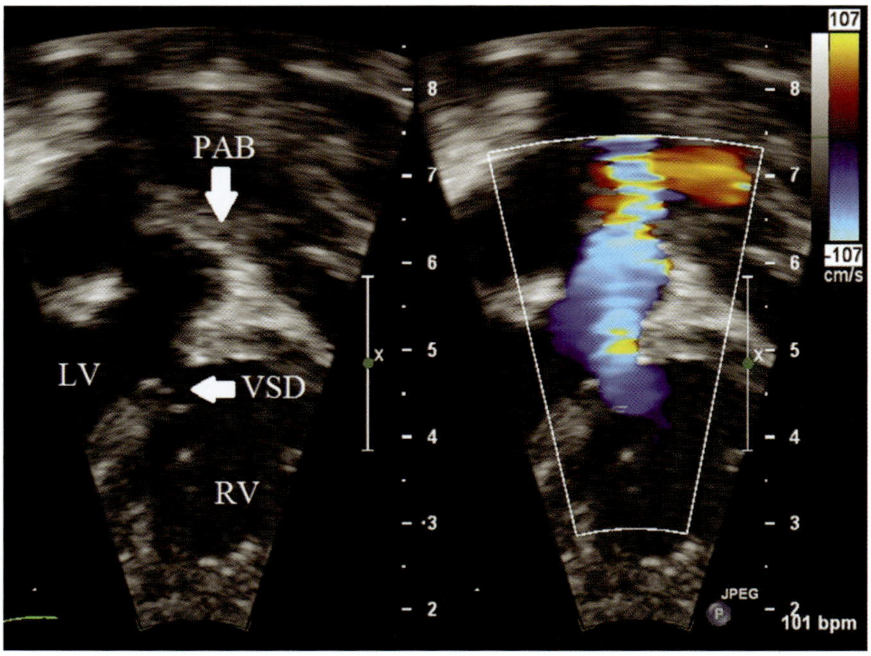

Figure 31.4 A 2D echocardiography subcostal coronal view in color compare mode. A ventricular septal defect is present, which has been palliated using a pulmonary artery band. LV, left ventricle; PAB, pulmonary artery band; VSD, ventricular septal defect; RV, right ventricle.

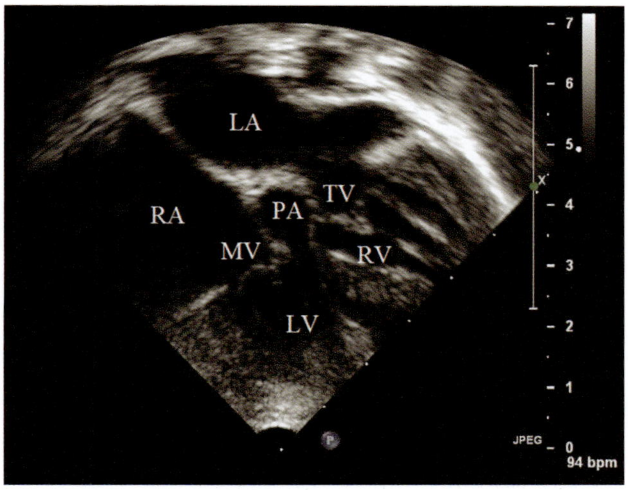

Figure 31.5 Subcostal coronal echocardiography view at the level of the atrioventricular valves. The pulmonary artery, lacking a subpulmonary conus, is wedged between the atrioventricular valves, in this case leading to subpulmonary stenosis. Mitral–pulmonic fibrous continuity is present. LA, left atrium; LV, left ventricle; MV, mitral valve; PA, pulmonary artery; RA, right atrium; RV, right ventricle; TV, tricuspid valve.

or dysplastic. This is characterized by the atrialization of the inlet of the morphologically right ventricle with frequent tricuspid regurgitation (Figure 31.6).

Clinical Presentation

Patients with CCTGA sometimes present late because they often are well oxygenated. Typically, a neonate comes to medical attention as a result of associated malformations. For example, those with a VSD may have a murmur and develop symptomatic congestive heart failure. Cyanosis and heart murmur may be the presenting symptoms if there is significant pulmonary stenosis. Typically, an electrocardiogram can show some key findings there is left access deviation, and Q-waves in the right precordial leads but not in the left precordial leads (Figure 31.7). Congenital complete atrioventricular block may be observed in utero or develop postnatally. A chest X-ray is not typically helpful in this situation; however, it may show the absence of a straight left heart border which might reflect a more anterior–posterior relationship between the great arteries (Figure 31.8).

Echocardiography remains the modality of choice in the diagnosis of CCTGA and its associated lesions, especially in the neonate. One of the more helpful views is the apical four-chamber view which shows the more trabeculated morphologic right ventricle on the left side and the smoother walled morphologic left ventricle on the right (Figure 31.2). The morphologic tricuspid valve should be carefully imaged to ensure there are no abnormalities such as an Ebsteinoid tricuspid valve or frank Ebstein malformation (Figure 31.6). Careful sweeps of the ventricular septum in the parasternal long and short-axis views can help to reveal VSDs. Both the left and right ventricular outflow tracts should be carefully examined to rule out any outflow tract abnormalities such as pulmonary valve or subvalvar stenosis. Care should also be taken to assess the aortic arch as coarctation of the aorta is known to occur (Figure 31.9). Cardiac magnetic resonance imaging (MRI) does not add much in the neonate, but certainly has a crucial role in these patients as they age, especially in quantitative assessment of the systemic right ventricular function.

Figure 31.6 Apical four-chamber echocardiography view in color compare mode. Ebstein malformation of the tricuspid valve is depicted – the morphologic tricuspid valve is displaced apically and is dysplastic with poor coaptation leading to severe valve regurgitation. Note the coarsely trabeculated morphologically right ventricle. LA, left atrium; RV, right ventricle; TV, tricuspid valve.

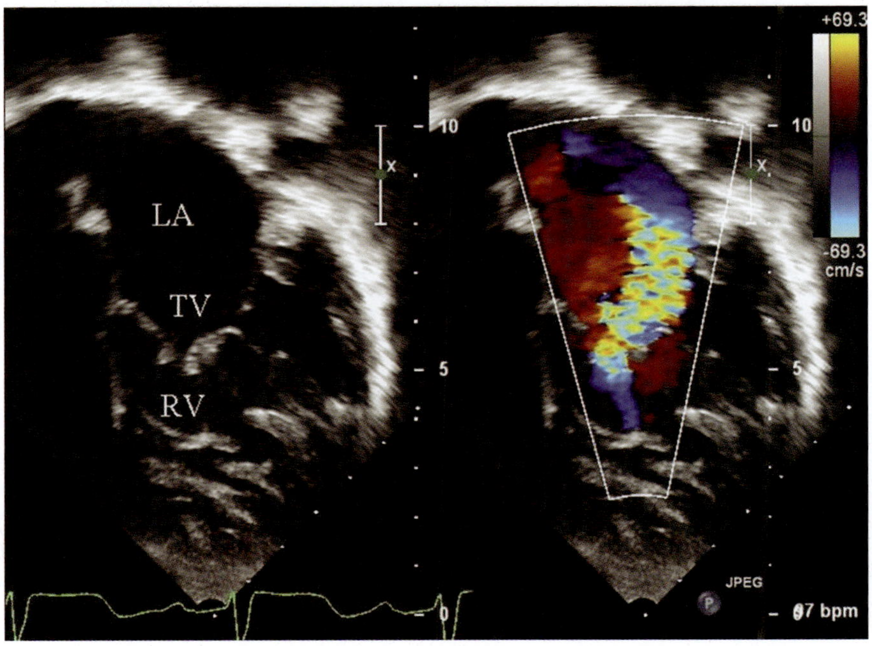

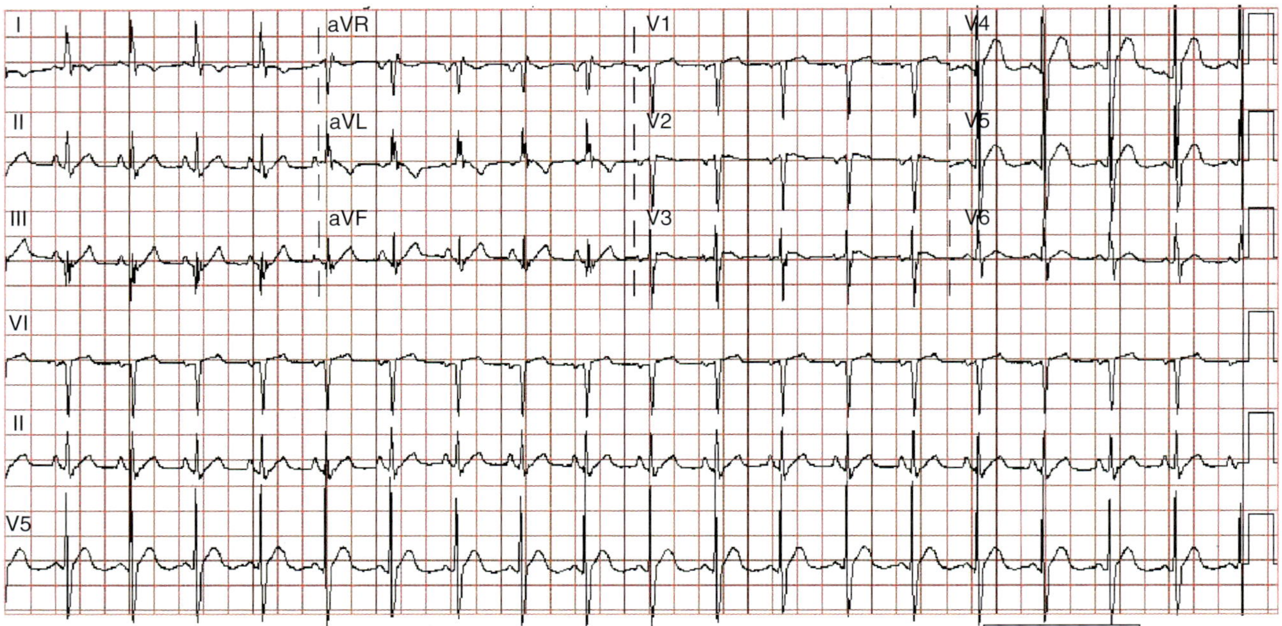

Figure 31.7 An electrocardiogram in a neonate with congenitally corrected transposition of the great arteries (CCTGA) showing left access deviation and Q-waves in the right precordial leads, but not in the left precordial leads.

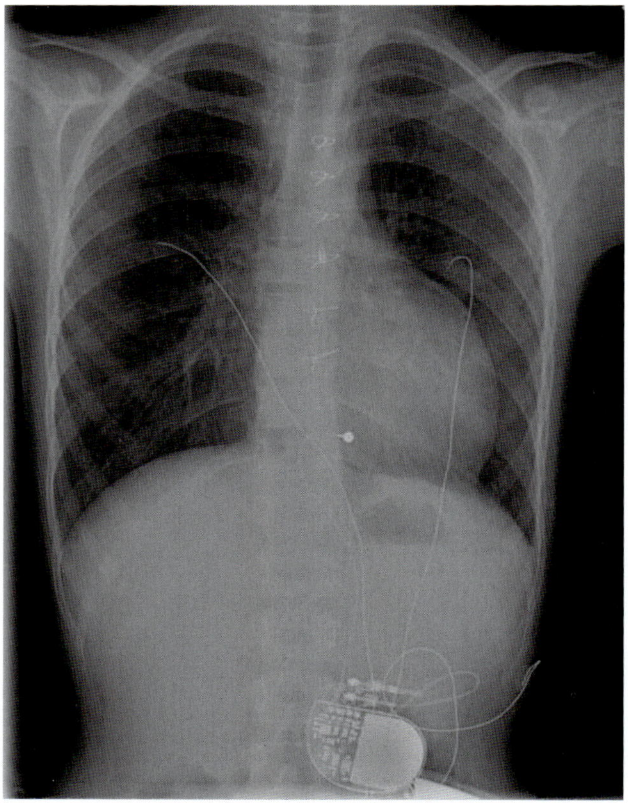

Figure 31.8 Single view anterior–posterior chest X-ray. Note the straight left heart border, sternal wires, and single lead epicardial pacemaker.

Outcomes and Interventions

Much of the impact on outcome in CCTGA is derived from the presence and severity of associated malformations. In uncomplicated CCTGA it is possible for the right ventricle to supply systemic circulation for decades, with rare cases when it has first been picked up in the fifth to seventh decade of life. However, most patients will develop progressive right ventricular dysfunction. A study of adults with CCTGA showed that systemic right ventricular dysfunction and congestive heart failure are common by the third decade of life [4]. Approximately 10% of infants born with congenital transposition have complete heart block, and the risk of developing it later increases to 30% by adulthood [5, 6].

Medical management in CCTGA typically involves managing the failing systemic right ventricle which can develop over time [7]. Occasionally, the patient also needs a pacemaker in the setting of advanced second or third degree AV block. When CCTGA is diagnosed clinically this does not necessarily mean immediate surgery. Clearly, if a neonate has a significant VSD, this will need to be addressed. An approach is to simply close the VSD and leave the right ventricle as the systemic ventricle. However, as more studies are showing concerns about the long-term reliability of the systemic right ventricle, a new approach is currently being

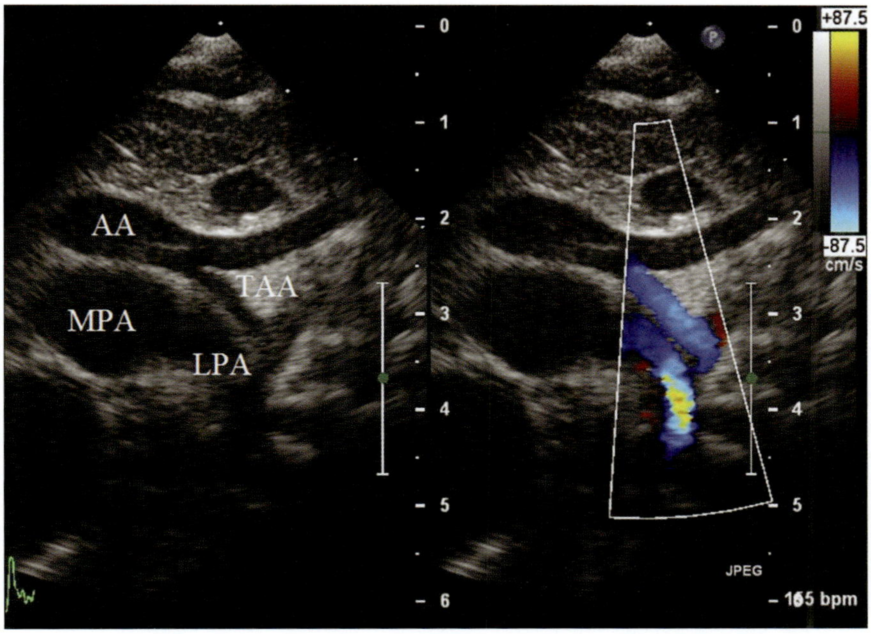

Figure 31.9 Suprasternal notch long-axis echocardiography view in color compare mode. The great vessels are parallel in proximal configuration with the aorta anterior. This patient has a hypoplastic aortic arch with coarctation. AA, ascending aorta; LPA, left pulmonary artery; MPA, main pulmonary artery; TAA, transverse aortic arch.

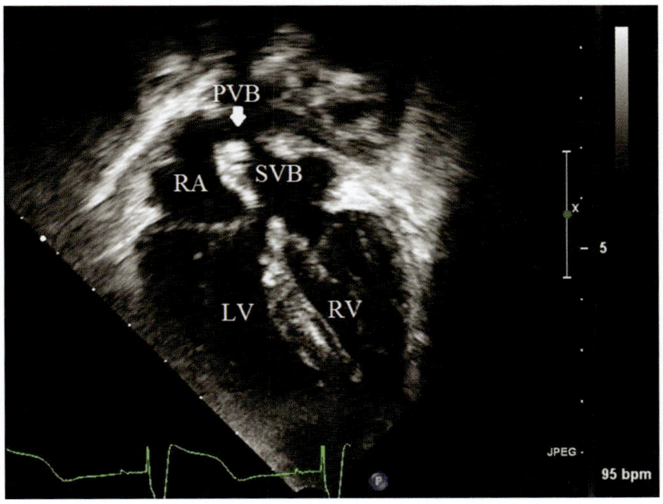

Figure 31.10 A 2D echocardiography apical four-chamber view. The atrial switch component of the double switch procedure is detailed: note the pulmonary venous baffle cascading over the systemic venous baffle toward the right atrium and right-sided morphologic left ventricle. Systemic venous blood is baffled right to left toward the morphologic right ventricle. LV, left ventricle; PVB, pulmonary venous baffle; RA, right atrium; RV, right ventricle; SVB, systemic venous baffle.

applied at many centers. This is described as "anatomic correction" or the "double switch" operation. This is essentially re-routing of the pulmonary venous return to the morphologic left ventricle and aorta and the systemic venous return to the morphologically right ventricle and pulmonary arteries; thus achieving a normal anatomic path of circulation. This involves a Senning-type baffling of systemic venous inflow to the left atrium or atrial switch (Figure 31.10) and an arterial switch operation to reroute the ventricular outflows (Figure 31.11). Thus, the neonate with CCTGA and a large VSD might undergo a pulmonary artery band at a month of age, followed by a double switch operation at around 10 months of age.

Recent research has shown that performing a double switch operation can produce good intermediate results with early mortality currently reported at approximately 5%, survival at 10 years of up to 95%, and survival at 20 years of 83% [8, 9]. Close follow-up by a pediatric cardiologist is needed through the childhood years, with compulsive transition to adult care by a specialist in adult congenital heart disease. The more typical long-term course for a systemic right ventricle is progressive decline in function and worsening tricuspid insufficiency, so the double switch operation does appear to offer some advantages. However, the jury is still out regarding this being the optimum strategy and further research is needed on long-term outcomes.

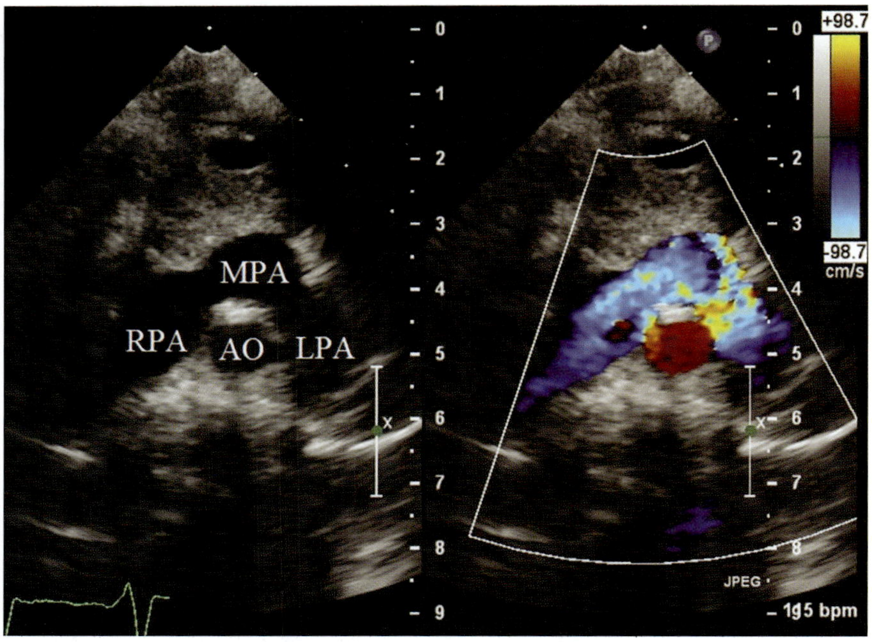

Figure 31.11 Suprasternal short-axis echocardiography view in color compare mode. Postoperative (double switch procedure) study showing the anatomy status post Lecompte maneuver. The main pulmonary artery has been brought forward and the branch pulmonary arteries now drape around the newly constructed ascending aorta. AO, aorta; LPA, left pulmonary artery; MPA, main pulmonary artery; RPA, right pulmonary artery.

References

1 Ferencz C, Rubin JD, McCarter RJ, *et al.* (1985) Congenital heart disease: prevalence at livebirth. The Baltimore-Washington Infant Study. *Am J Epidemiol*, **121** (1), 31–36. PubMed PMID: 3964990.

2 [No authors listed] (1980) Report of the New England Regional Infant Cardiac Program. *Pediatrics*, **65** (2 Pt 2), 375–461. PubMed PMID: 7355042.

3 Warnes CA. (2006) Transposition of the great arteries. *Circulation*, **114** (24), 2699–2709. PubMed PMID: 17159076.

4 Graham TP Jr, Bernard YD, Mellen BG, *et al.* (2000) Long-term outcome in congenitally corrected transposition of the great arteries: a multi-institutional study. *J Am Coll Cardiol*, **36** (1), 255–261. PubMed PMID: 10898443.

5 Friedberg DZ, Nadas AS. (1970) Clinical profile of patients with congenital corrected transposition of the great arteries: a study of 60 cases. *N Engl J Med*, **282** (19), 1053–1059. PubMed PMID: 5438426.

6 Huhta JC, Maloney JD, Ritter DG, Ilstrup DM, Feldt RH. (1983) Complete atrioventricular block in patients with atrioventricular discordance. *Circulation*, **67** (6), 1374–1377. PubMed PMID: 6851033.

7 Graham TP Jr, Markham L, Parra DA, Bichell D. (2007) Congenitally corrected transposition of the great arteries: an update. *Curr Treat Options Cardiovasc Med*, **9** (5), 407–413. PubMed PMID: 17897570.

8 Langley SM, Winlaw DS, Stumper O, *et al.* (2003) Midterm results after restoration of the morphologically left ventricle to the systemic circulation in patients with congenitally corrected transposition of the great arteries. *J Thorac Cardiovasc Surg*, **125** (6), 1229–1241. PubMed PMID: 12830039.

9 Hiramatsu T, Matsumura G, Konuma T, *et al.* (2012) Long-term prognosis of double-switch operation for congenitally corrected transposition of the great arteries. *Eur J Cardiothorac Surg*, **42** (6), 1004–1008. PubMed PMID: 22551964.

32

Common Arterial Trunk (Truncus Arteriosus)

Michael C. Mongé, Osama Eltayeb, Andrada Popescu, and Carl L. Backer

Division of Cardiovascular-Thoracic Surgery, Ann & Robert H. Lurie Children's Hospital of Chicago, and Department of Surgery, Northwestern University Feinberg School of Medicine, Chicago, IL, USA

Common arterial trunk (CAT, truncus arteriosus) is a rare congenital heart defect that occurs when a single arterial trunk overrides the interventricular septum and supplies the systemic, pulmonary, and coronary circulations. Nearly all patients have an associated non-restrictive ventricular septal defect (VSD). During embryologic development, the truncus arteriosus fails to separate and spiral into an anterior pulmonary artery and posterior aorta. As with other conotruncal malformations, CAT is associated with *22q11* microdeletion and DiGeorge syndrome.

Collett and Edwards' [1] original classification of CAT (1949) (Figure 32.1, upper row) was based on the origin of the pulmonary arteries. In type I, the main pulmonary artery arises from the left side of the trunk. Separate but closely positioned pulmonary arteries arise from the posterior trunk in type II. In type III, the pulmonary arteries are widely separated, arising laterally. In Van Praagh's 1976 classification (Figure 32.1, lower row) [2], type A1 is the same as Collett's type I. Collett's type II (pulmonary arteries arising separately from the posterior portion of the truncus) and type III (pulmonary arteries arising separately from the lateral walls of the truncus) are grouped as a single Van Praagh A2. Type A3 represents atresia of one of the pulmonary arteries with collateral flow to that lung. Type A4 is truncus associated with interrupted aortic arch.

More recently, Russell *et al.* [3] proposed simplifying the definition of CAT as either aortic or pulmonary artery dominant and we currently utilize that classification (Figure 32.2). This simple and practical approach reconciles the existing disparate categorizations of patients having common arterial trunks and it emphasizes the principal morphologic determinant of surgical outcome.

The truncal valve is usually trileaflet (60%), but may be quadricuspid (25%) or bicuspid (5%). The VSD is subarterial. In 25% of patients with CAT the aortic arch is right-sided, usually with mirror-image branching of the brachiocephalic arteries. A patent ductus arteriosus is usually absent and, when found, is often associated with interrupted aortic arch (commonly type B). Anomalous origin and distribution of the coronary arteries may be seen, often with the left coronary artery having a high origin, near the pulmonary artery take-off. A single coronary artery ostium may also be present.

The predominant pathophysiologic feature of CAT is a large left-to-right shunt, which increases as the pulmonary vascular resistance falls. Mixing of arterial and venous blood occurs at the level of the VSD. Pulmonary vascular obstructive disease can develop as early as 6 months because of pressure and volume overload of the pulmonary vasculature, in conjunction with both systolic and diastolic shunting. Truncal valve regurgitation is present in 25% of patients and is severe in 5% of patients, impacting the already volume-overloaded ventricles. Diastolic run-off via both the truncal regurgitation and low-resistance pulmonary circuit can cause poor systemic and coronary perfusion. Additionally, the elevated ventricular end-diastolic pressure will further compromise subendocardial perfusion. Truncal valve stenosis occurs rarely, although physiologic stenosis can be seen prior to repair because of increased flow across the truncal valve.

Patients often present within the first weeks of life with murmur, tachypnea, and dyspnea. Cyanosis is usually absent, but if present can indicate that pulmonary vascular resistance (PVR) is elevated. Diaphoresis and failure to thrive can be seen with progressive congestive heart failure. A pansystolic murmur can be auscultated at the left sternal border. If significant truncal regurgitation is present, a diastolic murmur may be present. The second heart sound is single. A bounding pulse may be appreciated, in addition to findings of congestive heart failure, such as hepatomegaly. A chest X-ray will show cardiomegaly and pulmonary plethora. If long-standing pulmonary

Visual Guide to Neonatal Cardiology, First Edition. Edited by Ernerio T. Alboliras, Ziyad M. Hijazi, Leo Lopez, and Donald J. Hagler.

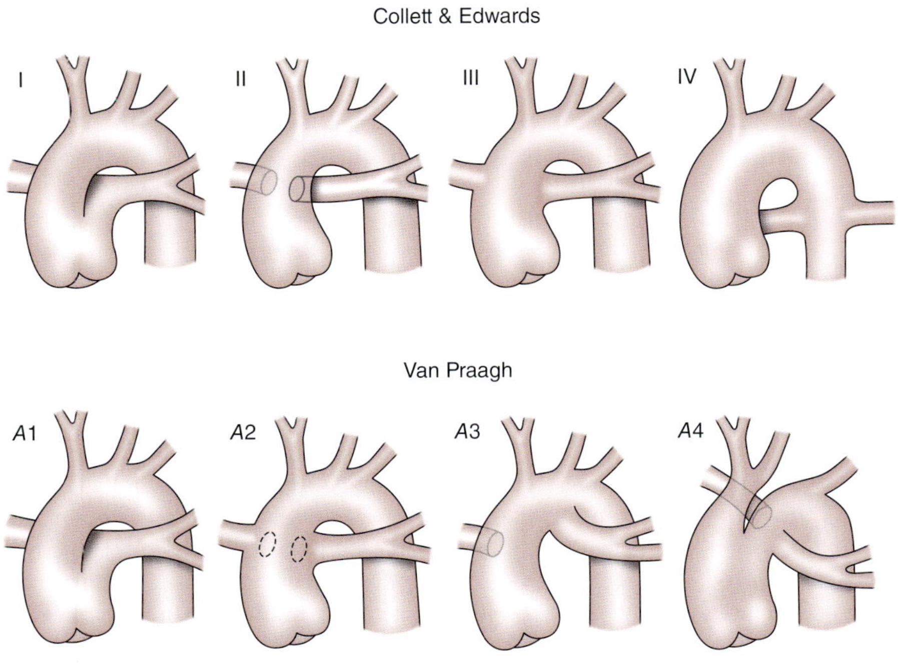

Figure 32.1 (Upper) Collett and Edwards 1949 classification of common arterial trunk (truncus arteriosus). (Lower) Van Praagh 1976 classification of common arterial trunk.

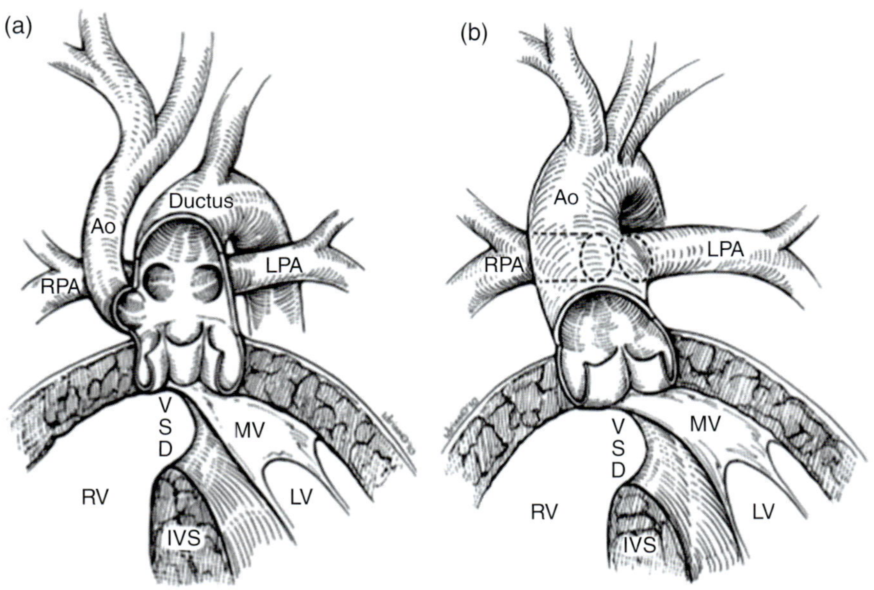

Figure 32.2 Russell's simplified classification of common arterial trunk. The diagram shows the essential features of pulmonary versus aortic dominance as observed in our autopsied specimens with common arterial trunk. (a) Interruption of the aortic arch. Only in this setting, and in hearts with severe aortic coarctation, did we find origin of the pulmonary arteries from either side of the intrapericardial pulmonary trunk. (b) The salient features of aortic dominance, with the pulmonary arteries arising separately but next to each other from the leftward and dorsal aspect of the common trunk. We also found pulmonary arteries arising more anteriorly, and then crossing as they extended toward the pulmonary hila. Ao, aorta; LPA/RPA, left/right pulmonary artery; PA, pulmonary artery; RV, right ventricle; VSD, ventricular septal defect.

vascular obstructive disease is present, there may be decreased pulmonary markings. The electrocardiogram will show biventricular hypertrophy. Right ventricular forces can predominate if pulmonary vascular obstructive disease develops.

An echocardiogram will provide information on the type of CAT and the characteristics of the truncal valve. Overriding of the VSD by the large truncal valve can be seen in the parasternal long-axis view. The origin of the coronary arteries and their proximity to the pulmonary trunk may be ascertained. In addition, the presence of a thymus should be noted. Advance medical imaging (CTA) techniques can provide more accurate anatomic details of the pulmonary artery origins and coronary artery locations, which can aid in operative planning. Cardiac catheterization may be warranted in the case of late presentation in order to measure the PVR.

Repair of CAT was first reported by McGoon at the Mayo Clinic in 1968 [4]. This is commonly referred to as a "Rastelli" repair (VSD closure with right ventricle to pulmonary artery conduit). Based on the work of Ebert *et al.* [5], early surgical intervention is now recommended.

We repair all patients with CAT in the neonatal period prior to hospital discharge. The repair is performed via a median sternotomy approach with the use of hypothermic cardiopulmonary bypass [6]. Bicaval venous cannulation is achieved with placement of a vent in the right superior pulmonary vein. Upon commencing cardiopulmonary bypass, the right and left pulmonary arteries are snared to prevent diastolic run-off into the lungs. After appropriate cooling, cold blood cardioplegia is administered. The origin of the pulmonary arteries from the CAT is ascertained. The pulmonary arteries are detached from the CAT (Figure 32.3). The resultant opening in the ascending aorta is closed with a pericardial patch tanned with glutaraldehyde. Occasionally, this maneuver is facilitated by completely transecting the ascending aorta. While the aorta is open, the truncal valve is inspected. Through the truncal valve, a small right angle can be placed to identify a site on the anterior surface of the right ventricle for the ventriculotomy. The ventriculotomy is then performed. After a second dose of cardioplegia has been administered (once the aorta has been repaired), the VSD is baffled from the left ventricle to the common truncal valve. In neonates, we have used a glutaraldehyde tanned pericardial patch for this portion of the procedure. The operation is completed by a homograft conduit from the right ventriculotomy to the transected pulmonary arteries (Figure 32.4). We have often used a pulmonary homograft from an appropriately sized donor. If this is not available, the Contegra graft (bovine jugular vein graft) has been used. Sometimes, the chest must be left open with a silastic skin patch for several days. Figure 32.5 demonstrates the repair technique for truncus arteriosus with interrupted aortic arch.

Postoperative management emphasizes control of PVR. We keep these patients ventilated and paralyzed for 24–48 hours and expectantly treat all of them with nitric oxide therapy. A small atrial fenestration is useful as a potential site for right-to-left shunting should the patient have elevated PVR in the postoperative period. Reoperation is required for conduit replacement and in some instances to repair truncal valve insufficiency. The overall mortality rate is 9% for isolated CAT repair, 24% for CAT repair with interrupted aortic arch, 30% for CAT repair with truncal valve surgery, and 60% for interrupted aortic arch with valve surgery. The greatest impact on postoperative mortality has been the association of interrupted aortic arch and severe truncal valve insufficiency.

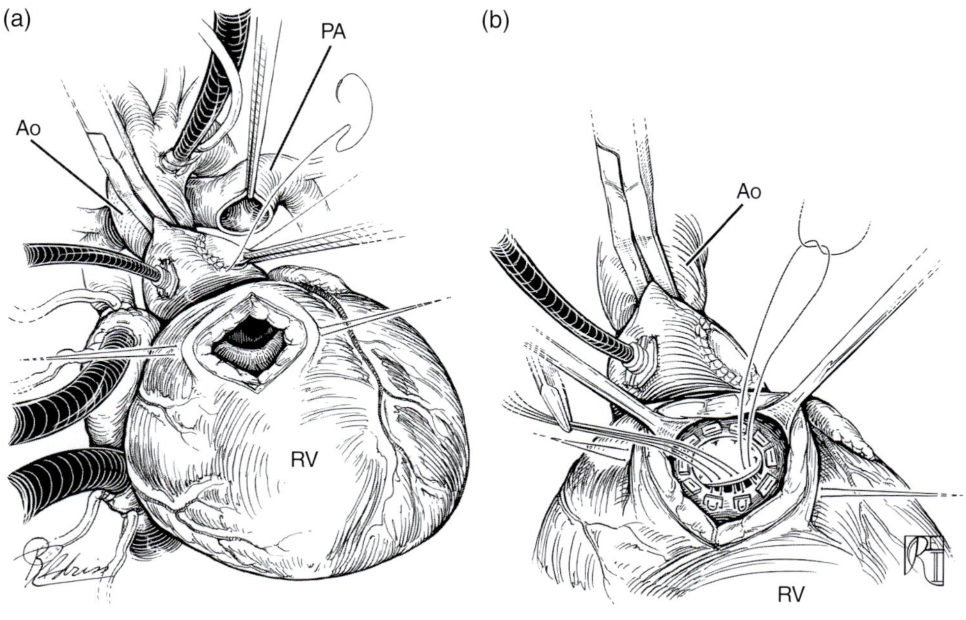

Figure 32.3 (a) Pulmonary artery has been disconnected from the arterial trunk, and the aorta has been reconstructed with a polytetrafluoroethylene (PTFE) patch to avoid coronary flow complications. (b) Transventricular closure of the ventricular septal defect is shown with interrupted pledgeted sutures and a Dacron patch. Ao, aorta; PA, pulmonary artery; RV, right ventricle.

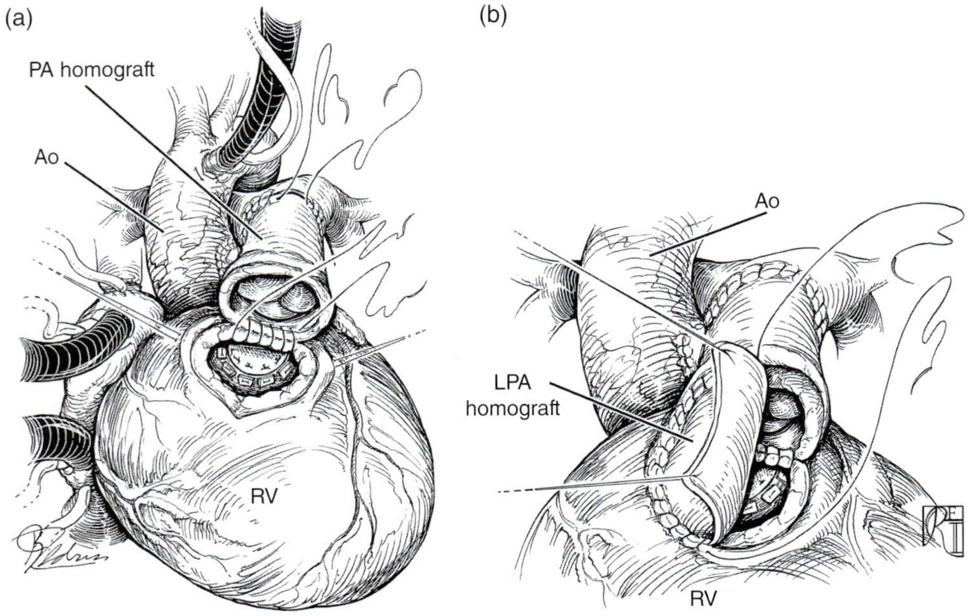

Figure 32.4 (a) Distal pulmonary homograft is sutured to the pulmonary artery (PA), and the posterior one-third portion of the homograft annulus is sutured directly to the superior rim of the right ventriculotomy. (b) Homograft hood technique. The previously harvested left pulmonary artery homograft segment is sutured. Ao, aorta; LPA, left pulmonary artery; RV, right ventricle.

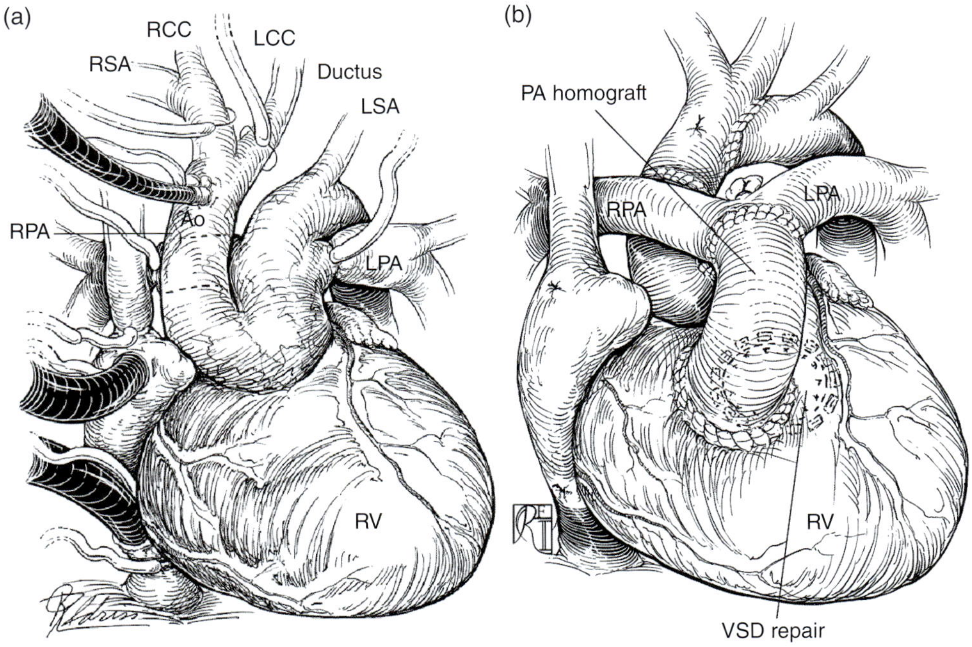

Figure 32.5 (a) Aorto-bicaval cardiopulmonary bypass is established with bilateral pulmonary artery constriction (enforced snuggers). Lower extremity flow is accomplished through the patent ductus arteriosus. (b) Completed repair of truncus arteriosus with interrupted aortic arch. Direct aortic reconstruction is performed without foreign material. The maneuver of Lecompte facilitates right ventricular-to-pulmonary artery continuity. Ao, aorta; LCC/RCC, left/right common carotid artery; LPA/RPA, left/right pulmonary artery; LSA/RSA, left/right subclavian artery; PA, pulmonary artery; RV, right ventricle; VSD, ventricular septal defect.

References

1 Collett RW, Edwards JE. (1949) Persistent truncus arteriosus: a classification according to anatomic types. *Surg Clin North Am*, **29**, 1245–1270.

2 Van Praagh R. (1976) Classification of truncus arteriosus communis (TAC). *Am Heart J*, **92**, 129–132.

3 Russell HM, Jacobs ML, Anderson RH, *et al.* (2011) A simplified categorization for common arterial trunk. *J Thorac Cardiovasc Surg*, **141**, 645–653.

4 McGoon DC, Rasteli GC, Ongley PA. (1968) An operation for the correction of truncus arteriosus. *JAMA*, **205**, 69–73.

5 Ebert PA, Turley K, Stanger P. (1984) Surgical treatment of truncus arteriosus in the first 6 months of life. *Ann Surg*, **200**, 45–456.

6 Russell HM, Pasquali SK, Jacobs JP, *et al.* (2012) Outcomes of repair of common arterial trunk with truncal valve surgery: a review of the society of thoracic surgeons congenital heart surgery database. *Ann Thorac Surg*, **93**, 164–169.

33

Mitral Valve Apparatus Abnormalities

Shubhika Srivastava

Division of Pediatric Cardiology, Mount Sinai Medical Center, New York, NY, USA

Mitral valve (MV) abnormalities rarely occur is isolation and have a reported echocardiographic incidence of 0.5% and 0.42% of all congenital cardiac defects in autopsy series [1]. The MV received its name from Andreas Vesalius who likened its bifoliate appearance to an episcopal mitre [2].

Normal Mitral Valve Complex

The **annulus** separates the left atrium (LA) from the left ventricle (LV). It is divided into an anterior portion, which is in fibrous contiguity with the aortic annulus, and a larger posterior portion that occupies two-thirds of the annular perimeter and is prone to dimensional change in response to stress. It is saddle-shaped, with the peaks located anteriorly and posteriorly and the valley at the lateral commissures [3].

The MV is an asymmetric bi-leaflet structure that is comprised of an aortic or anterior leaflet (AL), which is contiguous with the left and non-coronary cusp of the aorta, and the scalloped posterior or mural leaflet (PL).

The **anterior leaflet** extends along the anterior one-third of the circumference and contributes to two-thirds of the total leaflet cross-sectional area and forms the floor of the left ventricular outflow tract (LVOT). It does not have scallops or clefts. The coapting surface is divided into three corresponding segments designated as A1, 2, and 3.

The **posterior leaflet** extends across two-thirds of the perimeter, is shallow, and has two natural clefts that divide it into three scallops. The scallops are numbered from lateral to medial as P1, 2, and 3.

The **commissure** is the plane or semicircular line defined by the coapting surface of the MV leaflets. It is divided into an anterolateral or superior (smaller) and posteromedial or inferior commissure.

The **chordae** connect the leaflets to the papillary muscle and, unlike the tricuspid valve, have no attachment to the ventricular septum (except when associated with a cleft in anterior leaflet or with straddling). The first order chords connect the free margin of the leaflets to the papillary muscle beneath them and are essential to coaptation; second order Strut chords insert to the rough zone on the ventricular aspect and are essential for leaflet geometry; and third order basal chords of the PL attach to the LV posterior wall and are essential to ventricular geometry and are annular.

Two **papillary muscle** groups are situated under their corresponding commissures and receive chordal attachments from both leaflets. The posteromedial papillary muscle group has two or more heads or fascicles and is supplied by the right coronary artery. The anterolateral papillary muscle group is usually a single fascicle and is more proximal or superior in location and receives a dual blood supply from the left anterior descending and circumflex coronary arteries.

Embryology

MV formation begins in the fourth week of gestation. The PL develops from the lateral endocardial cushions and the AL from the apposition of the left part of the superior and inferior cushions. Chordae also originate from the endocardial cushions. The papillary muscles are derived from the ventricular myocardium.

Abnormalities of Mitral Valve Apparatus

Abnormality of Leaflet

Mitral Valve Prolapse

Mitral valve prolapse (MVP) is defined by the leaflets extending into the LA beyond the annular plane during ventricular systole. It is rare in infancy and patients present with insufficiency in neonatal Marfan syndrome. MVP can be seen secondary to papillary muscle infarction and LV dysfunction with anomalous origin of left coronary from the pulmonary artery and can be seen

Visual Guide to Neonatal Cardiology, First Edition. Edited by Ernerio T. Alboliras, Ziyad M. Hijazi, Leo Lopez, and Donald J. Hagler.

in children with right ventricular (RV) volume overload (e.g., atrial septal defects) secondary to distortion of the geometry of the MV annulus.

Echocardiography: secondary to the saddle shape of the annulus, erroneous diagnosis of prolapse may be made in the apical four-chamber view. Diagnosis of prolapse requires the position of the MV leaflets above the annular plane in parasternal long axis (PLAX) in ventricular systole.

Cleft Mitral Valve

Cleft MV leaflet is often seen in association with atrioventricular canal defect or with other complex congenital heart disease (CHD) such as transposition of the great arteries. Isolated cleft of the anterior MV leaflet is rare. The attachment of the cleft can result in LVOT obstruction. When associated with canal defects, the cleft is oriented towards the inlet ventricular septum (Figure 33.1). The cleft is directed towards the aortic root when seen in isolation or in association with other non-canal defects (Figure 33.2). Orientation of the cleft more anteriorly towards the right coronary cusp is associated with LVOT obstruction.

Rarely, a cleft may be noted in the PL and it may involve any segment of the leaflet but is reported to often occur within the middle scallop or P2 [4, 5].

Echocardiography: parasternal or subxiphoid short-axis (PSAX) imaging will define the presence and orientation of the cleft and regurgitation through it.

Double Orifice Mitral Valve

This is rarely seen in isolation but often noted with canal defects and other left-sided obstructive lesions. It is defined as a single annulus divided into two annuli with two orifices opening into the LV (Figure 33.3). The two orifices are usually equal (Figure 33.4), with normal function in 15%. A smaller posteromedial orifice was noted in 44% of cases in one series [4] and a predominance of a smaller anterolateral orifice in a different echocardiographic series of MV abnormalities [1]. In more than one-third it is of no functional consequence, regurgitation is noted in 43%, stenosis in 13%, and both in 6.5% [6].

Supramitral Ring

This lesion was initially described as part of the Shone complex (coarctation of aorta, subaortic stenosis, parachute MV) and is usually seen in association with other CHDs such as ventricular septal defect (VSD) and left-sided obstructive lesion. It is rarely seen in isolation. It is a fibrous membrane that originates within the MV and below the left atrial appendage. There are two types. The first type arises from the mitral annular ring. This

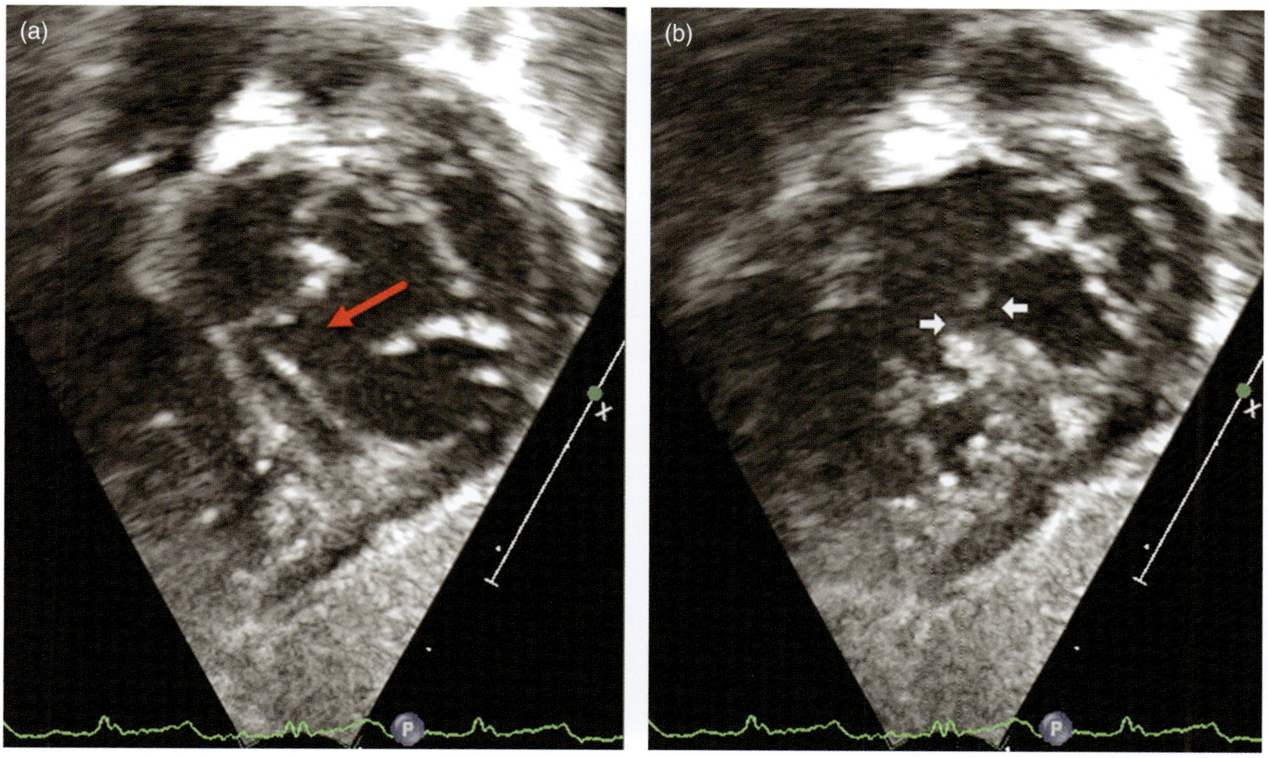

Figure 33.1 (a) Typical cleft in anterior mitral valve (MV) leaflet during diastole (red arrow). (b) Typical cleft in anterior MV leaflet during systole (white arrows).

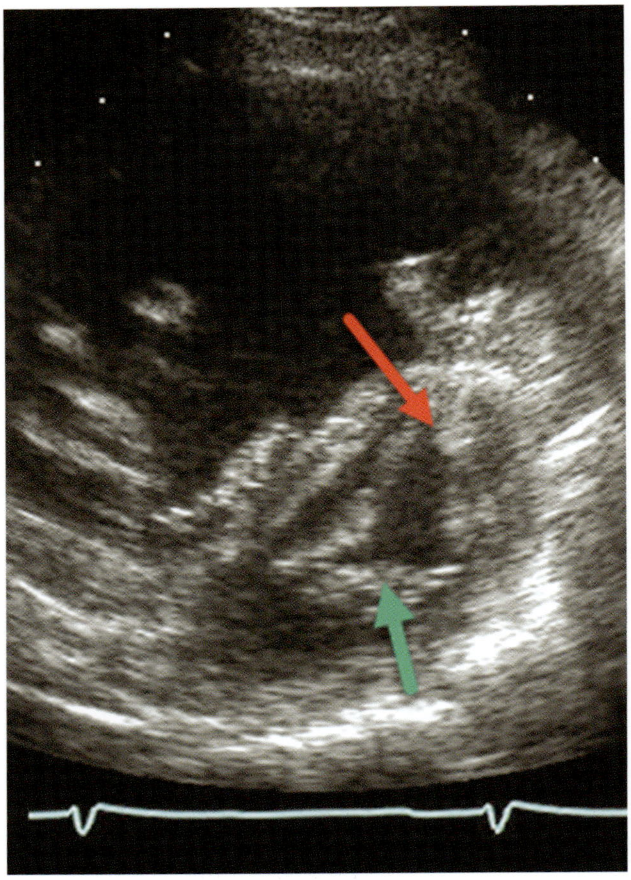

Figure 33.2 Atypical cleft of anterior MV leaflet (red arrow). The direction of the cleft is towards the plane of the left ventricular (LV) outflow tract. The posterior leaflet is shown by the green arrow.

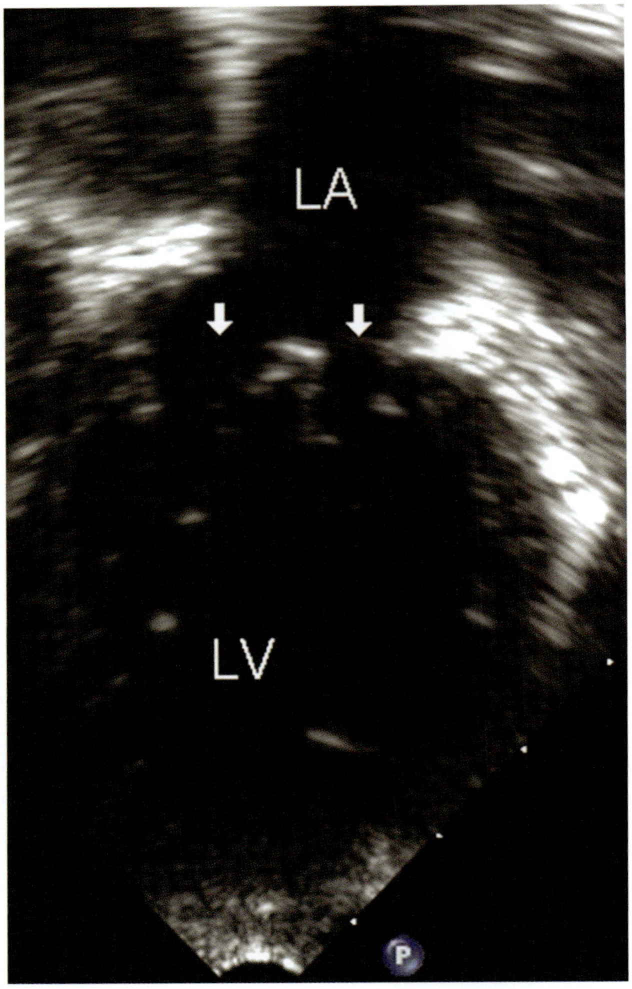

Figure 33.3 Apical four-chamber view showing a double orifice MV with the two orifices marked by white arrows. LA, left atrium; LV, left ventricle.

should be distinguished from cor triatriatum in which the membrane arises above the annular plane, dividing the LA into two chambers, with the left atrial appendage (LAA) below the dividing membrane (Figure 33.5). The second type of supramitral ring is more intramitral and is a thin membrane located within the funnel inflow of the MV leaflets and is always associated with an abnormal MV apparatus, parachute MV (Figure 33.6) [7]. The ring can be complete, circumferential, or partial, and usually results in progressive stenosis.

Ebstein Malformation of Mitral Valve

The first case of Ebstein malformation of a morphologic MV was described in 1976 by Ruschhaupt [4]. This affects the PL exclusively and the atrialized portion of the LA is not thinned out and patients present with mitral regurgitation (MR).

Accessory Mitral Valve

Accessory tissue is seen in association of the anterior MV leaflet and often results in LVOT and MR.

Mitral Valve Duplication

This is a very rare anomaly that differs from double orifice mitral valve by the presence of two separate adjoining MV apparatus inclusive of annuli, leaflets, and the supporting tensor apparatus. Patients present with MR more often than mitral stenosis.

Anomalies of the Chordae and Papillary Muscles (Tensor Apparatus)

Chordal Anomalies

Arcade or Hammock Mitral Valve

MV arcade is defined by either very short chordae or direct insertion of the leaflets into the papillary muscles (Figure 33.7). It appears like a hammock from the LA aspect when viewed by the surgeon. The abnormal chordae result in limited valve leaflet excursion and development of both stenosis and regurgitation [8, 9].

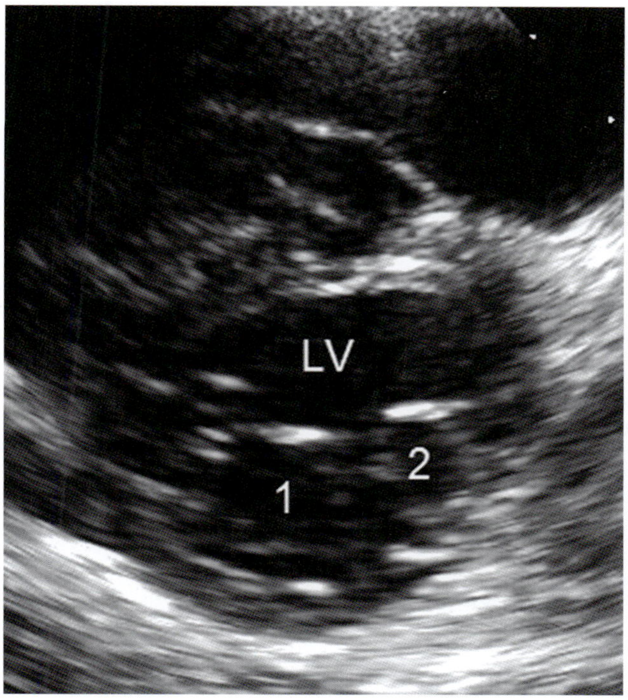

Figure 33.4 Parasternal short-axis view showing the two orifices (labeled 1 and 2) of the double orifice mitral valve. LV, left ventricle.

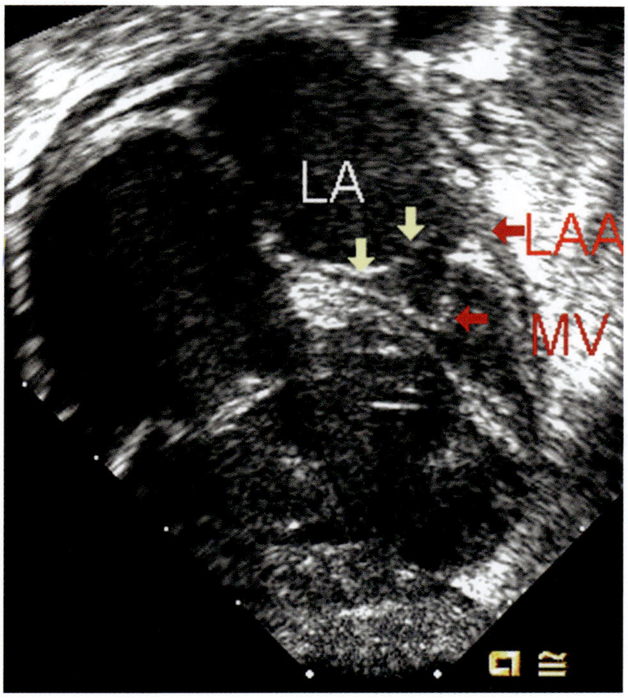

Figure 33.5 A membranous cor triatriatum is seen (yellow arrows) above the mitral annulus, dividing the left atrium. The left atrial appendage (LAA) is below the dividing membrane.

Straddling Mitral Valve

Straddling MV is defined by attachments of the supporting chordae to both the ventricles. This is seen is association with malalignment or outlet VSD defects and conotruncal abnormalities like double outlet RV or transposition. It is often associated with LV hypoplasia (Figure 33.8). It should be distinguished from overriding MV in which the MV inflow is shared by both ventricles with normal MV chordal attachments only to the LV.

Anomalies of the Papillary Muscles (Most Common of All Described Abnormalities)

Parachute Mitral Valve

This is characterized by chordal attachments from both MV leaflets to one papillary muscle group or to a single fused papillary muscle (Figure 33.9). The posteromedial papillary muscle group is usually the dominant one when both papillary muscle groups are present. It is often seen in association with other left-sided obstructive lesions and supramitral rings. When it occurs in isolation, the mitral stenosis is progressive in the majority of patients. Complete common AV canal defects may be associated with one papillary muscle by the lateral LV wall or two lateral papillary muscles with narrow interpapillary distance.

Congenital Mitral Stenosis

An incidence of 0.18% has been reported on echocardiography [1]. Congenital mitral stenosis is a combination of thickened MV leaflets with limited excursion and diastolic doming, with short chordae associated with closely spaced papillary muscles (mitral arcade) and LV endocardial fibroelastosis. In its extreme form it is seen in association with severely hypoplastic annulus in hypoplastic left heart syndrome [10, 11].

Echocardiographic Assessment of Mitral Stenosis The z score of the mitral annular diameter can determine valvar adequacy and postoperative prognosis. The degree of mitral stenosis by color and Doppler echocardiography may be masked by the presence of an atrial communication and overestimated in the setting of VSD. Transmitral flow and hence gradients are influenced by LA and LV function, compliance, stroke volume, and heart rate.

Quantification of mitral stenosis by mean gradients has been shown to correlate only modestly with the transmitral gradient obtained by cardiac catheterization in children. Assessment of the valve area using pressure half time has a very poor correlation with MV area using the Gorlin formula [1]. Assessment of severity and timing of intervention needs to be guided by clinical symptoms and presence of pulmonary hypertension.

Echocardiographic Assessment of Mitral Regurgitation There are no current pediatric guidelines for quantification of MR. The complex mechanism of MR and

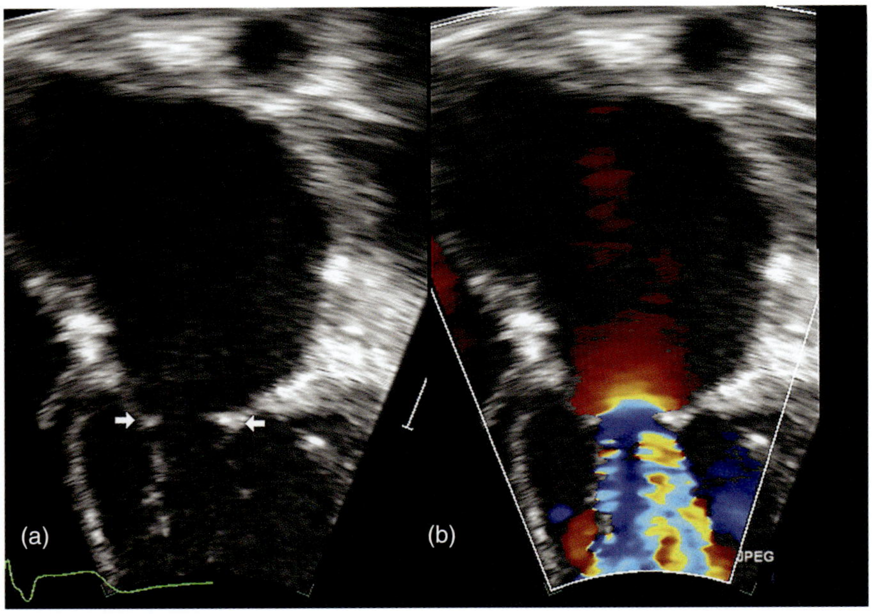

Figure 33.6 (a) Supramitral ring (white arrows) along the atrial surface of the mitral leaflet. LAA, left atrial appendage; MV, mitral valve. (b) Color Doppler demonstrating aliased flow velocity during diastole consistent with stenosis.

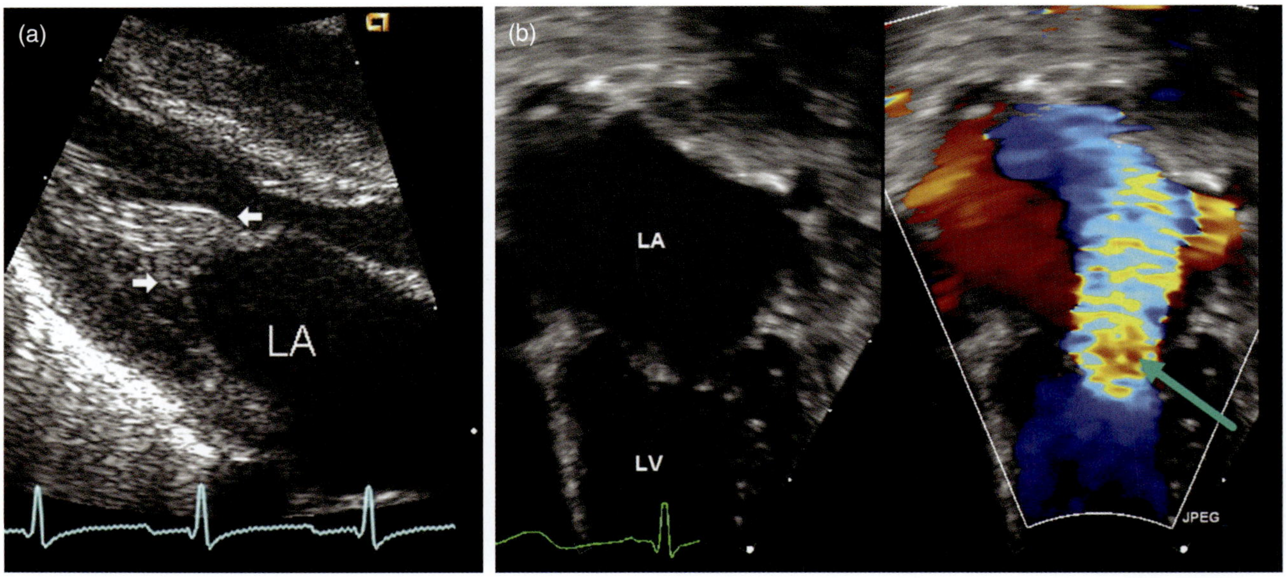

Figure 33.7 (a) Parasternal long-axis echocardiographic view in MV arcade showing direct insertion of valve leaflets into the papillary muscles through short or absent chordae (arrows). LA, left atrium. (b) Apical echocardiographic view in MV arcade showing a 2D image in the left and color flow Doppler demonstrating severe mitral regurgitation in the right.

multiple regurgitant jets challenge the application of current American Society of Echocardiography guidelines [12]. LA and LV systolic function and compliance also impact the degree of MR.

Detailed echocardiographic assessment of the mechanism of MR, LA, and LV size in correlation with assessment of pulmonary hypertension, LV wall stress, and clinical symptoms can be used to guide timing of intervention.

Conclusions

In summary, the MV apparatus is a complex dynamic unit. Abnormality in embryologic development of the annulus can range from annular hypoplasia to supramitral ring. Anatomic leaflet abnormalities can result in prolapse, flail, cleft MV, MV arcade, or parachute MV. Straddling MV results from tensor apparatus abnormalities. Most MV apparatus structural abnormalities are

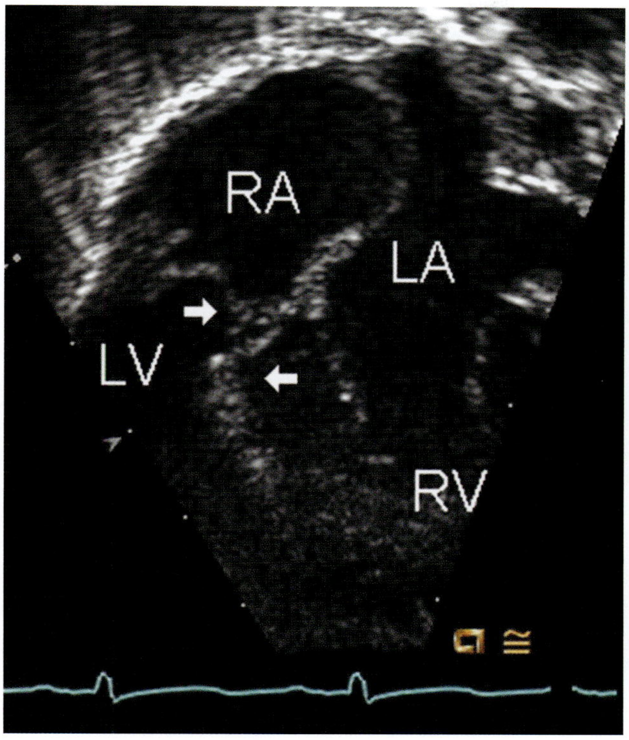

Figure 33.8 Apical four-chamber view in congenitally corrected transposition of great arteries with ventricular septal defect demonstrating an overriding and straddling right-sided mitral valve (white arrows). Note chordal attachments to the left-sided right ventricle.

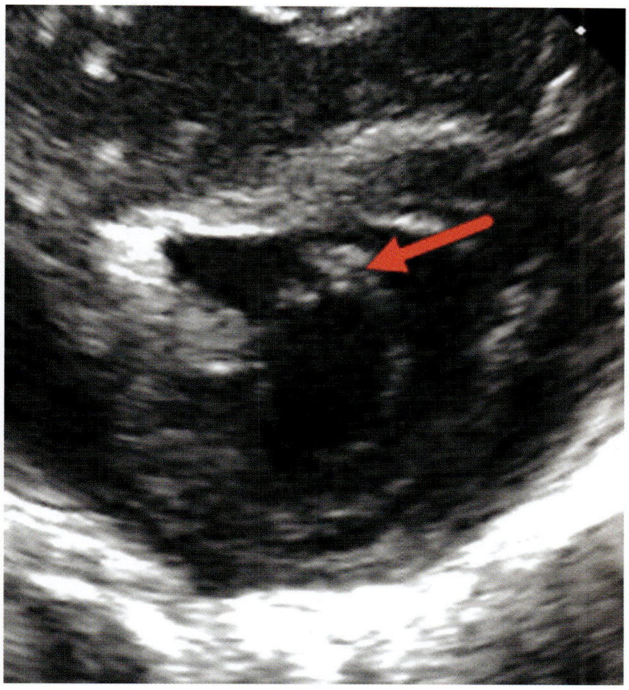

Figure 33.9 Parasternal short-axis echocardiographic view showing a parachute MV with crowding and chordal attachments to one anterior papillary muscle group (red arrow).

noted in conjunction with other CHD and patients often present with regurgitation (72%) rather than stenosis (13%) or both (15%), and this has a significant impact on morbidity and mortality [4]. MV repair rather than replacement remains the surgical option of choice with age at presentation, presence of pulmonary hypertension, and type of MV apparatus abnormality having a significant impact on outcomes [10, 13].

References

1 Banerjee A, Kohl T, Silverman NH. (1995) Echocardiographic evaluation of congenital mitral valve anomalies in children. *Am J Cardiol*, **76** (17), 1284–1291.

2 Asante-Korang A, O'Leary PW, Anderson RH. (2006) Anatomy and echocardiography of the normal and abnormal mitral valve. *Cardiol Young*, **16** (Suppl 3), 27–34.

3 Silbiger JJ. (2012) Anatomy, mechanics, and pathophysiology of the mitral annulus. *Am Heart J*, **164** (2), 163–176.

4 Seguela PE, Houyel L, Acar P. (2011) Congenital malformations of the mitral valve. *Arch Cardiovasc Dis*, **104** (8–9), 465–479.

5 Seguela PE, Brosset P, Acar P. (2011) Isolated cleft of the posterior mitral valve leaflet assessed by real-time 3D echocardiography. *Arch Cardiovasc Dis*, **10** (5), 365–366.

6 Zalzstein E, Hamilton R, Zucker N, Levitas A, Gross GJ. (2004) Presentation, natural history, and outcome in children and adolescents with double orifice mitral valve. *Am J Cardiol*, **93** (8), 1067–1069.

7 Anderson RH. (2009) When is the supravalvar mitral ring truly supravalvar? *Cardiol Young*, **19** (1), 10–11.

8 Remenyi B, Gentles TL. (2012) Congenital mitral valve lesions: correlation between morphology and imaging. *Ann Pediatr Cardiol*, **5** (1), 3–12.

9 Parr GV, Fripp RR, Whitman V, Bharati S, Lev M. (1983) Anomalous mitral arcade: echocardiographic and angiographic recognition. *Pediatr Cardiol*, **4** (2), 163–165.

10 del Nido PJ, Baird C. (2012) Congenital mitral valve stenosis: anatomic variants and surgical reconstruction. *Semin Thorac Cardiovasc Surg Pediatr Card Surg Annu*, **15** (1), 69–74.

11 Ruckman RN, Van Praagh R. (1978) Anatomic types of congenital mitral stenosis: report of 49 autopsy cases with consideration of diagnosis and surgical implications. *Am J Cardiol*, **42** (4), 592–601.

12 Zoghbi WA, Enriquez-Sarano M, Foster E, et al. (2003) Recommendations for evaluation of the severity of native valvular regurgitation with two-dimensional and Doppler echocardiography. *J Am Soc Echocardiogr*, **16** (7), 777–802.

13 Selamet Tierney ES, Pigula FA, Berul CI, et al. (2008) Mitral valve replacement in infants and children 5 years of age or younger: evolution in practice and outcome over three decades with a focus on supra-annular prosthesis implantation. *J Thorac Cardiovasc Surg*, **136** (4), 954–961, 961.e1–3.

34

Hypoplastic Left Heart Syndrome

Aaron Bell and Hannah Bellsham-Revell

Department of Paediatric Cardiology, Evelina Children's Hospital, London, UK

Hypoplastic left heart syndrome (HLHS) describes a spectrum of underdevelopment wherein the left heart is incapable of supporting the systemic circulation [1]. Without corrective surgery this is universally fatal with most neonates dying within 30 days. The incidence is 0.16–0.27 per 1000 live births [2, 3]. The etiology is poorly understood but thought to be multifactorial. Genetic associations have been described, including trisomies 13 and 18 [4, 5], Turner syndrome (45 X0), and Jacobsen syndrome (terminal 11q deletion). It is also associated with a family history of bicuspid aortic valve [6].

Anatomy

In classic HLHS, there is either stenosis or atresia of the mitral and aortic valves with left ventricular (LV) hypoplasia (Figure 34.1a). The most extreme type involves mitral and aortic atresia, often with no discernible LV on echocardiography (the rudimentary ventricle can sometimes be found during dissection) and complete absence of forward flow through the left heart. The ascending aorta is usually rudimentary but gives rise to the coronary arteries. Severe aortic hypoplasia or atresia may also be seen in unbalanced atrioventricular septal defect (Figure 34.1b) and double outlet right ventricle (RV) with mitral stenosis/atresia and ventricular septal defect (VSD; Figure 34.1c).

Mitral stenosis with aortic atresia involves some LV filling during fetal development, resulting in a hypoplastic but hypertrophied and often globular LV. Mitral and aortic valve stenosis is associated with less marked LV hypoplasia, but the LV will still be insufficient to support the systemic circulation. This is often described as the "borderline left heart" and is associated with fibrous changes of the LV endocardium (endocardial fibroelastosis). Figure 34.2 demonstrates these three subtypes.

In virtually all cases, the ascending aorta and transverse aortic arch are abnormal. When there has been little or no forward flow, the ascending aorta is diminutive, measuring 1–2 mm in diameter. When there is antegrade aortic flow, the ascending aorta may be larger but still hypoplastic. The transverse arch is usually hypoplastic, and there may be discrete coarctation.

Other forms of congenital heart disease also effectively result in HLHS. For example, an atrioventricular septal defect can be unbalanced with a small left-sided inlet valve and LV (with or without aortic obstruction), occasionally precluding intracardiac biventricular repair and requiring HLHS treatment. Mitral atresia or stenosis can also exist with a double outlet RV and VSD. Here there is little or no forward flow into the LV, which is almost always hypoplastic, but there is often forward flow into the aorta arising from the RV through the VSD. Ultimately, these children will require HLHS treatment because of the insufficient mitral valve and LV.

Other structural abnormalities can be seen. Approximately 10% of patients with HLHS have bilateral superior caval veins [7]. This may not be important with neonatal management but becomes relevant when considering further palliative interventions. Most patients have normal pulmonary venous drainage, but abnormalities can become relevant when considering surgical treatment. As there is absent or limited flow through the mitral valve to the LV, it is essential that the pulmonary venous flow reach the RV, making an unrestrictive atrial communication necessary. Occasionally, small coronary artery fistulae to the LV can be seen, usually in the setting of mitral stenosis and aortic atresia. In addition to ascending aorta and transverse arch hypoplasia, other arch abnormalities can be seen, such as an anomalous right subclavian artery.

Visual Guide to Neonatal Cardiology, First Edition. Edited by Ernerio T. Alboliras, Ziyad M. Hijazi, Leo Lopez, and Donald J. Hagler.

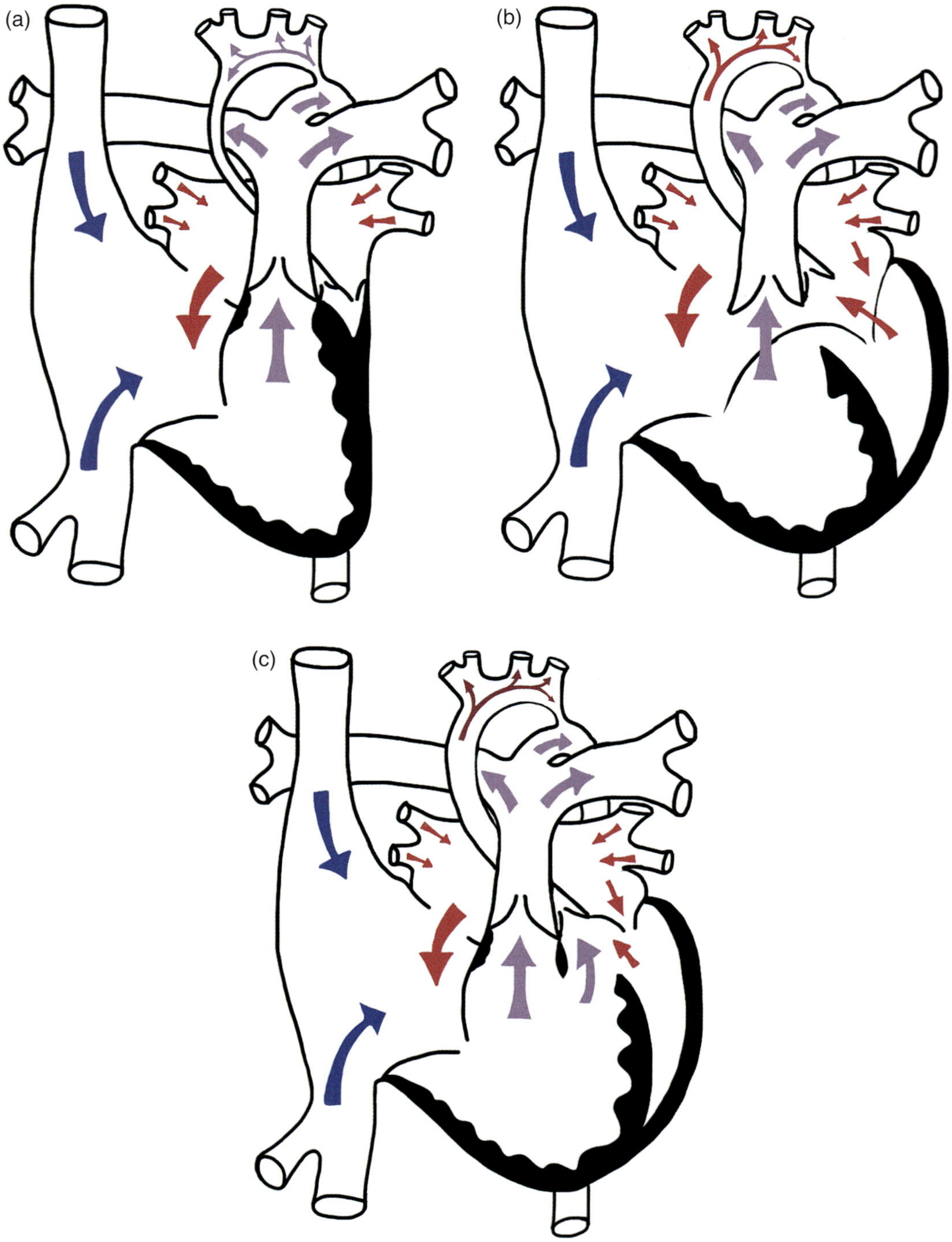

Figure 34.1 (a) Unoperated classic hypoplastic left heart syndrome (HLHS); (b) unbalanced atrioventricular septal defect; (c) mitral atresia/stenosis with a ventricular septal defect and a double outlet right ventricle.

Physiology

Following delivery, in order to maintain the cardiac output, there must be adequate flow across the arterial duct and atrial septum. Ductal patency is maintained with prostglandin E2 infusion, which can be instituted immediately after birth if a fetal diagnosis has been made. If the arterial duct constricts prior to diagnosis, systemic flow will be reduced, resulting in impaired organ perfusion, acidosis, shock, and even death if untreated. Rarely, the atrial communication is inadequate. This too will result in low cardiac output, desaturation, and

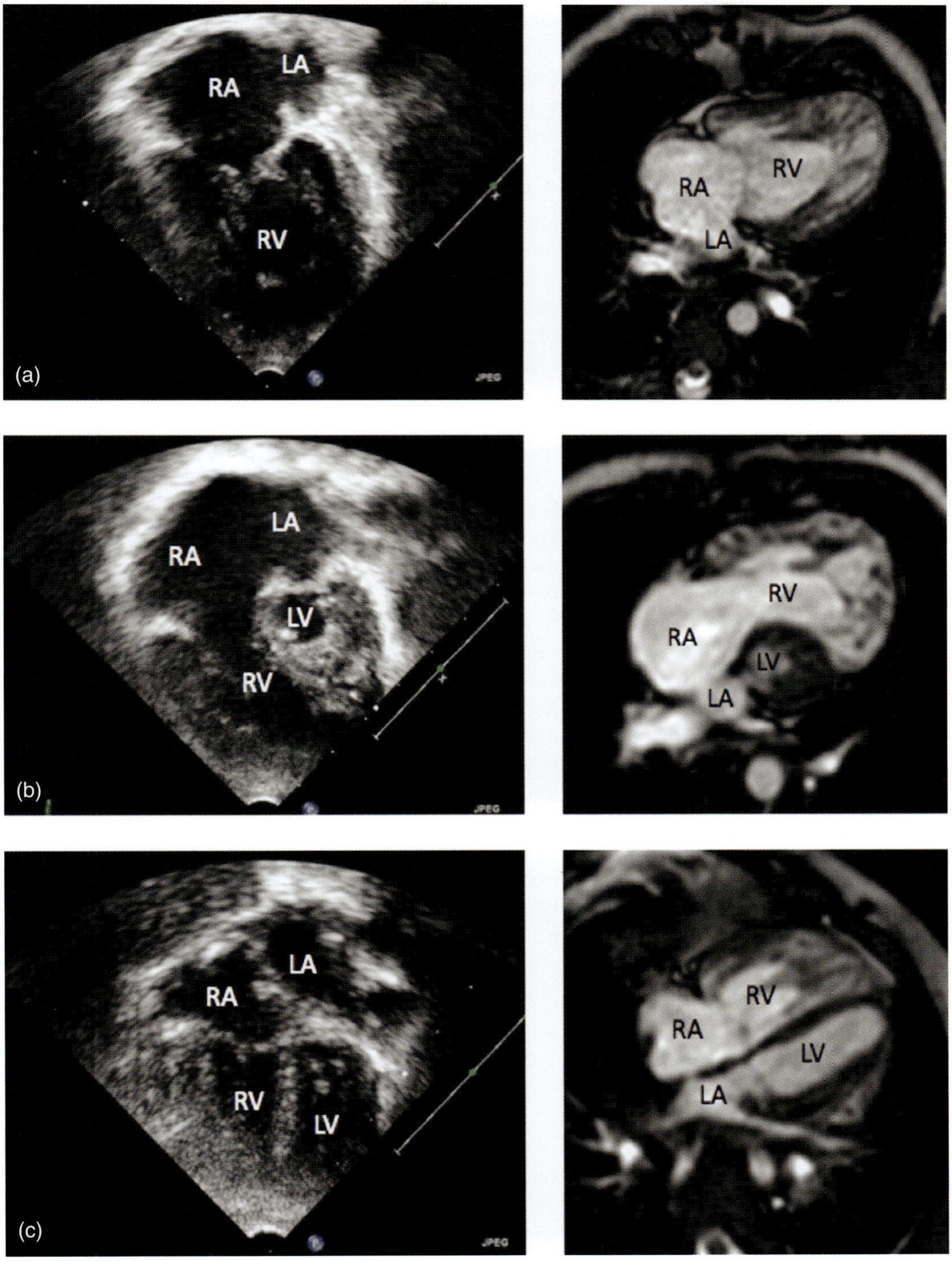

Figure 34.2 The different morphologic subtypes seen in HLHS as depicted by echocardiography (left column) and MRI (right column): (a) slit-like or no visible LV, usually associated with mitral and aortic atresia; (b) globular LV, usually associated with mitral stenosis and aortic atresia; and (c) the "borderline" left heart with mild LV hypoplasia and mitral and aortic stenosis. LA, left atrium; LV, left ventricle; RA, right atrium; RV, right ventricle.

shock. An inadequate or restrictive atrial communication can be diagnosed by fetal echocardiography [8], requiring appropriate delivery and immediate postnatal treatment.

Immediately after birth, the pulmonary and systemic vascular resistances are similar, and blood flow between the pulmonary and systemic circulations is balanced. As pulmonary vascular resistance falls, pulmonary blood flow increases at the expense of systemic flow. Reduced systemic flow will impair end organ function, and reduced coronary artery flow will result in myocardial ischemia, RV dysfunction, and further reduction in cardiac output.

When pulmonary blood flow increases this is described as "pulmonary overcirculation". Early clinical indicators of this include high systemic oxygen saturations, tachypnea, and low diastolic pressure, eventually progressing to reduced peripheral perfusion, hypotension, acidosis, and shock. Measures that reduce the pulmonary vascular resistance, such as oxygen administration, should be avoided. When pulmonary overcirculation is evident, it may be necessary to control ventilation, manipulate pulmonary resistance with permissive hypercapnia, and use inotropic support.

Diagnosis

Antenatal diagnosis of HLHS is becoming increasingly common and allows for prenatal counseling and treatment planning, including delivery in a center with the appropriate management expertise [9]. After birth, the patient may present during routine screening; for example, with clinical signs or abnormal four-limb oxygen saturations. However, presentation often occurs as cardiovascular collapse after arterial duct closure. These infants usually have a short history of reduced feeding and breathlessness.

Box 34.1 describes the main clinical signs in HLHS. Cardiovascular examination reveals globally reduced pulses with poor perfusion. The second heart sound is usually single with no added murmurs. If there is some forward flow through the left heart or a small arterial duct, a murmur may be heard. Four-limb blood pressures will be globally reduced. Oxygen saturations can also be reduced with differential saturations if there is forward flow across the aortic valve.

The electrocardiogram usually shows RV dominance and strain (although similar patterns can be seen in the normal young neonate) and may show signs of ischemia.

The chest X-ray may be normal or show pulmonary plethora and cardiomegaly, depending upon the balance of the circulation and cardiac function.

Echocardiography is the mainstay of diagnosis (Figure 34.3). A segmental structured approach is recommended (Box 34.2), with specific attention to the systemic and pulmonary venous connections, atrial communication, and arterial duct as well as RV function and tricuspid valve regurgitation, both of which are associated with increased mortality [10]. Assessment of RV function is important, not only in the neonatal period, but throughout life, and it is even more challenging in HLHS than in a normal heart. The most commonly employed method is subjective visual assessment, but this has significant limitations, and its value depends on operator experience [11]. Other methods to assess RV function are available but have not been validated, and normal reference values are limited (Figure 34.4).

Cardiac magnetic resonance imaging (MRI) or computed tomography scanning is not routinely indicated for the initial investigation and diagnosis of HLHS. However, the additional information can be useful for surgical planning, as in cases of abnormal pulmonary venous drainage or aortic arch anatomy (Figure 34.5).

Box 34.1 Clinical features of hypoplastic left heart syndrome

Tachypnea and respiratory distress
Globally reduced pulses
Impaired systemic perfusion
Precordial signs often absent, but often single second heart sound
Saturations may be reduced or normal, differential saturations if forward flow across aortic valve

End-organ damage:

- Renal and hepatic impairment
- Seizures
- Necrotizing enterocolitis

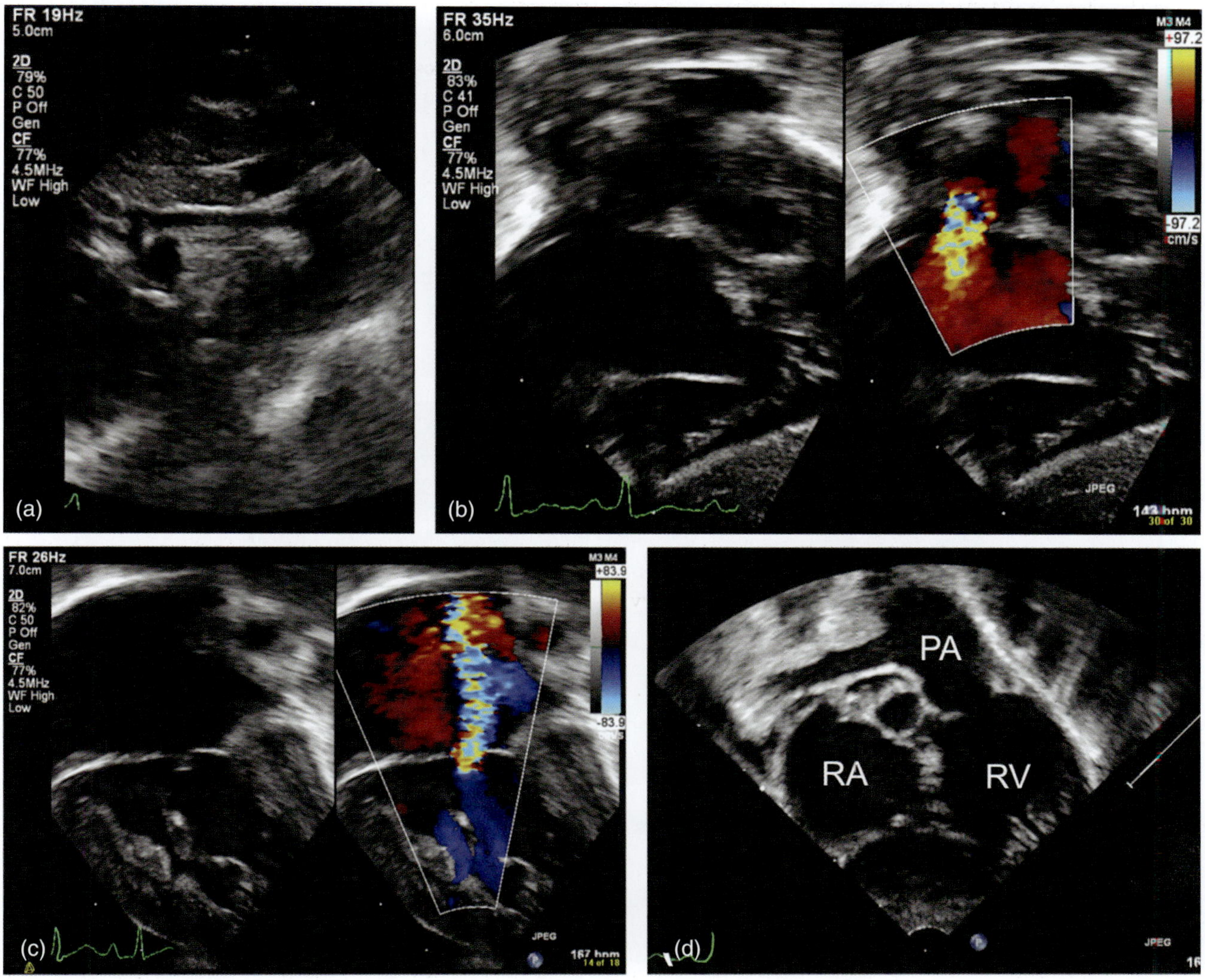

Figure 34.3 Echocardiographic assessment of HLHS depicting: (a) diminutive ascending aorta; (b) turbulent flow through a restrictive atrial communication; (c) severe tricuspid regurgitation; (d) subcostal oblique view of the right ventricle. PA, pulmonary artery; RA, right atrium; RV, right ventricle.

Box 34.2 Echocardiographic assessment of hypoplastic left heart syndrome.

Systemic and pulmonary venous connections and drainage

Atrial communication

Left heart structures: mitral valve, left ventricle, aortic valve, ascending aorta:

- Structure
- Size
- Function
- Endocardial fibroelastosis

Tricuspid valve:

- Morphology
- Function

Systolic function of right ventricle (Figure 34.4):

- Subjective assessment
- Tricuspid annular plane systolic excursion, fractional area change
- Advanced techniques: tissue Doppler, speckle tracking, three-dimensional echocardiography

Pulmonary valve:

- Stenosis/regurgitation

Branch pulmonary artery size

Ductal patency and direction of flow

Aortic arch anatomy and size

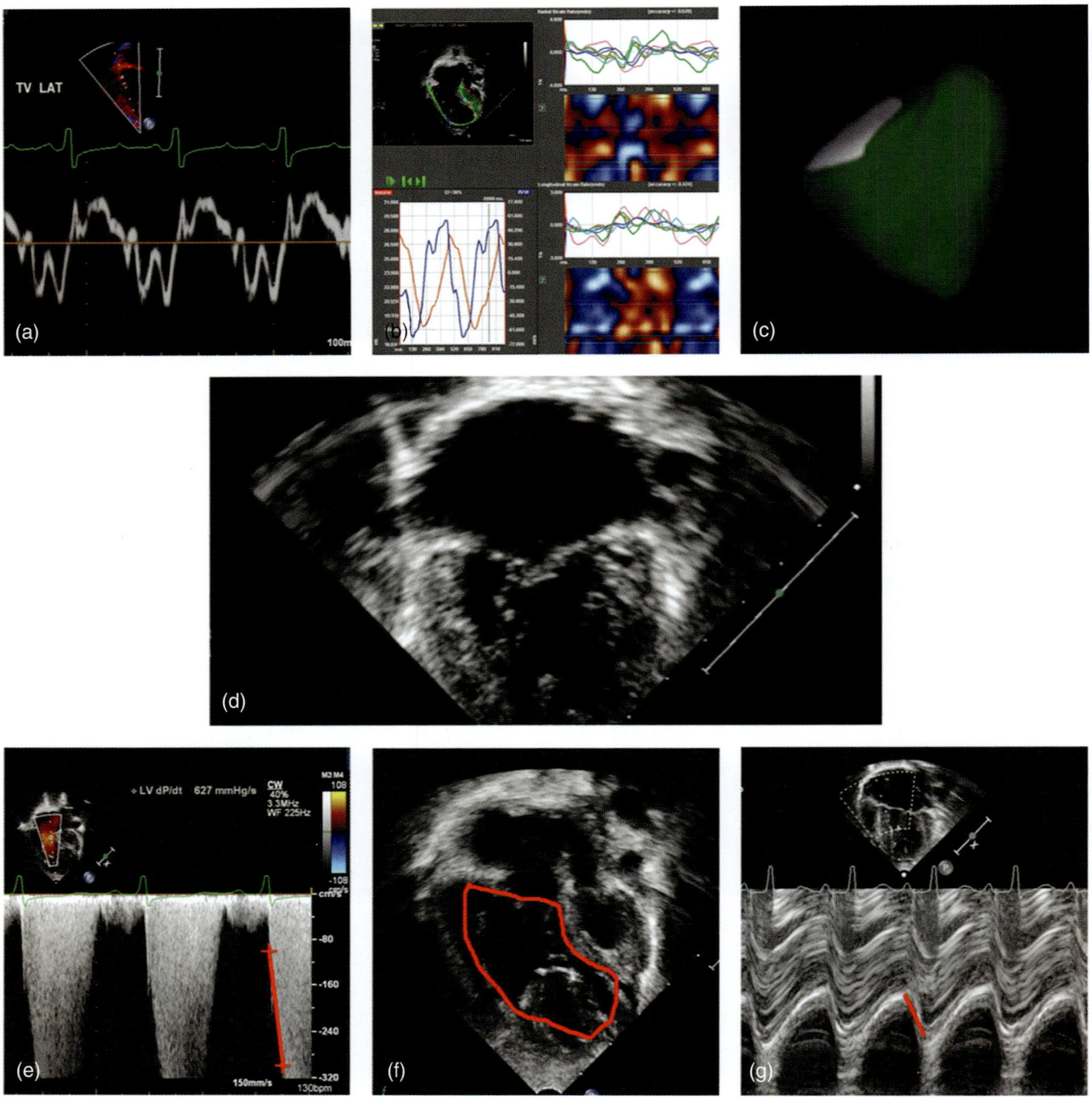

Figure 34.4 Methods for the assessment of RV function in HLHS: (a) tissue Doppler; (b) speckle tracking; (c) three-dimensional echocardiography; (d) subjective visual assessment; (e) change in pressure by time (dP/dT); (f) fractional area change (FAC); (g) tricuspid annular plane systolic excursion (TAPSE).

Management

Given the severity of HLHS, the high risk of mortality or other significant morbidities, and an uncertain prognosis, some parents choose not to continue with the pregnancy if discovered antenatally. Others may not wish for active intervention post-delivery and opt for compassionate comfort care. The mainstay of surgical management for HLHS is the Norwood procedure and subsequent progression to the Fontan circulation. Cardiac transplantation in the neonate remains an option but is severely limited by organ availability and therefore not considered a viable treatment option in many countries.

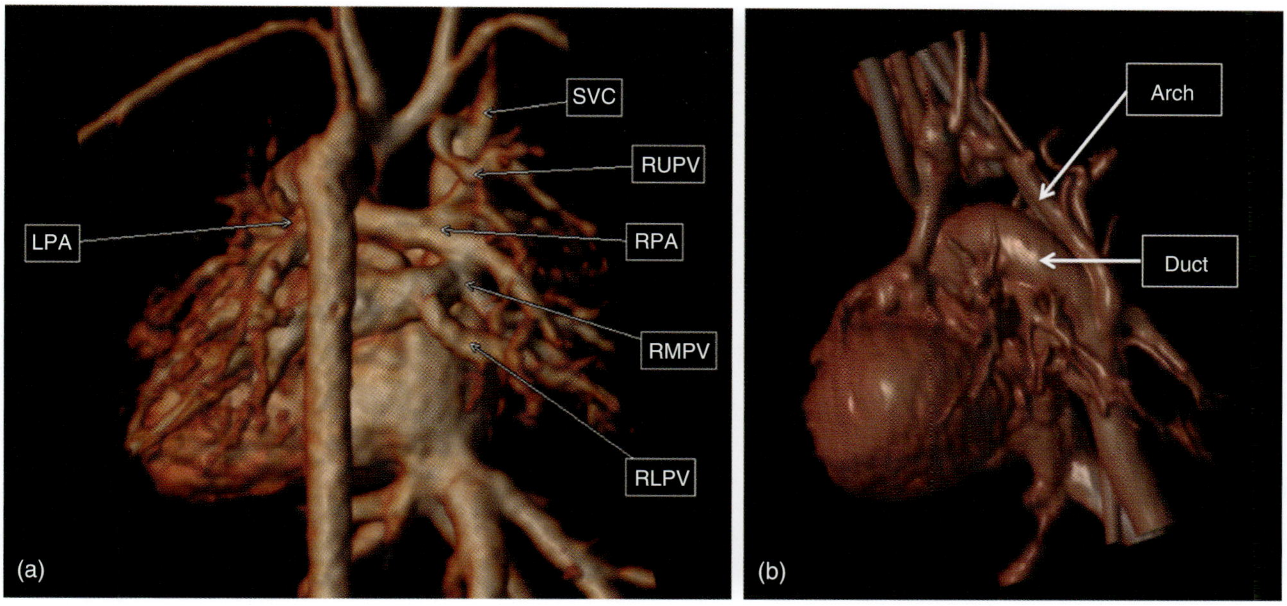

Figure 34.5 (a) MRI of anomalous drainage of the right upper pulmonary vein to the superior caval vein prior to the Norwood procedure; (b) CT demonstrating very abnormal aortic arch anatomy. LPA, left pulmonary artery; RLPV, right lower pulmonary vein; RMPV, right middle pulmonary vein; RPA, right pulmonary artery; RUPV, right upper pulmonary vein; SVC, superior caval vein.

The Norwood procedure (Figure 34.6a) was developed in the early 1980s and allows the RV to become the systemic ventricle. This consists of an aortic reconstruction where the pulmonary artery, having been disconnected from the branch pulmonary arteries, is anastomosed to the aortic arch with augmentation using homograft tissue (formation of the neo-aorta). In order to preserve coronary blood flow, the native aorta is anastomosed to the neo-aorta in the Damus–Kaye–Stansel anastomosis. An atrial septectomy allows for free flow across the atrial septum. Pulmonary blood flow is then established with either a modified Blalock–Taussig shunt from the innominate artery to the right pulmonary artery or through a non-valved conduit from the RV to the pulmonary artery (the Sano modification; Figure 34.6b).

An alternative strategy to the Norwood procedure as a primary palliation has been utilized more recently. The hybrid procedure consists of maintaining ductal patency with an arterial duct stent and limiting pulmonary blood flow with bilateral branch pulmonary artery bands (Figure 34.6c). The procedure is performed via a sternotomy but has the advantage of avoiding the need for cardiopulmonary bypass. This may be of particular advantage to babies of low birth weight or those who have had cardiovascular collapse. It may also provide an interim solution in those patients with a borderline left heart in whom it is hoped a full biventricular repair may be possible [12]. When children will not achieve a biventricular circulation, a Norwood procedure will ultimately need to be performed, whether this is as a stand-alone procedure or combined with a superior cavopulmonary connection. After the Norwood procedure or a hybrid, children will have common mixing of their circulations. Their saturations will be dependent on the ratio of pulmonary to systemic blood flow, but should ideally be around 75–85%.

Ultimately, the aim is for completion of a Fontan circulation involving connection of the superior and inferior caval veins directly to the pulmonary arteries (Figure 34.6d,e,f). This is usually performed as two separate operations, the first at 3–6 months of age and the second at 2–5 years of age, depending on institutional variation. Assessments are required prior to each surgical stage, usually involving clinical evaluation, echocardiography, and either MRI (Figure 34.7) or cardiac catheterization [13]. Prior to Fontan completion, it is necessary to evaluate pulmonary artery pressures, either with direct measurement at cardiac catheterization or from a central venous pressure (internal jugular) at MRI [7, 14].

Prognosis

HLHS remains an extremely serious congenital cardiac problem with significant mortality and morbidity. After birth, acute collapse from circulatory imbalance can be life-threatening, and some infants will not survive to undergo their first palliation. Initial palliation carries a

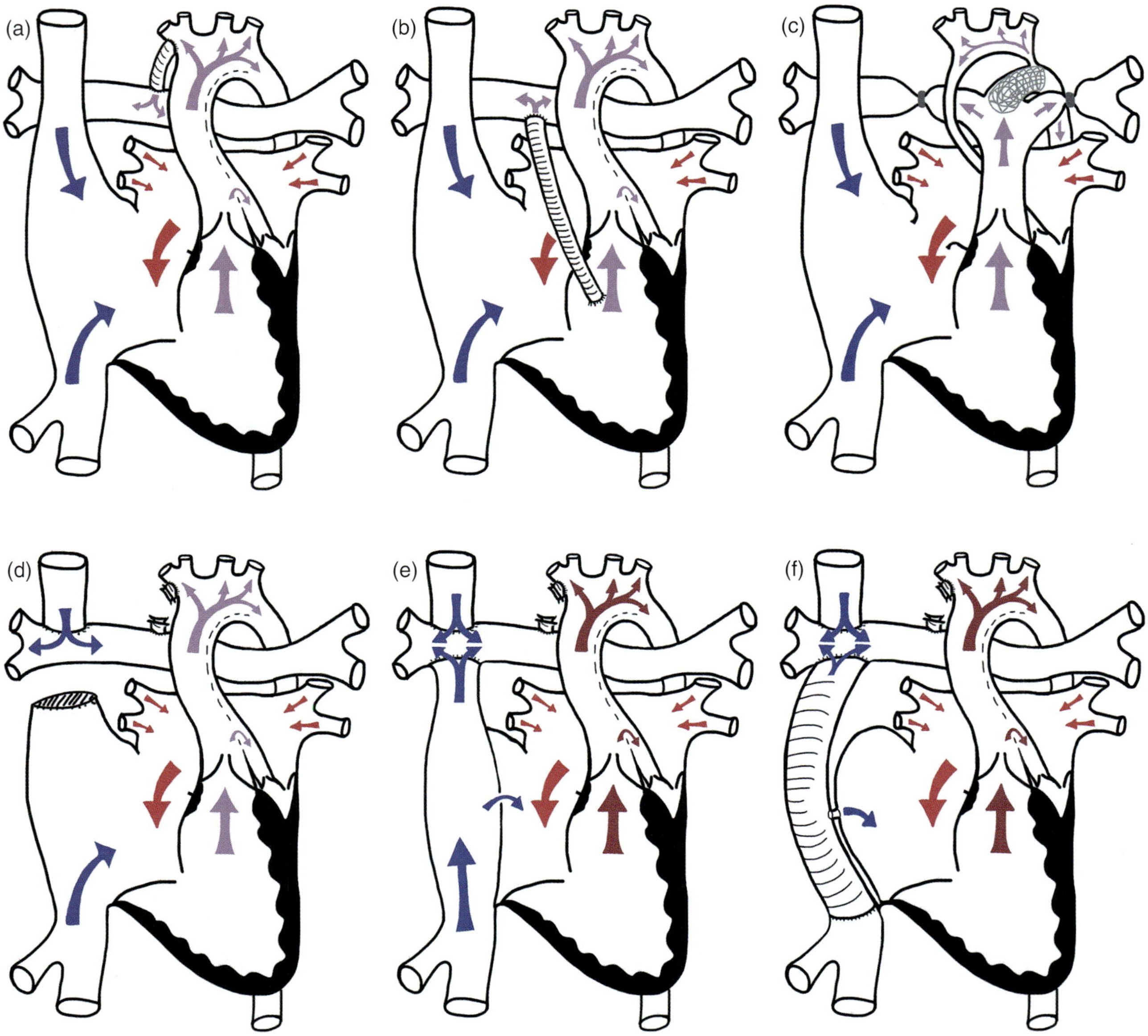

Figure 34.6 The surgical management of HLHS: (a) classic Norwood procedure; (b) Norwood procedure with the Sano modification; (c) hybrid procedure; (d) superior cavopulmonary anastomosis; (e) completion of the Fontan circulation with lateral tunnel; (f) completion of the Fontan circulation with an extracardiac conduit.

substantial procedural mortality of around 10–35% [1]. Given the precarious nature of the circulation following a Norwood or hybrid procedure, children are at risk for sudden death prior to the superior cavopulmonary connection. The mechanism of this may be acute shunt occlusion, a loss of circulatory balance resulting in pulmonary overcirculation, and/or progressive myocardial dysfunction. Procedure-related mortality for the superior cavopulmonary connection and completion of Fontan is low.

Staged palliation for HLHS results in a single systemic RV. The RV is not anatomically or physiologically designed to support the high-pressure systemic circulation for a prolonged period of time and will fail with time. However, it is impossible to predict in any individual when this may occur. Many children after Fontan live through to teenage years. Exercise intolerance is common, and other Fontan complications such as arrhythmias, thrombosis, protein losing enteropathy, and plastic bronchitis can also be seen. Cardiac transplantation remains an option for patients with failing RV and failed Fontan circulations, but outcomes are poor when compared with transplantation for other causes.

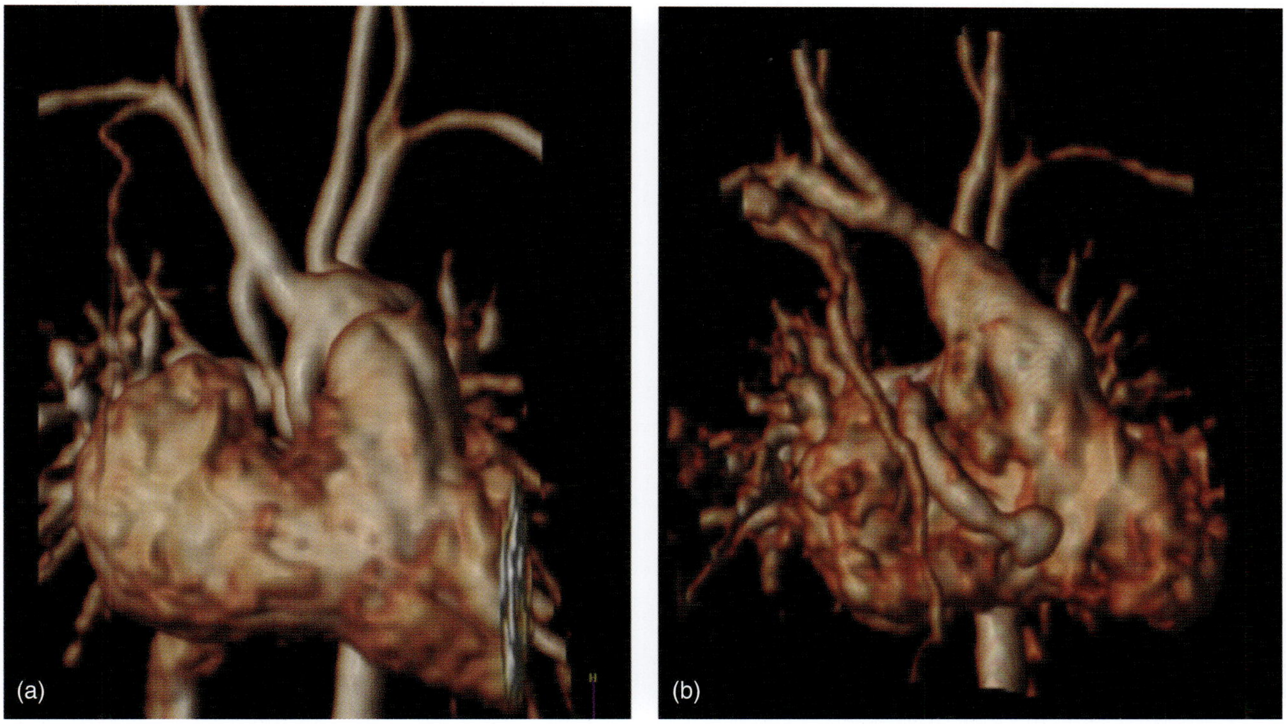

Figure 34.7 MRI prior to superior cavopulmonary anastomosis in a patient after: (a) classic Norwood; and (b) Sano modification.

References

1 Barron DJ, Kilby MD, Davies B, Wright JGC, Jones TJ, Brawn WJ. (2009) Hypoplastic left heart syndrome. *Lancet*, **374**, 551–564.

2 Botto LD, Correa A, Erickson JD. (2001) Racial and temporal variations in the prevalence of heart defects. *Pediatrics*, **107**, E32.

3 Hoffman JI, Kaplan S. (2002) The incidence of congenital heart disease. *J Am Coll Cardiol*, **39**, 1890–1900.

4 Allan LD, Sharland G, Milburn A, *et al.* (1994) Prospective diagnosis of 1,006 consecutive cases of congenital heart disease in the fetus. *J Am Coll Cardiol*, **23**, 1452–1458.

5 Raymond R, Simpson J, Sharland G, Ogilvie Mackie C. (1997) Fetal echocardiography as a predictor of chromosomal abnormality. *Lancet*, **350**, 930.

6 Hinton R, Martin L, Rame-Gowda S, *et al.* (2009) Hypoplastic left heart syndrome lins to chromosomes 10q and 6q and is genetically related to bicuspid aortic valve. *J Am Coll Cardiol*, **53**, 1065–1071.

7 Bellsham-Revell HR, Tibby S, Bell A, *et al.* (2013) Serial magnetic resonance imaging in hypoplastic left heart syndrome gives valuable insight into ventricular and vascular adaptation. *J Am Coll Cardiol*, **61** (5), 561–570.

8 Vida V, Bacha EA, Larrazabal LA, *et al.* (2007) Hypoplastic left heart syndrome with intact or highly restrictive atrial septum: surgical experience from a single center. *Ann Thorac Surg*, **84**, 581–585.

9 Kipps AK, Feuille C, Azakie A, *et al.* (2011) Prenatal diagnosis of hypoplastic left heart syndrome in current era. *Am J Cardiol*, **108**, 421–427.

10 Altmann K, Printz BF, Solowiejczky DE, *et al.* (2000) Two-dimensional echocardiographic assessment of right ventricular function as a predictor of outcome in hypoplastic left heart syndrome. *Am J Cardiol*, **86**, 964–968.

11 Bellsham-Revell HR, Simpson J, Miller O, Bell A. (2012) Subjective evaluation of right ventricular systolic function in hypoplastic left heart syndrome: how accurate is it? *J Am Soc Echocardiogr*, **26**, 52–56.

12 Venugopal PS, Luna KP, Anderson DR, *et al.* (2010) Hybrid procedure as an alternative to surgical palliation of high-risk infants with hypoplastic left heart syndrome and its variants. *J Thorac Cardiovasc Surg*, **139**, 1211–1215.

13 Muthurangu V, Taylor AM, Hegde SR, *et al.* (2005) Cardiac magnetic resonance imaging after stage I Norwood operation for hypoplastic left heart syndrome. *Circulation*, **112**, 3256–3263.

14 Fogel MA. (2005) Is routine cardiac catheterization necessary in the management of patients with single ventricles across staged Fontan reconstruction? No! *Pediatr Cardiol*, **26**, 154–158.

35

Aortic Stenosis

Salwa Gendi[1] and Ra-id Abdulla[2]

[1] University of Mississippi Medical Center, Jackson, MS, USA
[2] Department of Pediatrics, Section of Pediatric Cardiology, Rush University Medical Center, Chicago, IL, USA

Aortic Valve Stenosis

Definition

Aortic valve stenosis (AVS) is the most common form of left ventricular outflow tract (LVOT) obstruction. Other LVOT obstruction lesions include subvalvular and supravalvular aortic stenosis. Congenital AVS presenting in the neonatal period may be isolated, or part of a syndrome affecting other left heart components such as Shone complex or hypoplastic left heart syndrome.

Incidence

Aortic stenosis is more common in childhood and adolescence than in infancy. It occurs in 0.004–0.34% of live births and ranks 16th among critical congenital heart diseases in infants. Incidence increases with age to become the second most common congenital heart disease after ventricular septal defect in the third decade of life.

Pathology

AVS results from attenuation of the aortic valve orifice because of diminished aortic valve annulus, fusion of the aortic valve cusps, or thickening of these cusps. In many instances it results from a combination of these pathologic changes.

The commissures of the aortic valve may be fused, rendering the orifice small and at times eccentric. In addition, the aortic valve ring is occasionally hypoplastic. The valve is commonly bicuspid in aortic stenosis and the leaflets are asymmetric in 40% of cases. There is occasionally more than one level of obstruction in the LVOT or supravalvar region alongside the AVS. Ten percent of patients with aortic stenosis have subvalvar aortic stenosis. Aortic regurgitation is seen in 50% of patients with AVS. A small percentage of patients with bicuspid aortic valve will develop aortic stenosis, while the majority will not. Therefore, most patients with aortic stenosis are born with this lesion and it is not a result of progression of bicuspid aortic valve. Fusion between aortic valve cusps resulting in a right-to-left commissural fusion is noted to have a worse prognosis in bicuspid aortic than anteroposterior commissures in developing aortic stenosis. Eccentric orifices have a worse prognosis than central orifices in developing aortic stenosis.

Pathophysiology

Aortic stenosis causes a pressure gradient across the aortic valve, thus elevating left ventricular pressures. This will lead to hypertrophy of the left ventricle later in life and eventually can cause strain of the left ventricle from hypoxia as a result of increase in muscle mass with reduced coronary blood flow.

The ascending aorta can become dilated because of the forceful jet of blood as it crosses the aortic valve. Patients with bicuspid aortic valve are known to develop aortic root dilation; this may not be associated with aortic stenosis and the etiology in these cases is not clear but may be related to abnormal wall architecture of the ascending aorta.

Aortic regurgitation, occasionally noted with aortic stenosis, will hasten the development of left ventricular dilation and failure as it causes volume overload to the left ventricle on top of the pressure overload caused by aortic stenosis [1].

Natural History

Mild cases usually do not progress, while moderate and severe cases usually progress in severity. Subacute bacterial endocarditis occurs in 0.3% of patients. Sudden death can occur in any patient with aortic stenosis but mainly in more severe and symptomatic patients.

Visual Guide to Neonatal Cardiology, First Edition. Edited by Ernerio T. Alboliras, Ziyad M. Hijazi, Leo Lopez, and Donald J. Hagler.

Clinical Manifestations

Newborn infants with AVS usually have no symptoms. A heart murmur is the most common presenting sign suggesting aortic valve disease.

Symptoms are limited to patients with severe aortic stenosis caused by reduced cardiac output manifesting as easy fatigability (poor feeding in neonates), shortness of breath, pallor and sweating with exertion, and cool and clammy extremities.

Patients with critical AVS present with poor cardiac output and heart failure early in life, requiring immediate treatment to relieve the obstruction to blood flow through balloon dilation of the valve or surgical intervention.

Aortic valve leaflets are typically thick and may be gelatinous with small aortic valve rings, such as in critical aortic stenosis. The left ventricle may be small and in some instances smaller than compatible with adequate cardiac output. The ascending aorta is usually small or hypoplastic in critical aortic stenosis. Coarctation of aorta may also be present.

There may also be endocardial fibroelastosis which impacts left ventricular compliance, further reducing its effectiveness in producing an adequate cardiac output. Patent foramen ovale will allow left-to-right shunting to vent the left heart at the expense of reducing cardiac output. Patent ductus arteriosus (PDA) allows right-to-left shunting which if present results in improving cardiac output, even though it may cause cyanosis.

In an older child, severe aortic stenosis rarely causes heart failure. The child may experience chest pain, lightheadedness, or fainting spells particularly associated with exercise. Severe aortic stenosis is a rare, but well-documented, cause of sudden death during strenuous sports activities.

Physical examination can reveal a palpable thrill, particularly over the suprasternal notch as well as the right second intercostal space. On auscultation, the first heart sound is normal, followed by a systolic ejection click preceding a harsh systolic crescendo–decrescendo type murmur (Figure 35.1). The second heart sound (S_2) is normal except with severe aortic stenosis where the aortic valve closure (A_2) will be delayed secondary to prolonged left ventricular systole causing reversed splitting or single S_2. Half of patients with AVS also have a decrescendo early diastolic murmur caused by aortic regurgitation.

Electrocardiography

The electrocardiogram (ECG) is typically normal in the presence of mild-to-moderate aortic stenosis. With severe aortic stenosis, the ECG shows enlargement of the left ventricle and may even show evidence of left

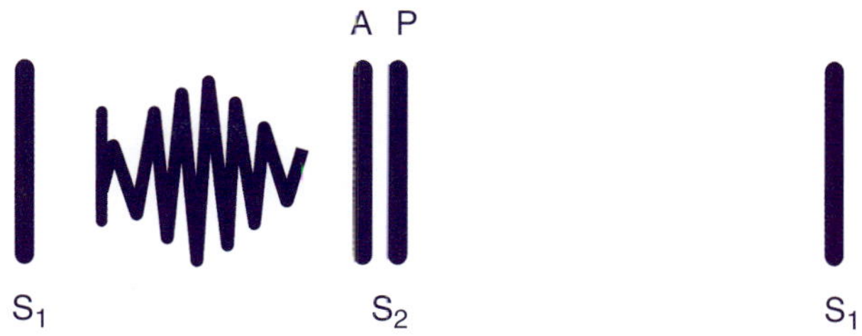

Figure 35.1 Auscultation in aortic stenosis is characterized by a normal first heart sound (S1), systolic ejection click followed immediately by a systolic crescendo decrescendo harsh murmur, usually 3/6 in intensity or louder. Second heart sound (S2) is usually normal, except in severe or critical aortic stenosis where the aortic component of S2 may be delayed or absent. Diastole is quiet unless there is aortic regurgitation as well resulting in an early decrescendo type murmur. If the systolic murmur is 4/6 or louder in intensity a precordial thrill will also be felt.

ventricular strain, particularly in the inferolateral leads (Figure 35.2).

The changes on the ECG reflects the chronic strain of the myocardium rather than the severity at rest in contrast with the severity measured through pressure gradient assessment at rest by echocardiography or cardiac catheterization.

Chest X-ray

Chest X-ray can be normal until left ventricular failure intervenes. Heart size is usually normal with rounding of the left ventricular border and apex. Post-stenotic dilatation of the aorta may be apparent.

Echocardiography

Parasternal short-axis view demonstrates the aortic valve annulus; this may be small in diameter. In addition, aortic valve cusp fusion may be noted with systolic doming of the valve (Figures 35.3 and 35.4). Fusion between the right and left coronary cusps will result in a right-to-left commissure and fusion of right and non-coronary cusps results in anteroposterior commissure. Color flow Doppler will show aliasing and disturbed flow across the valve (Figure 35.5). Left ventricular hypertrophy can also be seen in severe cases of aortic stenosis (Figure 35.6). A fusion of the left and non-coronary cusp is extremely rare. Assessment of pressure gradient across the aortic valve is best performed through apical five or three-chamber views, or from the suprasternal view (Figure 35.7). Aortic insufficiency can also be evaluated through echocardiography; this is best seen with color Doppler or Doppler flow from the apical five or three-chamber views as well as the parasternal long-axis view. The severity of aortic insufficiency is assessed by the width of the aortic regurgitation jet at the level of the valve cusps coaptation and not by how far the

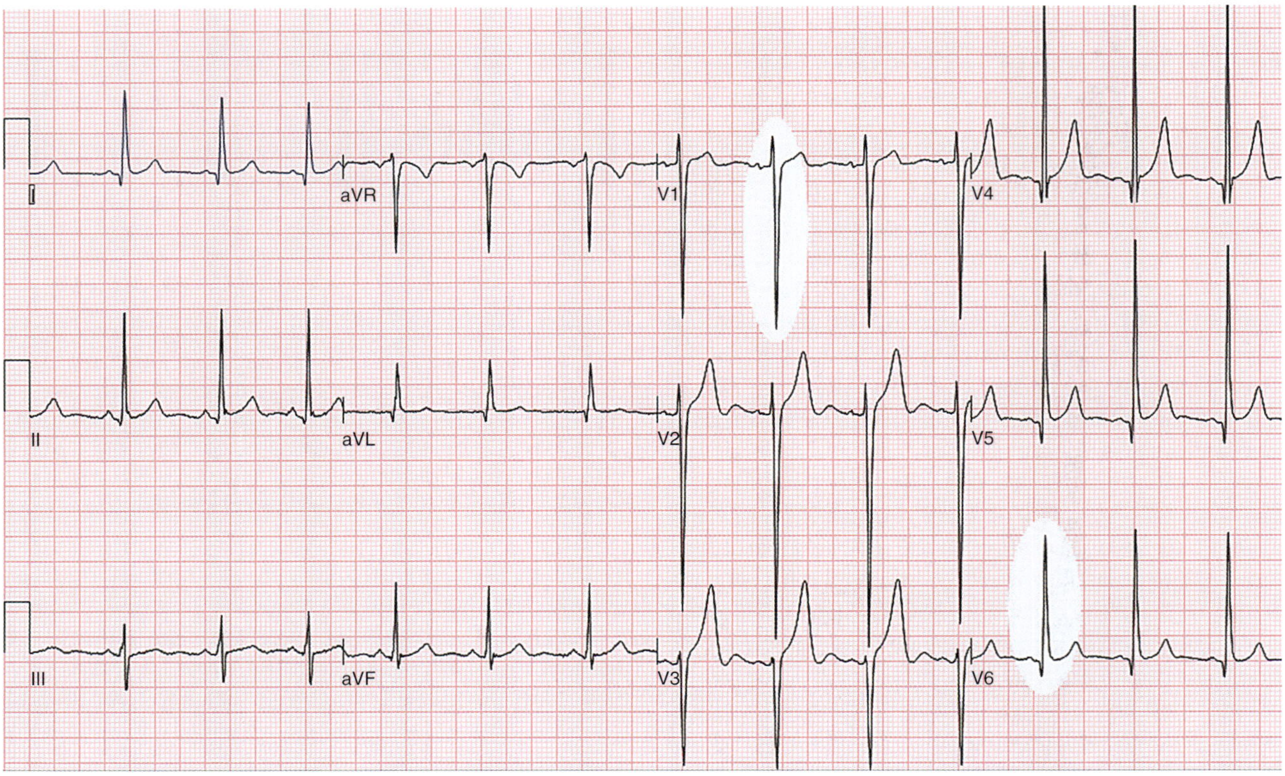

Figure 35.2 Patients with aortic stenosis develop left ventricular hypertrophy (LVH), typically manifesting as tall R wave in V6 and deep S wave in V1. Severe aortic stenosis may be accompanied with left ventricular strain pattern.

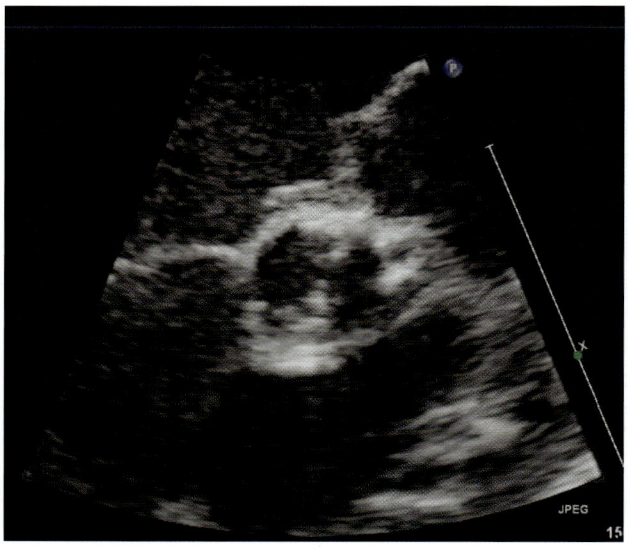

Figure 35.3 Parasternal short-axis view showing bicuspid aortic valve with thickened valve cusps. Bicuspid aortic valves may or may not be stenotic in early childhood. Bicuspid aortic valve results from fusion of two of the cusps, in the case demonstrated here the right and non-coronary cusps are fused to form a vertical slit-like orifice of the aortic valve.

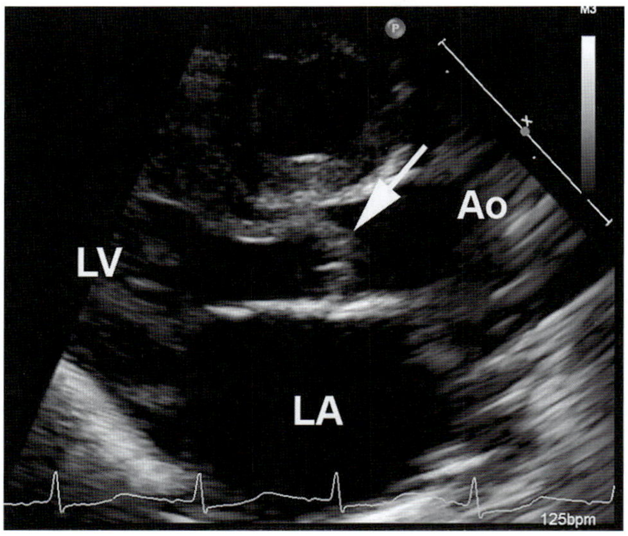

Figure 35.4 Parasternal long-axis echocardiography view showing the aortic valve cusps which are thickened (arrow), movie clip of this image is likely to show limited excursion of the aortic valve cusps. Ao, aorta; LA, left atrium; LV, left ventricle.

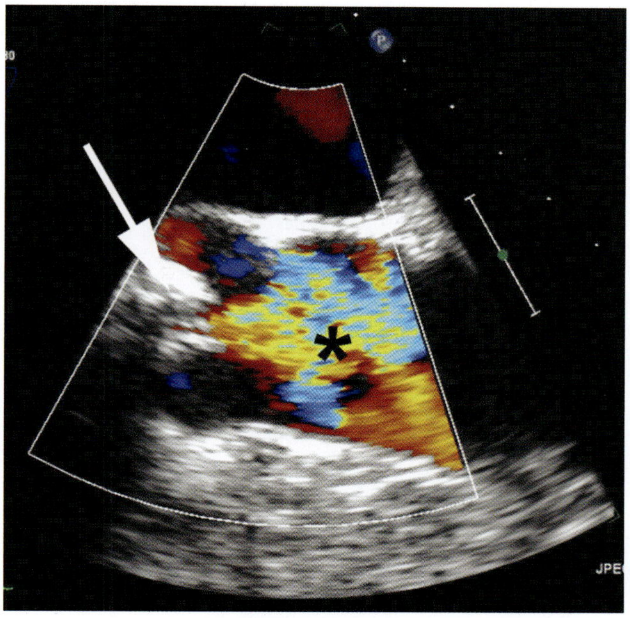

Figure 35.5 Color Doppler echocardiography parasternal long-axis view showing flow across the stenotic aortic valve (arrow). Color Doppler is turbulent as evident by the pixilation of the color (asterisk).

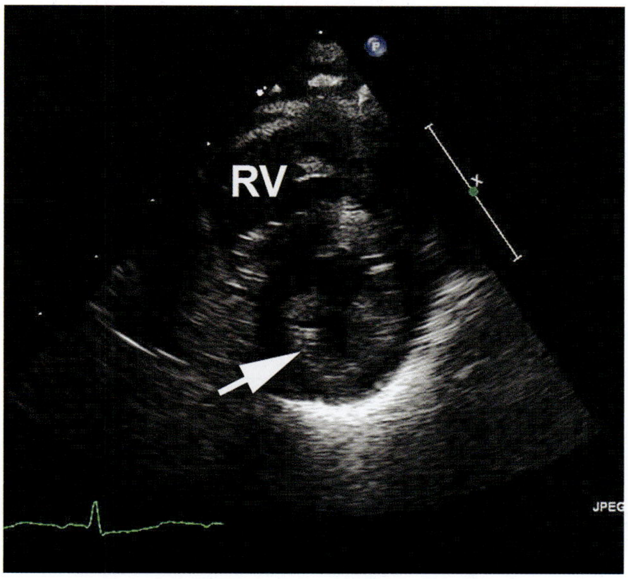

Figure 35.6 Parasternal short-axis view showing the right and left ventricles in short axis. The left ventricle (arrow) is significantly hypertrophied. RV, right ventricle.

regurgitation jet extends into the left ventricle. Diastolic reversal flow in the ascending aorta as assessed through Doppler flow provides another mean of assessing the severity of aortic regurgitation.

Cardiac Catheterization

Cardiac catheterization is not typically required for diagnostic purposes, but may be performed for therapeutic purposes to balloon dilate the aortic valve. Balloon dilation of aortic stenosis is performed when the pressure gradient is 50 mmHg or more. Balloon dilation of a stenotic valve is most effective when the dominant pathology is that of fusion of commissures of valve cusps (Figures 35.8 and 35.9). However, small aortic valve annulus or predominantly thickened cusps without commissural fusion respond less favorably to balloon dilation. Aortic regurgitation may worsen with balloon dilation and as such patients with moderate or severe aortic regurgitation are not well served by balloon dilation and may require surgical intervention [2].

Treatment

The first step in the management of aortic valve stenosis in the neonatal period is to ensure adequate cardiac output. Evidence of poor cardiac output is an indication for urgent relief of obstruction with balloon dilation or surgical intervention.

Balloon valvuloplasty is the method of choice for management of critical neonatal stenosis. In skilled hands, complications such as acute aortic regurgitation or injury to the mitral valve are exceedingly rare. On occasions, injury to a femoral or iliac vessel may necessitate surgical reconstruction of the injured vessel.

In cases of borderline left ventricle size, a scoring system is used to assess viability of left ventricle for a biventricular repair. The scoring system is based on a variety of left ventricular parameters. Biventricular repair is possible if the mitral valve area is more than 4.75 cm^2/m^2, long axis dimension of the left ventricle relative to the long axis of the heart is more than 0.8, diameter of the aortic root is more than 3.5 cm/m^2, and left ventricular mass is more than 35 g/m^2 [3].

Surgical intervention to enlarge left ventricular outflow and aortic valve annulus may be required for effective non-obstructed flow from the left ventricle [4].

Follow-up

Follow-up of patients with aortic stenosis is performed annually. In addition to clinical assessment, 12-lead ECG and echocardiography may be indicated. Holter monitor assessment of heart rhythm for 24 hours is used every few years to assess for occult arrhythmia.

Exercise testing is used as the child gets older and is able to undertake this study. Patients with residual AVS

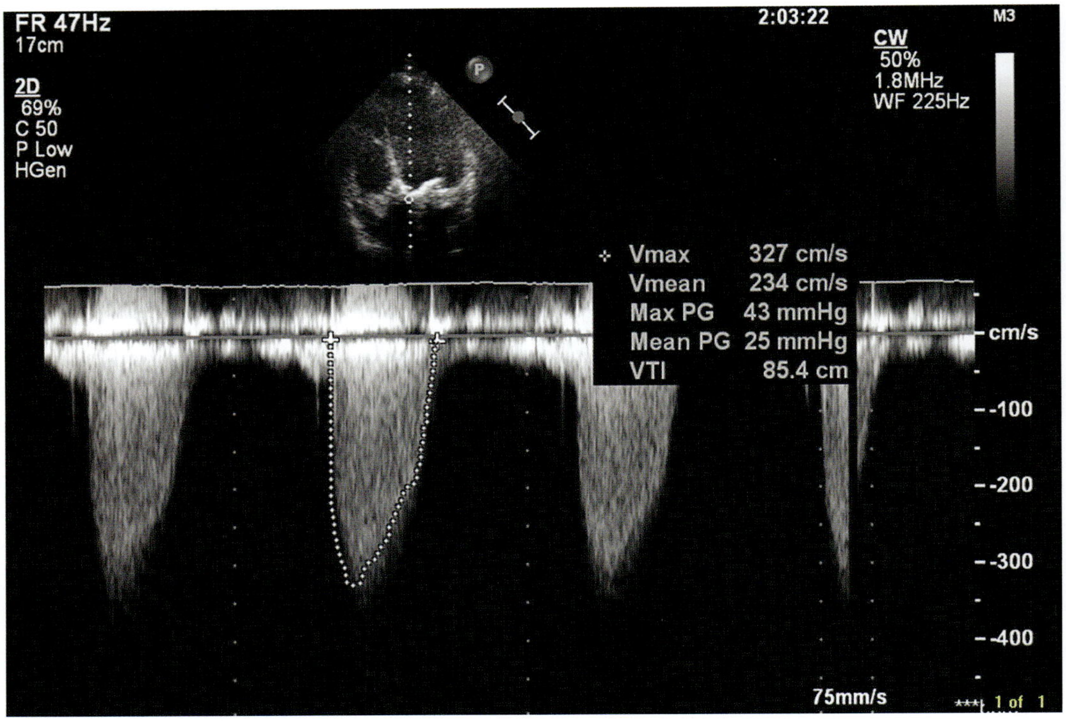

Figure 35.7 Continuous wave Doppler echocardiography. Doppler flow across stenotic aortic valve from the five-chamber view. The flow is accelerated (3.27 m/s) indicating a pressure gradient of 43 mmHg peak and 25 mmHg mean across the aortic valve.

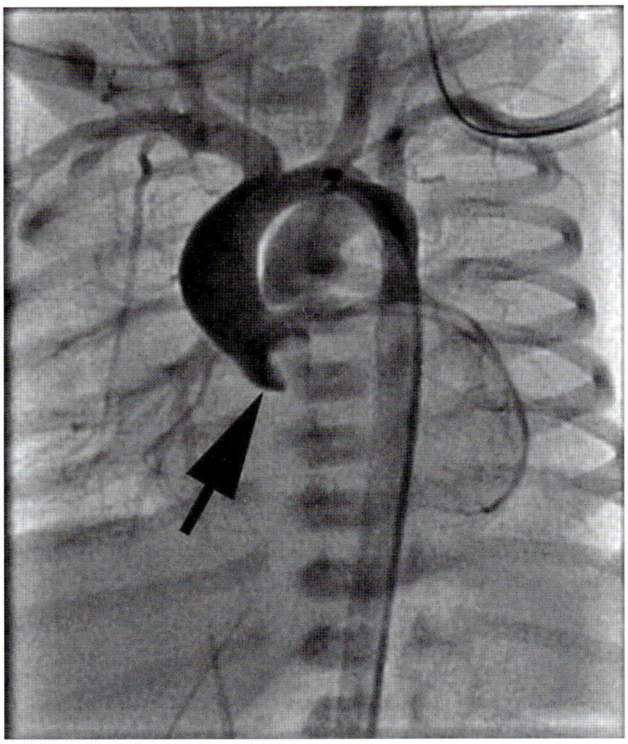

Figure 35.8 Aortic root angiogram in the anteroposterior projection. The aortic valve domes in an abnormal fashion indicating fusion of aortic valve cusps (arrow).

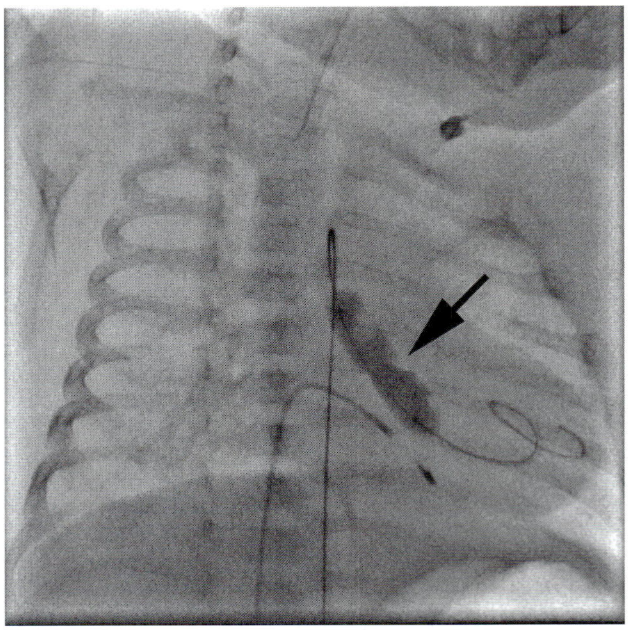

Figure 35.9 A balloon is inflated across the aortic valve to force opening of abnormally fused aortic valve cusps. The arrow points to the narrowing point of the inflated balloon which points to the level of the stenotic valve. Upon completion of inflation,the waist noted here disappears indicating successful dilation of valvar aortic stenosis.

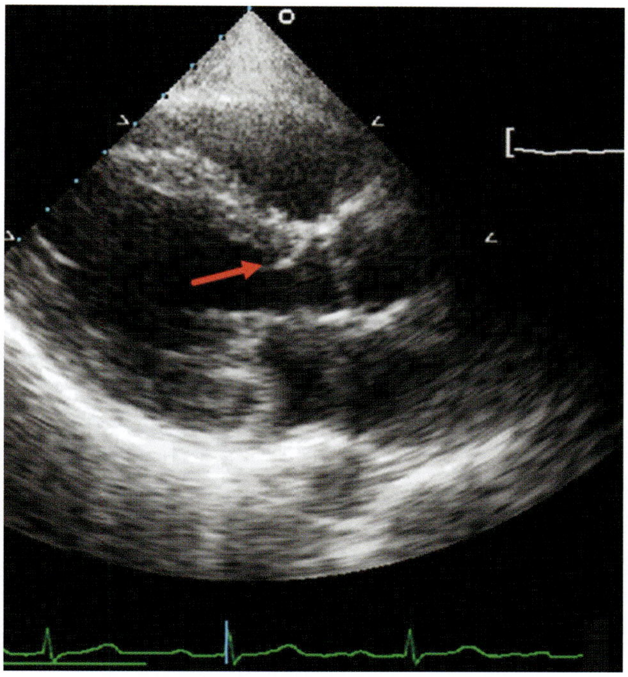

Figure 35.10 Parasternal long-axis view showing subaortic membrane.

may develop left ventricular strain noted by ST segment and T wave changes during exercise or develop ventricular arrhythmia induced by physical exertion.

Subaortic Stenosis

Subaortic stenosis is either caused by a discrete subaortic ridge (or membrane) or narrowing of the LVOT, also called tunnel-like LVOT obstruction. The latter can be caused by dynamic obstruction such as seen in patients with hypertrophic cardiomyopathy.

Discrete subaortic membrane is rare in the neonatal period and when present it typically causes only mild obstruction; however, this may become more severe as the child grows older. Echocardiography is diagnostic in these cases (Figure 35.10). It is particularly important to assess aortic valve competence as aortic regurgitation can result from the turbulent flow across the LVOT obstruction and if present surgical repair is indicated earlier rather than later. Surgical repair of LVOT obstruction is indicated when the pressure gradient across the LVOT is moderate to severe (pressure gradient more than

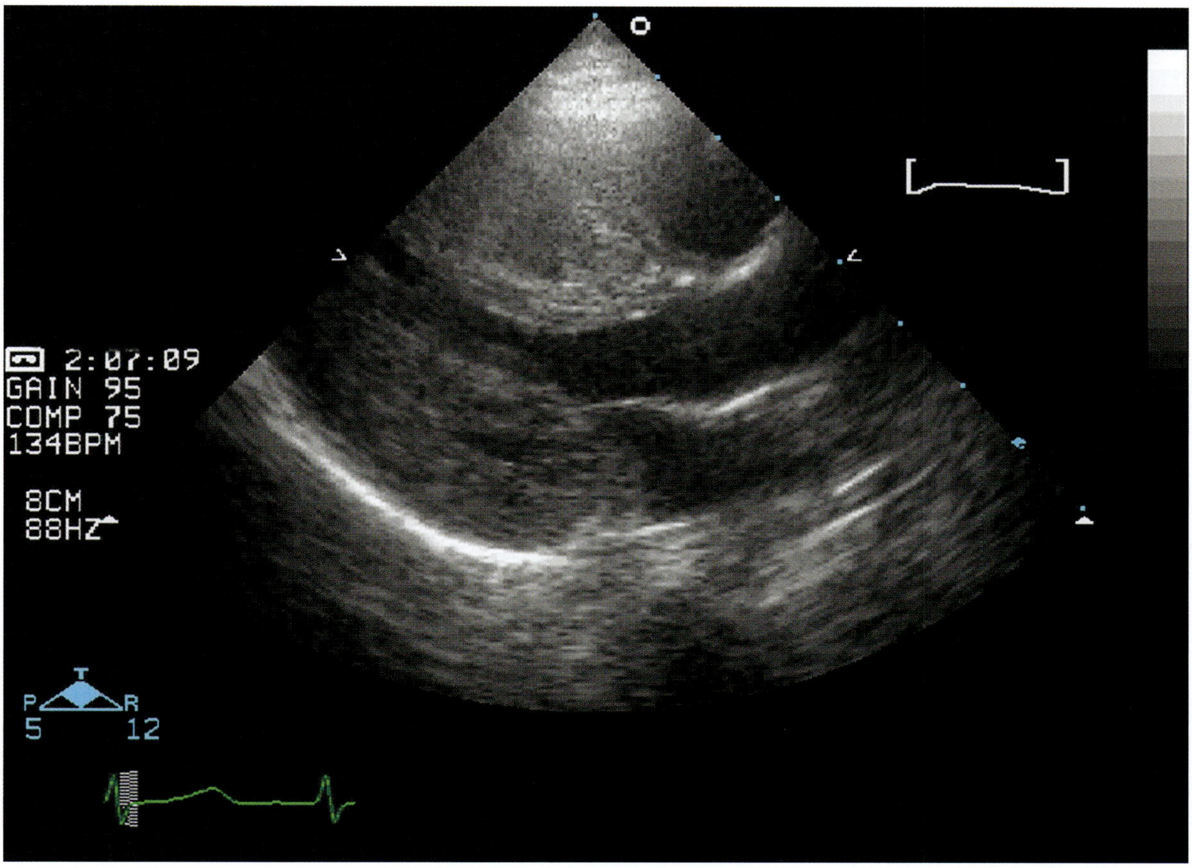

Figure 35.11 Parasternal long-axis view showing severe septal hypertrophy and mid cavity narrowing.

50 mmHg) or lower if there is documented appearance and progression of aortic valve insufficiency. The LVOT obstruction can be eliminated or reduced surgically if it is caused by a ridge (membrane) or hypertrophied muscles such as with hypertrophic cardiomyopathy (Figure 35.11). Small, tunnel-like LVOT obstruction can only be enlarged through a Kono procedure which requires enlargement of the LVOT obstruction through a patch, which may cause narrowing of the right ventricular outflow tract, which in turn will require patch enlargment.

Supravalvar Aortic Stenosis

Supravalvar aortic stenosis caused by narrowing of the sinotubular junction of the ascending aorta may occur in the neonatal period; however, this tends to be mild and worsens as child grows older. It is often associated with William syndrome. Echocardiography is diagnostic; however, cardiac catheterization is needed to assess the coronary arteries as the orifice of coronary arteries may be involved in the narrowing of the aorta. Balloon dilation is typically not effective and treatment is usually surgical.

References

1 Danford DA, Cronican P. (1992) Hypoplastic left heart syndrome: progression of left ventricular dilation and dysfunction to left ventricular hypoplasia in utero. *Am Heart J*, **123**, 1712–1713.

2 Lock JE, Keane JF, Perry SB. (2000) *Diagnostic and Interventional Catheterization in Congenital Heart Disease*, Kluwer Academic, Boston, p. 151.

3 Jonas RA, DiNardo J, Laussen PC, *et al.* (2004) *Comprehensive Surgical Management of Congenital Heart Disease*, Arnold, Hachette, UK, pp. 320–340.

4 Schwartz ML, Gauvreau K, Geva T. (2001) Predictors of of outcome of biventricular repair in infants with multiple left ventricular obstructive lesions. *Circulation*, **104**, 682–687.

Further Reading

Tworetzky W, Wilkins-Haug L, Jennings RW, *et al.* (2004) Balloon dilation of severe aortic stenosis in the fetus: potential for prevention of hypoplastic left heart syndrome: candidate selection, technique, and results of successful intervention. *Circulation*, **110** (15), 2125–2131.

36

Coronary Artery Anomalies

Grace Choi and Peter Koenig

Ann & Robert H. Lurie Children's Hospital of Chicago, Northwestern University Feinberg School of Medicine, Chicago, IL, USA

Coronary artery abnormalities, although relatively uncommon in neonates [1], may be life-threatening as isolated defects or important in the surgical management of other congenital heart defects [2]. In order to understand the types of coronary artery abnormalities that may be encountered in the neonatal period, it is useful to have an appreciation of the full spectrum of congenital heart abnormalities seen in the pediatric age group. Coronary abnormalities can be grouped into congenital or acquired (from another disease process). Congenital abnormalities can be further subdivided into groups. One such group consists of abnormalities of the origins either from the aorta (which may include a single or intramural origin of a coronary artery) or from the pulmonary artery, and stenosis or atresia of the ostia. Closely related to the latter include abnormalities of the course of the coronary arteries, such as interarterial, or anterior to the right ventricular outflow tract in patients with tetralogy of Fallot. There may also be abnormalities of the coronary artery terminations, namely, fistulae or coronary artery sinusoids. Coronary artery fistulae are discussed further in Chapter 38. Finally, congenital coronary arteries can also be seen as part of the findings of other congenital heart diseases. Coronary artery abnormalities associated with various types of congenital heart lesions are discussed in their respective chapters.

In the neonate, imaging consists mainly of echocardiography (2D and color) (Figure 36.1). Cardiac catheterization with coronary angiography (Figure 36.2) has also been used to demonstrate coronary artery origins as well as distribution. More recently, computed tomography (CT) has been utilized to demonstrate coronary artery anatomy in the neonate (Figures 36.3 and 36.4). Although advances have been made in cardiac magnetic resonance imaging (CMR), with improved resolution of coronary artery anatomy in older patients (Figure 36.5), the resolution required to image neonates and the higher heart rate that is typically involved make visualization of coronary artery anatomy in this patient population difficult. However, with continued advancements, CMR

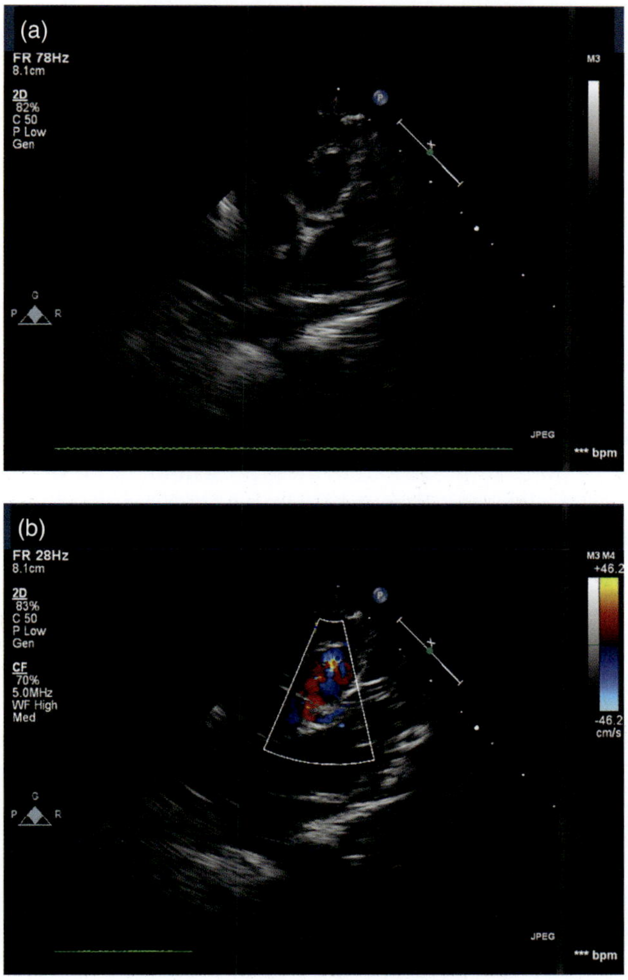

Figure 36.1 Anomalous origin of the left coronary artery from the pulmonary artery (ALCAPA). (a) Two-dimensional (2D) echocardiogram. Parasternal short-axis view of the anomalous left coronary artery arising from the posterior aspect of the pulmonary artery. (b) Color Doppler shows retrograde flow from the left anterior descending (LAD) coronary artery to the pulmonary artery (PA).

Visual Guide to Neonatal Cardiology, First Edition. Edited by Ernerio T. Alboliras, Ziyad M. Hijazi, Leo Lopez, and Donald J. Hagler.

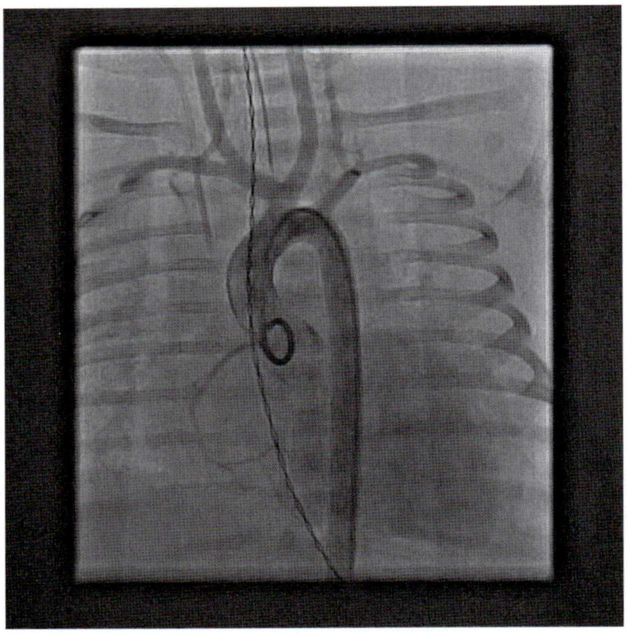

Figure 36.2 ALCAPA. Angiogram. Cardiac catheterization, with injection of contrast in the aortic root. The right coronary artery fills with contrast, which arises normally from the right sinus of Valsalva. The absence of the left coronary artery is noted.

will likely be a viable option for cross-sectional imaging of coronary arteries in the near future.

Anomalous origins of the coronary arteries are a rare congenital malformation, occurring in 0.17% of the pediatric population [3]. Rarely, these present in the newborn period. The most important primary or isolated coronary artery abnormalities are those with an abnormal origin of a coronary artery from the pulmonary artery (Figures 36.1, 36.2, and 36.6). Anomalous origin of the left coronary artery from the pulmonary artery (ALCAPA) typically presents in infancy, with an incidence of 0.023% of live births [4], or an incidence of 0.25–0.5% of children with congenital heart disease [5]. Anomalous origin of the left coronary artery (LCA) from the right pulmonary artery (RPA) have also been reported in neonates with AP window and tetralogy of Fallot [6, 7]. The incidence of anomalous origin of the right coronary artery from the pulmonary artery (ARCAPA) is even more rare, though this has been described [8]. The physiology of ALCAPA is one of coronary artery ischemia caused by decreased myocardial perfusion pressure which occurs with the decline of pulmonary vascular resistance. The history and laboratory findings are all consistent with an ischemic dilated cardiomyopathy. The main imaging modality is echocardiography. Additional imaging may be needed for confirmation, usually by angiography (Figure 36.4).

Less hemodynamically important congenital coronary artery lesions that may place patients at risk for sudden cardiac death include coronary artery origins from the opposite sinus of Valsalva. Symptoms do not typically arise in the neonatal period, though sudden death has been reported in infants [9]. An anomalous aortic origin of the coronary arteries (AAOCA) includes the right coronary artery from the left sinus of Valsalva and LCA from the right sinus of Valsalva. Invariably, these have an intramural course if there is a separate ostium and an interarterial course. Although echocardiography may provide the image of suspicion, confirmative imaging via CT or MRI can be performed when the child is older, when achieving a study with good anatomic resolution of the origins is possible and the need for sedation is no longer needed (Figures 36.3 and 36.4).

Myocardial ischemia from coronary ostial stenosis has also been described in neonates [10, 11]. This results in cardiac dysfunction with the associated signs and symptoms, and is a cause of early neonatal death. This may be suspected on echocardiography, but catheterization for coronary angiography may be needed to confirm the diagnosis (Figures 36.7, 36.8, and 36.9).

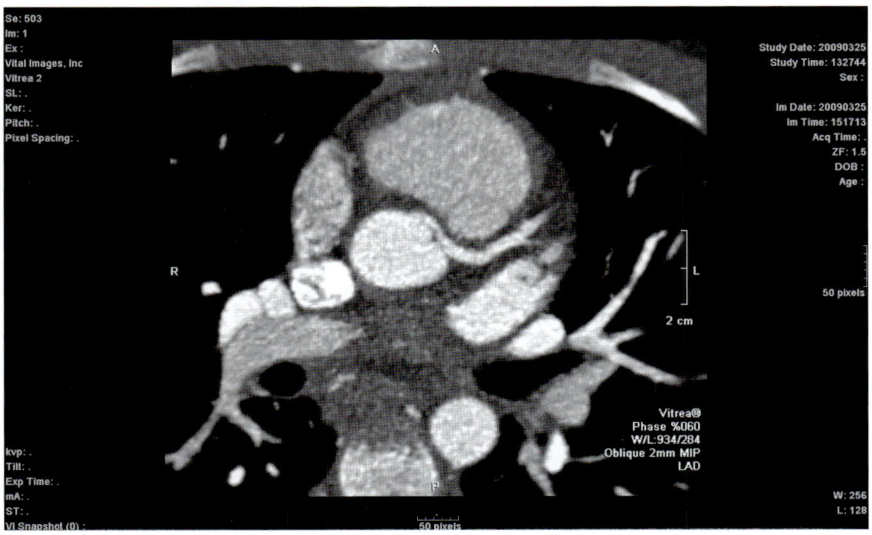

Figure 36.3 Computed tomography angiography (CTA) of anomalous aortic origin of the left coronary artery (LCA) from the right sinus of Valsalva.

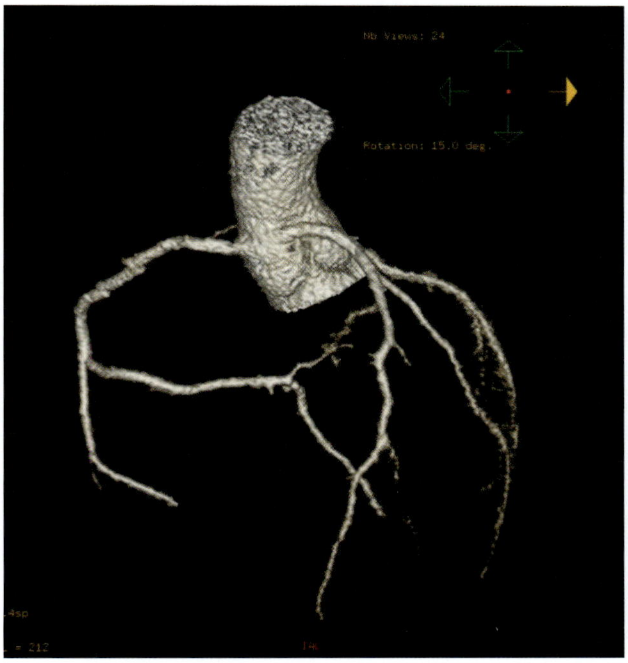

Figure 36.4 CTA with three-dimensional rendering of anomalous aortic origin of the LCA from the right sinus of Valsalva.

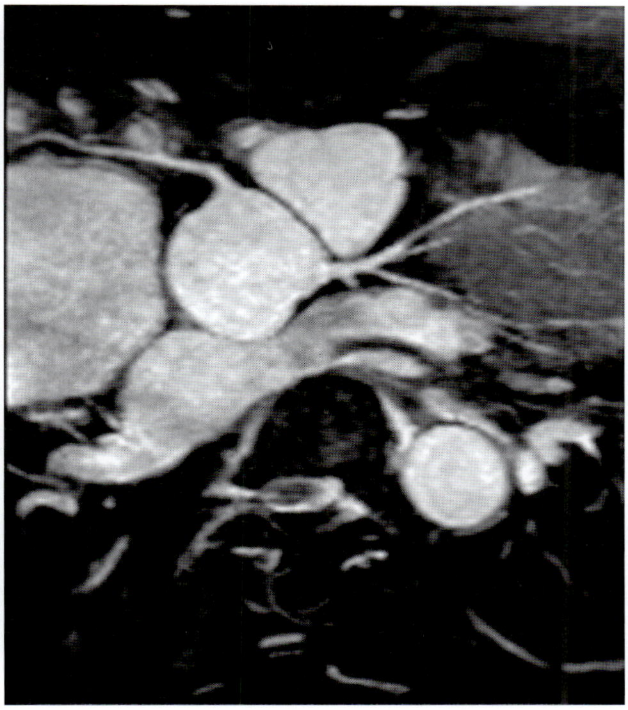

Figure 36.5 Normal coronary artery origins, as seen on cardiac MRI. The right and left coronary arteries arise from their respective sinuses of Valsalva.

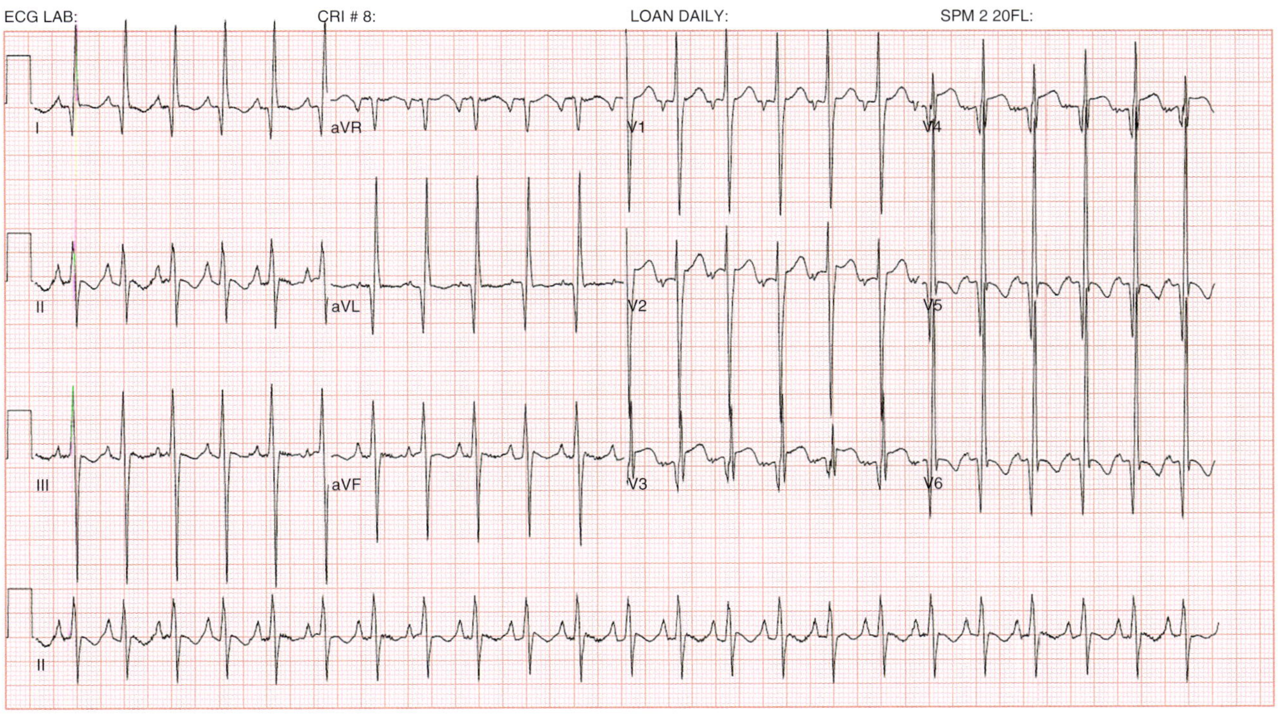

Figure 36.6 ALCAPA electrocardiogram. ECG demonstrates the typical pattern in an infant with ALCAPA. Q waves are present in leads I and AVF.

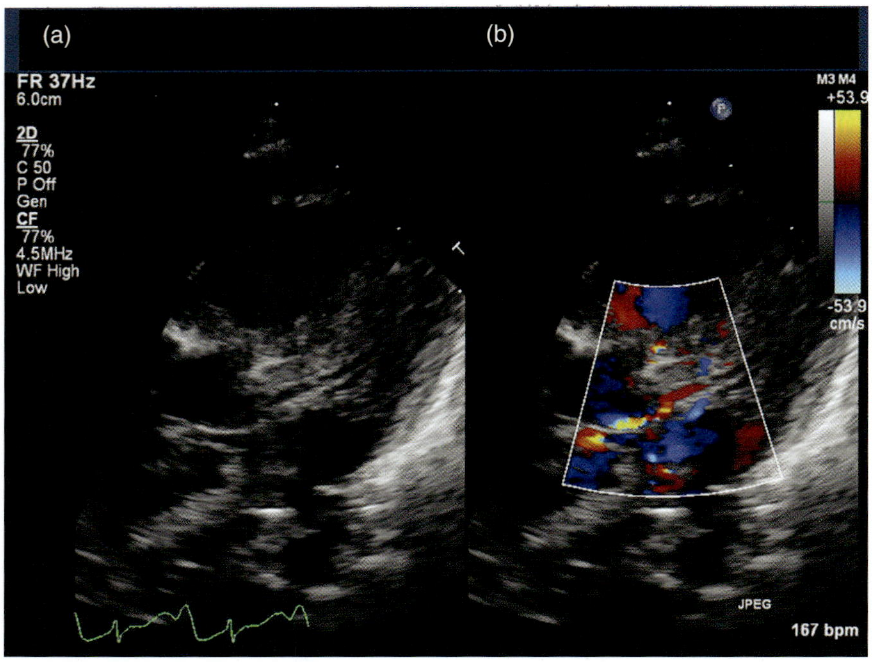

Figure 36.7 Left coronary artery stenosis. Echocardiogram in the short axis of the aortic root in: (a) 2D; and (b) with color Doppler. The left coronary artery ostium is located in the posterior aspect of the left sinus of Valsalva. Color Doppler shows turbulent flow across the LCA ostium, suggestive of ostial stenosis.

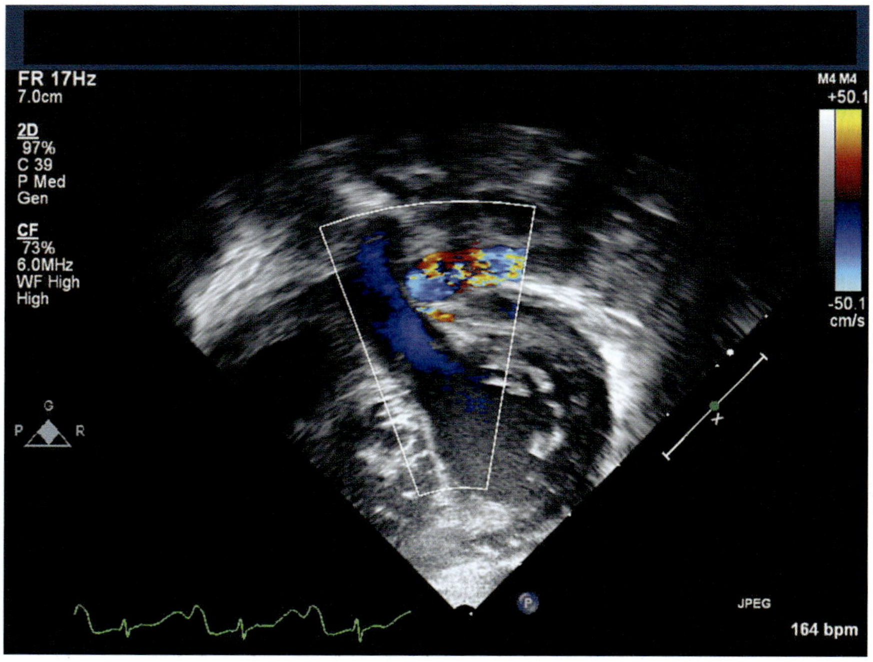

Figure 36.8 Echocardiogram of left coronary artery stenosis. Apical view of the aortic root. Turbulent flow across the proximal left coronary artery.

The acquired coronary artery abnormalities are unlikely to be encountered in neonates but should still be considered. Within each type of acquired abnormality, there are a number of causes including primary diseases which may be congenital. Examples of this are coronary thrombosis, disruption, narrowing after an intervention involving the coronary arteries, stenosis caused by a prior inflammatory illness (e.g., Kawasaki disease), or inborn error of metabolism. Although unlikely to be seen in the neonate, these are mentioned for completeness. Those associated with other congenital heart defects will most likely be diagnosed as part of the cardiac evaluation or caused by signs and symptoms of myocardial ischemia, including postsurgical complication of arterial switch for transposition of the great arteries involving transfer of the coronary arteries.

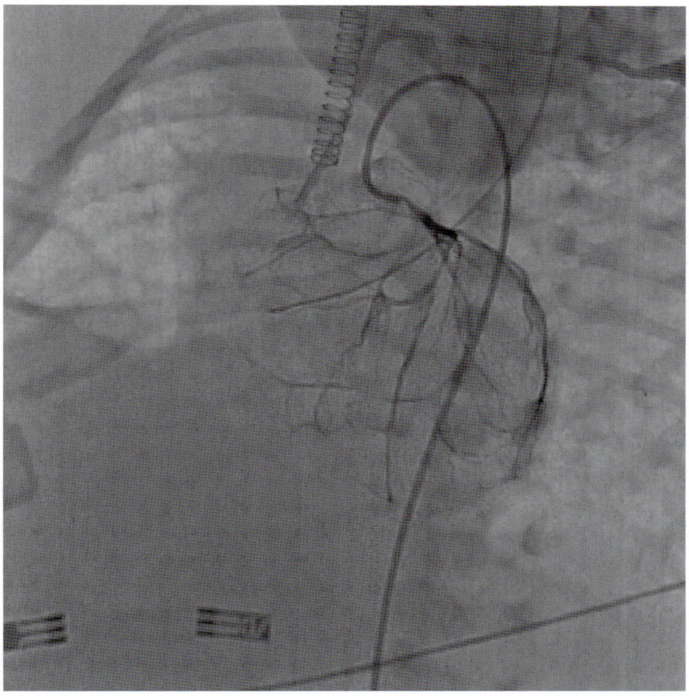

Figure 36.9 Left coronary artery stenosis. Cardiac catheterization with selective injection of the left coronary artery shows single left coronary artery. The proximal coronary artery is narrowed.

References

1 Kimbiris D, Iskandrian AS, Segal BL, Bemis CE. (1978) Anomalous aortic origin of coronary arteries. *Circulation*, **58**, 606.

2 Cieslinski G, Rapprich B, Kober G. (1993) Coronary artery anomalies: incidence and importance. *Clin Cardiol*, **16**, 717–715.

3 Davis JA, Cecchin F, Jones TK, Portman MA. (2001) Major coronary artery anomalies in a pediatric population: incidence and clinical importance. *J Am Coll Cardiol*, **37** (2), 593–597.

4 Brotherton H, Phillip RK. (2008) Anomalous left coronary artery from pulmonary artery (ALCAPA) in infants: a 5-year review in a defined birth cohort. *Eur J Pediatr*, **167** (1), 43–46.

5 Cherian KM, Bharati S, Rao SG. (1994) Surgical correction of anomalous origin of the left coronary artery from the pulmonary artery. *J Card Surg*, **9** (4), 386–391.

6 Morell VO, Feccia M, Cullen S, Elliot MJ. (1998) Anomalous coronarpy artery with tetralogy of Fallot and aortopulmonary window. *Ann Thorac Surg*, **66** (4), 1403–1405.

7 McMahon CJ, DiBardino DJ, Undar A, Fraser CD. (2002) Anomalous origin of the left coronary artery from the right pulmonary artery in association with tyupe III aortopulmonary window and interrupted aortic arch. *Ann Thorac Surg*, **74** (3), 919–921.

8 Williams IA, Gersony WM, Hellenbrand WE. (2006) Anomalous right coronary artery arising form the pulmonary artery: a report of 7 cases and a review of the literature. *Am Heart J*, **152** (5), 1004.

9 Liberthson RR, Gang DL, Custer J. (1983) Sudden death in an infant with aberrant origin of the right coronary artery from the left sinus of Valsalva of the aorta: case report and review of the literature. *Pediatr Cardiol*, **4**, 45-48.

10 Laux D, Bessieres B, Houyel L, *et al.* (2013) Early neonatal death and congenital left coronary abnormalities: ostial atresia, stenosis and anomalous aortic origin. *Arch Cardiovasc Dis*, **106** (4), 202–208.

11 Harada K, Fujiseki Y, Ryugin Y, Seki I, Sakurai I. (1980) Myocardial infarction and left coronary ostial stenosis in infancy simulating anomalous origin of the left coronary artery: a case report. *Jpn Heart J*, **21** (3), 435–442.

37

Aorto-Left Ventricular Tunnel

Patrick W. O'Leary

Division of Pediatric Cardiology, Mayo Clinic, Rochester, MN, USA

Aorto-ventricular tunnel is an abnormal, non-valved, extracardiac channel between the ascending aorta and a ventricular cavity [1]. Approximately 90% of these channels connect the aorta to the left ventricle (Figures 37.1 and 37.2). Such tunnels are rare cardiovascular malformations, representing less than 0.05% of all congenital heart defects. Tunnels allow flow of blood in both systole and diastole. As a result, systolic ventricular ejection occurs through both the semilunar valve and the tunnel. However, in diastole flow reverses and is directed from the aorta to the ventricle. Thus, the pathophysiology of aorto-left ventricular tunnel (AoLVT) mimics that of aortic valve regurgitation. Most tunnels are large and result in significant ventricular volume overload and infantile onset of congestive heart failure. Clinically, aorto-ventricular tunnel must be distinguished from other connections between the aortic root and adjacent structures, such as a ruptured sinus of Valsalva or aortopulmonary window. This chapter reviews the anatomy, associated cardiac anomalies, imaging manifestations, and treatment of the patient with aorto-ventricular tunnels, focusing on the more frequently encountered AoLVT.

Although it is not reviewed in detail, it should be noted that cases of aorto-right ventricular tunnel (AoRVT) have been reported, albeit very rarely. The patient with a large AoRVT will present with a large left-to-right shunt and severe right ventricular and/or pulmonary artery hypertension. Physical findings and hemodynamic consequences are similar to the patient with an aorto-pulmonary window (prominent aortic diastolic run-off, a murmur, and signs of pulmonary hypertension). However, both ventricles will be volume overloaded by the AoRVT, whereas the patient with aorto-pulmonary window will face additional volume to the left heart only. When the communicating AoRVT is smaller, the left-to-right shunt may be continuous, but in the absence of coexisting pulmonary outflow stenosis, the volume of left-to-right shunt flow will usually still be large.

Aorto-Left Ventricular Tunnel: Anatomic Characteristics

An AoLVT will have its aortic origin in the tubular portion of the ascending aorta (superior to the sinotubular junction; Figures 37.1, 37.2 and 37.3). Nearly 80% of these aortic orifices are centered above the right coronary sinus of Valsalva (Figure 37.3) [1]. Most of these orifices are large and have a large proximal extracardiac channel (Hovaguimian type 2 or 4; Figure 37.2). Those with smaller, elliptical aortic orifices present some restriction to flow and may have reduced or delayed symptom severity (Hovaguimian type 1 and 3; Figure 37.1). The mid-portion of the tunnel passes outside the heart, between the muscular subpulmonary infundibulum and the aortic sinuses (Figure 37.3). The ventricular orifice of the AoLVT is found on the left ventricular outflow septal surface beneath the left–right coronary commissure [1]. In contrast, rupture of a dilated sinus of Valsalva occurs below the sinotubular junction within the sinus itself. These ruptures tend to connect relatively directly to a cardiac chamber, usually the right atrium or ventricle (Figure 37.4). A ruptured sinus will usually have a tapering dimension (smaller exit than entrance) and may even have multiple exit orifices. The aorto-ventricular tunnel has a single orifice at the entrance and its exit. Tunnels arising above the left sinus have more varied ventricular exit points. In contrast to both a tunnel and a ruptured sinus, the aortopulmonary window has virtually no length and is best considered a failure of aortico-pulmonary septation (Figure 37.5). As a result, there is no shunt at the ventricular level, rather the shunt volume travels directly from the aorta to the pulmonary circulation.

Visual Guide to Neonatal Cardiology, First Edition. Edited by Ernerio T. Alboliras, Ziyad M. Hijazi, Leo Lopez, and Donald J. Hagler.

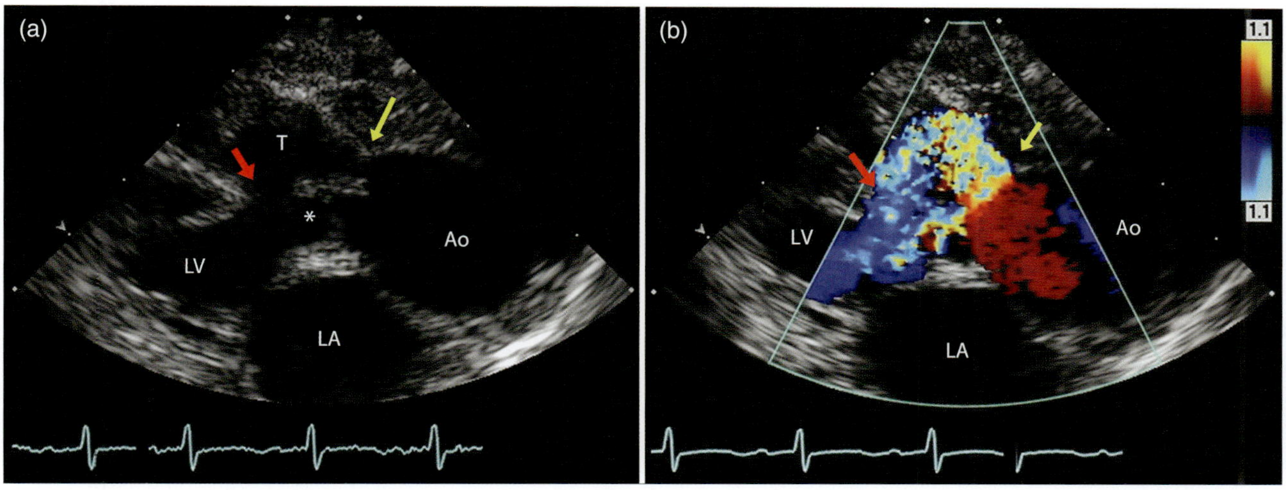

Figure 37.1 Parasternal long-axis images of a neonate with a type 3 (intraseptal aneurysm) aorto-left ventricular tunnel (AoLVT). (a) A two-dimensional anatomic scan; and (b) the prominent diastolic flow from the aorta, through the tunnel into the ventricular outflow tract using color flow Doppler. The yellow arrow indicates the aortic orifice of the tunnel, which in this case was elliptical and somewhat restrictive. The red arrow indicates the ventricular orifice which in this patient was quite large. The asterisk is positioned in the immediate subaortic portion of the left ventricular outflow tract. Ao, aorta; LA, left atrium; LV, left ventricle; T, aorto-ventricular tunnel.

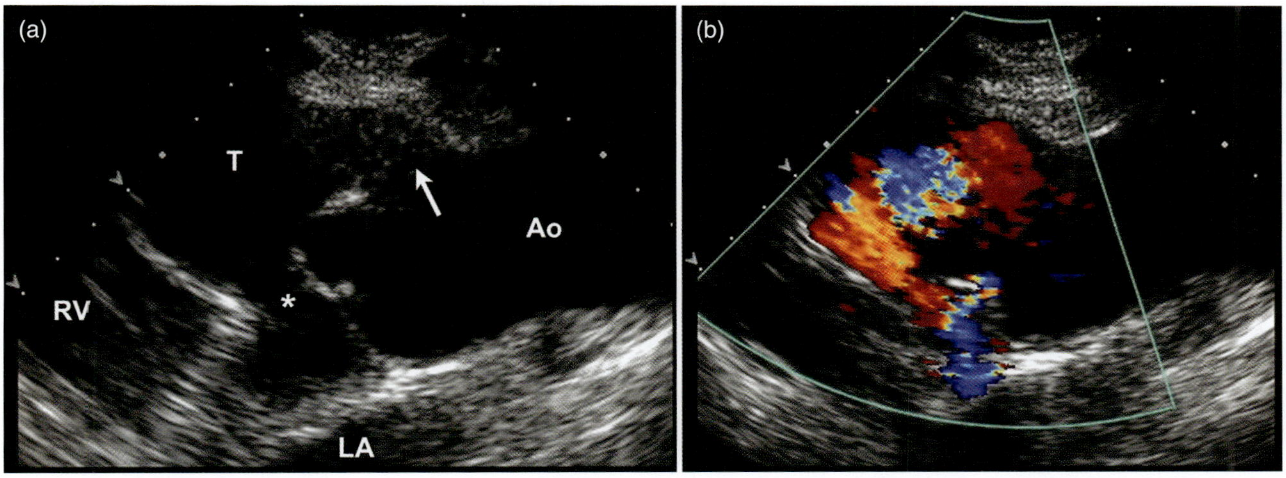

Figure 37.2 Echocardiographic long-axis images of a type 4 aorto-left ventricular tunnel. Both the aortic and ventricular orifice of this tunnel were large and the amount of diastolic flow was torrential (b). The arrow in (a) indicates the aortic orifice from the tubular ascending aorta, just above the sinotubular junction. The asterisk indicates the left ventricular exit orifice. Both the inlet and exit portions of this tunnel were severely dilated (T). The aortic valve had mild central regurgitation, but no stenosis. RV, right ventricle.

Associated Anomalies

Most AoLVTs occur without other congenital cardiac malformations. When additional abnormalities are present, they most often involve the semilunar valves and coronary arteries. Reports suggest that 25–45% of patients with an AoLVT will also have aortic valve abnormalities, most often involving leaflet dysplasia and stenosis [1, 2]. Pulmonary valve stenosis has been observed in less than 10% of cases. Patency of the ductus arteriosus was reported in almost 20%. However, this relationship may be skewed by the typically young age at which AoLVT presents. Coronary arterial abnormalities can coexist with these tunnels. The most common coronary malformation, occurring in about 5%, is anomalous origin of the right coronary artery from the body of the tunnel rather than from the aortic sinus. Presence of such an anomalous coronary origin will significantly impact the approach to repair.

Clinical Presentation

AoLVT is associated with widening of the aortic pulse pressure, and a loud "to and fro" murmur on physical examination. Most patients develop symptoms of heart

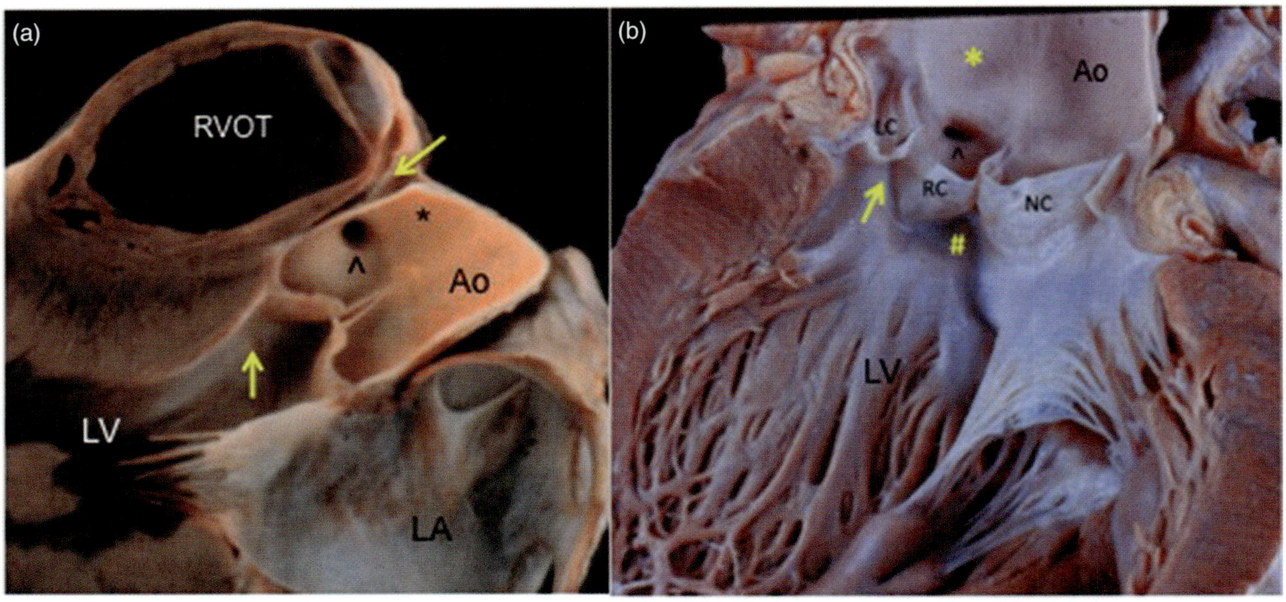

Figure 37.3 Two normal anatomic specimens that have been labeled to highlight the landmarks that are pertinent to aorto-left ventricular tunnel (AoLVT). (a) The left panel is presented in a manner analogous to a parasternal long-axis echocardiographic image. The right yellow arrow indicates the plane between the aorta and the right ventricular outflow tract/main pulmonary artery through which an AoLVT would "travel." The left arrow (more vertically oriented) indicates the area on the ventricular septum where most exit orifices tunnels would be found. The asterisk indicates the area of the tubular ascending aorta that gives rise to the aortic orifice. (b) The right panel is a specimen that is present in an inflow–outflow format and shows some of the same features of the internal ventricular and aortic anatomy. The arrow in (a) is oriented toward the right–left commissure of the aortic valve. This is area where the ventricular orifice of an AoLVT would be found. The "^" marks the orifice of the right coronary artery in both panels. Ao, aorta; LA, left atrium; LC, left coronary leaflet of the aortic valve; LV, left ventricle; NC, non-coronary leaflet of the aortic valve; RC, right coronary leaflet of the aortic valve; RVOT, right ventricular outflow tract; # indicates the membranous ventricular septum.

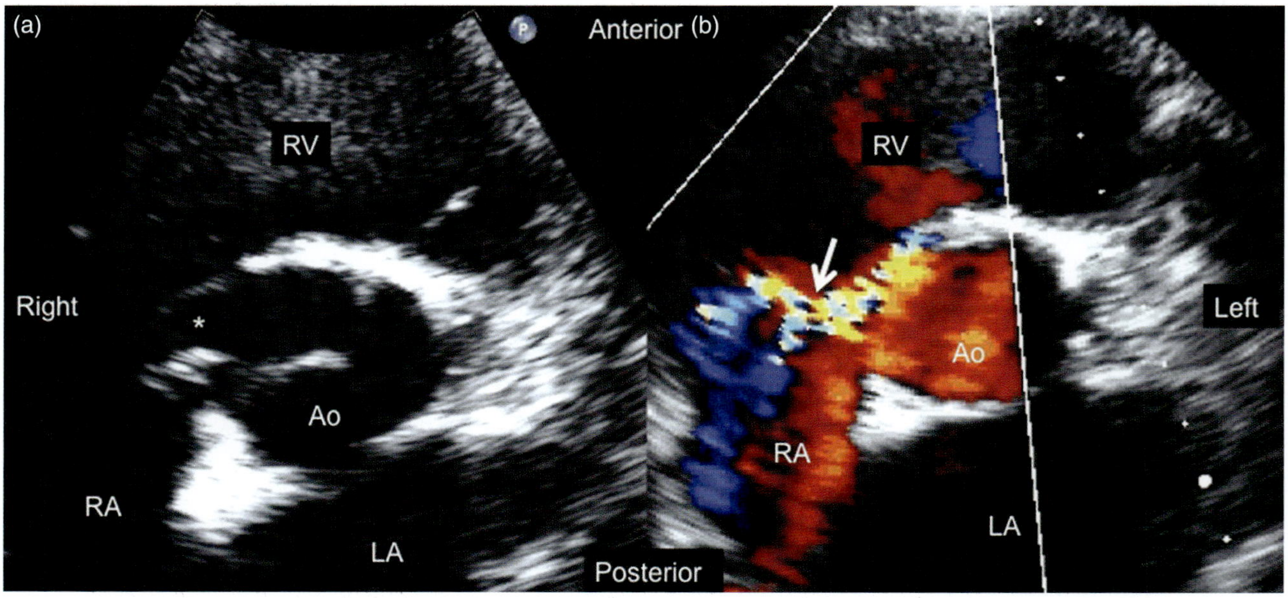

Figure 37.4 Ruptured right aortic sinus of Valsalva. (a) A two-dimensional, short-axis echocardiographic image of a ruptured sinus of Valsalva aneurysm. Note the tapering of the aneurysm from the aortic end to its right atrial exit (*). (b) A color flow Doppler diastolic image showing the aortic to right atrial shunt (arrow). Note that there are actually two defects (ruptures) in the distal sinus, creating a "Y-shaped" color jet. The exit was into the right atrium, so the shunt flow was continuous in this case. Ao, aorta; LA, left atrium; RA, right atrium; RV, right ventricle.

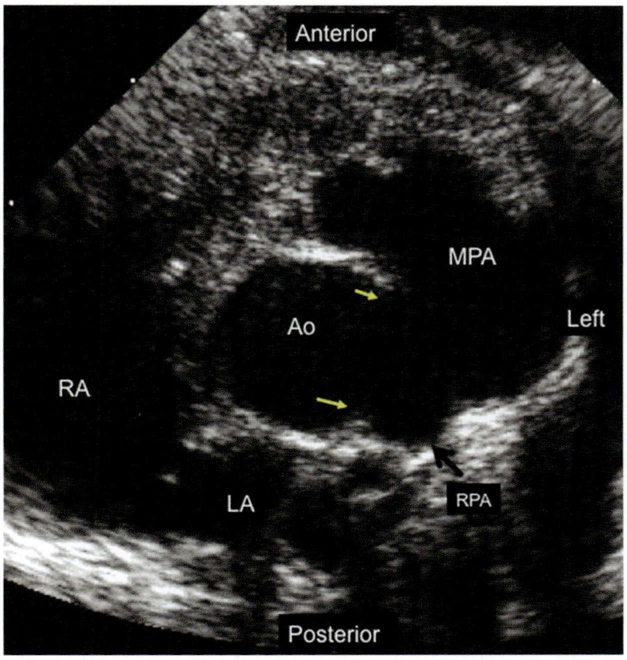

Figure 37.5 Aorto-pulmonary window. This is a horizontal (short axis) plane echocardiographic image demonstrating the proximal ascending aorta (Ao) in cross-section and the main pulmonary artery (MPA). The yellow arrows indicate the anterior and posterior edge of a large communication between the Ao and the MPA, an aorto-pulmonary window. In contrast to both an aorto-ventricular tunnel and a ruptured sinus of Valsalva aneurysm, this malformation has no "length." Rather, it is essentially an absence of the walls separating the two great arteries. LA, left atrium; RA, right atrium; RPA, right pulmonary artery origin.

failure during the first year of life, although isolated adult presentations of smaller tunnels have been reported. The course and severity of heart failure is variable; ranging from prenatal hydrops, to the typical infantile onset of heart failure with a prominent systolic/diastolic murmur, to rapid neonatal hemodynamic collapse (combined regurgitation and obstructive physiology), to years of compensated function without symptoms [2]. Those with the most rapid decline and demise tend to be patients with large tunnels and severe aortic outflow obstruction.

Prenatal presentation carries a worst prognosis. Early reports suggested greater than 50% mortality in those detected by fetal echocardiography. A more recent series has shown improved survival, but this likely represents an enhanced ability to detect less severe cases. The outlook remains very poor for the fetus with prenatal onset of heart failure resulting from an aorto-ventricular tunnel.

Diagnostic Methods

Echocardiography is the most common and useful imaging modality for the infant with aorto-ventricular tunnel. Standard transthoracic echocardiographic imaging is usually sufficient to detect the anomaly, define the pertinent anatomy and hemodynamics, as well as plan surgical interventions in neonates and infants (Figures 37.1, 37.2, 37.6, and 37.7). Cardiac magnetic resonance scanning and computed tomography can

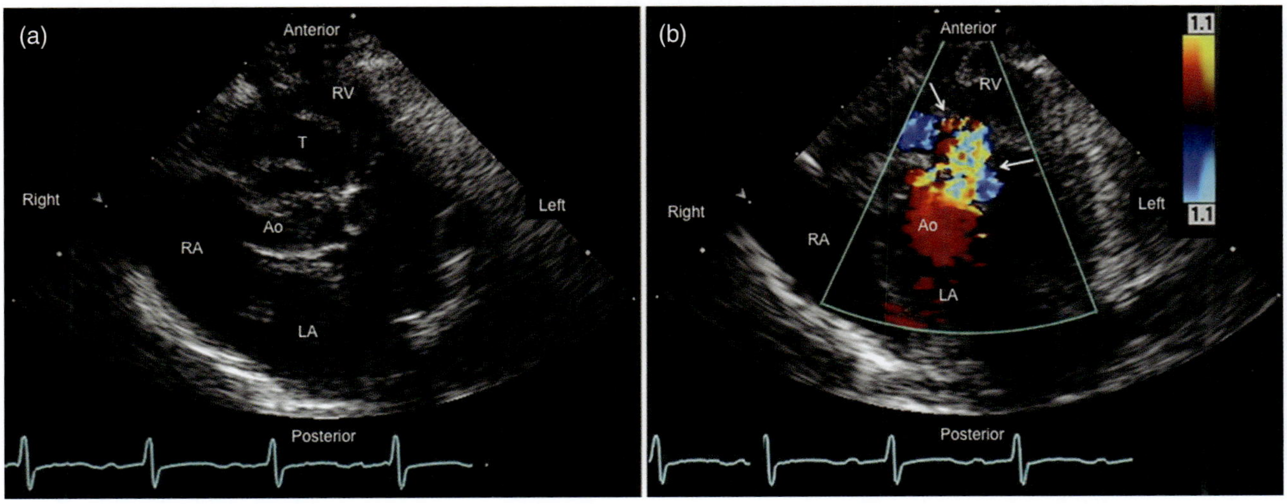

Figure 37.6 Parasternal short-axis views of a neonate with an aorto-left ventricular tunnel (AoLVT). (a) A two-dimensional anatomic scan and (b) color Doppler image highlights the diastolic flow from the aorta into the tunnel's aortic orifice (arrows). The body of the tunnel lies between the right aortic sinus of Valsalva and the right ventricular outflow tract (RV) and penetrates the upper ventricular septum to empty into the left ventricular outflow tract (out of plane, see Figure 37.1). Ao, aorta; LA, left atrium; RA, right atrium; T, aorto-ventricular tunnel.

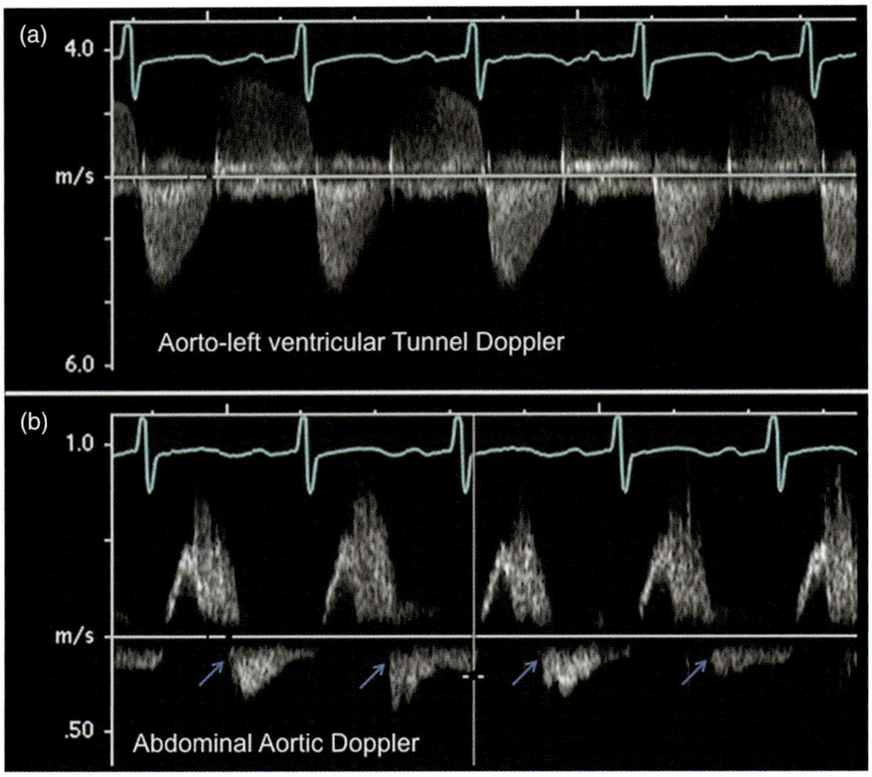

Figure 37.7 A Doppler evaluation of a neonate with an aorto-left ventricular tunnel (AoLVT). (a) A continuous wave Doppler tracing of the flow through the AoLVT itself. The diastolic signal (above the baseline) represents the "regurgitant" flow traveling from the aorta, through the tunnel, and into the left ventricle. The systolic ejection signal (below the baseline) has an increases maximum velocity, consistent with a moderate pressure gradient between the ventricle and the aorta due to "stenosis" of both the aortic valve and the AoLVT (type 3). (b) The lower image shows the pulsed wave Doppler signal taken from the patient's abdominal aorta. In addition to normal systolic forward flow (above the baseline), there is also prominent, holodiastolic reversal of flow (arrows). This reversed flow is secondary to the large diastolic flow through the AoLVT into the ventricle and is indistinguishable from the pattern created by severe aortic valve regurgitation.

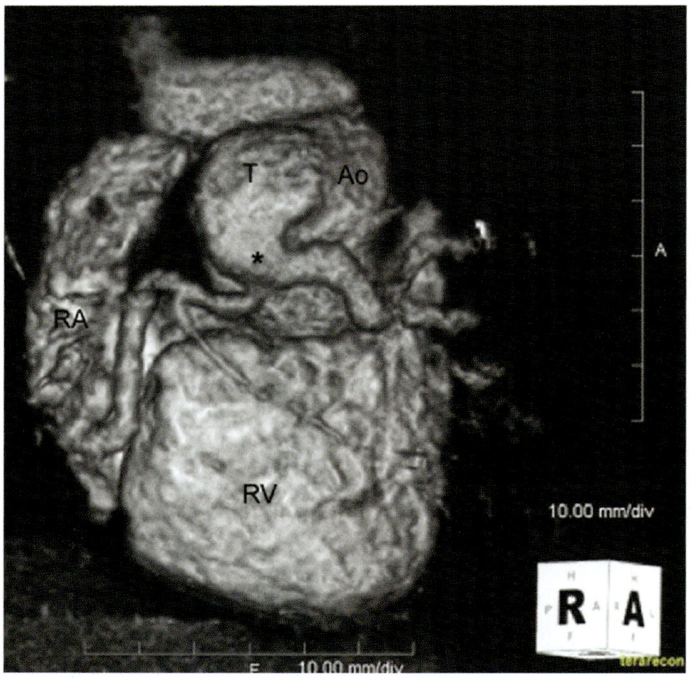

Figure 37.8 Aorto-left ventricular tunnel (AoVLT) and anomalous origin of the right coronary artery. This image is a surface rendered three-dimensional reconstruction created during a cardiac CT scan of a patient with a type 4 AoLVT. The AoLVT (T) arose from the tubular ascending aorta (Ao) and emptied into the left ventricle in the usual manner. This image reveals that the right coronary artery (*) originates from the distal aspect of the tunnel. The unbranched segment is short with a large anterior branch and a small right/posterior branch noted immediately beyond the asterisk. A, anterior; R, right; RA, right atrium; RV, right ventricle.

be used in select cases to address issues that were not resolved by the initial echocardiographic evaluation (Figure 37.8). These alternative imaging strategies can be very helpful in defining the origin of the right coronary artery, especially in the older patient. Invasive studies (cardiac catheterization with angiocardiography) are rarely necessary, unless it is not possible to define coronary arterial anatomy by any other means.

The images in Figures 37.1, 37.2, and 37.6 illustrate the typical echocardiographic appearance of a large AoLVT. Prenatal detection of AoLVT requires a high index of suspicion, especially when the physiology of aortic

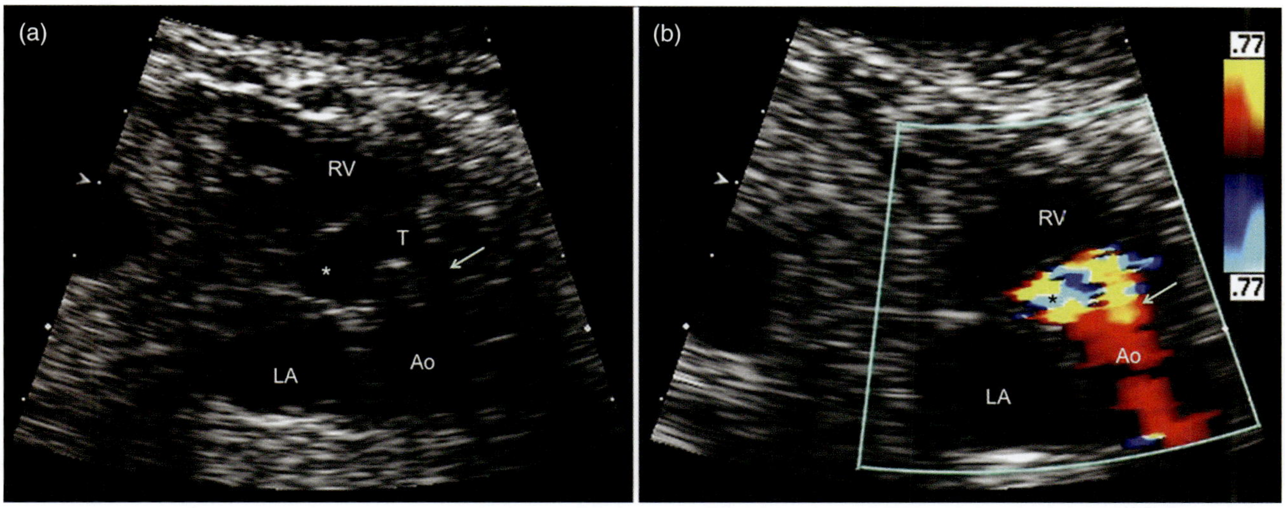

Figure 37.9 These images were taken during a prenatal echocardiogram performed because the fetus was thought to have truncus arteriosus with truncal valve regurgitation. The images oriented similar to parasternal long-axis transthoracic echocardiographic images. There was a normal pulmonary valve and no ventricular septal defect, eliminating truncus arteriosus as a possible diagnosis.
(a) An extracardiac, paravalvar connection between the ascending aorta (Ao) and the left ventricular outflow tract (white asterisk), confirming the presence of an aorto-left ventricular tunnel (AOLVT). (b) Color flow Doppler imaging revealed not only significant diastolic flow through the AoLVT (arrow), but also aortic valve regurgitation (black asterisk). Despite the combination of these two abnormalities, the fetus did not develop hydrops. He did require neonatal repair of both the AoLVT and the aortic valve with eventual aortic valve replacement later in childhood. He continues to do well postoperatively. LA, left atrium; RV, right ventricle; T, aorto-ventricular tunnel.

regurgitation is present (Figure 37.9). Cross-sectional imaging from the parasternal long (Figures 37.1, 37.2, and 37.9) and short-axis positions (Figure 37.6) usually provide most of the anatomic insights into the tunnel and its adjacent structures. In modified long-axis views, the body of the AoLVT will appear as a vascular space anterior to the aorta and penetrating the basal portion of the interventricular septum to empty into the left ventricular cavity (Figures 37.1, 37.2, and 37.9). Tunnels that open into the right ventricle are more optimally visualized in the short-axis view, because the body of the tunnel lies more parallel to the transverse axis of the heart.

Color Doppler imaging will confirm the presence of to and fro flow within or through the tunnel (Figures 37.1, 37.2, 37.6, and 37.9). Coexisting aortic valve and coronary arterial abnormalities can also be detected in these views. Apical, subcostal, and suprasternal images can provide additional confirmation of the hemodynamic significance of the tunnel. Doppler flow mapping illustrates the abnormal physiology (analogous to severe aortic regurgitation) and can be used to define the severity of aortic outflow obstruction (Figure 37.7).

Management

Medical therapy provides only temporary palliation for heart failure symptoms. Surgery to eliminate a tunnel with significant blood flow should be undertaken without delay, even in asymptomatic patients. Such early intervention is warranted as the risk of surgery is low and likelihood of long-term ventricular dysfunction is increased if repair occurs after 6 months of age. Repair consists of closing the tunnel in a way that supports the aortic valve, and does not impair ventricular outflow or coronary blood flow. This is usually accomplished by transaortic patch closure of both aortic and ventricular orifices of the AoLVT. Closure of the ventricular orifice, in addition, supports the right coronary leaflet and theoretically reduces the incidence and severity of late regurgitation. When a coronary artery arises directly from the tunnel, more complex repairs are required. Most often, the anomalous coronary artery is surgically "transferred" and reattached to the ascending aorta (similar to the technique used in the arterial switch operation). Catheter-based interventions (device closure) are not usually appropriate because of the small size of most of these patients, and the fact that such devices do not give the extra support to the aortic valve that is gained with surgical closure. Associated abnormalities should be treated as clinically indicated, either separately or at the time of repair.

Aortic valve dysfunction is the primary late concern after successful repair. Aortic valve regurgitation can progress, with up to half of patients reported to need aortic valve replacement later in life. Significant progression of aortic root enlargement has also been reported [3]. It is not clear whether aortic enlargement after repair carries an increased risk of dissection in adulthood. However, the histopathology in patients with AoLVT and severe root dilation results in findings similar to cystic medial degeneration.

Conclusions

AoLVTs are rare cardiac malformations that most often cause early onset heart failure. Patients present with signs and symptoms similar to those for severe aortic valve regurgitation. Echocardiography will detect an anterior extracardiac channel connecting the tubular ascending aorta to the left ventricular outflow tract in most of these patients. Treatment involves early surgical closure and results in excellent short and intermediate term outcomes. Progressive aortic valve regurgitation is the most common late problem, highlighting the potential benefit to patch closing both the aortic and ventricular orifices of the tunnel in an effort to provide added support to the aortic valve leaflets.

References

1 McKay R, Anderson RH, Cook AC. (2002) The aorto-ventricular tunnels. *Cardiol Young*, **12**, 563–580.
2 Martins JD, Sherwood MC, Mayer JE Jr, *et al.* (2004) Aortico-left ventricular tunnel: 35-year experience. *J Am Coll Cardiol*, **44**, 446–450.
3 Honjo O, Ishino K, Kawada M, *et al.* (2006) Late outcome after repair of aortico-left ventricular tunnel: 10-year follow-up. *Circ J*, **70**, 939–941.

38

Coronary Cameral Fistulas

Gareth J. Morgan[1] *and Shakeel A. Qureshi*[2]

[1] *Children's Hospital of Colorado; University of Colorado School of Medicine, Aurora, CO, USA*
[2] *Evelina London Children's Hospital, London, UK*

Definition

Coronary cameral fistulas (CCFs) are a group of conditions in which an abnormal connection (fistula) exists between a coronary artery and one of the cardiac chambers. The morphology, origin, and exit points are variable, allowing potential connections between any coronary artery branch and any cardiac chamber, venous channel, or pulmonary artery [1].

Etiology

The vast majority of CCFs are congenital but fistulous communications can also be created following surgical or percutaneous interventions. The abnormal coronary connections that course from the ventricles in the setting of pulmonary atresia with intact ventricular septum or hypoplastic left heart syndrome should be discussed in the context of their primary disease entity and will not be discussed further here [2].

Embryologically, CCFs arise because of incomplete regression of the primordial vessels, which supply blood to the developing myocardium prior to the establishment of the true coronary arteries. This accounts for the wide distribution of the anomalies throughout the coronary tree [3].

Pathophysiology and Natural History

Although rare, CCF is the most common congenital coronary anomaly. The incidence is unknown; however, it is likely to be between 1 in 100 000 and 1 in 10 000. Approximately 60% arise from the right coronary artery; 20% from the left descending coronary artery; and 20% from the left main stem or circumflex artery. The anatomy of CCF varies from a short connection arising proximally and discretely from a coronary artery as a side branch (Figure 38.1), to one that is large, tortuous, and distal, effectively an abnormal extension of the native coronary artery itself (Figure 38.2). Patients with small tortuous CCFs can remain completely asymptomatic and undetected throughout life, while large, short, window-like fistulas can present in infancy with heart failure and/or coronary ischemia [4, 5].

Patients with CCFs may present with:

1) *Incidental murmur:* the auscultatory findings depend on the exit chamber and the pressure difference between the coronary artery and that chamber during the cardiac cycle. The typical murmur is continuous, peaking in diastole when the pressure gradient is maximal.
2) *Heart failure:* presentation with heart failure requires a significant left-to-right shunt with coronary blood entering the pulmonary circulation. The clinical features are the same as any other cause of left-to-right shunt causing heart failure.
3) *Coronary ischemia:* occurs because of syphoning of blood away from the coronary circulation into a sump provided by the pulmonary circulation. CCFs presenting in neonatal life with ischemia and dysfunction have been known to regress with only non-specific supportive management [6].
4) *Arrhythmia and sudden death:* patients with CCFs having unexplained ventricular arrhythmias and sudden death have been reported, although this is extremely rare [7].

Diagnosis

Presentation with the symptoms and signs above should prompt investigation with ECG and echocardiography. The key echocardiographic features include a larger than normal coronary artery brought about by increased flow into the low pressure exit chamber. The fistulous exit point can be identified by color Doppler flow mapping.

Visual Guide to Neonatal Cardiology, First Edition. Edited by Ernerio T. Alboliras, Ziyad M. Hijazi, Leo Lopez, and Donald J. Hagler.

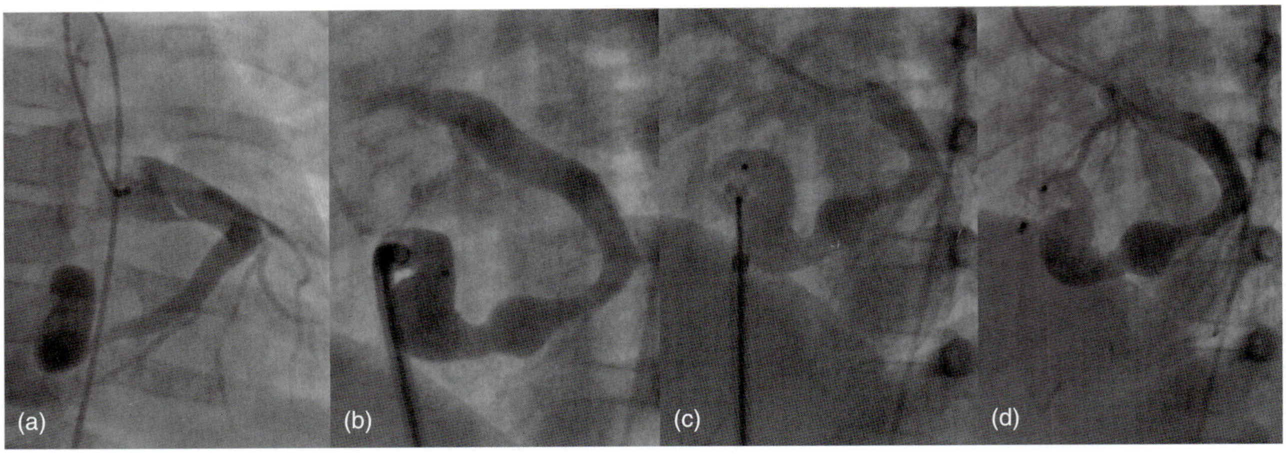

Figure 38.1 This large circumflex artery fistula drains into the right atrium, seen here during occlusion with a device designed for the ductus arteriosus. (a) Right anterior oblique projection shows selective injection into the dilated left coronary artery with contrast exiting into the atrium. (b) Left anterior oblique projection shows an injection through the delivery sheath for the occluder, which is positioned at the exit point of the fistula. This position was achieved by first forming a guide wire loop through the fistula from the native coronary artery. (c,d) Left anterior oblique projections show the device just before release and then after release. The device is defined by a radio-opaque marker on either end; best seen in (d).

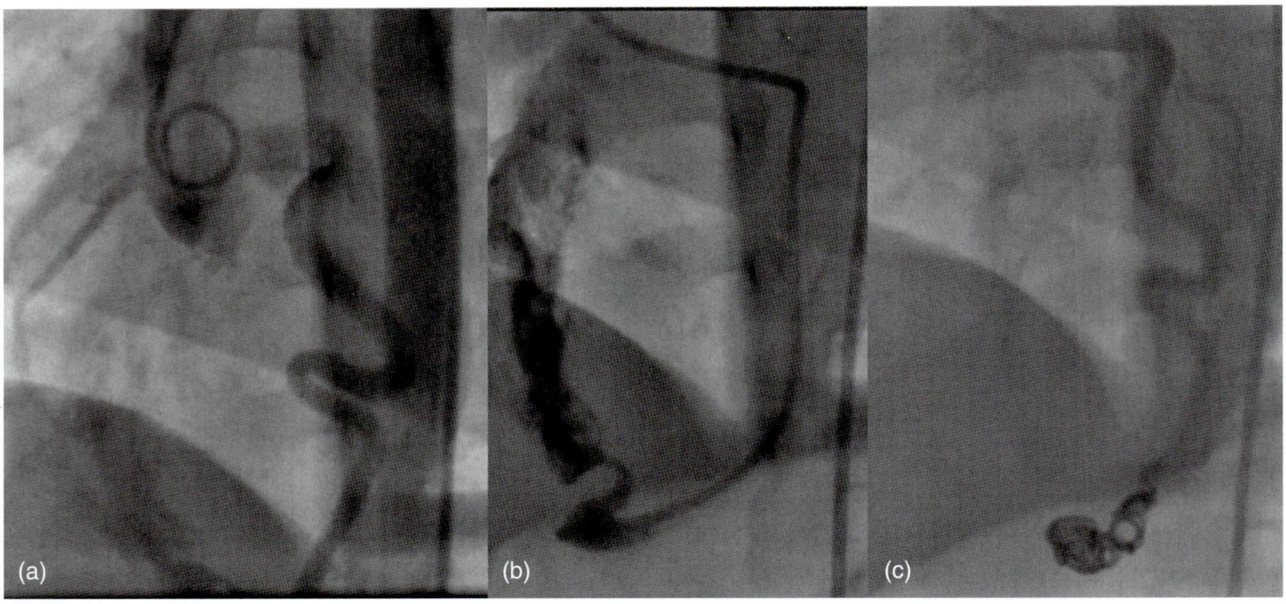

Figure 38.2 This distal left coronary artery fistula drains into the right ventricle. Occlusion here was achieved using coils which were deployed directly from a catheter placed through the length of the coronary artery. All three panels show left anterior oblique projections. (a) An aortic root injection that delineates a dilated left coronary artery system with a distal fistulous connection into the right ventricle. (b) An injection in the coronary artery at the point at which it becomes fistulous. This describes the area at which occlusive coils are then deployed (c).

The course of the fistula can sometimes be traced from the origin to the exit by color Doppler, allowing appreciation of the degree of tortuosity and relationship to standard coronary branches. Pulsed and continuous wave Doppler interrogation should show a continuous trace with more prominent diastolic than systolic flow. The diastolic predominance is because the aortic root (the origin of the coronary fistula flow) usually has the highest diastolic pressure in the circulation, resulting in a pressure gradient to the exit chamber. The exact nature of the flow pattern will depend on the exit chamber involved and its pressure profile.

Following echocardiographic diagnosis, a decision needs to be made about further diagnostic imaging. In some cases, it may be appropriate to proceed straight to cardiac catheterization with a view to occlusion of the defect at the same procedure. However, a more staged approach with diagnostic angiography, computed tomography (CT), or magnetic resonance imaging (MRI) may be taken [8, 9].

Management Strategies

The management strategy depends on symptoms or evidence of deleterious effects on the heart and circulatory function. Evidence of chamber dilation or an increase in pulmonary artery pressure should be sought. In these cases, standard medical management to control heart failure should be instituted alongside contemplation of definitive treatment [10].

Symptomatic coronary ischemia or evidence of ischemia on electrocardiogram in an infant with a CCF should prompt consideration of definitive management. Patients presenting with ventricular or atrial arrhythmias should have careful exclusion of other causes of the arrhythmia before focusing management on what may be an incidental CCF [11, 12].

Standard indications for definitive surgical or interventional therapy consist of:

1) Symptomatic from heart failure, arrhythmia, or coronary ischemia;
2) Asymptomatic but with echocardiographic evidence of a significant left–right shunt;
3) Asymptomatic but with ECG evidence of ischemia at baseline or on provocative testing;
4) Asymptomatic but with Holter monitoring evidence of significant arrhythmia.

Interventional Catheterization

Currently, interventional catheterization is the mainstay of definitive management. Consideration should be given to CT or MRI imaging for procedural planning. Such imaging can also be used to decide whether an interventional approach is feasible or if a surgical strategy should be adopted. Radiation dosage, need for general anesthesia, and the relative tachycardia of young patients need to be taken into consideration [8, 9]. Many patients will undergo catheterization without prior cross-sectional imaging. The primary goal in catheter therapy is complete occlusion of the fistula at the most distal point, to limit the risk of occlusion of an important coronary branch [13]. There is usually no need to intervene in a small baby unless heart failure cannot be controlled. It is technically easier to close the CCF when the child is older.

The initial approach is based around angiographic delineation of the coronary circulation: the origin, course, and exit point of the fistula and the relationships of the fistula. This is usually by selective injection in each coronary artery (Figures 38.1a and 38.2a). Because of the individual variations such as multiple feeding vessels, it is important to delineate the non-fistulous as well as the fistulous coronary artery. Multiple angiographic injections and angulations may be required to achieve the most useful views to plan an intervention. Achieving the ideal angiographic projection can be simplified if a CT or MRI scan has been performed before the procedure. Three-dimensional rotational angiography in a modern catheterization laboratory is particularly useful in long tortuous vessels [14].

Depending on patient characteristics and the individual anatomy of the fistula, the occlusive devices can be delivered either retrogradely from the native coronary artery (Figure 38.2c) or antegradely by engaging the exit point of the fistula (Figure 38.1c,d).

If the fistula is to be occluded via a delivery catheter placed along the course of the normal coronary artery, then occlusion is usually with coils, which can be passed through a 2 or 3 French microcatheter without impairing the flow through the coronary artery (Figure 38.2) [15].

Occlusive plugs such as patent ductus arteriosus closure device (PDA) or other similar devices and vascular plugs have to be delivered from an "exit point" approach because of their relatively large caliber and often stiffer delivery systems. This is often accomplished by passing a guidewire from the native coronary artery through the fistula and out of the exit point. This is then advanced into the superior vena cava or the pulmonary artery, where it is captured with a snare, placed via a femoral vein. Thus, an arteriovenous guidewire circuit is formed, which allows a larger delivery catheter or sheath to be coaxially railroaded over the guidewire from the venous side into a position to allow delivery of an appropriate device [6].

In either case, the goal is to occlude the vessel at the most distal site possible, allowing maintenance of flow in all the normal coronary side branches, which lie proximal to the fistulous connection.

Following occlusion, antiplatelet therapy is given, in particular in large dilated vessels, to avoid propagation of thrombus back along the coronary vessel and occlusion of important side branches. The duration of antiplatelet therapy is usually at least 3 months; however, there is no evidence to support this and it may be given for longer [16].

Surgical Therapy

In the modern era, surgical treatment is usually reserved for patients in whom interventional catheterization has either failed or is not an option because of anatomic constraints, such as the relation of the CCF to important coronary branches, or technical constraints from patient and equipment size discrepancies.

Conclusions

CCFs are a variable pathologic entity, in terms of vessel distribution and natural history. The treatment of choice is catheter intervention to occlude the abnormal vessel, although occasionally patients may need a surgical approach.

References

1 Shriki JE, Shinbane JS, Rashid MA, *et al.* (2012) Identifying, characterizing and classifying congenital anomalies of the coronary arteries. *Radiographics*, **32** (2), 453–468.
2 Anderson RH, Spicer D. (2010) Fistulous communications with the coronary origins in the setting of hypoplastic ventricles. *Cardiol Young*, **20** (Suppl 3), 86–91.
3 Ratajska A, Czarnowska E, Ciszek B. (2008) Embryonic development of the proepicardium and coronary vessels. *Int J Dev Biol*, **52** (2–3), 229–236.
4 Gowda ST, Forbes TJ, Singh H, *et al.* (2013) Remodeling and thrombosis following closure of coronary artery fistula with review of management: large distal coronary artery fistula – to close or not to close? *Catheter Cardiovasc Interv*, **82** (1), 132–142.
5 Khan MD, Qureshi SA, Rosenthal E, Sharland GK. (2003) Neonatal transcatheter occlusion of a large coronary artery fistula with Amplatzer duct occluder. *Catheter Cardiovasc Interv*, **60** (2), 282–286.
6 Malcic I, Belina D, Gitter R, *et al.* (2009) Spontaneous closure of fistula between right coronary artery and right ventricle in an infant. *Lijec Bjesn*, **131** (3–4), 65–68.
7 Bartoloni G, Giorlandino A, Calafiore AM, *et al.* (2012) Multiple coronary artery–left ventricular fistulas causing sudden death in a young woman. *Hum Pathol*, **43** (9), 1520–1523.
8 Natarajan A, Khokhar AA, Kirk P, Patel HH, Turner D. (2013) Coronary–pulmonary artery fistula: value of 64-MDCT imaging. *Q J Med*, **106** (1), 91–92.
9 Parga JR, Ikari NM, Bustamante LN, *et al.* (2004) Case report: MRI evaluation of congenital coronary artery fistulae. *Br J Radiol*, 77 (918), 508–511.
10 Latson LA. (2007) Coronary artery fistulas: how to manage them. *Catheter Cardiovasc Interv*, **70** (1), 110–116.
11 Suzuki T, Shirota K, Yokoyama E, Osaka T, Nakamura H. (2009) Coronary artery fistula into the right atrium complicated by atrial flutter: report of a case. *Kyobu Geka*, **62** (12), 1081–1084.
12 Corvaja N, Moses JW, Vogel FE, *et al.* (1999) Exercise-induced ventricular tachycardia associated with coronary arteriovenous fistula and correction by transcatheter coil embolization. *Catheter Cardiovasc Interv*, **46** (4), 470–472.
13 Armsby LR, Keane JF, Sherwood MC, *et al.* (2002) Management of coronary artery fistulae. Patient selection and results of transcatheter closure. *J Am Coll Cardiol*, **39** (6), 1026–1032.
14 Panzer J, Taeymans Y, De Wolf D. (2008) Three-dimensional rotational angiography of a patient with pulmonary atresia intact septum and coronary fistulas. *Pediatr Cardiol*, **29** (3), 686–687.
15 Qureshi SA, Reidy JF, Alwi MB, *et al.* (1996) Use of interlocking detachable coils in embolization of coronary arteriovenous fistulas. *Am J Cardiol*, **78** (1), 110–113.
16 Gowda ST, Latson LA, Kutty S, Prieto LR. (2011) Intermediate to long-term outcome following congenital coronary artery fistulae closure with focus on thrombus formation. *Am J Cardiol*, **107** (2), 302–308.

39

Aortopulmonary Window

Carl L. Backer[1,2], *Michael C. Mongé*[1,2], *Andrada Popescu*[1,2], *and Osama Eltayeb*[1,2]

[1] *Division of Cardiovascular-Thoracic Surgery, Ann & Robert H. Lurie Children's Hospital of Chicago, Chicago, IL, USA*
[2] *Department of Surgery, Northwestern University Feinberg School of Medicine, Chicago, IL, USA*

Aortopulmonary window (APW) is defined as a communication between the main pulmonary artery and the ascending aorta in the presence of two separate semilunar valves. The embryologic etiology is failure of fusion of the two opposing conal truncal ridges that are responsible for separating the common arterial trunk into the aorta and pulmonary artery. APW can occur as an isolated lesion or, in 30–50% of cases, is associated with other cardiac abnormalities. The most common associated lesion is interrupted aortic arch. In the presence of a large APW, the right pulmonary artery may arise from the rightward aspect of the ascending aorta, leading to a distinct syndrome: Berry syndrome.

The classification scheme suggested by the Society of Thoracic Surgeons is shown in Figure 39.1. The four types are: type 1, proximal; type 2, distal; type 3, total; type 4, intermediate. The presentation of patients with an APW is similar to other patients with a large left to right shunt, such as a large patent ductus arteriosus. Presentation usually occurs within the first several weeks of life when the pulmonary vascular resistance drops and increased pulmonary blood flow develops. The patients have tachypnea, poor feeding, diaphoresis, and failure to thrive.

Diagnosis is primarily made with echocardiogram. The echocardiogram will indicate the location and size of the defect and should be able to rule out other anomalies such as interrupted aortic arch, transposition of the great arteries, ventricular septal defect, and origin of the right pulmonary artery from the ascending aorta. We recently have used computed tomography (CT) imaging with three-dimensional reconstruction to image the precise location of the APW (Figure 39.2). Cardiac catheterization is not usually required, unless there is a question regarding the reversibility of pulmonary vascular obstructive disease in an older child. Of interest, the diagnosis is rarely made prenatally because of the equal pressures in the ascending aorta and pulmonary root in the fetus. Once the diagnosis is made, the patient should undergo operative intervention as there is no advantage to waiting. APW can be repaired via an incision through the window itself, through the ascending aorta, or through the main pulmonary artery. Our preference has been to repair the window through an incision in the ascending aorta, as illustrated in Figure 39.3.

After median sternotomy, cardiopulmonary bypass is initiated with a single venous cannula and a distal aortic cannula. The aorta must be cannulated distally enough that there is adequate room for placement of a cross-clamp. Immediately upon initiation of cardiopulmonary bypass, the right and left pulmonary arteries are occluded with snares. A vent is placed in the right superior pulmonary vein. After adequate cooling has been achieved, the aorta is cross-clamped and cold blood cardioplegia is injected into the aortic room. The aorta is opened with an anterior vertical incision oriented between the non-coronary sinus and the aortic cross-clamp. The APW is identified posteriorly (Figure 39.4). Care must be taken to identify the coronary artery orifices which can be in unusual locations and close to the APW. The cusps of the aortic valve and the origin and course of both right and left pulmonary arteries should be identified. We have utilized patch closure of the defect with a 0.4 mm thickness Gore-Tex cardiovascular patch (W.L. Gore & Associates, Flagstaff AZ, USA). The patch is anchored with a running suture. Suturing technique places all the knots for the sutures on the outside of the vessels. The anterior aortotomy is then closed with a running polypropylene suture. The heart is carefully de-aired and the patient warmed and weaned from cardiopulmonary bypass. One of the primary advantages of this approach is the lack of bleeding following the procedure, as the only site of potential bleeding is the aortotomy.

Other surgeons have had good results repairing the defect with an incision directly through the APW. After the initial incision is made, the patch is secured posteriorly to the junction between the ascending aorta and

Visual Guide to Neonatal Cardiology, First Edition. Edited by Ernerio T. Alboliras, Ziyad M. Hijazi, Leo Lopez, and Donald J. Hagler.

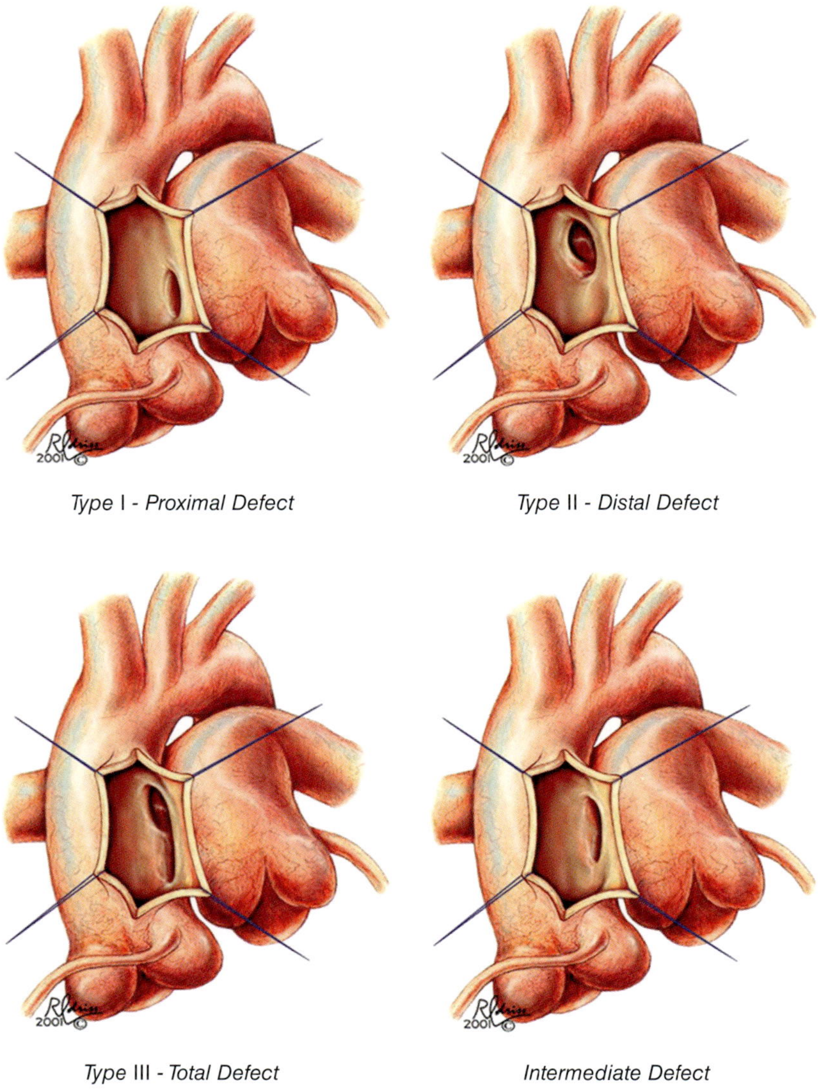

Figure 39.1 Classification scheme recommended by the Society of Thoracic Surgeons Congenital Heart Surgery Database Committee for aortopulmonary window. Type I is a proximal APW located just above the sinus of Valsalva, a few millimeters above the semilunar valve. Proximal defects are noted to have little inferior rim separating the APW from the semilunar valves. Type II is a distal APW located in the uppermost portion of the ascending aorta. This would correspond to the Richardson type 2 lesion, where the defect overlies a portion of the right pulmonary artery. Distal defects are noted to have a well-formed inferior rim but little superior rim. Type III is a total defect involving the majority of the ascending aorta. Type IV is the intermediate defect. These defects have adequate superior and inferior rims and are the group most suitable for possible device closure. *Source*: Backer and Mavroudis 2002 [1]. Reproduced with permission of Oxford University Press.

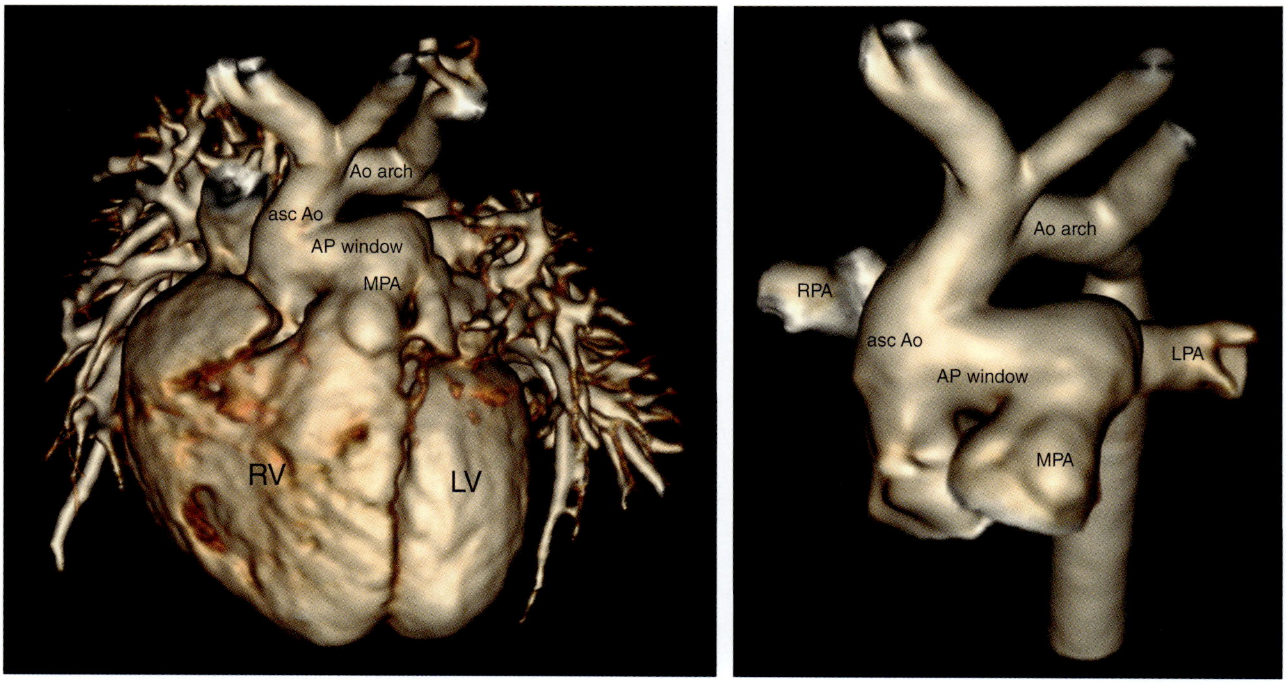

Figure 39.2 CT images demonstrating the location of aortopulmonary window (APW). Ao arch, aortic arch; AP, aortopulmonary; asc Ao, ascending aorta; LPA, left pulmonary artery; LV, left ventricle; MPA, main pulmonary artery; RPA, right pulmonary artery; RV, right ventricle.

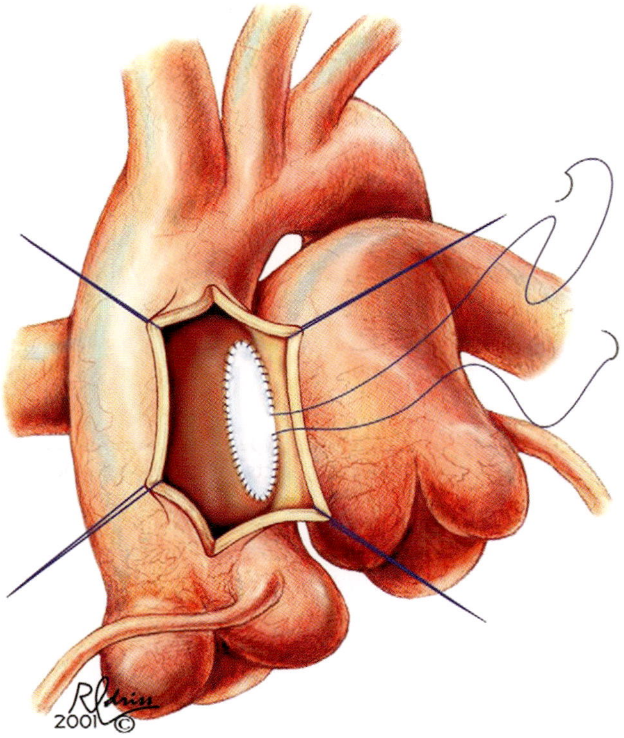

Figure 39.3 Operative closure of a type III total defect. Not illustrated are the aortic cross-clamp and CPB cannulas. The ascending aorta has been opened with a vertical aortotomy extending from the base of the innominate artery to a point between the non-coronary and right coronary cusps. This aortotomy helps avoid the orifice of the right coronary artery. The defect has been closed with an oval-shaped Gore-Tex cardiovascular patch that has been anchored with a running polypropylene suture. The final suture placement will be such that the knot is tied outside the circulation. *Source*: Backer and Mavroudis 2002 [1]. Reproduced with permission of Oxford University Press.

the main pulmonary artery. The anterior portion of the patch is sandwiched between the aorta and pulmonary artery, completing the closure (Figure 39.5).

The approach to the patient with APW and interrupted aortic arch is more complex. The initial approach is the same as for a simple APW. Interestingly, because of the large aortopulmonary communication, a single arterial cannula can be used. Flow to the lower half of the body is through the APW and then via the patent ductus arteriosus. We cool the patient to a core temperature of 18°C. During the cooling period, the ascending aorta, head vessels, patent ductus arteriosus, pulmonary arteries, and descending thoracic aorta are mobilized. After reaching the target temperature, circulatory arrest is established. The head vessels are snared. A spoon-shaped clamp is placed on the descending aorta. Cardioplegia solution is infused via the arterial cannula. Alternatively, continuous cerebral perfusion can be used. The ductus arteriosus is ligated

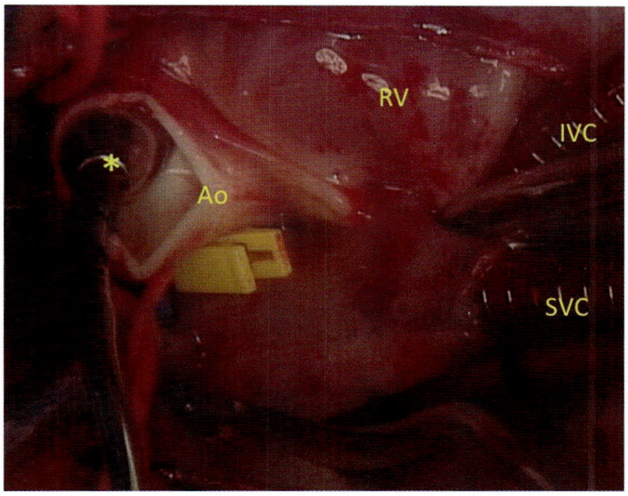

Figure 39.4 Intraoperative photo of a 7-mm dilator in aortopulmonary window (*). Ao, aortotomy; IVC, inferior caval vein cannula; RV, right ventricle; SVC, superior caval vein cannula.

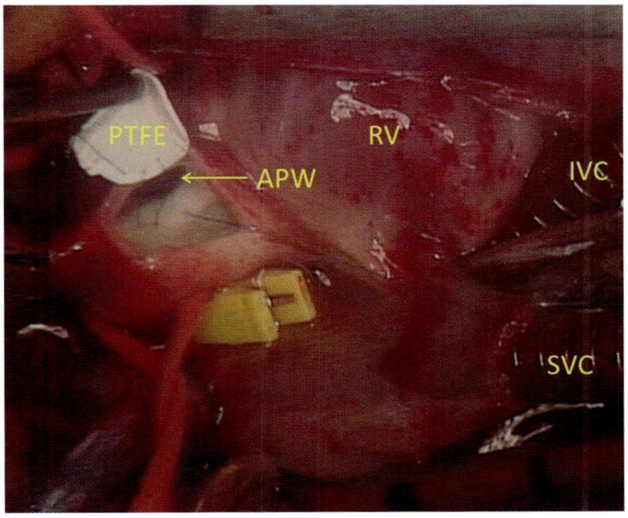

Figure 39.5 Intraoperative photo of PTFE patch closure of aortopulmonary window. Yellow atraumatic vascular clip is on the right pulmonary artery. APW, aortopulmonary window; IVC, inferior caval vein cannula; PTFE, polytetrafluoroethylene patch; RV, right ventricle; SVC, superior caval vein cannula.

and all ductal tissue is excised. The aorta is separated from the pulmonary artery leaving an opening in both. An extended end-to-end anastomosis can be created between the ascending and descending aorta with a homograft patch used to augment this anastomosis. The resulting opening in the pulmonary artery is patched with homograft or polytetrafluoroethylene.

In the postoperative period, patients with APW should be managed expectantly, observing them for potential pulmonary hypertensive crises in the postoperative period. We have kept these patients intubated, ventilated, and under neuromuscular blockade for the first 24 hours postoperatively. Nitric oxide therapy is used if there is significant pulmonary hypertension.

Transaortic patch closure of simple APW in our series and others is associated with a very low mortality. Interrupted aortic arch and APW is associated with a 9% operative mortality in the Congenital Heart Surgeons' Society study and an 84% survival at 10 years. Long-term follow-up is necessary to watch for branch pulmonary artery stenosis. We have not had to re-operate on any of the patients in our series having patch repair via aortotomy.

Reference

1 Backer CL, Mavroudis C. (2002) Surgical management of aortopulmonary window: a 40-year experience. *Eur J Cardiothorac Surg*, **21**, 773–779.

Further Reading

Bagtharia R, Trivedi KR, Burkhart HM, *et al*. (2004) Outcomes for patients with an aortopulmonary window, and the impact of associated cardiovascular lesions. *Cardiol Young*, **14**, 473–480.

Barnes ME, Mitchell ME, Tweddell JS. (2011) Aortopulmonary window. *Semin Thorac Cardiovasc Surg Ped Card Surg Annu*, **14**, 67–74.

Berry TE, Bharati S, Muster AJ, *et al*. (1982) Distal aortopulmonary septal defect, aortic origin of the right pulmonary artery, intact ventricular septum, patent ductus arteriosus and hypoplasia of the aortic isthmus: a newly recognized syndrome. *Am J Cardiol*, **49**, 108–116.

Jacobs JP, Quintessenza JA, Gaynor JW, Burke RP, Mavroudis C. (2000) Congenital Heart Surgery Nomenclature and Database Project: aortopulmonary window. *Ann Thorac Surg*, **69** (Suppl), S44–S49.

Konstantinov IE, Karamlou T, Williams WG, *et al*; for the Congenital Heart Surgeons' Society. (2006) Surgical management of aortopulmonary window associated with interrupted aortic arch: A Congenital Heart Surgeons' Society study. *J Thorac Cardiovasc Surg*, **131**, 1136–1141.

40

Anomalous Origin of a Branch Pulmonary Artery From the Ascending Aorta (Hemitruncus)

Michael C. Mongé[1,2], *Osama Eltayeb*[1,2], *Andrada R. Popescu*[1,2], *and Carl L. Backer*[1,2]

[1] *Division of Cardiovascular-Thoracic Surgery, Ann & Robert H. Lurie Children's Hospital of Chicago, Chicago, IL, USA*
[2] *Department of Surgery, Northwestern University Feinberg School of Medicine, Chicago, IL, USA*

Anomalous origin of a branch pulmonary artery from the ascending aorta (AOPAA), first described by Fraentzel in 1868, is an extremely rare congenital heart defect in which one branch pulmonary artery arises from the ascending aorta with normal origin of the other pulmonary artery from the right ventricle. There are two distinct great vessels arising from the ventricular mass, both of which are guarded by semilunar valves. An interventricular communication is not obligatory as in common arterial trunk (truncus arteriosus). Despite the similarity of the name, hemitruncus does not fall within the hierarchy of common arterial trunk and thus the term is discouraged in favor of AOPAA.

As with other conotruncal anomalies, pleuripotent neural crest cells contribute to the embryologic development of AOPAA. AOPAA has been reported to exist with tetralogy of Fallot, interrupted aortic arch, aortopulmonary window, isthmic hypoplasia, and ventricular septal defects. Although the pathophysiology and clinical presentation are similar, AOPAA should be distinguished from patients with a ductal origin of a discontinuous branch pulmonary artery.

Right pulmonary artery origin from the ascending aorta (AORPA) occurs from abnormal migration of the right sixth aortic arch. The right pulmonary artery (RPA) usually arises near the sinotubular junction from the right or posterior aspect of the ascending aorta. Twenty percent of patients with AORPA have no associated anomalies. Patent ductus arteriosus (PDA) is present in 50% of patients. Curiously, left pulmonary vein stenosis may also be present. AORPA is 4–8 times more common than anomalous origin of the left pulmonary artery (AOLPA).

AOLPA occurs when the left pulmonary artery (LPA) arises from the persistent aortic sac as a result of absence of the left sixth arch with persistence of the left fifth arch. AOLPA is often associated with a right aortic arch. Unlike in AORPA, tetralogy of Fallot is the most common associated finding. Given the common embryologic derivation of the LPA and ductus arteriosus from the left sixth aortic arch, complete absence of a ductus remnant in AOLPA is not unexpected.

Pulmonary overcirculation occurs for two reasons. First, the normally positioned pulmonary artery receives the entire cardiac output from the right ventricle. Second, the anomalous pulmonary artery is exposed to unrestricted systemic blood flow and pressure from the aorta. Because of the pressure and volume overload, pulmonary vascular obstructive disease can occur early and in both lungs.

Patients often present early in life with respiratory distress and heart failure. AOPAA has no typical auscultatory findings. ECG findings may be indicative of biventricular hypertrophy. Chest X-ray frequently demonstrates cardiomegaly with bilateral pulmonary plethora. However, if tetralogy of Fallot is present, differential pulmonary blood flow may be demonstrated.

The diagnosis is reliably made by echocardiography. Advanced medical imaging with computed tomography angiography (CTA) or magnetic resonance imaging (MRI) is quite useful for operative planning. Cardiac catheterization can measure the pulmonary vascular resistance in the normally connected lung which can guide operability in the older patient. However, as pulmonary flow will also pass through the reimplanted lung, a level of resistance above what may be normally acceptable for other shunting lesions should still be considered for repair.

If AOPAA is left untreated, 30% 1-year survival has been reported. Early repair of AOPAA is recommended to prevent the sequelae of pulmonary hypertension. Retroaortic direct reimplantation of the AORPA was first described by Kirkpatrick and King in 1967 at Indiana University.

The repair is performed via a median sternotomy approach with the use of hypothermic cardiopulmonary bypass. The ascending aorta is mobilized from the pulmonary trunk. Positioning of the aortic cannula

Visual Guide to Neonatal Cardiology, First Edition. Edited by Ernerio T. Alboliras, Ziyad M. Hijazi, Leo Lopez, and Donald J. Hagler.

should allow placement of the aortic clamp distal to the anomalous pulmonary artery origin. Bicaval venous cannulation is achieved with placement of a vent in the right superior pulmonary vein. Immediately after establishing cardiopulmonary bypass, the anomalous pulmonary artery is snared to prevent diastolic run-off into the lung. The ductus arteriosus is dissected and ligated. The aorta is cross-clamped and cold blood cardioplegia is administered. The pulmonary artery, which has been thoroughly mobilized, is excised from the ascending aorta. The defect in the aorta is closed with an autologous pericardial patch or with polytetrafluoroethylene (PTFE). Complete transection of the aorta with primary repair, following the pulmonary anastomosis, may also be performed. After retraction of the aorta anteriorly and leftward, the pulmonary trunk is brought beneath the aorta. An appropriate site is selected on the main pulmonary artery and the anomalous pulmonary artery is reimplanted in a tension-free manner. Several techniques of aortic and/or pulmonary arterial flaps for lengthening of the RPA have been implemented when direct reimplantation is not feasible.

Postoperative management emphasizes control of pulmonary vascular resistance. We keep these patients ventilated and paralyzed for 24–48 hours and expectantly treat them in the current era with nitric oxide therapy. Hospital mortality has been reported to be in the range of 0–21%, with good late survival. The most commonly reported late complication is stenosis at the pulmonary artery anastomosis which can usually be managed by balloon angioplasty. The need for re-intervention ranges 10–33%. Long-term follow-up with echocardiograms and differential lung perfusion scans (nuclear scintigraphy) is recommended.

Further Reading

Abu-Sulaiman RM, Hashmi A, McCrindle BW, Williams WG, Freedom RM. (1998) Anomalous origin of one pulmonary artery from the ascending aorta: 36 years' experience from one centre. *Cardiol Young*, **8**, 449–454.

Amir G, Frenkel G, Bruckheimer E, *et al.* (2010) Anomalous origin of the pulmonary artery from the aorta: early diagnosis and repair leading to immediate physiological correction. *Cardiol Young*, **20**, 654–659.

Kirkpatrick SE, Girod DA, King H. (1967) Aortic origin of the right pulmonary artery: surgical repair without a graft. *Circulation*, **36**, 777–782.

Nathan M, Rimmer MS, Piercey BS, del Nido PJ, Mayer JE. (2007) Early repair of hemitruncus: excellent early and late outcomes. *J Thorac Cardiovasc Surg*, **133**, 1329–1335.

Peng EW, Shanmugam G, Macarthur KJ, Pollock, JC. (2004) Ascending aortic origin of a branch pulmonary artery: surgical management and long-term outcome. *Eur J Cardiothorac Surg*, **26**, 762–766.

Talwar S, Meena A, Choudhary SK, *et al.* (2014) Anomalous branch of pulmonary artery from the aorta and tetralogy of Fallot: morphology, surgical techniques, and results. *Eur J Cardiothorac Surg*, **46**, 291–296.

41

Interrupted Aortic Arch

Michael C. Mongé, Hyde M. Russell, and Carl L. Backer

Division of Cardiovascular-Thoracic Surgery, Ann & Robert H. Lurie Children's Hospital of Chicago, Chicago, IL, USA; Department of Surgery, Northwestern University Feinberg School of Medicine, Chicago, IL, USA

Interrupted aortic arch (IAA) is the loss of luminal continuity between the ascending and descending aorta. Celoria and Patton devised an anatomic classification system based on the location of the discontinuity. Type A interruption occurs at the aortic isthmus and is found in 28% of patients. Type B has interruption between the left carotid and left subclavian arteries and is present in 70% of patients. Type C has interruption between the innominate and left carotid arteries (Figure 41.1) [1, 2].

A ventricular septal defect (VSD), usually of malalignment-paramembranous type, is present in nearly all patients with IAA, except when an aortopulmonary window exists. In patients with a VSD, posterior malalignment of the conal septum contributes to left ventricular outflow tract (LVOT) obstruction (Figure 41.2). An aberrant right subclavian artery originating from the descending aorta is found in approximately 25% of patients with type A interruption (Figure 41.3). In these patients, there is an increased risk of subaortic obstruction from the relatively greater proportion of blood that must travel through the ductus arteriosus as opposed to the LVOT during fetal development. Transposition of the great arteries occurs in 2–10% of infants with IAA. These infants may present with cyanotic upper extremities and pink lower extremities. A common arterial trunk is seen in 10% of patients with IAA and a functionally single ventricle is seen in 3% [2].

Children with IAA often have a microdeletion of chromosome 22q11, particularly type B and C interruption. In patients with IAA, 15–30% have DiGeorge syndrome, characterized by hypoparathyroidisim, thymic aplasia with altered immunity, cleft lip and palate, and developmental delay. Infants with IAA should be tested with fluorescence in situ hybridization (FISH) analysis for chromosomal microdeletion.

An increasing number of patients with IAA are diagnosed with prenatal ultrasonography. In those not diagnosed prenatally, IAA may become apparent only after ductal closure begins. These patients may present with a mottled or gray appearance of the lower body, lethargy, and oliguria progressing to profound shock with multiple organ dysfunction. Blood pressure and oxygen saturation differentials between the upper and lower extremities may not exist if an aberrant right subclavian artery is present. Following birth, if ductal patency persists, congestive heart failure may ensue as the pulmonary vascular resistance decreases.

Echocardiography is the primary diagnostic modality (Figure 41.4). The site and length of the aortic interruption and the origins of the branch vessels should be established. Atrial and ventricular septal defects, if present, should be characterized. An assessment of the LVOT and left-sided structures should be performed. However, the degree of left-sided obstruction may be underestimated in the presence of a large ductus. Detailed echocardiographic evaluation will help to rule out or establish the presence of coexistent anomalies. Finally, the absence of the thymus should be ascertained because of its association with microdeletion of chromosome 22 and DiGeorge syndrome.

In some situations, cardiac catheterization is a useful diagnostic and therapeutic adjunct. Although care should be taken when the already compromised patient undergoes invasive diagnostic testing, angiography can confirm the diagnosis of discontinuous pulmonary artery branches and assess anomalous pulmonary venous connections. It may be helpful to delineate the source of coronary blood flow in patients presenting with aortic atresia and IAA. Balloon atrial septostomy may be considered in those presenting with transposition of the great arteries and IAA. In addition, some have reported successful stenting of the ductus as a temporizing measure prior to definitive repair. More recently, magnetic resonance angiography and computed tomography have emerged as useful non-invasive modalities to clarify anatomic details of complex cardiac anomalies and aid in operative planning (Figures 41.5–41.7, and 41.8).

Visual Guide to Neonatal Cardiology, First Edition. Edited by Ernerio T. Alboliras, Ziyad M. Hijazi, Leo Lopez, and Donald J. Hagler.

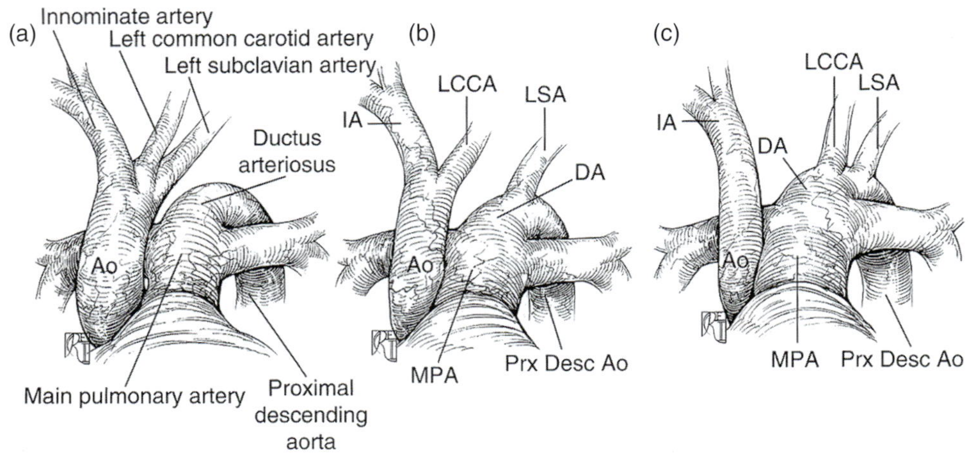

Figure 41.1 Anatomic types of interrupted aortic arch. (a) Type A, interruption distal to the left subclavian artery. (b) Type B, interruption between the left subclavian and left carotid arteries. (c) Type C, interruption between the left carotid and innominate artery. Ao, aorta; DA, ductus arteriosus; IA, innominate artery; LCCA, left common carotid artery; LSA, left subclavian artery; MPA, main pulmonary artery; Prx Desc Ao, proximal descending aorta. *Source*: Jonas 2013 [4]. Reprinted with permission of John Wiley & Sons.

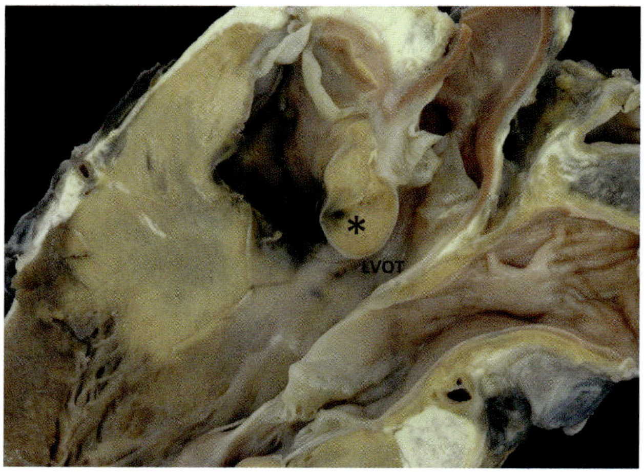

Figure 41.2 Anatomic specimen demonstrating posterior deviation of outlet septum (*) into left ventricular outflow tract (LVOT). Ventricular septal defect patch has been removed.

In patients suspected of having IAA, prostaglandin E1 infusion should be initiated to maintain ductal patency. Pulmonary vascular resistance should be maximized, through the use of low levels of inspired oxygen and the avoidance of respiratory alkalosis, in order to improve lower body perfusion. Intubation, with sedation and paralysis, may be required. Myocardial function is frequently depressed, so inotropic support with dopamine may be required. A milrinone infusion can be used to improve myocardial function while also decreasing systemic vascular resistance. Laboratory assessment of end-organ perfusion, including renal and hepatic function and a coagulation profile, should be performed; metabolic acidosis should be aggressively corrected. Genetic testing and family counseling can be initiated during this resuscitation period.

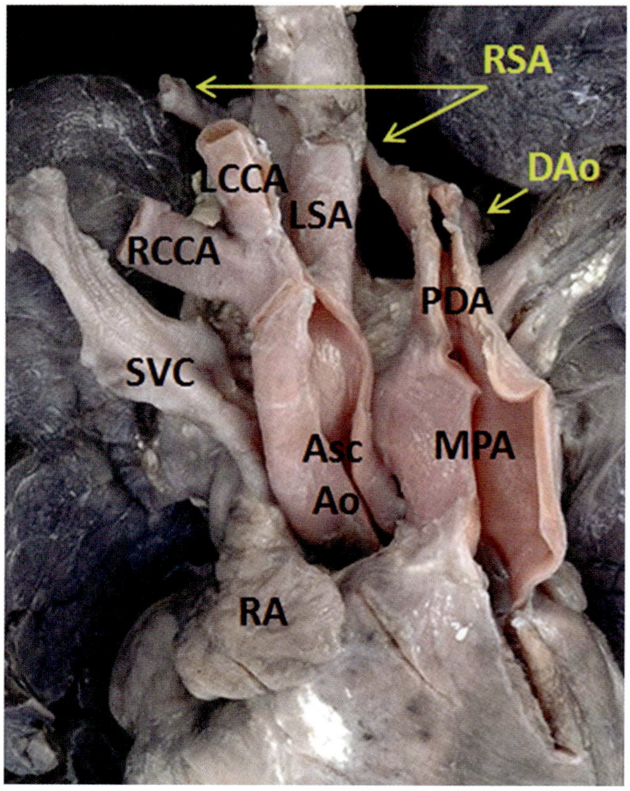

Figure 41.3 Anatomic specimen demonstrating type A interrupted aortic arch with retroesophageal aberrant right subclavian artery. Asc Ao, ascending aorta; DAo, descending aorta; PDA, patent ductus arteriosus; RA, right atrium; RCCA, right common carotid artery; SVC, superior vena cava.

Surgery is undertaken following recovery of hepatic and renal function and resulting resolution of acidosis, coagulopathy, and fluid and metabolic imbalances. Most commonly in the current era, a single-stage repair of IAA

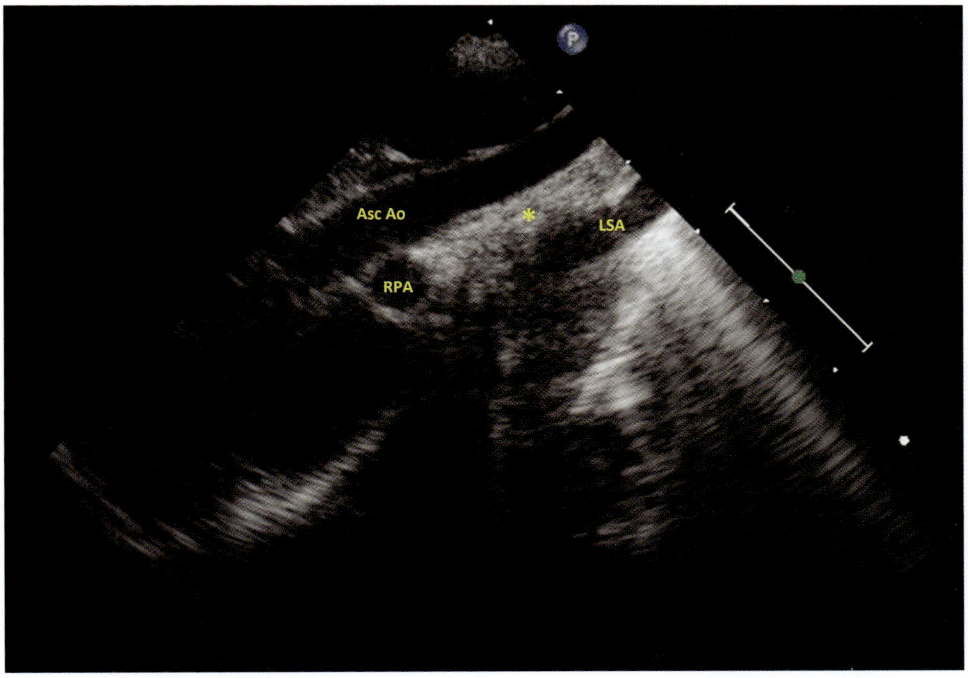

Figure 41.4 Transthoracic echocardiogram of type B interrupted aortic arch. Asterisk marks the site of interruption.

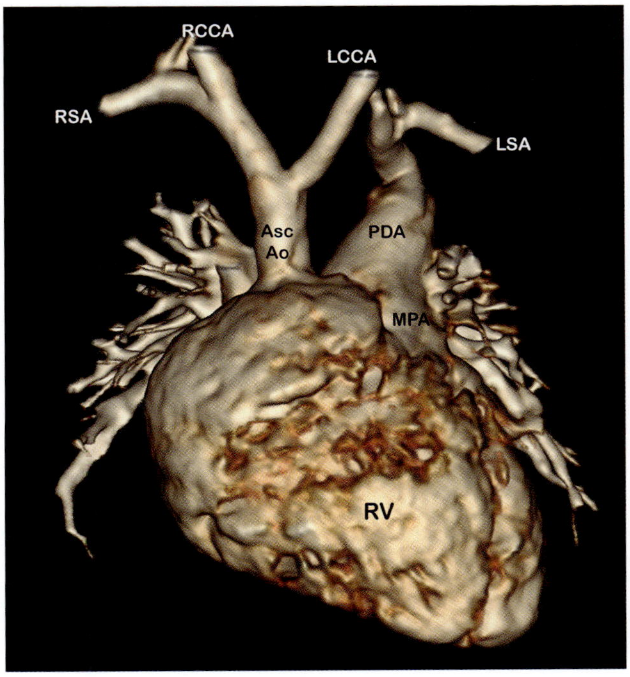

Figure 41.5 Computed tomographic three-dimensional (3D) reconstruction of type B interrupted aortic arch. RV, right ventricle.

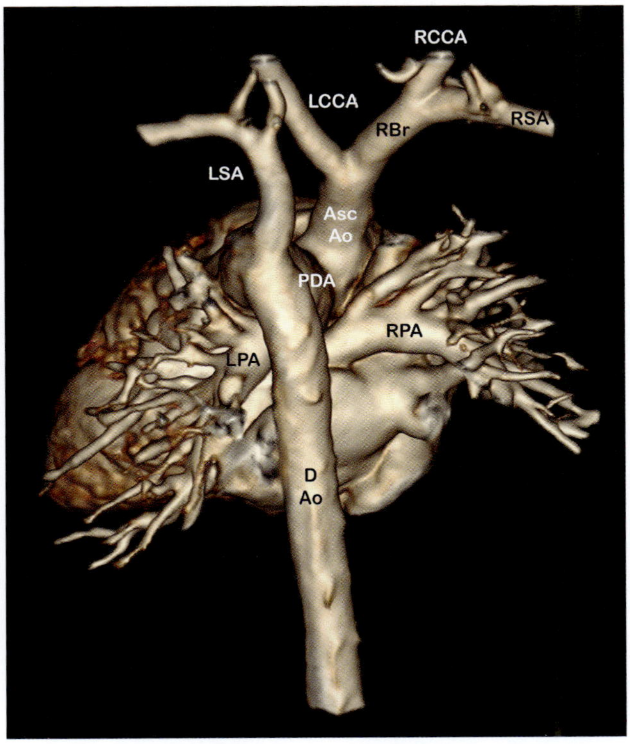

Figure 41.6 Computed tomographic reconstruction (posterior view) of type B interrupted aortic arch demonstrating origin of descending aorta from patent ductus arteriosus. RBr, right brachiocephalic artery; RPA, right pulmonary artery.

and intracardiac defects is performed with a direct aortic arch anastomosis [3]. Blood pressure monitoring should be performed above and below the arch anastomosis. A median sternotomy is performed. The thymus, if present, is excised. Arterial cannulation of the ascending aorta or innominate artery (if modified cerebral perfusion is to be employed) and the ductus arteriosus (for lower body perfusion) is established (Figure 41.9). Following initiation of cardiopulmonary bypass and cooling to a

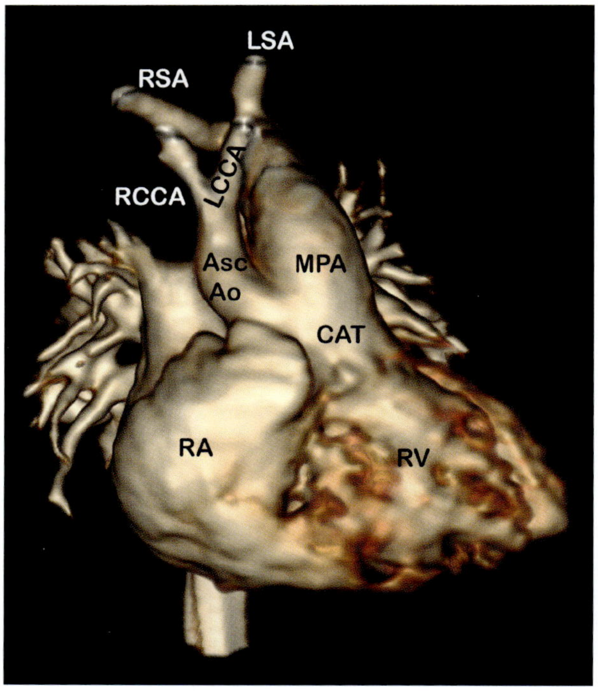

Figure 41.7 Computed tomographic 3D reconstruction of common arterial trunk (CAT) with type B interrupted aortic arch and aberrant right subclavian artery (RSA).

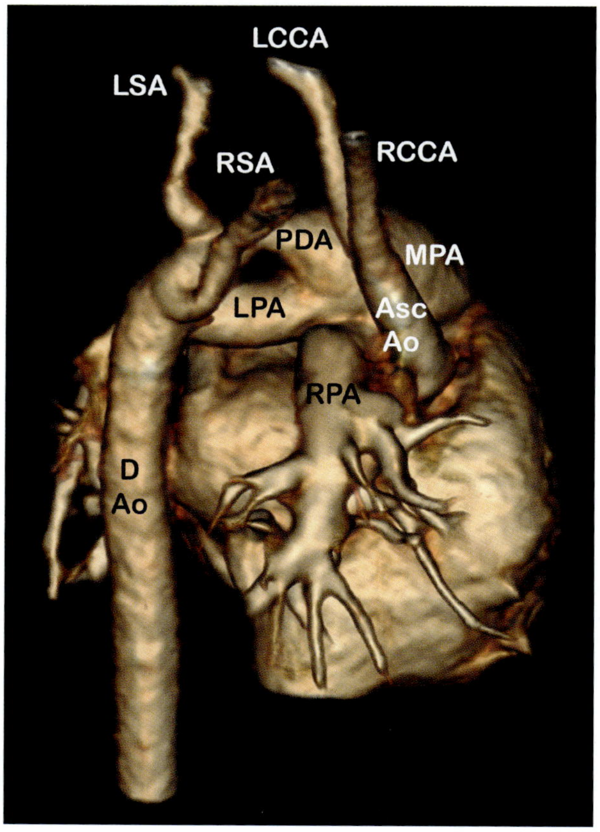

Figure 41.8 Computed tomographic 3D reconstruction (posterior view) of type B interrupted aortic arch with aberrant right subclavian artery.

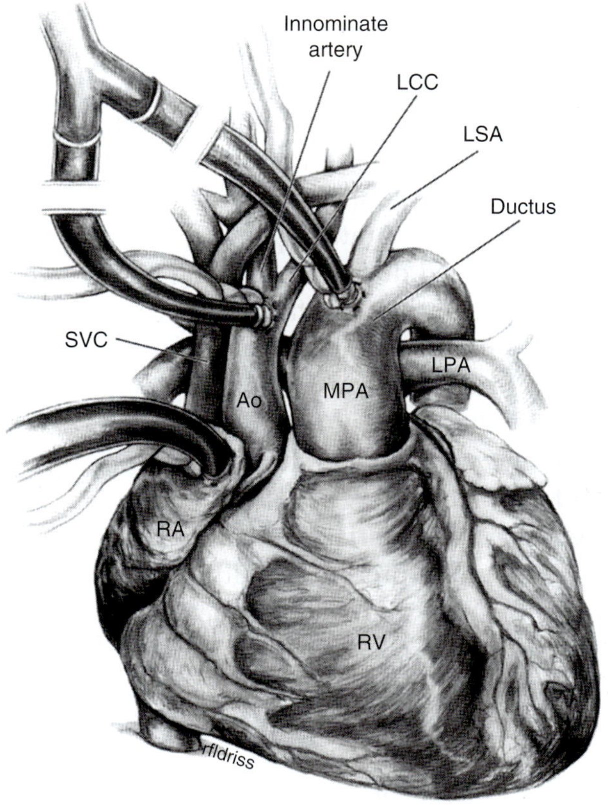

Figure 41.9 Arterial cannulation for repair of interrupted aortic arch. An 8-Fr cannula is inserted on the right side of the small ascending aorta. A second cannula is inserted into the ductus arteriosus. The pulmonary arteries are controlled with tourniquets after commencing cardiopulmonary bypass. *Source*: Jonas 2013 [4]. Reprinted with permission of John Wiley & Sons.

core temperature of 18°C, the proximal ductus arteriosus is ligated. Extensive mobilization of the ascending aorta, aortic arch, arch vessels, and descending aorta is performed. An aberrant right subclavian artery, if present, is ligated and divided. An aortic cross-clamp is applied and cardioplegia delivered. A period of deep hypothermic circulatory arrest with or without modified cerebral perfusion is then established. The ductus is ligated and divided, and any residual ductal tissue excised. An aortotomy is created on the lateral aspect of the ascending aorta. A direct end-to-side aortic anastomosis between the descending and ascending aorta is performed. Some patients may benefit from a homograft patch augmenting this anastomosis. Full cardiopulmonary bypass flow is re-established and warming commenced. The VSD repair is then performed, often via a transpulmonic approach because of the associated hypoplasia of the conal septum. After standard venting maneuvers, the aortic cross-clamp is removed [4].

Following repair of IAA, the possibility of late post-operative arch obstruction should be evaluated by serial examination. Invariably, all patients who have undergone neonatal repair of IAA with an interposition graft will develop late obstruction. Some patients having undergone direct aortic anastomosis will develop late obstruction. In the multi-institutional Congenital Heart Surgeons' Society (CHSS) study, freedom from reintervention for arch obstruction was 86% at 3 years in those who had direct arch anastomosis [1]. Moreover, in a study by Sell *et al.* [5], more than 60% of children undergoing direct aortic anastomosis had a gradient of greater than 30 mmHg within 18 months of surgery. Fortunately, balloon dilatation can successfully relieve the anastomostic gradient in the majority of children who have undergone direct arch anastomosis.

LVOT obstruction is an important late sequelae following repair of interrupted aortic arch. In the CHSS study, freedom from reintervention for LVOTO was 77% at 3 years [1]. Occasionally, the LVOT obstruction can be alleviated by resection of the posteriorly deviated conal septum. Alternatively, a Norwood procedure with a Damus–Kaye–Stansel (DKS) anastomosis may be performed [6]. The CHSS study suggested that conal septal resection or a pulmonary to aortic (DKS) anastomosis for LVOT obstruction during neonatal correction of IAA carried a greater risk of early death than simple repair [1], but single-center studies have demonstrated that the Norwood procedure or conal resection during IAA repair can be performed with acceptable mortality at high-volume centers [7, 8]. A modified Konno procedure may be required if there is tunnel subaortic stenosis.

If a direct aortic anastomosis is performed, left bronchial obstruction from bowstringing of the inadequately mobilized aorta over the left main bronchus can occur following repair of IAA. Hyperexpansion of the left lung from air trapping may be seen on X-ray. The diagnosis can be confirmed with bronchoscopy and advanced medical imaging. An interposition graft placed between the ascending and descending aorta may be needed to alleviate this condition.

IAA is a complex constellation of anomalies requiring preoperative stabilization with PGE_1 followed by neonatal repair. Advanced medical imaging facilitates planning of operative strategy. Lifelong follow-up is needed to diagnose and manage late complications of arch obstruction and LVOT obstruction.

References

1 Jonas RA, Quaegebeur JM, Kirklin JW, Blackstone EH, Daicoff G. (1994) Outcomes in patients with interrupted aortic arch and ventricular septal defect: a multiinstitutional study. Congenital Heart Surgeons' Society. *J Thorac Cardiovasc Surg*, **107**, 1099–1113.

2 McCrindle BW, Tchervenkov CI, Konstantinov IE, *et al.* (2005) Risk factors associated with mortality and interventions in 472 neonates with interrupted aortic arch: a Congenital Heart Surgeons' Society study. *J Thorac Cardiovasc Surg*, **129**, 343–350.

3 Oosterhof T, Azakie A, Freedom RM, Williams WG, McCrindle BW. (2004) Associated factors and trends in outcomes of interrupted aortic arch. *Ann Thorac Surg*, **74**, 1696–1702.

4 Jonas RA. (2003) Interrupted aortic arch, in, *Pediatric Cardiac Surgery*, 3rd edn. (eds C Mavroudis, CL Backer), Mosby, Philadelphia, pp. 273–282.

5 Sell JE, Jonas RA, Mayer JE, *et al.* (1988) The results of a surgical program for interrupted aortic arch. *J Thorac Cardiovasc Surg*, **96**, 864–877.

6 Yasui H, Kado H, Nakano E, *et al.* (1987) Primary repair of interrupted aortic arch and severe aortic stenosis in neonates. *J Thorac Cardiovasc Surg*, **93**, 539–545.

7 Suzuki T, Ohye RG, Devaney EJ, *et al.* (2006) Selective management of the left ventricular outflow tract for repair of interrupted aortic arch with ventricular septal defect: management of left ventricular outflow tract obstruction. *J Thorac Cardiovasc Surg*, **131**, 779–784.

8 Brown JW, Ruzmetov M, Okada Y, *et al.* (2006) Outcomes in patients with interrupted aortic arch and associated anomalies: a 20-year experience. *Eur J Cardiothorac Surg*, **29**, 666–674.

42

Coarctation of the Aorta

Hitesh Agrawal[1], John W. Bokowski[2], and Damien Kenny[3]

[1] Texas Children's Hospital, Houston, TX, USA
[2] Rush Center for Congenital and Structural Heart Disease, Chicago, IL, USA
[3] Our Lady's Children's Hospital, Crumlin, Dublin, Ireland

Pathophysiology

The aortic arch and its branches develop during the fourth to eighth weeks of gestation. Abnormalities in the development of left fourth and sixth embryonic aortic arch are thought to be implicated. Various theories have been proposed to explain how coarctation develops. Ductal theory states that ductal tissue surrounds the aortic arch in a circumferential fashion, thus causing narrowing of the aorta when ductal tissue constricts. This is supported by the fact that coarctation most commonly occurs at the site of ductal insertion and often manifests after ductal closure. However, aortic coarctation (CoA) can occur away from the insertion of ductus arteriosus, which cannot be explained solely by ductal theory. Developmental theory hypothesizes that coarctation develops as a result of hemodynamic disturbances that reduce the volume of blood flow through the fetal aortic arch, and it may be that CoA cannot be explained by a single pathophysiologic mechanism.

Clinical Manifestation

Newborns with CoA are usually asymptomatic at birth, when the ductus arteriosus is open, or if the narrowing is mild. After ductal closure, newborns present with dusky color, poor feeding, tachypnea, and often in a shock-like state if severe coarctation is present. Cases with milder degrees of narrowing may be missed until childhood or adulthood and can be brought to attention by the presence of an ejection systolic click from an associated aortic valve anomaly or a systolic ejection murmur in the aortic area, a continuous murmur arising from collateral formation, upper extremity hypertension, and diminished or delayed femoral pulses.

Prior to ductal closure, a difference in pulse oximetry between the upper (higher saturation) and lower extremity (lower saturation) can be the earliest clue. This results from shunting of deoxygenated blood through the patent ductus arteriosus. Hence, the American Academy of Pediatrics recommends that all healthy newborns be screened with pulse oximetry readings at 24–48 hours of birth, taken in the right hand and either foot. A screen result is considered positive if:

1) Any oxygen saturation measure is <90%;
2) Oxygen saturation is <95% in both extremities on three measures, each separated by 1 hour; or
3) There is a 3% absolute difference in oxygen saturation between the right hand and foot on three measures.

A positive screen warrants further cardiac evaluation [1]. The most useful clinical test is absence or reduction in the intensity of the femoral pulses. Further investigation is always warranted in this setting. Blood pressure difference between the upper (higher pressure) and lower extremities (lower pressure) has also been used to evaluate for CoA. However, there are limitations with this approach in newborn infants and therefore it should not be relied upon if other clinical correlates suggest CoA.

Investigations

Antenatal diagnosis of coarctation can be suspected on the basis of fetal echocardiography showing ventricular disproportion with right ventricular dilation (Figure 42.1; Box 42.1). The coarctation site itself is not easily identifiable because of the lack of flow through the isthmus and the presence of the arterial duct that overlies it [2]. Recent reports recommend serial measurements of isthmal z scores and isthmal-to-ductal ratios by

Visual Guide to Neonatal Cardiology, First Edition. Edited by Ernerio T. Alboliras, Ziyad M. Hijazi, Leo Lopez, and Donald J. Hagler.

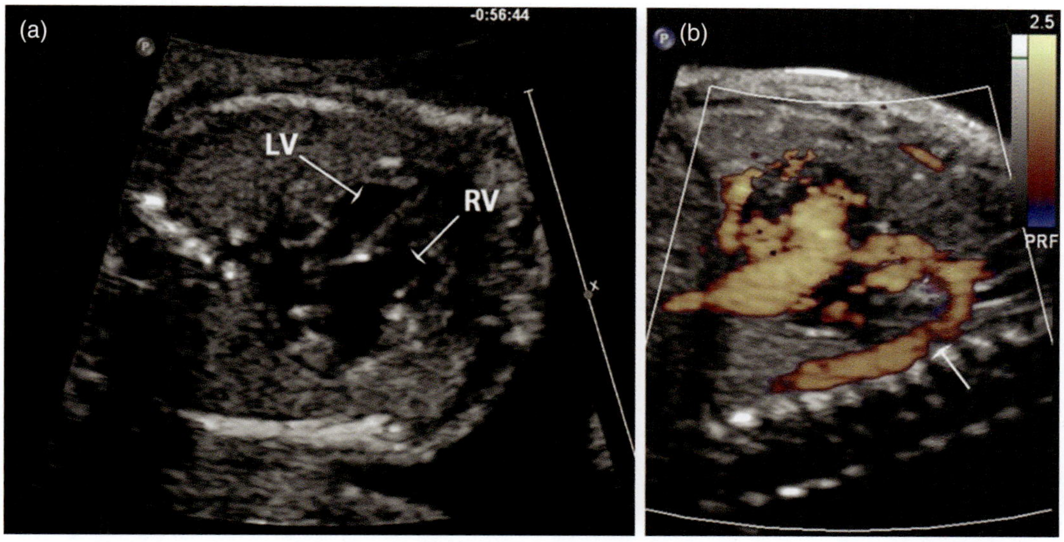

Figure 42.1 (a) Fetal echocardiogram showing ventricular disproportion with right ventricular dilatation; (b) power Doppler showing the area of coarctation marked by an arrow. LV, left ventricle; RV, right ventricle.

Box 42.1 Summary for diagnostic approach to coarctation of aorta

Antenatal echocardiography showing:

- Ventricular disproportion with right ventricular dilation
- Serial isthmal z scores and isthmal-to-ductal ratios

Postnatal diagnosis:

- Absent or reduced femoral pulses
- Discrepancy between upper and lower limb oxygen saturations
- Echocardiography showing narrowed aortic segment, with pressure gradient across it (and ductal patency with dominant right-to-left shunt)
- Cardiac catheterization to delineate the anatomy before balloon angioplasty, and stent placement

echocardiography in such high-risk cases to increase the sensitivity of screening [3]. Postnatal echocardiogram can delineate the anatomy of the narrowed segment of aorta, ductal patency, and can demonstrate the pressure gradient across the narrow segment using spectral Doppler (Figure 42.2). Electrocardiogram may show signs of right ventricular hypertrophy. Chest X-ray is usually normal, unless the neonate presents in cardiac failure where radiographic evidence of cardiomegaly with increased pulmonary vascular markings caused by pulmonary venous congestion may be seen. Cardiac catheterization is reserved for cases requiring rescue balloon angioplasty, palliative stent placement, or to further characterize other cardiac lesions (Figure 42.3). Karyotype may be considered, especially in female infants where there is an association with Turner syndrome.

Management

When there is a strong antenatal suspicion of CoA, the fetus should be delivered in a pediatric cardiology center and a prostaglandin infusion commenced immediately to maintain ductal patency. The early echocardiogram is revealing for anatomic variants and associations, and prostaglandin is maintained until surgical repair a few days later. Neonates who collapse and present in shock are resuscitated and prostaglandin is given in an attempt to reopen the arterial duct to buy time until the surgical repair [2].

Palliative ballooning or stenting can be used in those neonates with multiorgan failure and for those who do not respond to medical treatment. This can serve as a bridge to surgery in seriously ill patients. Native CoA in the neonatal period is managed surgically (Figure 42.4), as recoarctation and aneurysm rates are higher with balloon angioplasty in this age group. Two standard surgical approaches are currently used. First, resection and end-to-end (or end-to-side) anastomosis (extended end-to-end or end-to-side technique if with associated transverse arch hypoplasia), which is most the commonly used contemporary technique, and, second, subclavian flap repair, which involves ligation of the subclavian artery to use the proximal portion to overlay patch the

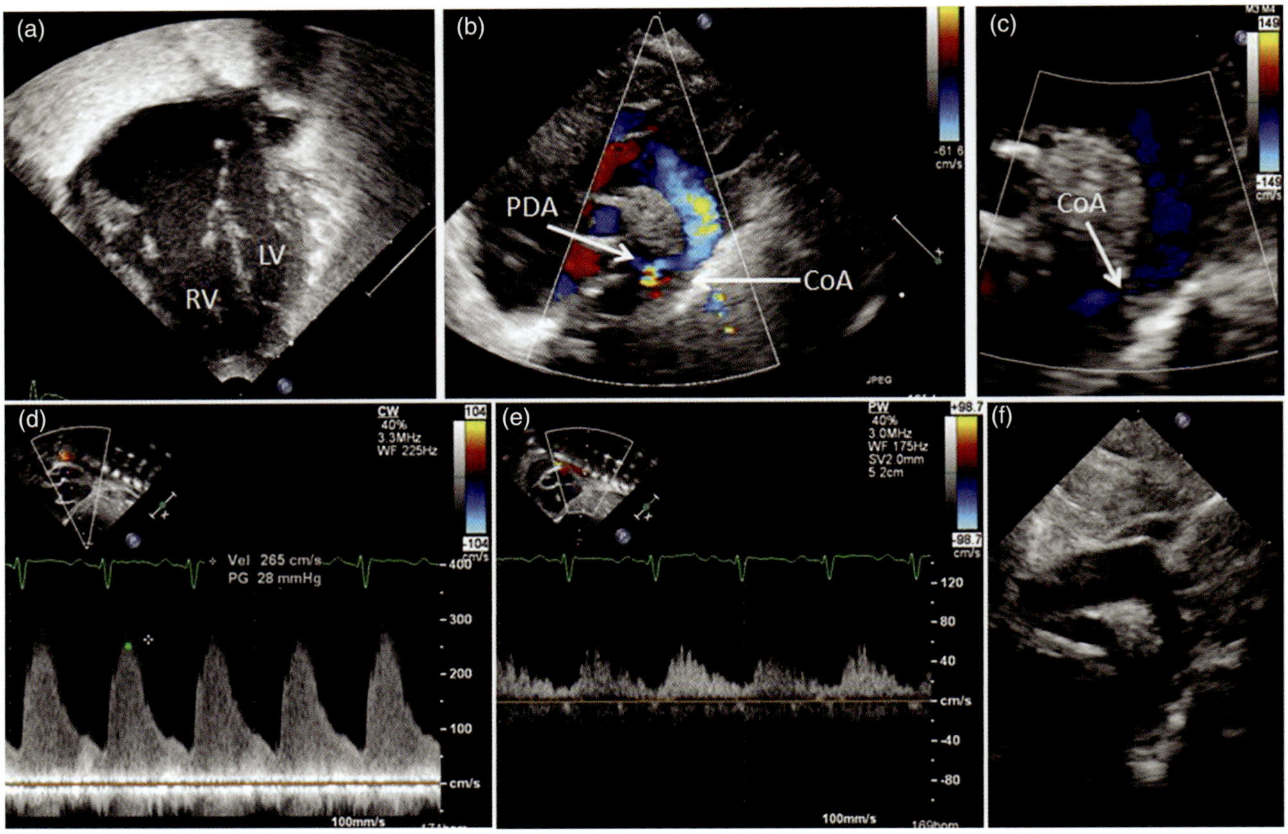

Figure 42.2 Series of postnatal echocardiography images from a patient with coarctation of the aorta (CoA): (a) four-chamber view with marked right ventricular dilation; (b) color flow mapping showing narrowing of the isthmus, patent ductus arteriosus (PDA), and posterior shelf; (c) magnified image of the narrowed segment showing the posterior shelf; (d) spectral Doppler at the site of narrowing with a significant pressure gradient and diastolic tail; (e) spectral Doppler of the abdominal aorta showing low velocity flow, increase in deceleration time, and diastolic tailing; (f) aortic arch status after extended end-to-end anastomosis repair.

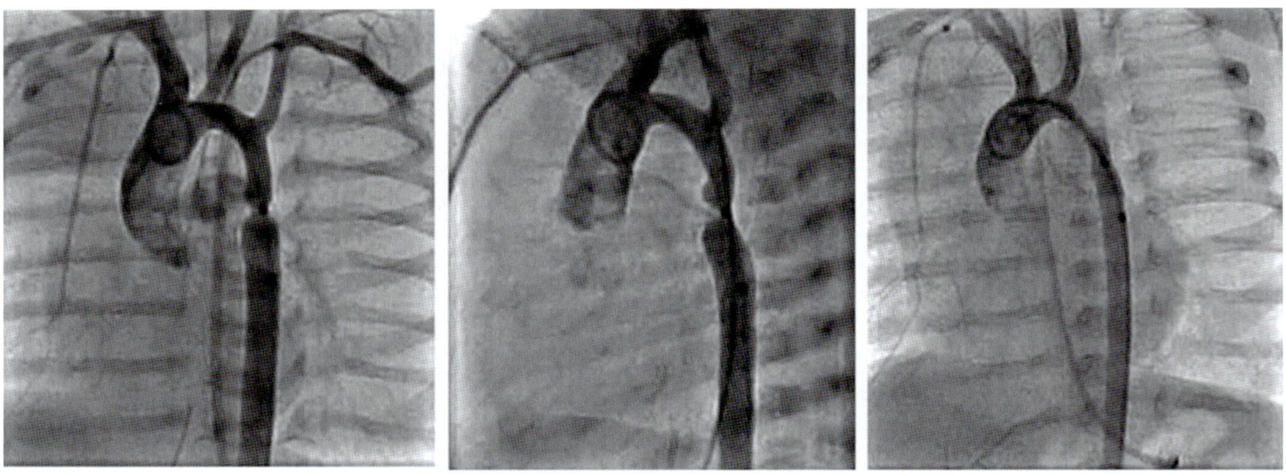

Figure 42.3 (a,b) Anteroposterior and lateral angiographic images of a late-preterm term infant showing an area of discrete narrowing of the mid-thoracic descending aorta at the insertion point of the arterial duct. The infant underwent extended end-to-end anastomosis repair 2 days later. (c) Oblique angiographic image taken 6 weeks following surgical repair showing significant long-segment recoarctation. The narrowed descending aortic arch is irregular in outline and the left subclavian artery has been sacrificed. (d) Ballooning of the descending aortic arch with 6 × 20 mm Tyshak II balloon. (e,f) Oblique and lateral angiographic images after successful ballooning demonstrating improvement in the diameter of the narrowed aortic segment with no aneurysm formation seen. More aggressive ballooning was not pursued at this time as the trans-CoA gradient had dropped significantly, to less than 20 mmHg.

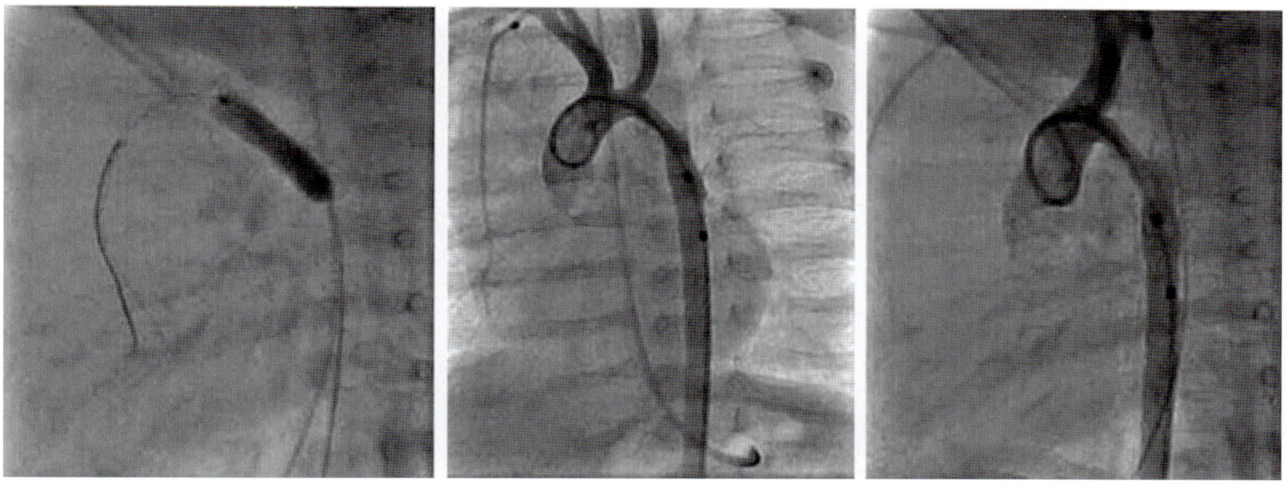

Figure 42.3 (*Continued*)

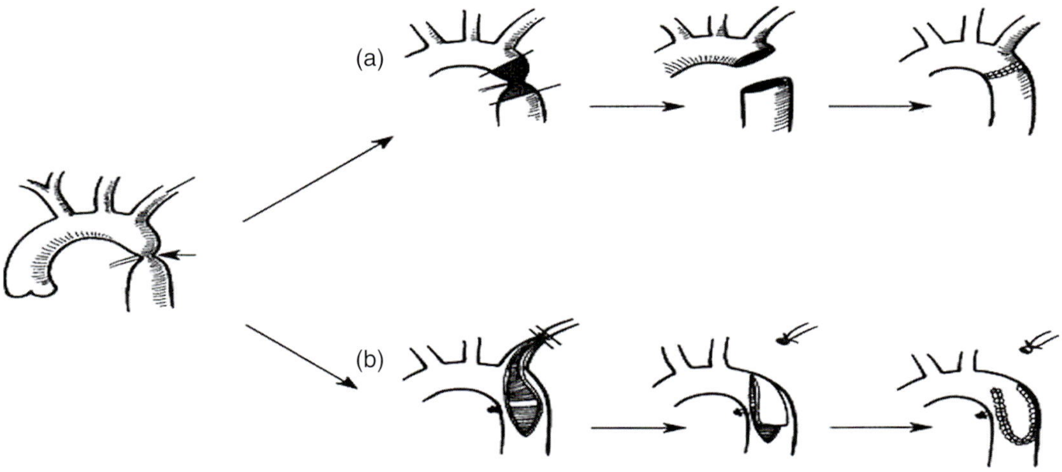

Figure 42.4 Schematic diagrams showing surgical techniques: (a) resection and end-to-end anastomosis; (b) subclavian flap repair.

coarctated segment [4]. In the latter approach, the left upper extremity is supplied by collateral arteries that develop over time, so atrophy of left upper extremity is rare in this circumstance. Following surgical repair, patients are at lifelong risk of developing recoarctation (15–20%), which can be treated by balloon angioplasty with possible stent placement across the coarcted segment if the patient is large enough for a stent inflatable to an adult size (usually >20 kg).

Smaller absolute transverse arch diameter and younger age are risk factors for recoarctation. However, with contemporary surgical approaches low birth weight is thought not to be a significant risk factor and it is recommended not to delay repair in relatively low birth weight infants [5]. Aneurysm formation has also been reported at the site of surgical repair. However, rates are significantly lower with current surgical techniques. Magnetic resonance imaging (MRI) assessment of the aortic arch is useful to evaluate for aneurysm formation in adolescence and early adulthood. Although early surgery can prevent or delay the onset of hypertension, approximately 30% of children will be hypertensive by adolescence despite early surgery, and it is now arguable that hypertension is the single most important outcome variable in patients with repaired CoA [4]. Attentive serial blood pressure evaluation and aggressive early medical management are important to avoid accelerated coronary artery disease, heart failure, and stroke.

References

1 Kemper AR, Mahle WT, Martin GR, *et al.* (2011) Strategies for implementing screening for critical congenital heart disease. *Pediatrics*, **128**, 1259–1267.

2 Rosenthal E. (2005) Coarctation of the aorta from fetus to adult: curable condition or life long disease process? *Heart*, **91**, 1495–1502.

3 Matsui H, Mellander M, Roughton M, Jicinska H, Gardiner HM. (2008) Morphological and physiological predictors of fetal aortic coarctation. *Circulation*, **118**, 1793–1801.

4 Kenny D, Hijazi ZM. (2011) Coarctation of the aorta: from fetal life to adulthood. *Cardiol J*, **18**, 487–495.

5 McElhinney DB, Yang SG, Hogarty AN, *et al.* (2001) Recurrent arch obstruction after repair of isolated coarctation of the aorta in neonates and young infants: is low weight a risk factor? *J Thorac Cardiovasc Surg*, **122**, 883–890.

43

Vascular Rings and Pulmonary Slings

Donald J. Hagler[1] *and Jessica Bowman*[2]

[1] Division of Cardiovascular Surgery, Mayo Clinic, Rochester, MN, USA
[2] Nationwide Children's Hospital, Columbus, OH, USA

Anomalies of the aortic arch and pulmonary artery slings represent a diverse group of anomalies that often present with airway or esophageal obstruction. Double aortic arch was described as early as 1737 by Hommel [1]. Kommerell [2] first described the radiologic findings of anomalous origin of the right subclavian artery in 1936.

Vascular rings are formed when one or more anomalies of the aortic arch or brachiocephalic branches, in the presence of a patent ductus arteriosus or ligamentum, forms a ring that completely encircles the trachea and esophagus producing symptoms of tracheal or esophageal obstruction.

Pulmonary artery slings are produced by anomalous origin of the left pulmonary artery from the right pulmonary artery and its subsequent course posterior to the trachea and anterior to the esophagus, most often resulting in tracheal compression.

Anomalies of the Aortic Arch

A review of the embryology of the aortic arch development is helpful in understanding the variety of possible arch anomalies.

Embryology

Anomalies of the aortic arch and great vessels are best appreciated in the context of the normal embryology of the aortic arch and the theoretical embryonic pathogenesis of aortic arch and pulmonary artery anomalies [3, 4]. The aortic arch initially exists as paired arteries originating from the aortic sac on the ventral surface of the embryo and coursing superiorly, then turning and pursuing a dorsal and caudal course (Figure 43.1). The aortic arches develop and regress with the development of the pharyngeal pouches. The left fourth aortic arch persists to contribute to the mature aortic arch, while the right fourth arch becomes the proximal right subclavian artery (Figures 43.1b and 43.2). The sixth aortic arch persists on the left as the ductus arteriosus and contributes to the main pulmonary artery while the right sixth arch contributes to the right pulmonary artery. It is possible to explain most aortic arch anomalies by postulating persistence or regression of various segments of the primitive hypothetical double aortic arch. Normally, the left aortic arch occurs with the regression of segment eight (region 1) of the right dorsal aorta and persistence of the left eighth segment (region 3) (Figure 43.3a). A right aortic arch would occur with regression of segment eight of the left dorsal aorta and persistence of the right eighth segment.

The normal left aortic arch crosses over the left main stem bronchus on the left side of the trachea. The normal brachiocephalic branching pattern includes the innominate artery as the first branch dividing into the right subclavian and the right carotid arteries. The left carotid and the left subclavian arteries are the second and third branches, respectively. A patent ductus arteriosus or ductal ligament descends from its origin near the left subclavian to the dome of the main pulmonary artery. A right aortic arch crosses over the right main stem bronchus and on the right side of the trachea. Mirror image brachiocephalic branching has a left innominate artery as the first branch dividing into the left subclavian and left carotid arteries. The mirror image right carotid and right subclavian are the second and third branches. A right aortic arch typically descends on the right side of the thoracic spine but may cross to the left near the diaphragm (Figure 43.3b).

Vascular Rings

Vascular rings can be best described as aortic arch vascular structures, which completely surround both the trachea and the esophagus. Clinically, vascular rings compress the trachea and esophagus resulting

Visual Guide to Neonatal Cardiology, First Edition. Edited by Ernerio T. Alboliras, Ziyad M. Hijazi, Leo Lopez, and Donald J. Hagler.

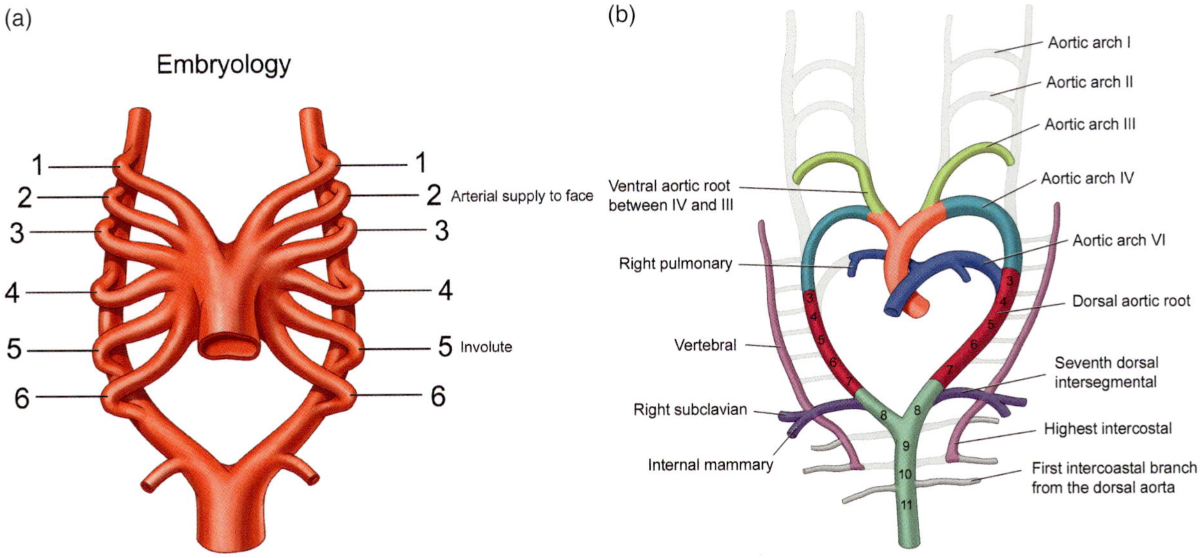

Figure 43.1 (a) The embryonic aortic arch complex in the human embryo. The first and second arches will eventually disappear. The third arches form the carotid arteries. The left fourth arch will remain as a part of the normal left aortic arch connecting to the aorta. The right fourth will form the most proximal portion of the right subclavian artery. The fifth arches disappear while the distal portion of the left sixth arch will remain as the left ductus arteriosus and a portion of the left pulmonary artery. The right sixth arch will contribute to the proximal portion of the right pulmonary artery. (b) The primitive arches that disappear and those that persist as portion of the aortic arch or patent ductus.

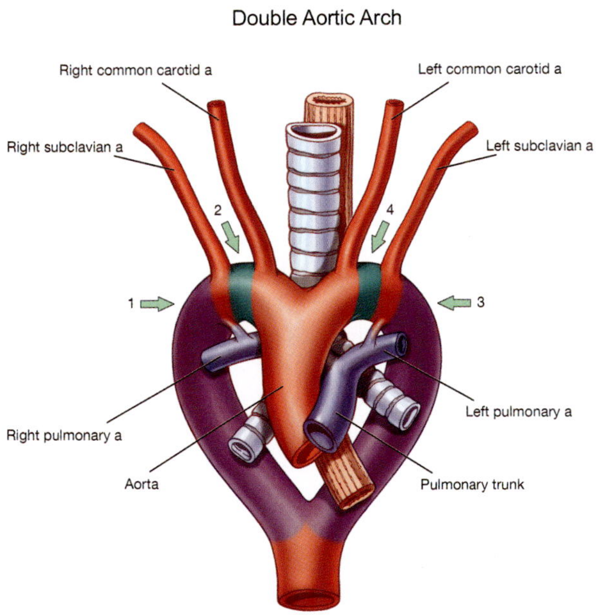

Figure 43.2 Edwards hypothetic double aortic arch and bilateral ducti arteriosi. The ascending and descending aorta are each depicted in midline positions. Arrows point to the four key location where regression occurs and are numbered 1–4. Arrow 1 indicates the eighth segment of the right dorsal aortic root; arrow 2, the right fourth arch; arrows 3 and 4, the corresponding two positions on the left.

in dysphagia and respiratory distress including stridor, wheezing, bronchitis, and pneumonia. Not all components of the vascular ring are patent as they may only be ligamentous structures. An excellent classification of vascular rings has been proposed by Stewart *et al.* [3]. Box 43.1 lists the various components of this classification. They proposed a hypothetical double aortic arch (Figure 43.2), which provided an embryologic explanation for the anticipated features of various vascular rings.

Double Aortic Arch

Double aortic arch represents the most common and most complex form of vascular ring. Double aortic arch results from persistence of both paired dorsal aortic arches with a failure of regression of the right eighth segment of the right dorsal aorta. One or both arches may be patent as observed in Figure 43.4. If one arch is not patent, an atretic zone results from only partial regression. The atretic segment can occur in any of the four dorsal aortic arch segments. More often the left arch is hypoplastic or atretic. Although the ductus arteriosus is not necessary to complete the vascular ring with double aortic arch, the right ductus arteriosus usually regresses but may persistent bilaterally.

The common feature of double aortic arch is the presence of both a left and right aortic arch, regardless of size and patency of the arches. The ascending aorta arises anterior to the trachea and divides into two arches which then pass posteriorly on either side of the trachea and esophagus. There is no innominate artery. Each arch gives rise to its common carotid and subclavian arteries, respectively. Both arches join to form the upper descending aorta behind the esophagus either to the right or left of midline. The first subgroup includes patency of

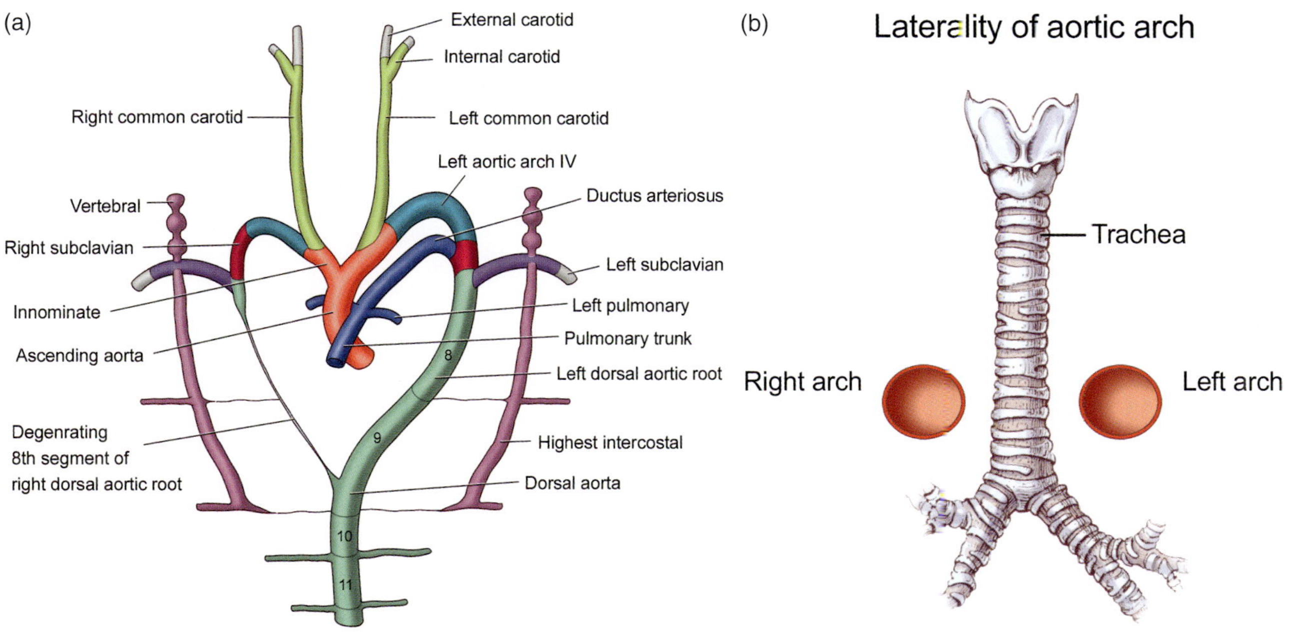

Figure 43.3 (a) The final remaining segments of the normal left aortic arch. (b) The location of left or right aortic arches identified by their relative location to the trachea.

Box 43.1 Major classification of vascular ring and related abnormalities

Each of the subgroups may have left, right, or bilateral ducti arteriosi.

1) Group I. Double aortic arch (left or right upper descending aorta)
   A. Both arches patent
   B. One arch atretic
2) Group II. Left aortic arch (left or right upper descending aorta)
   A. Both arches patent
   B. One arch atretic
3) Group III. Right aortic arch (left or right upper descending aorta)
   A. Mirror-image branching
   B. Aberrant left subclavian artery
   C. "Isolation" of left subclavian artery from aorta

both arches and in the second subgroup one arch is not patent. The most common type is that both arches are patent with the right being larger than the left and in which there is a left ductus arteriosus and the upper descending aorta is on the left. Division of the smaller arch distal to the subclavian or between the carotid and the subclavian is the treatment of choice.

Anomalous Subclavian Artery (Kommerell diverticulum)

During arch formation, if there is bilateral persistence of the eighth segments of the dorsal arches but regression of either the second or fourth arch segments, there is resultant anomalous origin of the subclavian artery from the descending aorta. Part of the persistent eighth segment results in a pouch-like diverticulum at the origin of the subclavian artery as described by Kommerell. The pouch-like diverticulum and the subclavian artery course posterior to the esophagus establishing the major segments of a vascular ring (Figure 43.5). The ring may be completed by a patent ductus arteriosus or ligamentum from the ipsilateral subclavian artery. This description of anomalous origin of the subclavian artery from the descending aorta can be applied either with its association with a left or right aortic arch. The most common anomaly would be associated with a left aortic arch. With a left-sided ductus arteriosus, there is not a true vascular ring. However, if there is persistence of the Kommerell diverticulum, significant esophageal compression and symptoms can result. Persistence of a right-sided patent ductus or ligamentum would be necessary to complete the vascular ring.

A left aortic arch with a right-sided descending aorta in association with a right-sided patent ductus

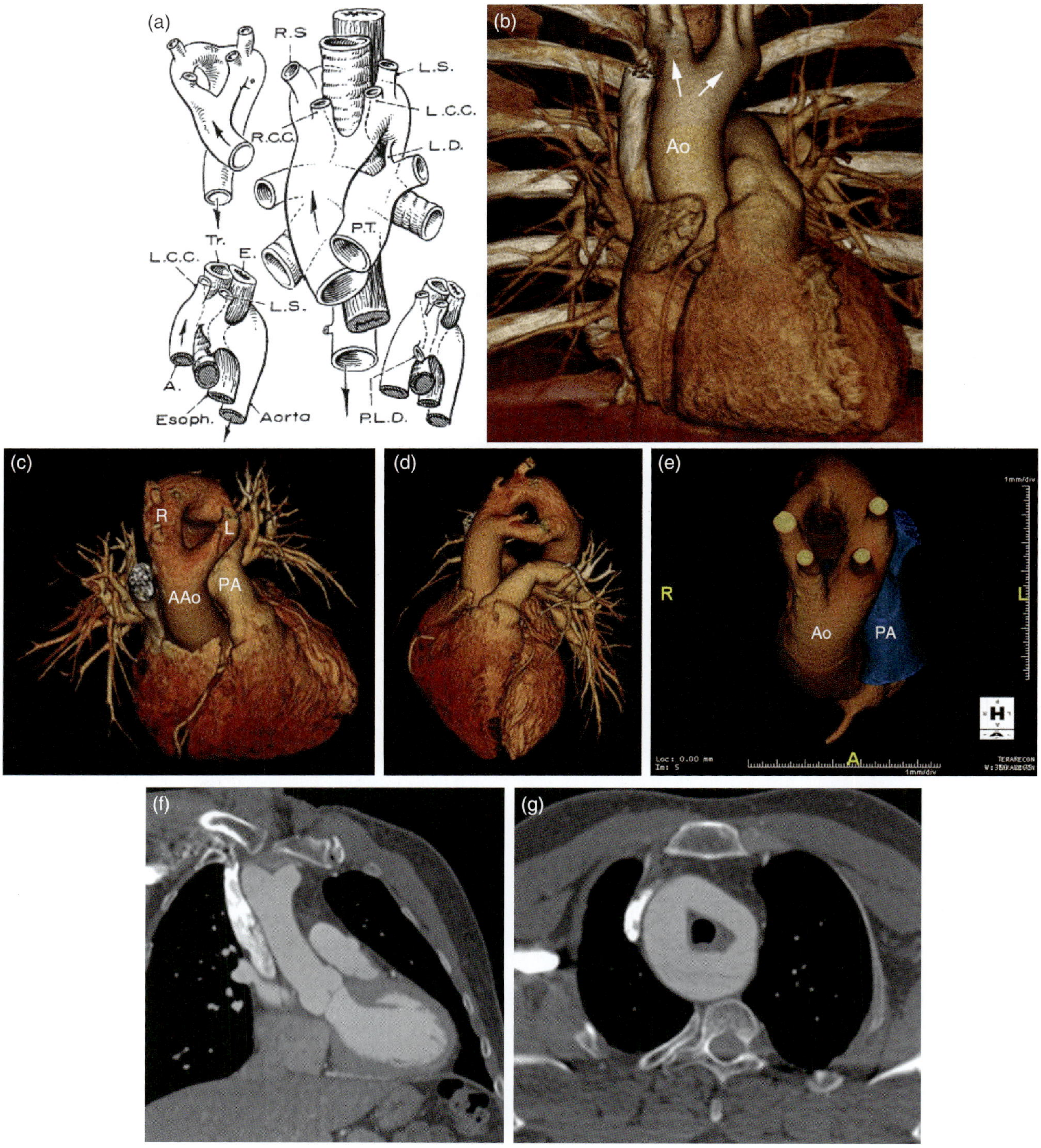

Figure 43.4 (a) Various segments of a double aortic arch. The upper left diagram shows the vascular ring from the front with other structures removed. The lower diagrams illustrate the malformation from the left side. On the lower left a patent left ductus (PLD) is shown. Esoph, E., esophagus; L.C.C., left common carotid; L.D., left ductus; L.S., left subclavian; P.T., pulmonary trunk; R.S., right subclavian; Tr., trachea. (b) CT 3D reconstruction of double aortic arch. Arrows illustrate the course both aortic arches. Ao, aorta. (c) CT 3D reconstruction of double aortic arch view from above with the trachea and esophagus removed. The left (L) arch as in this example is often somewhat hypoplastic compared to the right (R) arch. AAo, ascending aorta; PA, pulmonary artery. (d) Lateral view of the same CT 3D reconstruction. (e) CT 3D reconstruction of a double aortic arch viewed from above. Note the separate origin of all four brachiocephalic branches. In this example the left arch is dominate with some hypoplasia of the right arch. A, anterior; Ao, aorta; L, left; PA, main pulmonary artery; R, right. (f) MRI frontal plane view of double aortic arch illustrating the division of the aorta into two arches. (g) MRI short-axis image of a double aortic arch showing the circular constriction of the esophagus and the trachea.

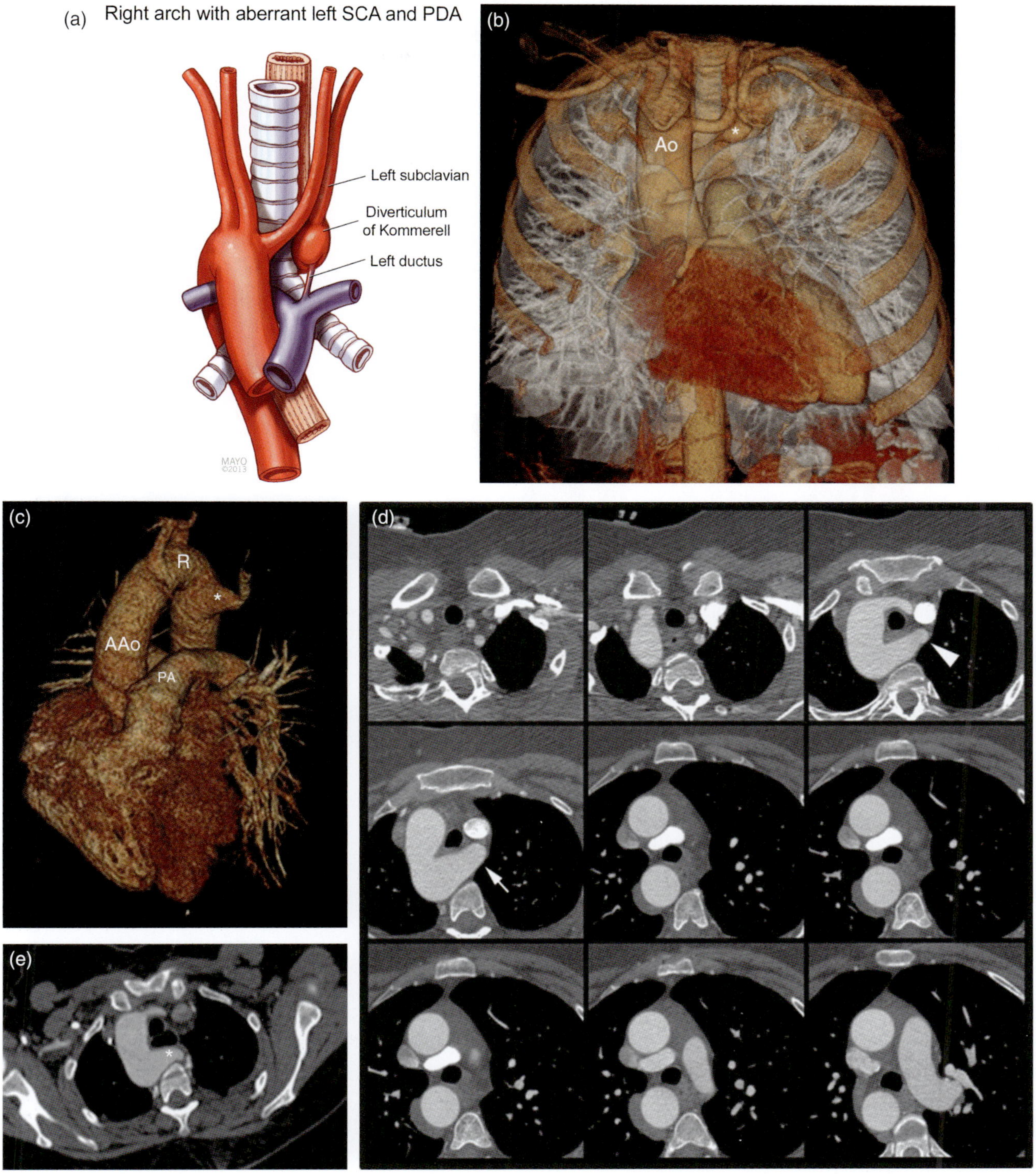

Figure 43.5 (a) Anatomy of a typical vascular ring comprised of a right aortic arch, Kommerell diverticulum with anomalous origin of the left subclavian artery, and a left ductus arteriosus which may be represented simply by a ligament. (b) CT 3D reconstruction illustrating this type of vascular ring with a very prominent Kommerell diverticulum (asterisk). Ao, aorta. (c) CT 3D lateral view of this vascular ring associated with a large Kommerell diverticulum. AAo, ascending aorta; PA, pulmonary artery; R, right aortic arch. (d) Sequential MRI short-axis cuts from the cranial aspect and inferiorly demonstrating the right aortic arch and Kommerell diverticulum (arrow). The arrowhead point to the origin of the left subclavian artery from the diverticulum. (e) MRI short-axis image of the vascular ring and Kommerell diverticulum (asterisk) as it encircles both trachea and esophagus.

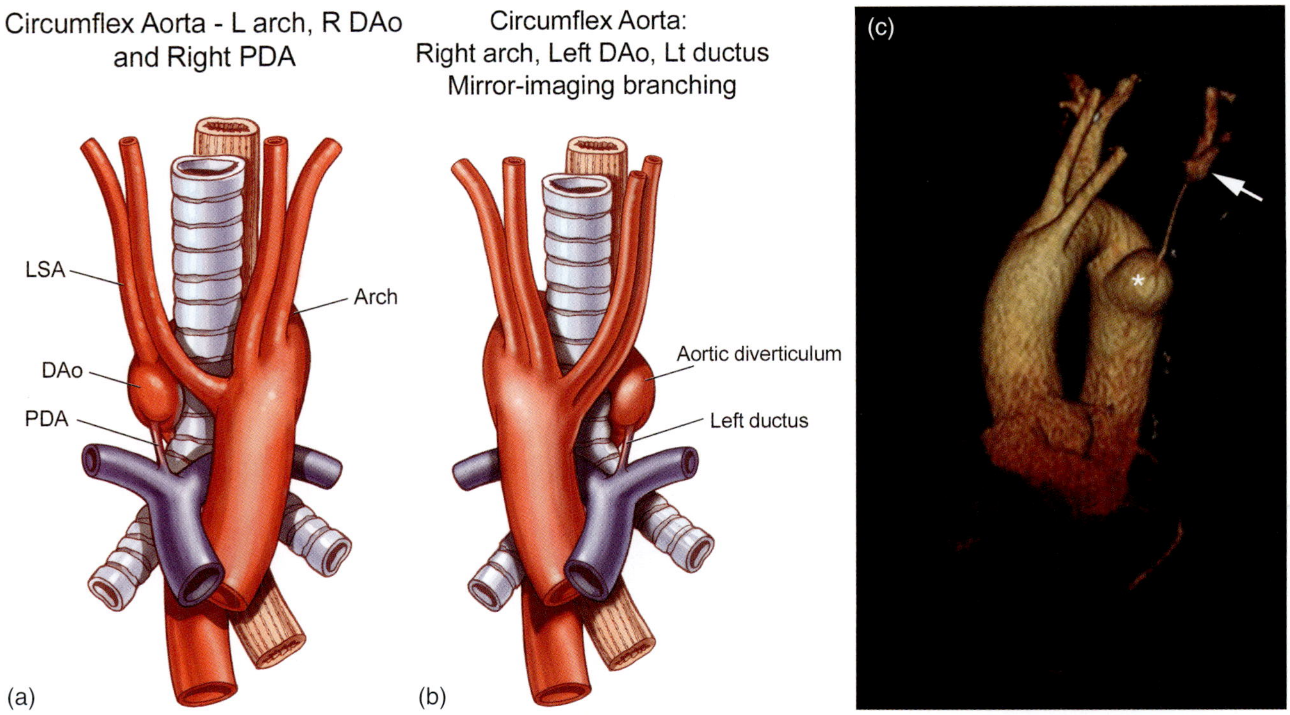

Figure 43.6 (a) The typical anatomic features of a "circumflex aorta." A left aortic arch with the descending aorta coursing behind the esophagus to the right and a right patent ductus arteriosus to create a vascular ring. (b) Anatomic features of a "circumflex aorta" with a right aortic arch and left descending aorta with a left patent ductus arteriosus. (c) CT 3D reconstruction of a right aortic arch, diverticulum of Kommerell, and "isolation" of the left subclavian artery with a long atretic segment originating from diverticulum (asterisk).

or ligamentum also produces a vascular ring because of the retroesophageal course of the descending aorta (Figure 43.6a). A true left aortic arch is present in this anomaly, so surgical correction would be performed from a right thoracotomy or midline approach in order to remove the right patent ductus or ligamentum. The reverse observation can be noted with right aortic arch and left descending aorta and left patent ductus (Figure 43.6b).

The more typical vascular ring results from regression of the primitive left aortic arch segment with resultant right aortic arch and anomalous origin of the left subclavian artery from the descending aorta (Figure 43.5a). A rare form of this occurs with origin of the innominate artery from the descending aorta (retroesophageal innominate artery). The presence of a left-sided patent ductus arteriosus or ligamentum would complete the vascular ring to produce symptoms. The right aortic arch with retroesophageal diverticulum of Kommerell is the second most common form of vascular ring.

"Isolation" of the subclavian artery is a subgroup of groups II and III. The right subclavian loses continuity with the aorta in group II with interruption of both regions 1 and 2 of the primitive double aortic arch. In group III, the left subclavian is no longer connected to the aorta with interruption of regions 3 and 4 (Figure 43.6c). Right, left, or bilateral ductus arteriosus can be present in both subgroups.

Diagnosis

Barium esophagram (Figure 43.7) in a patient with vascular ring will demonstrate a large posterior indentation in the lateral view, while a smaller posterior esophageal indentation may be observed with anomalous origin of the subclavian artery. Kommerell diverticulum will also produce a larger posterior esophageal indentation. A bilateral indentation of the esophagus may be observed in the anteroposterior projection in double aortic arch.

Magnetic resonance imaging (MRI) or computed tomography (CT) provides the most complete diagnostic information to allow appropriate surgical intervention.

Echocardiography may be helpful in recognizing the presence of an anomalous subclavian artery from the descending aorta by the absence of the typical bifurcation of the innominate artery or first branch of the aortic arch. Occasionally, the anomalous subclavian may be visualized as it originates from the descending aorta. A right aortic arch and anomalous left subclavian artery can be suggestive of the presence of a vascular ring and prompt further imaging investigation such as MRI.

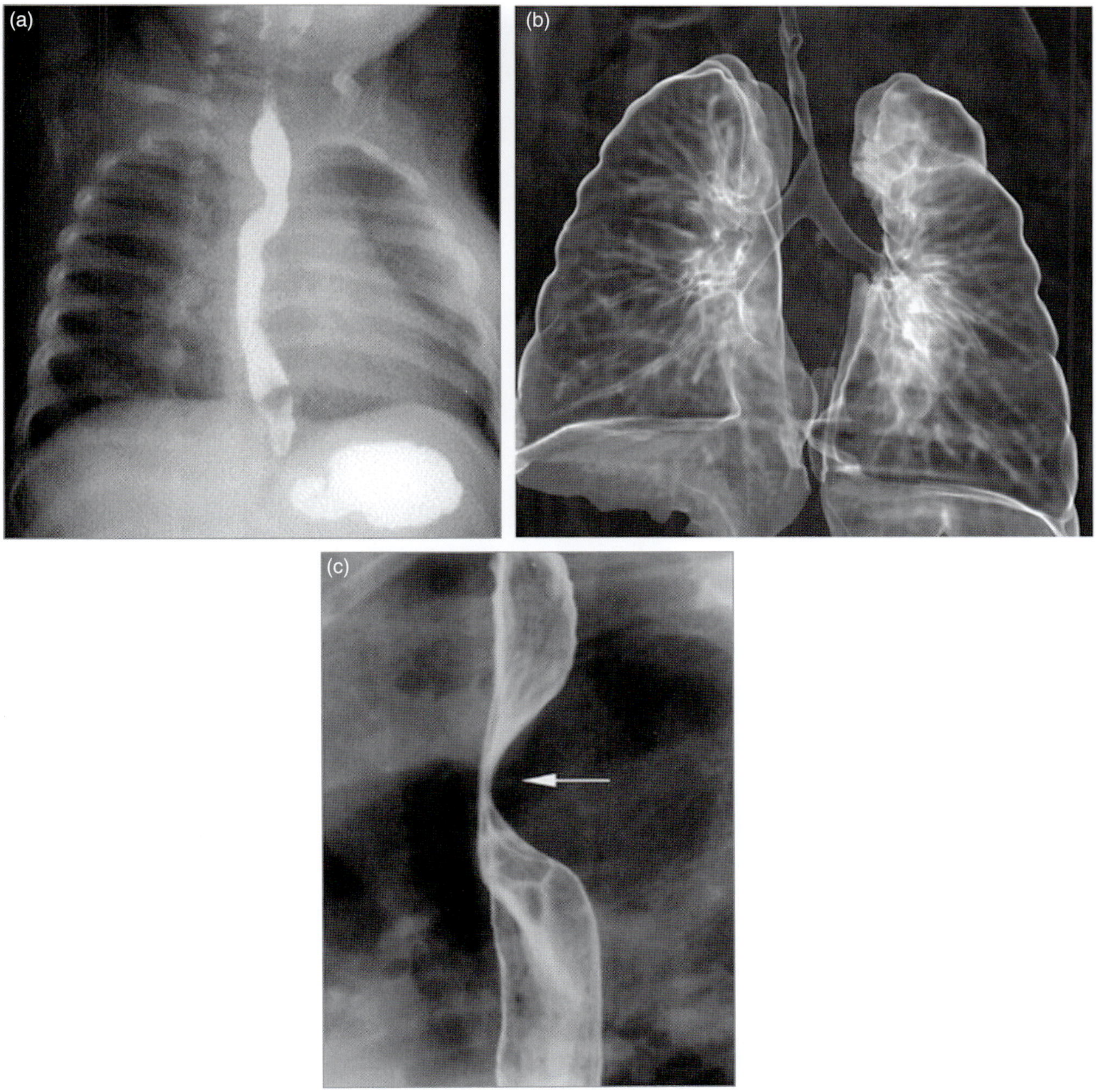

Figure 43.7 (a) AP view of barium esophagram in a patient with double aortic arch which produces a bilateral indentation of the esophagus. (b) Dynamic tracheal obstruction demonstrated by multidetector CT angiography. (c) Lateral view of barium swallow showing posterior esophageal indentation secondary to a Kommerell diverticulum and anomalous origin of the left subclavian artery.

Pulmonary Artery Slings

Anomalous origin of the left pulmonary artery from the right pulmonary artery (pulmonary artery sling) results from abnormal regression of the proximal left sixth aortic arch. This is also the embryonic cause for origin of the left pulmonary artery from the ascending aorta, and absence of the left pulmonary artery.

Anomalous origin of the left pulmonary artery from the right pulmonary artery (pulmonary artery sling) is the only condition in which a major vascular structure passes between the trachea and the esophagus. Patients frequently present in the neonatal period with severe tracheobronchial obstruction and respiratory distress (Figure 43.8). This anomaly can also be associated with tracheal stenosis secondary to complete cartilaginous

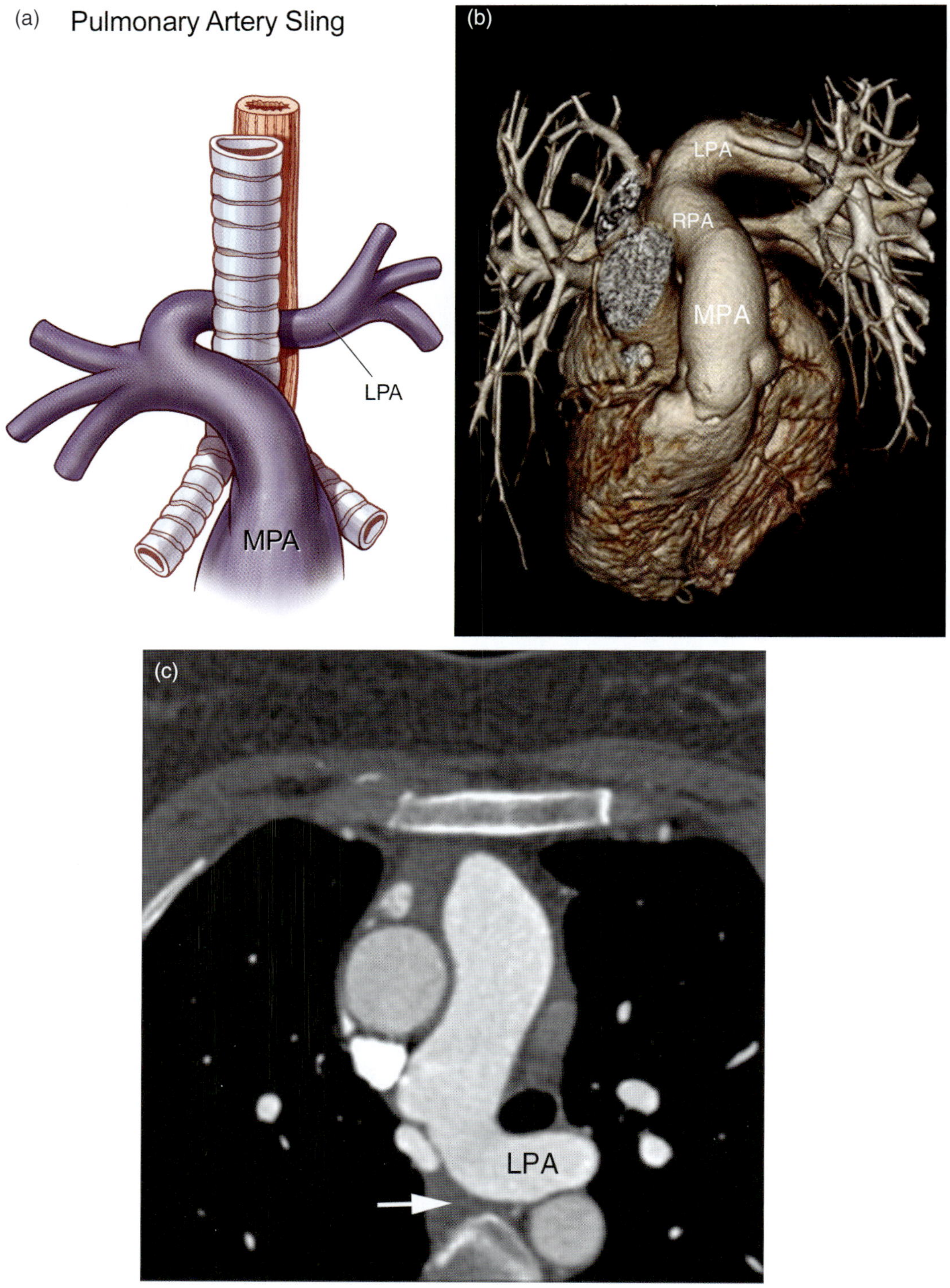

Figure 43.8 (a) The typical anatomic features of a left pulmonary artery sling. Note the course of the left pulmonary artery between the trachea and the esophagus. (b) CT 3D reconstruction of a pulmonary artery sling with anomalous origin of the left pulmonary artery from the right pulmonary artery. LPA, left pulmonary artery; MPA, main pulmonary artery; RPA, right pulmonary artery. (c) MRI short-axis image showing similar anatomy with the left pulmonary artery coursing behind the trachea and in front of the esophagus (arrow).

tracheal rings. The anomaly usually develops as an isolated defect but occasionally can be associated with cardiac defects such as tetralogy of Fallot. Often, the diagnosis can be made with barium swallow where there is a classic anterior compression of the esophagus by the left pulmonary artery. However, MRI and CT studies will be helpful in making a more definitive diagnosis and to define the tracheal anatomy.

Surgical repair is best achieved with division of the left pulmonary artery and reimplantation to the main pulmonary artery in front of the trachea. If complete tracheal rings are present, tracheal reconstruction may be necessary. Late follow-up should be recommended to monitor for recurrent left pulmonary artery stenosis.

References

1 Hommel W. (1737) Commercium literarium norimbergae. *Hebdom*, **21**, 162.

2 Kommerell B. (1936) Verlagerung des Osophagus durch eine abnorm verlaufende Arteria subclavian dextra (Arteria lusoria). *Fortschr Rontgenstr*, **54**, 590–595.

3 Stewart JR, Kincaid OW, Edwards JE. (1964) *An Atlas of Vascular Rings and Related Malformations of the Aortic Arch System*. Charles C. Thomas, Springfield, IL.

4 Edwards, JE. (1953) Malformations of the aortic arch system manifested as “vascular rings.” *Lab Invest*, **2**, 56–75.

44

Double Outlet Right Ventricle

Irene D. Lytrivi and H. Helen Ko

Division of Pediatric Cardiology, Mount Sinai Medical Center, New York, NY, USA

The diagnostic term double outlet right ventricle (DORV) is used for a spectrum of congenital cardiac anomalies that share the type of their ventriculo-arterial alignment where both great arteries arise exclusively or predominantly from the right ventricle [1]. A ventricular septal defect (VSD) is almost always present and serves as the outflow of the left ventricle. The presence of a well-developed conus beneath both great arteries was initially considered a prerequisite for the diagnosis [2]. However, the currently accepted definition is broader and encompasses lesions with variable arrangements of the subarterial conus [1, 3]. This chapter provides an overview of the classification of the different anatomic types of DORV and focuses on the subtypes that frequently manifest clinically in the newborn.

DORV is an uncommon congenital heart defect, ranking 12th in frequency in the Baltimore-Washington Infant study (2% of all cases) [4]. The incidence is estimated at 127 per million live births [5]. Most DORV cases are sporadic. When the diagnosis is made in utero, genetic testing should be recommended, as DORV has been associated with trisomies 13 and 18, and deletion of *22g11* (DiGeorge syndrome) [6, 7]. Maternal pregestational diabetes and exposure to solvents have also been implicated [8, 9].

Although the most common classification scheme is based on the VSD location, it is important to understand that in the majority of cases the VSD location is constant and located between the anterior and posterior limbs of the septal band. It is characterized as subaortic (40–57% of cases; Figure 44.1), subpulmonary (24–37% of cases; Figure 44.2), or doubly committed (3–12% of cases; Figure 44.3), depending on the relationship of the great arteries to each other and on the infundibular morphology and position. The VSD can also be remote to the semilunar valves (9–19% of cases) or absent (exceedingly rare) [10]. Remote VSDs are located in the inlet septum, as in a complete atrioventricular (AV) canal defect (Figure 44.4), or in the trabecular portion of the muscular septum. Commonly associated lesions vary depending on the VSD location: subaortic VSDs are frequently associated with pulmonary stenosis, whereas subpulmonary VSDs have a higher rate of subaortic obstruction, aortic coarctation, or interrupted aortic arch.

Eighty-six percent of surgical patients with DORV have concordant AV connections [11]. AV discordance is present in 11% [12]. There may be atrial situs solitus, situs inversus, or heterotaxy syndrome, especially when DORV is associated with AV canal defects [13, 14]. Another morphologic variation that needs to be ascertained during the diagnostic evaluation of the newborn is the presence of a well-developed infundibulum or conus beneath the great arteries. It is currently accepted that bilateral conus is not a prerequisite of the definition of DORV, and DORV can exist with bilaterally present (Figure 44.5), bilaterally absent (Figure 44.6), only subaortic, or only subpulmonary infundibulum. Moving to the next cardiac segment, the great artery relationship also needs to be precisely described. The great arteries can either be normally related with the aortic trunk posteriorly and to the right of the pulmonary trunk and spiraling around each other or be in parallel arrangement. When the great arteries are parallel in situs solitus, the aorta can be rightward and side-by-side with the pulmonary artery, rightward and anterior, directly anterior, or leftward and anterior. The aorta can be leftward and posterior to the pulmonary trunk in situs inversus totalis.

Additional associated abnormalities with important implications in planning the surgical repair are: atrial septal defects, persistent left superior vena cava to the coronary sinus or directly to the left atrium, leftward juxtaposition of the right atrial appendage, anomalous pulmonary venous connections, abnormal AV valve attachments through the VSD (Figure 44.7), straddling AV valves (Figure 44.8), parachute mitral

Visual Guide to Neonatal Cardiology, First Edition. Edited by Ernerio T. Alboliras, Ziyad M. Hijazi, Leo Lopez, and Donald J. Hagler.

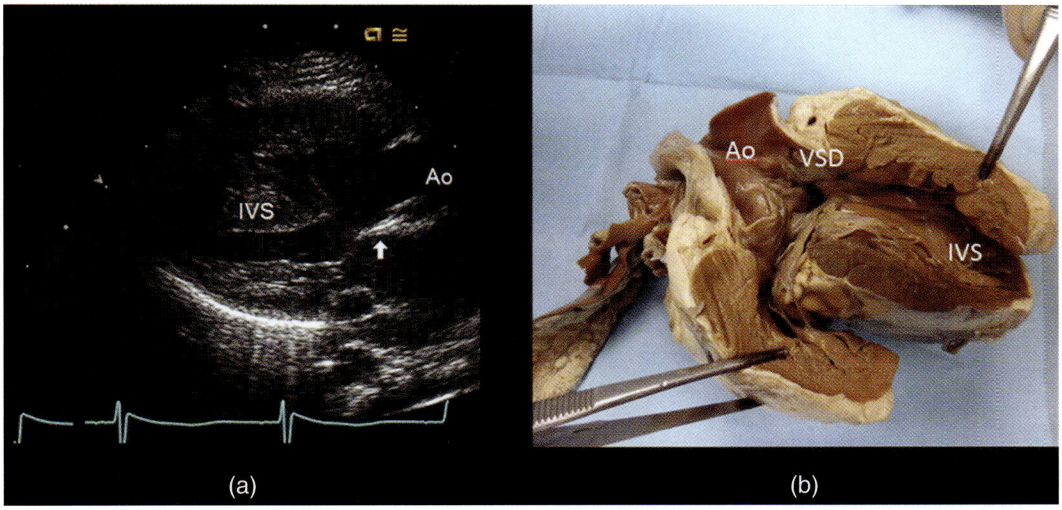

Figure 44.1 (a) Parasternal long-axis view of double outlet right ventricle (DORV) with subaortic ventricular septal defect (VSD). Note the subaortic conus (arrow) and the extreme dextroposition of the aorta, features that differentiate this DORV type from tetralogy of Fallot. (b) "En face" view of the interventricular septum from the right ventricular side showing a pathology specimen of DORV with subaortic VSD. Ao, aorta; IVS, interventricular septum.

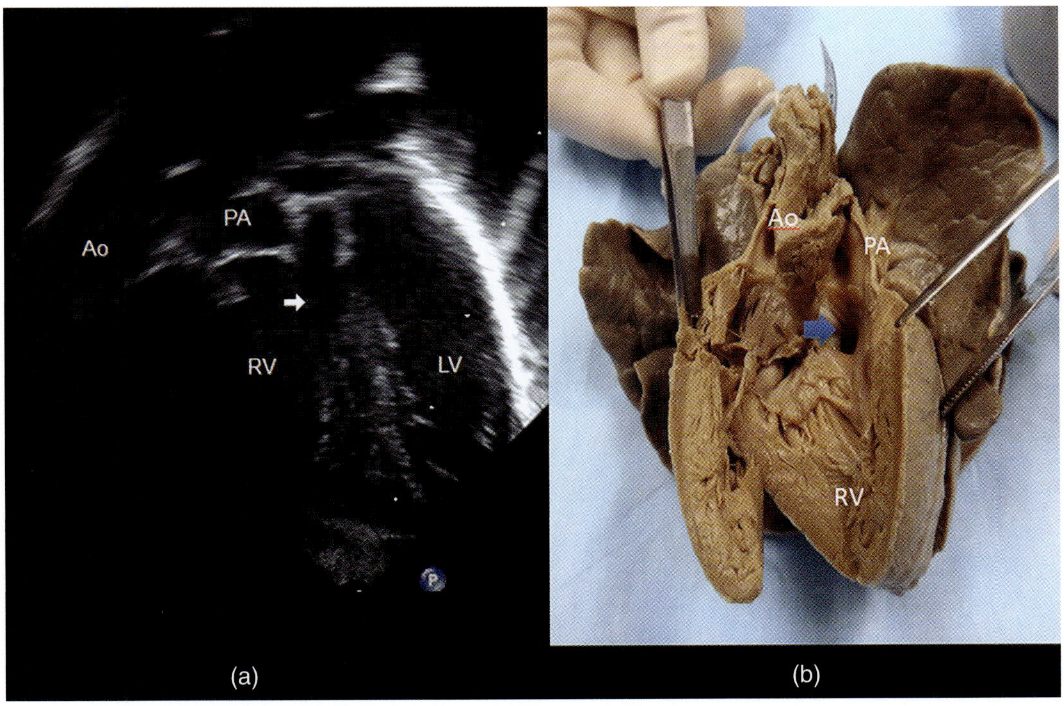

Figure 44.2 (a) Modified apical view angled anteriorly showing the subpulmonary VSD (arrow). (b) Pathology specimen also showing the origin of both great arteries from the right ventricle and the relationship of the VSD to the pulmonary artery. Ao, aorta; LV, left ventricle; PA, pulmonary artery; RV, right ventricle.

valve, supramitral ring, ventricular hypoplasia, and coronary artery anomalies. Abnormal coronary artery anatomy has been described in up to 30% of DORV patients [15], occurring more frequently in those with a subpulmonary VSD and side-by-side great arteries (Figure 44.9). Of particular importance for surgical management are those with coronary arteries crossing anteriorly to the right ventricular outflow tract, such as the left anterior descending coronary artery arising anomalously from the right coronary artery and crossing anteriorly to the interventricular groove, or the right coronary artery crossing anteriorly to the right

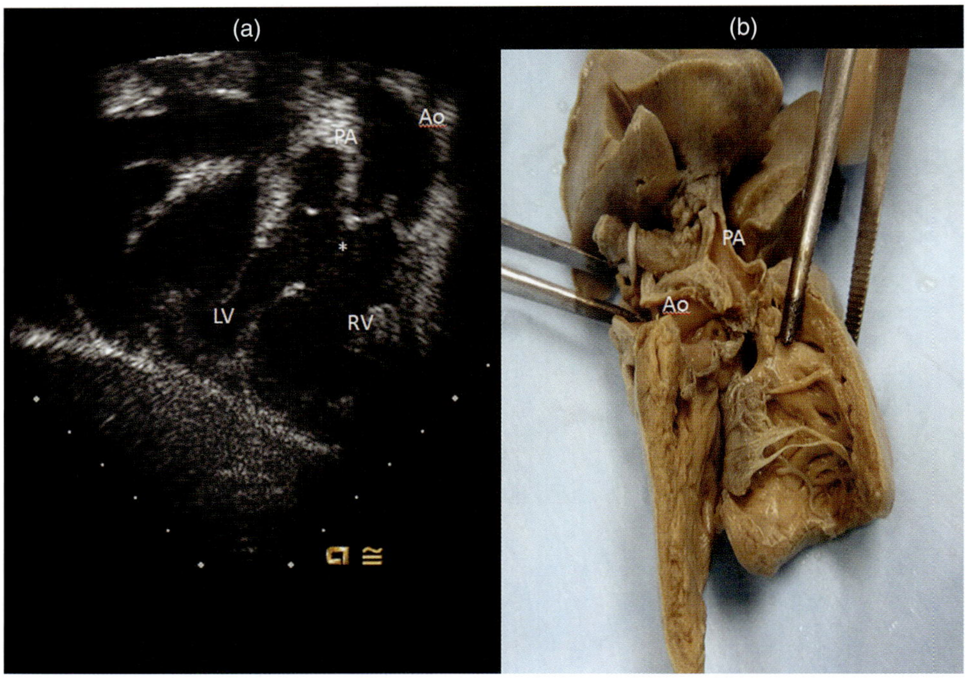

Figure 44.3 (a) Modified subxiphoid long-axis (LAO) view of DORV in the setting of dextrocardia and L-looped ventricles with a large doubly-committed VSD (*). (b) Large doubly-committed subarterial VSD and absence of subarterial conus as viewed from the right ventricular side in a pathology specimen.

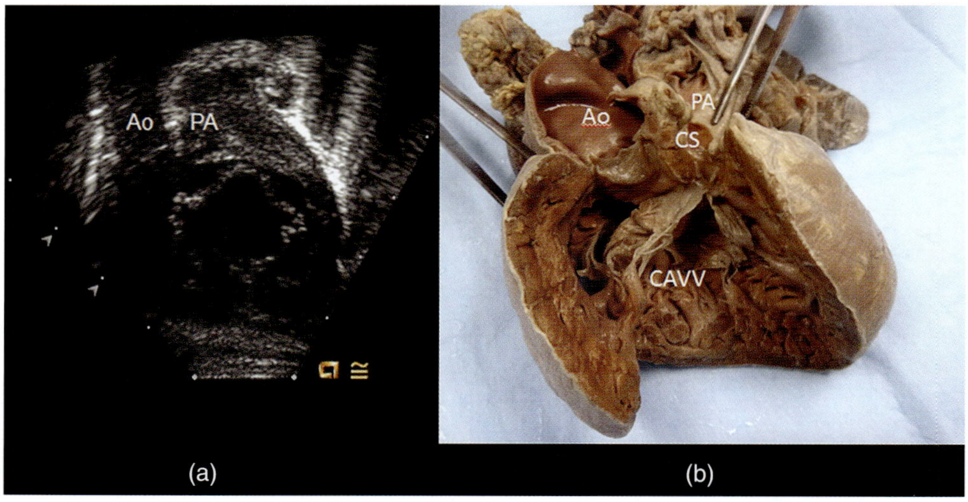

Figure 44.4 (a) Subxiphoid long-axis view of DORV associated with complete atrioventricular canal (CAVC) defect. The common AV valve is captured in diastole. (b) Pathology specimen showing the remote VSD of this case of DORV with CAVC defect and a well-developed conal septum. CAVV, common atrioventricular valve; CS, conal septum.

AV groove in cases of L-malposed aorta. Regardless of the anatomic variations, the different pathophysiologic presentations of DORV can be categorized as shown in Table 44.1.

Neonatal presentation occurs when accompanying lesions cause either cyanosis as a result of severe obstruction to pulmonary blood flow or transposition physiology, or systemic hypoperfusion caused by aortic coarctation or aortic arch interruption.

The most common form of DORV with subaortic VSD can occur in a neonate if the pulmonary outflow is small, leading to cyanosis. Obstruction is usually subvalvar but it can also be valvar and accompanied by hypoplasia of the main and branch pulmonary arteries. The examination reveals visible cyanosis, a single second heart sound (S2), and a loud systolic murmur, frequently with a thrill at the left upper sternal border and radiation to the lung fields. The chest X-ray can be similar to that seen with

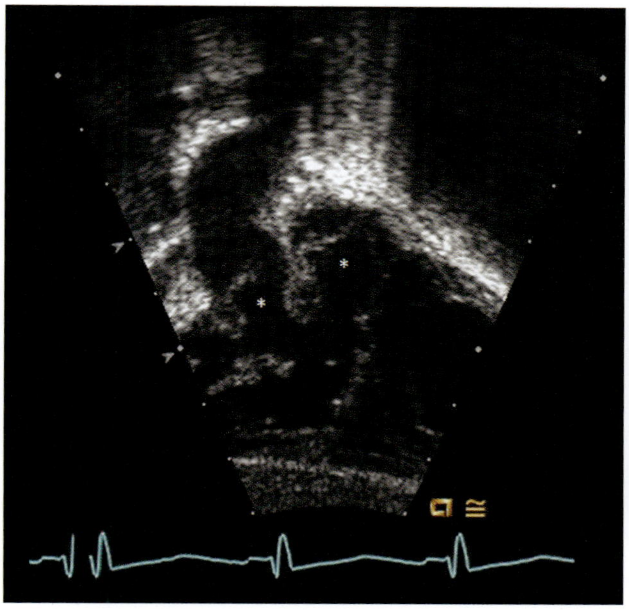

Figure 44.5 Subxiphoid long-axis view of DORV demonstrating the great arteries arising exclusively from the right ventricle (RV) with bilateral conus (asterisks).

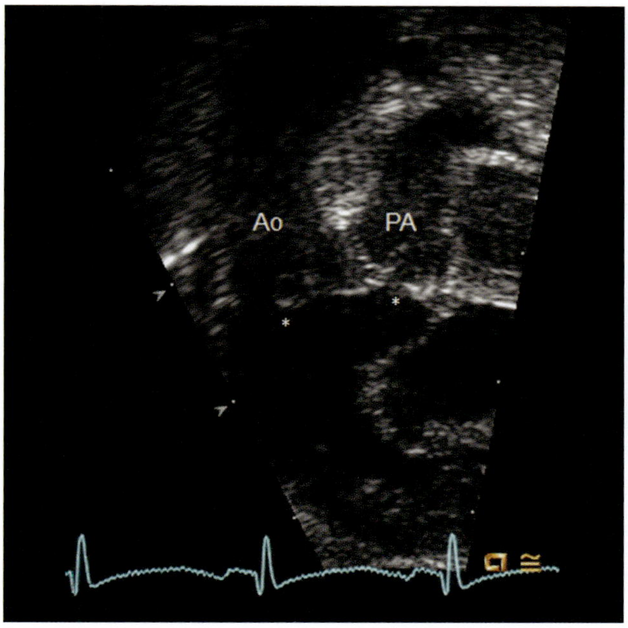

Figure 44.6 Subxiphoid long-axis view of DORV focused on the great arteries demonstrating bilaterally absent conus (asterisks).

tetralogy of Fallot with concave left upper cardiac border caused by varying degrees of hypoplasia of the central pulmonary arteries. Surgical repair consists of creation of a tunnel through the VSD to connect the left ventricle to the aorta and relief of the pulmonary outflow obstruction with techniques similar to those used for repair of tetralogy of Fallot.

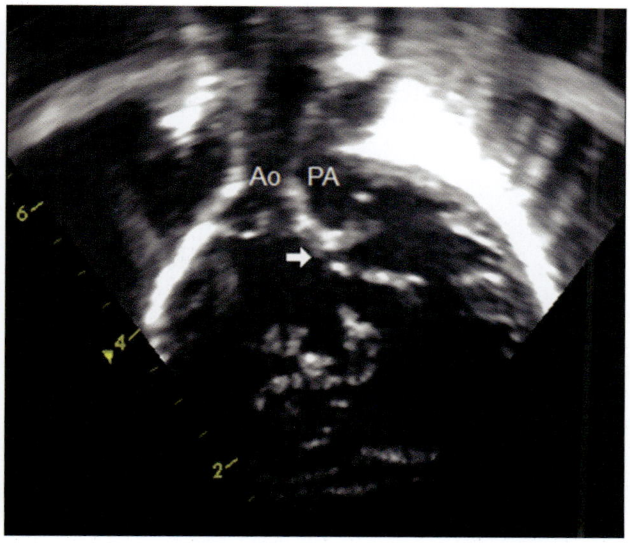

Figure 44.7 Subxiphoid short-axis image showing straddling attachments of the mitral valve to the conal septum (arrows), interfering with the potential LV–Ao pathway.

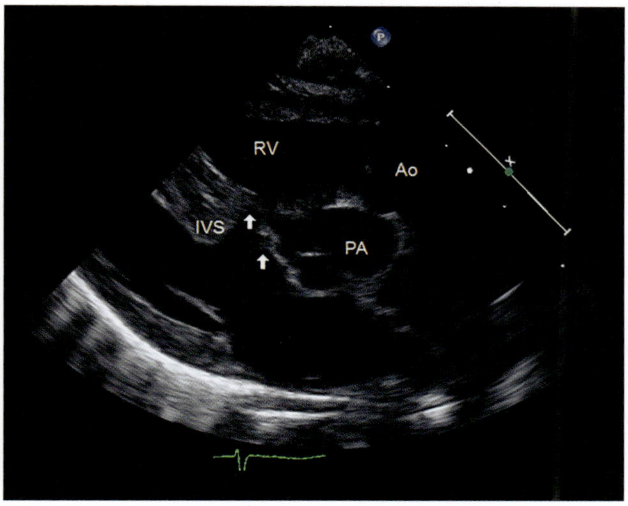

Figure 44.8 Parasternal long-axis view demonstrating straddling of the mitral valve (arrows) through the VSD, obstructing the subpulmonary area. Ao, aorta; IVS, interventricular septum; PA, pulmonary artery; RV, right ventricle.

DORV with a subpulmonary VSD usually presents early in life with transposition physiology caused by preferential streaming of oxygenated blood to the pulmonary artery. Infants are cyanotic, with a single, loud S2 caused by the proximity of the anterior aorta to the chest wall. In patients with no pulmonary stenosis (which represents the overwhelming majority of DORV patients with subpulmonary VSD), severe heart failure signs and symptoms coexist with cyanosis. With associated coarctation, the femoral pulses are diminished or absent. Finally, in the rare cases of coexistent pulmonary

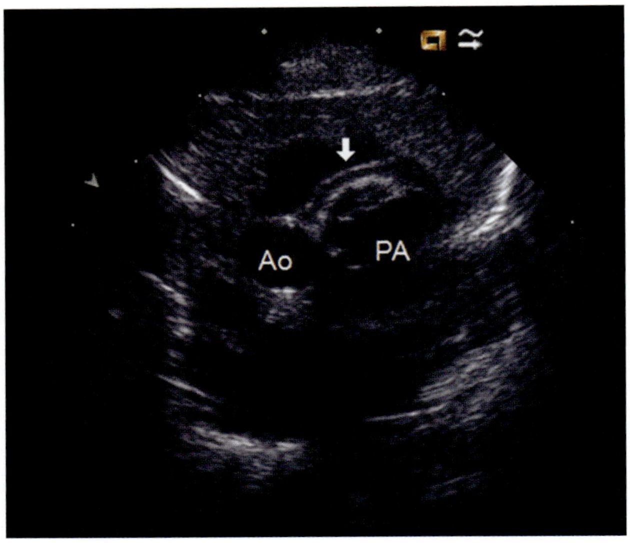

Figure 44.9 Parasternal short-axis view demonstrating side-by-side great arteries with the left coronary artery crossing the pulmonary outflow tract anteriorly (arrow). Ao, aorta; PA, pulmonary artery.

stenosis, there is a loud systolic murmur at the left upper sternal border.

The most common surgical approach to DORV with subpulmonary VSD is the arterial switch operation in combination with tunnel closure of the VSD to the pulmonary artery. Alternatively, when the aorta is rightward and side-by-side to the pulmonary artery, an intraventricular tunnel connecting the left ventricle to the aorta can be employed. This repair connects the LV to the aorta via a tunnel that runs posteriorly to the pulmonary artery between the pulmonary and tricuspid valves. Resection of the conal septum is often necessary in order to create an unobstructed pathway. In this repair, the distance between the tricuspid and pulmonary valve annuli is of major importance; unless the distance measures at least the same as the aortic valve annulus the pathway may become obstructed. In patients with pulmonary obstruction in whom the arterial switch cannot be performed, more complex intraventricular tunnel repairs such as the *réparation à l'etage ventriculaire* (REV) and Nikaidoh procedures need to be employed [16, 17].

DORV with non-committed VSD can have variable clinical presentations depending on the associated anomalies. When AV valve or other associated abnormalities preclude biventricular repair, staged palliation is performed. Newborns frequently undergo systemic-to-pulmonary shunts to increase pulmonary blood flow and alleviate cyanosis. Alternatively, in patients with no pulmonary stenosis, pulmonary artery banding can be performed to prevent pulmonary vascular disease until definitive repair is undertaken at an older age.

Surgical mortality of neonatal biventricular repair has recently been reported at 4–6% [18]. Survival at 15 years is in the range of 90–96% and freedom from reoperation is 72–87%, depending on the type of operation [19]. Long-term residual lesions are variable and specific to the type of repair performed, and these include subaortic stenosis, residual arch obstruction, pulmonary stenosis or conduit obstruction, and neo-aortic root dilation and regurgitation.

Acknowledgments

The authors thank Margret S. Magid, MD, Division of Pediatric Pathology, Icahn School of Medicine at Mount Sinai, who provided the specimens and helped with obtaining the images.

Table 44.1 Clinical presentations of double outlet right ventricle (DORV).

Pathophysiology	Clinical presentation	Example	Time of onset
VSD physiology	Signs of congestive heart failure	Subaortic or doubly committed subarterial VSD	First 4–6 weeks of life
Tetralogy of Fallot physiology	Cyanosis caused by pulmonary stenosis	Subaortic VSD	Neonatal period
Transposition physiology	Cyanosis caused by reduced effective pulmonary blood flow	Subpulmonary VSD, e.g. Taussig–Bing anomaly with subpulmonary VSD and bilateral conus	Neonatal period
Systemic outflow obstruction	Signs of low cardiac output	Subpulmonary VSD with aortic arch obstruction	Neonatal period
Single ventricle physiology	Cyanosis with complete mixing of blood	DORV in the setting of heterotaxy	Neonatal period

VSD, ventricular septal defect.

References

1 Walters, HL, Mavroudis C, Tchervenkov CI, *et al.* (2000) Congenital Heart Surgery Nomenclature and Database Project: double outlet right ventricle. *Ann Thorac Surg*, **69**, 249–263.

2 Neufeld HN, DuShane JW, Edwards JE. (1961) Origin of both great vessels from the right ventricle. II: with pulmonary stenosis. *Circulation*, **23**, 603.

3 Van Praagh S, Davidoff A, Chin A, *et al.* (1982) Double-outlet right ventricle: anatomic types and developmental implications based on a study of 101 cases. *Coeur (Paris)*, **12**, 389–439.

4 Perry LW, Neill CA, Ferencz C, *et al.* (1993) Infants with congenital heart disease: the cases, in, *Perspectives in Pediatric Cardiology*, Vol. 4: *Epidemiology of Congenital Heart Disease: The Baltimore-Washington Infant Study 1981–1989* (eds C Ferencz, JD Rubin, CA Loffredo, CA Magee), Futura, Mount Kisco, NY, pp. 33–62.

5 Hoffman JI, Kaplan S. (2002) The incidence of congenital heart disease. *J Am Coll Cardiol*, **39**, 1890–1900.

6 Vuillemin M, Pexieder T, Winking H. (1991) Pathogenesis of various forms of double outlet right ventricle in mouse fetal trisomy 13. *Int J Cardiol*, **33**, 281–304.

7 Van Praagh S, Truman T, Firpo A, *et al.* (1989) Cardiac malformations in trisomy 18: a study of 41 postmortem cases. *J Am Coll Cardiol* **13**, 1586–1597.

8 Ferencz C, Rubin JD, McCarter RJ, Clark EB. (1990) Maternal diabetes and cardiovascular malformations: predominance of double outlet right ventricle and truncus arteriosus. *Teratology*, **41**, 319–326.

9 Ferencz C, Correa-Villasenor A, Loffredo CA, Wilson PD. (1997) Malformations of the cardiac outflow tract, in, *Perspectives in Pediatric Cardiology*, Vol. 5: *Genetic and Environmental Risk Factors of Major Cardiovascular Malformations The Baltimore–Washington Infant Study 1981–1989* (eds C Ferencz, A Correa-Villasenor, CA Loffredo, PD Wilson), Futura, Armonk, NY, pp. 59–102.

10 Pandit SP, Shah VK, Daruwala DF. (1987) Double-outlet right ventricle with intact interventricular septum: a case report. *Indian Heart J*, **39**, 56–57.

11 Sondheimer HM, Freedom RM, Olley PM. (1977) Double-outlet right ventricle: clinical spectrum and prognosis. *Am J Cardiol*, **39**, 709–714.

12 Tabry IF, McGoon DC, Danielson GK, *et al.* (1978) Surgical management of double-outlet right ventricle associated with atrioventricular discordance. *J Thorac Cardiovasc Surg*, **76**, 336–344.

13 Danielson GK, Tabry IF, Ritter DG, *et al.* (1978) Successful repair of double-outlet right ventricle, complete atrioventricular canal, and atrioventricular discordance with dextrocardia and pulmonary stenosis. *J Thorac Cardiovasc Surg*, **78**, 710–717.

14 Alfieri O, Crupi G, Vanini V, *et al.* (1978) Successful surgical repair of double-outlet right ventricle with situs inversus, l-loop, l-malposition, and subaortic VSD in a 16 month-old patient. *Eur J Cardiol*, **7**, 40–47.

15 Wilcox BR, Ho SY, Macartney FJ, *et al.* (1981) Surgical anatomy of double-outlet right ventricle with situs solitus and atrioven–tricular concordance. *J Thorac Cardiovasc Surg*, **82**, 405–417.

16 Sakata R, Lecompte Y, Batisse A, *et al.* (1988) Anatomic repair of anomalies of ventriculoarterial connection associated with ventricular septal defect. I. Criteria of surgical decision. *J Thorac Cardiovasc Surg*, **95**, 90–95.

17 Nikaidoh H. (1984) Aortic translocation and biventricular outflow tract reconstruction: a new surgical repair for transposition of the great arteries associated with ventricular septal defect and pulmonary stenosis. *J Thorac Cardiovasc Surg*, **88**, 365–372.

18 Artrip JH, Sauer H, Campbell DN, *et al.* (2006) Biventricular repair in double outlet right ventricle: surgical results based on the STS-EACTS International Nomenclature classification. *Eur J Cardiothorac Surg*, **29**(4), 545–550.

19 Brown JW, Ruzmetov M, Okada Y, *et al.* (2001) Surgical results in patients with double outlet right ventricle: a 20-year experience. *Ann Thorac Surg*, **72** (5), 1630–1635.

45

Double Outlet Left Ventricle

Sarah Chambers Gurson[1] *and Leo Lopez*[2]

[1] *Pediatric Cardiology Associates PC, Fairfax, VA, USA*
[2] *Nicklaus Children's Hospital; Herbert Wertheim College of Medicine Florida International University, Miami, FL, USA*

Double outlet left ventricle (DOLV) is a very rare form of congenital heart disease in which the great vessels arise completely or almost completely from the left ventricle. DOLV was historically thought to be an anatomic impossibility. The first case was reported in 1967 with many more cases reported subsequently in the literature. It has been suggested that DOLV makes up 5% of all hearts with double outlet ventriculo-arterial connections, corresponding to an incidence of less than 1 in 100 000 births [1]. DOLV is usually seen with a ventricular septal defect (VSD), but it can also be seen with an intact ventricular septum. When a VSD is present, DOLV is subject to the same debates relating to diagnosis and nomenclature as seen with double outlet right ventricle (DORV), especially when an overriding semilunar valve is related to both the left and the right ventricles.

Etiology

A basic understanding of the embryogenesis of the outflow tracts helps one to understand the development of the normal ventricular outflow tracts and the possible ways in which DOLV might arise. After cardiac looping – in which the bulbus cordis becomes the right ventricle and the primitive ventricle becomes the left ventricle – the conotruncal outflow relates directly to the right ventricle. The process of separation of the conotruncus into the main pulmonary artery and aorta then begins, with spiraling internal tissue cushions and neural crest-derived cells dividing the outflow into two great arteries. More proximal tissue cushions form the semilunar valves and then fuse to separate the subaortic and the subpulmonary outflow tracts, both of which are still related to the right ventricle. These fused proximal cushions become the conal septum. The endocardial cushion and the muscular ventricular septum then meet the conal septum to fully separate the right and left ventricles. This results in a separate subpulmonary conus (or infundibulum) and subaortic conus and commits the aorta to the left ventricle and the pulmonary artery to the right ventricle. The subaortic conus regresses, ultimately resulting in fibrous continuity between the mitral and aortic valves.

There have been multiple proposed mechanisms to explain the development of DOLV. Initial reports suggested that DOLV results from bilaterally absent conus; however, this has been shown to be only one among several types of conal morphology in DOLV. Anderson *et al.* [2] have theorized that DOLV arises from abnormalities of the regression of the conal septum with varied conal morphology types such as single subaortic or subpulmonary conus, bilateral conus, and bilaterally absent conus [3]. Studies in the chick embryo suggest that DOLV results from a malalignment of the conal septum anterior to both semilunar valves, separating the right ventricular outflow tract from the pulmonary and aortic valves and keeping both semilunar valves related to the left ventricle [4].

Morphology

As with DORV, it is important to describe in detail the anatomy of each individual DOLV heart in order to decide upon the most appropriate surgical repair. Most cases of DOLV have two well-developed ventricles and most have a VSD (most commonly in the subaortic position). However, there is wide variation in the segmental anatomy, VSD location, and associated cardiac lesions in DOLV hearts.

Van Praagh and his colleagues have reported multiple patterns of segmental anatomy in patients with DOLV. The most common pattern of segmental anatomy is {S,D,D}: visceral and atrial situs solitus, D-looped ventricles (with atrioventricular concordance), and the aortic valve rightward of the pulmonary valve. However, they also report cases of almost every type of segmental

Visual Guide to Neonatal Cardiology, First Edition. Edited by Ernerio T. Alboliras, Ziyad M. Hijazi, Leo Lopez, and Donald J. Hagler.

anatomy possible, including visceroatrial situs solitus with L-looped ventricles, visceroatrial situs inversus with L- or D-looped ventricles, and multiple combinations of great artery relationships. The great artery relationships seen in DOLV are the same as those seen in DORV: side-by-side (aortic valve rightward), D-malposition with the aortic valve rightward and anterior or the aortic valve rightward and posterior (as in normally related great arteries), and L-malposition with the aortic valve leftward and anterior.

There are certain associated cardiac lesions that are commonly seen with DOLV. Pulmonary or aortic outflow tract obstruction, usually brought about by deviation of the conal septum, can be seen in combination with certain types of VSD. Other cardiac lesions that can be seen in association with DOLV include right ventricular hypoplasia (often with tricuspid valve anomalies), mitral atresia, double inlet left ventricle, and heterotaxy syndrome. The same types of VSD are seen in DOLV as are seen in DORV [3, 5]:

- *Subaortic VSDs* are the most common, occurring in 70–75% of all DOLV hearts. They are located under the aortic valve, far from the pulmonary valve. Deviation of the conal septum into the pulmonary outflow tract can cause associated subvalvar and valvar pulmonary stenosis.
- *Subpulmonary VSDs* are the second most common type of VSD, occurring in 15–17% of DOLV hearts (Figures 45.1 and 45.2). They are located under the pulmonary valve, far from the aortic valve. Deviation of the conal septum can cause subaortic stenosis in these patients (Figure 45.2), which in turn can lead to aortic coarctation or interruption of the aortic arch.

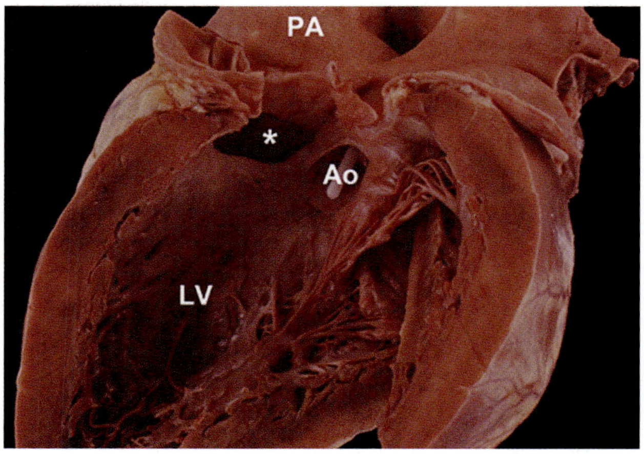

Figure 45.1 Pathologic specimen of a double outlet left ventricle with a subpulmonary ventricular septal defect (asterisk) and subaortic stenosis secondary to deviation of the conal septum into the subaortic region. Ao, aorta; LV, left ventricle; PA, pulmonary artery.

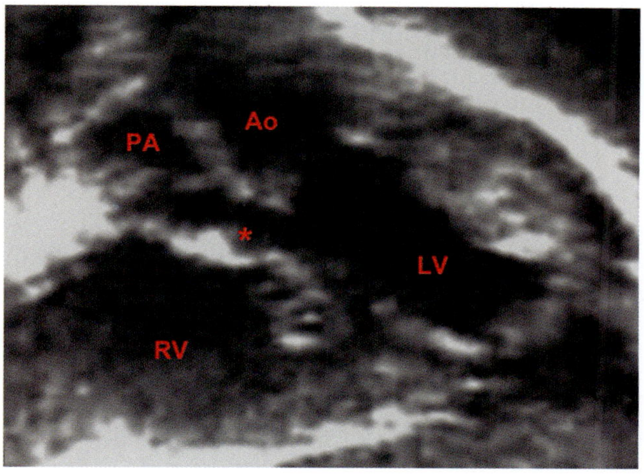

Figure 45.2 Subcostal long-axis image of a double outlet left ventricle with a subpulmonary ventricular septal defect (asterisk). Ao, aorta; LV, left ventricle; PA, pulmonary artery; RV, right ventricle.

- *Doubly committed VSDs*, seen in 6–9% of DOLV hearts, are close to both semilunar valves resulting from complete or almost complete absence of the conal septum. These cases can be difficult to distinguish from DORV with a doubly committed VSD and are sometimes termed "double outlet both ventricles" [3]. There is usually no outflow tract obstruction, although there are reports of aortic outflow obstruction in a few patients.
- *Remote VSDs*, seen in only 2% of DOLV hearts, are located far from the semilunar valves in the atrioventricular canal (inlet) septum or in the muscular septum.
- *Intact ventricular septum* is reported in 1–2% of patients with DOLV.

Pathophysiology

The pathophysiology of DOLV depends on the hemodynamics that result from the underlying anatomy *vis a vis* the amount of pulmonary blood flow and degree of outflow tract obstruction. The most common presentation is cyanosis in patients with a subaortic VSD, a rightward aorta, and pulmonary outflow tract obstruction (tetralogy of Fallot-like physiology). Patients with a subaortic VSD, a leftward aorta, and no pulmonary outflow tract obstruction will present with a transposition-type physiology. Other patients, such as those with a doubly committed VSD or a subpulmonary VSD without aortic obstruction will present with pulmonary overcirculation, similar to patients with a large VSD. Yet other patients, such as a DOLV with a subpulmonary VSD, aortic outflow obstruction, and aortic coarctation or interruption, will present with ductal-dependent systemic circulation.

Surgical Repair

As might be expected with such a heterogeneous lesion, the surgical options are varied and must be tailored to the individual anatomy of each patient. In the majority of patients with two well-developed ventricles, a biventricular repair is considered optimal. This usually involves patch closure of the VSD (if present) with placement of a conduit or homograft from the right ventricle to the pulmonary artery, direct translocation of the pulmonary artery root to the right ventricle (*réparation à l'etage ventriculaire* or REV procedure), or baffling of the right ventricle to the pulmonary artery. Cases that are not amenable to biventricular repair (such as double-inlet double-outlet left ventricle or DOLV with right ventricular hypoplasia) undergo single ventricle palliation (Fontan palliation). Because of the extreme rarity of DOLV, it is difficult to estimate surgical and long-term survival accurately, but one series reports a 70–75% survival for 19 patients with DOLV seen at a single tertiary care center from 1960 to 2008 [6].

Long-term Outcomes

Patients who have undergone DOLV repair, like any other congenital heart surgery patient, require lifelong cardiology follow-up. The long-term issues in patients with repaired DOLV depend on the individual lesion and surgical repair, but include residual VSDs, residual aortic or pulmonary outflow tract obstruction, obstruction along the conduit from the right ventricle to the pulmonary artery, pulmonary regurgitation, coronary perfusion abnormalities (in patients after arterial switch procedure), and arrhythmia. Patients with a Fontan palliation are subject to the additional mortality and morbidity associated with single ventricle circulation.

References

1 Wilkinson J. (2002) Double outlet ventricle, in, *Paediatric Cardiology*, 2nd edn (eds RH Anderson, EJ Baker, FJ Macartney, *et al.*), Churchill Livingstone. London, pp. 1353–1381.

2 Anderson R, Gibson R, G Miller. (1974) Double outlet left ventricle. *Br Heart J*, **36**, 554–558.

3 Lopez L. (2009) Double-outlet ventricle, in, *Echocardiography in Pediatric and Congenital Heart Disease From Fetus to Adult* (eds WW Lai, LL Mertens, MS Cohen, T Geva), Blackwell Publishing, Oxford, pp. 417–438.

4 Manner J, Seidl W, Steding G. (1997) Embryological observations on the formal pathogenesis of double-outlet left ventricle with a right-ventricular infundibulum. *Thorac Cardiovasc Surg*, **45** (4), 172–177. PubMed PMID: 9323818.

5 Menon SC, Hagler DJ. (2008) Double-outlet left ventricle: diagnosis and management. *Curr Treat Options Cardiovasc Med*, **10** (5), 448–452. PubMed PMID: 18814835.

6 Imai-Compton C, Elmi M, Manlhiot C, *et al.* (2010) Characteristics and outcomes of double outlet left ventricle. *Congenit Heart Dis*, **5** (6), 532–536. PubMed PMID: 21106011.

46

Single Ventricle and Biventricular Hearts with Hypoplasia of One Ventricle

Denise A. Hayes[1], *Sujatha Budde*[2], *and Wyman W. Lai*[3]

[1] Hofstra Northwell School of Medicine, Cohen Children's Medical Center, Queens, NY, USA
[2] Seattle Children's Hospital; University of Washington School of Medicine, Seattle, WA, USA
[3] Children's Hospital of Orange County, Orange, CA, USA

The term "single ventricle" encompasses a broad spectrum of pathology. Together the most common forms of functionally single ventricles make up about 7% of congenital heart defects (CHDs), and about 0.06% of live births [1]. While every lesion in this heterogeneous group can be classified as a "univentricular" heart, each has its own unique set of characteristics that alter management, surgical considerations, and outcomes.

Functionally univentricular CHDs may be right ventricular (RV) dominant, left ventricular (LV) dominant, or may have two adequately-sized ventricles but associated lesions that preclude biventricular repair (Box 46.1). The underdeveloped ventricle may be deficient in a specific region, diffusely small, or even rudimentary. Univentricular physiology involves complete mixing of systemic and pulmonary venous return, and ejection of this mixed blood to the systemic and pulmonary arterial circulations (one of which may be supplied entirely, or in part, by the ductus arteriosus).

Embryology and Genetics

Growth of cardiovascular structures before and after birth relies largely on the shear stress of blood flowing through cardiac chambers, valves, and vessels [2]. Thus, a popular theory of single ventricle development is that of flow dynamics, in which altered blood flow perturbs the normal shear stresses that trigger cardiovascular growth and differentiation [2]. A "downstream" obstruction (such as a stenotic aortic valve that leads to arrested LV development) or an "upstream" obstruction (such as a deviated atrial septum that hinders fetal blood flow through the foramen ovale toward the LV) can result in ventricular hypoplasia [3]. In addition, early aberrations in formation of the conotruncus or atrioventricular (AV) region can result in certain single ventricle lesions. Genetics also has an important role, and a number of disorders such as Turner syndrome, trisomy 21, and heterotaxy syndromes are associated with single ventricle CHD [4].

Prenatal Circulation

The single ventricle, although often incompatible with long-term survival, rarely causes a problem in utero or immediately after birth. Patency of the foramen ovale and ductus arteriosus permits fetal survival, but dramatic changes in the first hours, days, and weeks of life can result in cyanosis or circulatory collapse if the disease goes unrecognized.

Dominant Right Ventricle

In the fetus with a dominant RV (Figures 46.1, 46.2, and 46.3), there may be varying degrees of hypoplasia of the left atrium, mitral valve, and LV [5]. The aortic arch and coronary arteries may receive little to no antegrade flow, and be supplied by retrograde flow from the ductus arteriosus. In dominant RVs with transposition of the great arteries (TGA), the pulmonary outflow (which is associated with the small LV) may be obstructed, and the pulmonary arteries (PAs) may be significantly hypoplastic and supplied by reverse ductal blood flow.

Dominant Left Ventricle

In the fetus with a dominant LV, systemic venous return reaches the LV by passing right to left across the foramen ovale (as in tricuspid atresia; Figure 46.4), or by flowing through an AV valve directly into the LV (as in double

Visual Guide to Neonatal Cardiology, First Edition. Edited by Ernerio T. Alboliras, Ziyad M. Hijazi, Leo Lopez, and Donald J. Hagler.

Box 46.1 Functionally single ventricle lesions.

Dominant right ventricle:
- Hypoplastic left heart syndrome ± ventricular septal defect
- Shone complex
- Complex DORV
- RV-dominant complete CAVC

Dominant left ventricle:
- Tricuspid atresia
- Pulmonary atresia with intact ventricular septum
- Double inlet left ventricle
- DOLV
- LV-dominant complete CAVC
- Severe Ebstein anomaly

No ventricular dominance:
- Balanced complete CAVC with complex AV valve attachments
- DORV/DOLV with complex AV valve attachments
- Complex criss-cross heart

AV, atrioventricular; CAVC, common atrioventricular canal; DOLV, double outlet left ventricle; DORV, double outlet right ventricle; LV, left ventricle; RV, right ventricle.

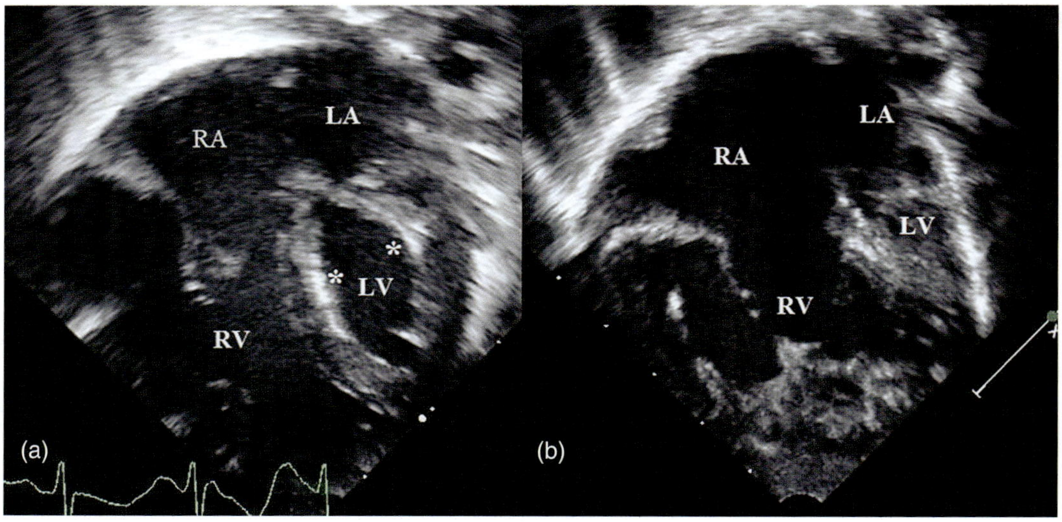

Figure 46.1 Hypoplastic left heart syndrome, apical view. The spectrum of disease ranges from (a) mitral and aortic stenosis with a moderately hypoplastic left ventricle (LV) to (b) valvar atresia and a rudimentary LV. Note the echogenic LV endocardium (*) consistent with endocardial fibroelastosis. LA, left atrium; LV, left ventricle, RA, right atrium; RV, right ventricle.

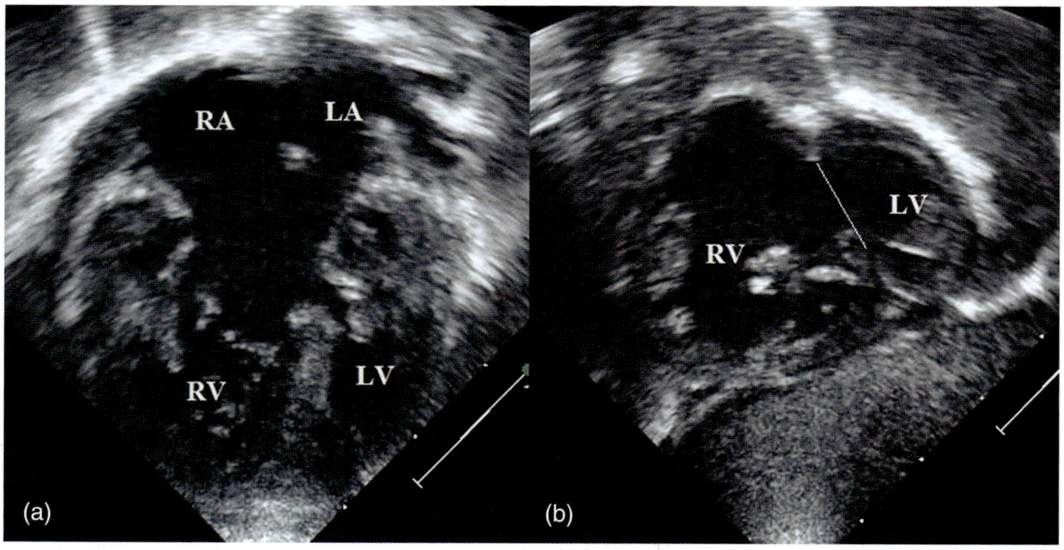

Figure 46.2 RV-dominant complete common atrioventricular canal: (a) apical; and (b) subxiphoid short axis views. In an "unbalanced" defect, the common atrioventricular valve is positioned predominantly over one ventricle, with hypoplasia of the other. LA, left atrium; LV, left ventricle; RA, right atrium; RV, right ventricle. Solid line represents plane of ventricular septal defect, emphasizing the LV hypoplasia.

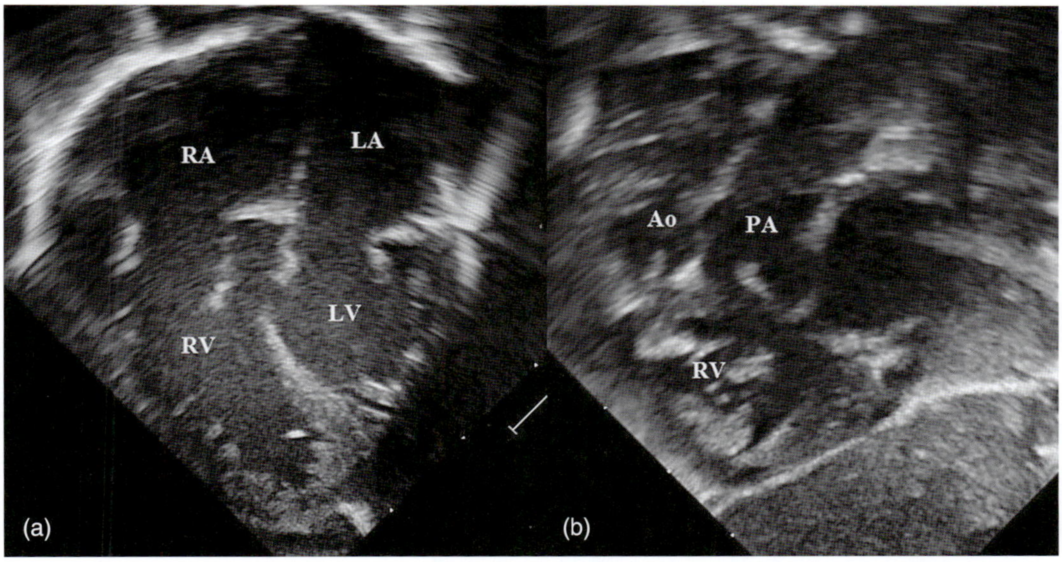

Figure 46.3 Double outlet right ventricle (DORV): (a) apical and (b) subxiphoid short axis views. While most are amenable to biventricular repair, some complex DORVs have significant LV hypoplasia requiring single ventricle palliation. Ao, aorta; LA, left atrium; LV, left ventricle; PA, pulmonary artery; RA, right atrium; RV, right ventricle.

Figure 46.4 Tricuspid atresia, apical view. LA, left atrium; LV, left ventricle; RA, right atrium. Asterisk represents atretic tricuspid valve.

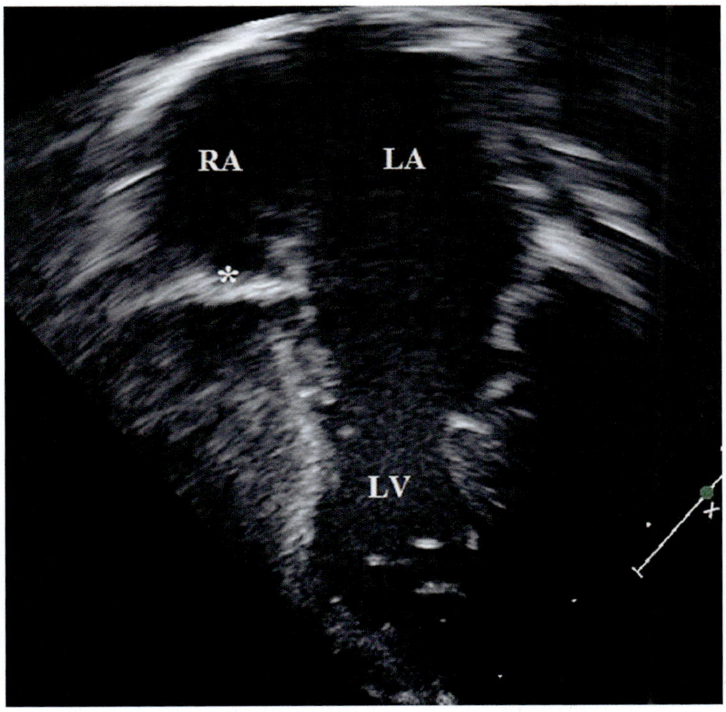

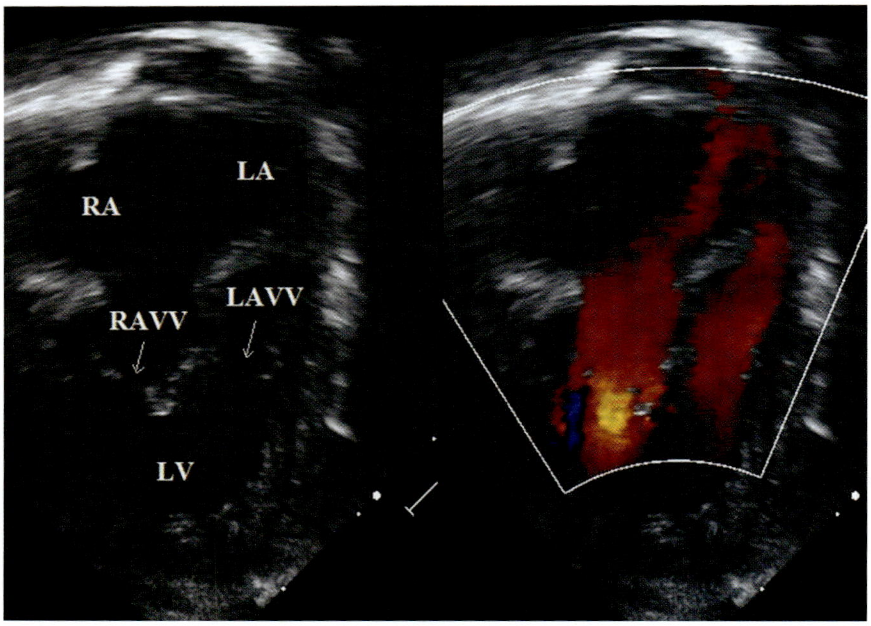

Figure 46.5 Double inlet left ventricle, apical view in color compare mode. LA, left atrium; LAVV, left atrioventricular valve; LV, left ventricle; RA, right atrium; RAVV, right atrioventricular valve.

inlet LV; Figure 46.5). Again, the ventriculo-arterial relationship often determines the type of outflow tract obstruction. Normally-related great vessels tend to be associated with PA hypoplasia and TGA tends to result in aortic arch obstruction, but other factors such as crowding of outflow tracts by accessory AV valve tissue can reverse this trend.

Postnatal Circulation and Clinical Presentation

Immediately after birth the lungs expand, separation from the placental circulation occurs, and the pulmonary vascular resistance (PVR) falls. Effective circulation in a functionally single ventricle depends on egress of atrial blood from the hypoplastic side (e.g., through an unrestrictive patent foramen ovale, PFO) and adequate pulmonary and systemic blood flow (which may require a persistent patent ductus arteriosus, PDA).

In the current era, most univentricular CHD is diagnosed prenatally, and implementation of routine pulse oximetry screening in newborns can help identify others [6]. However, in the undiagnosed infant, restriction or closure of the PFO and PDA can result in rapid clinical deterioration. Symptoms within the first days to weeks of life are often a result of restriction of the PDA, and depend on the type of outflow obstruction (cyanosis in those with ductal-dependent pulmonary blood flow, and cardiogenic shock with ductal-dependent systemic blood flow). Undiagnosed patients who survive the neonatal period tend to be those without significantly obstructed outflow tracts. These infants may present with a murmur, or with tachypnea and failure to thrive as PVR drops and blood from the single ventricle is ejected preferentially toward the low-resistance pulmonary circulation. Signs of hemodynamic instability immediately after birth are rare but indicate the presence of complicating factors such as a restrictive atrial communication (in those that depend on this shunt as an atrial outlet), obstructed total anomalous pulmonary venous return (TAPVR), ventricular dysfunction, or arrhythmias.

Preoperative Evaluation

Transthoracic echocardiography is the gold standard for diagnosis of the single ventricle and associated anomalies. Functional assessment and detailed measurements of all valves and chambers will help determine candidacy for biventricular repair. Cardiac magnetic resonance imaging can be utilized to more clearly define ventricular volumes and vascular abnormalities. In addition, cardiac catheterization may be necessary to clarify the details of complex extracardiac anatomy, and allows for hemodynamic assessment and transcatheter intervention if necessary.

Preoperative screening for genetic or extracardiac anomalies is important in neonates with single ventricle, as they have been shown to adversely affect outcomes [7]. Chromosomal analysis, fluorescence in situ hybridization for microdeletions, renal and head ultrasonography, and evaluation of the intestinal tract may be warranted. Severe extracardiac abnormalities or a life-threatening genetic syndrome can alter decisions about the infant's care.

Management

Prostaglandin E1

The management of a newborn with single ventricle CHD is focused on the need to artificially mimic fetal circulation while awaiting surgery. Intravenous prostaglandin E1 maintains ductal patency in the patient whose pulmonary or systemic blood flow depends on it, and may be started prior to echocardiographic diagnosis if the suspicion is high.

Balloon Atrial Septostomy

Many types of univentricular CHD have an obligatory atrial shunt, and fortunately a highly restrictive or intact atrial septum is relatively rare. While 5–15% of infants with atresia of the right-sided AV valve will demonstrate restriction of the atrial shunt [8], symptoms of right-sided congestion (hepatomegaly, edema) and the need for emergent balloon atrial septostomy in the newborn period are far less common. In contrast, up to 15% of patients with hypoplastic left heart syndrome (HLHS) may require preoperative left atrial decompression [9]. Recognizing signs of atrial septal restriction (such as profound cyanosis, pulmonary edema, and poor perfusion) is critical, and mobilizing the interventional cardiology team may be life-saving.

Other Medical Therapies

Other therapies can be indicated for the neonate awaiting palliation of functionally single ventricle CHD. Ventilation strategies must account for the unique physiology of the individual lesion, and critically ill neonates may require careful PVR manipulation to achieve appropriate balance between systemic and pulmonary blood flow. Inotropes are useful for patients with ventricular dysfunction. Afterload reduction is sometimes used in those with significant systemic AV valve regurgitation, and pulmonary vasodilators such as oxygen or nitric oxide may be indicated for those with elevated PVR.

Surgical Strategies

Biventricular Repair

The surgical strategy for an infant with hypoplasia of one ventricle depends on whether recruitment of the smaller ventricle is feasible (Figure 46.6). Given the life-long complications of the Fontan circulation and the likely need for subsequent cardiac transplantation, there is increasing interest in pursuing biventricular repair for patients with borderline ventricular hypoplasia. However, some authors have pointed out that a two-ventricle repair is not always superior to single-ventricle palliation, and in the face of certain morphologic findings can actually worsen outcomes [10–13].

The strategy of recruiting a hypoplastic ventricle should be initiated early, and in some centers may even begin prenatally (in select cases of systemic outflow obstruction) with fetal aortic balloon valvuloplasty. Although there is risk of maternal morbidity and fetal demise, some evidence suggests that improved prenatal

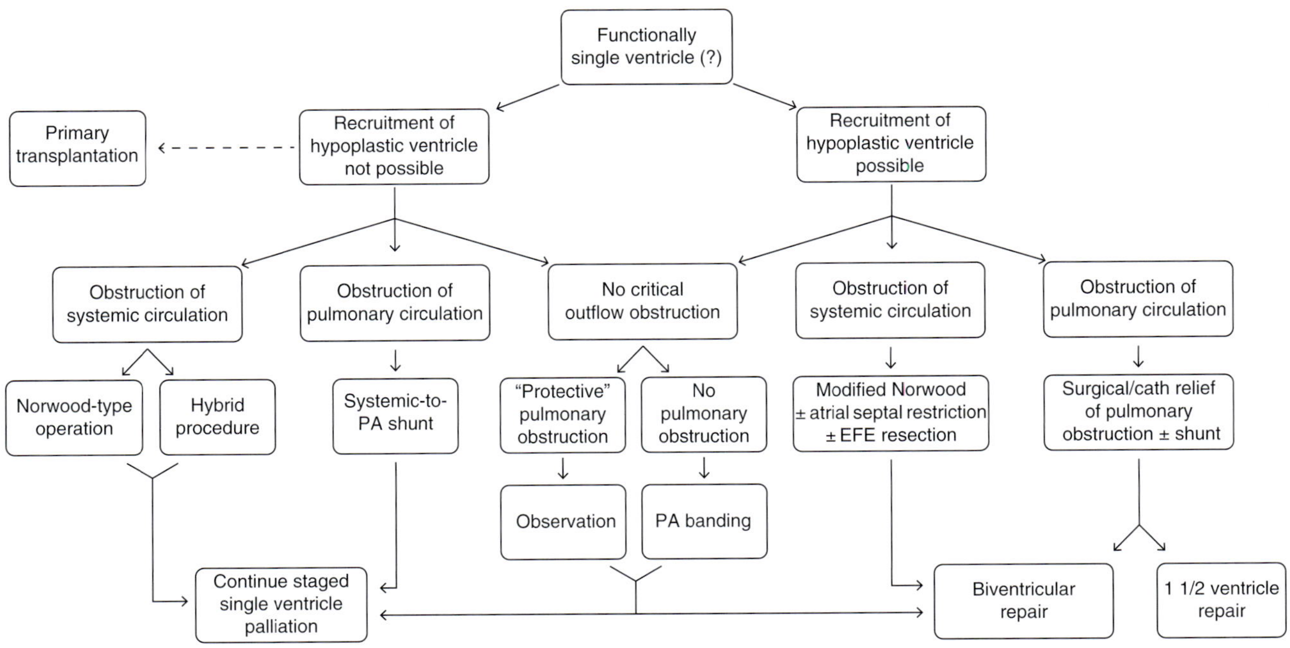

Figure 46.6 Surgical strategies for the neonate with a possible functionally single ventricle. EFE, endocardial fibroelastosis.

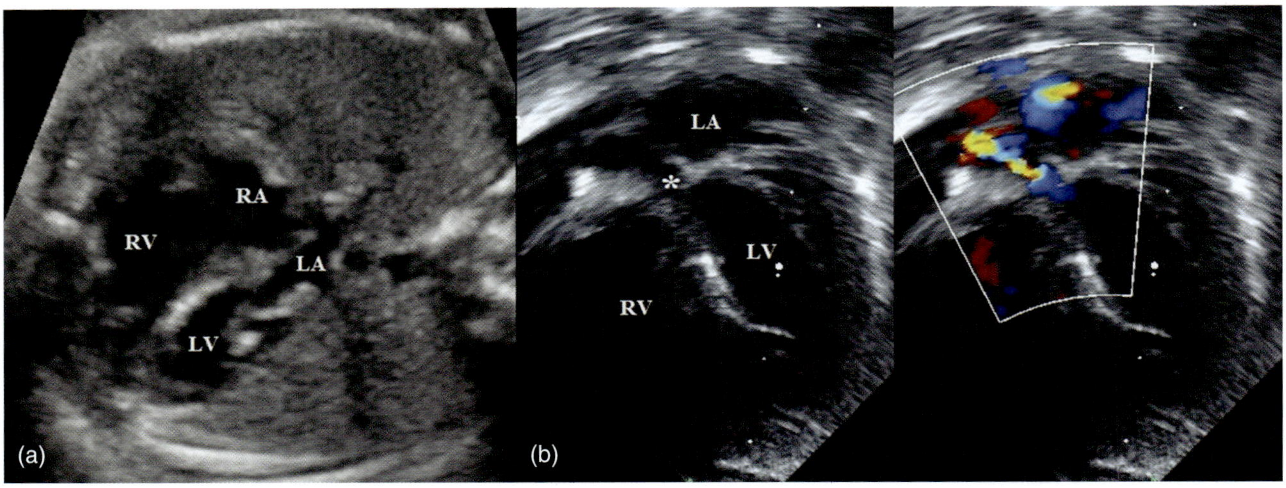

Figure 46.7 Severe aortic stenosis: (a) prior to in utero aortic balloon valvuloplasty and (b) postnatally. Significant residual aortic valve obstruction and LV hypoplasia is present after the fetal intervention. LA, left atrium; LV, left ventricle; RA, right atrium; RV, right ventricle. Asterisk represents stenotic aortic valve.

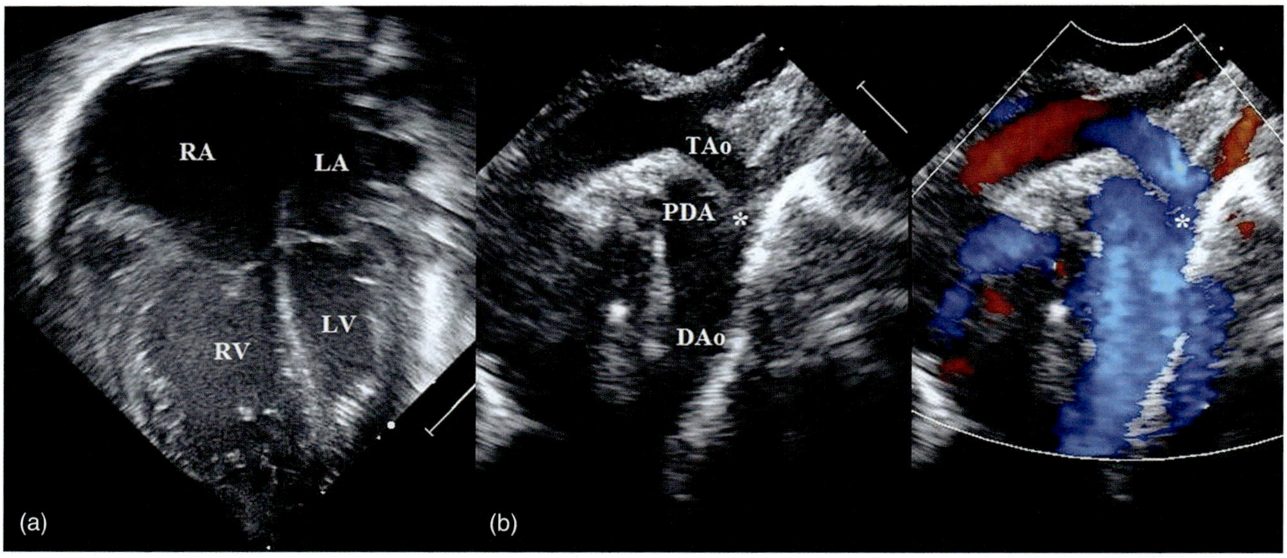

Figure 46.8 (a) Shone complex in apical view demonstrating mitral valve and LV hypoplasia, and (b) in suprasternal notch view in color compare demonstrating mild discrete juxtaductal aortic coarctation. DAo, descending aorta; LA, left atrium; LV, left ventricle; PDA, patent ductus arteriosus; RA, right atrium; RV, right ventricle; TAo, transverse aortic arch. Asterisk represents area of coarctation.

growth of the mitral and aortic valves can be achieved (Figure 46.7) [3].

If the postnatal morphologic findings are favorable, biventricular repair may be attempted. For RV-dominant lesions such as Shone complex (Figure 46.8), staged LV recruitment involving concomitant procedures to promote left heart growth can be considered during stages 1–3 of palliation [14]. These procedures include mitral and aortic valvuloplasty, restriction of the atrial septal defect to force left atrial blood across the mitral valve, and resection of restrictive LV endocardial fibroelastosis. If sufficient growth of the left heart is achieved, a biventricular conversion can be attempted at any stage [14]. The mitral valve annulus size is often the limiting factor in dominant RVs, and can prohibit biventricular repair regardless of LV dimensions. If the aortic valve is the primary problem, the Ross procedure (which replaces the hypoplastic aortic valve with the patient's own pulmonary valve) can be considered [15]. Biventricular options for LVs with borderline hypoplasia and TGA (with pulmonary outflow obstruction), include the Rastelli, Nikaidoh, and *réparation à l'etage ventriculaire* (REV) procedures [16].

LV-dominant lesions such as pulmonary atresia with intact ventricular septum and unbalanced common atrioventricular canal (CAVC) defects are amenable to biventricular repair if the RV and right AV valve annulus sizes are deemed adequate, although the dimensions of these structures are quite variable in patients who ultimately undergo successful two-ventricle repair [13]. Surgical or transcatheter relief of pulmonary outflow obstruction may be attempted in anticipation of future biventricular repair, or a "one-and-a-half ventricle" palliation (which maintains antegrade pulmonary blood flow from the RV and adds a superior cavopulmonary Glenn anastomosis). Finally, a "biventricular" repair occasionally employed in cases of double inlet LV utilizes a large patch to septate the single chamber into two ventricles [17].

No Critical Outflow Obstruction

Critical outflow obstruction can be averted during the development of some functionally single ventricles, including those with large ventricular septal defects (VSDs) and adequate flow to each outflow tract, or those in which early biventricular repair is precluded only by additional anatomic complexities. In these cases, the combined ventricular output enters the competing pulmonary and systemic circulations, and the flow ratio depends on their relative resistances. Occasionally, there is enough pulmonary stenosis to "protect" the pulmonary vascular bed, and surgery can be delayed. However, in cases of unobstructed pulmonary outflow tracts, PA banding may be necessary to restrict flow until more definitive repair or palliation.

Single Ventricle Palliation

When recruitment of the hypoplastic ventricle is not possible, the surgical strategy depends primarily on the type and degree of outflow tract obstruction. For lesions in which there is obstruction to systemic outflow, a series of palliative surgeries begins in the neonatal period with a Norwood-type operation. This procedure and its modifications establish reliable systemic blood flow by anastomosis of the native aorta to the pulmonary trunk, with patch augmentation as indicated to create the "neo-aorta." The PAs, now isolated from the heart, are supplied by a modified Blalock–Taussig shunt or RV-to-PA shunt [18, 19]. An atrial septectomy permits unobstructed left atrial egress. The next two surgical steps include the bidirectional Glenn operation (typically at 4–6 months of age), and the Fontan completion (typically at 2–4 years of age).

The "hybrid" procedure is a stage 1 alternative in some institutions (Figure 46.9). Most often reserved for neonates with complicating factors such as prematurity or low birth weight, this approach involves PDA stenting and bilateral PA banding without cardiopulmonary bypass [20]. This is followed later by a comprehensive stage 2 (essentially combining the Norwood and bidirectional Glenn operations), and finally the Fontan completion.

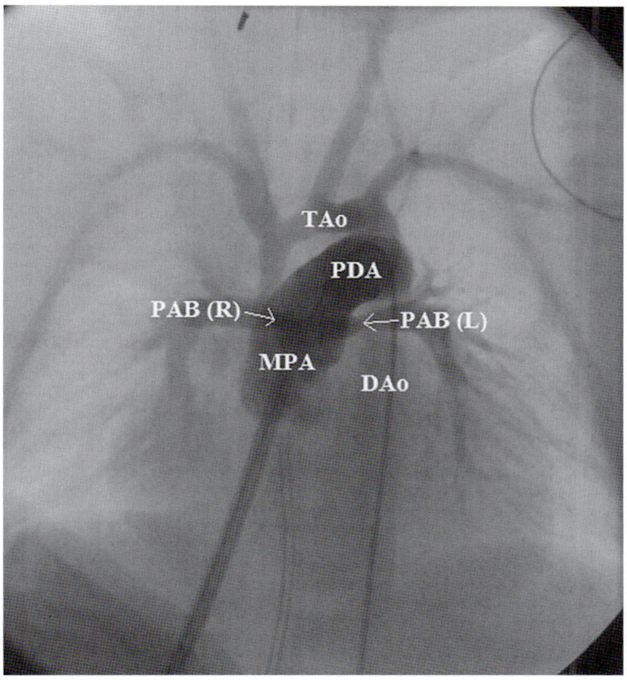

Figure 46.9 The "hybrid" approach. On this angiogram of a patient with hypoplastic left heart syndrome, contrast fills the main pulmonary artery (MPA), the banded left (L) and right (R) pulmonary arteries, the stented patent ductus arteriosus (PDA), and the descending aorta (DAo). The hypoplastic transverse aorta (TAo) fills in a retrograde manner. PAB, pulmonary artery band.

Similar to the single ventricle with systemic outflow obstruction, those with pulmonary outflow obstruction require staged palliation culminating in the Fontan operation. Palliation typically begins with a systemic-to-PA shunt, a less challenging first step than the Norwood operation.

When the single ventricle demonstrates significant myocardial dysfunction, major coronary abnormalities, or severe AV valve regurgitation deemed irreparable, the tactic of primary cardiac transplantation can be employed. Donor shortage and improved outcomes after single ventricle palliation have caused this option to fall out of favor [18].

Outcomes

Operative survival has improved greatly over the past two decades. Many centers report 84% or greater hospital survival after Norwood stage 1 [21], the most complex of the palliative options for single ventricle. Various predictors of mortality during Norwood hospitalization (specifically for RV-dominant lesions) have been identified, including the need for extracorporeal membrane oxygenation [19], lower birth weight [18], and genetic abnormalities

[18, 19]. The higher incidence of TAPVR [22] or heterotaxy [23] in certain forms of univentricular CHD can also negatively influence outcomes.

Late mortality remains an important consideration in univentricular CHD, and largely depends on the function of the dominant ventricle and complexities of the individual cardiac malformation. The LV is naturally equipped to function as the systemic ventricle, and there is evidence that survival is improved after palliation for single LV compared to single RV lesions (85% 10-year survival vs. 60%, respectively) [5, 23].

Outcomes of biventricular repair in borderline cases do not always validate the perception that "two ventricles are better than one" [10–13]. On the contrary, choosing the wrong surgical strategy can be a grave error, and in patients with LV hypoplasia who ultimately fail biventricular repair (including those in which salvage was attempted by transplant or conversion to a univentricular circulation), mortality rates of almost 80% have been reported [10]. This highlights the importance of meticulous preoperative evaluation and careful surgical decision-making. In cases of hypoplastic LV, multiple predictors of failure of biventricular repair (including a moderate-to-large VSD and lower mitral valve z score) [10], and of death after biventricular repair (including a smaller LV outflow tract diameter, echocardiographic evidence of endocardial fibroelastosis, and LV dysfunction) [11] have been identified. In cases of hypoplastic RV, determinants of candidacy for biventricular repair (including tricuspid valve z score and the degree of coronary fistulae) and predictors of death (including severe tricuspid regurgitation) have been reported [13]. In borderline cases with various combinations of these unfavorable findings, recruiting the hypoplastic RV or LV into a biventricular circulation can result in lower survival than those with more favorable morphology [11, 13]. Scoring systems incorporating detailed morphologic assessment can be valuable in determining candidacy for biventricular repair, and help to improve outcomes in this complex population.

Conclusions

The neonate with "functionally single ventricle" CHD is part of a large, heterogeneous group of patients with unique anatomic variations. The preoperative management and surgical strategies vary widely, and understanding the physiology of the individual lesion is crucially important in the care of these infants.

References

1 Hoffman JI, Kaplan S. (2002) The incidence of congenital heart disease. *J Am Coll Cardiol*, **39** (12), 1890–1900.

2 Hickey EJ, Caldarone CA, McCrindle BW. (2012) Left ventricular hypoplasia: a spectrum of disease involving the left ventricular outflow tract, aortic valve, and aorta. *J Am Coll Cardiol*, **59** (1), S43–54.

3 McElhinney DB, Marshall AC, Wilkins-Haug LE, *et al.* (2009) Predictors of technical success and postnatal biventricular outcome after in utero aortic valvuloplasty for aortic stenosis with evolving hypoplastic left heart syndrome. *Circulation*, **120** (15), 1482–1490.

4 Natowicz M, Chatten J, Clancy R, *et al.* (1988) Genetic disorders and major extracardiac anomalies associated with the hypoplastic left heart syndrome. *Pediatrics*, **82** (5), 698–706.

5 Daebritz SH, Nollert GD, Zurakowski D, *et al.* (2000) Results of Norwood stage I operation: comparison of hypoplastic left heart syndrome with other malformations. *J Thorac Cardiovasc Surg*, **119** (2), 358–367.

6 Frank LH, Bradshaw E, Beekman R, *et al.* (2013) Critical congenital heart disease screening using pulse oximetry. *J Pediatr*, **162** (3), 445–453.

7 Baker K, Sanchez-de-Toledo J, Munoz R, *et al.* (2012) Critical congenital heart disease-utility of routine screening for chromosomal and other extracardiac malformations. *Congenit Heart Dis*, **7** (2), 145–150.

8 Tzifa A, Gauvreau K, Geggel RL. (2007) Factors associated with development of atrial septal restriction in patients with tricuspid atresia involving the right-sided atrioventricular valve. *Am Heart J*, **154** (6), 1235–1241.

9 Hoque T, Richmond M, Vincent JA, *et al.* (2013) Current outcomes of hypoplastic left heart syndrome with restrictive atrial septum: a single-center experience. *Pediatr Cardiol*, **34**, 1181–1189.

10 Schwartz ML, Gauvreau K, Geva T. (2001) Predictors of outcome of biventricular repair in infants with multiple left heart obstructive lesions. *Circulation*, **104**, 682–687.

11 Hickey EJ, Caldarone CA, Blackstone EH, *et al.* (2007) Critical left ventricular outflow tract obstruction: the disproportionate impact of biventricular repair in borderline cases. *J Thorac Cardiovasc Surg*, **134**, 1429–1437.

12 Bradley TJ, Karamlou T, Kulik A, *et al.* (2007) Determinants of repair type, reintervention, and mortality

in 393 children with double-outlet right ventricle. *J Thorac Cardiovasc Surg*, **134**, 967–973.

13 Ashburn DA, Blackston EH, Wells WJ, *et al.* (2004) Determinants of mortality and type of repair in neonates with pulmonary atresia and intact ventricular septum. *J Thorac Cardiovasc Surg*, **127** (4), 1000–1008.

14 Emani SM, McElhinney DB, Tworetsky W, *et al.* (2012) Staged left ventricular recruitment after single-ventricle palliation in patients with borderline left heart hypoplasia. *J Am Coll Cardiol*, **60** (19), 1966–1974.

15 Elder RW, Quaegebeur JM, Bacha EA, *et al.* (2013) Outcomes of the infant Ross procedure for congenital aortic stenosis followed into adolescence. *J Thorac Cardiovasc Surg*, **145** (6), 1504–1511.

16 Hu SS, Liu ZG, Li SJ, *et al.* (2008) Strategy for biventricular outflow tract reconstruction: Rastell, REV, or Nikaidoh procedure? *J Thorac Cardiovasc Surg*, **135** (2), 331–338.

17 Margossian RE, Solowiejczyk D, Bourlon F, *et al.* (2002) Septation of the single ventricle: revisited. *J Thorac Cardiovasc Surg*, **124** (3), 442–447.

18 Gaynor JW, Mahle WT, Cohen MI, *et al.* (2002) Risk factors for mortality after the Norwood procedure. *Eur J Cardiothorac Surg*, **22** (1), 82–89.

19 Jacobs JP, O'Brien SM, Chai PJ, *et al.* (2008) Management of 239 patients with hypoplastic left heart syndrome and related malformations from 1993 to 2007. *Ann Thorac Surg*, **85** (5), 1691–1696, discussion 1697.

20 Bacha EA, Daves S, Hardin J, *et al.* (2006) Single-ventricle palliation for high-risk neonates: the emergence of an alternative hybrid stage I strategy. *J Thorac Cardiovasc Surg*, **131** (1), 163–171e2.

21 Tabbutt S, Ghanayem N, Ravishankar C, *et al.* (2012) Risk factors for hospital morbidity and mortality after the Norwood procedure: a report from the Pediatric Heart Network Single Ventricle Reconstruction trial. *J Thorac Cardiovasc Surg*, **144** (4), 882–895.

22 Owens GE, Gomez-Fifer C, Gelehrter S, *et al.* (2009) Outcomes for patients with unbalanced atrioventricular septal defects. *Pediatr Cardiol*, **30** (4), 431–435.

23 d'Udekem Y, Xu MY, Galati JC, *et al.* (2012) Predictors of survival after single-ventricle palliation: the impact of right ventricular dominance. *J Am Coll Cardiol* **59** (13), 1178–1185.

47

Dextrocardia and the Heterotaxy Syndromes

Sowmya Balasubramanian and Rajesh Punn

Division of Pediatric Cardiology, Department of Pediatrics, Stanford School of Medicine, Stanford, CA, USA

Heterotaxy Syndrome

The term heterotaxy is derived from the Greek words *heteros* (other) and *taxis* (order). Heterotaxy syndrome describes disorders involving abnormal lateralization of the abdominal and thoracic viscera in which structures that typically manifest right–left asymmetry are positioned ambiguously. It is often associated with complex cardiac malformations. In fact, "heterotaxy syndrome is the Murphy's Law of congenital heart disease in that almost anything that can go wrong will" [1]. This chapter focuses on the accepted classification systems, commonly associated non-cardiac and cardiac anomalies, and management options.

Heterotaxy syndrome involves either the absence of the spleen or presence of multiple spleens. The classification system developed by Van Praagh and colleagues divides patients into asplenia and polysplenia syndromes [2, 3]. An alternate classification system based on atrial appendage morphology stratifies hearts as either bilateral right atrial (RA) appendages (RA isomerism) or bilateral left atrial (LA) appendages (LA isomerism) [4]. Neither classification system is all-encompassing. Thus, we advocate for a detailed description of the cardiac structures instead.

Definitions

Asplenia syndrome involves congenital absence of the spleen most commonly associated with an intact inferior vena cava (IVC), unroofed coronary sinus, totally anomalous pulmonary venous connection (APVC), common atrioventricular (AV) canal defect, double outlet right ventricle (RV) or transposition of the great arteries, and pulmonary stenosis or atresia [3]. Polysplenia syndrome involves a cluster of multiple spenuli or a single large spleen with multiple small ones associated, commonly associated with an interrupted IVC, totally or partially APVC, complete or partial AV canal defect, and normally related great arteries [3].

Isomerism refers to the similarity of bilateral structures that are normally dissimilar, such as the bronchi and lungs [5]. RA isomerism involves bilateral structures with morphologic right characteristics, such as bilateral morphologic right bronchi and bilateral trilobed lungs. LA isomerism involves bilateral structures with morphologic left characteristics, such as bilateral morphologic left bronchi and bilateral bilobed lungs [5].

Levocardia occurs when the majority of the heart lies to the left of midline. Dextrocardia occurs when the heart is

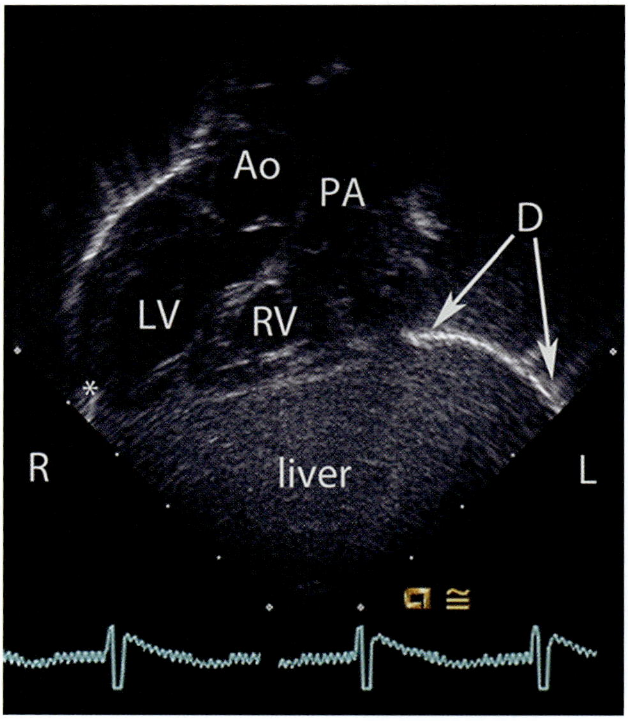

Figure 47.1 Subxiphoid coronal echocardiographic image showing the cardiac apex (asterisk) pointing rightward (R) with a right-sided left ventricle (LV) and a right-sided right ventricle (RV) giving rise to the aorta (Ao) and main pulmonary artery (PA), respectively. Notice the diaphragm (D) is intact on the left side (L) of this neonate.

Visual Guide to Neonatal Cardiology, First Edition. Edited by Ernerio T. Alboliras, Ziyad M. Hijazi, Leo Lopez, and Donald J. Hagler.

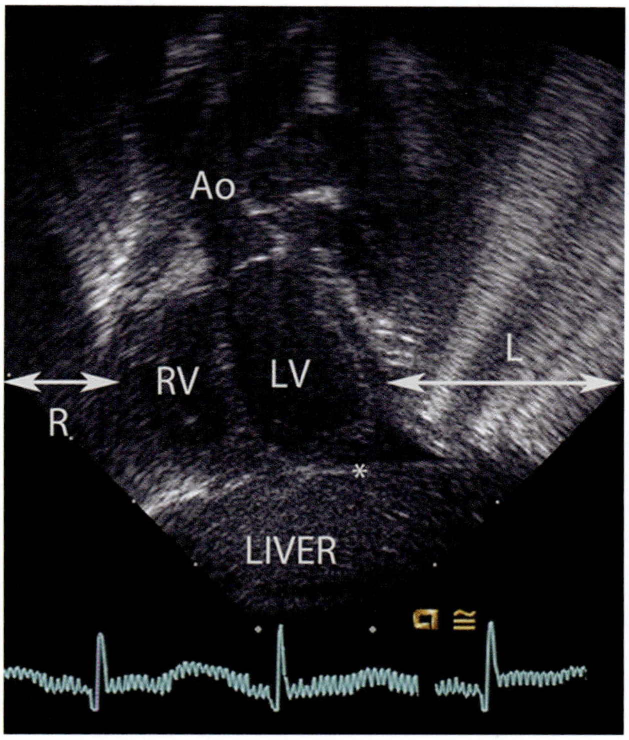

Figure 47.2 Subxiphoid coronal echocardiographic image showing the cardiac mass shifted rightward because the left arrow (L) is larger than the right (R). The cardiac apex in this example remains leftward (asterisk). Ao, ascending aorta; LV, left ventricle; RV, right ventricle.

in the right chest with a rightward apex (Figure 47.1) [6]. Mesocardia involves a midline heart extending equally into the right and left thoraxes, possibly representing a variation of normal when the ventricular looping is normal [5]. Dextroposition occurs in an otherwise normal heart that is shifted rightward because of an extracardiac factor such as eventration of the left diaphragm [6]. The apex of the heart points leftward (Figure 47.2). Some would dismiss the term dextroposition and designate hearts at the right of the chest as dextrocardia, mentioning the direction of the apex as a different entity. Situs solitus, derived from the Latin words for site or position and normal or usual, involves normal arrangement of the viscera and atria with a right-sided RA and a left-sided LA.

Associated Non-Cardiac Anomalies

Normal lung morphology is asymmetric: the right lung is formed with three lobes while the left lung consists of two. The bronchial anatomy is also asymmetric: the left bronchus is 1.5–2 times longer than the right bronchus to their first branch. The right bronchus courses over the right pulmonary artery (eparterial) while the left bronchus travels under the left pulmonary artery (hyparterial). In heterotaxy syndrome, the lungs and bronchi are usually abnormally symmetric. In a postmortem series of 109 patients with asplenia syndrome, 81% had bilateral trilobed lungs and 95% had bilateral eparterial bronchial course. Among those with polysplenia syndrome, 72% had bilateral bilobed lungs and 68% had hyparterial course (Figure 47.3) [3].

The spleen is almost always affected. Though there is significant variability in cardiac malformations, there is syndromic clustering that corresponds to the type of splenic malformation [3]. RA isomerism is usually associated with the absence of a spleen while LA isomerism is usually associated with multiple, poorly functioning spleens. Assessment of splenic function is important in patients with heterotaxy syndrome.

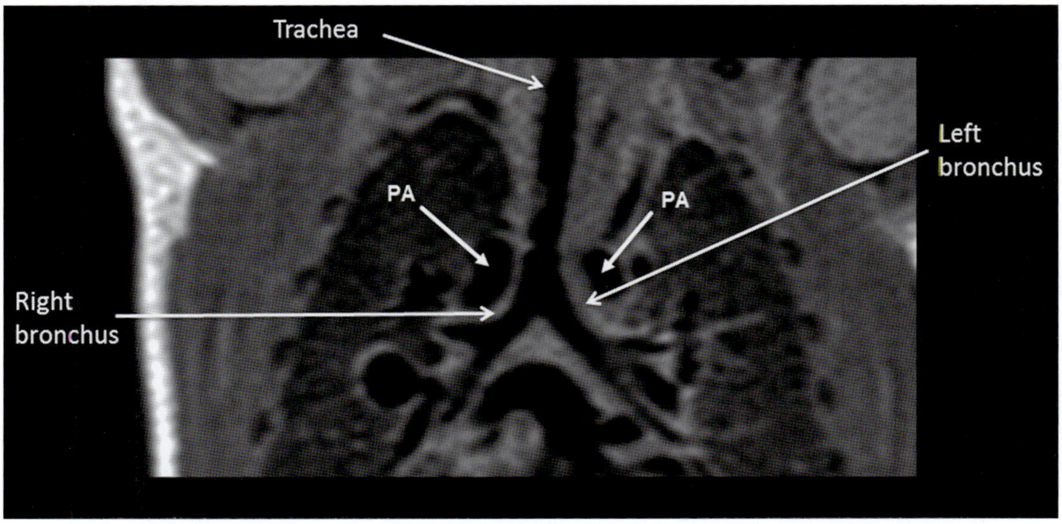

Figure 47.3 ECG-gated breath hold turbo spin echo double inversion recovery sequence magnetic resonance image in the coronal projection demonstrating bilateral left-sided bronchi. Note the right and left bronchi having only two branches consistent with a bilaterally left lung morphology. The right PA and left PA are seen above the bronchi (hyparterial bronchi).

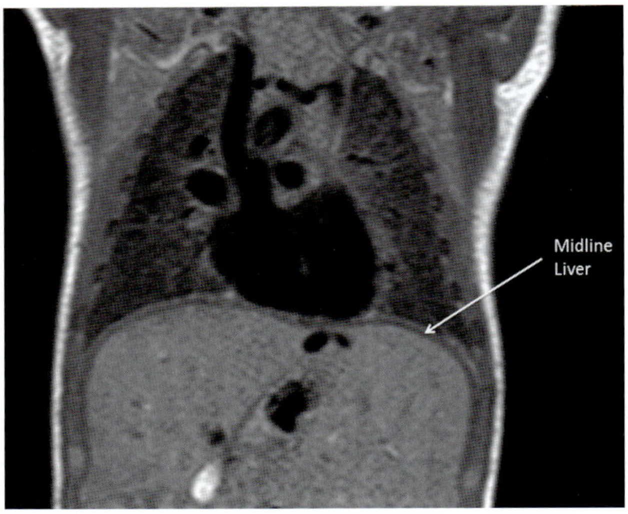

Figure 47.4 ECG-gated breath hold turbo spin echo double inversion recovery sequence magnetic resonance image in the coronal projection demonstrating a midline liver.

In contrast to a normal right-sided trilobed liver, the liver can be symmetric and midline in heterotaxy syndrome (Figure 47.4). Absent gallbladder or extrahepatic biliary atresia has been found in patients with visceral heterotaxy. Malrotation of the gut is common. A barium contrast study is used for diagnosis, although universal screening is not standard practice. With malrotation, a prophylactic Ladd procedure is recommended to prevent volvulus of the midgut.

Associated Cardiac Anomalies

Cardiac assessment should involve a segmental approach that includes the venoatrial connections, atria, AV junction, ventricular topology, and relationship of the great arteries. The orientation of the cardiac apex in the thorax and arrangement of the thoracoabdominal organs (including the spleen, lungs, and intestines) should be described.

A transverse subxiphoid echocardiographic view demonstrates the relationship of the aorta, IVC, and abdominal viscera relative to the spine. Abdominal situs solitus involves a right-sided liver and left-sided stomach. The IVC is to the right of the spine while the descending aorta is to the left. In abdominal situs ambiguous with asplenia syndrome, the liver is midline and the IVC and abdominal aorta travel together on the same side of the vertebral column.

Identifying features of a RA include the limbus of the fossa ovalis, large pyramidal appendage, crista terminalis, and the presence of pectinate muscles. The chamber that incorporates the right side of the sinus venosus is the RA. The right horn of the sinus venosus includes the orifices of the superior vena cava (SVC) and IVC and the smooth atrial wall in between. The mouth of the coronary sinus opens into the sinus venosus component of the RA. In contrast, the LA is identified by the finger-like atrial appendage and usually receives the pulmonary veins.

Anomalous venoatrial connections are common in heterotaxy syndrome. Only a few instances have normal or mirror-imaged venoatrial connections. Certain patterns permit the differentiation between asplenia and polysplenia syndromes (Table 47.1). In asplenia syndrome, the coronary sinus is often absent, bilateral SVC occurs in 50–80%, and absent intrahepatic IVC is rare [7]. In polysplenia syndrome, the coronary sinus is absent in only 30–55%, and 40–50% have bilateral SVC [8]. An interrupted IVC with drainage to the azygos vein occurs in ~80% of patients with polysplenia (Figure 47.5) [8]. APVC is seen occurring in 60–87% of patients with asplenia syndrome (Figure 47.6) and in only 2% with polysplenia syndrome [3]. In most polysplenia patients, the pulmonary veins are situated normally behind the LA while malposition of the atrial septum results in anomalous drainage of the pulmonary veins to the ipsilateral atria [3].

Table 47.1 Associated cardiac findings in asplenia and polysplenia syndromes.

	Asplenia (%)	Polysplenia (%)
Systemic veins		
Intact IVC	100	20
Interrupted IVC		80
Bilateral SVC	70	50
Pulmonary veins		
Totally anomalous pulmonary venous connection	60	2
Partial anomalous pulmonary venous connection		+++
Ventricles		
Balanced CAVC	44	63
Right dominant CAVC	28	24
Left dominant CAVC	11	11
Cardiac position		
Levocardia	72	67
Dextrocardia	36	33
Conduction		
Dual sinus nodes	+++	
Complete heart block		+++

Adapted from Van Praagh 2006 [3]. Numbers based on 101 postmortem cases. CAVC, complete atrioventricular canal; IVC; inferior vena cava; SVC, superior vena cava.

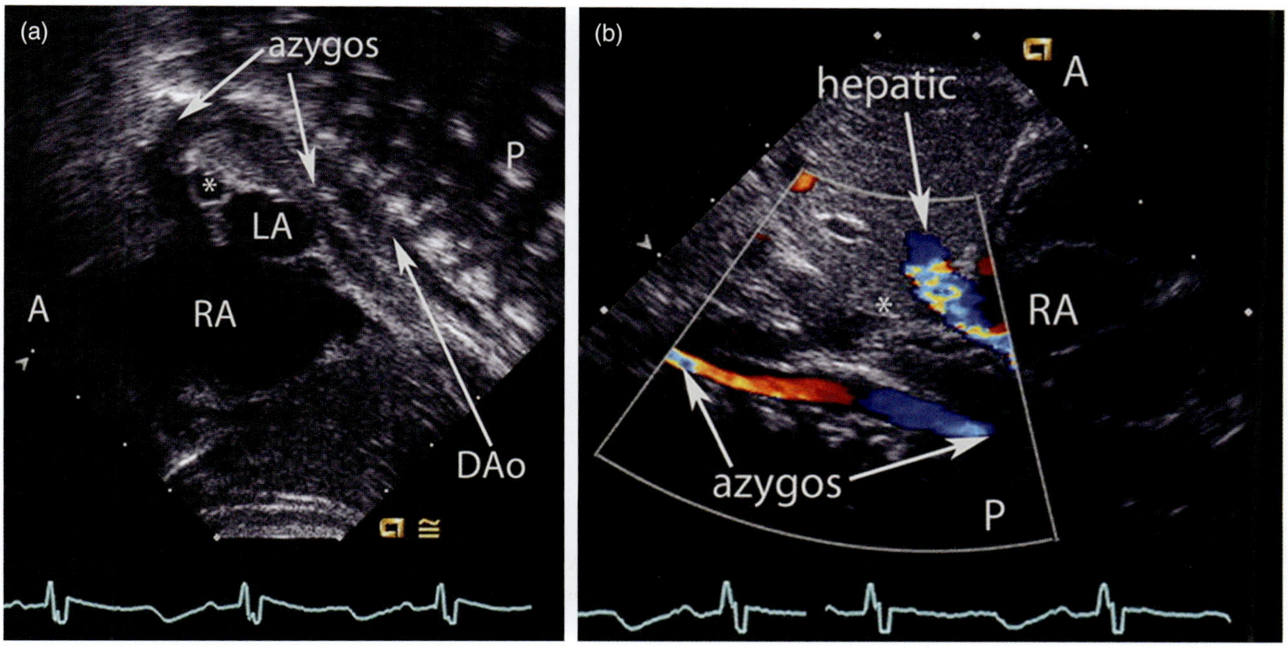

Figure 47.5 (a) Subxiphoid sagittal image of the azygos vein arching over the right pulmonary artery (asterisk) before connecting to the superior vena cava and draining into the right atrium (RA). (b) Subcostal image showing absence of an inferior vena cava (asterisk) joining the hepatic vein as it enters the RA. Instead, an azygos vein travels behind the heart. A, anterior; DAo, descending aorta; LA, left atrium; P, posterior.

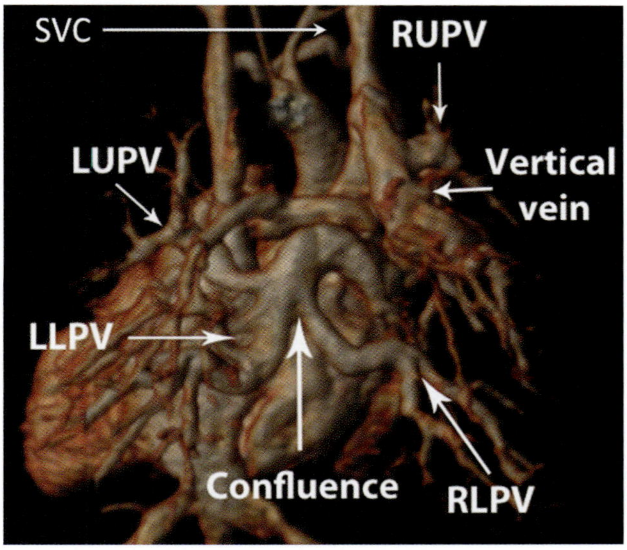

Figure 47.6 3D reconstruction of gadolinium-enhanced magnetic resonance angiogram demonstrating pulmonary veins forming a confluence which gives rise to a vertical vein draining into the superior vena cava (SVC). LUPV, left upper pulmonary vein; LLPV, left lower pulmonary vein; RLPV, right lower pulmonary vein; RUPV, right upper pulmonary vein.

A common AV valve is seen in 70% of patients with asplenia syndrome and only 33% of patients with polysplenia syndrome [3]. In contrast, <10% of patients with asplenia syndrome have normal AV valves and 35% with polysplenia syndrome have normal AV valves [3]. An isolated cleft mitral valve without a ventricular septal defect is the next most common anomaly [5]. A balanced AV canal defect with well-developed right and left ventricles was seen in 45% of asplenic patients and 63% of polysplenic patients [3]. Unbalanced AV canal defects are usually right-dominant [5]. A morphologic single ventricle occurs more frequently with asplenia syndrome [3].

Normal ventricular looping results in an anterior rightward RV and a posterior leftward LV (D-looped ventricles). In heterotaxy syndrome, the ventricles are usually D-looped without significant differences between asplenia and polysplenia syndromes in postmortem studies [3]. Ventricular myocardial non-compaction has been reported in patients with polysplenia syndrome [9].

The subpulmonary conus in a normal heart is the muscular ring located below the pulmonary valve. The ventriculo-arterial relationship in heterotaxy syndrome is markedly variable. A subaortic conus does not exist in a normal heart. An anterior right-sided aorta, along with a subaortic or bilateral conus, is most often seen in heterotaxy syndrome. Pulmonary outflow obstruction is less common (~20%) in patients with polysplenia. In contrast, systemic outflow obstruction (including aortic atresia or coarctation) occurs in 20–45% of patients with polysplenia [10].

The relationship between aorta and pulmonary artery is also significantly variable. In postmortem studies, only 9% were noted to have normally-related great arteries [3].

In asplenia syndrome, 85% have some form of pulmonary stenosis or atresia with accompanying ductal-dependent pulmonary circulation. The ventriculo-arterial relationship can be single or double outlet with discordant connections in more than 90% [10].

The sinus node is situated at the right SVC–RA junction. In polysplenia syndrome, the sinus node is absent or hypoplastic and an ectopic atrial rhythm occurs frequently. Complete heart block is seen in 20% of patients and carries significant morbidity and mortality in the fetus [11]. In 41 fetuses with polysplenia syndrome, 41% had complete heart block; the intrauterine demise rate was 17% [12]. The vast majority of patients with asplenia syndrome have normal sinus rhythm [13].

Management

Both medical and surgical therapy depend on the specific anatomy and splenic status. Asplenic patients usually have more severe heart defects, often precluding biventricular repair and necessitating staged single ventricle palliation. Biventricular circulation is more common in polysplenia syndrome given less severe lesions.

The infant with asplenia syndrome and ductal-dependent pulmonary circulation will become progressively cyanotic with ductal constriction. Prostaglandin E1 (PGE1) is needed to ensure pulmonary blood flow until reliable pulmonary blood flow is established by surgery or interventional catheterization. If accompanied by obstructed pulmonary veins resulting in severe hypoxemia, PGE1 may be detrimental by increasing pulmonary blood flow and causing worse pulmonary edema. Here, standard intensive care stabilization and immediate surgical repair may be necessary.

The infant with polysplenia syndrome rarely presents with cyanosis as pulmonary blood flow obstruction is rare. Rather, they present with heart failure and metabolic acidosis related to left heart obstruction with possible pulmonary overcirculation. Standard treatment for severe left-sided obstruction is employed. Complete AV block causing ventricular bradycardia can cause neonatal symptoms [12].

Surgical treatment of patients with heterotaxy syndrome is complex and first requires a decision whether biventricular repair is feasible. Most patients with asplenia syndrome initially require a stable source of pulmonary blood flow. Some also require correction of APVC. Mortality is increased if the initial palliation is performed at a younger age or if there is pulmonary venous obstruction [14]. Regurgitation of the AV valve is common and often worsened by an aortopulmonary shunt. An early bidirectional cavopulmonary anastomosis may be beneficial. The staged palliation culminates in the Fontan circulation, though mortality and morbidity is higher with asplenia syndrome at this stage when compared with other single ventricular lesions [14]. Improved outcomes in most recent studies may reflect better surgical tehcniques as well as better postoperative management [14]. Biventricular repair is more common in patients with polysplenia syndrome, though 50–70% require single ventricle palliation. Risk factors for poor outcomes in patients with polysplenia syndrome include biliary atresia, low birth weight, complete heart block, coarctation, and single ventricle physiology [11].

Some patients will eventually need cardiac transplantation, occurring more frequently after single ventricle palliation. The associated cardiac malposition and/or abnormal systemic and pulmonary venous anatomy can be challenging, but do not preclude successful transplantation.

Outcomes

Patients with asplenia and polysplenia syndromes have variable prognosis depending on the severity of the specific lesion(s). The natural history can be dire, and asplenic patients usually have worse outcome than patients with polysplenia [15]. Spontaneous intrauterine death occurs 3–4 times more frequently in fetuses with polysplenia syndrome, likely because of rhythm disturbances and ventricular dysfunction [16]. However, prenatal diagnosis of heterotaxy syndrome does not appear to affect survival when compared with other prenatally diagnosed single ventricle hearts [16].

Conclusions

Heterotaxy syndrome represents a complex group of anomalies involving the thoracoabdominal viscera. Classification systems are based on splenic anatomy (asplenia and polysplenia syndromes) or on the atrial appendages (RA and LA isomerism). Cardiac malformations are rarely singular and often occur as a constellation of abnormalities specifically associated with the disorders of laterality. More complex cardiac lesions are seen in patients with asplenia syndrome. However, there is significant mortality and morbidity associated with polysplenia syndrome because of the high incidence of conduction abnormalities. Prognosis depends largely on the underlying cardiac lesion. However, patients with heterotaxy syndrome carry a worse prognosis than those with comparable isolated cardiac lesions.

References

1 Cohen MS, Anderson RH, Cohen MI, *et al.* (2007) Controversies, genetics, diagnostic assessment, and outcomes relating to the heterotaxy syndrome. *Cardiol Young*, **17** (Suppl 2), 29–43.
2 Van Praagh R, Van Praagh S. (1990) Atrial isomerism in the heterotaxy syndromes with asplenia, or polysplenia, or normally formed spleen: an erroneous concept. *Am J Cardiol*, **66** (20), 1504–1506.
3 Van Praagh S. (2006) Cardiac malpositions and the heterotaxy syndromes, in, *Nadas's Pediatric Cardiology*, 2nd edn (eds JF Keany, JE Locke, DC Fyler). Saunders Elsevier, Philadelphia, pp. 589–608.
4 Van Mierop LH, Wiglesworth FW. (1962) Isomerism of the cardiac atria in the asplenia syndrome. *Lab Invest*, **11**, 1303–1315.
5 Perloff JK. (2011) The cardiac malpositions. *Am J Cardiol*, **108** (9), 1352–1361. PubMed PMID: 21861958. Epub 2011/08/25. eng.
6 Grant RP. (1958) The syndrome of dextroversion of the heart. *Circulation*, **8** (1), 25–36.
7 Van Praagh S, Kreutzer J, Alday L, Van Praagh R. (1990) Systemic and pulmonary venous connections in visceral heterotaxy, with emphasis on the diagnosis of the atrial situs: a study of 109 postmortem cases, in, *Developmental Cardiology Morphogenesis and Function* (eds EB Clark, A Takas), Futura, New York.
8 Sharma S, Devine W, Anderson RH, Zuberbuhler JR. (1987) Identification and analysis of left atrial isomerism. *Am J Cardiol*, **60** (14), 1157–1160.
9 Arunamata A, Punn R, Cuneo B, Bharati S, Silverman NH. (2012) Echocardiographic diagnosis and prognosis of fetal left ventricular noncompaction. *J Am Soc Echocardiogr*, **25** (1), 112–120.
10 Shinebourne EA, Macartney FJ, Anderson RH. (1976) Sequential chamber localization: logical approach to diagnosis in congenital heart disease. *Br Heart J*, **38** (4), 327–340. PubMed PMID: 1267978.
11 Gilljam T, McCrindle BW, Smallhorn JF, Williams WG, Freedom RM. (2000) Outcomes of left atrial isomerism over a 28-year period at a single institution. *J Am Coll Cardiol*, **36** (3), 908–916.
12 Lopes LM, Tavares GM, Damiano AP, *et al.* (2008) Perinatal outcome of fetal atrioventricular block: one-hundred-sixteen cases from a single institution. *Circulation*, **118** (12), 1268–1275.
13 Di Donato R, di Carlo D, Squitieri C, *et al.* (1987) Palliation of cardiac malformations associated with right isomerism (asplenia syndrome) in infancy. *Ann Thorac Surg*, **44** (1), 35–39.
14 Cetta F, Feldt RH, O'Leary PW, *et al.* (1996) Improved early morbidity and mortality after Fontan operation: the Mayo Clinic experience, 1987 to 1992. *J Am Coll Cardiol*, **28** (2), 480–486.
15 Foerster SR, Gauvreau K, McElhinney DB, Geva T. (2008) Importance of totally anomalous pulmonary venous connection and postoperative pulmonary vein stenosis in outcomes of heterotaxy syndrome. *Pediatr Cardiol*, **29** (3), 536–544.
16 Cohen MS, Schultz AH, Tian ZY, *et al.* (2006) Heterotaxy syndrome with functional single ventricle: does prenatal diagnosis improve survival? *Ann Thorac Surg*, **82** (5), 1629–1636.

48

Ectopia Cordis and Thoracopagus Twins

Sawsan Awad

Rush University Medical Center, Chicago, IL, USA

Ectopia Cordis

Ectopia cordis (EC) is a cardiac malposition wherein the heart is partially or completely outside the thorax. The name stems from the Greek word "*ektopos*" which means departure from the appropriate place of origin. It is a rare congenital abnormality, occurring in 5.5–7.9 per 1 million live births [1]. The abnormality is thought to be caused by failure of fusion of the two sternal islands that form the sternum at around 9–10 weeks' gestation. Sternal fusion defects can occur as an isolated finding. When associated with the heart outside the chest, the condition is called EC.

EC is classified into five types:

1) Cervical;
2) Cervicothoracic;
3) Thoracic;
4) Thoracoabdominal; and
5) Abdominal.

The thoracoabdominal type of EC is also called pentalogy of Cantrell. The full spectrum of pentalogy of Cantrell consists of five anomalies:

1) Defect in the lower sternum;
2) Midline supraumbilical abdominal wall defect;
3) Deficiency of the anterior diaphragm;
4) Defect in the diaphragmatic pericardium; and
5) Various congenital intracardiac abnormalities [2].

Diagnosis of EC is made by fetal ultrasound (Figures 48.1 and 48.2), with great accuracy as early as first trimester. Early diagnosis of EC and its associated fetal anomalies, most commonly omphalocele (Figure 48.1), allows for early family counseling [3]. The diagnosis, if not made by fetal ultrasound and fetal echocardiography, is evident on inspection of the infant at birth. It is essential to determine any intracardiac defects by sterile careful epicardial echocardiography.

Surgical correction includes four important steps: coverage of the naked heart; palliation or complete repair of major intracardiac defects; placement of the heart into the thoracic cavity; and sternal or thoracic reconstruction. Survival of this condition with or without surgery depends to great extent on the type of EC [4].

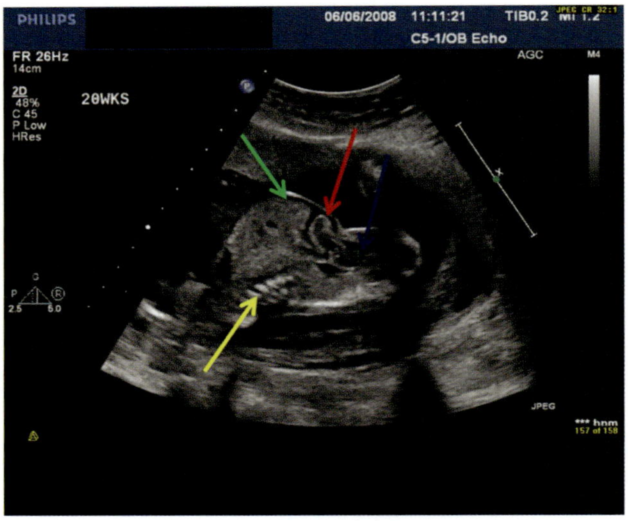

Figure 48.1 Fetal echocardiogram demonstrating a long-axis view of the thorax and abdomen. Note the abdominal wall defect presenting as a large omphalocele (green arrow) with the abdominal contents outside the cavity and partially covered by a sac. There is protrusion of the apical portion of the heart (red arrow) outside the chest cavity (blue arrow). Fluid accumulation is seen outside the heart and between the sac and the liver. The yellow arrow points to the fetal spine.

Thoracopagus Twins

Conjoined twins (CT) occur in about 1% of monochorionic twin pregnancies, with a 3 : 1 female predominance [5]. CT are attached through homologous sites, and the clinical classification is based on the most prominent site of union of the twins followed by the suffix -pagus [6], which is a Greek word meaning "that which is fixed."

Visual Guide to Neonatal Cardiology, First Edition. Edited by Ernerio T. Alboliras, Ziyad M. Hijazi, Leo Lopez, and Donald J. Hagler.

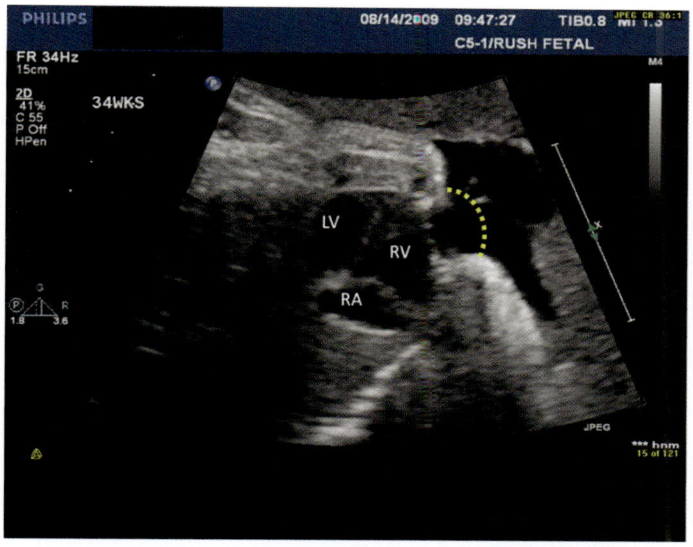

Figure 48.2 Fetal echocardiogram: cross-section of thorax in a fetus with sternal cleft and no omphalocele. Notice the sternal defect (dashed yellow connector). The heart protrudes through the sternal defect in real-time during respiratory movements. LV, left ventricle; RA, right atrium; RV, right ventricle.

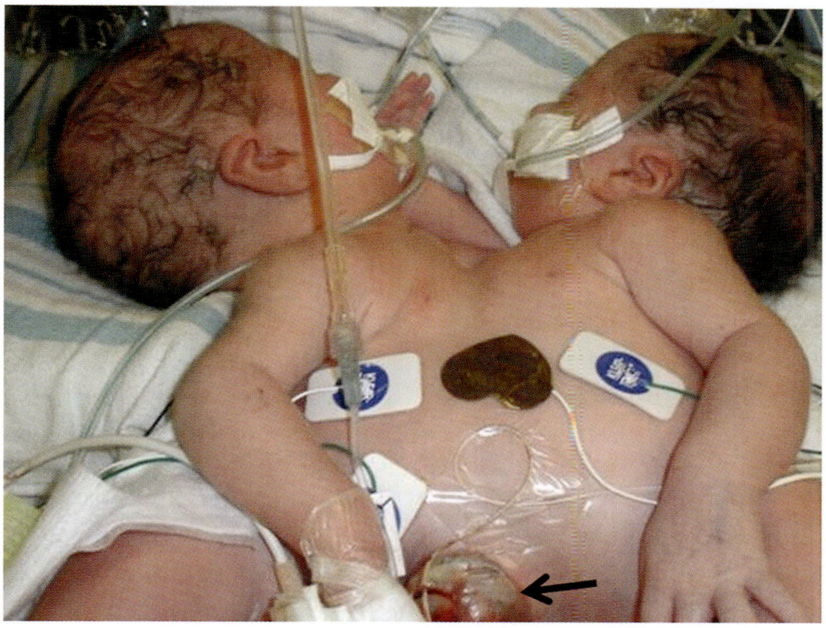

Figure 48.3 Thoracopagus twins at 1 day of age. Notice the associated omphalocele (black arrow).

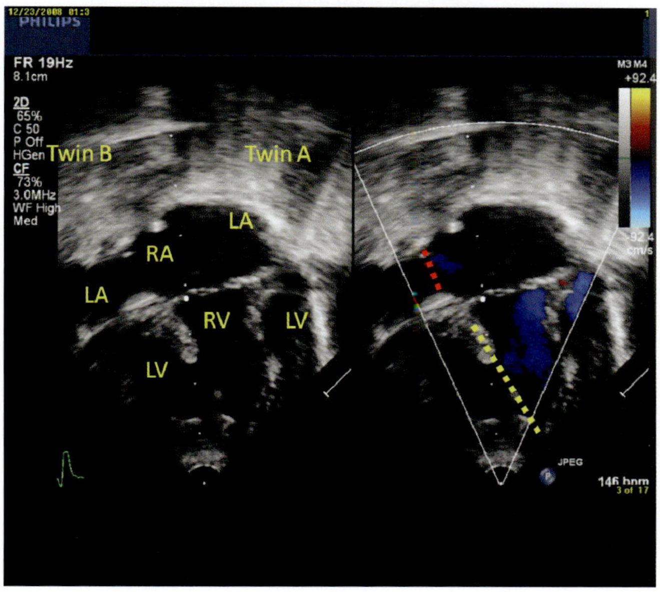

Figure 48.4 Postnatal transthoracic 2D and color Doppler echocardiography of thoracopagus conjoined twins in Figure 48.3. There are eight heart chambers. The twins' hearts are connected via RV of twin A and LV of twin B. Dashed yellow line denotes area of ventricular connection between twins' hearts. The dashed red line is the line of atrial connection between the twins' hearts. Intracardiac lesions include ventricular septal defect in twin A (not shown) and atrial septal defect in twin A and twin B (not shown). LA, left atrium; LV, left ventricle; RA, right atrium; RV, right ventricle.

Spencer [6] also divided the twins into three major groups:

1) Twins with a ventral union:
   - Cephalopagus (head);
   - Thoracopagus (chest);
   - Omphalopagus (umbilicus); and
   - Ischiopagus (hip).
2) Twins with a dorsal union; and
   - Pygopagus (sacrum);
   - Rachipagus (spine); and
   - Craniopagus (cranium).
3) Twins with a lateral union:
   - Parapagus (side) [7].

Thoracopagus is the most common type of presentation (20–70%) (Figure 48.3) [5]. Complex cardiac fusion is the most critical determinant of surgical separation and survival [8, 9]. An accurate transthoracic echocardiographic examination is crucial although may be challenging because of the thoracoabdominal connection of twins (Figure 48.4). Associated intracardiac

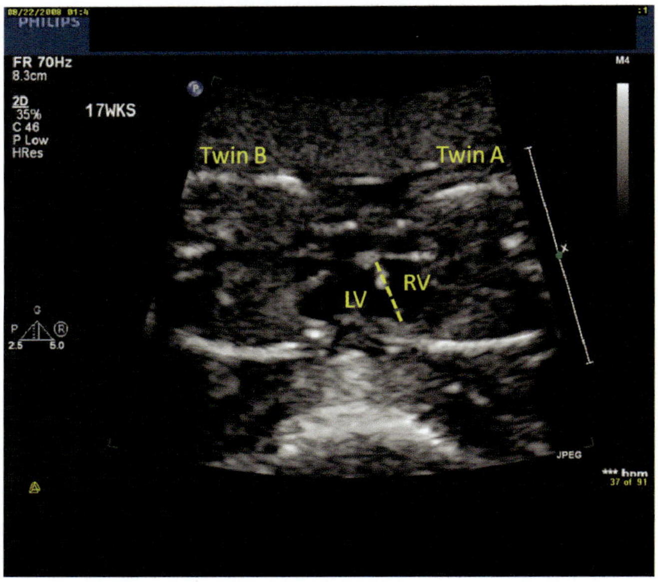

Figure 48.5 Fetal echocardiography of thoracopagus twins shown in Figure 48.3, at 17 weeks' gestation. The yellow dashed line demarcates the site of connection of the two hearts between the right ventricle (RV) of twin A and the left ventricle (LV) of twin B.

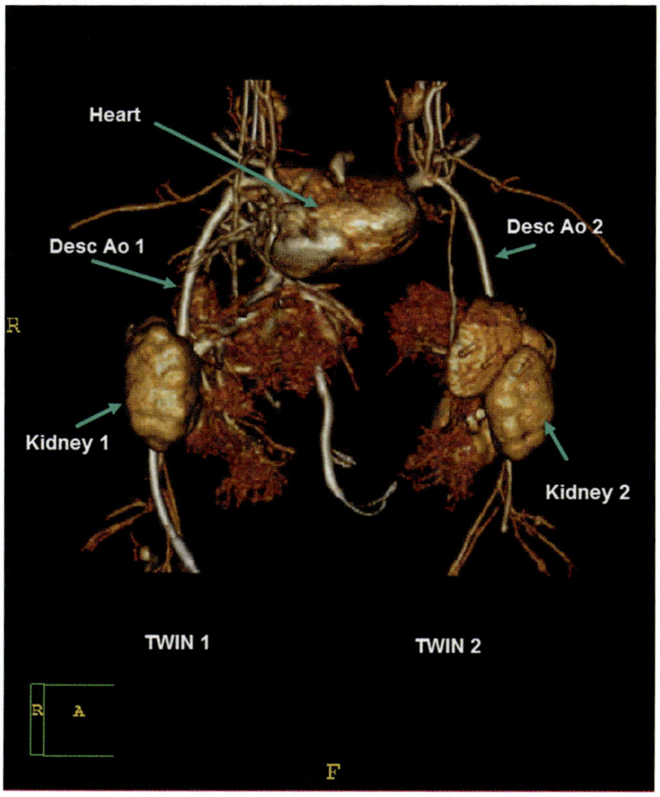

Figure 48.6 Computerized tomographic angiography with 3D reconstruction of thoracopagis twins with complex cardiovascular anatomy.

abnormalities are major determinants of feasibility of postnatal surgical separation of the twins and in counseling the parents regarding prognosis [10, 11]. Fetal echocardiographic evaluation is considered to be an important tool in early diagnosis and meaningful counseling of parents of conjoined twins fetuses (Figure 48.5). Computerized tomography with three-dimensional (3D) reconstruction can help provide salient details important in surgical planning and prognostication (Figure 48.6).

McMahon and Spencer [12] have summarized the cardiac anomalies found in more than 1200 pairs of conjoined twins reported in the literature. Their review included 192 cases that had some degree of cardiac fusion, with only three sets of twins surviving surgical separation. The patients who survived separation had only an interatrial communication as the extent of cardiac fusion.

References

1 Hornberger LK, Colan SD, Lock JE, *et al.* (1996) Outcome of patients with ectopia cordis and significant intracardiac defects. *Circulation*, **94**, 32–37.

2 Mallula KK, Sosnowski C, Awad S. (2013) Spectrum of Cantrell's pentalogy: case series from a single tertiary care center and review of the literature. *Pediatr Cardiol*, **34** (7), 1703–1710.

3 Hannoun A, Usta IM, Sawaya F, *et al.* (2011) First trimester sonographic diagnosis of ectopia cordis: a case report and review of the literature. *J Matern Fetal Neonatal Med*, **24** (6), 867–869.

4 Amato JJ, Douglas WI, Desai U, *et al.* (2000) Ectopia cordis. *Chest Surg Clin N Am*, **10** (2), 297–316, vii.

5 Lopes LM, Brizot ML, Schultz R, *et al.* (2013) Twenty-five years of fetal echocardiography in conjoined twins: lessons learned. *J Am Soc Echocardiogr*, **26** (5), 530–538.

6 Spencer R. (1996) Anatomic description of conjoined twins: a plea for standardized terminology. *J Pediatr Surg*, **31**, 941–944.

7 Tannuri AC, Batatinha JA, Velhote MC, Tannuri U. (2013) Conjoined twins: twenty years' experience at a reference center in Brazil. *Clinics (Sao Paulo)*, **68** (3), 371–377.

8 Spitz L. (2005) Conjoined twins. *Prenat Diagn*, **25**, 814–819.

9 Spitz L, Kiely EM. (2002) Experience in the management of conjoined twins. *Br J Surg*, **89**, 1188–1192.

10 Andrews RE, McMahon CJ, Yates RWM, *et al.* (2006) Echocardiographic assessment of conjoined twins. *Heart*, **92**, 382–387.

11 Sanders SP, Chin AJ, Parness IA, *et al.* (1985) Prenatal diagnosis of congenital heart defects in thoracoabdominally conjoined twins. *N Engl J Med*, **313**, 370–374.

12 McMahon CJ, Spencer R. (2006) Congenital heart defects in conjoined twins: outcome after surgical separation of thoracopagus. *Pediatr Cardiol*, **27**, 1–12.

49

Patent Ductus Arteriosus

Robert Puntel

Division of Cardiology, Phoenix Children's Hospital, Phoenix, AZ, USA

The ductus arteriosus is critical in fetal life as a shunt from high pressure in the pulmonary arterial system to the descending aorta. It connects the main pulmonary artery (MPA) with the descending aorta (Figure 49.1) or rarely a subclavian artery. In the embryo it is the distal left sixth primitive aortic arch that persists and forms the ductus arteriosus.

In fetal cardiac anatomy, less oxygenated blood returning from mainly the superior vena cava courses through the right side of the heart to the MPA through the ductus arteriosus to the lower body. More oxygenated and nutrient-rich blood flows from the placenta through the ductus venosus and is directed mainly through the patent foramen ovale by the Eustachian valve via the left ventricle to the developing brain and upper body.

Premature constriction of the fetal ductus arteriosus can lead to isolated right ventricular hypertrophy. However, clinical outcomes range from mild symptoms to lethal respiratory insufficiency [1]. The etiology is often unknown, but is associated with the use of maternal non-steroidal anti-inflammatory drugs in the third trimester [2].

With normal fetal ductal flow, the ductal anatomy assumes an arch facing inferiorly (Figure 49.2). If the right ventricular outflow tract flow is limited, the ductus arteriosus is often long and tortuous with a concave aspect superiorly. This "reverse-oriented ductus" can indicate intervention is needed to increase pulmonary blood flow after delivery (Figure 49.3).

The ductus arteriosus closes spontaneously in most term infants by 3 days of age [3]. Persistence of the ductus arteriosus, or patent ductus arteriosus (PDA) occurs after birth for many reasons including prematurity, low oxygen tension, and infections such as maternal rubella. It is common, with 40–55% of PDA persisting in babies born less than 29 weeks' gestation. The clinical changes are most often because of left to right

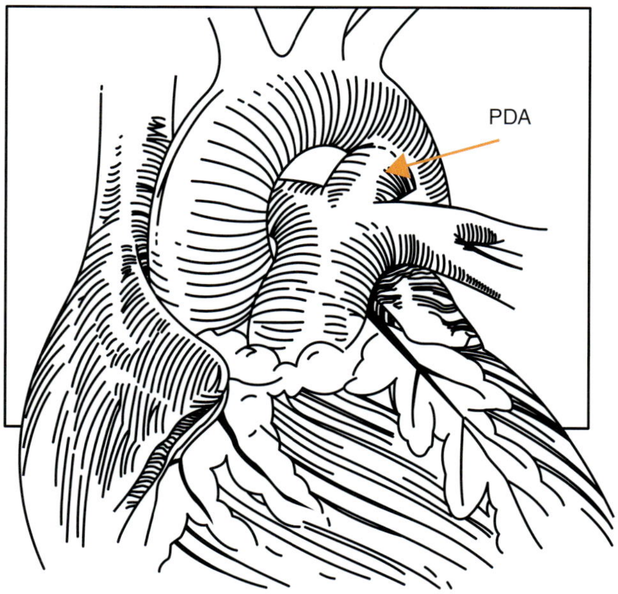

Figure 49.1 Drawing of a heart with a large patent ductus arteriosus (PDA) conncting the main pulmonary artery with the aorta.

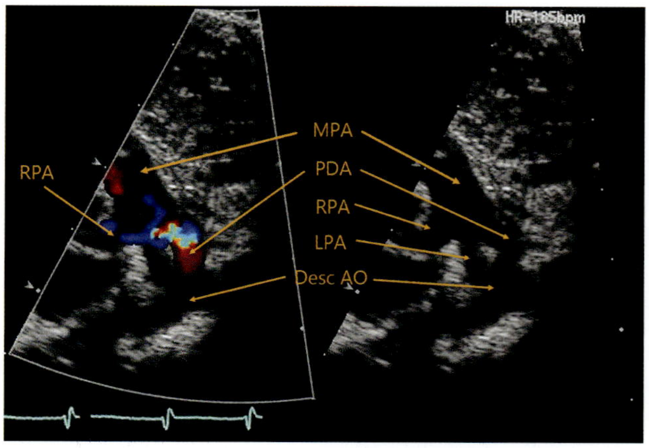

Figure 49.2 High left parasternal echocardiographic long-axis view of the cardiac vessels demonstrating the relationship of the PDA to the main pulmonary artery (MPA), left pulmonary artery (LPA), right pulmonary artery (RPA), and descending aorta (Desc Ao).

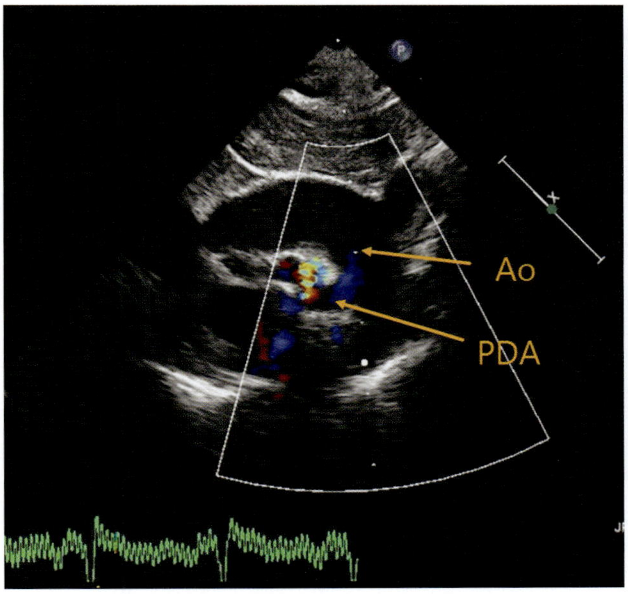

Figure 49.3 Suprasternal echocardiographic view of the aortic arch (Ao) and a PDA in a patient with a ductal dependent cyanotic heart defect. The PDA is tortuous and has a cranially directed concavity ("reverse-oriented" PDA).

shunting in very low birth weight (VLBW) and premature infants. This can lead to pulmonary overcirculation and edema which can lead to systemic hypoperfusion and/or need for increased ventilator management. It can be associated with renal hypoperfusion or necrotizing enterocolitis [3]. The natural history of PDA in preterm infants is unknown because it is often altered by medical treatments [4].

Echocardiography is the mainstay of detection and characterization of a PDA in the fetus and newborn. Spectral and color Doppler interrogation can be clinically valuable, and has been shown to be accurate in predicting the interplay of systemic and pulmonary vascular resistance.

With a left aortic arch the PDA connects the aortic isthmus and proximal left pulmonary artery–MPA junction (Figure 49.1). In a newborn with a PDA and significant pulmonary hypertension, the Doppler flow across the duct may be almost purely right to left (from pulmonary artery to aorta) during systole (Figure 49.4). In pulmonary hypertension with a restrictive PDA, there is usually pure right to left shunt peak at systole and continuing with a diastolic right to left runoff (Figure 49.5). As the pulmonary vascular resistance improves, with persistence of a PDA, the flow may be bidirectional, mainly right to left during systole and with a small left to right shunt during diastole (Figure 49.6). The amount of left to right shunt during diastole increases as pulmonary resistance decreases further (Figure 49.7). With normalization of pulmonary resistance, the flow across the PDA usually becomes a continuous left to right (Figure 49.8).

In right aortic arch (often associated with tetralogy of Fallot), the PDA can be between the right descending aorta and the right pulmonary artery–MPA junction, left-sided between the brachiocephalic trunk or proximal left subclavian artery, or bilateral. The most common form of right aortic arch is with mirror image branching and a left PDA or its ligamentum which results in a vascular ring [5, 6].

Aneurysm of the PDA is uncommon and is manifested by significant dilation of the PDA which can compress chest structures or develop thrombus which can migrate. This can be associated with connective tissue disorders or chromosomal anomalies [7].

The pathophysiology of the PDA is dependent upon the presence of congenital heart disease, gestational age, and

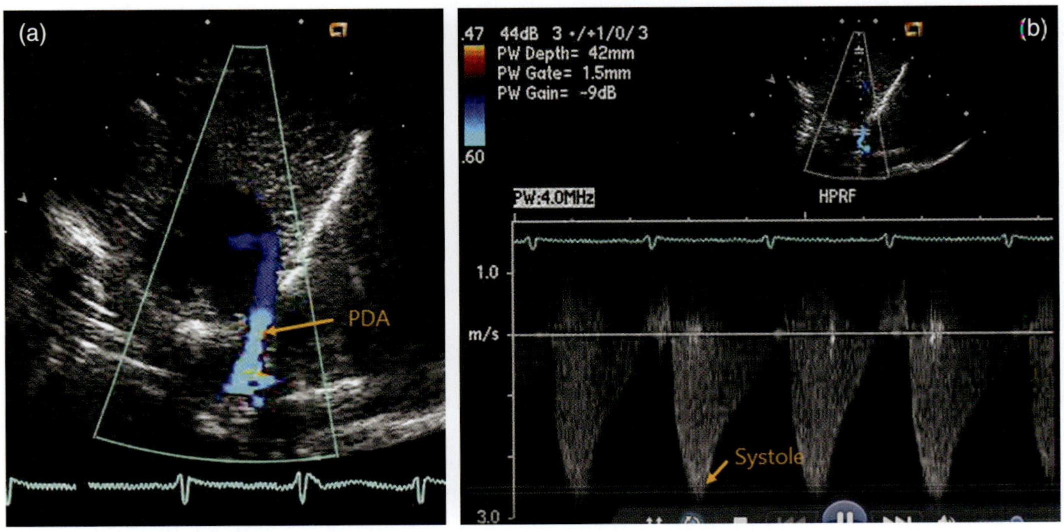

Figure 49.4 (a) Patient with pulmonary hypertension and a small PDA. (b) Spectral Doppler image demonstrates accelerated peak right to left systolic flow that terminates at mid-diastole.

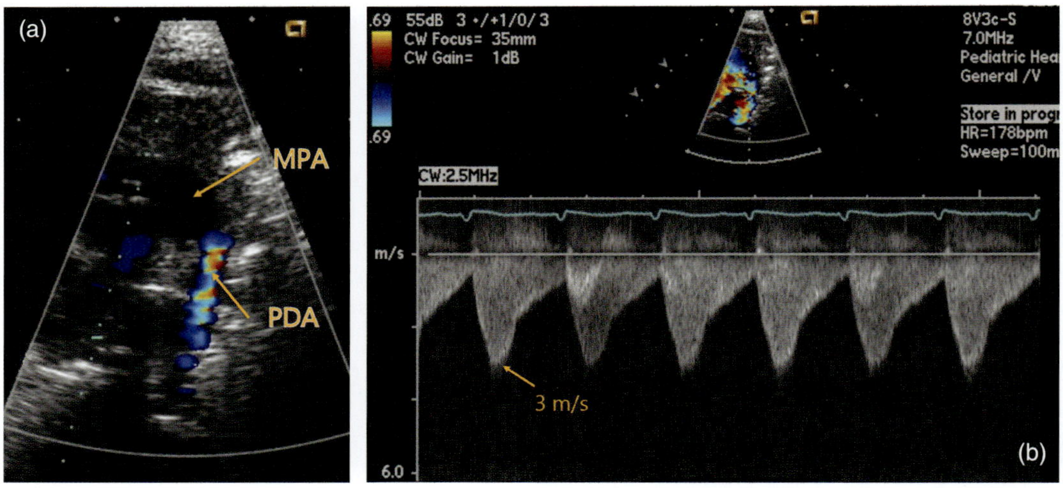

Figure 49.5 (a) Patient with pulmonary hypertension and a smaller PDA than in Figure 49.3. (b) Spectral Doppler image demonstrates a continuous systolic and diastolic right to left shunt, with systolic peaking. The Doppler profile is that of a saw-tooth pattern.

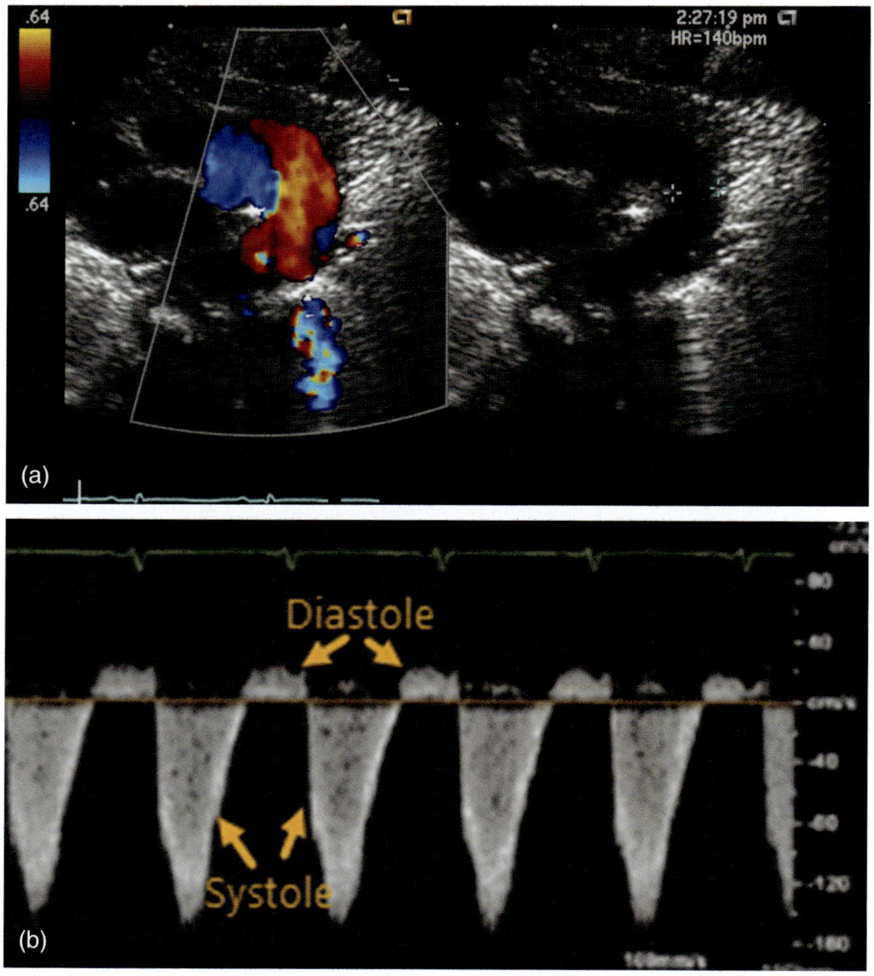

Figure 49.6 (a) Neonate with a large PDA and with elevated pulmonary resistance. (b) Spectral Doppler image demonstrates bidirectional shunt (right to left during systole and left to right during diastole) but with mainly a systolic shunt.

many hemodynamic and anatomic factors. Table 49.1 summarizes the common PDA flow directions.

The physiology of the PDA flow in term newborns and infants depends on the smallest cross-sectional area, the length of the PDA, and the systemic and pulmonary vascular resistance. A large PDA and large left to right shunt can result in pulmonary overcirculation, failure to thrive, and eventual pulmonary vascular disease. A small PDA can be hemodynamically insignificant but has an increased risk of endocarditis over a lifetime.

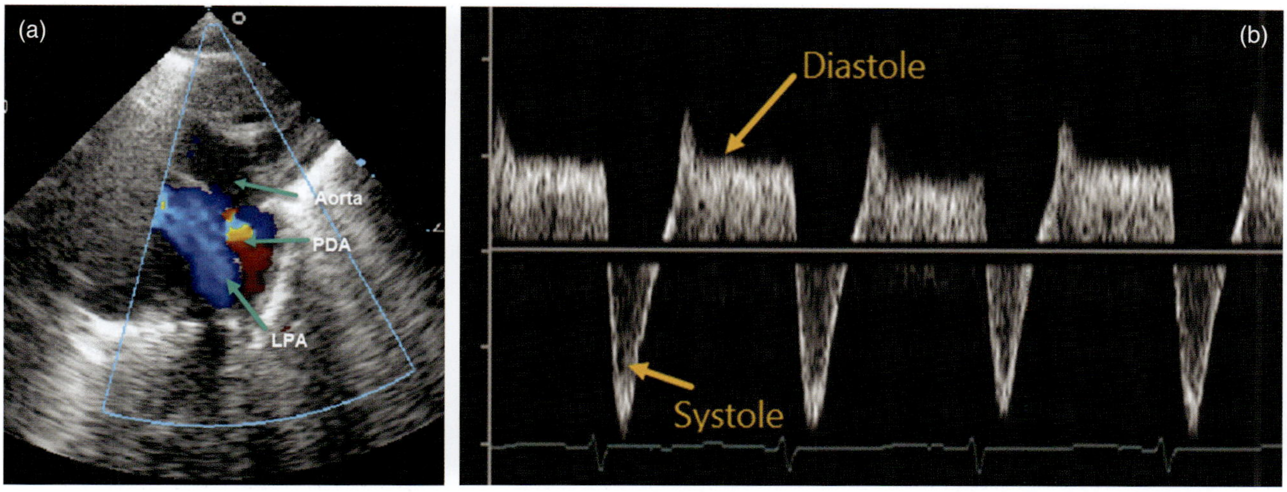

Figure 49.7 (a) Neonate with a moderate size PDA and with some degrees of elevated pulmonary resistance. (b) Spectral Doppler image also demonstrates bidirectional shunt (right to left during systole and left to right during diastole) but with this time with predominantly left to right shunt.

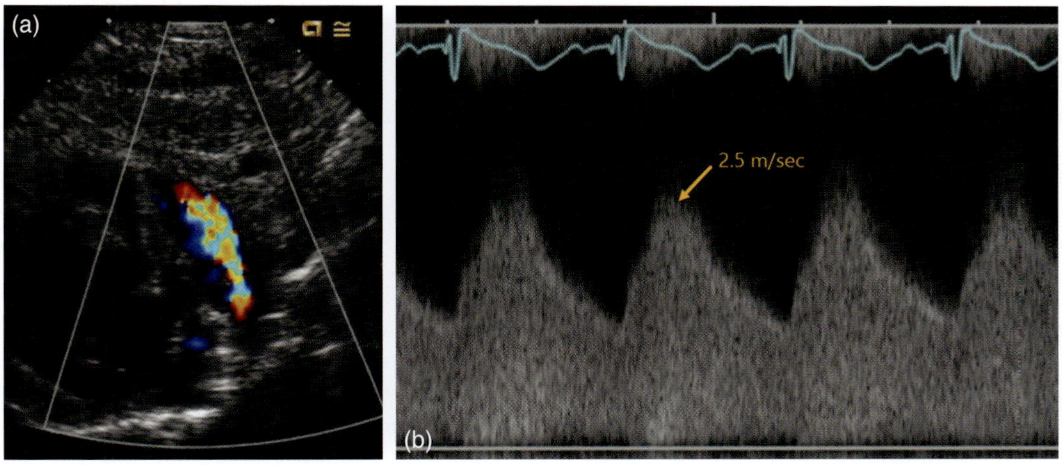

Figure 49.8 (a) Neonate with a small PDA and normal pulmonary resistance. (b) Spectral Doppler image demonstrates a continuous left to right shunt (from aorta to pulmonary artery). The peak flow occurs during systole.

Table 49.1 Significance of flow direction across the patent ductus arteriosus (PDA).

PDA flow	Right to left	Bidirectional	Left to right
PVR	Significantly elevated PVR	Elevated PVR	Normal PVR
Typical cardiac defects	Left heart obstructive lesions (e.g., hypoplastic left heart syndrome, coarctation of the aorta)	Often normal anatomy	Right heart obstructive lesions (e.g., pulmonary atresia)
Typical other findings	Cyanosis (lower body in coarctation) lower “post-ductal” pulse oximetry in lower extremity	Trisomy 21 Prematurity	Heart failure in normal anatomy (dilated left atrium and left ventricle) with large shunt and low PVR

PVR, pulmonary vascular resistance.

Table 49.2 Clinical and echocardiographic markers for staging.

Clinical findings	Echocardiographic findings
Mild Little oxygenation difficulty Respiratory support minimal Mild feeding intolerance CXR: increased pulmonary blood flow	*Small* PDA diameter <1.5 mm Restrictive PDA flow (Vmax >2 cm/s) Left atrial/aortic ratio <1.5 No left heart pressure loading Normal superior mesenteric and middle cerebral artery diastolic flow
Moderate Oxygenation difficulty Increasing ventilation requirements Feeding difficulty Oliguria Hypotension, requirement of inotropic support CXR: cardiomegaly/pulmonary edema Mild metabolic acidosis	*Moderate* PDA diameter 1.5–3 mm Unrestrictive pulsatile transductal flow (Vmax <2 cm/s) Left atrial : aortic ratio 1.5 to 2 : 1 Mild/moderate left heart pressure loading Decreased or absent diastolic flow in renal, middle cerebral, or superior mesenteric artery
Severe Significant oxygenation difficulty High ventilation requirement Pulmonary hemorrhage Suspected necrotizing enterocolitis Acute renal failure Hemodynamic instability requiring >1 inotropic agent Moderate to severe metabolic acidosis	*Large* PDA diameter >3 mm Unrestrictive pulsatile transductal flow Severe left heart volume loading Left atrial : aortic ratio >2 : 1 Severe left heart pressure loading Reversal of end-diastolic flow in superior mesenteric, middle cerebral, or renal arteries

CXR, chest X-ray; PDA, patent ductus arteriosus; Vmax, maximum velocity.
Source: Adapted from Sehgal and McNamara 2009 [8].

Patency of the ductus arteriosus is necessary in certain forms of congenital cardiac defects or ductal dependent lesions. Examples include hypoplastic left heart syndrome, interrupted aortic arch, pulmonary atresia, and transposition of the great arteries. Intravenous prostaglandin E1 infusion is at a rate of 0.05–0.1 μg/kg/minute.

Clinical Findings

Classically, with normal PVR there is a continuous murmur at the left upper sternal border with radiation to the left axilla and back. S2 is normal if there is no pulmonary hypertension. In the premature infant, the murmur can be atypical and appear as a systolic murmur only. Wide pulse pressure, bounding pulses, and other signs of congestive heart failure may be present.

Imaging

Chest X-ray can demonstrate dilated left heart and pulmonary arteries in proportion to the left to right shunt. Echocardiography is the mainstay of diagnosis and assessment. Color flow mapping displays shunt direction. Estimates of pulmonary artery pressure are determined by spectral Doppler assessment using tricuspid regurgitant jet and PDA velocity and direction. Cardiac catheterization is rarely used. Table 49.2 tabulates the clinical and echocardiographic markers for staging the significance of a PDA.

Management

Controversy exists in determining the size and degree of hemodynamic impact of a PDA, especially in premature newborns. In VLBW newborns weighing less than 1.5 kg, the presence of a PDA is usually treated. There is controversy in more mature newborns. Generally, three approaches are considered when treating a hemodynamically significant PDA, particularly in the premature infant: supportive therapy, medical closure with cyclooxygenase (COX) inhibitors (indomethacin or ibuprofen), or surgical ligation. Supportive therapy includes watchful waiting, fluid restriction, and diuretics. Indomethacin dosage is 0.1–0.2 mg/kg/dose at 12–24 hour intervals, generally for three doses. Ibuprofen dosage is 10 mg/kg followed by two 5 mg/kg doses at

24 hour intervals. A second course is given if there is failure to respond but response beyond age 10 days is unlikely. The side effects of COX inhibitorsinclude renal insufficiency, platelet dysfunction, and gastrointestinal perforation. They should not be used in ductal dependent congenital heart defects. There are no large randomized controlled trials to dictate best therapy; it is tailored to the individual and institution. Percutaneous catheter occlusion can be considered if the infant's weight is greater than 6 kg [9].

References

1 Gellewig M, Brown SC, Catte LD, *et al.* (2009) Premature foetal closure of the arterial duct: clinical presentations and outcome. *Eur Heart J*, **30** (12), 1530–1536.

2 Koren G, Florescu A, Costei AM, Boskovic R, Moretti ME. (2006) Nonsteroidal anti-inflammatory drugs during third trimester and the risk of premature closure of the ductus arteriosus: a meta-analysis. *Ann Pharmacother*, **40** (5), 824–829.

3 Gentile R, Stevenson G, Dooley T, *et al.* (1981) Pulsed Doppler echocardiographic determination of time of ductal closure in normal newborn infants. *J Pediatr*, **98**, 443–448.

4 Bose CL, Laughon MM. (2007) Patent ductus arteriosus: lack of evidence for common treatments. *Arch Dis Child Fetal Neonatal Ed*, **92** (6), F498–F502.

5 Craatz s, Kunzel E, Spanel-Borowski K. (2003) Right sided aortic arch and tetralogy of Fallot in humans: a morphologic study of 10 cases. *Cardiovasc Pathol*, **12**, 226–232.

6 Rao PS, Wagman AJ, Chen SC. (2001) Coil occlusion of patent ductus arteriosus associated with right aortic arch. *Catheter Cardiovasc Interv*, **52**, 79–82.

7 Wyman WL, Mertens LL, Cohen MS, Geva T. (2009) *Echocardiography in Pediatric and Congenital Heart Disease: From Fetus to Adult.* Wiley-Blackwell, Oxford, pp. 283–291.

8 Sehgal A, McNamara PJ. (2009) Echocardiographic markers of a haemodynamically significant ductus arteriosus. *Congenit Cardiol Today*, **7** (1), 1–10.

9 Philips JB, Garcia-Prats JA, Fulton DR, Kim MS. (2013) Management of patent ductus arteriosus in premature infants. *Up to Date,* February 27.

50

Neonatal Hypertrophic Cardiomyopathy and Syndromes with Infantile Cardiac Hypertrophy

J. Martijn Bos and Michael J. Ackerman

Windland Smith Rice Sudden Death Genomics Laboratory, Mayo Clinic, Rochester, MN, USA

Hypertrophic Cardiomyopathy

Hypertrophic cardiomyopathy (HCM) is a primary disease of the myocardium characterized by unexplained, mostly left ventricular hypertrophy (LVH) in the absence of inciting factors, such as aortic stenosis or systemic hypertension. Overall, its estimated incidence is 1 in 500 individuals. HCM is characterized by a wide variety in clinical course from a mild presentation that is asymptomatic throughout life to severely symptomatic needing surgical relief through cardiac myectomy. Common symptoms of HCM are chest pain, dyspnea, and syncope. Sometimes, the sentinel event is tragic, unexpected sudden cardiac death (SCD). The overall risk of SCD in HCM is approximately 1% per year. LVH is assessed by transthoracic echocardiography and defined as a maximum left ventricular wall thickness of >2 standard deviations above normal population mean for body surface area; for adolescents and adults this is ≥13 mm. While these pertains to HCM in all patients of all age-groups, unexplained cardiac hypertrophy during infancy is far different and most commonly part of a wider (genetic) syndrome for which the LVH is only a small, albeit sometimes primary, feature of the multiorgan disease.

Common Causes of Cardiac Hypertrophy in Neonates

A differential diagnosis for infantile cardiac hypertrophy can be abstracted from data from the Pediatric Cardiomyopathy Registry. Herein, among a large cohort of pediatric patients diagnosed with idiopathic HCM, approximately one-third of patients had identifiable causes for their hypertrophy [1].

In Chapter 2, Geiger and Moon-Grady mentioned that poorly controlled maternal diabetes increases the risk for fetal HCM, with a dose–response relationship between the degree of hyperglycemia and hypertrophy. There is negligible risk when HbA1C is maintained at <6%. Pregestational maternal diabetes is strongly associated with cardiac defects [2]. Infants with HCM associated with maternal diabetes tend to have asymmetric septal hypertrophy and yet have a good prognosis as hypertrophy generally regresses with time, usually within 6 months. HCM in infants of diabetic mothers (IDM) is associated with persistent hypoglycemia and macrosomia. HCM has also been associated with congenital hyperinsulinism, a disorder of hypoglycemia arising from mutations in insulin secretion pathway genes, most commonly KATP channel mutations (SUR1 and Kir6.2) [3]. While most of these infants are asymptomatic, some with severe hypertrophy develop congestive heart failure because of reduced ventricular compliance and/or severe left ventricular outflow tract obstruction and require supportive care. Consideration of a presence of a primary idiopathic HCM should be made if there is non-regression of cardiac hypertrophy in these infants.

Overall, for those with isolated cardiac pathology, about 75% had idiopathic HCM, while the remaining patients had cardiac hypertrophy stemming from inborn errors of metabolism (IEM; 9%), malformation syndromes (MFS; 9%) or neuromuscular disorders (NMD; 7%). Among these subgroups, approximately 65% of patients with IEM or MFS were diagnosed before the age of 1 year, while only 35% of patients with idiopathic non-syndromic cardiac hypertrophy (i.e., HCM) and 5% of patients with NMD were diagnosed before the age of 1 year. Within each of these categories (IEM, MFS, and NMD), a single disease dominates the etiology of infantile cardiac hypertrophy: Pompe disease (35% of IEM), Noonan syndrome (~80% of MFS), and Friedreich ataxia (~90% of NMD). Because of the later onset of disease, cardiac hypertrophy secondary to Friedreich ataxia is rare in neonates. Other, less common causes of infantile cardiac hypertrophy are summarized and discussed in studies by the Pediatric Cardiomyopathy Registry (PCMR) [4, 5].

Visual Guide to Neonatal Cardiology, First Edition. Edited by Ernerio T. Alboliras, Ziyad M. Hijazi, Leo Lopez, and Donald J. Hagler.

Characteristics of Neonatal HCM and Syndromes with Concomitant Cardiac Hypertrophy

The data from the PCMR show that idiopathic non-IDM HCM, Noonan syndrome, and Pompe diseases should be evaluated carefully and considered in the differential diagnosis of infantile cardiac hypertrophy. Diagnostic evaluation of cardiac hypertrophy in neonates should include thorough personal and family history, echocardiographic examination, detailed dysmorphology and medical examination (to elucidate MFS), appropriate laboratory and histologic testing (to elucidate IEM) as well as personal history and echocardiographic screening of first-degree relatives.

Characteristics of non-IDM neonatal HCM, Noonan syndrome, and Pompe disease are summarized in Table 50.1. Although cardiac hypertrophy might be the primary expression, careful clinical evaluation can distinguish key symptoms or features aiding in the diagnosis and subsequent treatment of an underlying syndrome. Noonan syndrome is characterized by facial features, short stature, and/or skeletal abnormalities, such as scoliosis and pectus excavatum. Pompe disease expresses significant muscular abnormalities, such as muscle weakness and decreased muscle tone, cardiomegaly, hepatomegaly, failure to thrive, and breathing problems. An electromyogram (EMG) and skin biopsy measuring the GAA-enzyme activity in fibroblasts are the gold standard for a diagnosis of Pompe disease.

Table 50.1 Common causes, features, and genetics of the most common causes of non-infants of diabetic mothers (non-IDM) infantile cardiac hypertrophy.

Disease	Cardiac and extracardiac features	Echocardiographic features	Diagnostic test	Major genes
Idiopathic, non-syndromic LVH (i.e. HCM)	Unexplained cardiac hypertrophy, affecting left ventricle predominantly No extracardiac features	Asymmetric, cardiac (septal) hypertrophy with or without LVOT obstruction, systolic anterior motion mitral valve	Echocardiogram	Myosin binding protein C (*MYBPC3*), β-myosin heavy chain (*MYH7*), cardiac troponin I (*TNNI3*), cardiac troponin T (*TNNT2*), cardiac troponin C (*TNNC1*), α-cardiac actin (*ACTC1*), regulatory myosin light chain (*MYL2*), essential myosin light chain (*MYL3*), α-tropomyosin (*TPM1*)
Noonan syndrome	LVH, pulmonary valve stenosis Distinct facial features (hypertelorism, downward eye slant, and low-set ears), short stature, skeletal abnormalities, bleeding disorders	Asymmetric cardiac (septal) hypertrophy, pulmonary valve/artery stenosis, atrial/ventricular defects, mitral valve abnormalities	Echocardiogram	Tyrosine-protein phosphatase non-receptor type 11 (*PTPN11*), V-RAF-1 murine leukemia viral oncogene homolog 1 (*RAF1*), v-Ki-ras2 Kirsten rat sarcoma viral oncogene homolog (*KRAS*), Son of sevenless homolog 1 (*SOS1*), neuroblastoma RAS viral oncogene homolog (*NRAS*)
Pompe disease	LVH, cardiomegaly Muscle weakness (myopathy), poor muscle tone (myotony), hepatomegaly, failure to thrive, breathing problems	Asymmetric cardiac (septal) hypertrophy with or without LVOT obstruction, severe hypertrophy; Wolf–Parkinson–White syndrome	Echocardiogram, EMG, blood CK level, skin biopsy (absence of GAA-activity in fibroblasts)	Acid α-glucosidase (GAA)

EMG, electromyogram; HCM, hypertrophic cardiomyopathy; LVH, left ventricular hypertrophy; LVOT, left ventricular outflow tract.

Echocardiographically, all cardiac hypertrophy-associated diseases in infancy are characterized by asymmetric cardiac hypertrophy that can be mild to severe, with or without left ventricular outflow tract obstruction (Figures 50.1, 50.2, and 50.3). LVH is commonly most severe in patients with Pompe disease. In approximately 25% of infants with Noonan syndrome, the disease can be distinguished readily from neonatal HCM and Pompe disease by their additional congenital cardiac malformations which include pulmonary valve stenosis, atrial or ventricular septal defects, and mitral valve abnormalities. Echocardiograms of a patient with idiopathic HCM, a patient with Noonan syndrome and a patient with Pompe disease are shown in Figures 50.1–50.3. Echocardiographically these syndromes might be tough to distinguish, so it is the combination of clinical evaluation and additional testing that will help in making the correct diagnosis (Table 50.1). Additionally, genetic testing for disease-associated genes can shed light on the diagnosis and underlying etiology.

Genetics of Neonatal HCM, Noonan Syndrome, and Pompe Disease

The most common disease associated genes for the three syndromes are summarized in Table 50.1. Genetically, approximately 40–50% of idiopathic HCM can be explained by mutations in genes encoding for the myofilament proteins in the cardiomyocyte, with the majority of mutations found in *MYBPC3*-encoded myosin binding protein C and *MYH7*-encoded β-myosin heavy chain [6].

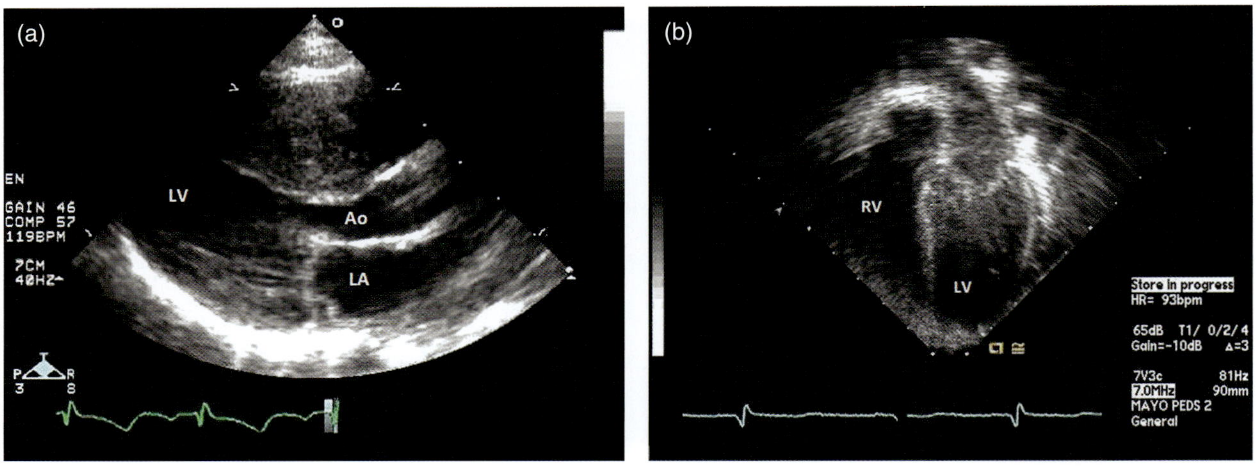

Figure 50.1 Echocardiogram of patient with non-syndromic, idiopathic left ventricular hypertrophy (LVH; i.e., hypertrophic cardiomyopathy, HCM). (a) Parasternal long-axis and (b) apical four-chamber views of patient with early onset HCM demonstrating severe concentric hypertrophy, thickened mitral valves, and hypertrophied papillary muscles. Ao, aorta; LA, left atrium; LV, left ventricle; RV, right ventricle.

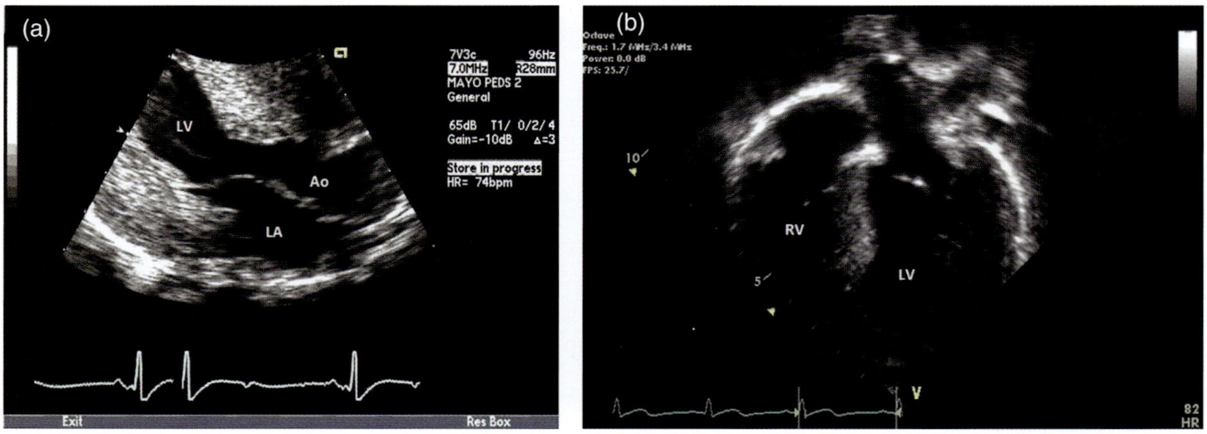

Figure 50.2 Echocardiograms of Noonan syndrome with left ventricular hypertrophy (LVH). (a) Parasternal long-axis and (b) apical four-chamber views of patient with (genotype negative) Noonan syndrome and LVH showing moderately increased concentric left ventricular wall thickness with maximum left ventricular wall thickness of 11 mm. There are no signs of pulmonary stenosis, valve abnormalities, or atrial or septal defects.

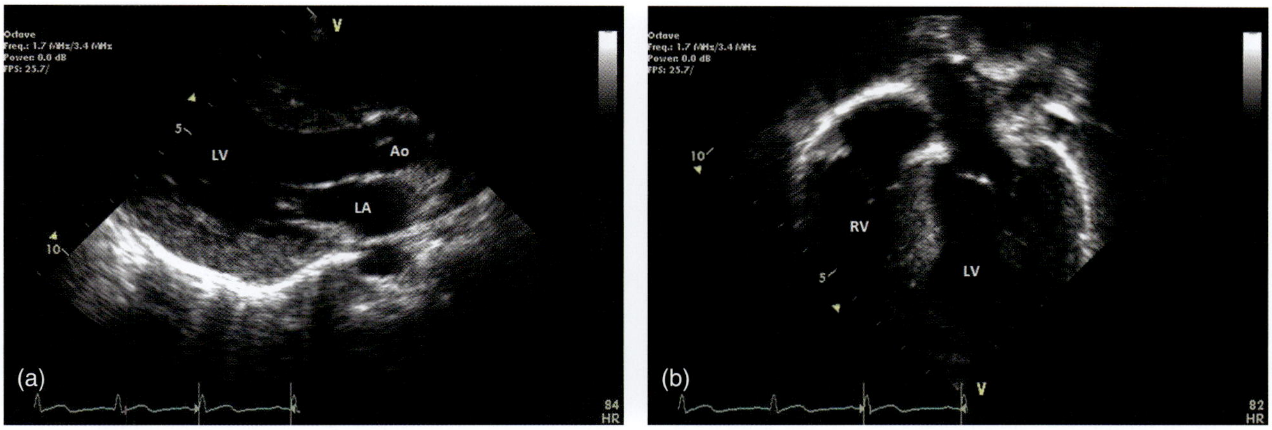

Figure 50.3 Echocardiograms of Pompe disease with left ventricular hypertrophy. (a) Parasternal long-axis and (b) apical four-chamber view of patient with Pompe disease with concomitant LV hypertrophy demonstrating concentric hypertrophy; maximum septal wall thickness 23 mm.

Overall, the yield of genetic testing in younger patients is significantly higher than patients with adult-onset HCM. Genetic testing can aid in identifying family members at risk for developing HCM and guide screening plans for affected family members [7, 8]. Furthermore, follow-up studies have shown that genotype-positive patients are more likely to develop systolic dysfunction, heart failure, or die from cardiovascular disease [9]. For idiopathic HCM, echocardiography can help to guide genetic testing based on cardiac septal morphology as patients with reverse-curve HCM are more likely to carry an HCM-associated sarcomeric mutation than patients with a septal hypertrophy with sigmoidal, neutral, or apical distribution (Figure 50.4).

Approximately 50% of Noonan syndrome is caused by mutations in *PTPN11*-encoded tyrosine-protein phosphatase non-receptor type 11; an additional set of genes account for a small percentage of genetics in Noonan syndrome (Table 50.1). Notably, although *PTPN11*-mediated Noonan syndrome is the most common subtype, it is rarely associated with cardiac hypertrophy and more likely to demonstrate pulmonary stenosis and atrial septal defects [8]. In fact, Noonan syndrome with LVH is most commonly attributed to Noonan syndrome with mutations in *SOS1* and *RAF1*. Both genes account for approximately 10% of genetic Noonan syndrome. Mutations in the other genes are rare and no specific genotype-phenotype have emerged

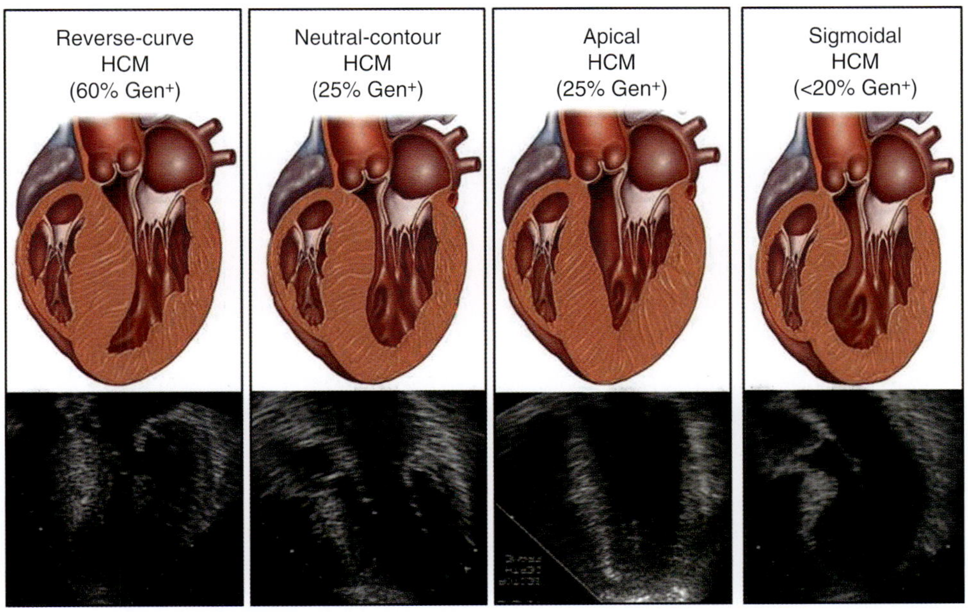

Figure 50.4 Septal shapes and yield of genetic testing for hypertrophic cardiomyopathy (HCM). The figure demonstrates the most common septal morphologies in HCM and yield of genetic testing for the most common HCM-associated genes.

for these subsets [10]. For Pompe disease, mutations are found in *GAA*-encoding acid alpha-glycosidase (also known as acid maltase).

Survival and Outcomes in Neonatal HCM and Syndromes with Concomitant LVH

Elucidating the root cause for the infant's cardiac hypertrophy is not only essential for monitoring and treatment, but also the outcome and survival of neonates with HCM or other LVH-associated syndromes are significantly different from adult-onset HCM. Patients with IDM HCM usually have a better prognosis than those with non-IDM HCM. Independent of the underlying cause of LVH, patients diagnosed before the age of 1 year have significantly worse survival rates than patients diagnosed over age of 1 year. Children with IEM like Pompe disease (55% survival) or MFM (82% survival) have significantly worse survival rates than patients with NMD (98% survival) or idiopathic HCM (94% survival) [2]. Patients with infantile non-syndromic HCM have worse survival rates than patients with idiopathic non-syndromic pediatric HCM diagnosed after age of 1 year (86 vs. 99% survival). Patients with idiopathic HCM who survive beyond the first year of life have a low annual mortality of 1.0 per 100 patient-years [2].

Conclusions

Ventricular hypertrophy is a common observation in IDM, and usually resolves in a few months. Non-IDM HCM is one of the most common heritable cardiovascular diseases. In neonates, careful evaluation is of utmost importance to distinguish idiopathic infantile HCM from several syndromes with concomitant LVH of which Noonan syndrome and Pompe disease are the most common. Considering that these diseases are so distinctive in their phenotype, outcomes, and interventions, the term HCM should be reserved for non-syndromic idiopathic LVH in an effort to minimize confusion and maximize clarity. Accordingly, an infant with Noonan syndrome and concomitant LVH should be referred precisely as such rather than referring to that patient as having HCM secondary to Noonan syndrome.

References

1 Cox GF, Sleeper LA, Lowe AM, *et al.* (2006) Factors associated with establishing a causal diagnosis for children with cardiomyopathy. *Pediatrics*, **118** (4), 1519–1531.

2 Loffredo CA, Wilson PD, Ferencz C. (2001) Maternal diabetes: an independent risk factor for major cardiovascular malformations with increased mortality of affected infants. *Teratology*, **64** (2), 98–106.

3 Huang T, Kelly A, Becker SA, Cohen MS, Stanley CA. (2013) Hypertrophic cardiomyopathy in neonates with congenital hyperinsulinism. *Arch Dis Child Fetal Neonatal Ed*, **98** (4), F351–354.

4 Colan SD, Lipshultz SE, Lowe AM, *et al.* (2007) Epidemiology and cause-specific outcome of hypertrophic cardiomyopathy in children: findings from the Pediatric Cardiomyopathy Registry. *Circulation*, **115** (6), 773–781.

5 Lipshultz SE, Orav EJ, Wilkinson JD, *et al.* (2013) Risk stratification at diagnosis for children with hypertrophic cardiomyopathy: an analysis of data from the Pediatric Cardiomyopathy Registry. *Lancet*, **382**, 1889–1897.

6 Bos JM, Towbin JA, Ackerman MJ. (2009) Diagnostic, prognostic, and therapeutic implications of genetic testing for hypertrophic cardiomyopathy. *J Am Coll Cardiol.* **54** (3), 201–211.

7 Gersh BJ, Maron BJ, Bonow RO, *et al.* (2011) ACCF/AHA Guideline for the Diagnosis and Treatment of Hypertrophic Cardiomyopathy: A Report of the American College of Cardiology Foundation/American Heart Association Task Force on Practice Guidelines Developed in Collaboration With the American Association for Thoracic Surgery, American Society of Echocardiography, American Society of Nuclear Cardiology, Heart Failure Society of America, Heart Rhythm Society, Society for Cardiovascular Angiography and Interventions, and Society of Thoracic Surgeons. *J Am Coll Cardiol*, **58** (25), e212–260.

8 Ackerman MJ, Priori SG, Willems S, *et al.* (2011) HRS/EHRA expert consensus statement on the state of genetic testing for the channelopathies and cardiomyopathies this document was developed as a partnership between the Heart Rhythm Society (HRS) and the European Heart Rhythm Association (EHRA). *Heart Rhythm*, **8** (8), 1308–1339.

9 Olivotto I, Girolami F, Ackerman MJ, *et al.* (2008) Myofilament protein gene mutation screening and outcome of patients with hypertrophic cardiomyopathy. *Mayo Clin Proc*, **83** (6), 630–638.

10 Roberts AE, Allanson JE, Tartaglia M, Gelb BD. (2013) Noonan syndrome. *Lancet*, **381**, 333–342.

51

Dilated Cardiomyopathy and Myocarditis

Jonathan N. Johnson

Division of Pediatric Cardiology, Mayo Clinic, Rochester, MN, USA

Pediatric cardiomyopathy has an estimated incidence of 1.13 cases per 100 000 children in the USA, of which half have dilated cardiomyopathy (DCM) [1]. The majority of patients with DCM have clinically silent disease in childhood and only present as adults, making the incidence of DCM in the neonate exceedingly rare [2, 3]. The central diagnostic features of DCM are those of cardiac dilation (Figures 51.1 and 51.2) and ventricular dysfunction.

Etiology

As in other age groups, DCM in the neonate represents a final common outcome for a diverse array of disease processes. Potential etiologies for DCM are listed in Table 51.1. In the neonate presenting with DCM, special attention should be given to ruling out causes of structural heart disease, including coronary anomalies such as anomalous origin of the left coronary artery from the pulmonary artery (ALCAPA), aortic arch anomalies, and any ductal-dependant lesion [4]. Common transient neonatal causes of reduced ventricular function include sepsis, hypoglycemia, and perinatal stress or hypoxia. Finally, familial cardiomyopathy or inborn errors of metabolism such as fatty acid oxidation disorders and organic acidemias should be considered [3].

Presentation

Presentation of DCM in the neonate can be varied. Patients can present with classic symptoms of heart failure and low cardiac output, including tachycardia, tachypnea, pallor, poor feeding, and poor weight gain. Complete cardiovascular collapse can occur. Those affected also present with more vague symptoms such as irritability. Physical examination can reveal a gallop rhythm, murmur of mitral regurgitation, hepatomegaly, and signs of poor perfusion.

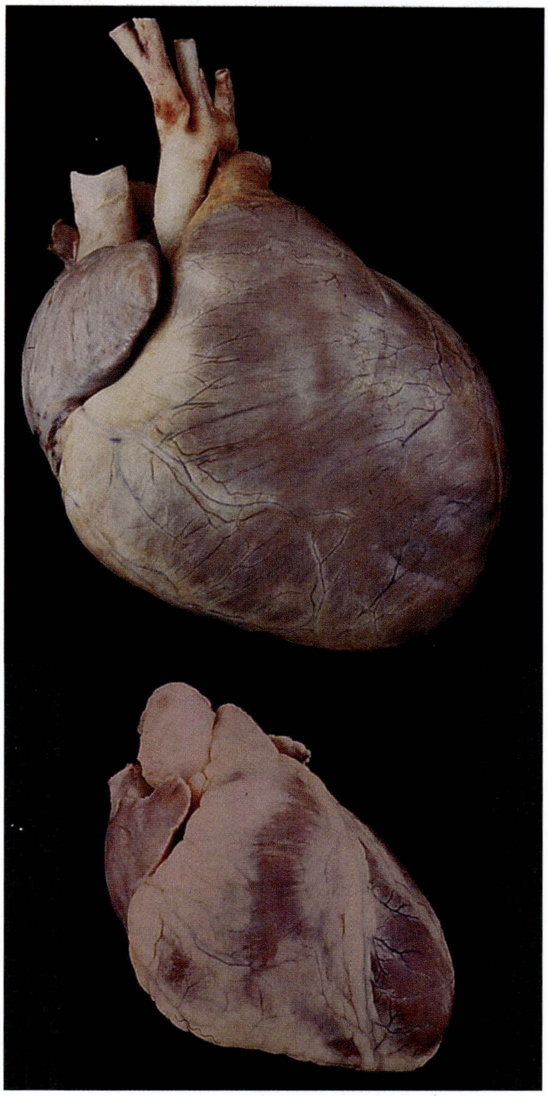

Figure 51.1 Dilated cardiomyopathy. Note the marked globoid cardiac enlargement of the affected heart (top) compared with a normal heart (bottom). Image courtsey of Dr. William D. Edwards, Division of Anatomic Pathology, Mayo Clinic, Rochester, MN, USA .

Visual Guide to Neonatal Cardiology, First Edition. Edited by Ernerio T. Alboliras, Ziyad M. Hijazi, Leo Lopez, and Donald J. Hagler.

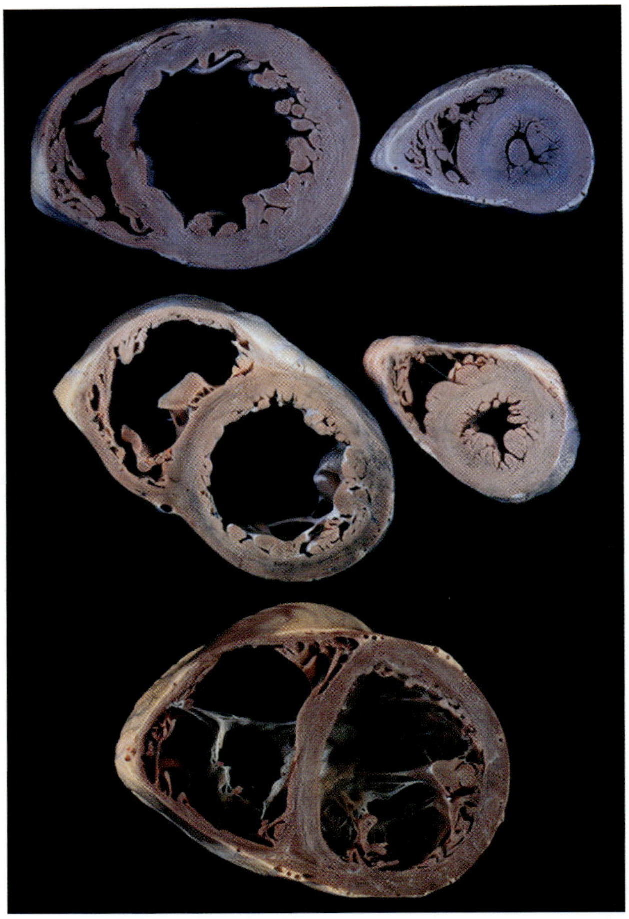

Figure 51.2 Patterns of dilation. Dilated cardiomyopathy can involve primarily the left ventricle (top), or it can involve both ventricles (middle). Each of the top two images are shown in comparison to a normal heart. Note that when the left ventricle is considerably dilated, the ventricular wall thickness will generally be normal, despite the substantial hypertrophy that is present (based on total heart weight). The bottom image demonstrates the atrioventricular valve support apparatus in the two ventricles; if the mitral and tricuspid valves become regurgitant, the heart will exhibit four-chamber dilation. Image courtsey of Dr. William D. Edwards, Division of Anatomic Pathology, Mayo Clinic, Rochester, MN, USA .

Testing

Chest radiography will often be performed in the setting of neonatal respiratory distress. In patients with DCM, radiography may show cardiomegaly (resulting from left ventricular and left atrial dilation) and pulmonary venous congestion (Figure 51.3). Left atrial enlargement can cause the left main stem bronchus to be elevated. Pleural effusions may be present. Not uncommonly, cardiomegaly is discovered incidentally on abdominal imaging performed for complaints of vomiting or poor feeding.

Echocardiography is the diagnostic test of choice in neonatal DCM. It can provide assessment of ventricular

Table 51.1 Possible causes of neonatal dilated cardiomyopathy and poor ventricular ejection fraction.

Acute myocarditis	See Table 51.2
Cardiac arrhythmia	Heart block, recurrent supraventricular or ventricular arrhythmias
Medications	Sympathomimetics, anthracyclines (older patients)
Endocrine	Hyper- or hypothyroidism, hypocalcemia, hypoglycemia, pheochromocytoma
Hereditary	Autosomal dominant, autosomal recessive, X-linked (Barth syndrome), mitochondrial
Inborn errors of metabolism	Fatty acid oxidation disorders, organic acidemias, mitochondrial disorders including Kearns–Sayre
Ischemic	Perinatal stress, hypoxia, anomalous coronary origins
Nutritional deficiencies	Thiamine, selenium, carnitine
Structural heart disease with ventricular dysfunction	Spongiform cardiomyopathy
Infectious	Sepsis
Neurologic	Cerebal or vein of Galen arteriovenous malformation

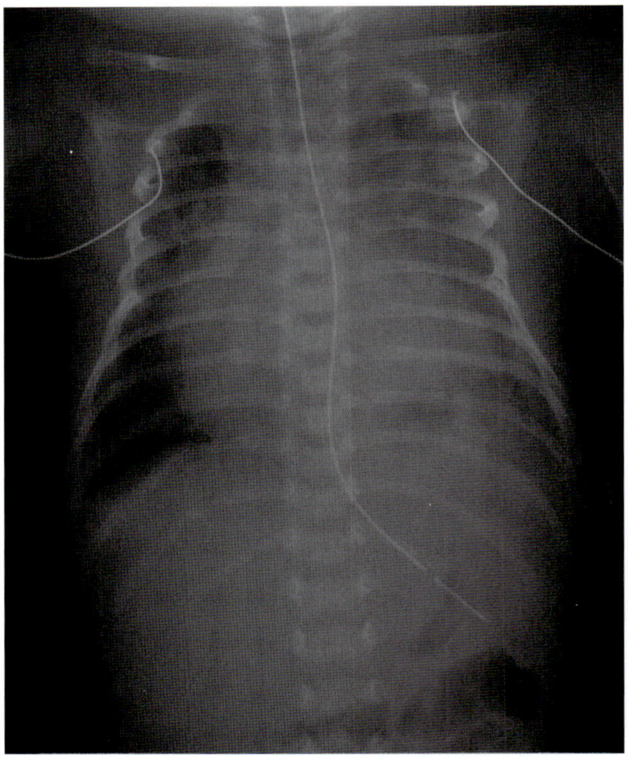

Figure 51.3 Chest X-ray obtained in a 15-day-old infant presenting with new onset respiratory distress. Note the marked cardiomegaly with pulmonary venous congestion and blunted left costophrenic angle.

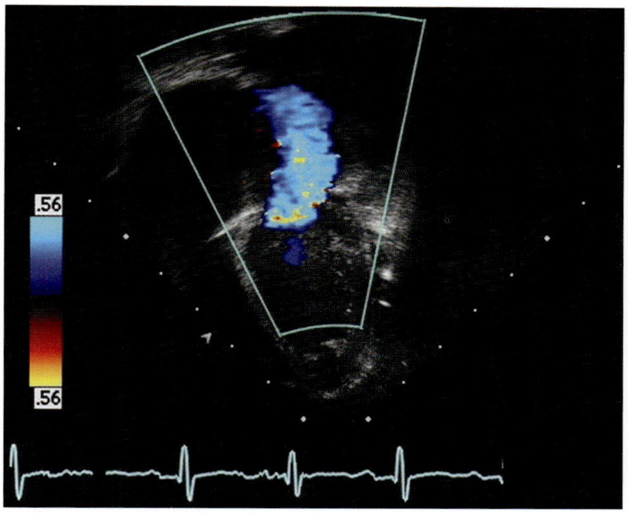

Figure 51.4 Echocardiography: four-chamber view obtained from a 15-day-old infant presenting with respiratory distress, with color Doppler. Note the significant degree of mitral regurgitation related to the ventricular dysfunction. In this case, the relatively normal appearing left ventricle (LV) size suggested an acute process causing the dysfunction.

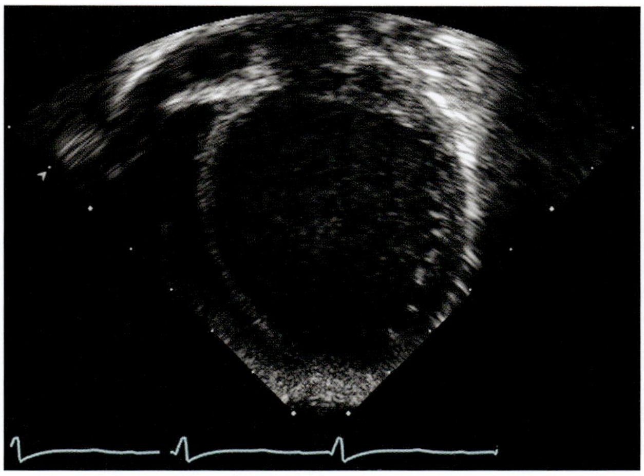

Figure 51.5 Echocardiography: four-chamber view obtained from a 1-month-old female presenting with poor growth, tachypnea, and sweating with feeds. The estimated ejection fraction was 15%. Note the marked LV enlargement. The patient's left atrium was also severely dilated.

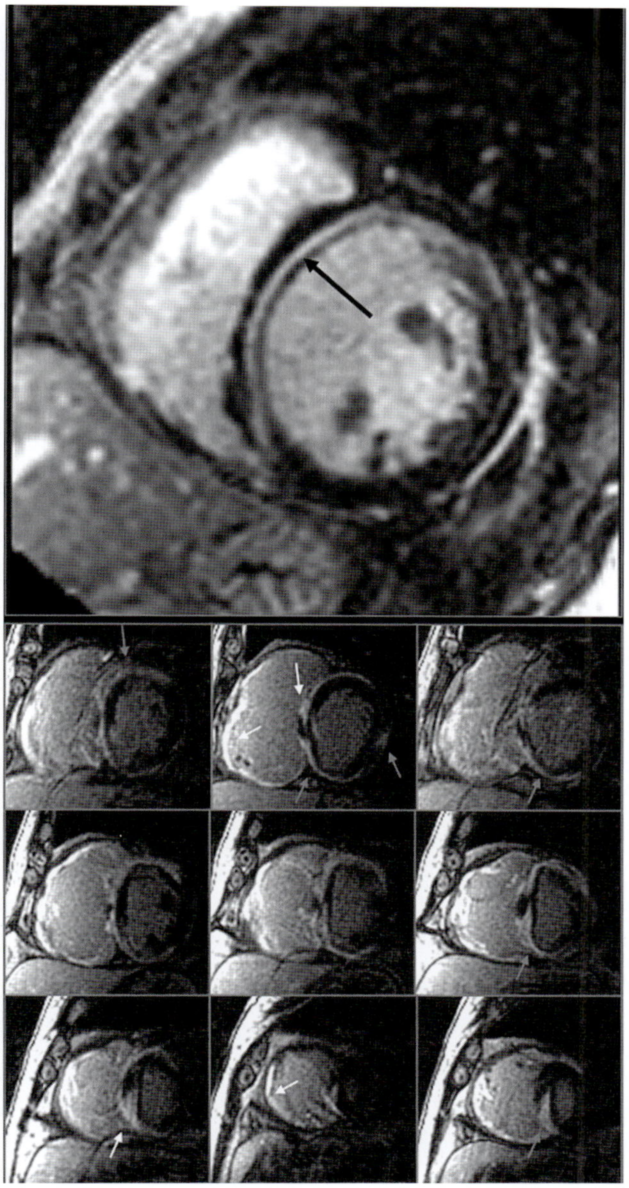

Figure 51.6 Cardiac magnetic resonance imaging (CMR). Top image: CMR utilizing a myocardial delayed enhancement sequence 10 minutes after administration of intravenous gadolinium. Patients with DCM most commonly have no delayed enhancement, while some may have a mid-myocardial stripe of delayed enhancement in the interventricular septum (black arrow). Bottom image: CMR utilizing a myocardial delayed enhancement sequence 10 minutes after administration of intravenous gadolinium. Short-axis imaging from base (upper left) to apex (lower right) demonstrates patchy areas of delayed enhancement in a non-coronary distribution with a predominantly subepicardial location (white arrows), consistent with myocarditis.

size and function as well as atrial size, with volume measurements indexed to body surface area. Valvular function can be characterized; in neonatal DCM, the mitral valve is often regurgitant secondary to ventricular dilation (Figures 51.4 and 51.5). Careful assessment of intracardiac and extracardiac anatomy should be performed to rule out alternate causes of ventricular dysfunction. Echocardiography can help predict patients with DCM at risk for sudden death [5]. Cardiac catheterization can be used if echocardiography is unable to rule out an anomalous coronary artery, or for purposes of endomyocardial biopsy.

Electrocardiography findings can be variable, but include sinus tachycardia, left ventricular hypertrophy, and left atrial enlargement. Arrhythmias such as supraventricular tachycardia or ventricular tachycardia occur secondary to atrial and ventricular dilation and dysfunction. Conversely, a tachycardia-induced cardiomyopathy can occur in patients with persistent arrhythmias; the cardiomyopathy may resolve after restoration of normal rhythm.

Cardiac magnetic resonance imaging (CMR) is a useful adjunctive tool in diagnosing patients with suspected myocarditis, but is less often performed in the neonatal population than older children and adults. The use of gadolinium contrast (looking for late gadolinium enhancement) can help distinguish myocardium that has had irreversible damage (necrosis and fibrosis; Figure 51.6) [6]. This can be a useful prognostic indicator for potential recovery of function.

Neonatal Myocarditis

Etiology

Myocarditis is characterized by inflammatory changes in the myocardium with resultant damage or necrosis of the myocytes involved. Most cases seen in the USA are viral in nature, primarily comprised of adenovirus, enteroviruses (including coxsackievirus), and parvovirus [7–11]. Infectious causes of myocarditis are listed in Table 51.2. Importantly, some medications cause a hypersensitivity reaction with resultant myocarditis, including antibiotics (penicillin, cephalosporins, and sulfonamides), diuretics (thiazide and loop diuretics) and dobutamine.

Incidence

Myocarditis occurs in a bimodal distribution, with peak incidence rates between 6 and 12 months of age and in adolescence [12]. Fortunately, myocarditis is rare in the neonatal population. The prognosis for neonates diagnosed with enteroviral myocarditis is poor, as high as 50% in some studies [13, 14]. The mortality for other viral causes of myocarditis in the neonatal period is not as well known but is presumed to be similarly high.

Table 51.2 Infectious causes of myocarditis.

Viral (most common)	Bacterial	Fungal
Enterovirus (including Coxsackie viruses)	Meningococcus	Actinomycosis
Parvovirus	Klebsiella	Coccidioidomycosis
Adenovirus	Streptococcus	Histoplasmosis
Cytomegalovirus	Mycoplasma	Candida
Herpesvirus	Brucella	
Varicella	Clostridia	**Other**
Rubella	Leptospira	Toxocara
Hepatitis B, hepatitis C	Legionella	Schistosomiasis
Rubeola	Salmonella	Cystericosis
Respiratory syncitial virus		Echinococcus
HIV	**Protozoal**	Heterophyiasis
Epstein–Barr virus	Trypanosoma cruzi	Trichinosis
Influenza	Amebiasis	Rickettsial diseases
	Toxoplasmosis	

Presentation

Similar to the initial presentation of DCM, the presentation of myocarditis in the neonate can vary from minimal non-cardiac symptoms (gastrointestinal discomfort) to

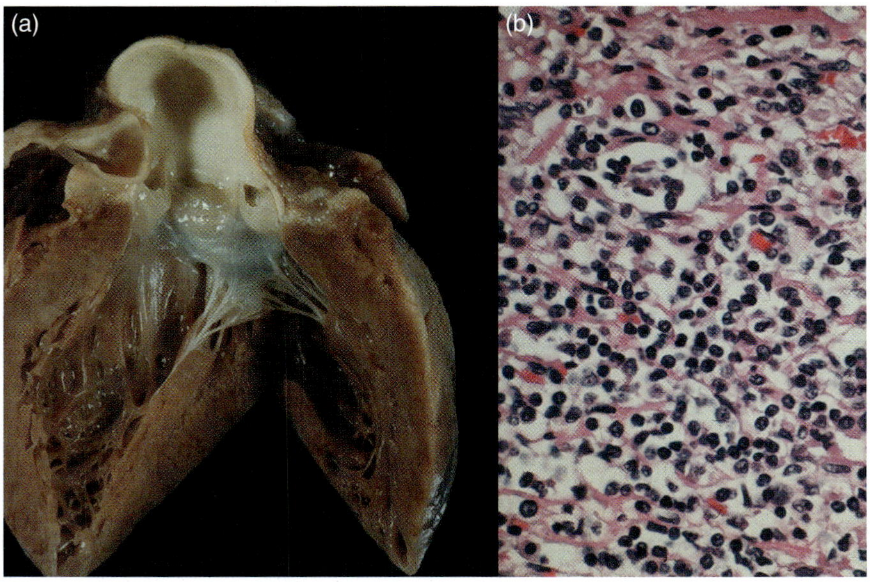

Figure 51.7 (a) Gross heart pathology specimen opened to the left ventricle and aortic valve, and (b) microscopic diffuse lymphocytic infiltration in the myocardium of an infant with viral myocarditis who died suddenly. Image courtesy of Dr. William D. Edwards, Division of Anatomic Pathology, Mayo Clinic, Rochester, MN, USA .

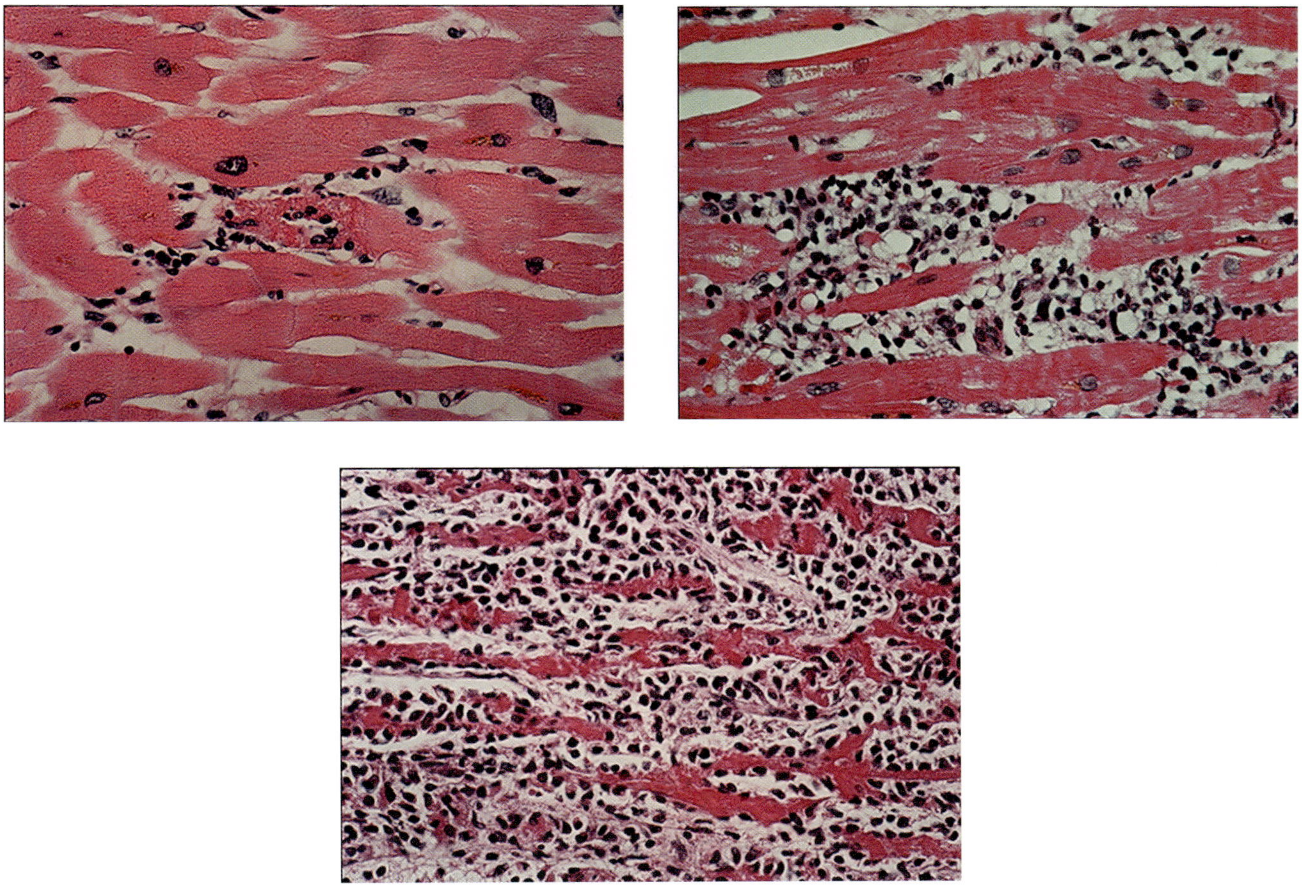

Figure 51.8 Myocardial biopsy samples with hematoxylin-eosin staining, demonstrating mild focal myocarditis (top), moderate focal myocarditis (middle), and severe diffuse myocarditis (bottom). Note the increasing amount of lymphocytic infiltration as the severity increases, with evidence of myocyte necrosis and fibrosis in the bottom panel. Image courtsey of Dr. William D. Edwards, Division of Anatomic Pathology, Mayo Clinic, Rochester, MN, USA .

cardiovascular collapse. The initial presentation can be sudden death, presumably from life-threatening arrhythmia (Figure 51.7). Parvovirus B19 infection in pregnant mothers is a well-established cause of fetal anemia, non-immune fetal hydrops in pregnancy, and myocarditis with subsequent heart failure.

Testing

Chest radiography, echocardiography, and cardiac catheterization are used in a similar manner to that described for DCM. The classic electrocardiographic pattern in patients with myocarditis is diffusely low-voltage QRS complexes. T waves may be inverted; in cases with significant myocardial involvement, a myocardial infarction pattern may be seen. Cardiac MRI can be utilized to document the specific location and extent of the myocardial inflammation (Figure 51.6). Additionally, it can be used as a follow-up study to examine for areas of fibrosis or scarring.

Endomyocardial biopsy is the gold standard test for diagnosis of myocarditis (Figures 51.7 and 51.8) [15]. However, biopsies in the setting of presumed myocarditis are not performed routinely at all centers, primarily because of low yield [16, 17]. Increasing the numbers of biopsy samples removed can help increase the yield [18]. When performed, biopsy helps provide prognostic information as well as specific diagnostic information, though its effect on clinical management is institution-dependent.

References

1 Lipshultz SE, Sleeper LA, Towbin JA, *et al.* (2003) The incidence of pediatric cardiomyopathy in two regions of the United States. *N Engl J Med*, **348**, 1647–1655.

2 Michels VV, Moll PP, Miller FA, *et al.* (1992) The frequency of familial dilated cardiomyopathy in a series of patients with idiopathic dilated cardiomyopathy. *N Engl J Med*, **326**, 77–82.

3 Towbin JA, Lipshultz SE. (1999) Genetics of neonatal cardiomyopathy. *Curr Opin Cardiol*, **14**, 250–262.

4 Schultz AH, Localio AR, Clark BJ, *et al.* (2008) Epidemiologic features of the presentation of critical congenital heart disease: implications for screening. *Pediatrics*, **121**, 751–757.

5 Pahl E, Sleeper LA, Canter CE, *et al.* (2012) Incidence of and risk factors for sudden cardiac death in children with dilated cardiomyopathy: a report from the Pediatric Cardiomyopathy Registry. *J Am Coll Cardiol*, **59**, 607–615.

6 Friedrich MG, Sechtem U, Schulz-Menger J, *et al.* (2009) Cardiovascular magnetic resonance in myocarditis: a JACC White Paper. *J Am Coll Cardiol*, **53**, 1475–1487.

7 Bowles NE, Bowles KR, Towbin JA. (2005) Viral genomic detection and outcome in myocarditis. *Heart Fail Clin*, **1**, 407–417.

8 Bowles NE, Towbin JA. (1998) Molecular aspects of myocarditis. *Curr Opin Cardiol*, **13**, 179–184.

9 Francalanci P, Chance JL, Vatta M, *et al.* (2004) Cardiotropic viruses in the myocardium of children with end-stage heart disease. *J Heart Lung Transplant*, **23**, 1046–1052.

10 Bowles NE, Ni J, Kearney DL, *et al.* (2003) Detection of viruses in myocardial tissues by polymerase chain reaction: evidence of adenovirus as a common cause of myocarditis in children and adults. *J Am Coll Cardiol*, **42**, 466–472.

11 Tschope C, Bock CT, Kasner M, *et al.* (2005) High prevalence of cardiac parvovirus B19 infection in patients with isolated left ventricular diastolic dysfunction. *Circulation*, **111**, 879–886.

12 Ghelani SJ, Spaeder MC, Pastor W, *et al.* (2012) Demographics, trends, and outcomes in pediatric acute myocarditis in the United States, 2006 to 2011. *Circ Cardiovasc Qual Outcomes*, **5**, 622–627.

13 English RF, Janosky JE, Ettedgui JA, *et al.* (2004) Outcomes for children with acute myocarditis. *Cardiol Young*, **14**, 488–493.

14 Bengtsson E, Lamberger B. (1966) Five-year follow-up study of cases suggestive of acute myocarditis. *Am Heart J*, **72**, 751–763.

15 Cooper LT, Baughman KL, Feldman AM, *et al.* (2007) The role of endomyocardial biopsy in the management of cardiovascular disease: a scientific statement from the American Heart Association, the American College of Cardiology, and the European Society of Cardiology. *Circulation*, **116**, 2216–2233.

16 Webber SA, Boyle GJ, Jaffe R, *et al.* (1994) Role of right ventricular endomyocardial biopsy in infants and children with suspected or possible myocarditis. *Br Heart J*, **72**, 360–363.

17 Mason JW, O'Connell JB, Herskowitz A, *et al.* (1995) A clinical trial of immunosuppressive therapy for myocarditis. The Myocarditis Treatment Trial Investigators. *N Engl J Med*, **333**, 269–275.

18 Chow LH, Radio SJ, Sears TD, *et al.* (1989) Insensitivity of right ventricular endomyocardial biopsy in the diagnosis of myocarditis. *J Am Coll Cardiol*, **14**, 915–920.

52

Cardiac Chamber Aneurysms and Diverticula

Lisa Hornberger

University of Alberta; Section Head of Pediatric Echocardiography, Stollery Children's Hospital, Edmonton, Alberta, Canada

Ventricular Diverticula and Aneurysms

An out-pouching of the ventricular wall is a rare form of congenital heart disease. Cardiac diverticula and aneurysms can occur in any part of the heart but are most commonly found in the left ventricle (Figure 52.1). It can occasionally be difficult to distinguish between them, but there are unique features for each.

Background and Anatomy

Ventricular diverticula are characterized by a relatively narrow base or entrance and can be more globular (Figure 52.1a) or appear as a finger-like projection from the ventricle. The diverticula contain all layers of cardiac muscle and as such tend to contract with the surrounding muscle during ventricular systole. Ventricular diverticula are always congenital, as apposed to aneurysms which are often acquired.

Ventricular diverticula can be divided into apical and non-apical. Non-apical diverticula are generally isolated defects without associated cardiac or non-cardiac defects. Apical ventricular diverticula, in contrast, are almost always associated with other defects, especially midline defects as described in Cantrell syndrome in which they may protrude through a diaphragmatic hernia (Figure 52.2) [1]. Associated cardiac conditions include ventricular septal defects, tetralogy of Fallot, and abnormalities of cardiac position (mesocardia and dextrocardia). Midline defects include sternal defects, umbilical hernias, and omphalocele [2].

Ventricular aneurysms are even more rare than ventricular diverticula (Figure 52.1b) [1]. Aneurysms usually have a broader based connection to the ventricle than diverticula (Figures 52.3 and 52.4). Ventricular aneurysms do not contain all of the usual tissue layers of cardiac muscle and may contain fibrous tissue or pericardium only. Because they do not contain cardiac muscle, aneurysms do not contract or can be hypocontractile during systole and this helps distinguish them from diverticula on echocardiography.

Ventricular aneurysms can be congenital, but are also commonly acquired. Acquired causes include trauma and infection. Ventricular aneurysms are usually isolated defects without associated cardiac or non-cardiac abnormalities.

Neonatal Presentation

As a result of improved fetal screening, especially at the 18–20 week morphology ultrasound, many of the more significant ventricular aneurysms and diverticula are diagnosed prenatally (Figures 52.2 and 52.3) [3]. The incidence and natural history of smaller or asymptomatic cardiac aneurysms or diverticula are unclear, as they do not tend to present to medical attention.

Apical congenital ventricular diverticula (CVD) are usually diagnosed in the setting of the associated cardiac and extracardiac anomalies. In some patients, an epigastric pulsation can be identified in the neonatal period. Non-apical CVD is commonly diagnosed prenatally and is otherwise often diagnosed during investigation for ventricular extrasystoles in the neonatal period [1].

Significant ventricular aneurysms are diagnosed prenatally in up to 50% of patients. Patients with symptomatic congenital ventricular aneurysm (CVA) in the neonatal period present with ventricular extrasystoles or, in the worst case, ventricular rupture [1]. If the CVA is large, it can lead to decreased heart function in fetal life and cardiac failure after birth.

Investigations

Transthoracic echocardiogram is the investigation of choice. In all cases, especially when an apical CVD is found, screening for associated non-cardiac structural defects should be performed.

Cardiac MRI (cMRI) can provide additional information when the exact nature and extent of the cardiac diverticula or aneurysm is not fully identified on echocardiogram. cMRI can identify the characteristics and motion of the tissue forming the defect and can

Visual Guide to Neonatal Cardiology, First Edition. Edited by Ernerio T. Alboliras, Ziyad M. Hijazi, Leo Lopez, and Donald J. Hagler.

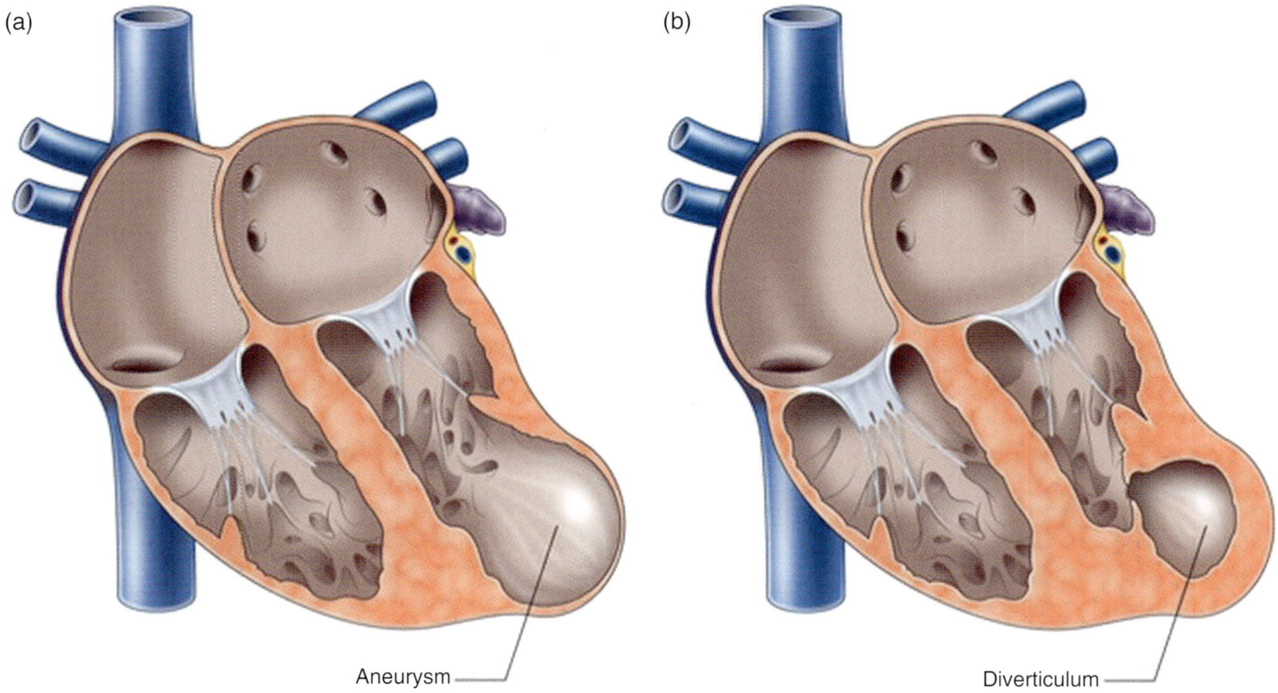

Figure 52.1 Ventricular diverticula and aneurysms. (a) A ventricular diverticulum is characterized by a narrow base and containing all layers of normal cardiac muscle. Apical diverticula, as shown in this image, are commonly associated with other midline defects. (b) A ventricular aneurysm usually has a broad base, is thin walled, and does not contain all layers of cardiac muscle. Aneurysms tend to be either hypocontractile or do not contract with ventricular systole.

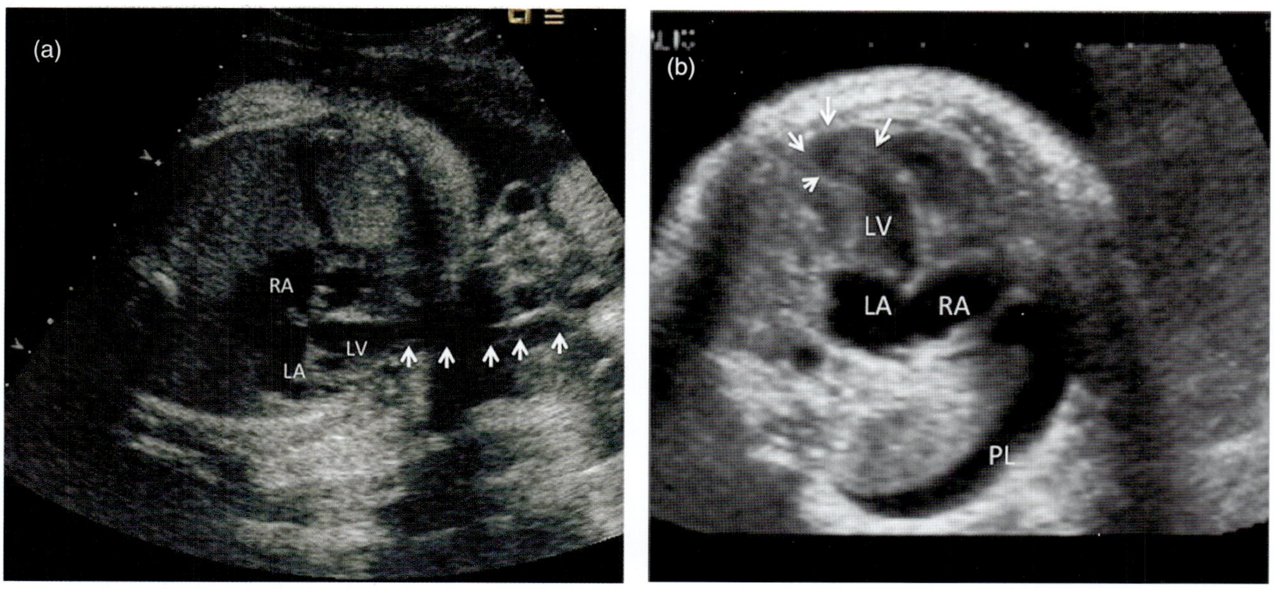

Figure 52.2 Left ventricular diverticula in two fetuses. (a) Diverticulum from the apex of the left ventricle in a fetus with a mild form of pentalogy of Cantrell. The diverticulum, which was finger-like and pulsatile, protruded through a midline diaphragmatic hernia and out through the umbilicus. The arrows demonstrate its course. Postnatally, the diverticulum was resected and the hernia repaired. (b) Diverticulum from the apex of the left ventricle in a mid-trimester fetus with biventricular hypertrophy. The diverticulum was of normal wall thickness and contracted similarly to the rest of the heart. LA, left atrium; LV, left ventricle; PL, pleural effusion; RA, right atrium.

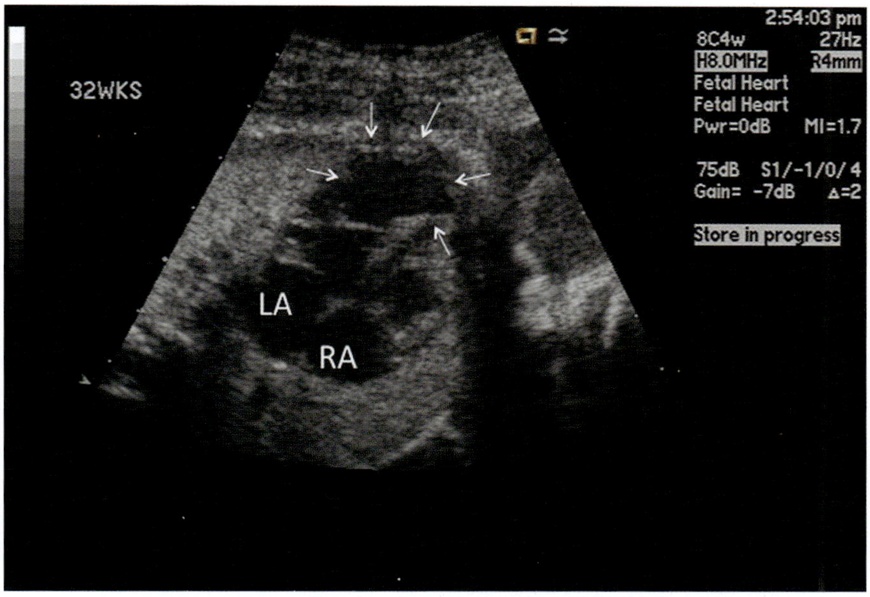

Figure 52.3 Left ventricular aneurysm in a 32-week fetus demonstrated in a four-chamber view. This aneurysm was thin-walled, had a wide communication with the rest of the left ventricular cavity, and was hypocontractile. LA, left atrium; RA, right atrium.

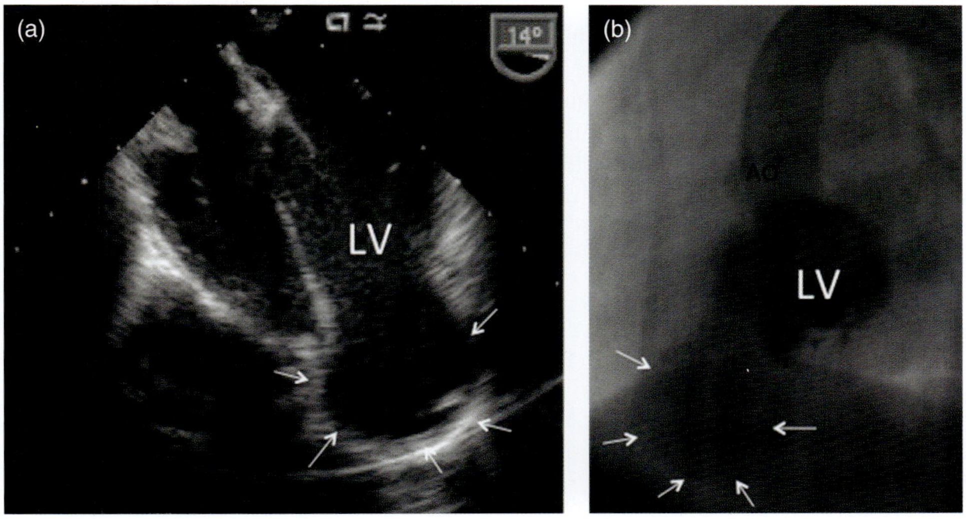

Figure 52.4 Left ventricular (LV) aneurysm identified in a 4-year-old immunodeficient girl. (Images reproduced from Jamshidi *et al.* 2009 [6]. Reproduced with permission of Elsevier.) (a) The echocardiogram suggested the presence of the aneurysm which was identified extending from the left ventricular apex (arrows). (b) Angiography was performed to exclude a coronary abnormality and further delineate the aneurysm (arrows). This child required surgical resection of the aneurysm after a small mural thrombus was identified.

be used to differentiate the muscle of a CVD from the fibrotic tissue of a CVA, for example, which is important for planning of surgical intervention.

ECG and Holter monitoring should be performed in all children with suspected cardiac aneurysm or diverticula to assess for cardiac arrhythmia.

Management

Management depends upon the clinical presentation and associated cardiac defects.

In cases of apical CVD, the diverticulum, if not involving a significant proportion of the ventricular volume, can often be successfully resected at the time of surgery for other associated cardiac defects. In cases of CVD without associated cardiac malformations, the decision whether to intervene surgically remains controversial. Although patients with asymptomatic CVD are at risk of thrombus formation, arrhythmia, and even ventricular rupture [4], generally the outlook without surgical intervention is very good, with even the possibility of complete regression over time [1].

In contrast, CVA is associated with a significantly worse prognosis than CVD. Ten-year mortality is reported to be as high as 80% [1]. There is risk of cardiac failure and death in those with large aneurysms involving significant portions of the left or right ventricle.

Aneurysm rupture and thrombus formation followed by stroke has been described [1]. In this setting, surgical resection of the aneurysm in asymptomatic patients may be considered more strongly than in patients with CVD.

Atrial Diverticula and Aneurysms

Atrial diverticula and aneurysms are extremely rare entities that are not often seen in the neonatal period. Right atrial defects include congenital enlargement of the right atrium, diverticula of the coronary sinus, and diverticula of the right atrium [5]. Left-sided defects often arise from the left atrial appendage, although any site in the left atrium is possible. Often, the diagnosis will come about after a routine chest radiograph demonstrates findings suggestive of an enlarged left or right atrium. Supraventricular tachycardia and its associated symptoms are the most common presenting features. Atrioventricular valve regurgitation and atrial thrombus are also seen in these conditions.

Treatment with surgical resection is usually indicated for arrhythmia in right-sided lesions [5]. Surgical resection in even asymptomatic patients with left-sided aneurysms or diverticula may be indicated because of the possibility of catastrophic stroke if thrombus forms.

References

1 Marijon E, Ou P, Fermont L, *et al.* (2006) Diagnosis and outcome in congenital ventricular diverticulum and aneurysm. *J Thorac Cardiovasc Surg*, **131**, 433–437.

2 Nam K, Kwon J, Son G, *et al.* (2010) Prenatally diagnosed left ventricular diverticulum with thoracoabdominal wall defect: a case and review of literature. *J Perinatol*, **30** (11), 760–762.

3 Hornberger L, Dalvi B, Benacerraf B. (1994) Prenantal sonographic detection of cardiac aneurysms and diverticula. *J Ultrasound Med*, **13** (1), 967–970.

4 Hamaoka K, Onaka M, Tanaka T, Onouchi Z. (1987) Congenital ventricular aneurysm and diverticula in children. *Pediatr Cardiol*, **8** (3), 169–175.

5 Binder T, Rosenhek R, Frank H, *et al.* (2000) Congenital malformations of the right atrum and the coronary sinus. *Chest*, **117** (6), 1740–1748.

6 Jamshidi R, Hornberger LK, Karl TR. (2009) Left ventricular aneurysm in a child with severe combined immunodeficiency syndrome. *Ann Thorac Surg*, **88** (5), 1678–1680.

53

Cardiac Tumors

Nadine Choueiter[1] *and Rebecca S. Beroukhim*[2]

[1] *Albert Einstein College of Medicine; Children's Hospital at Montefiore, Bronx, NY, USA*
[2] *Massachusetts General Hospital, Boston, MA, USA*

Cardiac tumors are rare in children. Most neonatal cardiac tumors are histologically benign and arise from intracardiac cellular precursors, including muscular (rhabdomyoma), ectopic (teratoma), fibrous (fibroma), and vascular (hemangioma) tissue (Table 53.1) [1].

Cardiac Rhabdomyoma

Cardiac rhabdomyoma is a hamartoma (excessive growth of striated muscle in the heart). Rhabdomyomas are well-circumscribed, firm, white or gray, rubbery nodules usually within the ventricle and interventricular septum (Figure 53.1). Histopathology reveals large glycogen-rich vacuoles, swollen myocytes, and strands of cytoplasm extending to the cell periphery ("spider cell") [2]. They are associated with tuberous sclerosis, an autosomal dominant disorder with non-malignant tumors of the heart, brain, kidneys, eyes, lungs, and skin. Multiple ventricular tumors seen on fetal or neonatal echocardiography are nearly pathognomonic and warrant exclusion of associated lesions [3]. They represent the most common primary cardiac tumors in fetuses and neonates [1, 4, 5], presenting in utero as single or multiple intramyocardial masses. Fetal demise may result from hydrops and/or arrhythmias [6, 7]. Neonates with severe outflow obstruction or extensive myocardial involvement can present with low output syndrome and heart failure. They may be associated with other lesions such as hypoplastic left heart syndrome (Figure 53.2). The most common arrhythmia is ventricular tachycardia (VT) [4]. The tumors usually regress within the first year of life with lower arrhythmia frequency.

Echocardiography reveals multiple homogeneous, well-circumscribed nodules in the ventricles (Figure 53.1a,c,d,e,f) and, rarely, in the atria (Figure 53.1b). They may be intramyocardial or sessile with irregular borders (Figure 53.1). Cardiac magnetic resonance (CMR) imaging aids in tissue characterization and differentiation from other tumors and is useful for solitary rhabdomyomas [8]. Most tumors regress spontaneously, so surgical resection is needed only for severe outflow obstruction or significant arrhythmias. Arrhythmias usually respond to medical treatment and eventually resolve with tumor regression. With minimal signs or symptoms, close echocardiographic follow-up is usually sufficient.

Table 53.1 Incidence of fetal and neonatal cardiac tumors.

Cardiac tumor	Fetal and neonatal No (%)
Total	224[a] (100)
Rhabdomyoma	120 (53.8)
Teratoma	40 (17.8)
Fibroma	28 (12.4)
Oncocytic cardiomyopathy	15 (6.6)
Vascular tumors	13 (5.8)
Myxoma	6 (2.7)
Malignant	2 (0.9)

Source: Isaacs 2005 [1]. Reproduced with permission of Springer.
a) Representation of 224 fetal and neonatal tumors collected from the literature.

Intrapericardial Teratoma

Intrapericardial teratoma is a rare primary cardiac tumor arising from primordial germ cells. Gross pathology reveals a large, encapsulated, cystic mass with fluid-filled cavities [9]. It is the second most common neonatal tumor [1, 9–12]. Prenatal diagnosis can be delayed because rapid tumor growth does not occur until 20–40 weeks' gestation [13], usually presenting as a large mass associated with pericardial effusion [14]. Neonatal presentation usually involves respiratory distress, cyanosis, and congestive heart failure [13].

Visual Guide to Neonatal Cardiology, First Edition. Edited by Ernerio T. Alboliras, Ziyad M. Hijazi, Leo Lopez, and Donald J. Hagler.

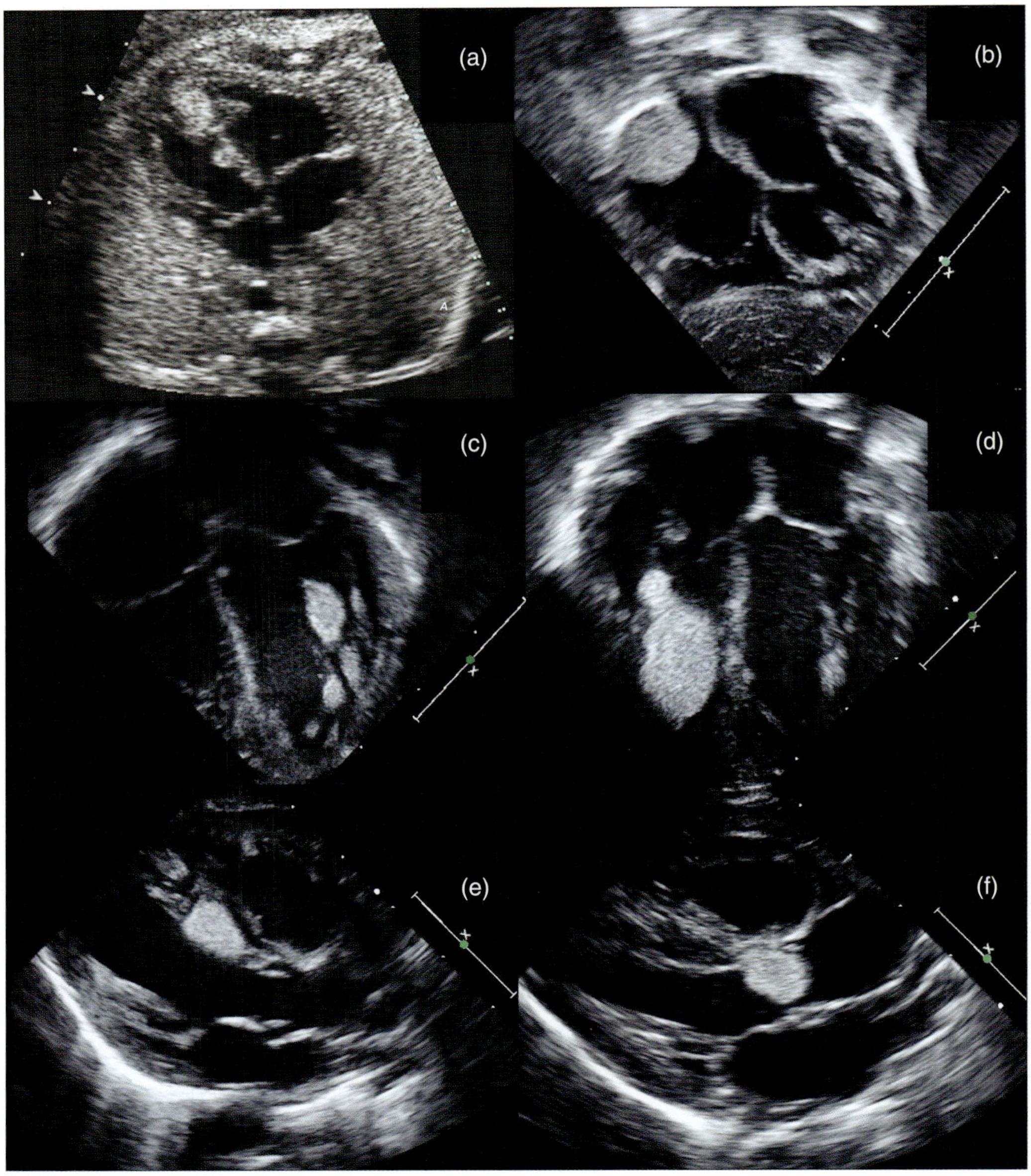

Figure 53.1 Rhabdomyomas associated with tuberous sclerosis: (a) fetal presentation of multiple homogenous tumors in the ventricular septum and free wall; (b) right atrial rhabdomyoma; (c) multiple left ventricular tumors; (d) large right ventricular tumor with multiple smaller tumors in the septum and left ventricle; (e) intramyocardial tumor within the ventricular septum; (f) obstructive tumor protruding into the left ventricular outflow tract.

Echocardiography, computed tomography (CT), and CMR reveal a solitary, inhomogeneous, multicystic intrapericardial mass, almost always associated with pericardial effusion (Figure 53.3). The tumors are usually in the right-sided pericardial cavity between the aorta and superior vena cava, occasionally compressing the superior vena cava, right atrium, and/or right ventricle. Prenatal management is guided by the presence or absence of hydrops, which is associated with a poor prognosis. Here, pericardiocentesis, pericardioamniotic shunting, or early delivery is recommended [14]. Postnatal resection shortly after birth can resolve clinical symptoms and reduce the risk of malignant metastasis.

Fibromas

Cardiac fibromas are large, connective tissue tumors composed of collagen and elastic tissue, occasionally with areas of central calcification and necrosis (Figure 53.4) [15, 16]. Gross pathology reveals a single, white, firm, non-encapsulated tumor commonly originating from ventricular septum or free wall. Giant tumors can obliterate the intracavitary space, causing inflow or outflow obstruction or atrioventricular valve disruption. There is no genetic or familial predisposition, but they have been associated with extracardiac malformations (e.g., Gorlin syndrome) [1]. They are the third most

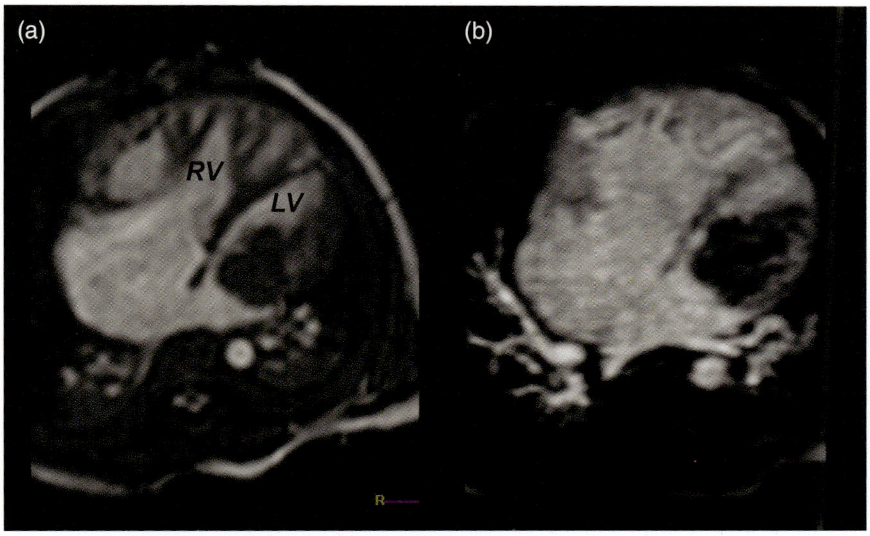

Figure 53.2 Cardiac magnetic resonance (CMR) images of a single rhabdomyoma obstructing left ventricular inflow and causing hypoplastic left heart syndrome with (a) isointense appearance relative to myocardium on cine imaging; and (b) hypoperfusion on magnetic resonance angiography.

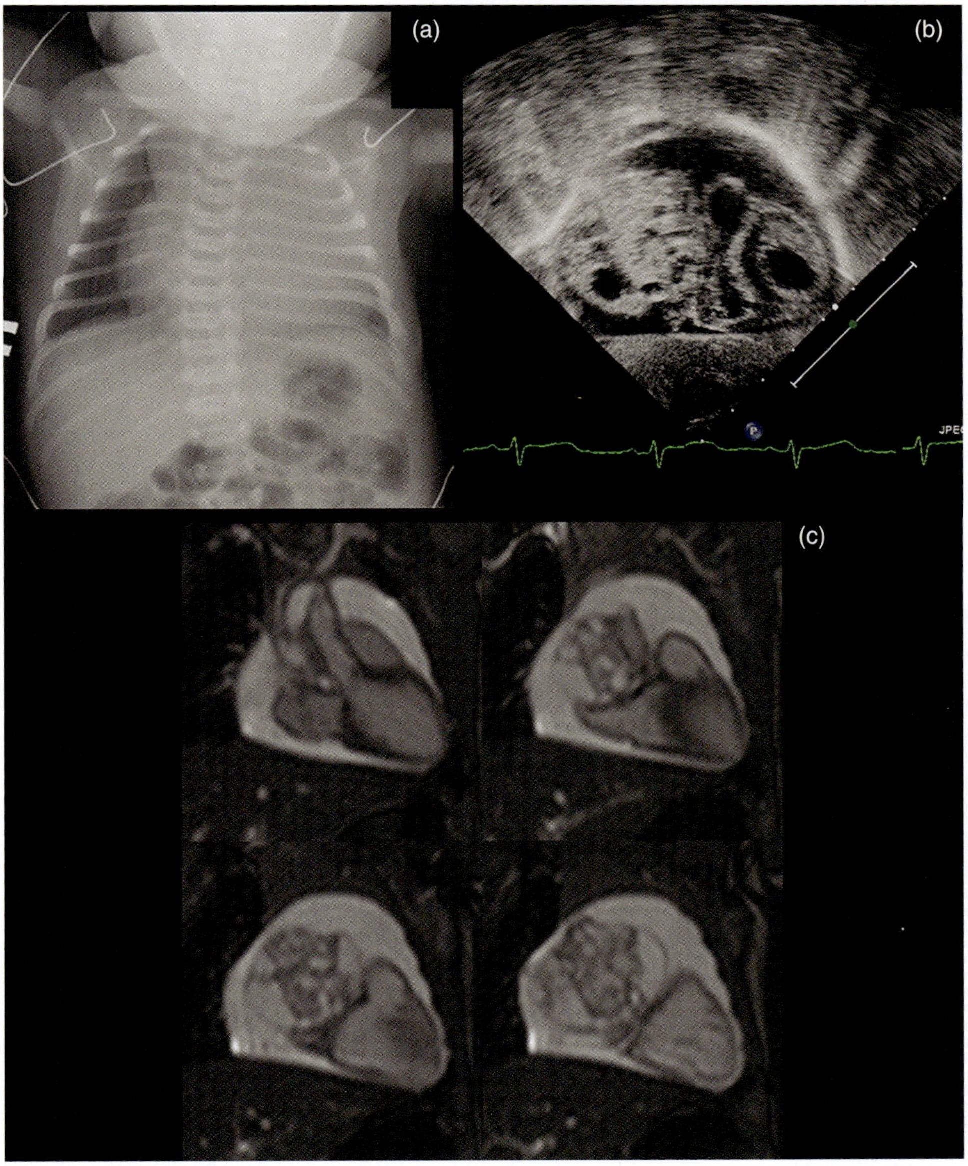

Figure 53.3 (a) Intrapericardial teratoma presenting with cardiomegaly on chest radiography; (b) large intrapericardial cystic mass compressing the right atrium and pericardial effusion on echocardiography; and (c) with CMR imaging.

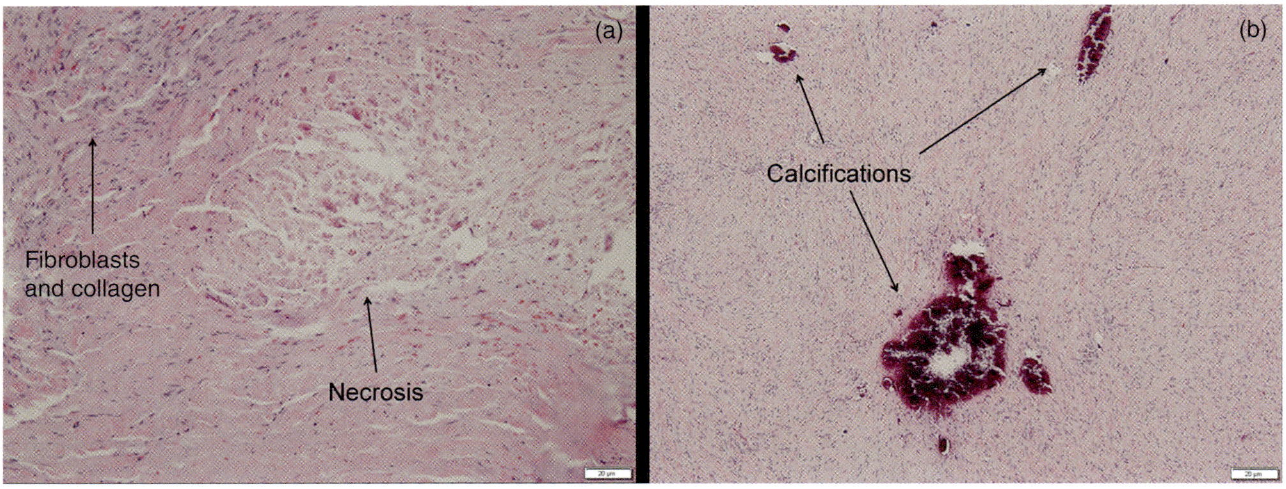

Figure 53.4 Histologic section of a fibroma, showing benign spindle cell proliferation with bland appearing fibroblasts and intervening collagen bundles as well as (a) focal necrosis and (b) areas of calcification localized at the tumor center.

common neonatal tumors (Table 53.1) [1], presenting frequently in the newborn period and occasionally in utero [17]. Symptoms include congestive heart failure, low cardiac output, cyanosis (for right ventricular tumors), and symptomatic arrhythmias [18], with VT as the most common arrhythmia (67%) and presenting clinical manifestation [4].

Cardiomegaly is typically seen on chest radiography. Echocardiography reveals a large, solitary, homogenous, intramyocardial mass in the ventricular septum or free wall or, rarely, in the atrium (Figure 53.5). CMR can identify marked hyperenhancement on myocardial delayed enhancement imaging. Central calcifications may be seen on chest radiography or CT (Figure 53.6). Resection is not necessary in asymptomatic infants without arrhythmia. Management includes antiarrhythmic and heart failure medications and/or surgical resection [5]. Surgical debulking or resection will abolish the arrhythmia in most patients with VT [4]. During infancy, fibromas may grow in size [5], eventually appearing smaller with somatic growth. Arrhythmias can persist but become less significant in unoperated survivors [4].

Cardiac Hemangioma

Cardiac hemangiomas result from proliferation of blood vessel endothelial cells. Histologically, they are identical to other hemangiomas [19] and classified based on their biochemical and histologic profiles (Box 53.1). Most are benign and classified as congenital or infantile [20, 21].

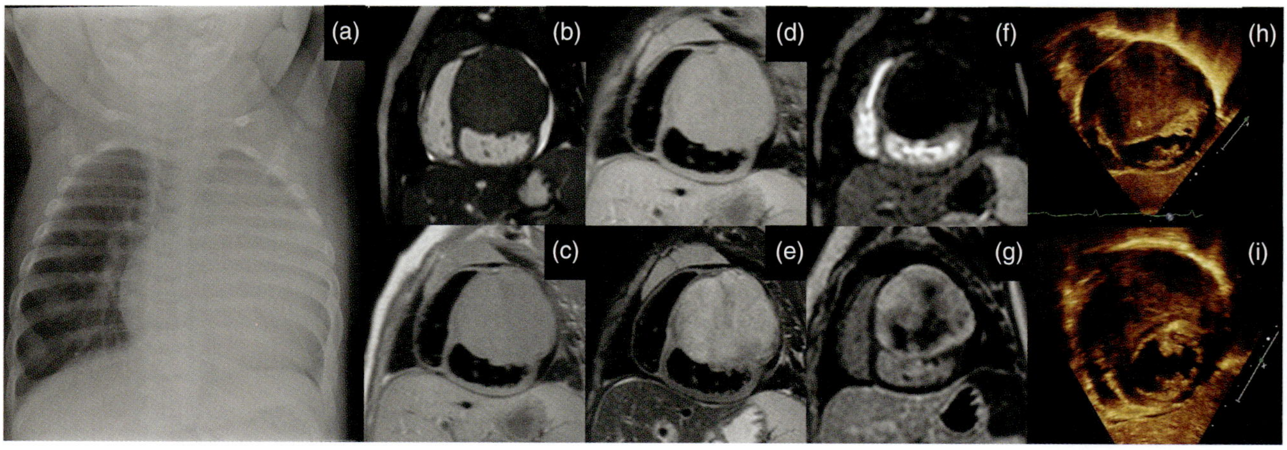

Figure 53.5 Large fibroma in the left ventricular anterior wall with (a) marked cardiomegaly on chest radiography; (b) isointense appearance by CMR using cine imaging, (c) T1-weighted imaging, and (d) T1-weighted imaging with fat suppression; (e) hyperintense and inhomogenous appearance using T2-weighted imaging; (f) hypointense appearance on first pass perfusion imaging; (g) hyperintense appearance with a central dark core on myocardial delayed enhancement imaging; (h) homogenous appearance in systole and (i) in diastole. A thin rim of normal myocardium surrounds the tumor; best seen in (e), (f), and (g).

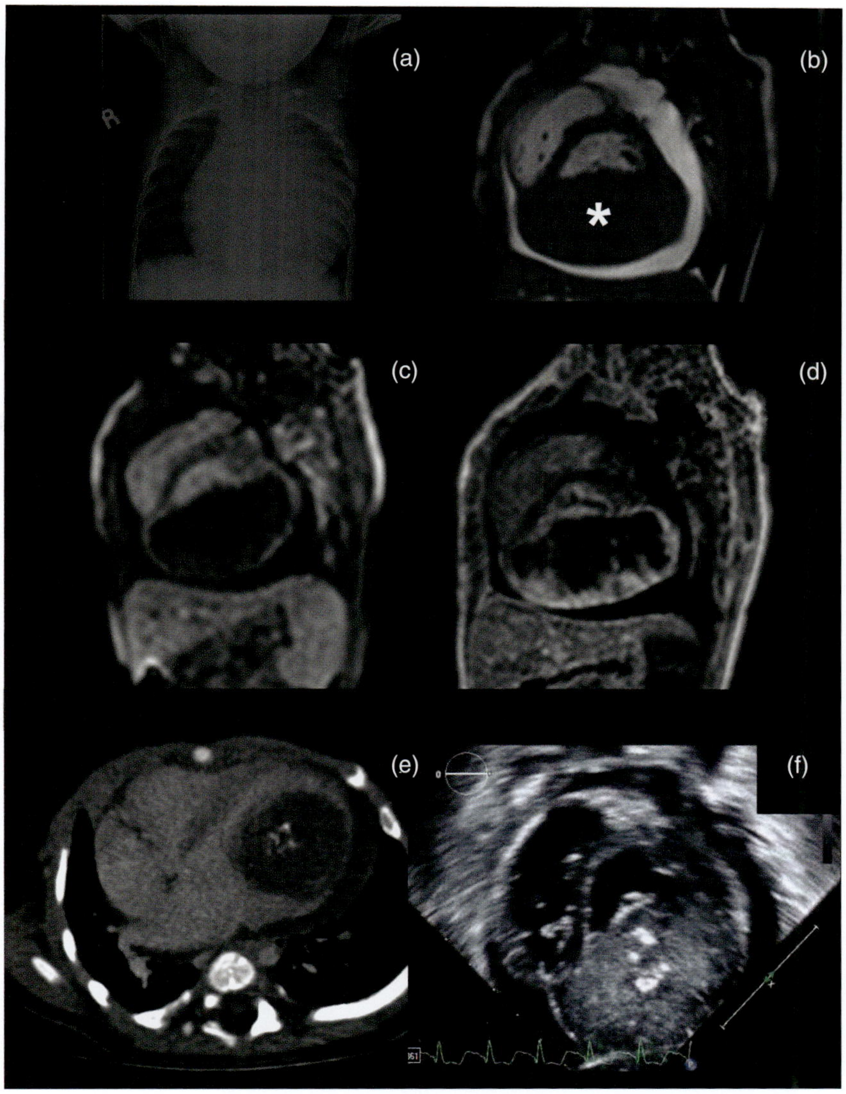

Figure 53.6 Large fibroma with central calcification located at the inferior wall of the left ventricle with (a) marked cardiomegaly on chest radiography; (b) isointense appearance by CMR using cine imaging; (c) hypoperfused appearance on first pass perfusion imaging; and (d) strong peripheral enhancement with a central dark core using on myocardial delayed enhancement imaging; (e) hypoperfusion and central calcifications with contrast CT; and (f) echo-bright calcifications within the tumor center by echocardiography (f).

Box 53.1 Classifications of cardiac hemangiomas

Benign vascular tumors

Congenital hemangioma (GLUT 1–)
- Rapidly involuting congenital hemangioma (RICH)
- Non-involuting congenital hemangioma (NICH)

Infantile hemangioma (GLUT 1+)
Intramuscular hemangioma
Miscellaneous (pleomorphic, etc.)

Neonates present with pericardial effusion and cardiac tamponade, respiratory distress, congestive heart failure, arrhythmia, sudden cardiac death, asymptomatic murmur, or ventricular fibrillation [19, 20].

Echocardiography usually reveals a right atrial mass with multiple irregular fluid components and occasionally with vascular channels, though they can be seen in other cardiac locations [20]. It may be confused with teratoma because of its inhomogenous appearance, size, and location (Figure 53.7) [8]. CMR can differentiate cardiac hemangiomas from non-vascular tumors as they have a strong signal on first pass perfusion imaging (Figure 53.8) [8]. Because most neonates are symptomatic, surgical excision usually results in a favorable outcome [20]. The natural history is not well known because of incorrect or variable terminology in the literature and lack of precise histologic diagnosis (which can predict spontaneous regression). The potential for malignancy usually determines the need for biopsy or surgical resection. No clear guidelines have been established regarding management of asymptomatic patients.

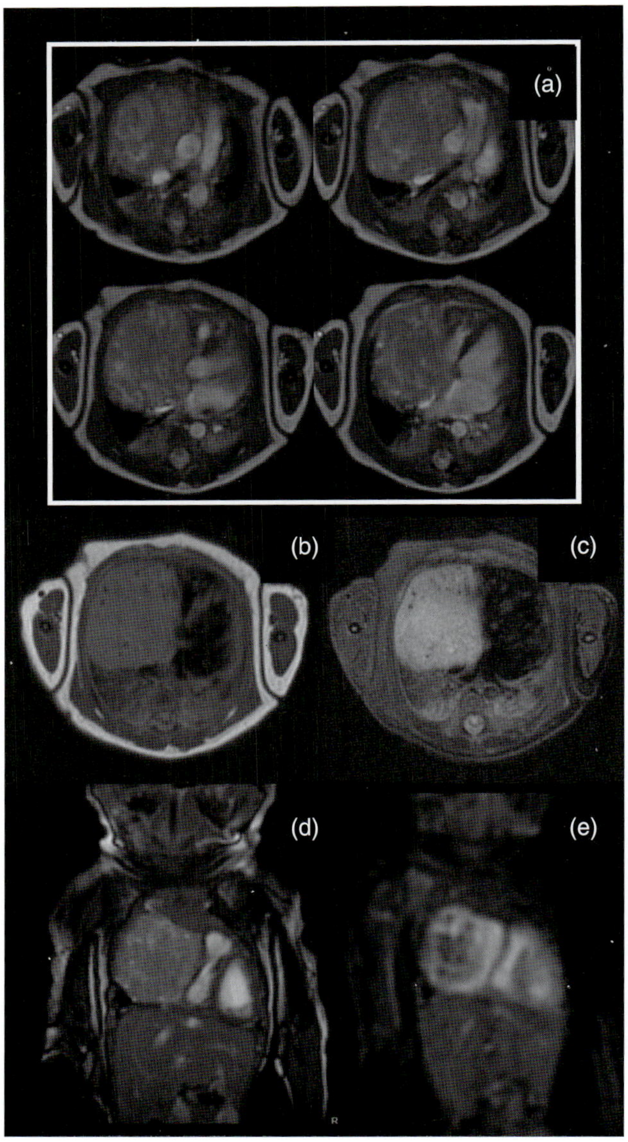

Figure 53.7 CMR images of a large right atrial hemangioma filling nearly the entire right hemothorax and compressing the right heart and superior vena cava with (a) an inhomogenous appearance by cine imaging; (b) an isointense appearance with T1-weighted imaging; and (c) a hyperintense appearance secondary to its highly vascular nature by T2-weighted imaging with fat suppression. (d) The tumor compresses the right ventricle by cine imaging in a coronal plane, and (e) it demonstrates intense perfusion with a central dark region, consistent with regions of high vascularity and intervening cystic tissue.

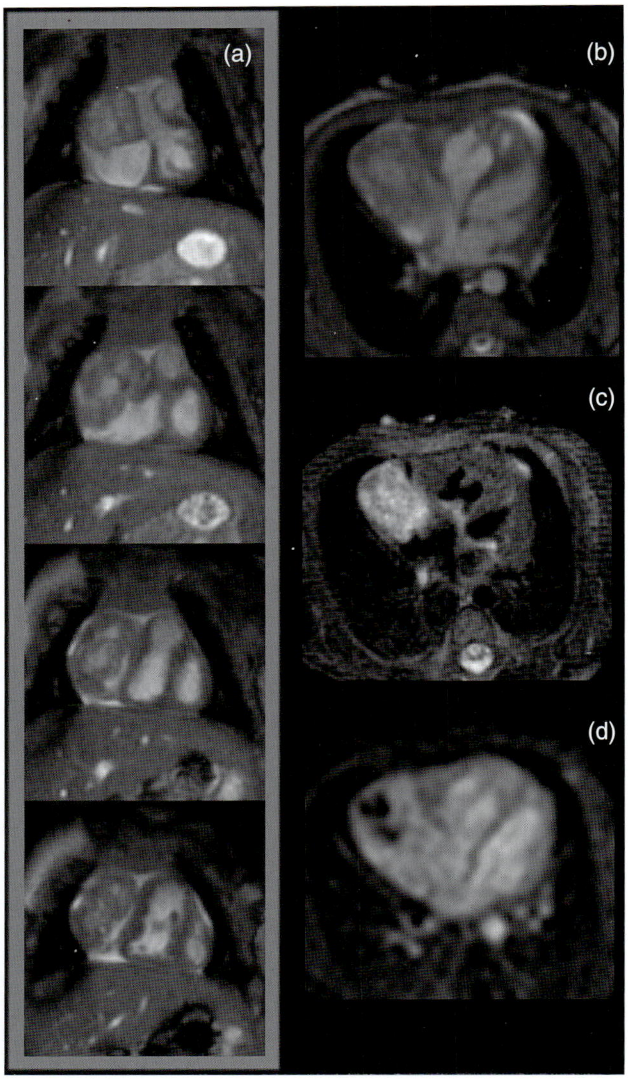

Figure 53.8 CMR images of a right atrial hemangioma causing mild right heart compression with (a,b) an inhomogenous appearance corresponding to either vascular channels or cysts by CMR; (c) a hyperintense appearance on T2-weighted imaging consistent with increased fluid content; and (d) profound enhancement on first pass perfusion imaging with the exception of a central dark area, likely corresponding to cysts.

References

1 Isaacs H Jr. (2004) Fetal and neonatal cardiac tumors. *Pediatr Cardiol*, **25** (3), 252–273.

2 Fletcher CDM. (1995) *Diagnostic Histopathology of Tumors*, Churchill Livingstone, Edinburgh.

3 Tworetzky W, McElhinney DB, Margossian R, *et al.* (2003) Association between cardiac tumors and tuberous sclerosis in the fetus and neonate. *Am J Cardiol*, **92** (4), 487–489.

4 Miyake CY, Del Nido PJ, Alexander ME, *et al.* (2011) Cardiac tumors and associated arrhythmias in pediatric patients, with observations on surgical therapy for ventricular tachycardia. *J Am Coll Cardiol*, **58** (18), 1903–1909.

5 Yinon Y, Chitayat D, Blaser S, *et al.* (2010) Fetal cardiac tumors: a single-center experience of 40 cases. *Prenat Diagn*, **30** (10), 941–949.

6 Sharma J, Inglis S, Cavalieri R, Udom-Rice I. (2011) Fetal demise secondary to massive rhabdomyoma in the early second trimester of pregnancy. *Pediatr Cardiol*, **32** (2), 243–244.

7 Geva T, Santini F, Pear W, Driscoll SG, Van Praagh R. (1991) Cardiac rhabdomyoma: rare cause of fetal death. *Chest*, **99** (1), 139–142.

8 Beroukhim RS, Prakash A, Valsangiacomo Buechel ER, *et al.* (2011) Characterization of cardiac tumors in children by cardiovascular magnetic resonance imaging a multicenter experience. *J Am Coll Cardiol*, **58** (10), 1044–1054.

9 Gonzalez M, Krueger T, Schaefer SC, Ris HB, Perentes JY. (2010) Asymptomatic intrapericardial mature teratoma. *Ann Thorac Surg*, **89** (6), e46–47.

10 Iacona GM, Barber MA, Medina M, Abella R. (2011) Intrapericardial teratoma in a low birth weight preterm infant: a successful multidisciplinary approach. *Interact Cardiovasc Thorac Surg*, **12** (2), 287–289.

11 Kalavrouziotis G, Konstantopoulou G, Stefanaki K, *et al.* (2010) Intrapericardial teratoma in a premature neonate: pre-delivery diagnosis and successful surgical removal. *Hellenic J Cardiol*, **51** (3), 278–280.

12 Laforgia N, Calderoni G, Di Mauro A, *et al.* (2011) A case of neonatal intrapericardial teratoma. Clinical and pathological findings. *Acta Paediatr*, **100** (8), e90–92.

13 Soor GS, Chakrabarti MO, Luk A, *et al.* (2010) Prenatal intrapericardial teratomas: diagnosis and management. *Cardiovasc Pathol*, **19** (1), e1–4.

14 Tomek V, Vlk R, Tlaskal T, Skovranek J. (2010) Successful pericardio-amniotic shunting for fetal intrapericardial teratoma. *Pediatr Cardiol*, **31** (8), 1236–1238.

15 Becker AE. (2000) Primary heart tumors in the pediatric age group: a review of salient pathologic features relevant for clinicians. *Pediatr Cardiol*, **21** (4), 317–323.

16 Nwachukwu H, Li A, Nair V, *et al.* (2010) Cardiac fibroma in adults. *Cardiovasc Pathol*, **20** (4), 146–152.

17 Gutberlet M, Abdul-Khaliq H, Stiller B, *et al.* (2002) Giant fibroma in the left ventricle of an infant: imaging findings in magnetic resonance imaging, echocardiography and angiography. *Eur Radiol*, **12** (Suppl 3), S143–148.

18 Kiaffas MG, Danias PG, Kaklamanis L, Rammos S. (2009) Fatal cardiac arrest due to an unusual fibroma of the pulmonary valve. *Pediatr Cardiol*, **30** (4), 536–539.

19 McAllister HA, Fenoglio JJ. (1978) *Tumors of the Cardiovascular System*, Armed Forces Institute of Pathology, Washington, pp. 141.

20 Mackie AS, Kozakewich HP, Geva T, Perez-Atayde AR, Mulliken JB. (2005) Vascular tumors of the heart in infants and children: case series and review of the literature. *Pediatr Cardiol*, **26** (4), 344–39.

21 Hassanein AH, Mulliken JB, Fishman SJ, Greene AK. (2011) Evaluation of terminology for vascular anomalies in current literature. *Plast Reconstr Surg*, **127** (1), 347–351.

54

Arteriovenous Malformations

Allison K. Cabalka

Division of Pediatric Cardiology, Mayo Clinic, Rochester, MN, USA

In the developing embryo, congenital arteriovenous malformations (AVM) form when the connections between the arterial and venous structures fail to differentiate from the common capillary network, leaving direct connections between the feeding arteries and draining veins. Clinical signs and symptoms are variable and are related directly to the location of the fistula and the size of the connections. In utero, the placenta is typically the lowest resistance part of the circulation, so fetuses may be protected from significant symptoms because of restriction of flow through the low resistance AVM. However, once delivery occurs and the low resistance placental circuit is removed, flow through these abnormal connections can increase rapidly and dramatically [1]. Intracranial and intrahepatic connections are the most common, but important AVM can exist in other locations. In the neonate, there are two primary clinical manifestations of significant fistula connections: congestive heart failure (most common) or cyanosis (less common).

Intracranial

Cerebral arteriovenous malformations are seen sporadically or as part of a systemic malformation syndrome, such as hereditary hemorrhagic telangiectasia. Approximately 5% of pediatric AVM will present in the neonate with congestive heart failure [1, 2]. A vein of Galen aneurysmal malformation (VGAM) is the most common type of intracranial AVM presenting in the neonatal population, responsible for approximately 40% of pediatric intracranial shunts [2, 3]. Other less common types include superficial (pial) or dural sinus malformation and dural arteriovenous fistula. VGAM usually involves multiple shunts at the choroid fissure that eventually enter a dilated vein.

Prenatal presentation can occur with non-immune hydrops, hydrocephalus, and intracranial hemorrhage. However, neonatal presentation is more common, with signs and symptoms of high output cardiac failure; as systemic vascular resistance increases postnatally the amount of shunt through the intracranial AVM can increase dramatically [1]. Craniomegaly and neurologic symptoms, such as seizures, can be seen, but these symptoms typically occur in the older patient.

Clinically, the neonate in high output congestive heart failure presents with tachycardia, tachypnea, bounding pulses, a hyperdynamic precordium, with a systolic outflow murmur and gallop on auscultation. An intracranial bruit may be appreciated [1, 2]. The amount of the shunt through the AVM will depend directly on the size of the communication, the number of communicating vessels, and the resistance of the systemic vascular circuit. If there is no outflow restriction (i.e., on the venous side of the lesion), the neonate will have very early and significant symptoms of high output congestive heart failure.

Cranial ultrasound is diagnostic (Figure 54.1) but detailed imaging, such as magnetic resonance imaging and angiography, will confirm the diagnosis and aid in assessment of cerebral changes and assist in planning technique and timing of therapeutic intervention [1]. Chest radiography reveals cardiomegaly (Figure 54.2a). Echocardiography shows dilated cardiac chambers, dilated head and neck vessels, with accentuated flow through the aortic arch and venous return from the superior vena cava (Figure 54.3a,b,c). Retrograde flow reversal in the descending thoracic aorta can be present if significant flow into the intracranial AVM is present (Figure 54.3d) [3, 4]. The intracardiac anatomy is most commonly normal, but pulmonary hypertension and a persistent patent ductus arteriosus are common associated features in the neonate. Persistent fetal circulation with high pulmonary artery pressure can also be predictive of the need for early intervention in the neonate with large intracranial AVM. One should be particularly suspicious of an intracranial AVM if these echocardiographic findings are present in a neonate who presents with congestive heart failure; imaging of the head should

Visual Guide to Neonatal Cardiology, First Edition. Edited by Ernerio T. Alboliras, Ziyad M. Hijazi, Leo Lopez, and Donald J. Hagler.

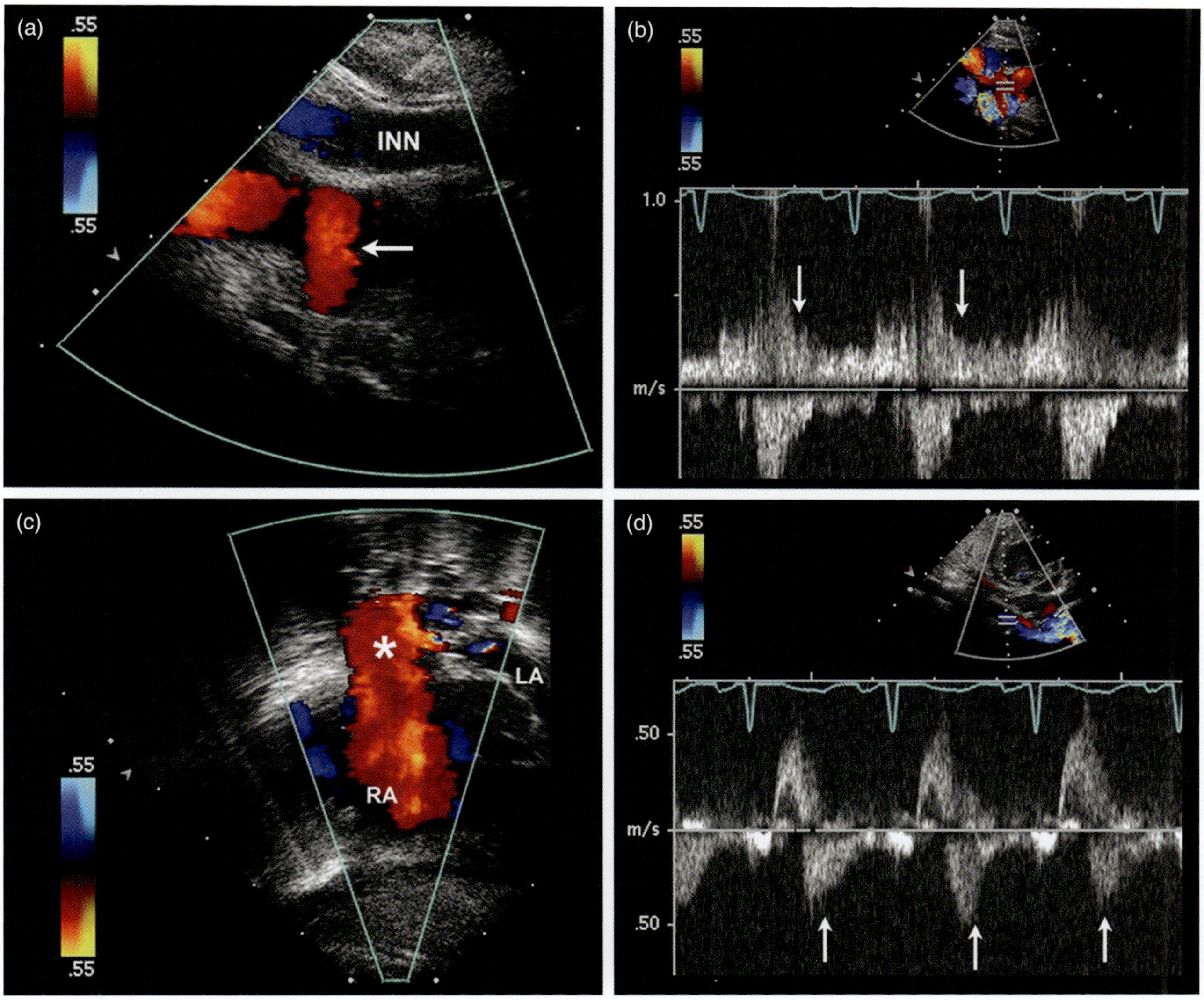

Figure 54.1 Characteristic echocardiographic findings in neonate with high output cardiac failure resulting from large vein of Galen aneurysmal malformation (VGAM). (a) Suprasternal notch image showing color flow toward the transducer, indicating flow reversal in proximal descending aorta (arrow). A dilated innominate vein (INN) is seen superior to the arch vessels. (b) Pulsed-wave Doppler interrogation of aortic arch vessels from suprasternal notch indicating holodiastolic flow toward the transducer, evidence of high flow into cerebral vessels (arrows). (c) Subcostal coronal imaging demonstrating a very dilated superior vena cava (asterisk) entering the right atrium (RA). The atrial septum is bowed toward the left atrium (LA). (d) Abdominal aorta Doppler shows diastolic flow reversal (arrows) consistent with proximal runoff from the large VGAM.

be performed. Associated congenital heart disease has been reported, such as sinus venosus type of atrial septal defect, coarctation of the aorta, partial anomalous pulmonary venous return, ventricular septal defect, and atrioventricular canal [4].

A multidisciplinary team approach is necessary for the care of these patients, including neonatology, cardiology, pediatric anesthesia, neurology, and interventional neuroradiology. Prognosis is very poor for the neonate presenting with a large VGAM and cardiac failure if no therapy is undertaken. However, if significant parenchymal abnormalities are present in the brain, only conservative therapy and comfort measures may be undertaken. The goal of therapy is to decrease the high flow through the AVM. If the neonate cannot be weaned from the ventilator or inotropic cardiac therapy, then early intervention will be required to control as much of the AVM as possible. Endovascular therapy is preferred and serial treatments may be needed. [1, 3]. Aggressive control of congestive heart failure will be needed, and the neonate will often require inotropic and ventilator support as the intracranial AVM is being treated. The ultimate outcome will depend entirely on the preservation of normal brain tissue and normal brain function. Cardiac function will normalize with control of the shunt through the AVM and successful embolization of the significant feeder arterial supply to the malformation (Figure 54.2b).

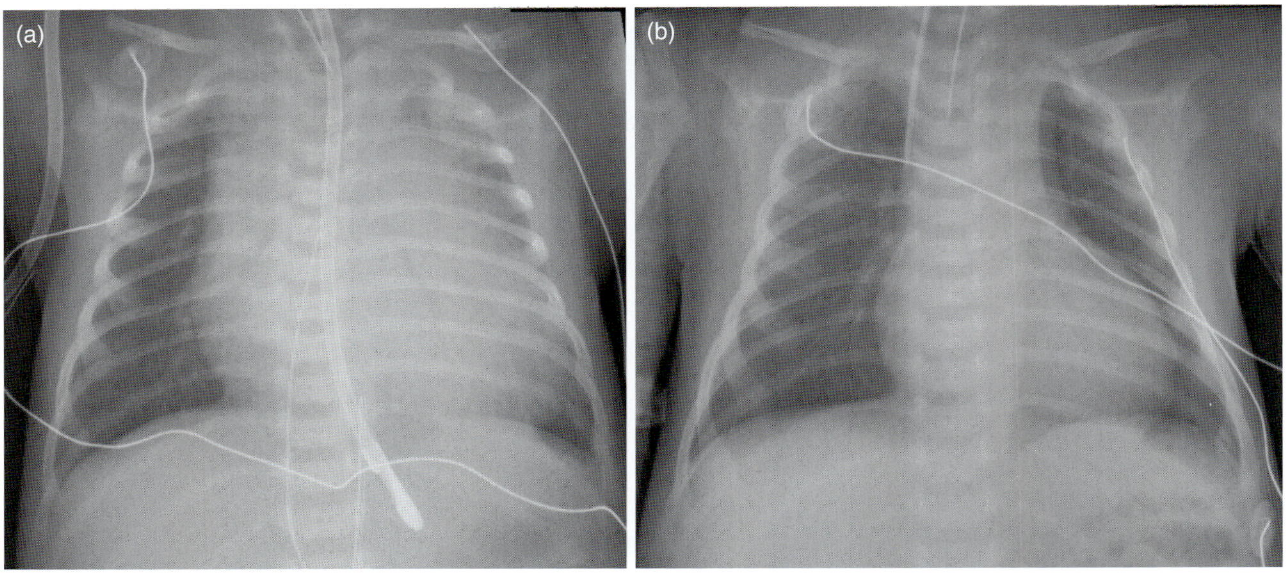

Figure 54.2 Chest radiograph in neonate with large vein of Galen aneurysmal malformation (VGAM). (a) Significant cardiomegaly is present at diagnosis on day of life 1. (b) Improvement in cardiac size after three sessions of embolization therapy with complete occlusion of the VGAM (endotracheal tube placed for interventional procedure), age 3 weeks.

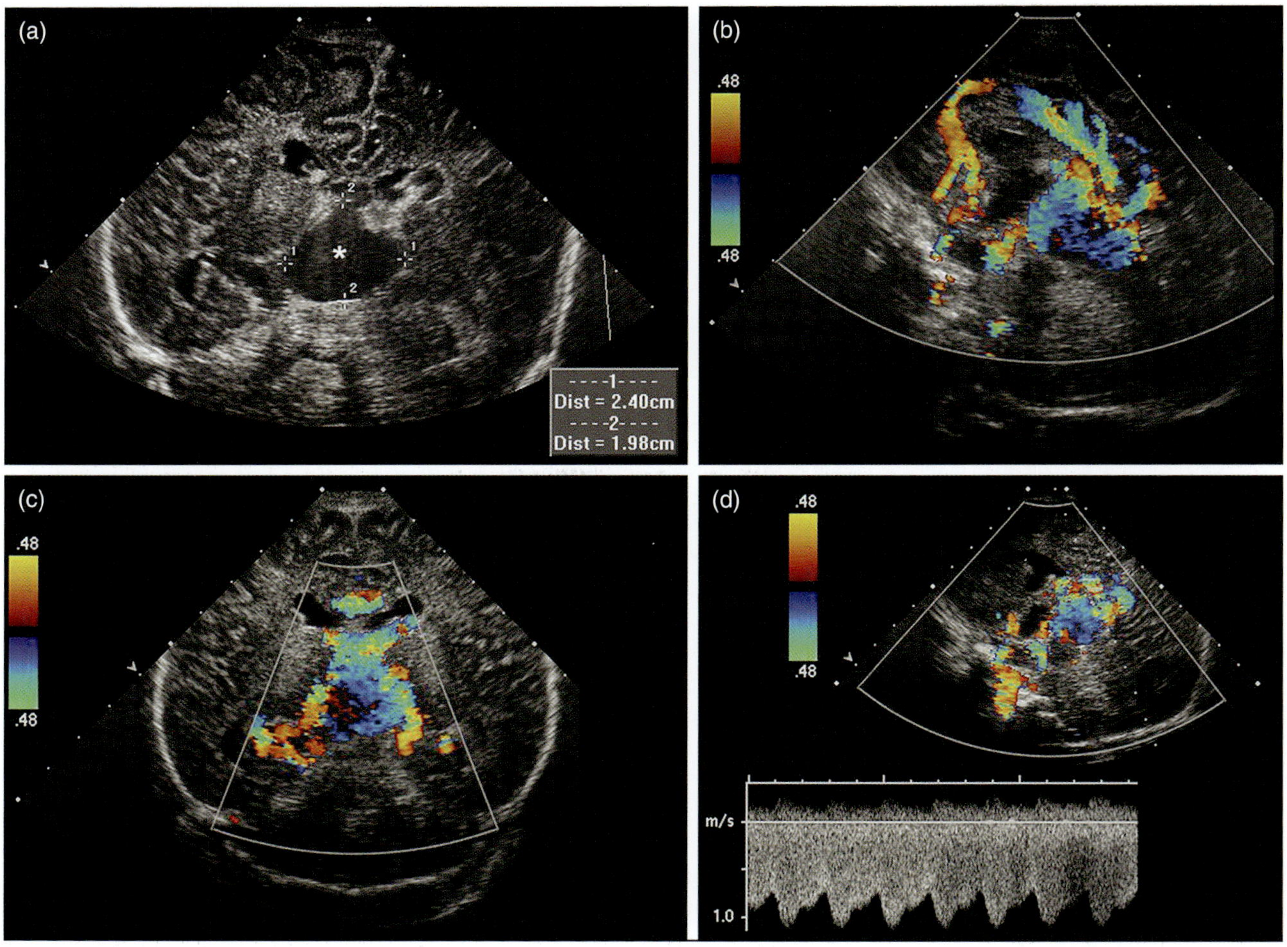

Figure 54.3 Neonate with large vein of Galen aneurysmal malformation (VGAM). (a) Coronal plane image depicting a dilated hypoechoic vascular structure (asterisk shows prosencephalic vein). (b) Sagittal plane image with color Doppler demonstrating increased vascular flow through multiple paramedian vessels. (c) Coronal plane image of structures depicted in (b). (d) Doppler interrogation shows continuous flow in the dilated vascular structures, consistent with a large VGAM.

Extracranial Arteriovenous Malformations

Intrahepatic

Similar to intracranial malformations, intrahepatic malformations will cause varying degrees of congestive heart failure. The neonate may not be as symptomatic as one with a large intracranial AVM, but symptoms progress over time, also related to the changes in systemic vascular resistance and size of the hepatic connections. The average age at presentation is approximately 2 months. Typical congestive heart failure symptoms are present (as described for intracranial AVM). Additionally, infants can have hepatomegaly, consumptive coagulopathy, portal hypertension, and/or anemia. The echocardiographic findings will also show significant chamber dilation; however, the flow returning to the right-sided chambers from the hepatic or inferior vena cava area will be most prominent, in contrast to the superior vena cava flow in the setting of an intracranial AVM (Figure 54.4). Continuous forward flow may be seen in the descending thoracic aorta if significant shunt is present into the hepatic AVM. Liver ultrasound will show the characteristic Doppler flow patterns of hepatic AVM; however, multislice detailed computerized tomographic imaging will be needed to outline the nature of the feeder arteries and supply to the AVM.

Surgical therapy was commonly employed in the late 1970s for treatment of hepatic AVM, but endovascular transcatheter embolization therapy is now recommended. If congestive heart failure can be controlled medically, the natural history of a hepatic AVM may be favorable in terms of spontaneous resolution, or diminution enough to relieve the burden of congestive heart failure symptomatology.

Other Systemic Arteriovenous Malformations

AVM can occur in other locations and produce significant early congestive heart failure symptoms because of

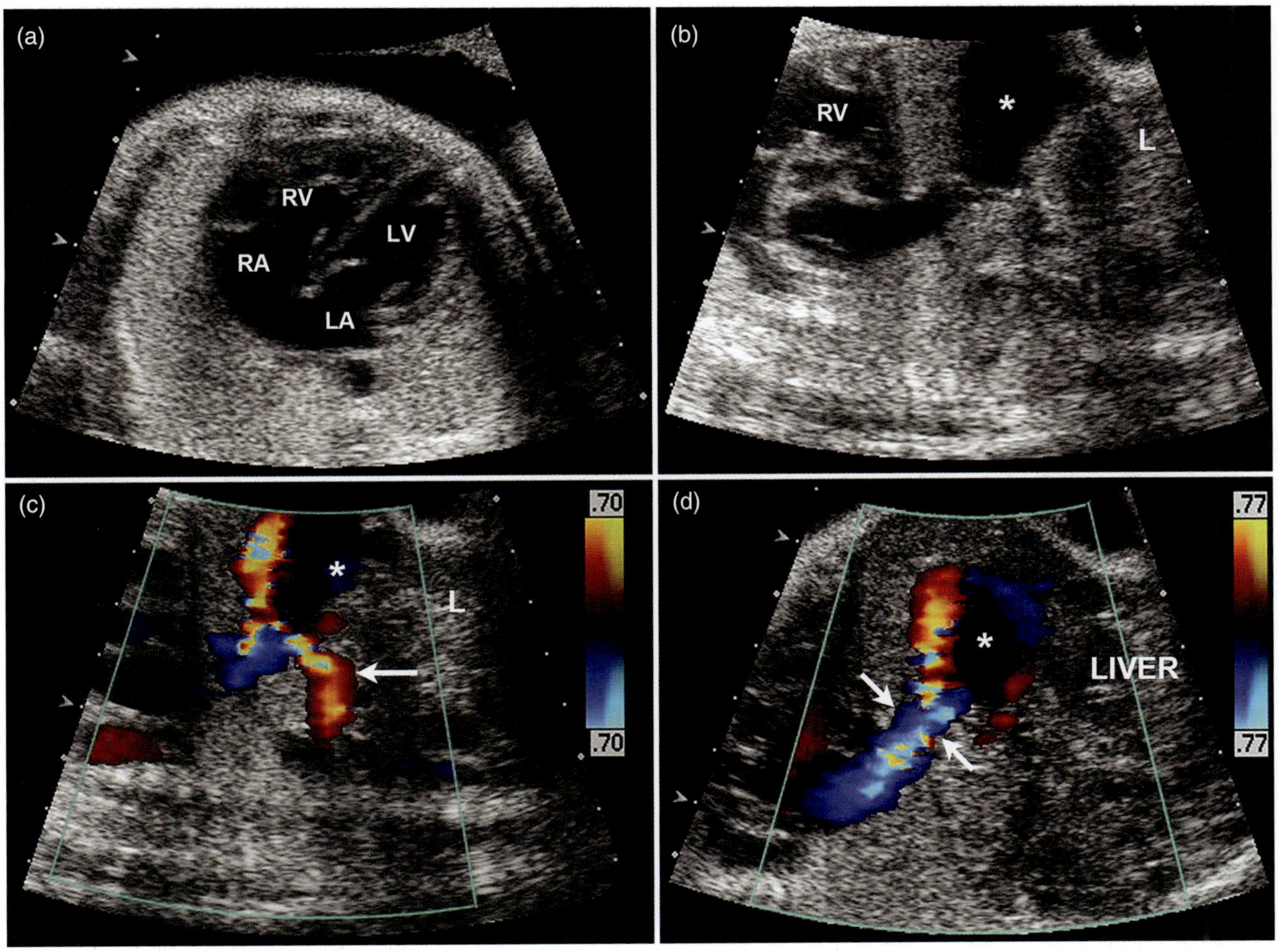

Figure 54.4 Fetal echocardiogram in fetus with large hepatic arteriovenous malformation (AVM). (a) Four-chamber view showing moderate cardiomegaly. (b) Sagittal scan depicting hepatic AVM as large echogenic space (asterisk) in liver (L). (c) Color Doppler flow of arterial supply into large hepatic AVM (asterisk). (d) Increased venous return (arrows) is present from the liver to the right atrium in this situation. LA, left atrium; LV, left ventricle; RA, right atrium; RV, right ventricle.

the continuous shunt between a systemic artery and vein. A communication between the subclavian artery and vein is rare, as is an internal mammary artery connection to the hepatic circulation. Clinical signs and symptoms are similar to the findings in a neonate with intracranial or intrahepatic AVM. On physical examination, the bruit will be located directly over the area of involvement (i.e., subclavian artery in the setting of subclavian artery to vein fistula).

Echocardiographic findings with respect to the intracardiac anatomy are similar to those seen in VGAM, and Doppler or color Doppler mapping can be used to locate and evaluate the significance of the fistulous connection. Catheter-based therapy to occlude the communication can be considered in systemic arteriovenous malformations but in some situations surgical ligation may be needed if the connection is very large and the arterial vessel is very small [5].

Pulmonary Arteriovenous Malformation

Pulmonary AVM is a rare cause of significant cyanosis in the neonate. The most common connection will be between the right pulmonary artery and the pulmonary veins or left atrium directly [6, 7]. Neonatal presentation is more unusual than presentation in the older child or even adult, and will typically only be seen when there is a large communication. The degree of cyanosis will be proportional to the size of the connection between the pulmonary artery (containing deoxygenated blood) and the pulmonary vein, returning this deoxygenated to the systemic circulation. Rarely, this type of connection may be recognized on fetal echocardiography; a severely dilated pulmonary artery and prominent flow in the pulmonary vein may be seen (Figure 54.5) and a very symptomatic neonate would be expected. More commonly, this will be recognized postnatally. The neonate will be cyanotic,

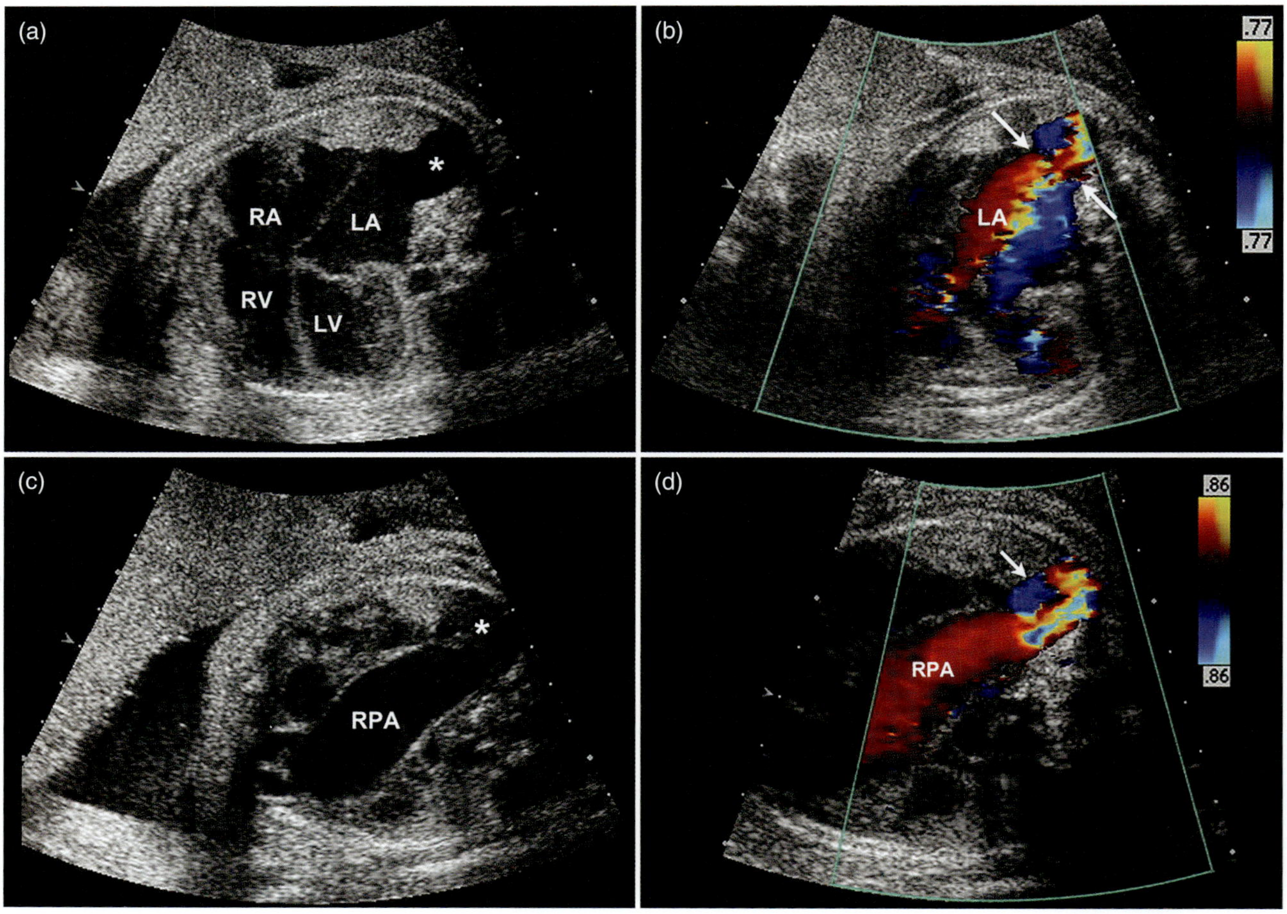

Figure 54.5 Fetal echocardiogram in large right pulmonary artery to pulmonary vein fistula. (a) Four-chamber view showing severe cardiomegaly with four-chamber dilation and aneurysmal appearance of right pulmonary vein (asterisk). (b) Color Doppler flow from fistulous communication into left atrium. (c) Dilated right pulmonary artery (RPA) with large connection to pulmonary vein (asterisk). (d) Color Doppler flow between RPA and right pulmonary vein in large fistulous connection. LA, left atrium; LV, left ventricle; RA, right atrium; RV, right ventricle.

and may have a continuous murmur appreciated on auscultation over the lung field that is involved.

Transthoracic echocardiography will demonstrate normal intracardiac anatomy, with dilation of the involved pulmonary artery and evidence of dilated left heart structures. Turbulent flow may be seen with color Doppler interrogation in the area of the fistulous connection; Doppler velocity will typically be very low with continuous flow present. Cardiac catheterization will be considered in the symptomatic cyanotic neonate and catheter-based embolization therapy of the primary feeding artery can be undertaken if the anatomy is suitable [6, 7]. Risks of leaving a significant intrapulmonary AVM untreated include congestive heart failure exacerbated by cyanosis, endocarditis, stroke, and bleeding.

Conclusions

The neonate with unexplained high output congestive heart failure or significant cyanosis in the presence of normal intracardiac anatomy should be carefully evaluated for the presence of an AVM. Detailed imaging includes evaluation of potential locations of such fistula/malformations, including intracranial, intrahepatic, intrapulmonary, or other vascular malformation. Endovascular therapy is most commonly employed to occlude important feeder arteries and connections with the goal of therapy being control of symptoms and preservation of normal vascular and brain function, especially in the setting of a significant intracranial AVM. A multidisciplinary team approach will be needed to care for these complex, often seriously ill, neonates.

Acknowledgement

The author would like to thank Carlen Fifer, MD, for providing additional fetal echocardiographic images.

References

1 Recinos P, Rahmathulla G, Pearl M, *et al.* (2012) Vein of Galen malformations: epidemiology, clinical presentations, management. *Neurosurg Clin N Am*, **1**, 165–177.

2 Karadeniz L, Coban A, Sencer S, *et al.* (2011) Vein of Galen aneurysmal malformation: prenatal diagnosis and early endovascular management. *J Chinese Med Assoc*, **74** (3), 134–137.

3 Berenstein A, Fifi J, Niimi Y, *et al.* (2012) Vein of Galen malformations in neonates: new management paradigms for improving outcomes. *Neurosurgery*, **5**, 1207–1213.

4 Musewe N, Smallhorn J, Burrows P, Izukawa T, Freedom R. (1988) Echocardiographic and Doppler evaluation of the aortic arch and brachiocephalic vessels in cerebral and systemic arteriovenous fistulas. *J Am Coll Cardiol*, **6**, 1529–1535.

5 Balakrishnan P, Guleserian K, Schuster J, Blalock S. (2011) Congenital arteriovenous malformation between the subclavian artery and superior vena cava presenting in neonatal heart failure. *Pediatr Cardiol*, **8**, 1204–1206.

6 Celebi A, Yücel I, Dedeoğlu R, Erdem A. (2013) Echocardiographic diagnosis and transcatheter occlusion of pulmonary arteriovenous fistula in cyanotic newborn. *Congenit Heart Dis*, **8** (6), E188–191.

7 Slack M, Jedeikin R, Jones J. (2000) Transcatheter coil closure of a right pulmonary artery to left atrial fistula in an ill neonate. *Catheter Cardiovasc Interv*, **3**, 330–333.

55

Pericardial Defects

Donald J. Hagler

Division of Cardiovascular Surgery, Mayo Clinic, Rochester, MN, USA

Congenital pericardial defects include a wide range of defects varying from minor partial defects to total absence of the pericardium [1].

Van Praagh *et al.* [2] noted the first report of congenital pericardial defects by Columbus in 1559. Although an uncommon lesion, congenital pericardial defects are difficult to diagnose clinically and are often first recognized at autopsy. Pericardial defects represent defective formation of the pleuropericardial membrane or, if diaphragmatic, defective formation of the septum transversum [3]. Most series reported left-sided congenital pericardial defects as the most common [1], and the classification by Ellis *et al.* [4] demonstrated the complete left-sided defect as by far the most common form, representing 56% of their cases. Right-sided, diaphragmatic, and total absence of the pericardium are rare. Approximately one-third of patients with total absence of the pericardium have associated pulmonary lesions such as bronchogenic cyst or sequestration and congenital heart lesions such as tetralogy of Fallot.

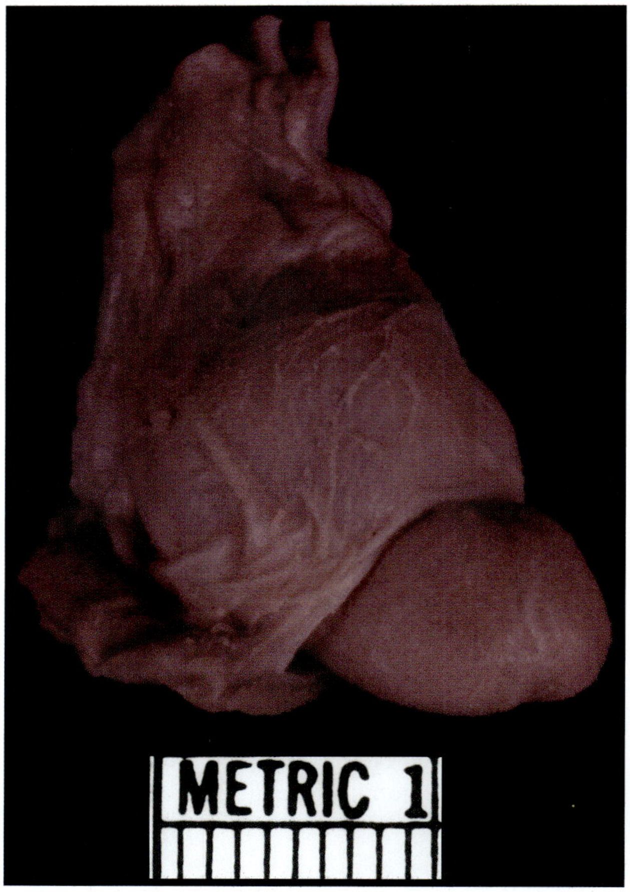

Figure 55.1 Pathologic specimen demonstrating strangulation of the apex of the left ventricle with a partial absence of the pericardium.

Manifestations

Associated anomalies can dominate the clinical presentation if the pericardial defect is associated with other congenital anomalies such as diaphragmatic hernia or congenital heart disease. Many patients with isolated pericardial defect are asymptomatic. Symptoms, when present, are non-specific, consisting of vague left chest discomfort, recurrent pulmonary infection, palpitations, and occasionally dizziness and syncope. Partial left-sided pericardial defects can be associated with herniation of the ventricles through the patent pleuropericardial foramen, resulting in strangulation of the ventricles and leading to death (Figure 55.1). Herniation and strangulation of the left atrial appendage also can occur. Obstruction of the superior vena cava can be associated with a right-sided pericardial defect secondary to herniation of the right lung into the pericardial space. Chest pain and the radiographic appearance of cardiomegaly can occur with diaphragmatic pericardial defect because the associated diaphragmatic defect allows herniation of the greater omentum into the pericardial space.

Visual Guide to Neonatal Cardiology, First Edition. Edited by Ernerio T. Alboliras, Ziyad M. Hijazi, Leo Lopez, and Donald J. Hagler.

Diagnosis

Physical examination may yield few abnormal signs. A crescendo–decrescendo systolic murmur at the left sternal border has been attributed to turbulent blood flow with an unusually mobile heart. The apical impulse may be hyperactive and displaced to the left.

The chest radiograph often provides the first clues to the diagnosis (Figure 55.2) [5]. With a complete left pericardial defect, the cardiac silhouette is displaced to the left and the left heart border has unusually prominent bulges at the aortic knob, the pulmonary artery, and the left ventricle. There may be insertion of a small portion of the lung between the aorta and the main pulmonary artery or between the left portion of the diaphragm and the inferior border of the heart. A diagnostic left pneumothorax results in pneumopericardium. A partial left pericardial defect can result in herniation of the left atrial appendage, and there may be prominence of the pulmonary artery segment or the atrial appendage or both. Computed tomography of the chest or magnetic resonance imaging (MRI) now permits better visualization of absence of the pericardium (Figures 55.3, 55.4, and 55.5).

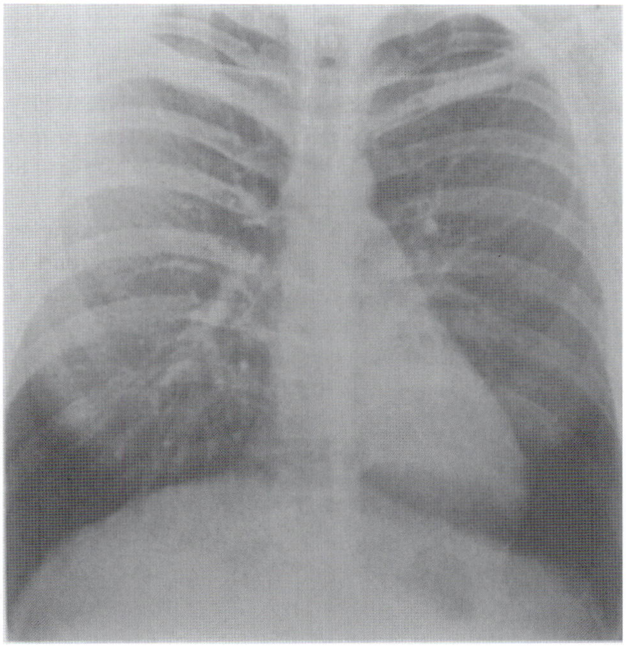

Figure 55.2 Chest X-ray demonstrating displacement of the cardiac silhouette to the left and flattened upper left cardiac border. *Source*: Van Son *et al*. 1993 [5]. Reproduced with permission of Elsevier.

Treatment

Complete absence of the pericardium is usually asymptomatic and requires no treatment. Only partial forms of pericardial defect (left-sided, right-sided, or diaphragmatic) require surgical treatment. Surgical treatment of partial pericardial defect has been of two types: enlargement, to avoid the risk of strangulation; and closure, usually with a flap of mediastinal pleura. The latter is considered preferable. A defect of the diaphragmatic pericardium requires reduction of the abdominal contents into the abdomen and repair of the diaphragmatic defect.

Ectopia Cordis

Ectopia cordis clearly represents a form of pericardial defect but is further characterized by partial or complete displacement of the heart outside the thorax. A strict interpretation of the term ectopia would

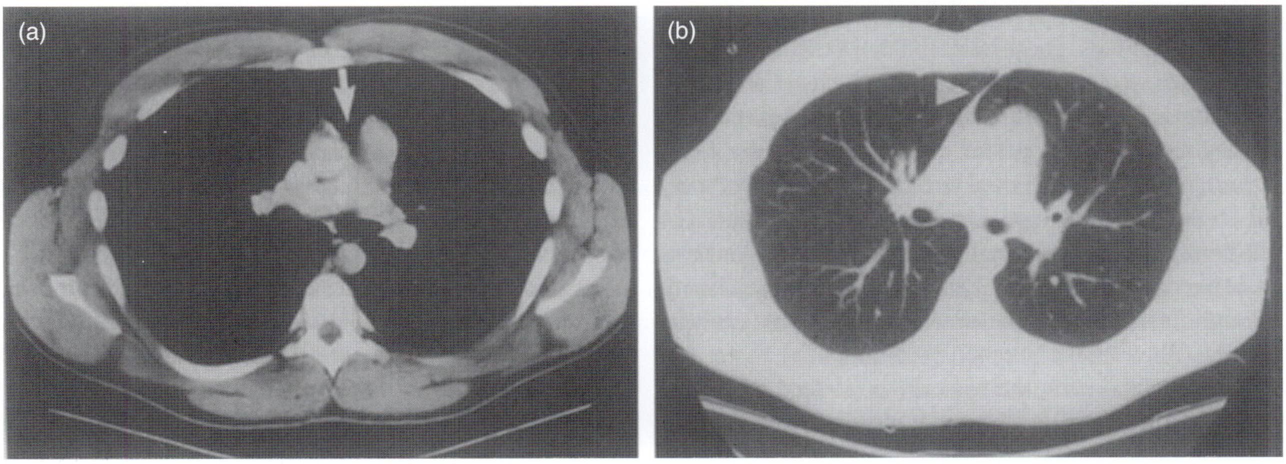

Figure 55.3 Computed tomography of the chest. (a) Scan at the level of the pulmonary artery demonstrates lung interposed between main pulmonary artery and the ascending aorta (arrow), a finding strongly suggestive of absent pericardium. (b) Lung setting at the same level demonstrates prominence of the sternopericardial ligament (arrowhead), which is evident when pericardium is absent. *Source*: Van Son *et al*. 1993 [5]. Reproduced with permission of Elsevier.

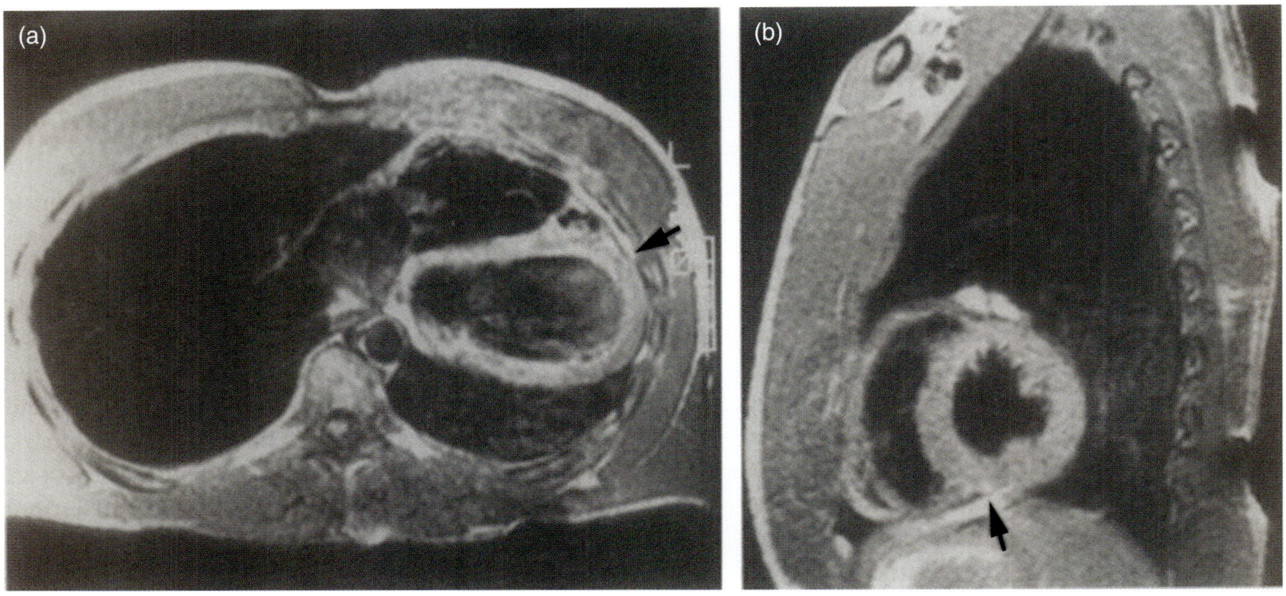

Figure 55.4 Magnetic resonance imaging scans of chest. (a) Axial scan through mid-ventricular level demonstrates pronounced leftward deviation of cardiac axis. Pericardial stripe terminates abruptly (arrow). (b) Sagittal view results in a short axis projection because of leftward deviation of heart. Note abrupt termination of pericardial stripe (arrow). *Source*: Van Son *et al*. 1993 [5]. Reproduced with permission of Elsevier.

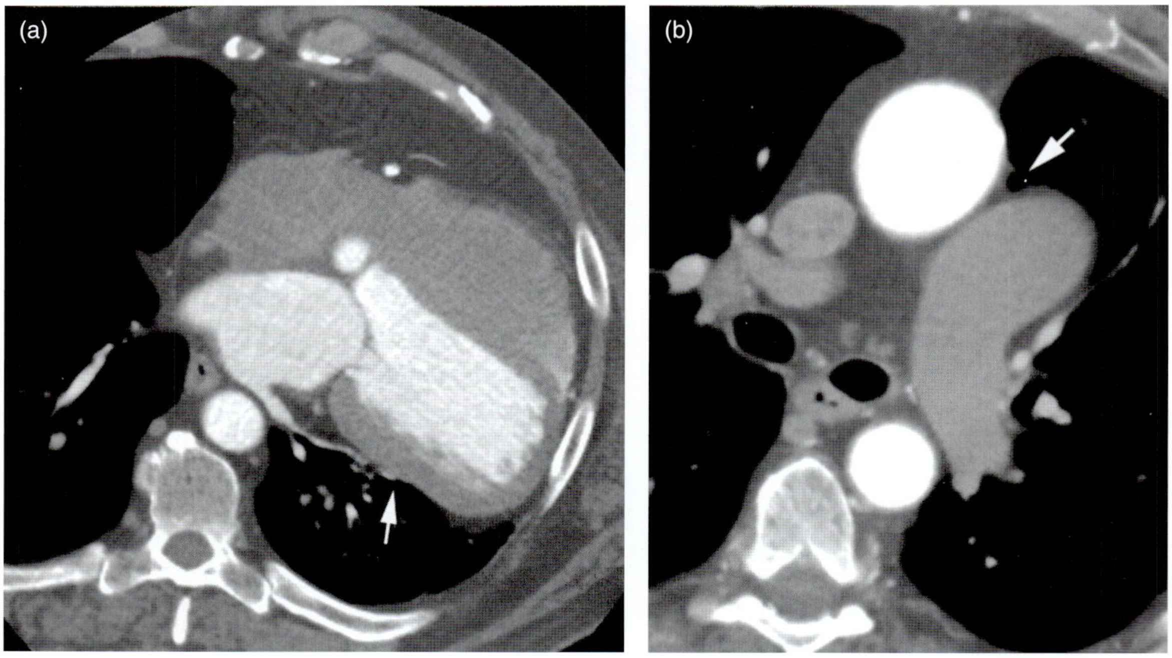

Figure 55.5 Computed tomography of the chest. (a) Scan demonstrating marked deviation of the heart into the left chest with indentation of the left ventricle secondary to the pericardial defect (arrow). (b) Short-axis image at the level of the pulmonary artery demonstrating typical interposition of the lung between the pulmonary artery and the aorta (arrow).

suggest a displacement or malposition and would include conditions such as dextrocardia. However, the classic definition of ectopia cordis has represented this entity as a congenital displacement of the heart outside the thoracic cavity. Kanagasuntheram and Verzin [6] suggested a classification including five types: cervical, thoracocervical, thoracic, thoracoabdominal, and abdominal. Van Praagh *et al.* [2] classified ectopia cordis as represented by four types (cervical, thoracic, thoracoabdominal, and abdominal) but suggested that for practical purposes only two types, thoracic and thoracoabdominal, are clearly represented clinically.

Tetralogy of Fallot has been reported in association with the thoracoabdominal form of ectopia cordis.

Cervical forms, usually observed with the sternum intact, were noted to be rare and may simply represent retention of the heart in its embryonic position in the neck. The review by Leca *et al.* [7, 8] noted 18 cases (8.5%) but included some cases with partial sternal defect. However, thoracocervical forms with the heart partially in the cervical region and with a defect in the superior end of the sternum appear to represent a distinct type of complete ectopia cordis not included in their review (Figure 55.6). The heart is completely outside the thoracic cavity, and there is a complete absence of parietal pericardium and a cephalic orientation of the cardiac apex. However, no omphalocele or abdominal diastasis was present. Pathologic examination and earlier echocardiographic identification during fetal evaluation now demonstrates more variation in ectopia cordis with recognition of classic complete as well as partial forms of ectopia.

The thoracic type is the classic form of ectopia cordis characterized by the following: a sternal cleft allowing protrusion of the heart outside the chest cavity; complete absence of the parietal pericardium; cephalic orientation of the cardiac apex; epigastric omphalocele or diastasis recti; and a small thoracic cavity. The thoracic type occurs in 80 cases (37%) in the review by Leca *et al.* [7]. A small thoracic cavity appears to be a significant etiologic agent as well as having significant implications for successful surgical correction of this defect. There can be congenital heart disease, most commonly tetralogy of Fallot but also including ventricular hypoplasia, transposition of the great arteries (TGA), and double outlet right ventricle.

Thoracoabdominal ectopia cordis appears to represent a partial form of ectopia cordis and is characterized by the following: partial absence or cleft of the lower sternum; a crescentic midline anterior diaphragmatic defect; a defect of the diaphragmatic parietal pericardium resulting in a free pericardioperitoneal communication; an omphalocele-like ventral abdominal defect or diastasis recti with partial displacement of the ventricular portion of the heart through the diaphragmatic defect into the epigastrium; and intracardiac congenital heart disease (Figure 55.7).

Treatment

Saxena [9] reported the first successful surgical repair of thoracic ectopia cordis. Although general surgical reports have demonstrated poor results for repair of this defect, most have advocated immediate surgery to correct the congenital heart disease and the anterior chest wall defect. Most advocate some form of prosthetic reconstruction of the chest wall and covering the heart with skin. Dobel *et al.* [10] advised a staged approach with enlargement of the posterior pericardial space by dividing posterior pericardial attachments to the rib margins.

Scott [11] reported the first successful surgical repair of thoracoabdominal ectopia cordis in 1950 by Brock. Repair in this case included repair of the diaphragmatic defect and of the epigastric hernia.

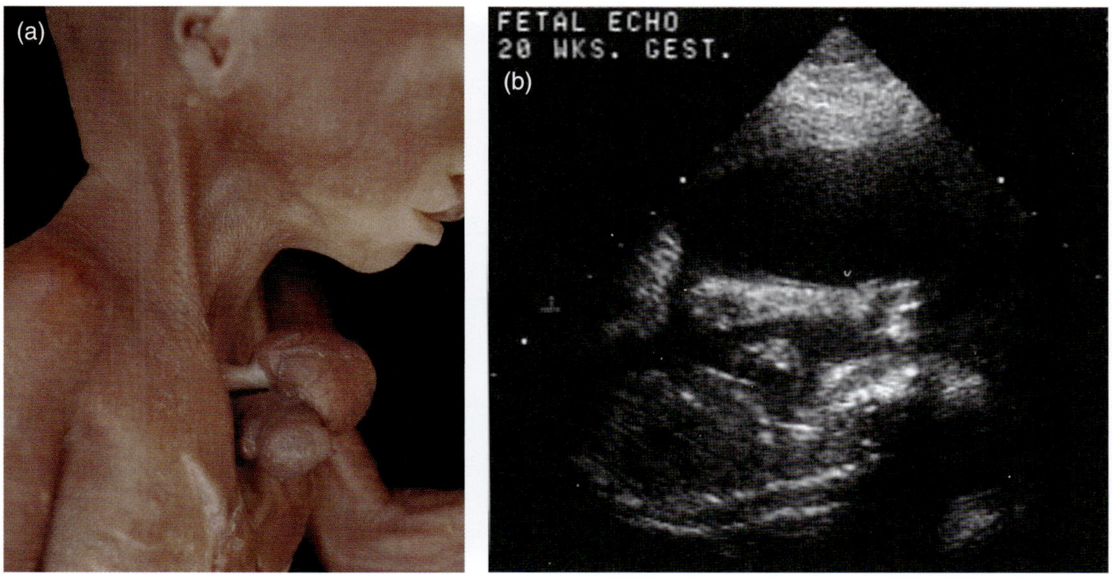

Figure 55.6 (a) Thoracocervical ectopia cordis in a 20 weeks' gestation fetus. There is a defect in the superior portion of the sternum. There is cephalic orientation of the cardiac apex and complete absence of the parietal pericardium. Double outlet right ventricle and left ventricular hypoplasia were present. Extracardiac defects were also present as evidenced by the bilateral cleft lip and palate. Chromosome analysis was normal. (Image courtesy of William D. Edwards). (b) Fetal echocardiogram demonstrating the findings noted in (a) with thoracocervical ectopia cordis.

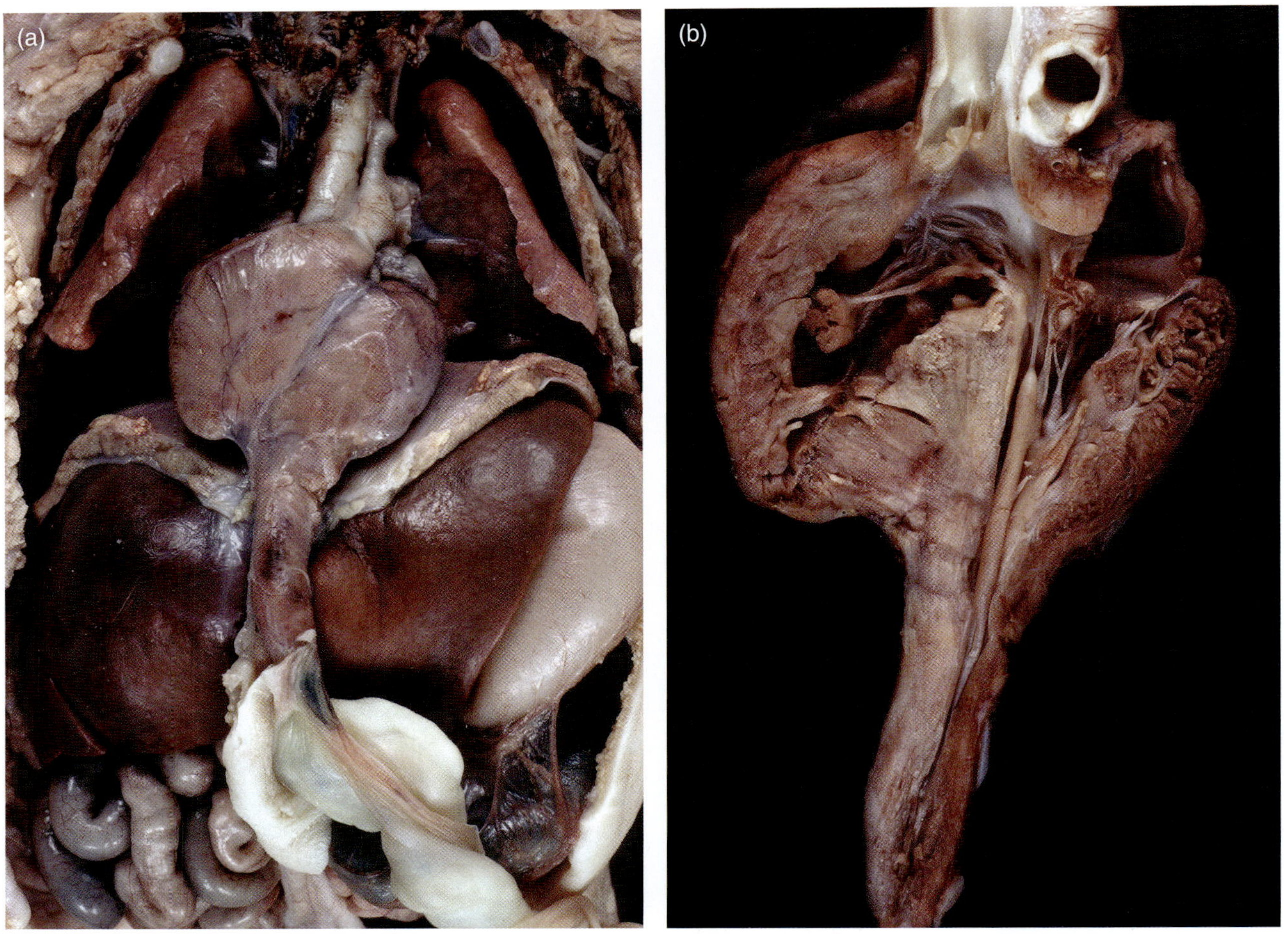

Figure 55.7 (a) Left ventricular apical diverticulum (opened thoracoabdominal cavities, viewed anteriorly). The diverticulum passes through an anterior midline diaphragmatic defect and down to the level of the umbilicus. As a result, the apical direction is inferiorly (representing mesocardia, with two distinct ventricular apexes).The pericardial defect is along the diaphragmatic (inferior) aspect of the pericardial sac. (b) Internal cardiac structures, after removal of anterior half of heart, showing a large ventricular septal defect and origin of the aorta from the right ventricle. The elongated left ventricular apical diverticulum extends toward the umbilicus. Note the markedly elongated posteromedial mitral papillary muscle that has been pulled down into the diverticulum as well.

References

1 Southworth H, Stevenson CS. (1938) Congenital defects of the pericardium. *Arch Intern Med*, **61**, 223–240.
2 Van Praagh R, Weinberg PM, Smith SD, *et al.* (1989) Malpositions of the heart, in, *Heart Disease in Infants, Children, and Adolescents*, 4th edn, (eds FA Adams, GC Emmanouilides, TA Riemenschneider), Williams & Wilkins, Baltimore, p. 530.
3 Cantrell JR, Haller JA, Ravitch MM. (1958) A syndrome of congenital defects involving the abdominal wall, sternum, diaphragm, pericardium, and heart. *Surg Gynecol Obstet*, **107**, 602.
4 Ellis K, Leeds NE, Himmelstein A. (1959) Congenital deficiencies in the parietal pericardium: a review with two new cases including successful diagnosis by plain roentgenography. *Am J Roentgenol Radium Ther Nucl Med*, **182**, 125.
5 Van Son JAM, Danielson GK, Schaff HV, *et al.* (1993) Congenital partial and complete absence of the pericardium. *Mayo Clin Proc*, **68**, 743–747.
6 Kanagasuntheram R, Verzin JA. (1962) Ectopia cordis in man. *Thorax*, **17**, 159–167.
7 Leca F, Thibert M, Khoury W, *et al.* (1989) Extrathoracic heart (ectopia cordis): report of two cases and review of the literature. *Int J Cardiol*, **22**, 221–228.
8 Toyama WM. (1972) Combined congenital defects of the anterior abdominal wall, sternum, diaphragm, pericardium, and heart: a case report and review of the syndrome. *Pediatrics*, **50**, 778.

9 Saxena NC. (1976) Ectopia cordis child surviving: prosthesis fails. *Pediatr News*, **10**, 3.
10 Dobel ARC, Williams HB, Long RW. (1982) Staged repair of ectopia cordis. *J Pediatr Surg*, **17**, 353.
11 Scott GW. (1955) Ectopia cordis: report of a case successfully treated by operation. *Guy's Hosp Rep*, **104**, 55.

56

Miscellaneous Chest Abnormalities Affecting the Heart: Diaphragmatic Hernia and Eventration; Congenital Cystic Adenomatoid Malformation of the Lung

Mark Wylam

Division of Pediatric Pulmonology and Critical Care Medicine, Department of Pediatric and Adolescent Medicine, Mayo Clinic, Rochester, MN, USA

Diaphragmatic Hernia

Congenital diaphragmatic hernia (CDH) is defined as the presence of an orifice in the diaphragm that permits herniation of abdominal contents into the thorax (Figure 56.1). The finding is more common on the left and located posterolaterally. The estimated incidence of CDH is 1 in 2000–5000 births [1]. Two percent of the cases are familial, and using high-resolution molecular cytogenetic 30% of the patients have been found to have a single gene or chromosomal abnormality [2]. About one-third of patients have cardiovascular malformations [3] and lesser proportions have skeletal, neural, genitourinary, gastrointestinal, or other defects. As many as 13% of CHD are undiagnosed in infancy. Ultimately, the severity of this pathology depends on the magnitude of pulmonary hypoplasia, degree of pulmonary hypertension, and non-pulmonary associated malformations.

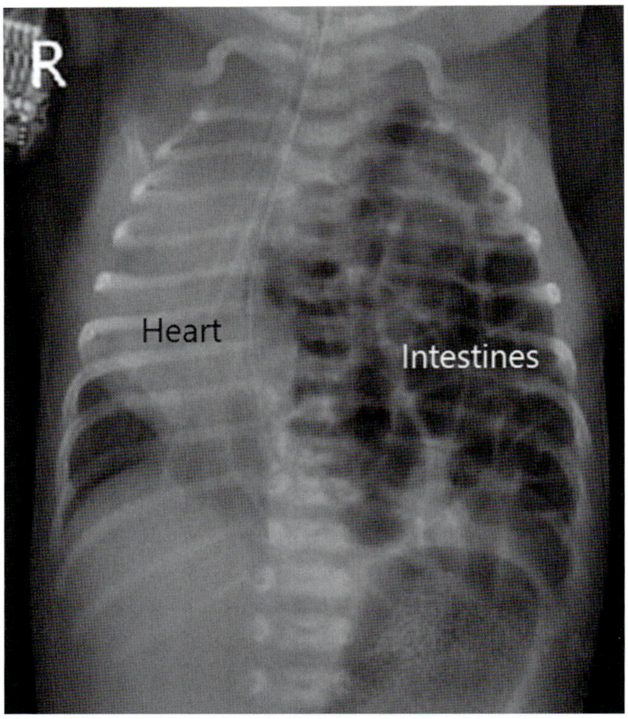

Figure 56.1 Frontal anteroposterior (AP) roentgenogram of an infant with a left-sided diaphragmatic hernia. Note the intestinal contents present in the left chest. The heart is deviated to the right chest by the herniated viscera.

Embryologic Development of the Diaphragm

The diaphragm muscle (DIAm) is the major muscle providing mechanical action of inspiration in mammals. The DIAm is also involved in several non-ventilatory motor behaviors such as coughing, defecation, emesis, micturition, parturition, sneezing, vocalization, and weight lifting.

The embryologic origin of the DIAm has been elucidated using molecular markers such as transcription factor *Mrg1,* a marker for the septum transverum [4], which reflects a common origin of the DIAm in the pleuroperitoneal fold [5]. The pleuroperitoneal fold forms a partition separating the coelomic cavity into thoracic (superior; containing the developing heart and pericardium) and abdominal (inferior; containing the future peritoneal cavity) portions. Growth of the embryonic axis causes a progressive caudal displacement of the pleuroperitoneal fold, with its anterior edge eventually becoming attached at the mid-thoracic level while its dorsal edge becomes attached at the lowest thoracic level [6]. Committed myoblasts migrate within the pleuroperitoneal fold and eventually differentiate to form DIAm myotubes and myofibers. Coincident with myoblast migration, the phrenic nerves exit the cervical spinal cord with phrenic motor axons and begin branching within the pleuroperitoneal fold as myoblasts radiate into the dorsocostal, sternocostal, and crural regions of the DIAm [7]. It remains clear that the musculature of the diaphragm has a distinct origin compared to the thoracic wall. In murine models, the receptor-protein encoded by c-met is essential for the delamination and

Visual Guide to Neonatal Cardiology, First Edition. Edited by Ernerio T. Alboliras, Ziyad M. Hijazi, Leo Lopez, and Donald J. Hagler.

migration of diaphragm myocytes yet its absence yields normal thoracic wall muscularization [8].

In humans, fetal breathing movements detected by ultrasonography begin at about 10 weeks' gestation. As these breathing movements alter fetal intrathoracic pressure they affect fluid movement within the trachea. Reduction in tracheal fluid movement elicits a significant reduction in fetal lung development. In fetuses with severe lung hypoplasia there is a significant reduction in displaced fluid. Accordingly, the assessment of tracheal fluid movement by prenatal Doppler ultrasound may be a useful predictor of outcome in CDH [9]. Eventually, the DIAm becomes rhythmically active during late fetal development (fetal respiratory movements), as at birth it must be ready to sustain ventilation.

Postnatal Anatomy and Physiology of the Diaphragm

The diaphragm is a dome-shaped structure, consisting of a central tendon (aponeurosis) which is perforated by the vena cava and is surrounded by a ring of predominantly radially oriented striated muscle, the musculus diaphragma. The muscular part of the diaphragm has crural (crus mediale and laterale) and sternocostal parts. The tendons of the crural diaphragm are joined with those the vertebral column. The crural diaphragm bears foramina for the esophagus and aorta. Except in pathologic situations, the diaphragm completely separates the paired pleural cavities from the abdomen. In general, it is obliquely oriented in the body cavity, the dorsal margin extending further caudally than the ventral one. Postnatally, the DIAm is one of the most active skeletal muscles, with a duty cycle (time active versus relaxed) of ~30–40%, compared to limb muscles (duty cycles ranging from 2 to 15%) [10].

Types of Congenital Diaphragmatic Hernia

Posterolateral (Bochdalek) hernias (95% of all CHD) are formed when abdominal contents fail to be excluded from the chest and the pleuroperitoneal canal remains open. Most commonly, this occurs on the left posterolateral side (80%) but is occasionally bilateral. The contents of the hernia include fat, omentum, or spleen, small or large intestine. Agenesis of the diaphragm is likely the severe end of the spectrum of Bochdalek hernia. Rarely, Bochdalek hernia can be discovered incidentally in adults, where 68% occur on the right side. Non-posterolateral (Morgagni) hernias (2% of all CHD) occur anteriorly (mostly on the right side) through a defect resulting from failure of the anterior pleuroperitoneal membrane to fuse with the sternum and costal cartilages. Most are accompanied by a hernia sac and are commonly asymptomatic. Much less common are anterior hernias associated with defects in the midline abdominal wall, lower sternum, and pericardium.

Etiology of CDH

Genetic defects have been identified in a minority of patients with CDH [11]. Maternal deficiency in vitamin A intake, genetic defects in retionoid signaling, and retinoid-dependent diaphragm genes are linked to risk of developing CDH. A CDH-like phenotype has been linked to a deficient maternal intake of vitamin A [12], genetic defects in retinoid signaling [13], and the expression of retinoid-related genes in the primordial diaphragm [14]. In humans, CDH has been linked to deleted or duplicated chromosomal regions that contain genes related to the vitamin A pathway (Klaassens *et al.* [11, 15], as well as a case–control study showing that below recommended dietary vitamin A intake was significantly associated with an increased risk of a child with CDH.

Congenital Heart Disease in CDH

Congenital heart disease is the most common lesion associated with CDH, occurring in 10–35% of patients with CDH. Though isolated CDH is more common in males, there is no sex-based difference in CDH associated with heart defects. Overall, atrial septal defects (34%) and ventricular septal defects (23%) are the most common types of congenital heart defects in CDG. In a review from the Children's Hospital of Philadelphia of 174 patients with CDH, the incidence of heart disease was 17.8%, with left heart obstruction (coarctation of the aorta, aortic arch hypoplasia, and hypoplastic left heart syndrome) accounting for 32% of the defects [16]. Of this group, 29% had significant non-cardiac or chromosomal anomalies. In contrast, only 11.1% of the CDH alone group had additional anomalies. The influence of comorbid congenital heart disease in CDH is both varied and significant. The apparent additional risk of death is 2.9 times greater for patients with congenital heart disease compared with those without the disease [16]. Some of this excess mortality was as a result of significant pulmonary hypoplasia.

In a larger series of 2636 collected from the CDH study group, survival was lower in patients with hemodynamically significant cardiac defects (n = 280; 11% of cohort) compared with those without cardiac defects (41% versus 70%) [17]. In that report, cardiac lesions included ventricular septal defects (n = 118), aortic arch obstruction (n = 42), single ventricle anatomy (n = 39), and tetralogy of Fallot variants (n = 31).

A more recent report from the CDH study group found that survival had not improved in 2006–2010 compared to 2000–2005 [18]. Moreover, factors that predicted lower survival were birth weight <2.5 kg, associated non-cardiac anomalies, single ventricle physiology, no sildenafil therapy, no CDH repair, and no cardiac repair. Survival was lowest in infants with transposition of great arteries (0%) and single ventricle physiology (16%). Survival of patients with CDH and CHD supported by extracorporeal membrane oxygenation (ECMO) have a better short-term prognosis than predicted above. Data from the Extracorporeal Life Support Organization revealed an overall survival to hospital discharge of 47% in 3343 cases of CDH with a 9.5% coincidence of CHD [19].

Newborn Pathophysiology in CDH

Infants born with CDH present with a multitude of problems. The affected lung is intrinsically abnormal, as all stages of lung development are affected. Lungs from fetuses and children with CDH have reduced numbers of airways and alveoli (pulmonary hypoplasia), abnormal differentiation of type II pneumocytes (surfactant deficiency), and reduced numbers of pulmonary arteries per unit lung volume (elevated pulmonary vascular resistance) [18]. Moreover, the intrapulmonary arteries become excessively muscularized during gestation with thickened adventitia and media; and this over-muscularization extends peripherally. These pulmonary vessels display an abnormal response to vasoactive substances and hypoxic pulmonary vasoconstriction (variable pulmonary hypertension) [18]. Taken together, these problems elicit hypoxemia, hypercapnia, and right heart limited cardiac output and shock. Not unexpectedly, these fundamental pathophysiologies contribute to persistent fetal circulation with right to left shunting at the level of patent foramen ovale and ductus arteriosus.

Diagnosis of CDH

Routine ultrasound scans of pregnant women in the second trimester have increased the antenatal detection rate of CDH. A recent European study reported a 59% antenatal detection rate; the average gestational age at diagnosis was 24.2 weeks [20]. Typical findings are the presence of the stomach or loops of bowel within the thoracic cavity and mediastinal shift away from the side of the lesion. Dedicated antenatal echocardiography is obligatory. The diagnosis can be missed if the stomach is not in the thorax and right-sided defects are more difficult to diagnose. Estimates of lung volume using three-dimensional ultrasound or magnetic resonance imaging (MRI) may reveal the degree of pulmonary hypoplasia, which strongly determines outcome [20]. The best fetal lung volume (FLV) ratio to predicted lung volume to predict mortality with 100% specificity was 30% of expected FLV.

Pre- and Postnatal Management of CDH

Recent advances in intensive neonatal care, including ECMO, nitric oxide inhalation, high-frequency ventilation, and delayed operative repair of the diaphragmatic hernia, have reduced mortality for full-term fetuses without liver herniation and a favorable lung: head ratio (above 1.4) at tertiary centers [21]. Anticipated survival approaches 80%. However, as pulmonary hypoplasia is a fundamental problem, in utero repair has been used to improve lung growth prior to birth. Direct anatomic repair of the hernia during open hysterotomy had high mortality and was abandoned. Alternatively, fetal surgery occluding the trachea with a detachable silicone balloon placed with a fetal bronchoscopy through a single 5-mm uterine port is designed to allow lung-derived amniotic fluid to maintain lung volume and growth which is otherwise limited by external lung compression by abdominal contents. This procedure is then followed at delivery using hysterotomy followed by the EXIT procedure (ex utero intrapartum treatment), to deflate and remove the intratracheal balloon and administer exogenous surfactant prior to delivery [22]. However, a recent randomized controlled trial of tracheal occlusion in fetuses with no liver herniation demonstrated no survival benefit over standard postnatal therapy [23]. Nevertheless, it is possible that severely affected fetuses with liver herniation are a subgroup that may benefit from this in utero intervention.

The beneficial effects of prenatal use of corticosteroids for infants with CDH remain unproven despite experimental studies involving CDH animal models having shown that corticosteroids result in accelerated synthesis and release of surfactant and improvement in lung morphology and compliance. To date, small case series have reported a favorable effect of steroid administration prior to birth in infants with CDH, but the potential benefits of improved lung function may not outweigh the risks to the development of other vital organs [24].

Initial post-delivery management begins with conventional open strategy protected lung conventional ventilation [25] to maintain the partial pressure of arterial carbon dioxide in the range of 45–60 mmHg (permissive hypercapnia) and preductal oxygen saturation of 90% or higher. If ventilation and oxygenation goals are not met, high frequency oscillation, inhaled nitric oxide, and ECMO are used. Permissive hypercapnia has supplanted aggressive hyperventilation to lower pulmonary vascular resistance (PVR). Surfactant therapy is commonly given but is not associated with a beneficial effect on survival, need for ECMO, or incidence of chronic lung disease in term infants with no other major anomalies [26].

Typically, the surgical repair of the CDH takes place only after the infant's respiratory status has stabilized

[21]. The infant remains sedated from birth until 24 hours after operative repair. The surgical approach to repair of live-born infants with CDH remains variable despite overwhelming use of open abdominal surgery. Minimally invasive surgical repair, both laparoscopic and more commonly thoracoscopic, has gained popularity. The need for ECMO is 33% and patch repair of the diaphragm 52% [27]. Delay in repair and preoperative stabilization results in surgery typically on day 6–7 of life.

Presentation of CHD after infancy, so-called delayed presentation, may be a result of the acute onset of respiratory distress or gastrointestinal symptoms [28]. Infection or incarceration of bowel contents in the chest may occur. The later the presentation, the less compensatory growth of lung volume is anticipated.

Outcome and Prognosis of CDH

Overall survival is 83%. Overall recurrence for CDH is 2.9%, and even higher if a patch repair is necessary. Several cross-sectional studies reveal peripheral airway obstruction in infants [29], children [30], and adults [31] with repaired CDH. Patients with CDH maintain increased airway reactivity compared with a healthy cohort but this decreases as the child gets older [32]. Thus, the presence of an asthma phenotype is increased in CHD. Total lung volumes are normal, with an elevated residual volume indicating air trapping. Although a normal total lung capacity (TLC) suggests the absence of residual lung hypoplasia in CDH, it cannot differentiate between normal lungs and hyperinflated hypoplastic lungs. Significantly increased RV/TLC and decreased levels of diffusing capacity of the lungs for carbon monoxide (DL_{CO}) in patients with CDH suggest persisting abnormal lung structure and decreased diffusion. This abnormal structure leads to an increase in alveolar size [33] and reduced pulmonary vascular bed. From ventilation–perfusion data [34] it is suggested that most of the lung growth in CDH populations between 0.1 to 13 years is caused by the expansion of already existing alveoli and not by increasing numbers of alveoli. Despite minor pulmonary function abnormalities, most children and adolescents with CHD have exercise capacities that do not differ from healthy matched control groups, indicating that the majority of patients do not have significant physical impairment [35].

Eventration and Diaphragm Paresis

Eventration

The diaphragm can be positioned abnormally high in the thorax without herniation. Congenital eventration results from inadequate development of the diaphragm contractile elements or, less commonly, the absence of the phrenic nerve. Acquired eventration is usually a result of injury to the phrenic nerve from traumatic birth or incidental to cardiac surgery for congenital heart disease (diaphragm paresis). Eventually, regardless of cause, some part of the diaphragmatic muscle is replaced by fibroelastic tissue.

Epidemiology of Eventration and Acquired Diaphragm Paralysis

The incidence of congenital eventration remains uncertain, although one study reported the condition to be minor in 4% of normal births and 0.1% in more complete eventrations [36]. Males are affected more than females and right-sided eventration is more frequent, or at least more symptomatic. Congenital eventrations can be isolated, although they are sometimes associated with other developmental defects such as cleft palate, congenital heart disease, situs inversus, or undescended testicle [37]. Paralysis of diaphragm on one or, exceptionally, both sides is a common cause of delayed recovery and excessive morbidity following pediatric cardiac surgery. The phrenic nerve can be injured by the ice cold slush used for myocardial protection. The left phrenic nerve can be damaged while removing thymus or during the dissection of the vertical pulmonary vein in patients undergoing repair of total anomalous pulmonary venous return. Trauma to the nerve can occur while dissecting near the superior vena or from adherent lung during re-operations. During pericardiectomy for constrictive pericarditis, accidental damage to sever the phrenic nerve on one or both sides can occur.

The incidence of diaphragm paralysis following surgery for CHD ranges from 0.28% to 5.6% [38]. The incidence is particularly high after the bidirectional Glenn or Fontan operations, systemic to pulmonary artery shunts particularly the classic or modified Blalock–Taussig (BT) shunt (11.1%), ventricular septal defect closure, surgery for tetralogy of Fallot (31.5%), and arterial switch operation (11.1%).

Pathogenesis of Eventration

In congenital eventration, the muscular defect can be either partial or diffuse [39]. In the former, the defect is localized; whereas in the latter, the diaphragm consists of a thin, diaphanous membrane that is attached peripherally to normal muscle. In one series, partial defects, mostly affecting the right anterior hemidiaphragm, occurred in 65% of children [40]. Diffuse defects tend to be unilateral but occur more commonly on the left side. In the acquired form, the central tendon is normal and the diaphragm consists of normally developed muscle that is atrophic. The phrenic nerve is typically small and both sides are affected equally.

Clinical Features of Eventration

Most adult patients are asymptomatic, especially when the eventration is localized [41]. In older children, unilateral diaphragmatic paralysis or complete eventration reduces forced vital capacity (FVC) by 25% and is usually well tolerated [42]. In infants, moderate or greater diaphragm elevation compresses the ipsilateral lung which is exacerbated by elevation and angulation of the stomach and worsened by feeding. In newborns, the degree of respiratory distress can be increased by congenital lung hypoplasia on the affected side and if the mediastinum is shifted, hypoplasia can also occur on the contralateral side. Acquired unilateral paresis may be sufficient to elicit respiratory failure in neonates whose relatively compliant chest wall is a mechanical disadvantage. Additionally, atelectic compression of the lung bases can promote bronchopneumonia. Although respiratory signs prevail, gastrointestinal issues such as feeding intolerance, gastric reflux, and vomiting often predominate.

Diagnosis of Eventration

The diagnosis of eventration or paresis should be considered in infants with respiratory distress or when incidentally noted on chest radiograph. Typically, the diagnosis is confirmed by fluoroscopy or ultrasonography. Diaphragm movement during breathing typically is minimal or the diaphragm may move paradoxically.

Management of Eventration

Congenital eventration is unlikely to improve acutely and traumatic diaphragm paresis has an unpredictable recovery. Following surgery for CHD, recovery is possible but may require 6–12 months, with 16% never recovering [43, 44]. The management of eventration depends upon the severity of respiratory distress. Mild distress can be managed supportively, including supplemental oxygen. Moderate distress can require nasogastric feeding to provide adequate nutrition. More severe respiratory distress may necessitate mechanical ventilation or surgical plication [45]. A plication procedure reduces the surface area of the diaphragm by surgical pleating. This procedure can reposition the diaphragm lower in the thorax, reducing atelectasis and improving functional residual capacity (FRC). It also minimizes paradoxical motion and improves ventilation generated by intercostal and abdominal muscles during breathing. Some recommend continuous positive airway pressure (CPAP) (8–10 cmH_2O) to identify patients who will respond to plication as CPAP reduces paradoxical motion and increases functional residual capacity [46].

In larger infants, video-assisted thoracic surgery can offer a less invasive approach because it avoids incision of the lower intercostal muscles, which may adversely affect ventilation. A few reports suggest the procedure may be performed in newborn infants with birth weights as low as 2.2 kg [47]. Early surgical intervention is recommended by some to improve lung growth and reduce the incidence of pneumonia, bronchiectasis, and pneumonia. Long-term outcomes following diaphragm plication are limited. There remains the possibility of phrenic nerve recovery (weeks to months) in patients with acquired eventration.

Congenital Cystic Adenomatoid Malformation of the Lung (Congenital Pulmonary Airway Malformation)

Congenital cystic adenomatoid malformations (CCAM) or congenital pulmonary airway malformation (CPAM) of the lung encompass a spectrum of cystic abnormalities resulting from dysembroygenesis of the end bronchioles with suppression of alveolar growth by a defect in lung embryogenesis [48]. In the modern era, cystic adenomatoid malformations are commonly diagnosed by prenatal ultrasound (Figure 56.2, arrows define the border of the CPAM/CCAM). Interestingly, regression of a CCAM on prenatal ultrasound scan is common, suggesting that the process does not continue after birth [49]. A normal chest X-ray does not indicate complete regression of a CCAM; a computed tomography (CT) scan is required to evaluate such patients, and will generally demonstrate a CCAM.

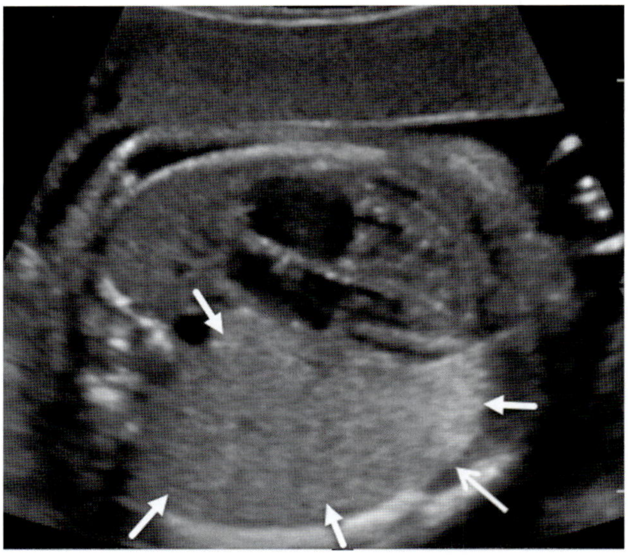

Figure 56.2 Short-axis view of a fetal chest showing the presence of a large left-sided congenital cystic adenomatoid malformation of the lung/congenital pulmonary airway malformation (CCAM/CPAM). The arrows define the border of the CCAM/CPAM. The heart is deviated to the right chest by the pulmonary abnormality.

CCAMs are classified according to type. These attempt to define the anatomic locus of dysembryogensis: type 0 bronchial; type 1 bronchial/bronchiolar; type 2 bronchiolar; type 3 bronchiolar/alveolar duct; and type 4 peripheral. These classification system may be useful as rare bronchioloalveolar carcinomas arise in association with type 1 CCAMs recurrence following resection. Type 4 CCAMs show histologic overlap with grade 1 pleuropulmonary blastomas (a pulmonary form of Wilms tumor spectrum) and distinction between these entities may not be possible on histology alone [50]. Controversy exists but current practice suggests that asymptomatic patients with a CCAM may be followed up non-operatively with no apparent adverse effects. Ensuring involution takes place while guarding against persistence and the rare malignant potential [51]. However, CCAM can cause respiratory symptoms if of sufficient size to compress normal lung or mediastinal structures. Fetal therapies are being performed at many centers for significant CPAM that manifests with fetal cardiovascular complications. These fetal therapeutic procedures include steroid therapy, catheter-based therapy, fetal resection, and the EXIT procedure.

Postnatally, physical examination often demonstrates signs of mediastinal shift with dyspnea, tachypnea, and cyanosis. Urgent lobectomy is indicated and often proves curative. CCAMs that present later in life are typically smaller, and patients present with obstructive pneumonia.

References

1 Torfs CP, Curry CJ, Bateson TF, Honore LH. (1992) A population-based study of congenital diaphragmatic hernia. *Teratology*, **4**, 555–565.

2 Veenma DC, de Klein A, Tibboel D. (2012) Developmental and genetic aspects of congenital diaphragmatic hernia. *Pediatr Pulmonol*, **47**, 534–545.

3 Lin AE, Pober BR, Adatia I. (2007) Congenital diaphragmatic hernia and associated cardiovascular malformations: type, frequency, and impact on management. *Am J Med Genet C Semin Med Genet*, **145C**, 201–216.

4 Dunwoodie SL, Rodriguez TA, Beddington RS. (1998) Msg1 and Mrg1, founding members of a gene family, show distinct patterns of gene expression during mouse embryogenesis. *Mech Dev*, **72**, 27–40.

5 Clugston RD, Greer JJ. (2007) Diaphragm development and congenital diaphragmatic hernia. *Semin Pediatr Surg*, **16**, 94–100.

6 Kluth D, Keijzer R, Hertl M, Tibboel D. (1996) Embryology of congenital diaphragmatic hernia. *Semin Pediatr Surg*, **5**, 224–233.

7 Babiuk RP, Zhang W, Clugston R, Allan DW, Greer JJ. (2003) Embryological origins and development of the rat diaphragm. *J Comp Neurol*, **455**, 477–487.

8 Birchmeier C, Brohmann H. (2000) Genes that control the development of migrating muscle precursor cells. *Curr Opin Cell Biol*, **12**, 725–730.

9 Kalache KD, Chaoui R, Hartung J, Wernecke KD, Bollmann R. (1998) Doppler assessment of tracheal fluid flow during fetal breathing movements in cases of congenital diaphragmatic hernia. *Ultrasound Obstet Gynecol*, **12**, 27–32.

10 Hussain SN, Roussos C, Magder S. (1989) Effects of tension, duty cycle, and arterial pressure on diaphragmatic blood flow in dogs. *J Appl Physiol*, **66**, 968–976.

11 Holder AM, Klaassens M, Tibboel D, *et al*. (2007) Genetic factors in congenital diaphragmatic hernia. *Am J Hum Genet*, **80**, 825–845.

12 Andersen DH. (1949) Effect of diet during pregnancy upon the incidence of congenital hereditary diaphragmatic hernia in the rat; failure to produce cystic fibrosis of the pancreas by maternal vitamin A deficiency. *Am J Pathol*, **25**, 163–185.

13 Mendelsohn C, Lohnes D, Decimo D, *et al*. (1994) Function of the retinoic acid receptors (RARs) during development (II): multiple abnormalities at various stages of organogenesis in RAR double mutants. *Development (Cambridge, England)*, **120**, 2749–2771.

14 Clugston RD, Zhang W, Greer JJ. (2008) Gene expression in the developing diaphragm: significance for congenital diaphragmatic hernia. *Am J Physiol Lung Cell Molec Physiol*, **294**, L665–675.

15 Klaassens M, van Dooren M, Eussen HJ, *et al*. (2005) Congenital diaphragmatic hernia and chromosome 15q26: determination of a candidate region by use of fluorescent in situ hybridization and array-based comparative genomic hybridization. *Am J Hum Genet*, **76**, 877–882.

16 Cohen MS, Rychik J, Bush DM, *et al*. (2002) Influence of congenital heart disease on survival in children with congenital diaphragmatic hernia. *J Pediatr*, **141**, 25–30.

17 Graziano JN, Congenital Diaphragmatic Hernia Study Group. (2005) Cardiac anomalies in patients with congenital diaphragmatic hernia and their prognosis: a report from the Congenital Diaphragmatic Hernia Study Group. *J Pediatr Surg*, **40**, 1045–1049; discussion 1049–1050.

18 Menon SC, Tani LY, Weng HY, *et al.* (2013) Clinical characteristics and outcomes of patients with cardiac defects and congenital diaphragmatic hernia. *J Pediatr*, **162**, 114–119 e2.
19 Dyamenahalli U, Morris M, Rycus P, *et al.* (2013) Short-term outcome of neonates with congenital heart disease and diaphragmatic hernia treated with extracorporeal membrane oxygenation. *Ann Thorac Surg*, **95**, 1373–1376.
20 Garne E, Haeusler M, Barisic I, *et al.* (2002) Congenital diaphragmatic hernia: evaluation of prenatal diagnosis in 20 European regions. *Ultrasound Obstet Gynecol*, **19**, 329–333.
21 Kesieme EB, Kesieme CN. (2011) Congenital diaphragmatic hernia: review of current concept in surgical management. *ISRN Surg*, **2011**, 974041.
22 Bouchard S, Johnson MP, Flake AW, *et al.* (2002) The EXIT procedure: experience and outcome in 31 cases. *J Pediatr Surg*, **37**, 418–426.
23 Harrison MR, Keller RL, Hawgood SB, *et al.* (2003) A randomized trial of fetal endoscopic tracheal occlusion for severe fetal congenital diaphragmatic hernia. *N Engl J Med*, **349**, 1916–1924.
24 Lally KP, Bagolan P, Hosie S, *et al.* (2006) Corticosteroids for fetuses with congenital diaphragmatic hernia: can we show benefit? *J Pediatr Surg*, **41**, 668–674; discussion 674.
25 Vitali SH, Arnold JH. (2005) Bench-to-bedside review: ventilator strategies to reduce lung injury – lessons from pediatric and neonatal intensive care. *Crit Care*, **9**, 177–183.
26 Van Meurs K. (2004) Is surfactant therapy beneficial in the treatment of the term newborn infant with congenital diaphragmatic hernia? *J Pediatr*, **145**, 312–316.
27 Bryner BS, West BT, *et al.*; Congenital Diaphragmatic Hernia Study Group (2009) Congenital diaphragmatic hernia requiring extracorporeal membrane oxygenation: does timing of repair matter? *J Pediatr Surg*, **44**, 1165–1171; discussion 1171–1172.
28 Kitano Y, Lally KP, Lally PA. (2005) Late-presenting congenital diaphragmatic hernia. *J Pediatr Surg*, **40**, 1839–1843.
29 Koumbourlis AC, Wung JT, Stolar CJ. (2006) Lung function in infants after repair of congenital diaphragmatic hernia. *J Pediatr Surg*, **41**, 1716–1721.
30 Peetsold MG, Heij HA, Nagelkerke AF, Deurloo JA, Gemke RJ. (2011) Pulmonary function impairment after trachea-esophageal fistula: a minor role for gastro-esophageal reflux disease. *Pediatr Pulmonol*, **46**, 348–355.
31 Peetsold MG, Vonk-Noordegraaf A, Heij HH, Gemke RJ. (2007) Pulmonary function and exercise testing in adult survivors of congenital diaphragmatic hernia. *Pediatr Pulmonol*, **42**, 325–331.
32 Nakayama DK, Mutich R, Motoyama EK. (1991) Pulmonary dysfunction in surgical conditions of the newborn infant. *Crit Care Med*, **19**, 926–933.
33 Thurlbeck WM, Kida K, Langston C, *et al.* (1979) Postnatal lung growth after repair of diaphragmatic hernia. *Thorax*, **34**, 338–343.
34 Hayward MJ, Kharasch V, Sheils C, *et al.* (2007) Predicting inadequate long-term lung development in children with congenital diaphragmatic hernia: an analysis of longitudinal changes in ventilation and perfusion. *J Pediatr Surg*, **42**, 112–116.
35 Peetsold MG, Heij HA, Nagelkerke AF, *et al.* (2009) Pulmonary function and exercise capacity in survivors of congenital diaphragmatic hernia. *Eur Respir J*, **34**, 1140–1147.
36 Chin EF, Lynn RB. (1956) Surgery of eventration of the diaphragm. *J Thorac Surg*, **32**, 6–14.
37 Smith CD, Sade RM, Crawford FA, Othersen HB. (1986) Diaphragmatic paralysis and eventration in infants. *J Thorac Cardiovasc Surg*, **91**, 490–497.
38 Talwar S, Agarwala S, Mittal CM, Choudhary SK, Airan B. (2010) Diaphragmatic palsy after cardiac surgical procedures in patients with congenital heart. *Ann Pediatr Cardiol*, **3**, 50–57.
39 Visouli AN, Mpakas A, Zarogoulidis P, *et al.* (2012) Video assisted thoracoscopic plication of the left hemidiaphragm in symptomatic eventration in adulthood. *J Thorac Dis*, **4**, 6–16.
40 Wayne ER, Campbell JB, Burrington JD, Davis WS. (1974) Eventration of the diaphragm. *J Pediatr Surg*, **9**, 643–651.
41 Laxdal OE, Mc DH, Mellin GW. (1954) Congenital eventration of the diaphragm. *N Engl J Med*, **250**, 401–408.
42 Robotham JL. (1979) A physiological approach to hemidiaphragm paralysis. *Crit Care Med*, **7**, 563–6.
43 Iverson LI, Mittal A, Dugan DJ, Samson PC. (1976) Injuries to the phrenic nerve resulting in diaphragmatic paralysis with special reference to stretch trauma. *Am J Surg*, **132**, 263–269.
44 Watanabe T, Trusler GA, Williams WG, *et al.* (1987) Phrenic nerve paralysis after pediatric cardiac surgery: retrospective study of 125 cases. *J Thorac Cardiovasc Surg*, **94**, 383–388.
45 Groth SS, Andrade RS. (2010) Diaphragm plication for eventration or paralysis: a review of the literature. *Ann Thorac Surg*, **89**, S2146–2150.
46 de Vries TS, Koens BL, Vos A. (1998) Surgical treatment of diaphragmatic eventration caused by phrenic nerve injury in the newborn. *J Pediatr Surg*, **33**, 602–605.
47 Slater BJ, Meehan JJ. (2009) Robotic repair of congenital diaphragmatic anomalies. *J Laparoendosc Adv Surg Tech A*, **19** (Suppl 1), 123–127.

48 Cangiarella J, Greco MA, Askin F, *et al.* (1995) Congenital cystic adenomatoid malformation of the lung: insights into the pathogenesis utilizing quantitative analysis of vascular marker CD34 (QBEND-10) and cell proliferation marker MIB-1. *Mod Pathol*, **8**, 913–918.

49 van Leeuwen K, Teitelbaum DH, Hirschl RB, *et al.* (1999) Prenatal diagnosis of congenital cystic adenomatoid malformation and its postnatal presentation, surgical indications, and natural history. *J Pediatr Surg*, **34**, 794–798; discussion 798–799.

50 MacSweeney F, Papagiannopoulos K, Goldstraw P, *et al.* (2003) An assessment of the expanded classification of congenital cystic adenomatoid malformations and their relationship to malignant transformation. *Am J Surg Pathol*, **27**, 1139–1146.

51 Aziz D, Langer JC, Tuuha SE, *et al.* (2004) Perinatally diagnosed asymptomatic congenital cystic adenomatoid malformation: to resect or not? *J Pediatr Surg*, **39**, 329–334; discussion 334.

57

Persistent Pulmonary Hypertension of the Newborn

Amish Jain[1,3] *and Mark K. Friedberg*[2,3]

[1] *Division of Neonatology, Department of Pediatrics, Mount Sinai Hospital, Toronto, Canada*
[2] *Division of Pediatric Cardiology, The Labatt Family Heart Center, Hospital for Sick Children, Toronto, Canada*
[3] *Department of Pediatrics, University of Toronto, Toronto, Canada*

Persistent pulmonary hypertension of the newborn (PPHN) is a circulatory disorder unique to the immediate neonatal period. Failure of reduction in the normally high fetal pulmonary vascular resistance (PVR) after birth results in a marked decline in pulmonary blood flow (PBF) and oxygenation capacity of the lungs leading to catastrophic clinical consequences for the neonate (Figure 57.1). A wide range of disorders can be associated with PPHN (Figure 57.2), but birth asphyxia, meconium aspiration syndrome, and sepsis account for the majority of acute cases [1]. Although improved obstetric care has reduced the incidence of these perinatal pathologies, PPHN remains a commonly encountered problem in tertiary neonatal units [2, 3].

Circulatory Pathophysiology

PPHN is a disorder of persistently high right ventricular (RV) afterload (i.e., PVR) resulting in an incompletely understood cycle of reduced PBF, hypoxemia, acidosis, and ventilation–perfusion mismatch (Figure 57.3). Depending on the disease severity, the clinical picture can be complicated by RV dysfunction and/or dilatation, which by virtue of adverse interventricular interactions can compromise left ventricular function [4]. If uncorrected, the clinical picture evolves into that of severe systemic hypoperfusion and shock.

Diagnostic Work-up

PPHN is almost always secondary to an underlying etiology. A careful appraisal of the clinical scenario including a detailed case history and thorough clinical examination provides important etiological clues (Figure 57.4). This is usually followed by a stepwise approach to investigations. While some investigations are standard, others need to be individualized based on the index of suspicion (Table 57.1). Echocardiography is the clinical investigation of choice to confirm the diagnosis of PPHN and to monitor disease progression or response to therapies (Figure 57.5) [5, 6].

Ruling out a critical congenital heart defect can be a decisive factor for infants with suspected PPHN, particularly when the symptoms fail to resolve with standard treatments or when extracorporeal membrane oxygenation (ECMO) is being considered. Many cardiac defects such as total anomalous pulmonary venous drainage, transposition of the great arteries, and Ebstein anomaly can present with hypoxic respiratory failure (HRF) after birth, and delay in appropriate referral can worsen patient outcomes [7, 8]. PPHN can also be an associated finding, thereby requiring a comprehensive echocardiography by an experienced operator (Figure 57.6).

Management Considerations

For neonates presenting with HRF, timely stabilization using standard neonatal resuscitation is necessary for trial of pulmonary vasodilator therapies (Figure 57.7). Most infants with significant PPHN will require invasive ventilatory support. While a short trial of non-invasive ventilation may be acceptable, close clinical monitoring is essential to ensure timely escalation. The goal of ventilation strategy should be to establish adequate alveolar recruitment and carbon dioxide clearance while avoiding lung hyperexpansion. Important concepts relevant to the management of PPHN are summarized in Figure 57.8 [9–11].

Visual Guide to Neonatal Cardiology, First Edition. Edited by Ernerio T. Alboliras, Ziyad M. Hijazi, Leo Lopez, and Donald J. Hagler.

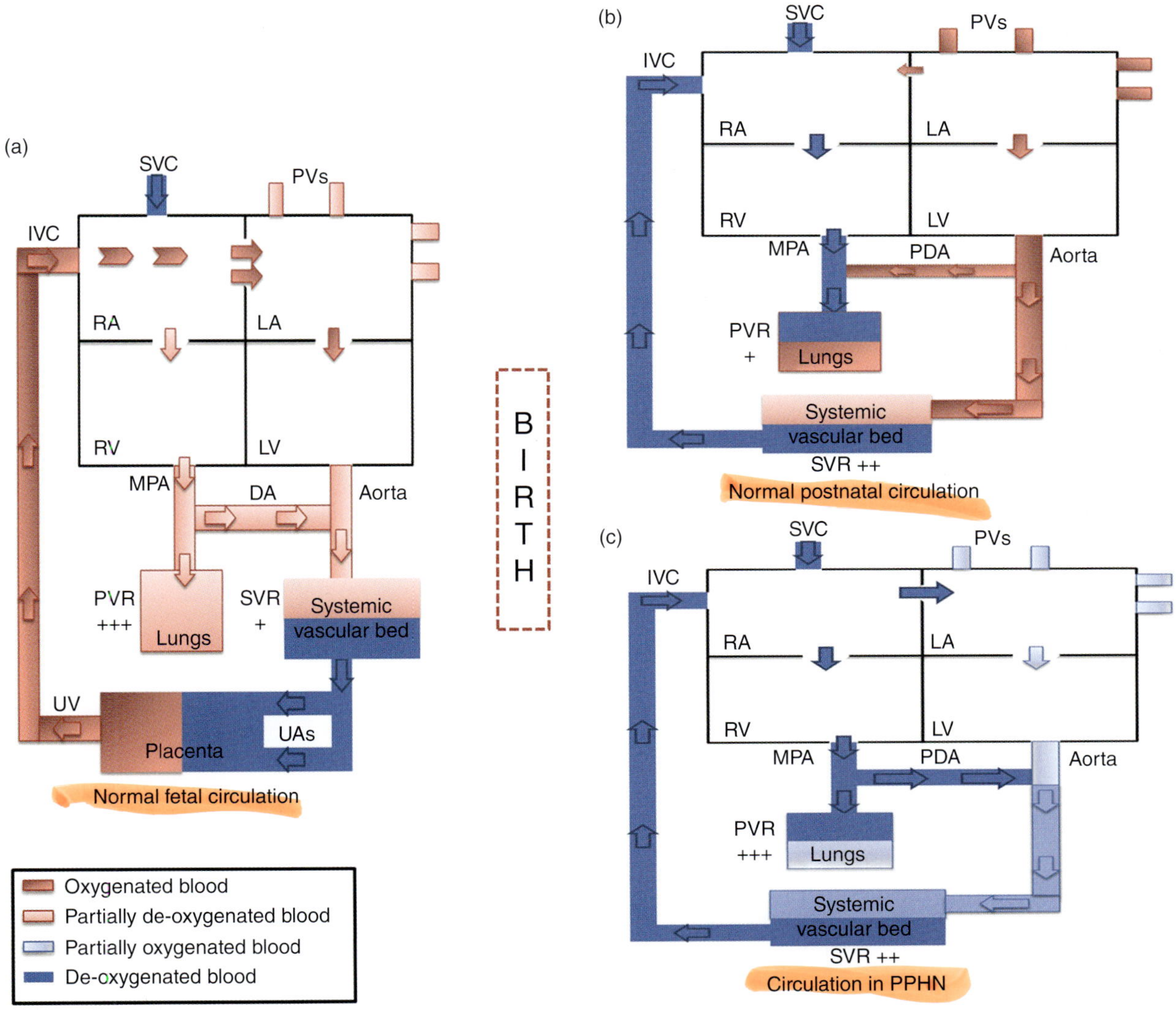

Figure 57.1 (a) In normal circulation during fetal life, high pulmonary vascular resistance (PVR) allows for shunting of oxygenated placental blood away from the pulmonary into systemic circulation at the atrial and ductal levels. (b) The immediate postnatal period is characterized by marked reduction in PVR with relatively mild increase in systemic vascular resistance (SVR). The fetal shunts may persist for days after birth but are rarely of hemodynamic significance. (c) Following birth in infants with PPHN, there is persistently high PVR, pulmonary-to-systemic shunting of deoxygenated blood, and markedly reduced lung function. DA, ductus arteriosus; IVC/SVC, inferior and superior vena cava; MPA, main pulmonary artery; PDA, patent ductus arteriosus; PV, pulmonary vein; PVR/SVR, pulmonary and systemic vascular resistance; RA/LA, right and left atrium; RV/LV, right and left ventricle; UV/UA, umbilical vein and artery.

Inhaled nitric oxide (iNO) is the only approved pulmonary vasodilator therapy for PPHN. Although it has reduced the need for ECMO, the mortality and long-term morbidities have not changed [3, 12]. Escalating costs and a high rate of non-responders (40–50%) have prompted investigators to explore other cellular pathways (Figure 57.9). Successful use of other agents has been reported, but none have been tested in large clinical trials. [13–16].

Conclusions

PPHN is a serious and complex circulatory problem of the neonatal period. It is imperative that clinicians familiarize themselves with the disease physiology and specific concepts to be able to avoid common pitfalls. Prompt recognition, exclusion of critical congenital heart disease, and early effective management is important to ensure optimal patient outcomes.

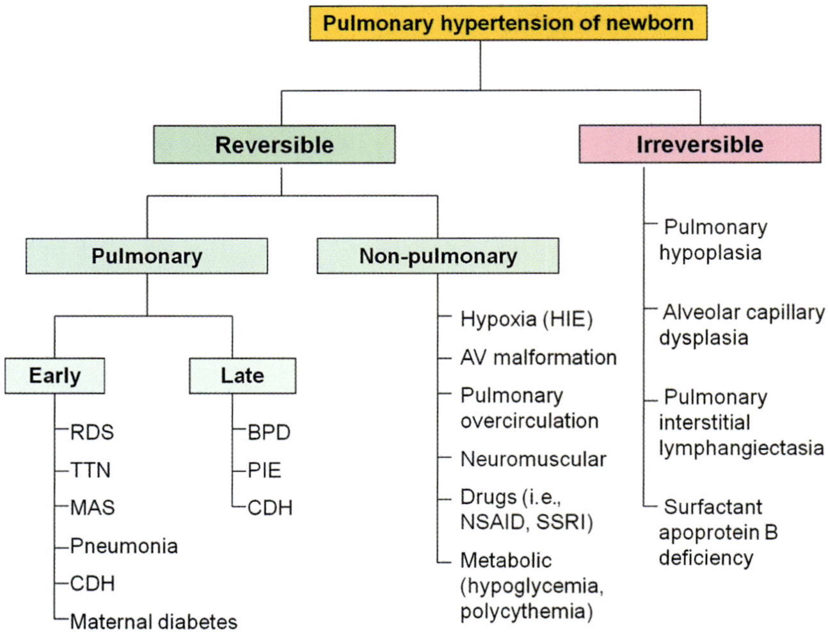

Figure 57.2 Pulmonary and extrapulmonary pathologies associated with pulmonary hypertension during the neonatal period. AV, arteriovenous; BPD, bronchopulmonary dysplasia; CDH, congenital diaphragmatic hernia; HIE hypoxic ischemic encephalopathy; MAS, meconium aspiration syndrome; NSAID, non-steroidal anti-inflammatory drug; PIE, pulmonary interstitial emphysema; RDS, respiratory distress syndrome; SSRI, selective serotonin reuptake inhibitor; TTN, transient tachypnea of newborn. *Source*: Jain and McNamara 2013 [1]. Reproduced with permission from Bentham Science Publishers.

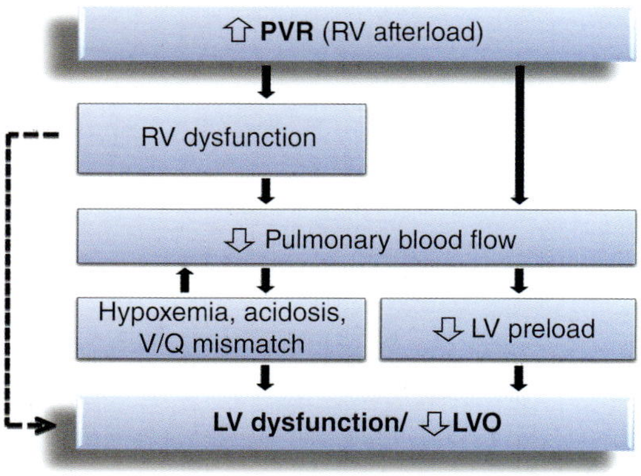

Figure 57.3 Pathophysiology and hemodynamic alterations associated with PPHN. LV, left ventricle; LVO, left ventricular output; PVR, pulmonary vascular resistance; RV, right ventricle; V/Q ventilation perfusion. *Source*: Jain and McNamara 2013 [1]. Reproduced with permission from Bentham Science Publishers.

History

Family history:
- Previous neonatal deaths
- Consanguinity

Current pregnancy:
- Maternal diseases – diabetes, depression
- Drug exposure – SSRI, NSAIDs, other prescribed or illicit drugs
- Maternal serum screen – trisomy 21
- Antenatal ultrasounds – structural anomalies (CDH, CHD, AVM); oligohydramnios (pulmonary hypoplasia); fetal growth (IUGR – polycythemia, hypoglycemia)

Perinatal events:
- Infection risks – PROM, GBS colonization, chorioamnioitis (maternal fever, uterine tenderness, raised WCC)
- Evidence of fetal distress on CTG
- Mode of delivery (elective CS)
- Green liquor (meconium aspiration, listeria sepsis)

Symptoms
- Respiratory distress – grunting, tachypnea, intercoastal and subcoastal recessions
- Excessive oral secretions (TTN; TEF)
- Lethargy
- Poor feeding
- Central cyanosis if hypoxemia severe

Signs
- Hypotonia, dysmorphism
- Lability – respiratory distress and hypoxemia worsens on handling
- Scaphoid abdomen (CDH)
- Meconium stained umbilical cord (MAS)
- Auscultation – Crepitations / reduced breath sounds (associated parenchymal lung disease)
- Heart sounds shifted to right (CDH)
- Rule out signs suggestive of CHD
- Low saturations on pulse oximetry
- Pre-ductal saturation higher than post-ductal (significant right to left shunt at the ductal level)
- Hepatomegaly (right heart pressure overload)
- Signs of circulatory failure – prolong CRT, weak peripheral pulses, hypotension

Figure 57.4 Systematic appraisal of clinical history and examination may point to underlying etiology. A positive family history may suggest a genetic etiology (such as surfactant protein deficiency syndromes, alveolar capillary dysplasia). Respiratory distress is a hallmark feature of PPHN and its absence in a hypoxemic neonate raises suspicion for alternate etiologies (such as cyanotic CHD, myopathies). AVM, arteriovenous malformation; CDH, congenital diaphragmatic hernia; CHD, congenital heart defect; CRT, capillary refill time; CS, caesarean section; CTG, cardiotocography; GBS, group B streptococcus; IUGR, intrauterine growth restriction; MAS, meconium aspiration syndrome; NSAID, non-steroidal anti-inflammatory drug; PROM, premature rupture of membranes; SSRI, selective serotonin reuptake inhibitor; TEF, tracheo-esophageal fistula; TTN, transient tachypnea of newborn; WCC, white cell count.

Table 57.1 Investigations and their rationale for infants suspected to have persistent pulmonary hypertension of the newborn (PPHN).

Investigations		Rationale
Blood – standard	Blood culture, C-reactive protein Complete blood count, blood group Blood glucose, electrolytes	Screen for sepsis Rule out anemia, hypoglycemia, electrolyte disturbances
	Serum lactate ABG	Evaluate systemic perfusion Rule out acidosis, hypercarbia
Blood – special cases	ABG with hyperoxia test	Screen for critical cyanotic heart defect
	Liver, renal function tests Coagulation screen (INR, PT, APTT) Serum ammonia	Evaluate for end-organ dysfunction (e.g., in sepsis, asphyxia) Rule out coagulopathy Metabolic screen
	Genetic testing Karyotyping Screen for specific mutations	Presence of dysmorphic features Suspicion of familial causes (surfactant protein deficiency, ACD)

(Continued)

Table 57.1 (Continued)

Investigations		Rationale
Imaging – standard	Chest X-ray	Position of endotracheal tube
	(with nasogastric or orogastric tube in situ)	Rule out pneumothorax
		Parenchymal lung disease (e.g., RDS, MAS)
		Structural lung defects (e.g., CDH, esophageal atresia)
		Abnormal heart shape (e.g., 'snowman' shape in TAPVD; narrow mediastinum with egg-shape heart in TGA; massive cardiomegaly in Ebstein anomaly)
		RVH – boot-shaped heart with apex 'lifted' from the diaphragm
	Abdominal X-ray	Confirm position of umbilical lines
	Echocardiogram	Confirm diagnosis and monitor progress
		Rule out CHD
Imaging – special cases	Cranial ultrasound	AVMs (vein of Galen malformation)
		Evidence of brain injury
	Chest CT scan	Pulmonary lymphangiectasia
Pathology	Lung biopsy	ACD; surfactant protein deficiency

ABG, arterial blood gas; ACD, alveolar capillary dysplasia; APTT, activated partial thromboplastin time; AVM, arteriovenous malformation; CDH, congenital diaphragmatic hernia; CHD, congenital heart defect; CT, computed tomography; INR, international normalized ratio; MAS, meconium aspiration syndrome; PT, prothrombin time; RDS, respiratory distress syndrome; RVH, right ventricle hypertrophy; TAPVD, total anomalous pulmonary venous drainage; TGA, transposition of great arteries.

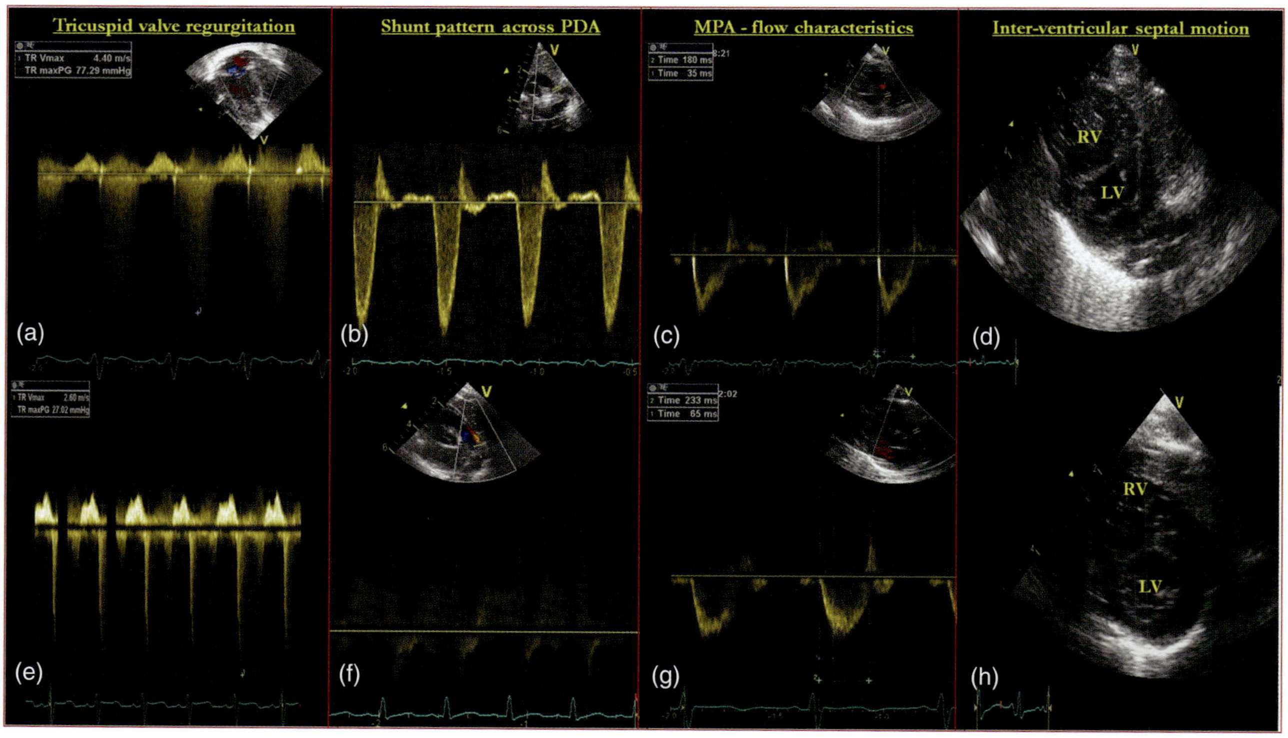

Figure 57.5 Echocardiography in an infant with PPHN before (a–d) and after successful treatment with inhaled nitric oxide (e–h). (a,e) Tricuspid regurgitation (TR) can quantify peak systolic pressure gradient across tricuspid valve (TRmaxPG). Peak systolic pulmonary artery pressure = TRmaxPG + estimated right atrial pressure. (b,f) Doppler of patent ductus arteriosus (PDA). In (b), the majority of shunting is from the main pulmonary artery to aorta during systole indicated by Doppler flow below the reference line (away from the transducer), suggesting suprasystemic systolic pulmonary artery pressure. (c,g) Doppler of the main pulmonary artery. Pulmonary artery acceleration time (PAAT, time 1 in figures) and right ventricular ejection time (RVET, time 2 in figures) can indirectly estimate pulmonary vascular resistance (PVR). High PVR is associated with short PAAT and high RVET : PAAT ratio. (d,h) Qualitative appraisal of the curvature of the interventricular septum in systole. The 'flat' septum in (d) indicates at least half systemic right ventricular (RV) pressure. Following treatment, the septum assumes a more leftward concavity (h) suggesting lower RV pressure.

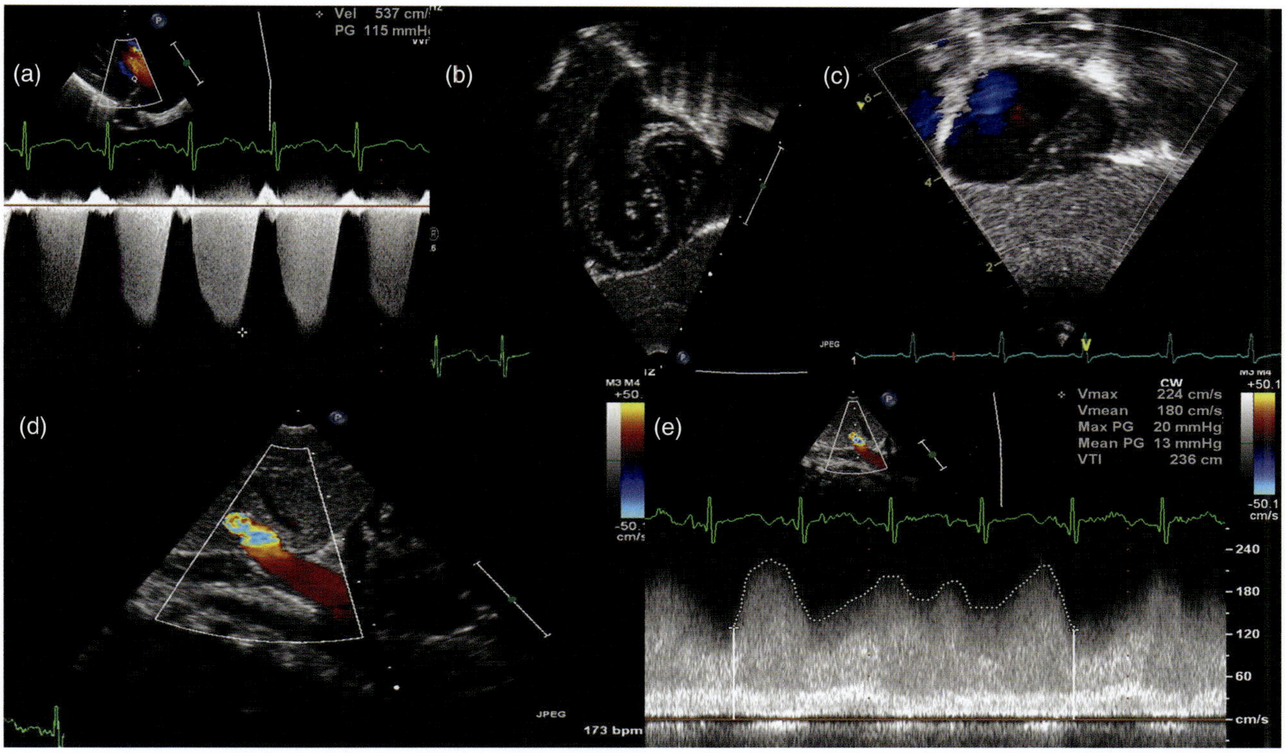

Figure 57.6 Typical echocardiogram in a newborn with PPHN who failed to respond to vasodilator therapy: (a) severe tricuspid regurgitation; (b) flat interventricular septum; (c) right to left atrial shunt. Further imaging revealed a vertical vein from all the pulmonary veins draining into the portal circulation. (d) Doppler interrogation showed an obstructed venous flow pattern. (e) Obstructed total anomalous pulmonary venous drainage can present as PPHN and must be excluded to ensure correct management.

Suggested management approach for infants presenting with HRF at birth

Resuscitation

Airway - assess patency
- Is the infant apneic?
- Visualize oral cavity for obstruction (secretions, meconium)

Breathing
- Are there signs of respiratory distress (mild, moderate or severe)?
- Obtain pre-ductal pulse oximetry (on right hand)
- Provide O_2 therapy to maintain SpO_2 in normal range (>95%)
- Establish - Is SpO_2 responsive to O_2 therapy?
  - FiO_2 reqired to maintain normal SpO_2
- Assess need for respiratory support - noninvasive (CPAP) vs. invasive (CMV/HFV)
- **Aim** for adequate lung expansion (indicated by CXR and normal $PaCO_2$)
- Persistent high FiO_2 - Apply additional post-ductal pulse oximetry (on foot)
- Establish - Is there a pre- and post-ductal SpO_2 difference? Is the infant labile?
  - Calculate oxygenation index [OI = (FiO_2 x MAP)/PaO_2]
  - Is a trial of surfactant therapy warranted (RDS, pneumonia, MAS)?

Circulation
- Assess for signs of circulatory inefficiency (CRT>3 seconds, week peripheral pulses, tachycardia, arterial lactate > 2)
- Provide fluid resuscitation as required (normal saline boluses to optimize preload)
- Assess need for inotropes if signs persist in spite of fluid therapy

Acquire history and perforrn a quick examination for possible clues to etiology

Presence of severe hypoxemia in an infant appearing well with minimal respiratory distress is highly suggestive of a critical cyanotic CHD

- Obtain CXR
- Establish i.v. access
- Obtain blood for investigations
- Consider antibiotic therapy

Vasodilator therapy

- HRF persists in spite of above measures and OI ≥ 15
- Ensure $PaCO_2$ within acceptable range (45–55mmHg) and correct acidosis it significant (arterial PH < 7.25 in spite of normal $PaCO_2$)
- Absence of clinical signs strongly suggestive of a critical CHD
- Inhaled nitric oxide is the first line agent of choice

Urgent echocardiogram to confirm diagnosis and rule out CHD

Consider referral to a regional ECMO center
- OI > 40 in spite of resuscitation measures
- Clinical suspicion of a critical CHD
- Infants unresponsive to vasodilator therapy with persistent high or worsening OI

Figure 57.7 Management approach for infants with hypoxic respiratory failure (HRF). Vasodilatory therapies are usually indicated when HRF persists despite resuscitation with restoration of adequate ventilation and correction of circulatory derangements. An echocardiogram is desirable in all infants with persistent HRF, but it is urgent for infants failing to respond to iNO or if ECMO is being considered. Neonatal treatment with iNO can reduce the need for ECMO only when the oxygenation index (OI) is between 15 and 40. Hence, ECMO referral should not be delayed for a "trial of iNO" if OI is persistently >40. CHD, congenital heart defect; CMV, conventional mechanical ventilation; CPAP, continuous positive airway pressure; CRT, capillary refill time; CXR, chest X-ray; ECMO, extracorporeal membrane oxygenation; FiO_2, fraction of inspired O_2; HFV, high frequency ventilation; i.v., intravenous; MAP, mean airway pressure; MAS, meconium aspiration syndrome; O_2, oxygen; $PaCO_2$/PaO_2, partial pressure of carbon dioxide and oxygen in arterial blood; RDS, respiratory distress syndrome; SpO_2, oxygen saturation measured using a pulse oximeter.

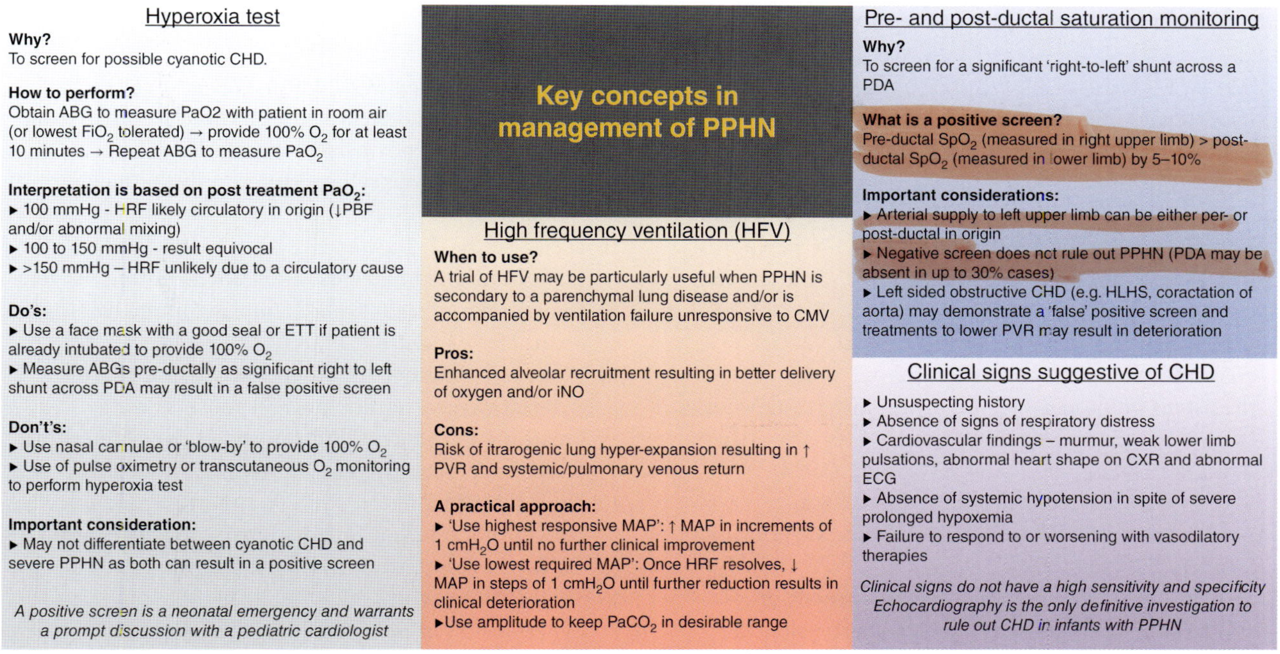

Figure 57.8 Important concepts in management of infants with PPHN. ABG, arterial blood gas; CHD, congenital heart disease; CMV conventional mechanical ventilation; ECG, electrocardiogram; ETT, endotracheal tube; FiO_2, fraction of inspired oxygen; HLHS, hypoplastic left heart syndrome; HRF, hypoxic respiratory failure; iNO, inhaled nitric oxide; MAP, mean airway pressure; $PaO_2/PaCO_2$ partial pressure of oxygen and carbon dioxide in arterial blood; PBF, pulmonary blood flow; PDA, patent ductus arteriosus; PPHN, persistent pulmonary hypertension of newborn; PVR, pulmonary vascular resistance; SpO_2, oxygen saturation measured by pulse oximetry.

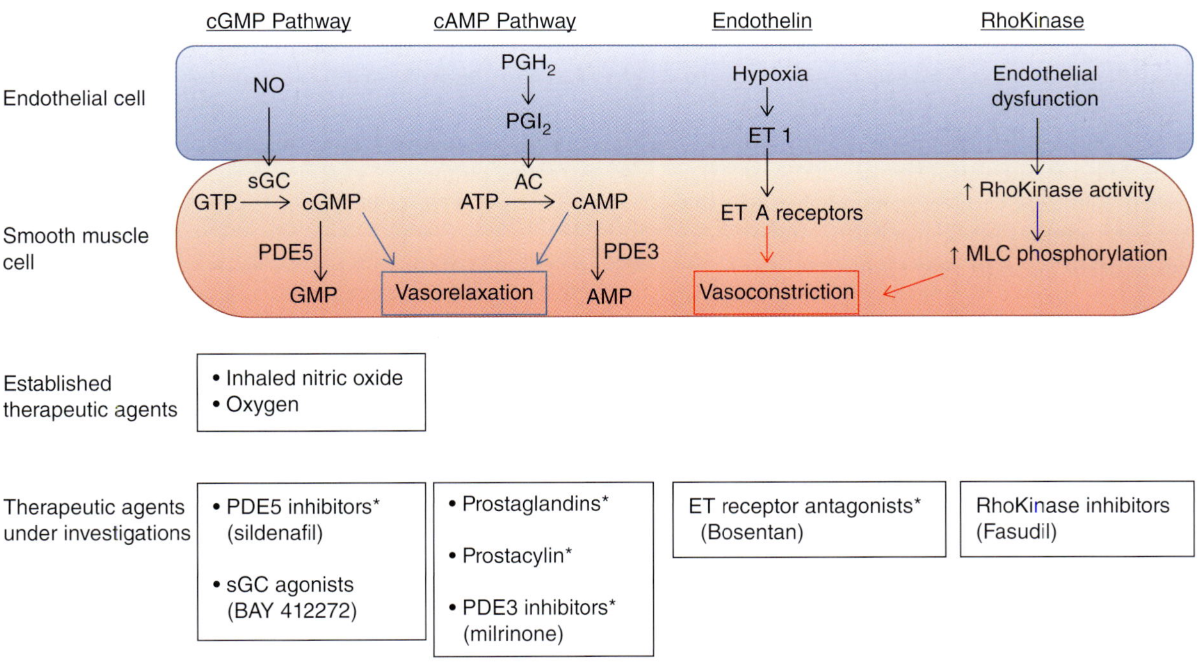

* Successful clinical use in neonates with PPHN has been reported but there are no large scale clinical studies to establish efficiency or safety in this population

Figure 57.9 Important cellular pathways involved in mediating pulmonary vascular tone and various therapeutic agents. Oxygen and iNO are the only established interventions for infants with PPHN and should be used as first line therapies. Agents under various stages of investigation are also shown. AC, adenyl cyclase; ATP, adenosine triphosphate; cAMP, cyclic adenosine monophosphate; cGMP, cyclic guanyl monophosphate; ET, endothelin; GTP, guanyl triphosphate; MLC, myosin light chain; NO, nitric oxide; PDE3, phosphodiestrase type 3; PDE5, phosphodiestrase type 5; PGH_2, prostaglandin; PGI_2, prostacyclin; sGC, soluble guanylate cyclase.

References

1 Jain A, McNamara PJ. (2013) Persistent pulmonary hypertension of the newborn: physiology, hemodynamic assessment and novel therapies. *Curr Pediatr Rev*, **9**, 55–66.
2 Walsh-Sukys MC, Tyson JE, Wright LL, *et al.* (2000) Persistent pulmonary hypertension of the newborn in the era before nitric oxide: practice variation and outcomes. *Pediatrics*, **105**, 14–20.
3 Lipkin PH, Davidson D, Spivak L, *et al.* (2002) Neurodevelopmental and medical outcomes of persistent pulmonary hypertension in term newborns treated with nitric oxide. *J Pediatr*, **140**, 306–310.
4 Hoffman D, Sisto D, Frater RW, *et al.* (1994) Left-to-right ventricular interaction with a noncontracting right ventricle. *J Thorac Cardiovasc Surg*, **107**, 1496–1502.
5 Henry GW. (1984) Noninvasive assessment of cardiac function and pulmonary hypertension in persistent pulmonary hypertension of the newborn. *Clin Perinatol*, **11**, 745–755.
6 Ochikubo CG, Waffarn F, Turbow R, *et al.* (1997) Echocardiographic evidence of improved hemodynamics during inhaled nitric oxide therapy for persistent pulmonary hypertension of the newborn. *Pediatr Cardiol*, **18**, 282–287.
7 Long WA. (1984) Structural cardiovascular abnormalities presenting as persistent pulmonary hypertension of the newborn. *Clin Perinatol*, **11**, 601–626.
8 Brown KL, Miles F, Sullivan ID, *et al.* (2005) Outcomes in neonates with congenital heart disease referred for respiratory extracorporeal membrane oxygenation. *Acta Paediatr*, **94**, 1280–1284.
9 Kinsella JP, Troug WE, Walsh WF, *et al.* (1997) Randomized, multicenter trial of inhaled nitric oxide and high-frequency oscillatory ventilation in severe, persistent pulmonary hypertension of the newborn. *J Pediatr*, **131**, 55–62.
10 Meier-stauss P, Bucher HU, Hürlimann R, *et al.* (1990) Pulse oximetry used for documenting oxygen saturation and right-to-left shunting immediately after birth. *Eur J Pediatr*, **149**, 851–855.
11 Jones RW, Baumer JH, Joseph MC, *et al.* (1976) Arterial oxygen tension and response to oxygen breathing in differential diagnosis of congenital heart disease in infancy. *Arch Dis Child*, **51**, 667–673.
12 Finer NN, Barrington KJ. (2006) Nitric oxide for respiratory failure in infants born at or near term. *Cochrane Database Syst Rev*, **4**, CD000399.
13 Shah PS, Ohlsson A. (2007) Sildenafil for pulmonary hypertension in neonates. *Cochrane Database Syst Rev*, **3**, CD005494.
14 McNamara PJ, Laique F, Muang-In S, *et al.* (2006) Milrinone improves oxygenation in neonates with severe persistent pulmonary hypertension of the newborn. *J Crit Care*, **21**, 217–223.
15 Nakwan N, Choksuchat D, Saksawad R, *et al.* (2009) Successful treatment of persistent pulmonary hypertension of the newborn with bosentan. *Acta Paediatr*, **98**, 1683–1685.
16 Evgenov OV, Kohane DS, Bloch KD, *et al.* (2007) Inhaled agonist of soluble guanylate cyclase induce selective pulmonary vasodilation. *Am J Respir Crit Care Med*, **176**, 1138–1145.

58

Hydrops Fetalis

James C. Huhta

Pediatric Cardiology Associates, St. Petersburg, FL, USA; Institute of Clinical Medicine, University of Tromso, Norway

Hydrops fetalis (HF) is a condition characterized by an abnormal collection of fluid with at least two of the following:

- Edema (fluid beneath the skin, more than 5 mm);
- Ascites (fluid in abdomen);
- Pleural effusion (fluid in the pleural cavity, the fluid-filled space that surrounds the lungs);
- Pericardial effusion (fluid in the pericardial sac, the covering that surrounds the heart).

In addition, HF is frequently associated with polyhydramnios and a thickened placenta (>6 cm).

Presentation

HF is typically diagnosed during ultrasound evaluation for other complaints such as polyhydramnios, size greater than dates, fetal tachycardia, decreased fetal movement, abnormal serum screening, or antenatal hemorrhage.

Causes

Czernik *et al.* [1] investigated the impact of medical progress on the diagnostic spectrum and outcome of infants with HF. They reviewed the charts of all live-born HF infants (n = 70) over a 16-year period (1993–2009). Data were compared with two published case series (Gainesville, Florida 1983–1992, n = 62 [2]; Glasgow, UK 1990–2004, n = 30 [3]). Only two cases were immune HF. The proportion of infants with unexplained HF (30%), lymphatic (24%), cardiac (17%), hematologic (6%), or chromosomal anomalies (6%) did not differ from the published case series. There was also no difference in overall mortality (57% vs. 55% or 67%, respectively). Low gestational age (< 34 weeks), low 5-min Apgar scores (< 4), and heart failure were independently associated with fatality. They concluded that the diagnostic spectrum and mortality of HF has changed little over the last 25 years [1].

HF is found in about 1 in 2000 births and is categorized as either immune or non-immune.

1) *Immune hydrops* (accounts for less than 10% of cases). Maternal antibodies against red cells of the fetus cross the placenta and coat fetal red cells, which are then destroyed (hemolysis) in the fetal spleen. The severe anemia leads to high-output congestive heart failure and increased red blood cell production by the spleen and liver leads to hepatic circulatory obstruction (portal hypertension). Anti-D, anti-E, and antibodies directed against other Rh antigens comprise the majority of antibodies responsible for hemolytic disease of the fetus or newborn. Less commonly encountered, antibodies include anti-K (Kell), anti-Fya (Duffy), and anti-Jka (Kidd) which can also cause hemolytic disease of the newborn.
2) *Non-immune hydrops* (accounts for 80–90% of cases; Box 58.1). By definition, non-immune hydrops is hydrops from any cause other than immune. In general, non-immune hydrops fetalis (NIHF) is caused by a failure of the interstitial fluid (the liquid between the cells of the body) to return into the venous system. This may because of cardiac failure (e.g., high output failure from anemia, sacrococcygeal teratoma, fetal adrenal neuroblastoma), impaired venous return (metabolic disorders), obstruction to normal lymphatic flow (thoracic malformations), increased capillary permeability (such as with infection), or decreased colloidal osmotic pressure (congenital nephrosis).

Some conditions involve more than one mechanism. For example, parvovirus can cause cardiomyopathy from myocarditis and anemia from marrow suppression. Randenberg [4] described NIHF as a condition in which excess fluid has accumulated in the fetal interstitial spaces as a result of one or more non-immune factors. A plethora of maternal, placental, and fetal disease

Visual Guide to Neonatal Cardiology, First Edition. Edited by Ernerio T. Alboliras, Ziyad M. Hijazi, Leo Lopez, and Donald J. Hagler.

Box 58.1 Conditions associated with non-immune hydrops fetalis

1) *Cardiac:*
   - Fetal arrhythmias (SVT, atrial flutter, heart block)
   - Cardiac anomalies associated with poor myocardial function (dilated cardiomyopathy)
   - Congenital heart disease with significant valvular regurgitation (mitral arcade, atrioventricular canal defect, Ebstein anomal, premature closure of the foramen ovale, acute constriction/closure of the ductus arteriosus)
   - Intracardiac tumors (rhabdomyomas, teratomas)
2) *Chromosomal/genetic syndromes:* trisomies 13, 18, and 21, XO (Turner syndrome), Noonan syndrome, multiple pterygium syndrome, Pena–Shokeir, arthrogryposis
3) *Fetal anemia:* alpha (α) thalassemia, parvovirus, fetal hemorrhage, G6PD deficiency
4) *Infection:* parvovirus, CMV, syphilis, coxsackie virus, rubella, toxoplasmosis, herpes,varicella, adenovirus, enterovirus, influenza, listeria
5) *Thoracic abnormalities:* congenital cystic adenomatoid malformation (CCAM), chylothorax, diaphragmatic hernia, mediastinal tumor, skeletal dysplasias. The mechanism of thoracic mass lesions may be obstruction of the thoracic duct or great vessels
6) *Twinning:* twin–twin transfusion. There is severe anemia in the donor twin or high-output failure in the recipient
7) *Tumors:* fetal sacrococcygeal teratoma, hemangiomas (hepatic, Klippel–Trenaunay syndrome), fetal adrenal neuroblastoma, placental tumors (chorioangioma) and other peripheral arteriovenous fistulae
8) *Miscellaneous:* cystic hygromas, inheritable disorders of metabolism (lysosomal storage diseases), maternal thyroid disease, congenital nephrotic syndrome

processes have been associated with NIHF. Knowledge of the various etiologies of NIHF and how the disease process affects fluid homeostasis is important for planning patient care and counseling families of patients diagnosed with NIHF [4].

Evaluation

Obtain maternal history (including pedigree).

Evaluation for Immune Hydrops

Obtain maternal indirect Coombs test to screen for antibodies associated with blood group incompatibility.

Evaluation for Non-immune Hydrops

1) Level II sonogram with Doppler measurement of the peak systolic velocity (PSV) in the fetal middle cerebral artery (MCA) to assess for fetal anemia. If there is evidence for anemia or equivocal result obtain:
2) Maternal blood counts and hemoglobin electrophoresis (with hemoglobin DNA analysis), Kleihauer–Betke stain, glucose 6-phosphate dehydrohgenase deficiency screen.
3) Maternal TORCH titers, rapid plasma reagin (RPR), listeria, parvovirus B19, coxsackie, adenovirus, and varicella IgG and IgM, as indicated.
4) Consider fetal heart rate monitoring with fetal echocardiogram for 12–24 hours if fetal arrhythmia is suspected. The cardiovascular profile score may be useful to identify fetuses with hydrops on a cardiac basis.
5) Amniocentesis for fetal karyotype and polymerase chain reaction (PCR) for infections *or* fetal percutaneous blood sampling for same and in addition fetal liver function; and metabolic testing if indicated.
6) In the presence of a family history of an inheritable metabolic disorder or recurrent NIHF, test for:
   - Storage disorders such as Gaucher, gangliosidosis, sialidosis, beta-glucuronidase deficiency, and mucopolysaccharidosis;
   - Enzyme analysis and carrier testing in parents and/or analysis of fetal or neonatal blood or urine;
   - Histologic examination of fetal tissues;
   - Maternal thyroid antibodies.

Faced with the fetus with NIHF, one must first determine if the hydrops is cardiac, inflammatory, or metabolic. Many cases of hydrops are attributed to fetal systemic infection. New markers are identifying etiologic agents such as parvovirus or adenovirus. The associated hepatitis with these infections can compromise the protein-producing capability of the fetus, thereby decreasing the fetal oncotic pressure. Immune hydrops must always be considered in the differential diagnosis, but other causes of anemia can also cause hydrops, such as hemoglobinopathies. Infections can cause hemolytic anemia, which can be treated by fetal transfusion.

Anemia can cause hydrops; however, ventricular shortening fraction did not significantly change among 111 fetuses with hemoglobin Bart disease with and without hydrops [5]. However, left and right ventricular shortening fraction were significantly decreased (mean z scores 5 standard deviations and 8 standard deviations below the mean, respectively) in 21 hydropic fetuses as a result of congenital heart defects ($P < 0.001$). These authors

Table 58.1 Treatment for fetal hydrops by cause.

Cause	Treatment
Fetal anemia	Fetal blood sampling followed by in utero transfusion
Fetal arrhythmia	Medications such as digoxin, sotalol, propanolol, flecainide, amiodarone
Intrinsic thoracic malformations	Thoracentesis or thoracoamniotic shunt for pleural effusions in select cases
Twin–twin transfusion	Fetoscopic laser ablation of communicating vessels
Fetal AV fistula or persistent R ductus venosus	Digoxin 0.25 mg PO BID

concluded that fetuses with HF secondary to cardiac defects and anemia have different patterns of shortening fraction. Defects develop with cardiac decompensation; whereas in fetal anemia, failure is probably caused by hypervolemia with cardiac decompensation occurring when the cardiac compensatory mechanism is exhausted. Fetal cardiomyopathy described as a case of isolated left ventricular non-compaction (LVNC), a severe congenital cardiomyopathy, which presented in the neonatal period as fetal hydrops has been described [6].

Treatment

Treatment of fetal cardiovascular problems can be classified into five groups based on the etiology of congestive heart failure:

1) Abnormal peripheral impedances causing redistribution of flow and growth failure;
2) High output caused by anemia or arteriovenous fistula;
3) Primary or secondary valvular regurgitation;
4) Heart failure caused by myocardial dysfunction; and
5) Tachycardia/bradycardia.

Interventions aimed at improving the effective cardiac output are also aimed at prolonging the pregnancy and preventing prematurity and prenatal asphyxia.

Treatment with digoxin for evidence of decreased ventricular shortening is controversial. Digoxin is known to decrease the catecholamine response to congestive heart failure, and if there is diastolic dysfunction in the fetus, this may lower filling pressures. If the afterload is high, then an increase in oxygen consumption could result from increased inotropy without improved myocardial perfusion. Terbutaline appears promising as an inotropic and chronotropic agent [7], but studies of the possible negative effects on the fetal myocardium are needed. Currently, we use digoxin for fetal cardiac failure caused by arrhythmias and high-output states, such as fistula and anemia. In a case of acardiac twinning, in which the normal fetus was supporting two circulations, digoxin appeared to improve cardiac function and result in a prolonged and successful gestation for the normal twin. Laser treatment of the twin–twin communications or cord ligation with acardiac twins could be performed to improve cardiac failure (Table 58.1).

Maternal Complications

The mother can develop edema, hypertension, and proteinuria during conservative management of hydrops, a condition known as Mirror syndrome (also known as pseudotoxemia or Ballantyne syndrome). Symptoms can persist after delivery.

Prognosis

In 2007, a retrospective review of a large national dataset showed a total of 253 651 discharges from 162 neonatal intensive care units; 598 patients were identified with a report of HF. The most common associated diagnoses were congenital heart problems (13.7%), abnormalities in heart rate (10.4%), twin–twin transfusion (9%), congenital anomalies (8.7%), chromosomal abnormalities (7.5%), congenital viral infections (6.7%), congenital anemia (5%), and congenital chylothorax (3.2%). Of those 598 neonates, 115 were transferred either to another hospital or to another service, 215 died before discharge, and 267 were discharged from the hospital. Mortality rates were highest among neonates with congenital anomalies (57.7%) and lowest among neonates with congenital chylothorax (5.9%). Factors that were associated independently with death in logistic regression analyses were younger gestational age, low 5-minute Apgar score, and need for high levels of support during the first day after birth (higher levels of inspired oxygen support and more often treated with high-frequency ventilation) [8].

Huang *et al.* [9] studied 28 live-born neonates with hydrops and most presented with pleural effusions

(21 of 28) and ascites (22 of 28). The majority of patients had hydrops resulting from cardiovascular diseases (7 of 28), hematologic disorders (6 of 28), lymphatic malformations (6 of 28), and idiopathic origins (6 of 28). The overall survival rate was 50% and was highest (83%) in infants with lymphatic malformations. By univariate analysis, risk factors for mortality are earlier ages at diagnosis and at birth, low Apgar scores, need for resuscitation in the delivery room, low serum albumin level, and severe acidemia. After using stepwise multiple logistic regression analysis, the most significant factors associated with fatality were younger gestational age at birth and lower serum albumin level. The authors concluded that HF remains a complex condition with a high mortality rate. Hydrops resulting from lymphatic malformations has a more favorable outcome. Preterm birth at less than 34 weeks and serum albumin concentration lower than 2 g/dL are two poor prognostic factors for survival [9].

Multiple mechanisms of hydrops can coexist and the primary cause may not be immediately obvious. Of more importance is the determination of the prognosis. This task would be aided by a semiquantitative measure of fetal heart failure.

Fetal Hydrops for the Perinatal Cardiologist

The challenge of hydrops assessment can be summarized by several questions for the perinatal cardiologist. Is hydrops from the heart? Is fetal heart failure a result of congenital heart disease? Is it becoming more severe? Is there fetal myocardial dysfunction [10–12]?

After birth, the prognosis will depend on the answers to these and many other questions. The long-term outcome is dependent on whether the insult is reversible and whether there were periods of ischemia and/or brain injury. There are several possible causes of heart failure in the fetus after ruling out fetal infection. The most useful predictor of perinatal death in fetal hydrops is the presence of umbilical venous pulsations [13] because the most common pathway of perinatal demise is compromised fetal cardiac output – fetal congestive heart failure. There follows a method to detect this entity and to determine which fetuses should be referred to a fetal center. Initially, the following data are collected during fetal echocardiography:

1) *Cardiac size : thoracic size (C : T):* cardiac divided by thoracic area ratio (normal 0.25–0.35) or C : T circumference ratio (normal < 0.5).
2) *Venous Doppler:* inferior caval (or hepatic venous; increased atrial reversal) and umbilical cord vein (pulsations).
3) *Four-valve Doppler:* any leak of the valve should be evaluated further. If there are abnormalities in any of these measurements, then there may be a cardiac cause or associated physiologic problem and detailed study is indicated to rule out serious cardiovascular involvement.

The cardiovascular system, which provides much information about the well-being of the fetus, is accessible because of rapid developments in non-invasive techniques, particularly ultrasound. For example, fetal heart rate monitoring by non-focused ultrasound can detect abnormal rate changes, and a lack of normal variability may be related to ischemia. The fetal biophysical profile is useful for detecting changes in fetal well-being [14]. The decision to deliver a fetus prematurely because of cardiac changes must be made with consideration of the risks both pre- and postnatally. Most associations of cardiovascular changes and other organ functions in the fetus have yet to be defined. Therefore, any assessment requires a coordinated team approach by perinatalogists, cardiologists, and neonatologists.

The definition of fetal congestive heart failure is similar to that after birth: inadequate tissue perfusion. Inadequate cardiac output results in a series of complex reflexes and adaptations to improve forward flow or to direct flow to vital organs. This state can be described as a deficiency of flow of blood to the tissues such that certain reflexes are triggered for the survival of the fetus.

One of these reflexes is the secretion of excess circulating catacholamines, which are produced in response to peripheral vascular detection of abnormal perfusion. Powerful hormonal reflexes are triggered, including those that control salt and water retention in an attempt to increase myocardial preload, and those that control adrenocorticoid excess, which mobilizes additional calories for the increased metabolic demand. The fetus is capable of producing cytokine activation as well as the secretion of endothelin, troponin T [15], tumor necrosis factor, and brain naturetic factor. The maturational changes of the systemic vascular bed with gestational age are not known, but at some point in the pregnancy it is thought that vasoconstriction of the fetal systemic resistance vessels occurs in response to stress. How this affects compensation in the fetal circulation is under investigation.

The diagnosis of fetal congestive heart failure must be addressed in a clinical fashion similar to that after birth. The classic clinical tetrad of cardiomegaly, tachycardia, tachypnea, and hepatomegaly has been used in neonates and children. This clinical state in the fetus can be characterized by findings in at least five categories that are obtained during the ultrasonographic examination. The following categories are each worth 2 points in a 10-point scoring system used quantitatively to assess the cardiovascular system: hydrops, umbilical venous Doppler, heart size, abnormal myocardial function, and arterial Doppler. Abnormalities in the cardiovascular profile score can occur prior to the clinical state of HF.

Within specific disease entities, more emphasis is placed on certain areas to predict the prognosis. This information can only comprise a portion of the total picture and must be integrated by the attending physician into the diagnostic and treatment plan for the patient.

The cardiovascular profile score gives a semi-quantitative score of fetal cardiac well-being and uses known markers by ultrasound that have been correlated with poor fetal outcome. This profile is normal if the score is 10 and signs of cardiac abnormalities result in a decrease of the score from normal. For example, if there is ascites but no other abnormalities, there would be a deduction of 1 point for hydrops (ascites but no skin edema) and no deductions for the other categories, for a score of 9 of 10.

Counseling

Long-term prognosis depends on underlying cause and severity of the heart failure. If the cause of NIHF cannot be determined, the perinatal mortality is approximately 50%. Prognosis is much poorer if diagnosed at less than 24 weeks and if pleural effusion is present, or structural abnormalities are present. Pulmonary hypoplasia is a common cause of death in neonates with pleural effusions. HF associated with a structural heart defect is associated with an almost 100% mortality rate. If hydrops is found early in pregnancy (less than 24 weeks) with no treatable cause, the option of termination may be a consideration. Recurrence is uncommon unless related to blood group incompatibility (isoimmunization) or inheritable disorder. A cardiovascular profile score less than 7 is associated with mortality.

Antepartum

Follow-up will depend on the gestational age of the fetus, and the mother's wishes regarding intervention. If treatment has been successful or hydrops is resolving spontaneously, the fetus may be followed with repeat sonograms every 1–2 weeks and antenatal testing. Patients treated for immune hydrops are usually delivered at 37 weeks' gestation or when fetal lung maturity has been confirmed. Consultation with the neonatologist helps to decide when it is appropriate to proceed with preterm delivery for possible postnatal treatment.

The mother should be evaluated frequently for signs of Mirror syndrome.

Delivery

The fetus should be delivered at a tertiary care center with a neonatologist and other appropriate specialists. There is no evidence that delivery by cesarean section has a marked effect on outcome. Cord blood should be obtained at delivery. A postmortem evaluation should be performed in all cases of hydrops that result in neonatal death. One study showed that a combined approach of a thorough antenatal assessment and autopsy was more likely to determine the cause of NIHF.

CV Profile Score in Hydrops

In early stages, HF develops with ascites, pleural effusion, pericardial effusion (Figures 58.1 and 58.2), or a combination of these findings. In advanced hydrops, there is generalized skin edema seen easily over the scalp and abdominal wall. In scoring hydrops for the cardiovascular profile score, 1 point is deducted for early hydrops and 2 points for skin edema.

Umbilical and Ductus Venous Doppler

Fetal venous blood velocities have been examined and investigations have been clinically promising [11]. Several studies have confirmed that normal flow in the inferior vena cava of the fetus has a pulsatile, triphasic pattern. The first forward wave begins to increase with atrial relaxation, reaches its peak during ventricular systole, and then declines to reach its nadir at the end of ventricular systole. The second forward wave occurs during early diastole and a reverse flow is usually present in late diastole with atrial contraction. In normal pregnancy, the peak velocities obtained during the first wave of systole are greater than the early diastolic values. The systolic: diastolic ratios do not appear to change with advancing gestational age, but a significant decrease in flow reversal with atrial contraction is evident.

Studies in the fetal lamb model have shown that this decrease in the percentage of reversed flow seen in normal pregnancy is related to the pressure gradient between the right atrium and the right ventricle during end diastole [16, 17]. It appears to be related to both ventricular compliance and ventricular end diastolic pressure and therefore is a reflection of central venous pressure. Recording venous blood velocity might thus give important information on fetal cardiac pump function. Studies in humans have shown that alterations in central venous blood velocity patterns accurately reflect abnormalities in cardiac hemodynamics [15, 18, 19]. The abnormal pulsatility pattern consisting of increased velocity of blood flow reversal away from the heart during atrial contraction has been reported in the fetus with

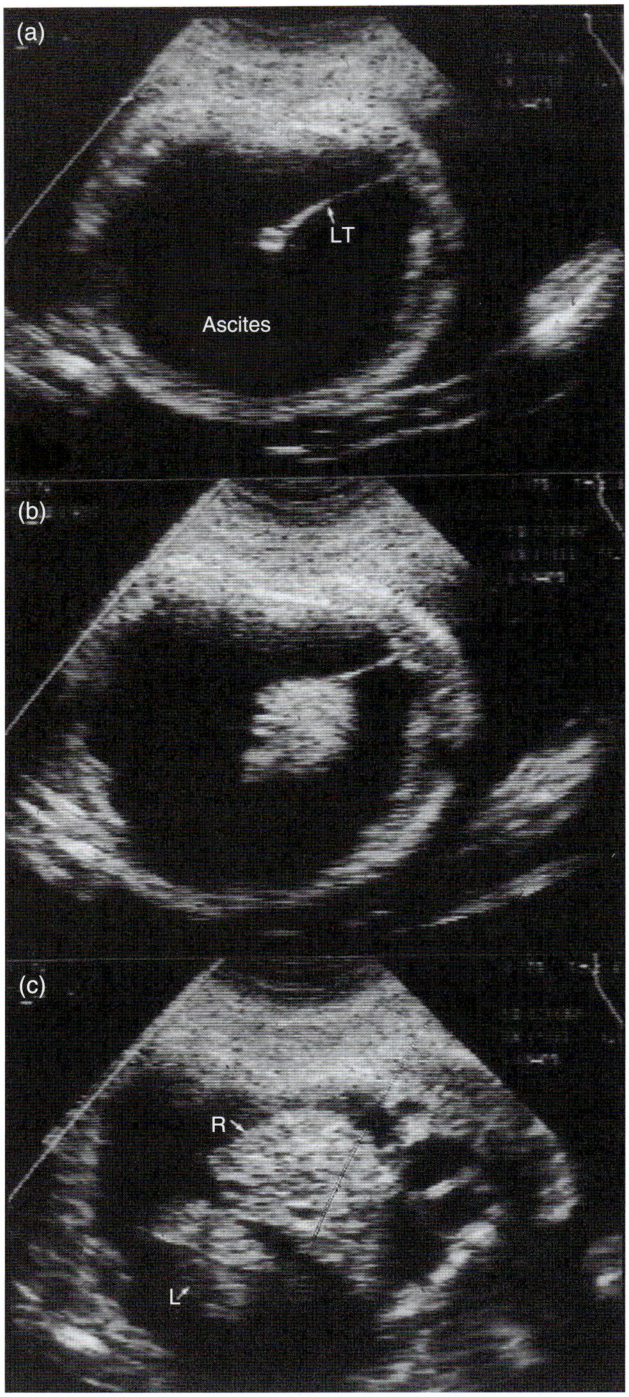

Figure 58.1 (a–c) Acites fluid in a fetus with hydrops fetalis showing the ligament teres (LT) and the right (R) and left (L) lobes of the liver.

congestive heart failure and may be a sign of increased end diastolic pressure in the ventricles of the failing heart. Abnormal inferior vena cava (IVC) flow velocity patterns have been described in several fetal pathologic conditions, including anemia, non-immune hydrops, and arrhythmias, and in severely growth-retarded fetuses

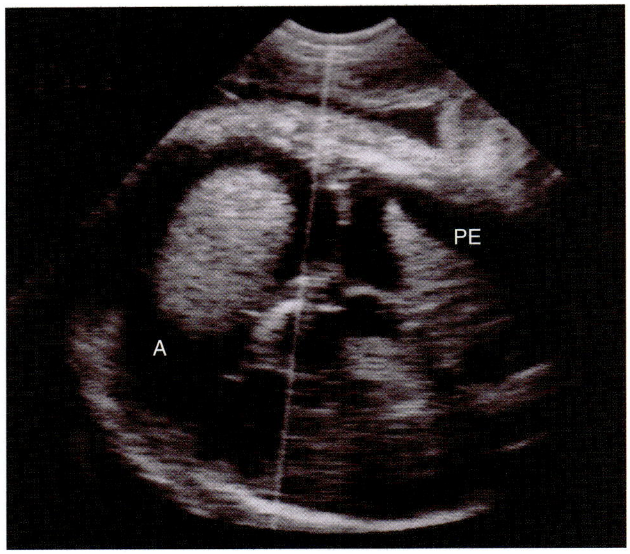

Figure 58.2 Fetal hydrops with pleural effusion (PE) and ascites (A).

characterized by the absence of end diastolic flow in the umbilical artery. The compromised fetus with acidosis is known to manifest abnormalities of venous Doppler, including increased atrial reversal in excess of normal in the IVC at the junction with the right atrium [20] and increased pulsatility in the ductus venosus. The prognostic importance of these abnormalities has been confirmed in the fetus with intrauterine growth retardation and in those with hydrops. An increased A : S ratio in the ductus venosus (peak atrial reversal divided by the peak filling wave during ventricular systole) appears to be the most useful sign for quantifying the increase in central venous pressure in fetuses with growth retardation. Normally, the ratio of the area of the atrial reversal to the entire forward flow area should be less than 7%.

Transmission of the venous pulsations into the portal and umbilical circulation correlates with increasing degrees of cardiac compromise. Tulzer *et al.* [18] studied the cardiac factors related to prognosis in hydrops and noted that umbilical venous pulsations could stand in for a number of cardiac variables in predicting prognosis, including ventricular shortening fraction, ejection velocities, and percentage IVC atrial reversal. Abnormal venous Doppler develops with increasing heart failure in the following order:

1) Increased atrial reversal in the IVC;
2) Ductus venosus atrial reversal;
3) Portal venous atrial pulsations;
4) Umbilical venous atrial pulsations.

To assess the venous system consistently, pulsed Doppler sampling is obtained in the IVC, the ductus venosus, the umbilical vein in the abdomen, and the umbilical cord vein as part of each serial examination.

The end stage finding of abnormal venous Doppler is atrial pulsations in the umbilical cord vein. This finding of diastolic block predicts perinatal mortality. Venous pulsations are not normal in the portal vein, and such a finding can precede the progression to umbilical venous pulsations. Transmission of the atrial reversal into the ductus venosus and later into the portal and cord vein sites over time suggests progression of heart failure. The cardiovascular profile score has deductions for abnormal venous Doppler as follows: ductus venosus atrial reversal, 1 point; umbilical venous atrial pulsations, 2 points. The maximum deduction in any category is 2 points.

Cardiomegaly

Enlargement of the cardiac chambers is a universal sign of heart failure. This is also true in the fetus, but few of the mechanisms are understood. It is likely that neural humoral reflexes are triggered, resulting in retention of extracellular volume leading to increased end diastolic volume of the ventricles. At some point, this increased ventricular size indicates increased end diastolic pressure. However, unlike in the postnatal human, it is uncommon to encounter persistent tachycardia with signs of catacholamine excess. It is possible that the levels of humoral agents are modified by the fetal–maternal exchange mechanisms, which exist when the placenta is functioning normally. The most common cardiac chamber that expresses enlargement as a sign of impending cardiac failure is the right atrium (RA). The reasons for this relate to the many causes of heart failure, but the RA is a final pathway for blood flow returning to the heart and will manifest enlargement in situations of relative foramen obstruction, volume overload, tricuspid valve regurgitation, and increased afterload. Increased RA size may be a result of increased right ventricle (RV) end diastolic pressure, which may be brought about by increased afterload or coronary insufficiency. The RV may be more susceptible to increased work because of the nature of the afterload and the resultant increased demands for oxygen in the face of increased chamber wall stress. It is generally believed that increased atrial wall stress without increased ventricular work does not lead to clinical difficulties in the fetus. The processes of cardiac ventricular remodeling with changes in loading are poorly understood. An early marker of cardiac decompensation is RV shape and size changes and may predispose to supraventricular arrhythmias.

Small heart size with external compression has been correlated with hydrops and poor outcome in fetuses with cystic adenomatoid malformation [21]. When heart size was less than 20% of the chest area, fetal outcome was affected. In fetuses with cystic adenomatoid malformation, a small C : T ratio (<0.2) is associated with a poor prognosis [21]. In utero, the heart area can be easily compared with the area of the thorax and the ratio should be less than one-third and greater than one-fourth in the presence of normal chest development. Cardiac size calculations are as follows:

1) C : T area ratio = cardiac area/chest area (normal 0.2–0.35); and
2) C : T circumference ratio = cardiac circumference/chest circumference (normal <0.5).

Cardiovascular profile scoring for cardiac size is as follows: normal heart : chest area ratio is less than 0.35 and greater than 0.20:

- Mild cardiomegaly: area ratio >0.35; deduct 1 point
- Severe cardiomegaly: area ratio >0.50; deduct 2 points
- Small heart ratio <0.2; deduct 2 points.

Maximum deduction is −2 points.

Abnormal Myocardial Function

The cardiac function is assessed indirectly by the global shortening (and thickening) of the walls of the ventricles and by the function of the atrioventricular and semilunar valves. The diameters of both the right and left ventricles should shorten more than 28% in systole compared to diastole. Measurements of cardiac dimensions with time are performed using M-mode echocardiography. The shortening fraction (FS) of a ventricle is calculated by taking the difference between the diastolic (DD) and systolic dimensions (SD) and dividing by the diastolic dimension:

$$\text{Fractional shortening (FS)} = \text{DD minus SD}/\text{DD normal} > 0.28.$$

An abnormal shortening fraction could reflect myocardial compromise or an increase in the fetal ventricular workload. Regardless, an increase in diastolic dimension is often related to a decrease in shortening fraction and should be regarded as an indication for more intensive monitoring.

The atrioventricular and semilunar valves are competent in the normal fetus, and if regurgitation is detected it is usually a sign of altered cardiovascular physiology. Respondek *et al.* [22] showed that 7% of fetuses who had a fetal echocardiogram displayed trivial (holosystolic) or significant tricuspid valve regurgitation. Most had some reason for this, such as constriction of the ductus arteriosus from indomethacin treatment of preterm labor, but 93% had no trace of regurgitation with state-of-the-art equipment and careful examination. Tricuspid valve regurgitation is common after birth, so we may speculate that the fetal RV is well adapted to systemic pressure work. Therefore, valvular competence is normal, and only in disturbances of cardiovascular physiology in which there is increased ventricular wall stress is tricuspid valve regurgitation present. Trace tricuspid regurgitation, defined as non-holosystolic regurgitation lasting at least 70 ms, is not normal. This may be the first sign of a problem but has little prognostic importance. Holosystolic tricuspid regurgitation is abnormal and indicates the need for further investigation [22]. When regurgitation is detected by color Doppler, it must be confirmed and graded by pulsed Doppler. With congenital diseases of the tricuspid valve, hydrops and fetal death can occur [23].

Regurgitation of tricuspid, mitral, aortic or pulmonary valves is usually a sign of more advanced congestive heart failure and can occur in the moribund fetus with acidosis and severe heart failure as a sign of myocardial compromise. Tricuspid valve regurgitation can be a reversible sign of heart failure because successful therapy for anemia or tachycardia in fetuses in utero has been performed. Progression to mitral valve regurgitation is a sign of fetal congestive heart failure and usually means that a significant increase in left ventricular wall stress is present.

With severe myocardial failure, the support for the semilunar valves is compromised and pulmonary or aortic valve regurgitation can occur. The nature of the velocity waveform of atrioventricular valvular regurgitation has prognostic value in the calculation of fetal ventricular dP/dt. With holosystolic tricuspid valve regurgitation, the time interval from one RV–RA pressure difference to another can be used to calculate the change in pressure over time or the dP/dt. A value of less than 800 mmHg/s is abnormal, and a value less than 400 mmHg/s predicts a poor fetal outcome [24]. This measurement requires continuous-wave Doppler and the peak velocity may be 2.5–4.5 m/s. We have found that the most useful range for dP/dt measurement in fetal tricuspid regurgitation is 0.5–2.5 m/s (i.e., a RV–RA gradient of 1–25 mmHg or a 24-mmHg difference). The fetal ventricles are at equal systemic pressure throughout gestation and therefore the blood pressure of the fetus is estimated using this technique. The filling pattern of the ventricles in diastole is an indicator of the diastolic function of the heart. Normal values show that the proportion of atrial filling during the atrial contraction is constant from 14 to 40 weeks' gestation [25]. Monophasic filling of the ventricles is a sign of compromised diastolic function and fetal heart failure.

Several disease states have been identified in which thickening of the ventricular chambers (myocardial hypertrophy) occurs in the absence of congenital ventricular outflow obstruction. This is assessed by measuring the end diastolic wall thickness of the left ventricle (LV) and comparing it with the normal values for age. Any LV posterior wall thickness greater than 4 mm is abnormal. The most severe cases of fetal hypertension are in the larger of twins in the syndrome known as twin–twin transfusion [26] in which a mortality rate higher than 70% for fetuses is common. Treatment strategies such as laser ablation of the vascular communications to prevent hydrops in the larger fetus result in improved survival [7].

Regardless of the etiology, thickening of the fetal ventricles can restrict the cardiac reserve before or after birth. Because cardiac hypertrophy can occur rapidly but takes weeks or months to resolve, its identification is an important marker of a cardiovascular system at risk. Abnormalities of diastolic function can be expected and should be excluded by comparing the filling patterns of the ventricles using pulsed Doppler to standardized normal values. A rule of thumb is that the A wave of the ventricular filling is always greater than the E wave. Monophasic filling of the ventricles occurs in severe diastolic dysfunction and with severe external cardiac compression.

Arterial Doppler Redistribution of Fetal Cardiac Output

It is well established that the blood velocities measured by Doppler echocardiography in the umbilical artery and in other peripheral vascular beds can be used as indirect indicators of the relative vascular impedances. Findings of an increased pulsatility index in the umbilical artery (UA) and descending aorta (DAo) and a decreased index in the middle cerebral artery (MCA) are non-invasive signs of redistribution of flow. It is important to recognize that a pulsed Doppler finding in one portion of the circulation is affected by changes in the rest of the circulation. For example, if there is significant aortic valvular regurgitation in the fetus, the diastolic reversal in the DAo and the increased pulsatility index in the UA are secondary to this change in the heart and do not reflect peripheral resistance only. The most common cause of elevated vascular resistance in the fetus is placental dysfunction secondary to vasculopathy leading to asymmetrical growth retardation. This complex pathophysiologic state is poorly understood but there is evidence that there is hypoxemia resulting from placental dysfunction and additional compromise of nutrition severe enough to impair growth. Once the normal pattern of growth is disturbed (usually asymmetrical such that the brain continues growing but the body does not), the fetus is at risk of organ damage from hypoxemic/ischemic injury. The umbilical artery manifests this problem with a loss or reversal of diastolic blood flow. There is redistribution of flow to the brain (brain sparing) by reflex vasodilatation of the cerebral vessels. This is manifested by a decrease in the pulsatility index (PI) in the MCA such that diastolic flow is relatively increased (PI <2 SD below the mean [27, 28]). In the fetus with hypoxemia, the peripheral fetal vessels are vasoconstricted and the larger arteries are suspected to be non-compliant compared with a healthy cohort with increased blood pressure. In other words, this is a physiologic state characterized by increased vascular resistances and, at end stage, decreased vascular compliance and cardiac output. Right ventricular enlargement occurs in some cases. Fetal brain sparing is a marker of cardiac output redistribution that is sensitive for the detection of significant hypoxemia and placental dysfunction. However, there is evidence that reversal of diastolic flow in the umbilical artery or in the aortic isthmus can be significant risk factors for abnormal outcomes. As a sign of fetal heart failure, the vasoconstriction resulting from decreased cardiac output and the compensatory sign of vasodilatation in the brain can be included in the cardiovascular profile score: absent end diastolic flow in the umbilical artery + brain sparing (increased MCA diastolic velocity), deduct 1 point, and reversed end diastolic flow in the umbilical artery, deduct 2 points.

Cardiovascular Profile Score

A cardiovascular profile score is calculated by assigning 2 points for each of the five categories and using the score in serial studies to provide a method of uniform physiologic assessment. By taking a multivariate approach, this type of multifactorial score can combine assessment of direct and indirect markers of cardiovascular (CV) function. Initial validation of the CV profile score in hydrops was shown by Falkensammer *et al.* [11]. Seven fetuses with hydrops, including three with congenital heart disease, had correlation of the CV profile score with the myocardial performance index (Tei index). RV and LV Tei indices were assessed in a control group and showed no change with gestational age. Hofstaetter *et al.* [29] measured the CV profile score in 59 hydrops fetuses. Mortality was 21/59. The median score in those who died pre- or postnatally was 5, whereas the median score in the survivors was 7.

Conclusions

Fetal cardiac findings must be integrated into the clinical management of the fetus with HF by the perinatologist. The CV profile score can be used by the perinatal cardiology team to assess the urgency of abnormalities and the prognosis. Serial studies using the CV profile score are necessary to obtain the value from this test. It can be used to plan uniform treatment strategies.

References

1 Czernik C, Proquitte H, Metze B, Buhrer C. (2011) Hydrops fetalis: has there been a change in diagnostic spectrum and mortality? *J Maternal Fetal Neonatal Med*, **24**, 258–263.

2 Wafelman LS, Pollock BH, Kreutzer J, Richards DS, Hutchison AA. (1999) Nonimmune hydrops fetalis: fetal and neonatal outcome during 1983–1992. *Biol Neonate*, **75**, 73–81.

3 Simpson JH, McDevitt H, Young D, Cameron AD. (2006) Severity of non-immune hydrops fetalis at birth continues to predict survival despite advances in perinatal care. *Fetal Diagn Ther*, **21**, 380–382.

4 Randenberg AL. (2010) Nonimmune hydrops fetalis part I: etiology and pathophysiology. *Neonatal Netw*, **29**, 281–295.

5 Tongsong T, Wanapirak C, Piyamongkol W, *et al.* (2011) Fetal ventricular shortening fraction in hydrops fetalis. *Obstetr Gynecol*, **117**, 84–91.

6 Richards A, Mao CY, Dobson NR. (2009) Left ventricular noncompaction: a rare cause of hydrops fetalis. *Pediatr Cardiol*, **30**, 985–988.

7 Quintero RA, Comas C, Bornick PW, Allen MH, Kruger M. (2000) Selective versus non-selective laser photocoagulation of placental vessels in twin-to-twin transfusion syndrome. *Ultrasound Obstet Gynecol*, **16**, 230.

8 Abrams ME, Meredith KS, Kinnard P, Clark RH. (2007) Hydrops fetalis: a retrospective review of cases reported to a large national database and identification of risk factors associated with death. *Pediatrics*, **120**, 84–89.

9 Huang HR, Tsay PK, Chiang MC, Lien R, Chou YH. (2007) Prognostic factors and clinical features in liveborn neonates with hydrops fetalis. *Am J Perinatol*, **24**, 33–38.

10 Chaoui R, Bollmann R, Goldner B, Heling KS, Tennstedt C. (1994) Fetal cardiomegaly: echocardiographic findings and outcome in 19 cases. *Fetal Diagn Ther*, **9**, 92–104.

11 Falkensammer CB, Paul J, Huhta JC. (2001) Fetal congestive heart failure: correlation of Tei index and cardiovascular score. *J Perinat Med*, **29**, 390–398.

12 Huhta JC. (1995) What is perinatal cardiology? (editorial). *Ultrasound Obstet Gynecol*, **5**, 145–147.

13 Gudmundsson S, Huhta JC, Wood DC, *et al.* (1991) Venous Doppler ultrasonography in the fetus with non-immune hydrops. *Am J Obstet Gynecol*, **164**, 33–37.

14 Manning FA, Harman CR, Morrison I, *et al.* (1990) Fetal assessment based on fetal biophysical profile scoring. *Am J Obstet Gynecol*, **162**, 703–709.

15 Rizzo G, Arduini D, Romanini C. (1992) Inferior vena cava flow velocity waveforms in appropriate and-small-for-gestational-age fetuses. *Am J Obstet Gynecol*, **166**, 1271–1280.

16 Reed KL, Appleton CP, Anderson CF, Shenker L, Sahn DJ. (1990) Doppler of vena cava flows in human fetuses. *Circulation*, **81**, 498–505.

17 Reuss ML, Rudolph AM, Dae MW. (1983) Phasic blood flow patterns in the superior and inferior venae cavae and umbilical vein of fetal sheep. *Am J Obstet Gynecol*, **145**, 70–78.

18 Tulzer G, Gudmundsson S, Wood DC, *et al.* (1994) Doppler in non-immune hydrops fetalis. *Ultrasound Obstet Gynecol*, **4**, 279–283.

19 Huhta JC. (2004) Guidelines for the evaluation of heart failure in the fetus with or without hydrops. *Pediatr Cardiol*, **25**, 274–286. DOI: 10.1007/s00246-003-0591-3.

20 Hecher K, Snijders R, Campbell S, Nicolaides K. (1995) Fetal venous, intracardiac, and arterial blood flow measurements in intrauterine growth retardation: relationship with fetal blood gases. *Am J Obstet Gynecol*, **173**, 10–15.

21 Mahle WT, Rychik J, Tian ZY, *et al.* (2000) Echocardiographic evaluation of the fetus with congenital cystic adenomatoid malformation. *Ultrasound Obstet Gynecol*, **16**, 620–624.

22 Respondek M, Kammermeier M, Ludomirsky A, Weil SR, Huhta JC. (1994) The prevalence and clinical significance of fetal tricuspid valve regurgitation with normal heart anatomy. *Am J Obstet Gynecol*, **171**, 1265–1270.

23 Hornberger LK, Sahn DJ, Kleinman CS, Copel JA, Reed KL. (1991) Tricuspid valve disease with significant tricuspid insufficiency in the fetus: diagnosis and outcome. *J Am Coll Cardiol*, **17**, 167–173.

24 Tulzer G, Gudmundsson S, Rotondo KM, *et al.* (1991) Doppler in the evaluation and prognosis of fetuses with tricuspid regurgitation. *J Matern Fetal Invest*, **1**, 15–18.

25 Tulzer G, Khowsathit P, Gudmundsson S. (1994) Diastolic function of the fetal heart during second and third trimester: a prospective longitudinal Doppler-echocardiographic study. *Eur J Pediatr*, **153**, 151–154.

26 Hecher K, Ville Y, Nicolaides KH. (1995) Fetal arterial Doppler studies in twin–twin transfusion syndrome. *J Ultrasound Med*, **14**, 101–108.

27 Rasanen J, Debbs RH, Huhta JC. (1997) Echocardiography in intrauterine growth restriction. *Clin Obstet Gynecol*, **40**, 796–803.

28 Rizzo G, Arduini D. (1991) Fetal cardiac function in intrauterine growth retardation. *Am J Obstet Gynecol*, **165**, 876–882.

29 Hofstaetter C, Hansmann M, Eik-Nes SH, Huhta JC, Luther SL. (2006) A cardiovascular profile score in the surveillance of fetal hydrops. *J Matern Fetal Neonatal Med*, **19** (7), 407–413.

Part V

Rhythm Disturbances in the Newborn

59

Structural, Metabolic, and Genetic Abnormalities Affecting the Neonatal Conduction System

Supaluck Kanjanauthai and Ira Shetty

Department of Pediatric Cardiology, Advocate Children's Hospital, Oak Lawn, IL, USA

The cardiac conduction system (CCS) is formed of specialized cells and networks that include the sinoatrial (SA) node, internodal tracts (connections between SA node and atrioventricular node, AVN), Bachmann bundle (interatrial communications), AVN and the His–Purkinje system. The functional components of the CCS can be broadly divided into the impulse-generating nodes and the impulse-propagating His–Purkinje system. Human diseases of the conduction system have been identified that alter impulse generation, impulse propagation, or both [1]. Detection of these abnormalities of CCS could be carried out in utero.

In those without abnormalities, the SA node is located at the junction of the superior vena cava and the upper lateral aspect of the right atrium. The AVN lies in the Koch triangle (the boundaries of which are the ostium of the coronary sinus medially, the anterior septal leaflet commissure of the tricuspid valve, and the tendon of Todaro, a tendinous structure connecting the valve of the inferior vena cava ostium to the central fibrous body, posteriorly). Structural abnormalities in the neonatal heart can affect not only the blood flow into and out of the heart, but also the location of the conduction system, thus affecting impulse generation and propagation (Figures 59.1–59.3, and 59.4). Tumors within the heart, depending on location and proximity to the CCS, can also cause a series of cardiac electrical abnormalities including intractable arrhythmias even after tumor resection.

Awareness of atrial appendage arrangement is important prior to surgery or interventional cardiac procedure. In situs inversus, the locations of all the structures described are expected to be reversed. In juxtaposed atrial appendages, the SA node moves more anteriorly in the right atrium. Right atrial isomerism (associated with asplenia) can often have "bilateral" SA nodes and/or two AVNs. One AVN tends to be more anterior and the other more posterior, leading to two distinct QRS morphologies. The AVNs may be connected by a Monckeburg sling [2], which can allow re-entrant arrhythmias. The patient with left atrial isomerism (polysplenia) is at risk for absence of a sinus node or one with a variable location, often presenting with sinus node dysfunction or ectopic atrial rhythms.

The position of the AVN and bundle of His are dependent on the location and interrelationship of the right and left ventricles along with any degree of underdevelopment of the right atrioventricular (AV) valve ring. With incomplete formation of the right ventricle as in tricuspid atresia, double inlet left ventricle, or straddling tricuspid valve, the AV conduction system always is located at the junction of the inferocaudal aspect of the ventricular septum carrying the bundle of His, and the AV junction where the AV node forms. In tricuspid atresia, the AVN is located on the floor of the blindly ending right atrium, with the remaining conduction system coursing into the crest of the muscular ventricular septum leading inferoposterior to the rim of the ventricular septal defect. In two very specific malformations, AV canal defect and congenitally corrected transposition of great arteries, the AVN is anatomically displaced outside the normal triangle of Koch [3]. Straddling tricuspid valve and AV canal defect have the AV conduction system located at the junction of the inferocaudal aspect of the ventricular septum carrying the bundle of His, and the AV junction where the AV node forms. However, the node in AV canal defect is outside the triangle of Koch with central fibrous body missing and a long His extending to the inferior rim of the muscular ventricular septum. In corrected transposition of great arteries, the AVN is positioned anteriorly near the atrial septum with a long bundle of His directed anterocephalad along the pulmonary outflow tract, passing anteriorly along the rim of the ventricular septal defect. Complete AV block at birth is seen in approximately 5% of corrected transposition and some have a progressive decline in conduction over the first two decades of life, with 20% requiring pacing for complete AV block by adulthood [4].

Metabolic disturbances (Table 59.1) such as electrolyte imbalance (Figure 59.5), acidosis, and thyroid

Visual Guide to Neonatal Cardiology, First Edition. Edited by Ernerio T. Alboliras, Ziyad M. Hijazi, Leo Lopez, and Donald J. Hagler.

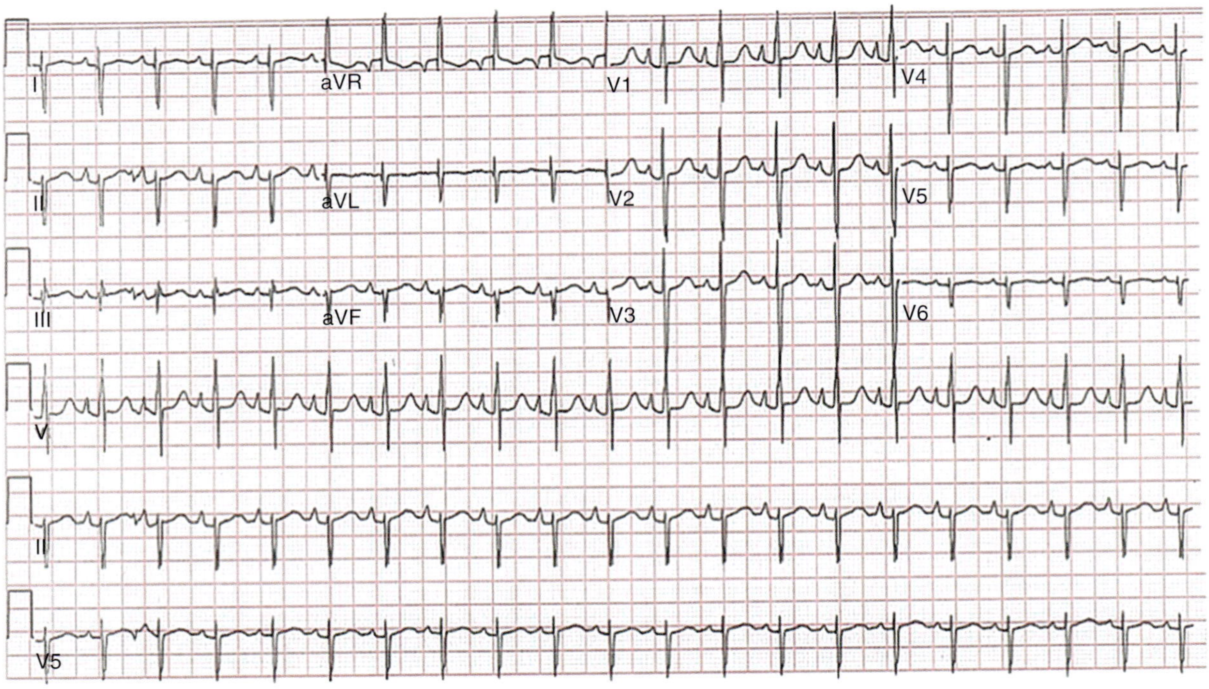

Figure 59.1 Complete atrioventricular canal defect (CAVCD) has an sinoatrial (SA) node in normal position and atrioventricular (AV) node is displaced inferiorly and posteriorly from normal position, with central fibrous body missing and a long non-penetrating bundle extending to the inferior rim of the ventricular septal defect. Shown is a corresponding ECG of a newborn with Down syndrome and CAVCD showing sinus rhythm with *northwest axis, counterclockwise vector* loop in frontal plane, right atrial enlargement, and prolonged PR interval for age.

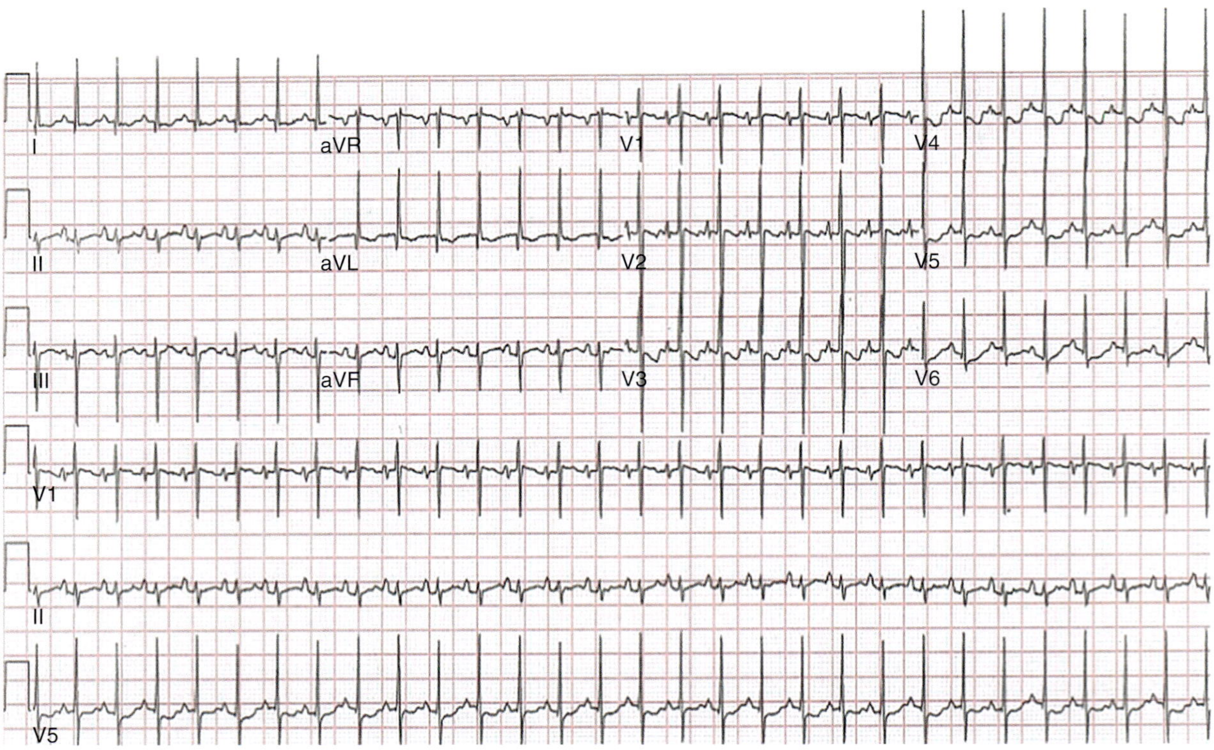

Figure 59.2 Tricuspid atresia has an SA node located in the normal position, but the AV node is located on the floor of the blindly ending right atrium with the remaining conduction system coursing into the crest of the muscular ventricular septum leading inferoposterior to the rim of ventricular septal defect. The corresponding ECG of newborn with tricuspid atresia with normally related great vessels shows sinus rhythm, *left axis deviation*, right atrial enlargement, and left ventricular hypertrophy.

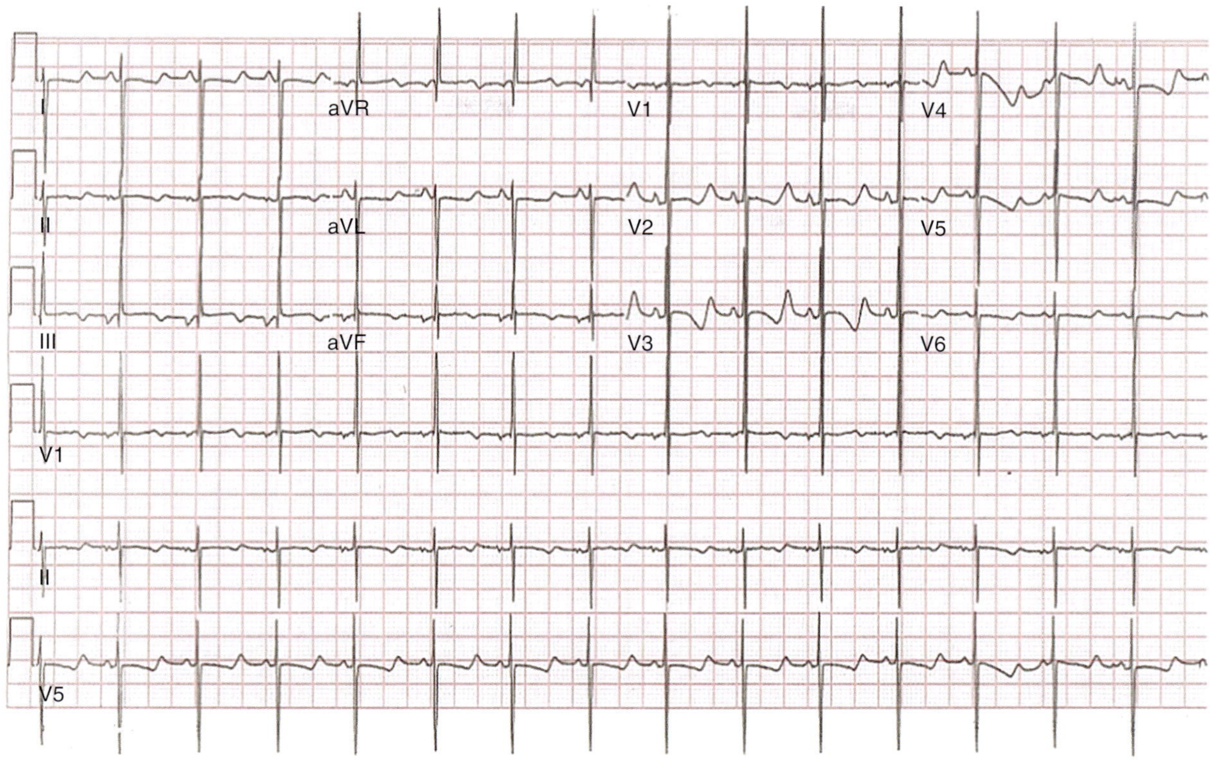

Figure 59.3 Left atrial isomerism (polysplenia) with interrupted inferior vena cava with azygos continuation, bilateral morphologic left atria, right dominant unbalanced CAVCD. The SA node is in abnormal position or absent while the AV node and the rest of the conduction system vary depending on the intracardiac lesions. The displayed ECG is of a newborn with left atrial isomerism and ventricular non-compaction showing low right atrial rhythm (inverted P wave in III and aVF), a heart rate at the lower limit for age, and an abnormal repolarization with prolongation of QT interval.

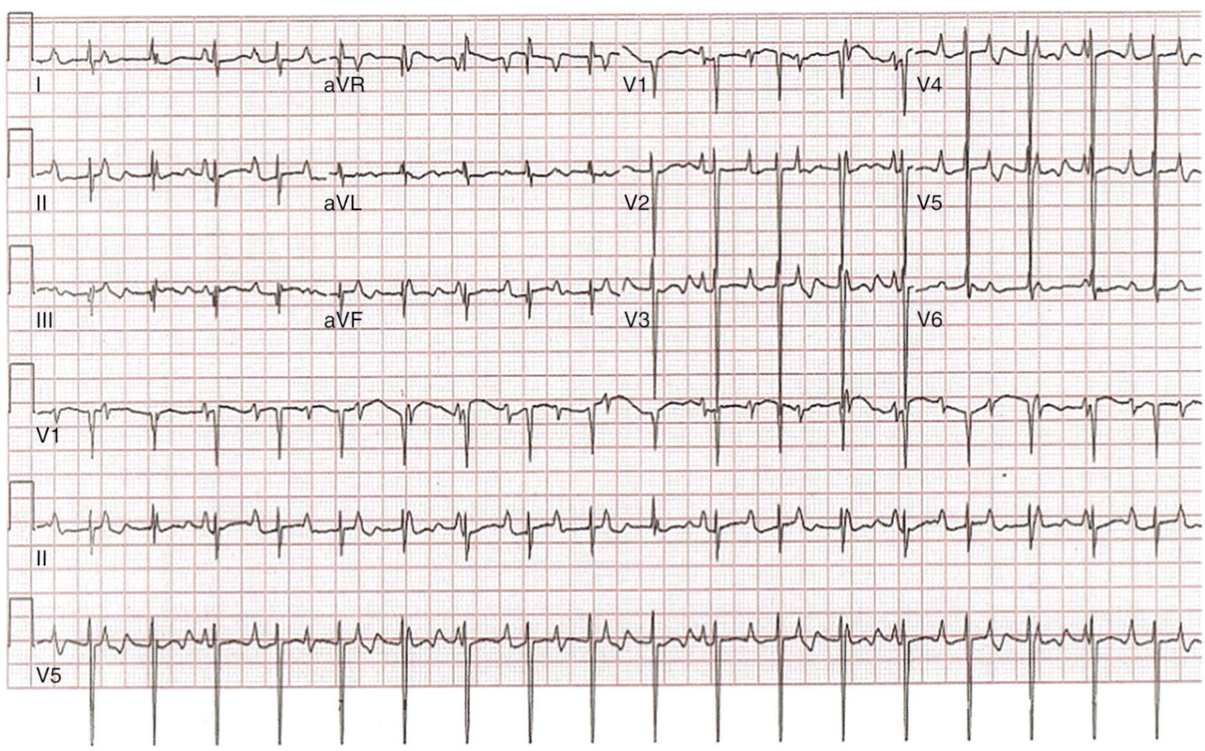

Figure 59.4 Congenitally corrected transposition of great vessels demonstrate atrioventricular and ventriculoarterial discordance. The SA node is situated in normal position while the AV node is displaced anteriorly and laterally giving rise to an elongated and fragile His bundle coursing across the anterior rim of the pulmonary valve (high risk for heart block). It continues superiorly bordering the septal defect if ventricular septal defect (VSD) is present. A corresponding ECG of a newborn shown demonstrates complete AV block (A rate 145 bpm, V rate 115 bpm), left axis deviation, and absence of septal Q wave (lateral precordial leads, I and aVL).

Table 59.1 Metabolic disturbances and cardiac conduction abnormalities.

Metabolic disturbances	Cardiac conduction effects	ECG findings
Hypokalemia	Premature atrial contractions, supraventricular tachycardia, junctional rhythm, first degree AV block, premature ventricular contraction, bidirectional ventricular tachycardia or ventricular fibrillation	Increase P-wave amplitude Increase QRS duration Prolongation in PR and QT intervals Flat or inverted T wave ST segment depression Prominent U wave Findings may not always correlate with the level of hypokalemia
Hyperkalemia (mEq/L)	Accelerated AV conduction (5.5–6) Slow AV conduction (≥7–7.5) Failure of cardiac capture by artificial pacemaker (6–7.5) Reversible fascicular block (6.5–7.5) Reentrant ectopic beats (7.5–8.5) Cardiac arrest or VF (>8)	Tent-shaped T wave and shortened QT (≥5.5) Increase QRS duration (≥6.5) Flat and broad P wave (7–7.5) Disappearing P wave, sine wave patterns of QRS (≥8–9)
Hypocalcemia	Only severe hypocalcemia or hypercalcemia cause dysrhythmia, sinoatrial block or AV block	No effect on P wave Prolongation of ST segment Prolongation of Q-onset T wave Less effect on QTc
Hypercalcemia		No effect on P wave Shortening of ST segment Shortening of Q-onset T wave Less effect on QTc
Hypomagnesemia	Usually associated with other electrolyte abnormalities (e.g., hypokalemia)	
Hypermagnesemia	If acute increase in levels can lead to asystole	
Hypothyroidism	Sinus bradycardia	Low-voltage P, QRS and T waves
Hyperthyroidism	Sinus tachycardia, atrial fibrillation or atrial flutter, rare paradoxical AV block, fascicular block or bundle branch block	Increase QRS and P waves amplitude (simulating left ventricular hypertrophy and P-pulmonale)
Hypothermia	Sinus bradycardia, junctional rhythm, atrial flutter, and atrial fibrillation Severe hypothermia <28°C may cause ventricular extrasystoles and ventricular fibrillation	Prolonged PR, QRS, and QTc intervals, and the Osborn waves (slowly inscribed camel-hump like deflections of the J point in the same direction as the QRS complexes)
Hyperthermia	Sinus tachycardia	ST depression and T-wave flattening
Acidosis	Rhythm disturbances may be secondary to associated abnormalities of potassium or calcium	Increased T-wave amplitude
Alkalosis		Flattening of T wave or T-wave inversion

dysfunction can also affect the conduction system of the newborn with a normal heart [5]. Complete heart block (CHB) can be seen in neonates with both normal and malformed hearts. In those with normal hearts, CHB is frequently related to maternal lupus erythematosus that allows transplacental passage of maternal autoantibodies to the fetus (Figure 59.6). In more than 95% of the patients, the autoantibodies found in the mother are anti-Ro, also known as Sjögren syndrome antibodies (SSA), anti-La (SSB) antibodies, and antiribonucleoprotein (RNP) antibodies. Affected newborns may also have ventricular dysfunction, sinus node disease, junctional rhythms, or systemic manifestations of neonatal lupus erythematosus (i.e., skin lesions on the face, scalp, and upper trunk, resembling the lesions of discoid lupus erythematosus) [6]. About 25% of infants

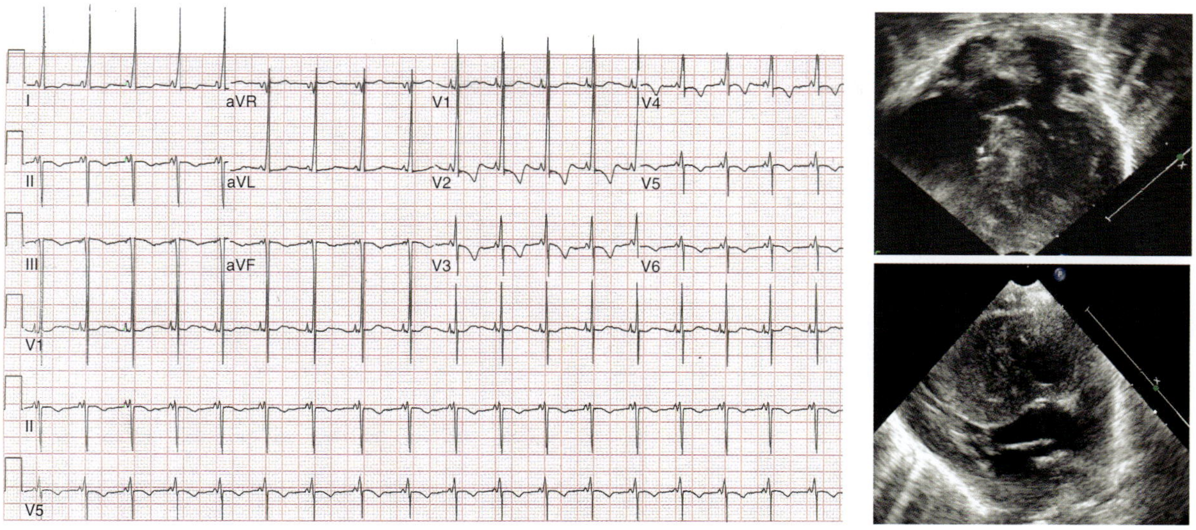

Figure 59.5 In hypocalcemia, cardiac action potential (top right figure) has prolongation of the plateau phase (phase 2) which resulted in prolongation of ST segment (bottom right figure). A corresponding ECG from neonate with hypocalcemia shows normal sinus rhythm with prolonged ST segment which later normalized after calcium level was corrected.

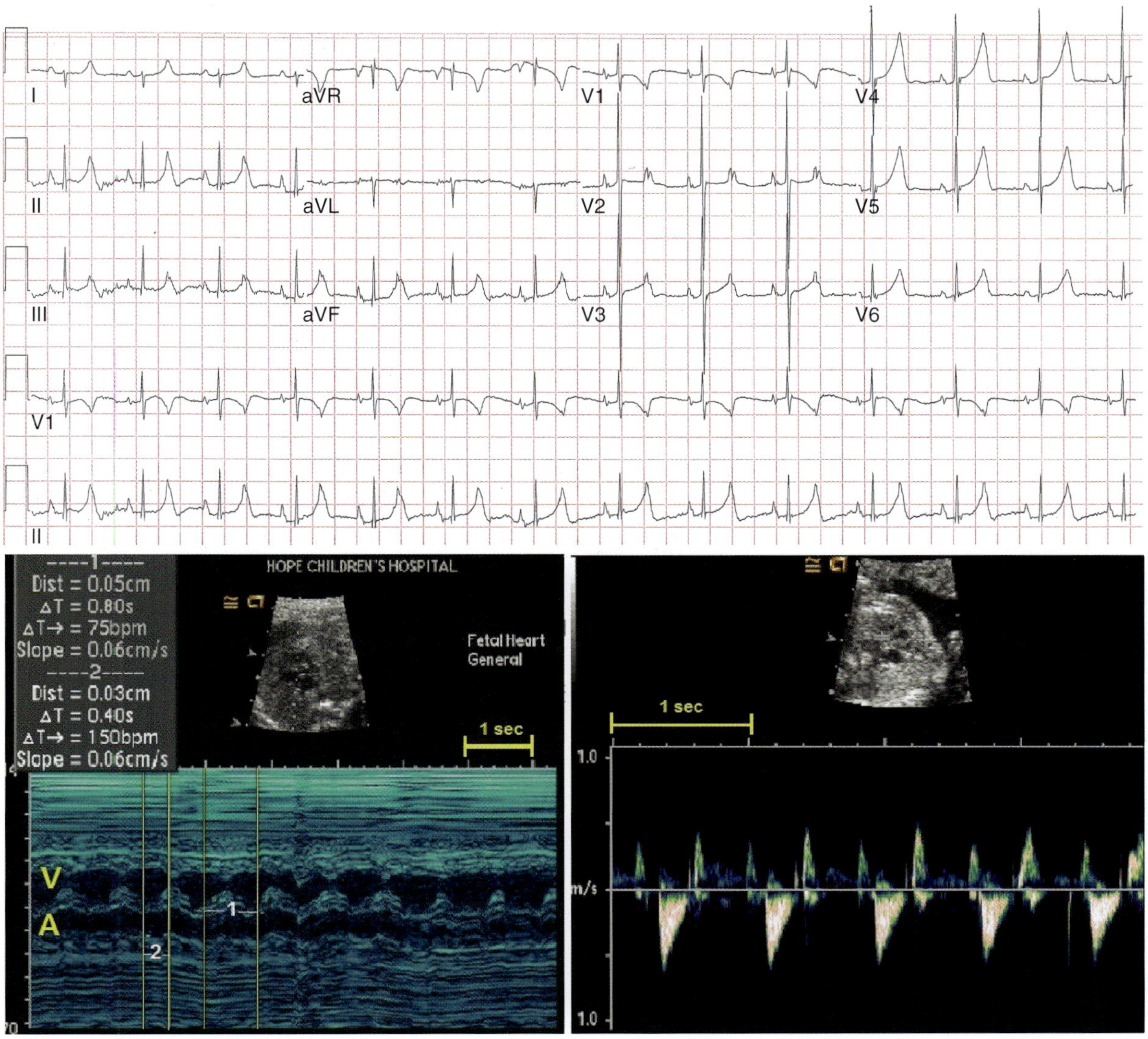

Figure 59.6 ECG of infant with maternal positive Sjögren syndrome antibodies (SSA) antibody showing 2 : 1 AV block (A rate 150 bpm; V rate 75 bpm). Note the difference in QT intervals compared with Figure 59.7 differentiating this from a pseudo 2 : 1AVB from LQTS. This patient was referred pre-delivery because of fetal bradycardia. Fetal echocardiogram (left lower panel) confirmed 2 : 1 AV block with M-mode across atria and ventricle (right lower panel); pulse wave Doppler sampling left ventricular outflow tract.

Table 59.2 Genetic and immulogic disorders.

Immunologic and genetic abnormalities (gene mutations)	Cardiac conduction disturbances	Other manifestations
Long QT syndrome (*KCNQ1, KCNQ2, SCN5A* most common)	Fetal bradycardia, sinus node dysfunction, AV block, ventricular tachycardia or fibrillation, torsades de pointes	Normal heart, SIDS
Catecholaminergic polymorphic ventricular tachycardia (*RYR2, CASQ2*)	Premature ventricular contractions, biventricular tachycardia, ventricular fibrillation	Normal heart, SIDS
Holt–Oram syndrome (*TBX5*)	Sinus bradycardia, AV block, bundle branch block	Skeletal abnormalities, ASD, VSD
Glycogen storage disease aka Pompe disease (*PRKAG2*)	AV block and Wolff–Parkinson–White syndrome	Ventricular hypertrophy
Maternal SSA, SSB antibodies	Congenital AV block (1–5%) Rarely sinus node dysfunction	ASD, VSD, transposition of great arteries and anomalous pulmonary venous drainage seen in up to 25% patients Ventricular dysfunction. Manifestation of neonatal lupus erythematosus including rash
Carnitine deficiency (*SLC22A5*)	Brady-dysrhythmic cardiac arrests, T-wave changes caused by DCM	Skeletal muscle weakness, episodic weakness, episodic hypoglycemia, encephalopathy
Hypertrophic cardiomyopathy (most common – β-myosin heavy chain)	Premature ventricular contractions, ventricular tachycardia, ventricular fibrillation or cardiac arrest	Stillbirth
Arrhythmogenic right ventricular dysplasia (Plakophilin-2, Desmoglein-2 Desmocollin-2 Desmoplakin Plakoglobin)	Ventricular tachycardia Epsilon waves	Rare in infant Right ventricular dilatation, aneurysms and or dysfunction

ASD, atrial septal defect; DCM, dilated cardiomyopathy; SIDS, sudden infant death syndrome; VSD, ventricular septal defect.

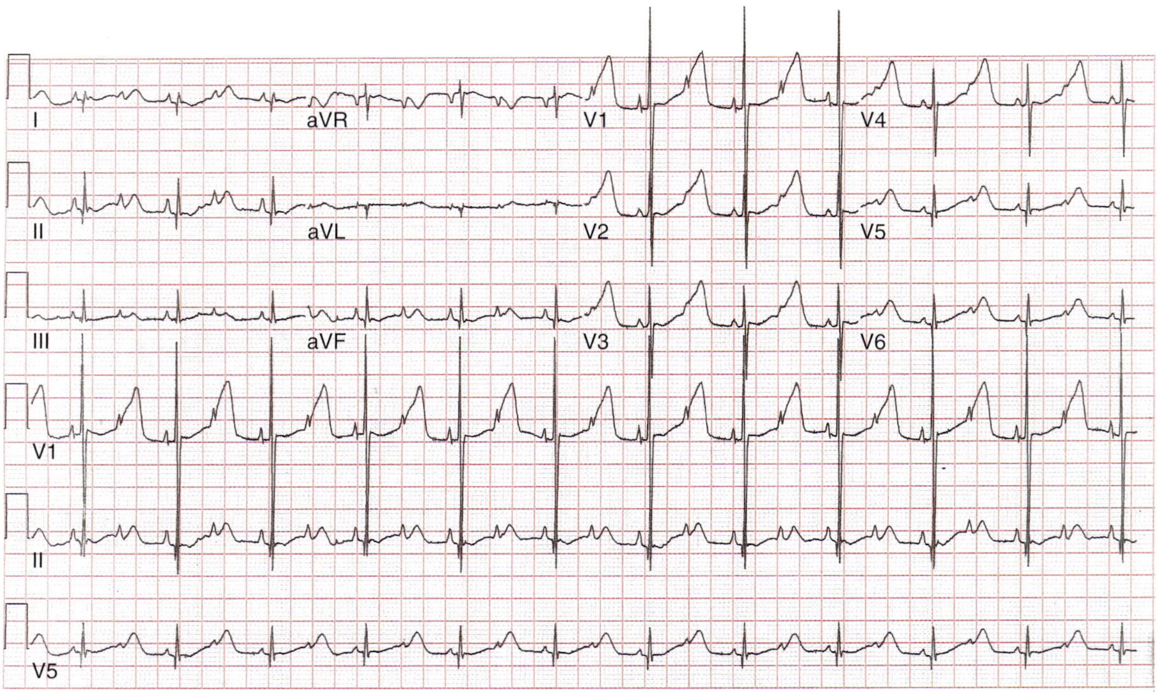

Figure 59.7 This ECG shows pseudo 2 : 1 AV block in a newborn patient with congenital long QT syndrome. Sinus rate was normal (A rate 150 bpm, V rate 70 bpm) but AV block occurred at the level of ventricular myocardium because of abnormally prolonged repolarization with measured corrected QT interval of 611 ms.

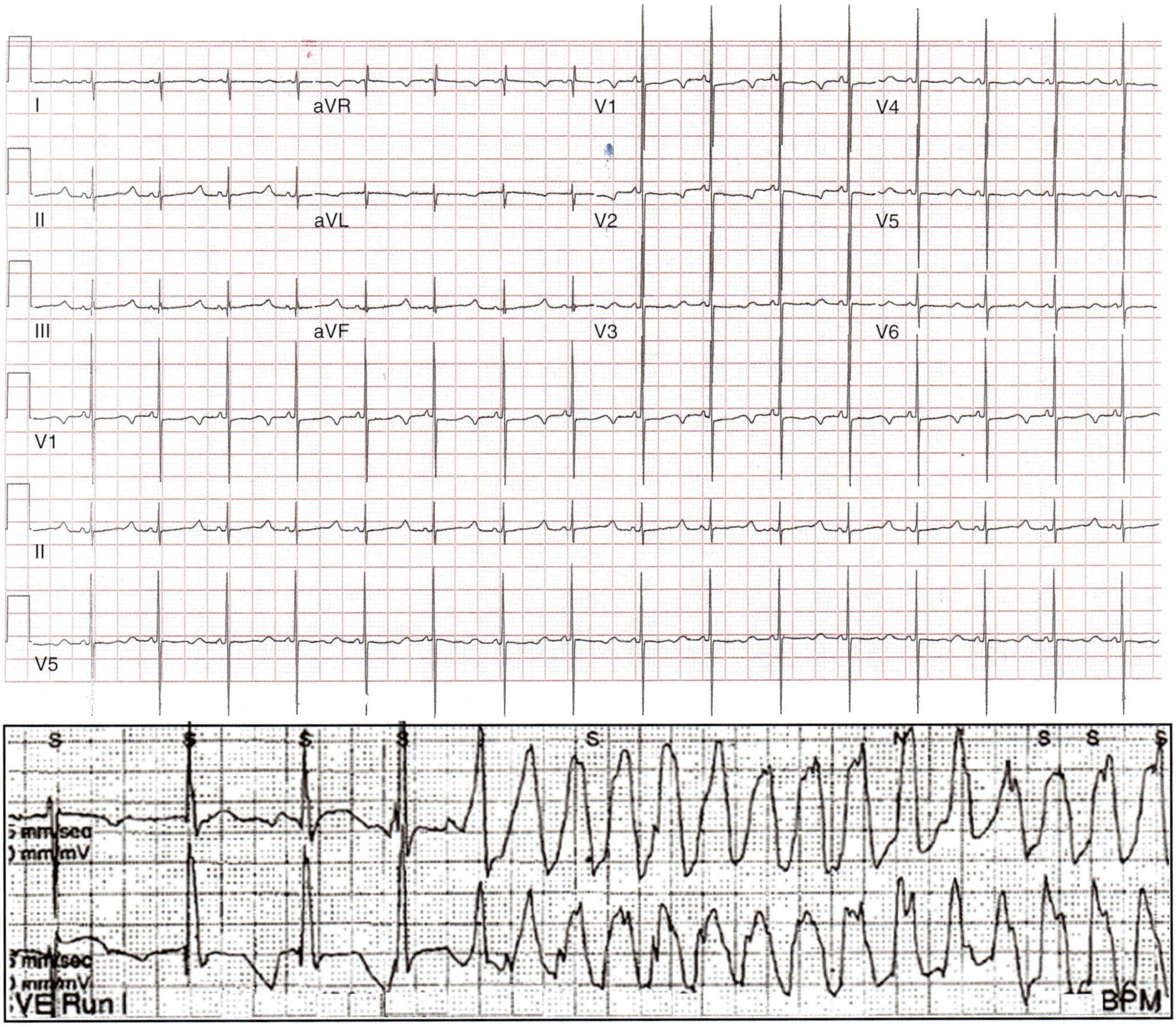

Figure 59.8 ECG of neonate with congenital long QT syndrome type 2 showing sinus bradycardia with prolonged corrected QT interval of 540 ms. This same patient developed multiple episodes of spontaneous polymorphic ventricular tachycardia, as shown in the rhythm strip below the 12-lead ECG. The patient received epicardial implantable cardiac defibrillator (ICD) along with antiarrhythmic medications.

with CHB have associated structural congenital cardiac anomalies such as atrial septal defect (ASD), ventricular septal defect, corrected transposition, or anomalous pulmonary venous return.

Cardiac conduction diseases caused by genetic disorders include abnormalities in ion channels, cellular proteins, transcription factors, or metabolic regulators (Table 59.2). They may manifest as long QT syndrome (Figures 59.7, 59.8, and 59.9), catecholaminergic polymorphic ventricular tachycardia, carnitine deficiency, familial hypertrophic cardiomyopathy, Holt–Oram syndrome (skeletal abnormalities, ASD with first degree AV block), or *PRKAG2* mutation (Pompe disease), all of which can be seen in the newborn. There are some other genetic disorders affecting conduction system that manifest in later life such as Brugada syndrome, arrhythmogenic right ventricular dysplasia (both presenting with life-threatening arrhythmias), LAMP2 (Danon's cardiomyopathy presenting with hypertrophic cardiomyopathy and pre-excitation; Figure 59.10), and *NKX2.5* gene mutation (ASD and later CHB) [7].

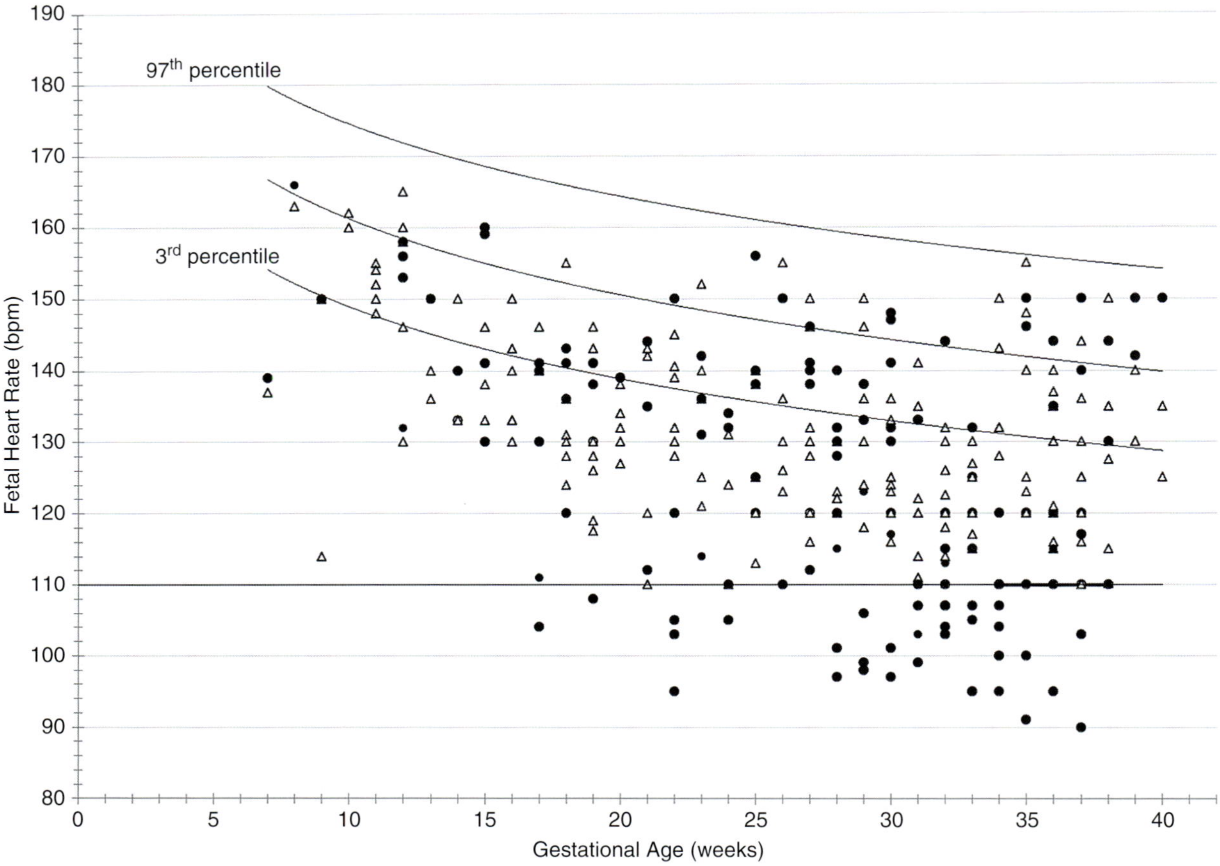

Figure 59.9 Relationship between fetal heart rates and gestational ages of genetically confirmed long QT (LQT) syndrome fetus cohorts. The triangles represent LQT fetuses referred due tor a family history of LQT syndrome and black circles represent LQT fetuses referred for abnormal fetal rhythms. Lines represent percentiles of normal fetal heart rate. Majority of long QT fetuses had heart rates lower than the third percentile of normal.

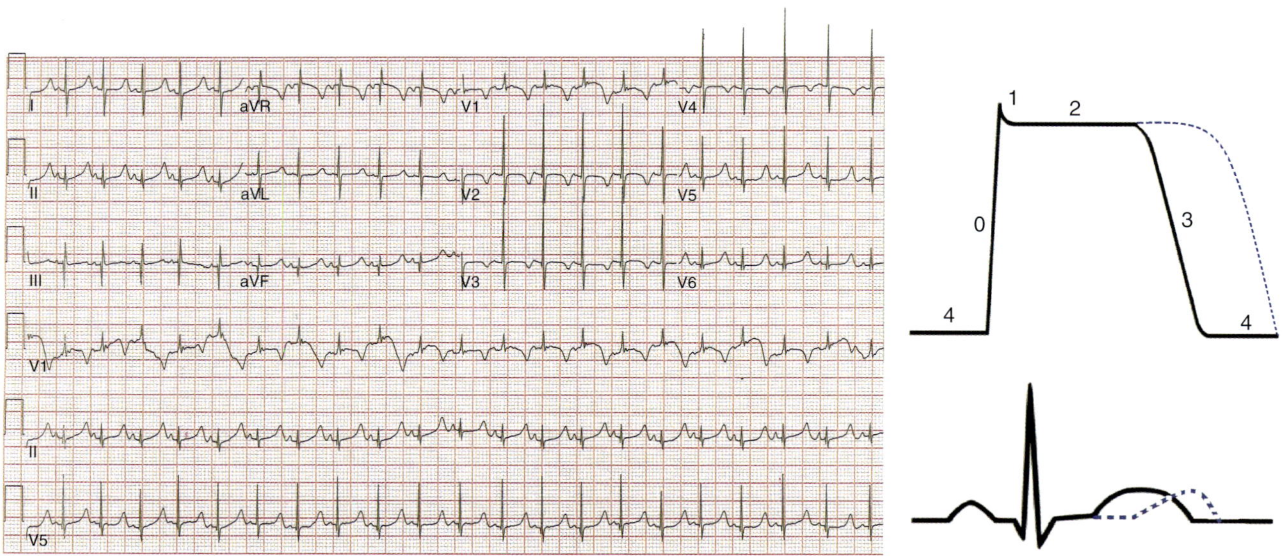

Figure 59.10 An echocardiogram still images from a neonate with hypertrophic cardiomyopathy without known metabolic disease. An apical four-chamber view (top right) and parasternal long-axis view (bottom right) show significant asymmetric septal hypertrophy with near obliteration of LV cavity during systole. The corresponding ECG of this patient showed sinus bradycardia (patient was on beta-blocker) with LVH (voltage criteria) and ventricular pre-excitation (Wolff–Parkinson–White), which was confirmed to be caused by abnormal atrioventricular accessory connection during an electrophysiologic study.

References

1 Park DS, Fishman GI. (2011) The cardiac conduction system. *Circulation*, **123**, 904–915.

2 Mönckeberg JG. (1913) Zur entwicklungsgeschichte des atrioventrikularsystems. *Verh Deutsch Path Ges*, **16**, 228–249.

3 Anderson RH, Ho SY. (1991) The disposition of the conduction tissues in congenitally malformed hearts with reference to their embryological development. *J Perinat Med*, **19**, 201–206.

4 Huhta JC, Maloney JD, Ritter DG, Ilstrup DM, Feldt RH. (1983) Complete atrioventricular block in patients with atrioventricular discordance. *Circulation*, **67**, 1374–1377.

5 Madias JE. (2010) 20 miscellaneous electrocardiographic topics, in, *Comprehensive Electrocardiology* (eds PW Macfarlane, A van Oosterom, O Pahlm, *et al.*), Springer-Verlag, London, pp. 863–883.

6 Gilbert-Barness E, Barness LA. (2006) Pathogenesis of cardiac conduction disorders in children genetic and histopathologic aspects. *Am J Med Genet A*, **140** (19), 1993–2006.

7 Park DS, Fishman GI. (2011) The cardiac conduction system. *Circulation*, **123**, 904–915.

60

Tachydysrhythmias

Barbara J. Deal

Ann and Robert H. Lurie Children's Hospital of Chicago; Northwestern University Feinberg School of Medicine, Chicago, IL, USA

The incidence of arrhythmias presenting in infancy was recently shown to be approximately 24 per 100 000 live births and was associated with structural heart disease in about 23% of babies [1]. Supraventricular tachycardia (SVT) accounts for about 84% of neonatal tachycardia, with a 2 : 1 male predominance. Almost half of neonatal SVT occurs on day 1 of life [2], with a mean heart rate of 270–280 beats per minute (bpm). Tachycardia can be detected incidentally during routine visits, usually by 3 weeks of age. Congestive heart failure is present in 30–48% of neonates presenting with SVT, usually manifesting as gastrointestinal symptoms [2, 3]. Medical therapy is associated with excellent outcomes in infants without structural heart disease. In contrast, sustained ventricular arrhythmias are highly uncommon in neonates, and can be life-threatening when associated with ion channel disorders.

Supraventricular Tachycardia

SVT refers to a typically narrow QRS tachycardia involving the atria, although bundle branch block is present in up to 15% of episodes. The incidence of SVT is estimated to be 1 in 200–250 babies. Structural heart disease is present in 7–46% of babies [2, 4, 5], with higher incidences reported from tertiary cardiology centers. Lesions more often associated with SVT include transposition of the great arteries, Ebstein anomaly, or hypertrophic cardiomyopathy [4]. Understanding the mechanisms of different types of SVT is important for therapy and prognosis, and can be inferred from the electrocardiogram (ECG) during tachycardia and in sinus rhythm.

SVT involves an accessory connection in almost three-quarters of neonatal SVT [6] and is termed atrioventricular reciprocating tachycardia. When the accessory connection is visible during sinus rhythm with a delta wave on ECG, the accessory connection is termed "manifest" or Wolff–Parkinson–White syndrome (Table 60.1). A delta wave is identified in 22–53% of initial ECGs in sinus rhythm among babies with neonatal SVT [2, 4, 5, 7, 8], although the accessory connection can quickly become "concealed" in many infants (delta wave not present on subsequent ECGs in sinus rhythm). SVT using an accessory connection most commonly proceeds from atria to the ventricles over the normal atrioventricular (AV) node, termed orthodromic reciprocating tachycardia (ORT), and returns via the accessory connection, often located along the left atrioventricular annulus (Figure 60.1a). In less than 10% of episodes of tachycardia, conduction proceeds from the atria over the accessory connection to the ventricles, termed antidromic reciprocating tachycardia (ART). The QRS complex is usually narrow, and a retrograde P wave follows the QRS with an average interval of 100 ms, appearing as a deflection in the T wave most readily seen in ECG leads II, III, or V1. At the onset of SVT, a wide QRS complex can be apparent from rate-related bundle branch block. The ORT re-entrant circuit requires the AV node for maintenance, and maneuvers producing block at the AV node will terminate tachycardia. The much less common ART produces a wide QRS tachycardia with a pre-excited appearing QRS complex; rapid conduction to the ventricles via the accessory connection triggers ventricular fibrillation. As digoxin accelerates conduction over an accessory connection, the use of digoxin is avoided in infants with manifest pre-excitation (delta waves) apparent on ECG during sinus rhythm.

A particular subset of ORT utilizes a slowly conducting, concealed accessory connection, commonly located in the posteroseptal region of the heart. Tachycardia is usually slower in rate, commonly 180–260 bpm, but incessant rather than paroxysmal in nature. This tachycardia (termed the permanent form of junctional reciprocating tachycardia, or PJRT) is characterized by a long QRS-P interval, and a relatively normal PR interval; the P wave is negative in the inferior ECG leads II, III, and aVF, and is often confused with a low atrial tachycardia. Tachycardia terminates with maneuvers producing AV

Visual Guide to Neonatal Cardiology, First Edition. Edited by Ernerio T. Alboliras, Ziyad M. Hijazi, Leo Lopez, and Donald J. Hagler.

Table 60.1 Types of tachydysrhythmias demonstrating electrocardiographic (ECG) appearance, their description and arrhythmia mechanism.

ECG	Description	Arrhythmia mechanism
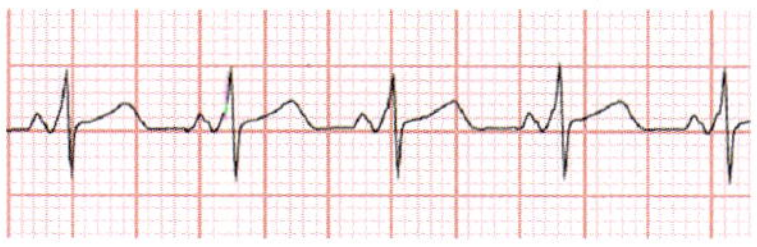	Short PR interval Slurred onset of QRS complex	Delta wave, manifest pre-excitation
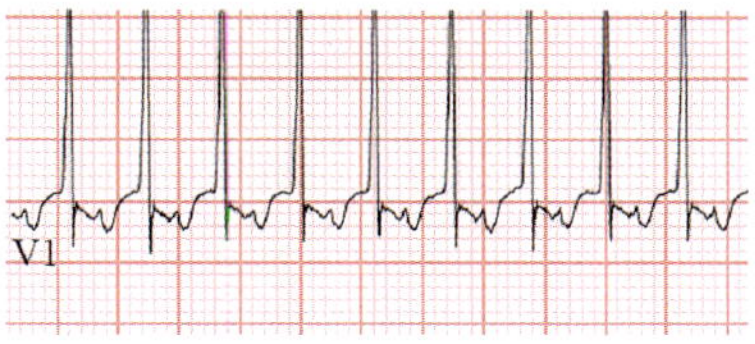	Narrow QRS complex 1 : 1 QRS: P, interval ≥70 ms Retrograde P waves seen within T wave	Orthodromic reciprocating tachycardia (ORT)
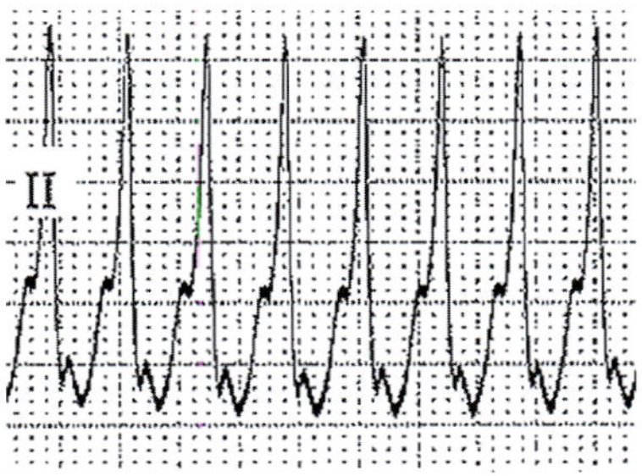	Wide QRS tachycardia 1 : 1 P-QRS relationship Pre-excited QRS appearance	Antidromic reciprocating tachycardia (ART)
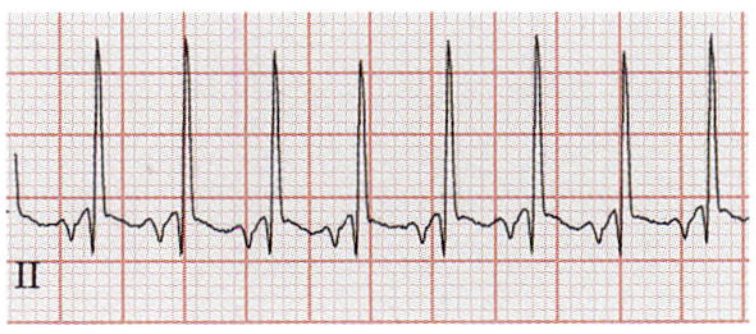	Narrow QRS tachycardia Long QRS-P interval Negative P waves in inferior leads II, III, aVF	Permanent form of junctional reciprocating tachycardia (PJRT)
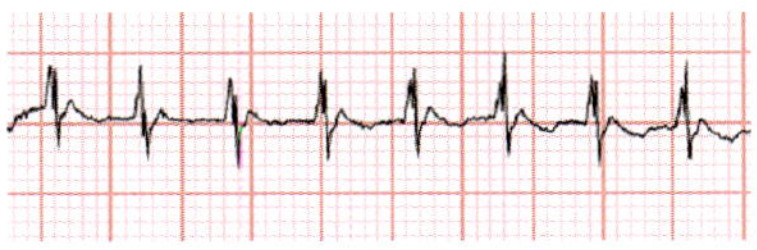	Narrow QRS tachycardia P waves not readily seen Rsr in lead V1	Atrioventricular nodal re-entrant tachycardia (AVNRT)
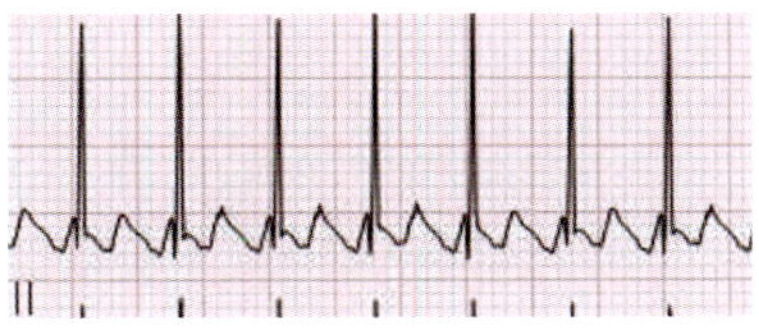	Sawtooth flutter waves in inferior leads Variable AV conduction	Atrial flutter
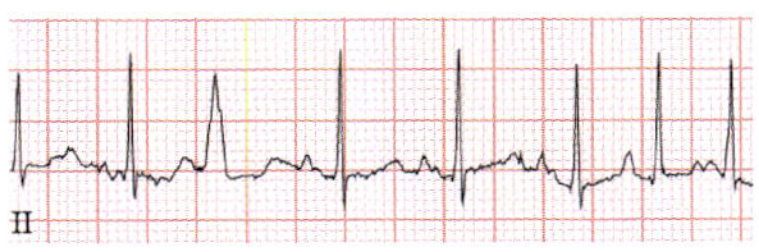	At least three distinct P-wave morphologies Some P waves blocked, some conducted with aberrancy	Multifocal atrial tachycardia
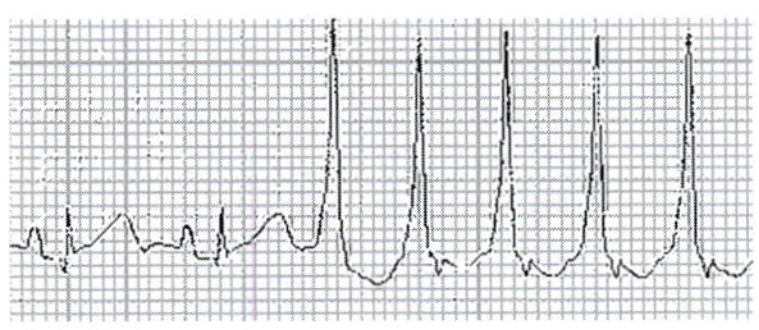	Wide complex rhythm Rate ~20 bpm faster than preceding sinus rate	Accelerated ventricular rhythm (AVR)
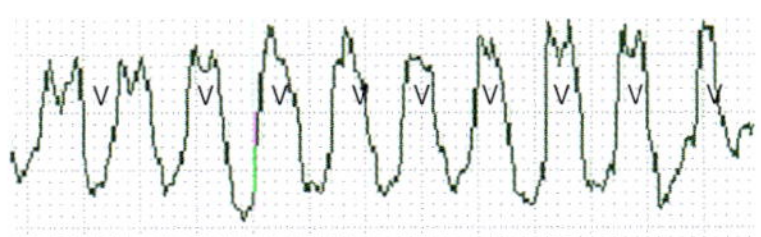	Wide complex tachycardia P-QRS dissociation Rate >180 bpm	Ventricular tachycardia (VT)

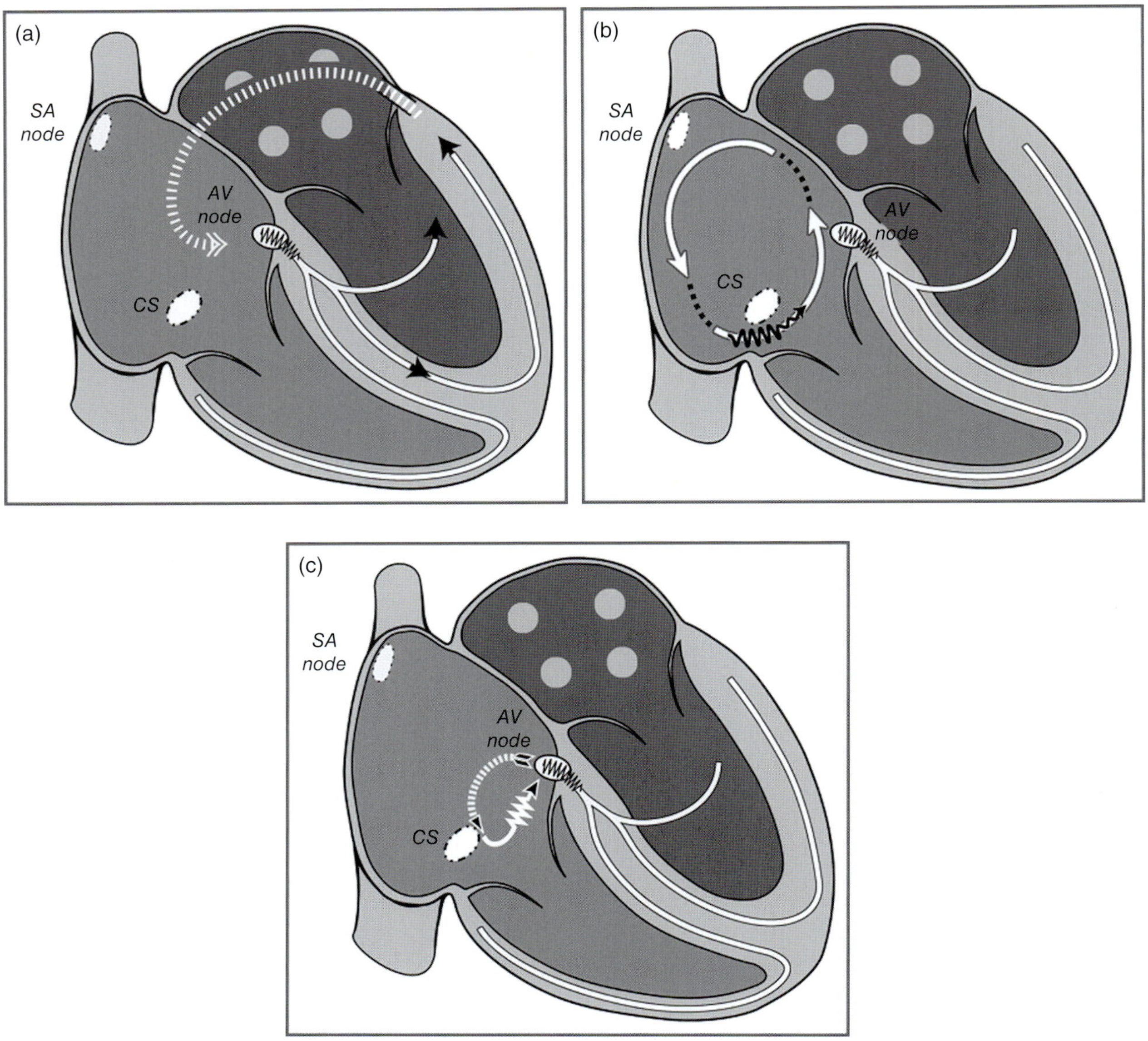

Figure 60.1 (a) Orthodromic reciprocating tachycardia. Re-entrant circuit with conduction proceeding from atria through atrioventricular node to ventricles, and returning via an accessory connection along the atrioventricular annulus. (b) Primary atrial tachycardia. Tachycardia circuit confined to atrial tissue, typically proceeding up atrial septum and down lateral atrial wall. Conduction to ventricles may be variable. (c) Atrioventricular nodal re-entry tachycardia. Re-entrant circuit occurs within atrioventricular nodal tissue, with conduction to atria and ventricles occurring simultaneously. *Source*: Mavroudis *et al.* 2008 [20]. Reprinted with permission of Elsevier.

block, but promptly resumes. Because of its incessant nature, congestive heart failure results. Pharmacologic control of this "refractory" tachycardia usually involves more than one medication, often including sotalol, flecainide, or amiodarone in addition to propranolol [4, 5, 9, 10].

The second most common mechanism of neonatal SVT is atrial flutter, with the re-entrant circuit confined to atrial tissue (primary atrial tachycardia), and conduction over the AV node is not critical to maintenance of tachycardia (Figure 60.1b). The atrial rate is usually about 300 bpm, with either 1 : 1, 2 : 1, or variable AV conduction. In the setting of atrial flutter at 300 bpm with 1 : 1 AV conduction, vagal maneuvers or adenosine can slow the ventricular response to 2 : 1 or 150 bpm, and may be confused with termination of SVT. Failure to recognize this occurrence can allow persistence of tachycardia and subsequent development of congestive heart failure. Adenosine administration can result in transiently slowed AV conduction and allow the flutter waves to become more readily apparent on ECG. Typical flutter waves have a "sawtooth" negative wave appearance in ECG leads II, III, and aVF (Table 60.1).

Other forms of primary atrial tachycardia in infancy include multifocal atrial tachycardia (MAT, sometimes referred to as chaotic atrial tachycardia), or a single ectopic focus of tachycardia often referred to as automatic atrial tachycardia (AAT). Careful analysis of P-wave morphology during tachycardia allows discrimination between these P waves and a normal sinus P wave which has a smooth upright P wave in ECG leads I, II, III, and aVF. When associated with sustained runs of rapid atrial tachycardia, treatment may be indicated to prevent the risk of developing heart failure. Because the tachycardia circuit is confined to atrial tissue, adenosine or vagal maneuvers are not usually successful in terminating primary atrial tachycardia.

Less commonly, atrioventricular nodal re-entry tachycardia (AVNRT) occurs in neonates, diagnosed in 5–12% of infants in the first year of life [4, 6]. As the name suggests, this tachycardia enters and exits the AV node towards both the atria and ventricles simultaneously, producing a QRS-P interval of less than 70 ms (Figure 60.1c). The surface ECG shows a narrow QRS tachycardia without apparent retrograde P waves, as the P wave is buried within the QRS complex giving the appearance of an rsr deflection in lead V1, or a slight broadening of the base of the QRS complex in leads II and III. Tachycardia terminates with vagal maneuvers or adenosine, and is highly responsive to treatment with either digoxin or propranolol. Recurrent tachycardia is uncommon after the first months of life, although studies are not available to assess recurrence risk in later childhood.

Evaluation and Treatment

SVT can be detected in utero or within the first 2 days of life in at least half of patients with neonatal tachycardia, appearing as a heart rate greater than 250 bpm on monitors. Hydrops can be present, although this is now usually detected prenatally. Heart failure is present in up to half of infants, and is more likely in those presenting at 2–4 weeks of life versus day 1 of life. Symptoms are non-specific, with tachypnea, poor feeding, gastrointestinal symptoms, or lethargy present in the first weeks of life; infrequently, the neonate presents to an emergency department in shock, and tachycardia as the etiology can be overlooked during resuscitation. Obtaining a 12-lead electrocardiogram while on tachycardia and prior to intervention is helpful, not only for distinguishing the mechanism of tachycardia, but also for guiding expectations for therapy and estimating the risk of recurrent tachycardia; this step is frequently overlooked.

Acute termination of SVT involving the AV node (the majority of neonatal SVT episodes) can be achieved with maneuvers that block conduction at the AV node: ice to the face, insertion of an intravenous line, or adenosine. Because of the bronchospasm associated with adenosine, pain can stimulate adrenalin release and re-initiate tachycardia after a brief termination; this re-initiation is not to be confused with "failure" of adenosine. Infants with congestive heart failure are less likely to respond to vagal maneuvers [3]. If vagal maneuvers produce AV block, and tachycardia does not terminate, the tachycardia is likely atrial in origin, and visible atrial activity without conduction to the ventricle should become apparent. Adenosine administration in this setting is diagnostic, rather than therapeutic. Initial therapy to prevent recurrences of SVT is commonly digoxin (in the absence of pre-excitation) or propranolol, with about 30% of infants on either drug having recurrences in the first 6 months of life [8]. Sotalol, amiodarone, or flecainide are predominantly used for babies with recurrent or refractory SVT [5, 9, 10].

Atrial flutter responds to oral or intravenous digoxin, transesophageal pacing, synchronized direct-current cardioversion, or spontaneously terminates during the first 24 hours. In the setting of heart failure or structural heart disease, procainamide, sotalol, or amiodarone can be required to prevent acute recurrences of tachycardia. The risk of recurrent atrial flutter after the neonatal period is quite low.

In the setting of congestive heart failure, particularly in the 2- to 4-week-old infant admitted from home, therapy can be quite complicated; these babies require expeditious transfer to a center with cardiac critical care and electrophysiology expertise. Usual efforts to treat heart failure such as intubation or fluid resuscitation can directly worsen the ventricular dysfunction, resulting in profound hypotension. Inotropic agents can provoke arrhythmia recurrences, and intravenous antiarrhythmic medications such as amiodarone are particularly potent negative inotropes in the setting of heart failure. The guidelines for amiodarone dosing in this setting can directly precipitate profound hemodynamic decompensation with extracorporeal membrane oxygenation support needed precipitously [11]. Short-acting esmolol or procainamide infusion [12] with transesophageal pace terminations as needed, or intermittent adenosine, may be effective. Transesophageal pacing is particularly advantageous in the setting of frequent recurrences of SVT in critically ill neonates.

Ventricular Tachydysrhythmias

Accelerated ventricular rhythm (AVR) is an infrequent form of runs of ventricular rhythm appearing in the neonate. The QRS complex is generally wide, with a left bundle branch block morphology, and occurs at a rate up to 15% faster than the preceding sinus rate [13]. There is often a recurring pattern of AVR alternating with sinus rhythm. The baby remains asymptomatic and hemodynamically stable during AVR. Antiarrhythmic treatment is rarely indicated, which is fortuitous as it is difficult to suppress this rhythm with medications. AVR typically resolves within the first few years of life.

Ventricular tachycardia is exceedingly uncommon in neonates, and when it occurs a careful search for underlying causes is required. The QRS complex is broad, and the rate of ventricular tachycardia is fast, usually greater than 180 bpm in the newborn. Associated predisposing conditions include myocarditis, cardiac rhabdomyomas, congenital heart disease, medication, or indwelling line-related and ion channelopathies. Babies who are asymptomatic during ventricular arrhythmia, with a structurally normal heart with normal ventricular function, and normal electrocardiograms for age during sinus rhythm (including absence of bradycardia, conduction delay, or QT prolongation) generally have an excellent prognosis with resolution of the arrhythmia during the first year of life [14, 15]. The decision to treat these low risk infants depends on the frequency of ventricular arrhythmia and rates of tachycardia.

Conversely, symptomatic ventricular tachycardia in the neonate is exceedingly rare, requires aggressive therapy and evaluation, and is often associated with significant risk and mortality. In the absence of structural heart disease or myocarditis/cardiomyopathy, the ECG during sinus rhythm and family history are helpful in assessing etiology. On ECG during sinus rhythm, the presence of bradycardia, conduction delay, AV block, or QT prolongation are strongly suggestive of ion channelopathies, including sodium channel disorders (SCN5A) and Brugada syndrome, and are associated with a high risk [16, 17]. Up to 10% of cases of sudden infant death syndrome can be attributed to heritable long QT syndrome gene variants [18]. There may be a family history of sudden cardiac death, seizure disorders, or miscarriages, and genotyping may ultimately be helpful.

Evaluation and Treatment

A careful assessment for predisposing causes of ventricular arrhythmias includes echocardiogram, ECG during sinus rhythm, 24-hour ECG monitor, electrolyte analysis, removal of indwelling cardiac lines, and detailed family history. Asymptomatic ventricular arrhythmias in the low-risk setting (normal echocardiogram and ECG, absence of predisposing causes, negative family history) only merit treatment if the frequency of ventricular arrhythmia is concerning for the development of ventricular dysfunction. In this setting, beta-blocker medication is often effective when necessary, for the first months of life.

Hemodynamically unstable ventricular tachycardia in the neonate is challenging to manage as it is likely to be recurrent and/or incessant. Direct current cardioversion followed by intravenous infusion of antiarrhythmic medications as dicated by the substrate is indicated. Pause-dependent bradycardia, as may be seen in long QT type 1 with AV block, can respond to isoproterenol infusion. More commonly, esmolol, lidocaine, procainamide, or amiodarone infusions are needed. Particularly in the setting of a structurally normal heart, infants with hemodynamically unstable VT are at high risk for cardiac arrest in their first 10 years of life [19], and may require defibrillator implantation in infancy.

References

1 Turner CJ, Wren C. (2013) The epidemiology of arrhythmia in infants: a population-based study. *J Paediatr Child Health,* **4**, 278–281.

2 Gilljam T, Jaeggi E, Gow RM. (2008) Neonatal supraventricular tachycardia: outcomes over a 27-year period at a single institution. *Acta Paediatr,* **97** (8), 1035–1039.

3 Deal BJ, Keane JF, Gillette PC, Garson A Jr. (1985) Wolff–Parkinson–White syndrome and supraventricular tachycardia during infancy: management and follow-up. *J Am Coll Cardiol,* **5** (1), 130–135.

4 Weindling SN, Saul JP, Walsh EP. (1996) Efficacy and risks of medical therapy for supraventricular tachycardia in neonates and infants. *Am Heart J,* **131** (1), 66–72.

5 Knudson JD, Cannon BC, Kim JJ, Moffett BS. (2011) High-dose sotalol is safe and effective in neonates and infants with refractory supraventricular tachyarrhythmias. *Pediatr Cardiol,* **32** (7), 896–903.

6 Ko JK, Deal BJ, Strasburger JF, Benson DW Jr. (1992) Supraventricular tachycardiamechanisms and their age distribution in pediatric patients. *Am J Cardiol,* **69** (12), 1028–1032.

7 Drago F, Silvetti MS, De Santis A, *et al.* (2008) Paroxysmal reciprocating supraventricular tachycardia in infants: electrophysiologically guided medical treatment and long-term evolution of the re-entry circuit. *Europace,* **10** (5), 629–635.

8 Sanatani S, Hamilton RM, Gross GJ. (2002) Predictors of refractory tachycardia ininfants with supraventricular tachycardia. *Pediatr Cardiol,* **23** (5), 508–512.

9 Price JF, Kertesz NJ, Snyder CS, Friedman RA, Fenrich AL. (2002) Flecainide andsotalol: a new combination therapy for refractory supraventricular tachycardia inchildren <1 year of age. *J Am Coll Cardiol,* **39** (3), 517–520.

10 Tavera MC, Bassareo PP, Neroni P, *et al.* (2010) Supraventricular tachycardia in

neonates: antiarrhythmic drug choice dilemma. *J Matern Fetal Neonatal Med,* **23** (Suppl 3), 30–33.

11 Salerno JC, Seslar SP, Chun TU, *et al.* (2011) Predictors of ECMO support in infants with tachycardia-induced cardiomyopathy. *Pediatr Cardiol,* **32** (6), 754–758.

12 Chang PM, Silka MJ, Moromisato DY, Bar-Cohen Y. (2010) Amiodarone versus procainamide for the acute treatment of recurrent supraventricular tachycardia in pediatric patients. *Circ Arrhythm Electrophysiol,* **3** (2), 134–140.

13 Freire G, Dubrow I. (2008) Accelerated idioventricular rhythm in newborns: a worrisome but benign entity with or without congenital heart disease. *Pediatr Cardiol,* **29** (2), 457–462.

14 De Rosa G, Butera G, Chessa M, *et al.* (2006) Outcome of newborns with asymptomatic monomorphic ventricular arrhythmia. *Arch Dis Child Fetal Neonatal Ed,* **91** (6), F419–422.

15 Levin MD, Stephens P, Tanel RE, Vetter VL, Rhodes LA. (2010) Ventricular tachycardia in infants with structurally normal heart: a benign disorder. *Cardiol Young,* **20** (6), 641–647.

16 Wang DW, Crotti L, Shimizu W, *et al.* (2008) Malignant perinatal variant of long-QT syndrome caused by a profoundly dysfunctional cardiac sodium channel. *Circ Arrhythm Electrophysiol,* **1** (5), 370–378.

17 Kanter RJ, Pfeiffer R, Hu D, *et al.* (2012) Brugada-like syndrome in infancy presenting with rapid ventricular tachycardia and intraventricular conduction delay. *Circulation,* **125** (1), 14–22.

18 Arnestad M, Crotti L, Rognum TO, *et al.* (2007) Prevalence of long-QT syndrome gene variants in sudden infant death syndrome. *Circulation,* **115** (3), 361–367.

19 Spazzolini C, Mullally J, Moss AJ, *et al.* (2009) Clinical implications for patients with long QT syndrome who experience a cardiac event during infancy. *J Am Coll Cardiol,* **54** (9), 832–837.

20 Mavroudis C, Deal BJ, Backer CL, Tsao S. (2008) Arrhythmia surgery in patients with and without congenital heart disease. *Ann Thorac Surg,* **86**, 857–868.

61

Bradydysrhythmias

Gregory Webster and Barbara J. Deal

Ann and Robert H. Lurie Children's Hospital of Chicago; Northwestern University Feinberg School of Medicine, Chicago, IL, USA

Neonatal bradycardia merits attention because of the rare life-threatening diseases that occur with slow heart rates in the first several months of life. There are few cardiac causes of bradycardia; most can be diagnosed with a history, physical examination, and 12-lead electrocardiogram (ECG), occasionally augmented with 24-hour rhythm monitoring or echocardiography. This chapter first enumerates the critical cardiac causes that cannot be missed and then reviews the non-cardiac causes that are important to consider once cardiac causes have been eliminated.

Normal heart rates on the standard 12-lead ECG are subdivided by day of life. Between the first week of life and 3 months of age, the minimum normal heart rate on ECG increases from 90 to 121 beats per minute (bpm) [1, 2]. This rise in expected heart rate is important when considering physiologic bradycardia. This transition is shown in Figure 61.1. These heart rates are based on the "resting" ECG, recognizing that babies may be fussy during the study and several attempts may be required to obtain a resting ECG.

The resting ECG is not optimal for assessing the degree or importance of bradycardia in an infant; continuous heart rate monitoring at various physiologic states is preferred, with at least 24 hours of recording being optimal. Obtaining this information requires inpatient telemetry or 24-hour "ambulatory" (Holter) monitors. On 24-hour monitors, mean and minimum heart rates should be evaluated. Normal mean heart rates in full-term infants on 24-hour monitors are from 95 bpm while asleep to 113 bpm while awake. Minimum heart rates below 60 bpm while asleep and 80 bpm while awake are abnormally slow [3, 4].

Whether the heart rate is obtained by 24-hour monitoring or by ECG, a slow heart rate is only an observation; the prognosis of bradycardia depends on the etiology. The purpose of this chapter is to review the most important causes of bradycardia in the neonate. It will review life-threatening cardiac causes first, including complete heart block, genetic causes, and congenital heart disease. These are not the most common causes encountered by the practicing neonatologist because non-cardiac causes predominate in practice. Non-cardiac causes are reviewed subsequently, followed by typical evaluation and treatment. A list of etiologies of neonatal bradycardia by estimated frequency of presentation is listed in Table 61.1.

Diagnosis of Abnormal Atrioventricular Conduction

If atrioventricular (AV) conduction is abnormal, the first task is to identify and classify the abnormality. First, second, and third degree block are defined by the relationship of the atrium to the ventricle. Third degree or "complete" heart block is complete failure of the p-waves to conduct from the atrium to the ventricle (antegrade dissociation). The p-wave usually occurs at the expected normal heart rate for age. The QRS complex occurs at a slower rate. The ventricular timing is entirely independent of the atrial timing and usually has a very regular pattern. The diagnosis can be unequivocal, with the p-wave marching through independently of the QRS complex in an obvious fashion. However, when the ECG of a newborn shows a slow ventricular rate, care must be taken to search diligently for hidden p-wave inscriptions, often buried in the QRS complex or in the T-wave. Buried p-waves may be especially challenging to see when the atrial rate is a multiple of the ventricular rate. This is critically important because complete heart block can be diagnosed as sinus bradycardia if the extra p-waves are not appreciated. As noted later, the therapy differs markedly.

In second degree block, AV conduction is intermittent. The p-wave typically occurs on schedule, at a usual heart rate for age. The AV node is able to conduct, but the conduction interval gets longer with each beat; therefore, the

Visual Guide to Neonatal Cardiology, First Edition. Edited by Ernerio T. Alboliras, Ziyad M. Hijazi, Leo Lopez, and Donald J. Hagler.

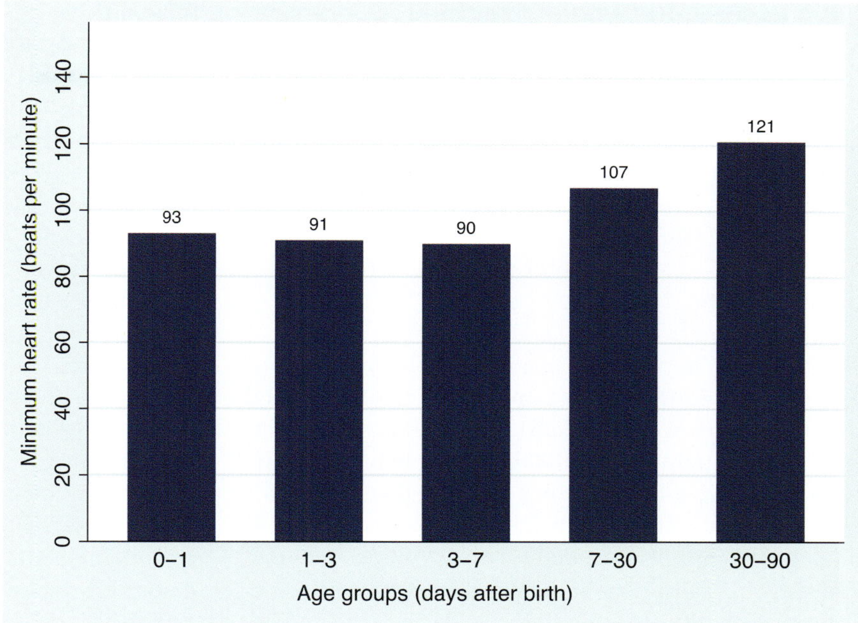

Figure 61.1 Minimum heart rates in beats per minute in infants. *Source*: Davignon *et al.* 1979 [1]. Reproduced with permission of Springer

Table 61.1 Etiologies of neonatal bradycardia, listed by frequency of presentation.

Frequency	Mechanism	Etiology
Common	Sinus bradycardia	Apnea and bradycardia of prematurity
		Gastroesophageal reflux
		Pulmonary disease
		Neurologic injury/head cooling
	Non-sinus mechanisms	Blocked premature atrial contractions
Uncommon	Sinus bradycardia	Metabolic causes[a)]
		Neonatal medications
		Congenital heart disease
		Long QT syndrome
Rare	Sinus bradycardia	Maternal medications
		Mechanical/iatrogenic
	Non-sinus mechanisms	Congenital heart block
		Post-surgical heart block
		Diptheria
		Tumors

Note that some etiologies may have both sinus and non-sinus mechanisms for bradycardia. Classification is based on the most common presentation.

a) See text for an enumeration of the most common metabolic causes of bradycardia.

PR interval gets longer as well. Eventually, the p-wave fails to conduct through the AV node for one beat. This variable conduction produces an irregular pattern of the QRS complex on an ECG with characteristic "grouped beating." The term "high-grade" AV block is used when some, but not all, of the normal sinus beats are conducted. It is typically used when the AV node is more abnormal than second degree block, but where the atrium and ventricle are not completely dissociated, which would imply complete heart block. Second degree AV block can be further subdivided into Mobitz type I and II block, but this is rarely of clinical significance in an infant. All second degree heart block should be recognized and merits further work-up.

First degree heart block is caused by delayed conduction in the atrium or in the AV node. On the first day of life, the PR interval may be as long as 160 ms. Over the first week, the upper limit of normal decreases to 140 ms and remains between 140 and 150 ms until 3 months of age when it begins to gradually increase [1].

Etiologies of Abnormal Atrioventricular Conduction

Third degree or complete atrioventricular heart block (CAVB) carries the highest mortality of all neonatal causes of bradycardia (Table 61.2). CAVB is rare, affecting approximately 1 in 20 000 live-born babies [5]. The natural history of the disease is associated with 14–34% early mortality, although much higher rates are reported when fetal demise is included [5, 6]. CAVB occurs most frequently in the setting of maternal autoimmune disorder (usually with a structurally normal heart) or complex congenital heart disease.

Maternal autoimmune work-up should be pursued in neonates with high-grade or complete heart block without structural heart disease. Maternal SSA/Ro and SSB/La antibodies are thought to provoke an inflammatory response in the fetal myocardium, with targeted cell death at or below the AV node, producing CAVB [7]. The AV block progresses over the first months of life, initially as first degree heart block or as intermittent or persistent second degree AV block, with the appearance of complete block not occurring until the child is older. The full mechanism of antibody-mediated CAVB is incompletely understood. Approximately 10% of neonates who are born with antibody-mediated heart block eventually develop cardiomyopathy, even if appropriate pacing is provided [8, 9]. For a mother whose newborn has congenital heart block because of maternal antibodies, the recurrence risk for heart block in the next pregnancy is 15% [10]. Maternal autoimmune disease resulting in neonatal AV block is often subclinical; the absence of maternal symptoms should not delay a thorough search for antibodies in the early postpartum period. Idiopathic congenital CAVB, unrelated to known maternal antibodies, also exists.

In series from cardiac tertiary care centers, over 90% of patients with CAVB will eventually receive a pacemaker, whether in infancy or in childhood [11]. Because ventricular escape rates tend to decline slowly with age, few patients with congenital CAVB emerge from adolescence without a device.

Table 61.2 Abnormalities of atrioventricular conduction.

ECG	Description	Arrhythmia mechanism
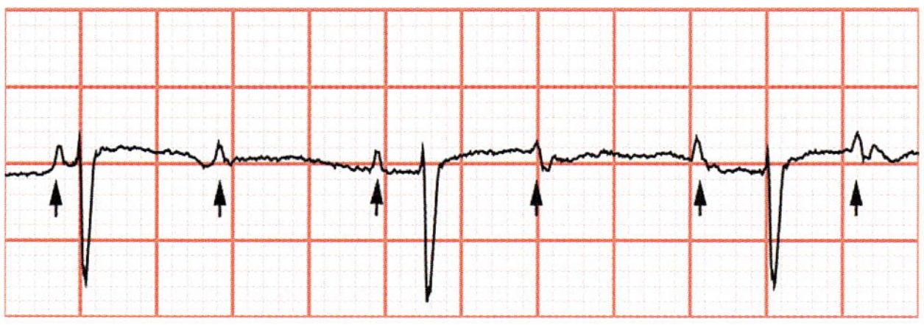	Atrial rate 143 bpm Ventricular rate 79 bpm	Complete heart block
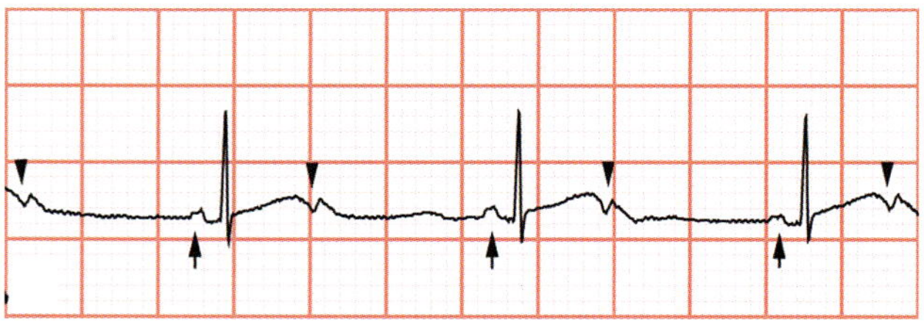	Downgoing, premature p-wave inscription Blocked conduction at the AV node	Blocked PACs are premature atrial contractions, not AV nodal dysfunction
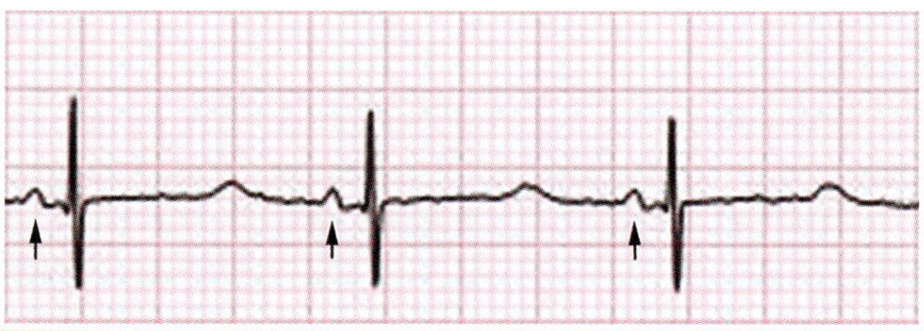	Atrial and ventricular rate are both 75 bpm QTc 580 ms	Prolonged QT interval and bradycardia secondary to cooling for neurologic protection

AV, atrioventricular; bpm, beats per minute; ms, milliseconds; QTc, corrected QT interval (see text for Bazett formula for rate correction). Upward arrows indicate the position of p waves with a sinus rhythm morphology. Downward arrowheads indicate premature atrial contraction.

Developmental abnormalities of the conduction system also cause neonatal AV block secondary to structural defects in the heart. A diagnostic echocardiogram is appropriate for all patients with second or third degree AV block to exclude structural heart disease as well as myocardial dysfunction. Although heart block is possible in multiple forms of structural congenital heart disease, the incidence is particularly high in {S,L,L} transposition of the great vessels, where there is AV discordance, and in heterotaxy syndromes with left atrial isomerism [12].

Post-surgical heart block is an important cause of neonatal heart block and bradycardia, but because it occurs after surgical intervention, the diagnosis is typically readily made in the operating room or the intensive care unit. Recovery can occur spontaneously and temporary pacing is often indicated, typically for at least 10 days to allow recovery of conduction. Permanent pacemaker implantation is necessary in 57% of patients with surgical AV block [13].

Mechanical iatrogenic causes of AV block are rare in the neonatal period, but include heart block after cardiac catheterization and bradycardia after placement of a central line. Sinus node suppression from central line placement is less common with current, soft central lines and typically resolves when the line is drawn back above the superior vena cava–right atrial junction.

Second degree AV block can be caused by the same etiologies as complete heart block (including antibody-mediated disease and structural heart disease), but second degree heart block is more commonly caused by drug toxicity, abnormal electrolytes, mechanical causes, or other transient phenomena. In particular, second degree heart block resulting from abnormal AV conduction must be differentiated from blocked premature atrial contractions. With blocked premature atrial contractions, the atrial impulse is blocked at the AV node because the impulse arrives too early for the AV node to conduct the impulse, not because the AV node itself is abnormal (Table 61.2). The etiology and management of premature atrial contractions are covered in Chapter 62.

Inherited Causes of Bradycardia

The long QT syndrome is a heterogeneous ion channelopathy with mutations described in 13 genes to date, usually involving potassium or sodium cellular flux [14]. The prevalence of long QT syndrome approaches 1 in 2000–2500 individuals, and can be a significant cause of sudden infant death syndrome [15]. Clinical long QT syndrome is associated with bradycardia [16, 17]. Heart rates tend to be only mildly decreased from normal mean values; however, fetal or neonatal bradycardia can be an early indicator of long QT syndrome [18]. For this reason, even mild neonatal bradycardia is an indication for a 12-lead surface ECG because the consequences of failing to detect congenital long QT syndrome are potentially severe.

The hallmark of long QT syndrome is a prolonged QT interval corrected for heart rate. The QT interval is measured in sinus rhythm and includes the period from the start of the QRS until the point where the T wave returns to the isoelectric baseline. The normal corrected QT interval in males is less than 450 ms, and less than 460 ms in females. In neonates during the first week of life, the QT interval can be mildly prolonged, up to 480–490 ms, but should attain normal intervals less than 450 ms by 2 weeks of life in more than 99% of babies [19]. Measurement of the QT interval is usually performed using leads II and V5 and can be taught to any level of independent practitioner. Measurement does not necessarily require a cardiologist for initial screening [20]. Correction of the QT interval for heart rate is performed using the Bazett formula (QT interval in milliseconds, divided by the square root of the preceding R-R interval, in milliseconds). Current ECG algorithms can overestimate the QTc interval, so the automated report can require correction. A QTc interval greater than 470 ms by 2 weeks of life is distinctly abnormal, and is associated with a positive genotype for long QT syndrome in up to 43% of babies [19].

In exceptional cases, the QT interval is sufficiently prolonged that ventricular repolarization is still occurring when the next atrial beat is presented to the ventricle. In this case, 2 : 1 AV conduction block will occur. The presence of 2 : 1 conduction block from ventricular repolarization is a marker of significant QT prolongation.

Although overall therapies for bradycardia are presented later in the chapter, therapy for long QT syndrome is particularly unique and is presented here. Pharmocologic therapy with beta-adrenergic receptor antagonists should be initiated at the time of diagnosis, including in the neonatal period. When recurrent life-threatening arrhythmias occur despite beta-blocker therapy, device implantation can be considered. Epicardial implantable cardioverter-defibrillator (ICD) therapy has been performed in the neonatal period. Because bradycardia-induced ventricular arrhythmia has been noted in long QT syndrome, pacemaker implantation (without a defibrillator) is occasionally an alternative therapy, allowing placement of a smaller generator. Pacing eliminates prolonged pauses that potentiate tachyarrhythmias [21, 22]. Antibradycardia pacing therapy needs to be balanced against the lack of high-voltage defibrillation therapy for tachyarrhythmias present in ICDs. Pacemakers have the advantage of requiring less hardware and have a lower side effect profile than epicardial ICD implantation, but expert consultation should be sought in neonatal cardiac rhythm device selection.

Complications of permanent pacing are more common in neonates, which can influence device choice.

Several rare genetic diseases have been described that have effects on cardiac conduction, including NKX2.5, HCN4, and Kearns–Sayre syndrome. These conduction disorders are not usually apparent during the neonatal period. The cardiac transcription factor *NKX2.5* has been associated with congenital heart disease and familial conduction system disorders [23]. Hyperpolarization-activated, cyclic nucleotide-gated (HCN) channels are involved in regulation of intrinsic cardiac pacemaker function. Mutations in the *HCN4* subtype have been seen in families with autosomal dominant sinus bradycardia [24, 25]. Kearns–Sayre syndrome is a rare disorder associated with deletions in mitochondrial DNA and can result in bradycardia, AV block, and proarrhythmia [26]. Presentation of clinical bradycardia in the neonatal period has not been reported yet in these diseases, which are rare and still incompletely described. Genetic causes of AV block or bradycardia should be considered in the presence of a family history of early sudden death or seizures and after thorough evaluation for other causes.

Non-Cardiac Causes of Bradycardia

Once cardiac causes of bradycardia have been excluded, attention can be turned to the more usual non-cardiac causes. Non-cardiac causes are, by far, the most common reasons for clinical presentation of neonatal bradycardia. In the preterm infant, immaturity of autonomic regulation and a hypervagal state can result in bradycardia [27]. Episodic apnea, hypoxia, and subsequent bradycardia are typical in the immature neonate and typically resolve by 37 weeks' gestation, although interim treatment with methylxanthines is common to prevent episodic apnea and bradycardia [28]. Other causes of hypoxia, including bronchopulmonary dysplasia, pneumonia, pulmonary hemorrhage, and pneumothorax, can cause acute or episodic bradycardia. Elevated intracranial pressure or cooling for neurologic protection can produce marked bradycardia and QT prolongation (Table 61.2).

Both neonatal and maternal medication lists should be carefully reviewed for potential bradycardic effects. Antiarrhythmic medications for neonatal tachyarrhythmias such as supraventricular tachycardia (SVT) frequently affect the sinus node as well as AV and accessory pathway conduction. Bradycardia is an important side effect of these medications, particularly digoxin in the neonate, and occasionally requires alteration of the pharmacologic plan for neonatal SVT. Morphine increases parasympathetic tone and can cause sinus bradycardia as well as, rarely, affecting AV nodal conduction. Maternal drugs can pass across the placenta and remain in the neonatal circulation even after birth, depending on the half-life of the drug. Transplacental effects can slow the neonatal sinus node and decrease AV nodal conduction. Mothers receiving pharmacologic therapy may also pass drugs to a breastfeeding baby. Maternal medications should be evaluated for safety during breastfeeding. Often, the offending maternal drug can be discontinued, the dosage can be decreased, or an alternative maternal drug can be found. In some uncommon scenarios, switching to formula feeding is required.

Neonatal hypothyroidism may lead to bradycardia, but heart rate effects are rare and occur only in the most severe cases. Infants with hypothyroidism detected by mass screening efforts do not have heart rates that are distinguishable from matched controls [29, 30]. Severe hypoglycemia and hyperkalemia can produce bradycardia [31]. Sinus node exit block, diphtheria, and cardiac tumors can cause bradycardia, but this presentation is rare in the newborn period [32, 33].

Evaluation

The history and physical examination are critical in the evaluation of neonatal bradycardia, with attention to maternal history (including prenatal and perinatal drug administration). Maternal medications or illicit drugs remain relevant postpartum if the baby is breastfeeding. Family history of bradycardia, sudden unexplained death in young relatives, AV block, device implantation, and a maternal history of autoimmune disease (especially lupus or Sjögren syndrome) should be elicited. A thorough physical examination should be completed; the cardiac examination, pulmonary examination, and a careful dysmorphology evaluation are high-yield.

Initial procedural evaluation requires a 12-lead ECG, run at standard settings, with care taken to use at least 150 Hz high-pass filter settings. While this filter setting is standard on most machines, occasionally an adult ECG machine will be set to 100 Hz, which can lead to incorrect measurements of neonatal intervals. Inpatient telemetry or a 24-hour continuous monitor is helpful to capture mean and minimum heart rates, to diagnose and quantify ectopy, and to evaluate intermittent AV conduction.

Invasive electrophysiology study to determine sinus node recovery time and intrinsic heart rate has been performed; however, invasive electrophysiology is rarely used for evaluation in neonatal bradycardia in current practice [34].

Management

In cases of non-cardiac bradycardia, treatment of the underlying cause usually results in improvement in

Table 61.3 Management strategies for symptomatic neonatal bradycardia.

Intervention	Advantages	Disadvantages
Intravenous isoproterenol infusion	Rapid initiation; increases sinus node rate; improves AV nodal conduction	Requires intravenous access and may cause peripheral vasodilation with diastolic hypotension
Transcutaneous pacing	Rapid initiation	Meticulous attention to evidence of ventricular capture is necessary
Transesophageal pacing	Technically straightforward	Effective for sinus node dysfunction only; no ventricular capture. Prolonged transesophageal pacing pacing may cause esophageal lesions
Temporary transvenous endocardial pacing	Temporary ventricular pacing is highly effective at maintaining heart rate	Often requires fluoroscopy in the neonate to minimize risk of performation
Permanent transvenous endocardial pacing	Permanent pacing is a definitive therapy	Technically challenging; concern for long-term sequelae of neonatal transvenous systems
Temporary epicardial pacing	Limited subxyphoid incision for temporary ventricular wires provides stable pacing	Small risk of infection or conversion to a more extensive procedure
Permanent epicardial pacing	Permanent pacing is a definitive therapy. Dual chamber pacing is optimal	Sternal incision, although often limited in scope

heart rate. For cardiac causes of bradycardia, treatment depends on the etiology and the severity of illness at the time of presentation.

Patients who are in bradycardic arrest should be managed according to resuscitation guidelines [35, 36]; infusions of isoproterenol or other sympathomimetic agents may be necessary. Other strategies for maintaining an adequate neonatal heart rate are listed in Table 61.3. Although pharmacologic management is the typical first line of therapy, emergent pacing may be needed. Immediate ventricular capture can be obtained with transcutaneous pacing; however, infant pads are necessary to avoid a short-circuit because of overlapping two large pads on a small chest. The pacing artifact and the skeletal muscle contractions induced by transcutaneous pacing make verification of ventricular muscle capture technically challenging and meticulous attention must be paid to monitoring arterial response, distal perfusion, and systemic signs of adequate perfusion in the setting of transcutaneous pacing. In the setting of sinus bradycardia, transesophageal pacing of the atria may be effective if AV conduction is intact.

Temporary chronotropic therapy can be provided via a temporary epicardial pacing wire on the ventricle, or a temporary transvenous pacing wire. Navigating an intravenous course in infants is technically challenging and cardiac perforation is possible; fluoroscopy is often helpful in ensuring correct placement.

Guidelines for permanent pacemaker therapy were published in 2008 and updated in 2012. Indications for pacing are categorized as Class I (universal agreement for therapy), Class II (therapy may be considered), and Class III (therapy not indicated). Class I indications for neonatal pacing include CAVB with a wide QRS escape rhythm, complex ectopy, ventricular dysfunction, or a ventricular rate less than 55 bpm. In patients with congenital heart disease, a ventricular rate less than 70 bpm is a Class I indication for pacing. Additional guidelines for implantation of a permanent pacemaker have been described [37]. Permanent transvenous pacemakers have been implanted in children under 10 kg, but concerns persist about technical challenges associated with placement of the pulse generator as well as long-term implications for venous thrombosis and difficulty in placing subsequent pacing systems [38, 39]. Epicardial dual-chamber pacing systems have low complication rates and have excellent system durability in infants [40]. When an indication for permanent pacemaker implantation exists during infancy, our institutional practice has been to implant an epicardial system. The need for permanent pacing in the neonate with structural heart disease is associated with high early mortality, approaching 40% in the first year of life [36].

Conclusions

Relative physiologic sinus bradycardia occurs in the first week of life; the minimum normal heart rate increases after the second week of life. Abnormally slow heart rates may be caused by sinus bradycardia or as abnormalities of AV conduction. Non-cardiac causes of sinus bradycardia predominate as the most common etiology of bradycardia, including autonomic immaturity, apnea, and bradycardia of premature infants, and secondary to medications or other illnesses. Neonatal sinus bradycardia can be the initial manifestation of long QT syndrome. AV block is not physiologic in the infant and requires thorough cardiac evaluation of the infant and maternal assessment for autoimmune antibodies. The presence of structural heart disease and neonatal complete AV block is associated with significant early mortality.

References

1 Davignon A, Rautaharju P, Boisselle E, *et al.* (1979) Normal ECG standards for infants and children. *Pediatr Cardiol*, **1**, 123–152.
2 Schwartz PJ, Garson A Jr, Paul T, *et al.* (2002) Guidelines for the interpretation of the neonatal electrocardiogram: a task force of the European Society of Cardiology. *Eur Heart J*, **23** (17), 1329–1344.
3 Richards JM, Alexander JR, Shinebourne EA, *et al.* (1984) Sequential 22-hour profiles of breathing patterns and heart rate in 110 full-term infants during their first 6 months of life. *Pediatrics*, **74** (5), 763–777.
4 Montague TJ, Taylor PG, Stockton R, Roy DL, Smith ER. (1982) The spectrum of cardiac rate and rhythm in normal newborns. *Pediatr Cardiol*, **2** (1), 33–38.
5 Buyon JP, Hiebert R, Copel J, *et al.* (1998) Autoimmune-associated congenital heart block: demographics, mortality, morbidity and recurrence rates obtained from a national neonatal lupus registry. *J Am Coll Cardiol*, **31** (7), 1658–1666.
6 Groves AM, Allan LD, Rosenthal E. (1996) Outcome of isolated congenital complete heart block diagnosed in utero. *Heart*, **75** (2), 190–194.
7 Hutter D, Silverman ED, Jaeggi ET. (2010) The benefits of transplacental treatment of isolated congenital complete heart block associated with maternal anti-Ro/SSA antibodies: a review. *Scand J Immunol*, **72** (3), 235–241.
8 Moak JP, Barron KS, Hougen TJ, *et al.* (2001) Congenital heart block: development of late-onset cardiomyopathy, a previously underappreciated sequela. *J Am Coll Cardiol*, **37** (1), 238–42.
9 Udink ten Cate FE, Breur JM, Cohen MI, *et al.* (2001) Dilated cardiomyopathy in isolated congenital complete atrioventricular block: early and long-term risk in children. *J Am Coll Cardiol*, **37** (4), 1129–1134.
10 Waltuck J, Buyon JP. (1994) Autoantibody-associated congenital heart block: outcome in mothers and children. *Ann Intern Med*, **120** (7), 544–551.
11 Jaeggi ET, Hamilton RM, Silverman ED, Zamora SA, Hornberger LK. (2002) Outcome of children with fetal, neonatal or childhood diagnosis of isolated congenital atrioventricular block: a single institution's experience of 30 years. *J Am Coll Cardiol*, **39** (1), 130–137.
12 Schmidt KG, Ulmer HE, Silverman NH, Kleinman CS, Copel JA. (1991) Perinatal outcome of fetal complete atrioventricular block: a multicenter experience. *J Am Coll Cardiol*, **17** (6), 1360–1366.
13 Weindling SN, Saul JP, Gamble WJ, *et al.* (1998) Duration of complete atrioventricular block after congenital heart disease surgery. *Am J Cardiol*, **82** (4), 525–527.
14 Webster G, Berul CI. (2013) An update on channelopathies: from mechanisms to management. *Circulation*, **127** (1), 126–140.
15 Schwartz PJ, Stramba-Badiale M, Segantini A, *et al.* (1998) Prolongation of the QT interval and the sudden infant death syndrome. *N Engl J Med*, **338** (24), 1709–1714.
16 Vincent GM. (1986) The heart rate of Romano–Ward syndrome patients. *Am Heart J*, **112** (1), 61–64.
17 Mitchell JL, Cuneo BF, Etheridge SP, *et al.* (2012) Fetal heart rate predictors of long QT syndrome. *Circulation*, **126** (23), 2688–2695.
18 Horigome H, Nagashima M, Sumitomo N, *et al.* (2010) Clinical characteristics and genetic background of congenital long-QT syndrome diagnosed in fetal, neonatal, and infantile life: a nationwide questionnaire survey in Japan. *Circ Arrhythm Electrophysiol*, **3** (1), 10–17.
19 Schwartz PJ, Stramba-Badiale M, Crotti L, *et al.* (2009) Prevalence of the congenital long-QT syndrome. *Circulation*, **120** (18), 1761–1767.
20 Postema PG, De Jong JS, Van der Bilt IA, Wilde AA. (2008) Accurate electrocardiographic assessment of the QT interval: teach the tangent. *Heart Rhythm*, **5** (7), 1015–1018.
21 Moss AJ, Liu JE, Gottlieb S, *et al.* (1991) Efficacy of permanent pacing in the management of high-risk patients with long QT syndrome. *Circulation*, **84** (4), 1524–1529.
22 Eldar M, Griffin JC, Abbott JA, *et al.* (1987) Permanent cardiac pacing in patients with the long QT syndrome. *J Am Coll Cardiol*, **10** (3), 600–607.
23 Konig K, Will JC, Berger F, Muller D, Benson DW. (2006) Familial congenital heart disease, progressive

atrioventricular block and the cardiac homeobox transcription factor gene NKX2.5: identification of a novel mutation. *Clin Res Cardiol*, **95** (9), 499–503.

24 Mehta AV, Chidambaram B, Garrett A. (1995) Familial symptomatic sinus bradycardia: autosomal dominant inheritance. *Pediatr Cardiol*, **16** (5), 231–234.

25 Laish-Farkash A, Glikson M, Brass D, *et al.* (2010) A novel mutation in the HCN4 gene causes symptomatic sinus bradycardia in Moroccan Jews. *J Cardiovasc Electrophysiol*, **21** (12), 1365–1372.

26 Lee KT, Lai WT, Lu YH, *et al.* (2001) Atrioventricular block in Kearns–Sayre syndrome: a case report. *Kaohsiung J Med Sci*, **17** (6), 336–339.

27 Scagliotti D, Deal BJ. (1986) Arrhythmias in the tiny, premature infant. *Clin Perinatol*, **13** (2), 339–350.

28 Henderson-Smart DJ, De Paoli AG. (2010) Methylxanthine treatment for apnoea in preterm infants. *Cochrane Database Syst Rev*, **12**, CD000140.

29 Yasuda T, Ohnishi H, Wataki K, *et al.* (1999) Outcome of a baby born from a mother with acquired juvenile hypothyroidism having undetectable thyroid hormone concentrations. *J Clin Endocrinol Metab*, **84** (8), 2630–2632.

30 Asami T, Suzuki H, Yazaki S, Sato S, Uchiyama M. (2001) Effects of thyroid hormone deficiency on electrocardiogram findings of congenitally hypothyroid neonates. *Thyroid*, **11** (8), 765–768.

31 Lista G, Bastrenta P, Castoldi F, Meneghin F, Zuccotti G. (2011) Severe bradycardia in an extremely low birth weight preterm infant with hyperkalaemia. *Resuscitation*, **82** (5), 640–641.

32 Nadas AS, Ellison RC. (1968) Cardiac tumors in infancy. *Am J Cardiol*, **21** (3), 363–366.

33 Stockins BA, Lanas FT, Saavedra JG, Opazo JA. (1994) Prognosis in patients with diphtheric myocarditis and bradyarrhythmias: assessment of results of ventricular pacing. *Br Heart J*, **72** (2), 190–191.

34 Miller MS, Shannon KM, Wetzel GT. (2000) Neonatal bradycardia. *Prog Pediatr Cardiol*, **11** (1), 19–24.

35 Kattwinkel J, Perlman JM, Aziz K, *et al.* (2010) Part 15: neonatal resuscitation: 2010 American Heart Association Guidelines for Cardiopulmonary Resuscitation and Emergency Cardiovascular Care. *Circulation*, **122** (18 Suppl 3), S909–919.

36 Kleinman ME, Chameides L, Schexnayder SM, *et al.* (2010) Part 14: pediatric advanced life support: 2010 American Heart Association Guidelines for Cardiopulmonary Resuscitation and Emergency Cardiovascular Care. *Circulation*, **122** (18 Suppl 3), S876–908.

37 Epstein AE, DiMarco JP, Ellenbogen KA, *et al.* (2013) 2012 ACCF/AHA/HRS focused update incorporated into the ACCF/AHA/HRS 2008 guidelines for device-based therapy of cardiac rhythm abnormalities: a report of the American College of Cardiology Foundation/American Heart Association Task Force on Practice Guidelines and the Heart Rhythm Society. *Circulation*, **127** (3), e283–352.

38 Kammeraad JA, Rosenthal E, Bostock J, Rogers J, Sreeram N. (2004) Endocardial pacemaker implantation in infants weighing $<$ or $=$ 10 kilograms. *Pacing Clin Electrophysiol*, **27** (11), 1466–1474.

39 Robledo-Nolasco R, Ortiz-Avalos M, Rodriguez-Diez G, *et al.* (2009) Transvenous pacing in children weighing less than 10 kilograms. *Pacing Clin Electrophysiol*, **32** (Suppl 1), S177–181.

40 Kelle AM, Backer CL, Tsao S, *et al.* (2007) Dual-chamber epicardial pacing in neonates with congenital heart block. *J Thorac Cardiovasc Surg*, **134** (5), 1188–1192.

62

Atrial and Ventricular Ectopies

Sabrina Tsao and Barbara J. Deal

Ann & Robert H. Lurie Children's Hospital of Chicago; Northwestern University Feinberg School of Medicine, Chicago, IL, USA

In older series, premature atrial or ventricular contractions are reported in less than 1% of electrocardiograms (ECGs) and about 11% of 24-hour monitoring recorded in neonates, and are predominantly supraventricular in origin [1–4]. With the dramatic changes in the last three decades in fetal and neonatal monitoring, arrhythmias are increasingly recognized in the perinatal period, but extensive data about natural history and management strategies are not yet available. The major risks posed by supraventricular premature beats include bradycardia caused by blocked contractions, and the risk of frequent atrial ectopy escalating into supraventricular tachycardia (SVT) and heart failure. For the much less common premature ventricular contractions, the goal is to identify potentially life-threatening underlying cardiac conditions and implement appropriate therapy.

Premature Atrial Contractions

Using 12-lead ECG for screening in 2030 babies aged 6–9 days old, Southall identified premature atrial contractions (PACs) in 0.4%, and SVT was detected in 0.09% [1, 2]. The same group reported Holter monitor studies in 134 infants in the first 10 days of life, and found extrasystoles in 14% of infants, thought to be supraventricular in origin. However, only 2.9% of babies had more than 50 PACs in the 24-hour period [3]. In another study of 63 newborns, at least one PAC was reported in about half of infants, but more than 50 PACs in 24 hours were present in only 1.5% of babies [5]. Thus, rare isolated PACs are present in 11–50% of infants, but fewer than 2% of babies will have more than 50 premature beats during a 24-hour timeframe.

More complex atrial ectopy consisting of couplets, triplets, or non-sustained atrial runs were not reported on normal infant Holter monitoring. Among fetuses noted to have complex or frequent PACs, it is estimated that the risk of developing SVT is about 0.5% [6]. As complex or more frequent PACs (>50 PACs/24 hours) are not normally present, and because of the small risk of progression to a sustained arrhythmia, it has been our practice to continue to monitor these infants over the first months of life. The frequency of monitoring varies based on the amount of atrial ectopy and other predisposing risk factors.

The etiology of the PACs is speculative, and may be related to remnants of neural crest cells in atrial myocardium [7], or autonomic nervous system immaturity. The neonatal nervous system matures rapidly during the first weeks of life, and is consistent with the usual observation of progressive resolution of premature beats within the first months of life. Atrial ectopy may be mechanical, caused by a prominent aneurysmal flap of the atrial septum, atrial myxoma, or presence of a central venous line. Rarely, PACs are the initial manifestation of atrial electrical disease, which can progress over years, ultimately developing into frequent palpitations, atrial tachycardia or fibrillation, or sinus node dysfunction.

Clinical Presentation

The PAC, by definition, does not arise from the normal sinus node, and thus has a slightly different P-wave morphology compared with the sinus P wave. This premature P wave may then conduct to the ventricles with a slightly prolonged PR interval. Most infants with PACs are asymptomatic and the arrhythmia is most commonly detected during fetal scanning or routine monitoring. Symptoms related to PACs occur when frequent PACs are present and either are not conducted, resulting in bradycardia, or are conducted without sufficient recovery of cardiac output, resulting in hypotension.

Isolated PACs occur as conducted PACs, non-conducted (or "blocked") PACs, or PACs conducted with aberrancy (widened QRS complex, bundle branch

Visual Guide to Neonatal Cardiology, First Edition. Edited by Ernerio T. Alboliras, Ziyad M. Hijazi, Leo Lopez, and Donald J. Hagler.

ECG	Description	Clinical	Treatment
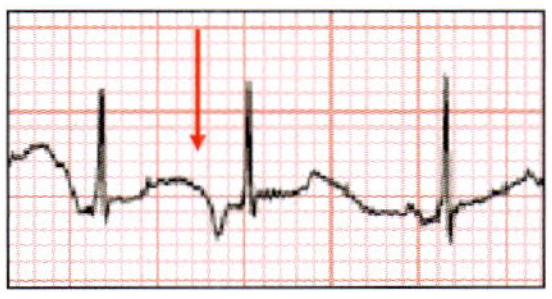	Conducted PAC. Premature beat from atrium, different P wave morphology to sinus beats	Common, usually isolated beats. PACs predispose to development of SVT in 1 in 200 infants	Rule out intracardiac catheters, rule out structural heart disease. Observe.
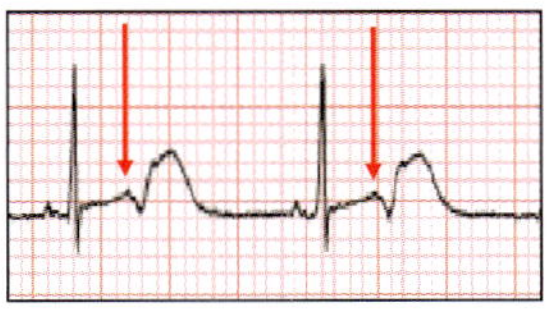	Blocked PAC. Premature beat from atrium, different P wave morphology, does not conduct to the ventricle. Abnormal T waves	Common, causes bradycardia due to blocked PAC in bigeminy.	Similar to conducted PAC.
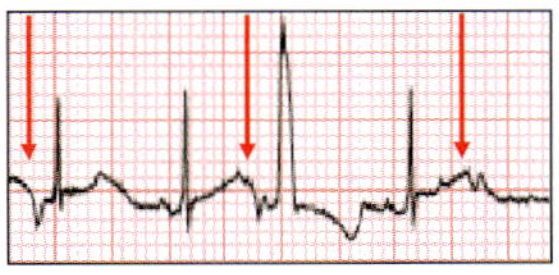	Conducted PAC, conducted PAC with aberrancy (not abnormal P wave in preceding T wave), and blocked PAC	Ashman phenomenon. Compensatory pause –alter sinus rhythm cycle length	Similar to conducted PAC

↓ PAC with different P wave morphology

Figure 62.1 Different types of premature atrial contractions (PACs).

block). Therefore, there are three clinical appearances of PACs (Figure 62.1):

1) *Irregular heart rhythm caused by conducted PACs:* a premature P wave with a different P-wave morphology compared with the sinus P wave, followed by a narrow QRS complex resembling the normal QRS. The PR interval of the premature complex may be prolonged. These beats can occur in a paired fashion with the preceding sinus beat, giving the appearance of atrial bigeminy.
2) *Aberrantly conducted PACs:* the premature P wave occurs slightly earlier and conducts to the ventricles with delay below the atrioventricular node, or bundle branch block (Ashman phenomenon; Figure 62.2). The premature wide QRS caused by conduction "aberrancy" is commonly mistaken for premature ventricular contractions (PVCs). In order to distinguish the aberrantly conducted PAC from a PVC, search for the premature P wave deforming the preceding T wave.
3) *Bradycardia caused by blocked PACs:* P waves that occur quite early following the sinus beat can fall within the preceding T wave, and fail to conduct to the ventricles. The premature P wave may not be distinctly apparent on monitor strips. The blocked PACs are most commonly mistaken for sinus bradycardia; the distinction is particularly important as prenatal "bradycardia" may be interpreted as fetal distress, and provoke unnecessary premature delivery (Figure 62.3).

Aberrant PAC

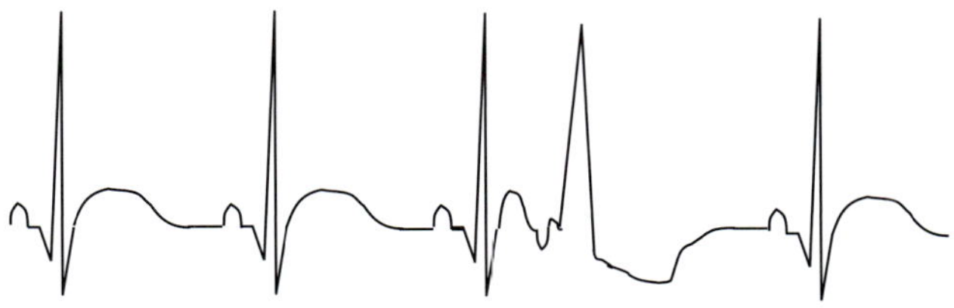

Figure 62.2 Aberrant PAC – Ashman phenomenon.

Evaluation

Initial evaluation of any arrhythmia includes assessment of hemodynamic stability, and identification of predisposing causes for arrhythmia. Maternal history of drug ingestion, including caffeine, bronchodilators, or cocaine use can cause atrial extrasystoles [8]. Administration of cardiac sympathomimetic medications in high doses or placement of venous lines reaching the atrium are common causes of premature beats in the neonatal intensive care setting.

A 12-lead ECG is obtained both to identify the premature P waves, and to exclude chamber hypertrophy or QTc prolongation suggesting underlying cardiac disease. For infants with venous lines, a chest radiograph locates the line within the atria and guides the amount of distance for line withdrawal if necessary.

For frequent premature beats, an echocardiogram is usually obtained to exclude atrial pathology, congenital

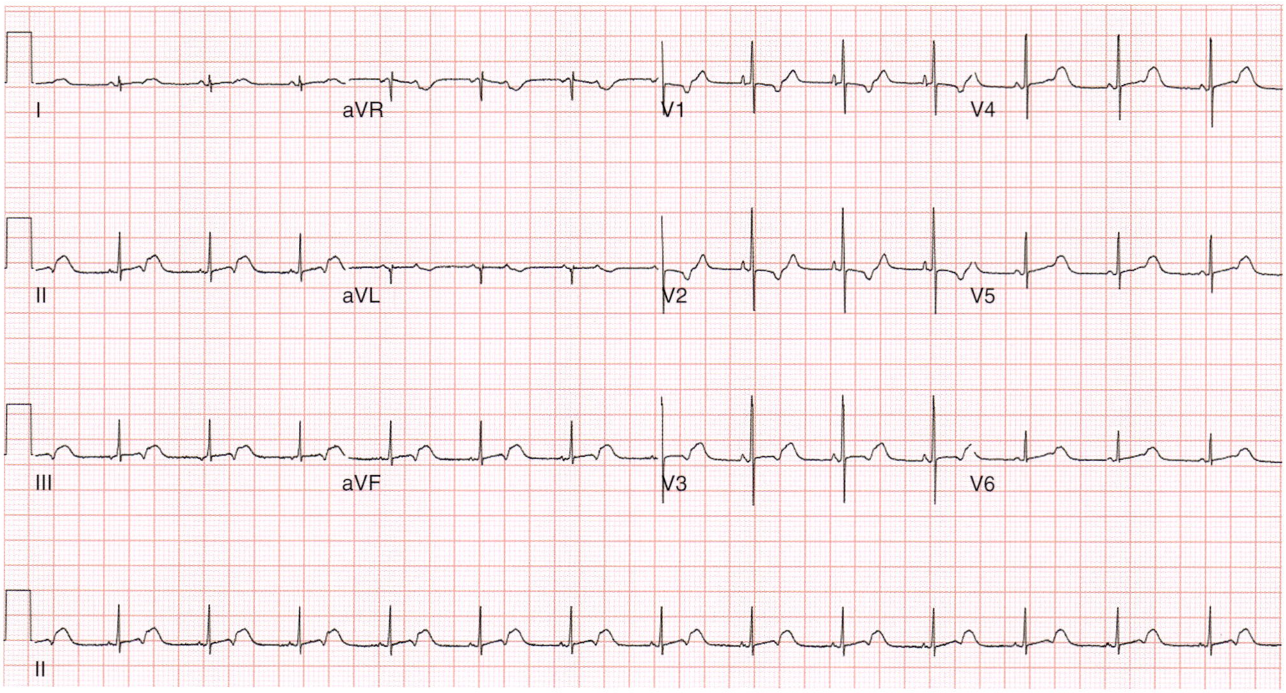

Figure 62.3 Electrocardiogram (ECG) of a 28 weeks' gestation infant delivered for fetal bradycardia. Note blocked PACs and sinus beat in bigeminy. Blocked PACs – negative inflection in the T wave – best seen in leads II, III, and aVF.

cardiac defects, assessment of contractility, and potential pericardial effusion. For frequent PACs, a 24-hour Holter monitoring is obtained to establish frequency of beats, and assess complex ectopy or possible SVT. Quantification of PACs as a percentage of total heart beats is useful in determining the potential need for medication, and assessing the frequency of follow-up needed.

Management

Undiagnosed blocked PACs can be mistaken for fetal distress and fetal bradycardia. Infants born with frequent blocked PACs resulting in symptomatic bradycardia may require transient treatment to increase the heart rate. In this setting, sympathomimetic medications improve conduction as well as augment the blood pressure. The use of digoxin can be considered in an attempt to reduce the frequency of atrial ectopy; there is not strong evidence to support this approach. Withdrawal of lines from within the atria may be necessary, as well as minimizing the use of stimulants thought to be contributing to ectopy, such as caffeine for apnea of prematurity.

The frequency of ongoing cardiac monitoring depends on the presence of complex atrial ectopy or runs, and the percentage of PACs noted in 24 hours. Our center uses an algorithm for follow-up (Figure 62.4). Most babies with more than 50–100 PACs in 24 hours receive follow-up monitoring in 2–4 weeks, and subsequently repeat monitoring depending on the progression of ectopy. The first 6–12 weeks of life are the highest risk period for developing SVT, and vigilance is highest during this time. Parents of infants with frequent atrial ectopy (more than ~1–2%) are taught how to count the heart rate, and the signs and symptoms associated with tachycardia such as poor feeding, increased respiratory rate, or lethargy, and instructed about the need for urgent follow-up if symptoms are noted.

Premature Ventricular Contractions

In the first week of life, Southall reported PVCs in about 0.5% of newborns seen on ECG [3]. Holter data on PVCs in neonates is limited, as premature beats have been typically categorized as "extrasystoles" without specifying supraventricular or ventricular origin. In one study of 63 newborns, at least one PVC in 24 hours was noted in 18%; notably, no infant had 50 or more PVCs by 24-hour monitoring [5]. The presence of more than a few isolated PVCs or any ventricular couplets in the newborn infant is considered abnormal, and requires further evaluation.

The etiology of ventricular ectopy is related to underlying cardiac or systemic disease, or related to the remnants of cardiac excitable tissue or immature nervous system as speculated for PACs. Cardiac etiologies include cardiac abnormalities such as rhabdomyoma, myocarditis, cardiomyopathy, and congenital long QT syndrome. A recent report [9] of multiform PVCs described as multifocal ectopic Purkinje-related premature contractions

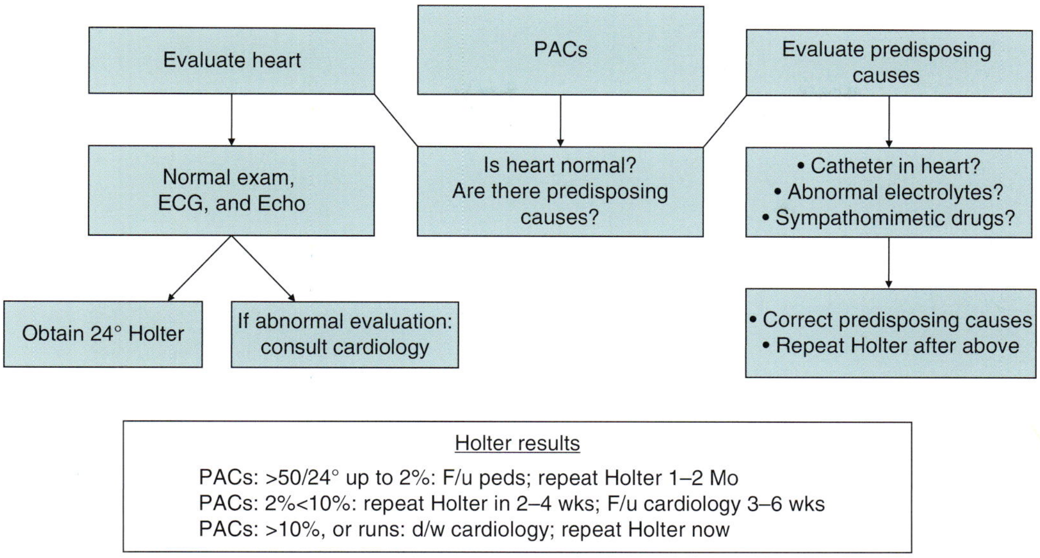

Figure 62.4 PAC management algorithm.

is caused by a gain of function of the sodium channel SCN5A. This mutation results in hyperexcitability of the fascicular-Purkinje system giving rise to multiform PVCs, which may present in infancy.

Clinical Presentation

Newborns with isolated PVCs are usually asymptomatic and present with an irregular heart rhythm noted during examination or on hospital monitoring. Isolated PVCs appear as premature (usually) wide QRS complex beats on ECG or telemetry monitoring. Of note, the duration of the QRS complex of PVCs in newborns can be narrower than in older children. Patients with multiform Purkinje-related PVCs present with sinus or junctional rhythm, or atrial arrhythmias in additional to multiform PVCs. Babies with systemic disease or underlying cardiac disease present with low cardiac output in the setting of PVCs noted on monitor.

Evaluation

Initial evaluation of any arrhythmia includes assessment of hemodynamic stability and identification of predisposing causes of arrhythmia. Maternal history of intercurrent illness, chorioamnionitis, or maternal lupus can cause infectious or immune-mediated myocarditis. Family history of sudden unexplained death, congenital deafness, drowning, or seizures heighten suspicion for congenital long QT syndrome. In symptomatic infants or babies with frequent PVCs, electrolytes are obtained to assess potassium, calcium, and magnesium levels, which might contribute to arrhythmia.

A 12-lead ECG (Figures 62.5, 62.6, and 62.7) is obtained to differentiate PVCs from aberrantly conducted PACs, to assess the QT interval and T-wave morphology, as well as chamber hypertrophy.

Similar to the evaluation of infants with PACs, a chest radiograph in patients with venous lines locates the line within the ventricle and guides the distance for line withdrawal.

An echocardiogram is recommended for infants with more than rare PVCs. This is to assess anatomy, ventricular size and contractility, and evaluate the presence of myocardial fibromas or pericardial effusion.

In infants with more than rare isolated PVCs, 24-hour Holter monitoring is obtained to establish frequency of beats, morphology of ventricular ectopy (uniform morphology indicating one ventricular focus; multiform morphologies indicate myocardial dysfunction or cardiac channelopathy) and detect runs of ventricular tachycardia (VT) that may not be apparent on telemetry.

Management

In general, isolated PVCs do not need treatment, other than addressing predisposing conditions. In the setting of shock or myocarditis, PVCs usually respond to treatment of the underlying pathology, and rarely require antiarrhythmic therapy other than maintenance of normal electrolytes. As the QT interval may be mildly prolonged in the first few days of life, babies with prolongation of the QT interval require serial ECGs; in most cases, the QTc shortens to <460 ms within 2–4 days. Sinus bradycardia associated with prolonged QT interval raises the index of suspicion for long QT syndrome [10]; these babies require frequent follow-up

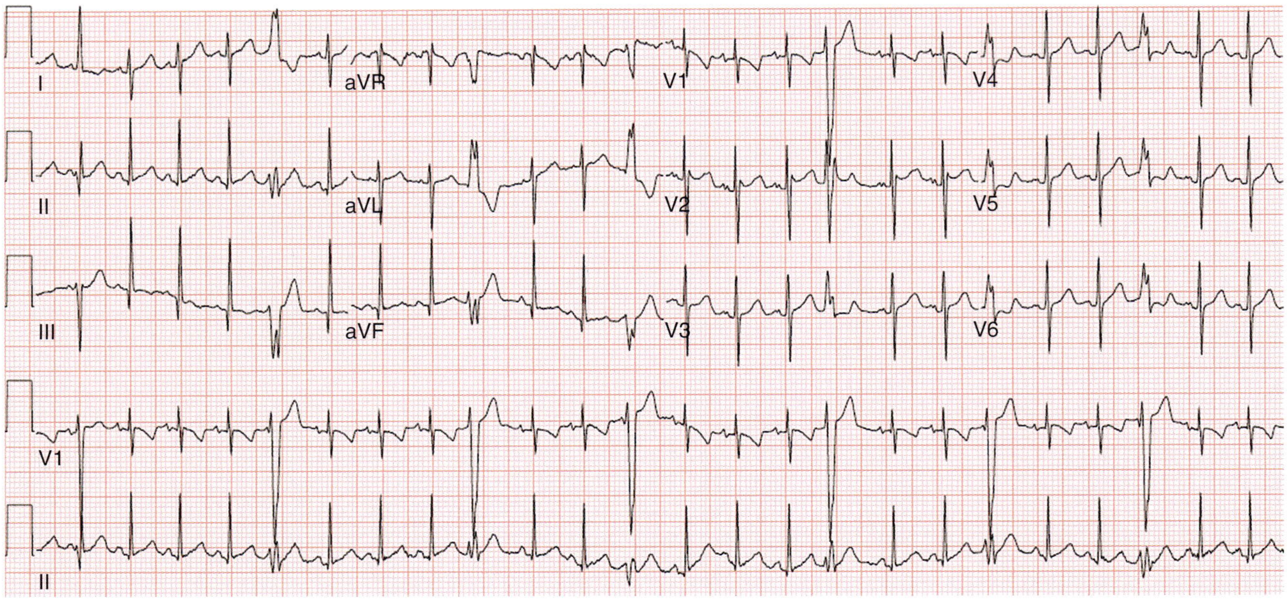

Figure 62.5 A 12-lead ECG with isolated uniform premature ventricular contractions (PVCs).

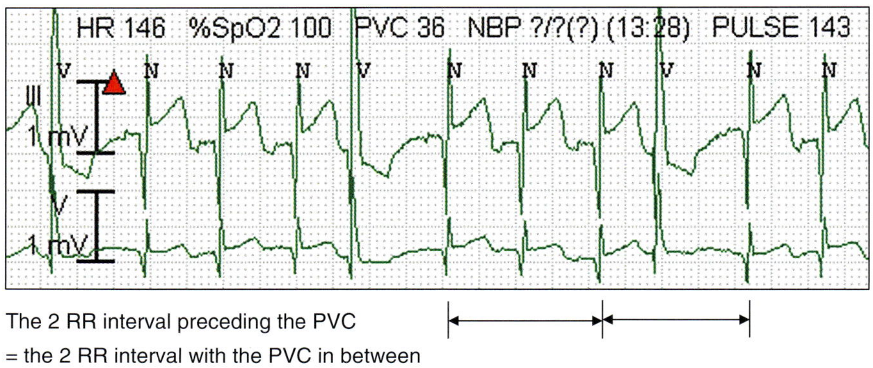

Figure 62.6 Telemetry strip showing PVCs.

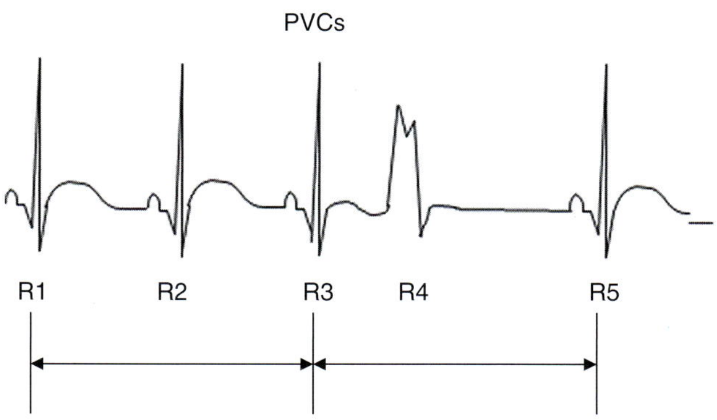

Figure 62.7 Premature ventricular contractions.

visits to monitor the QT interval in the first months of life. Should the QT be markedly prolonged or remain abnormal, decision-making regarding the likelihood of long QT syndrome ensues. Review of family ECGs and careful family history can aid this decision.

Certain scenarios prompt consultation with a pediatric electrophysiologist. Prolongation of the QT interval >490 ms by day 4–5 of life is abnormal, and can require beta-blocker initiation. Complex ventricular ectopy consisting of polymorphic PVCs, ventricular couplets, triplets or runs of non-sustained VT are very uncommon and require inpatient monitoring for a period of days while attempts to identify underlying causes proceed. In patients suspected to have multifocal Purkinje premature beats, a detailed family history should be obtained and family members screened if necessary. In this rare setting, flecainide can control atrial arrhythmias, and may reduce the amount or risk of VT.

Assuming that the heart is structurally normal, with a normal ECG, and no other concurrent conditions, our center uses a management protocol based on the frequency and complexity of PVCs on the initial Holter monitoring (Figure 62.8). With isolated PVCs accounting for <2% of total beats, the baby has a repeat 24-hour ambulatory monitor as an outpatient within 1–2 weeks;

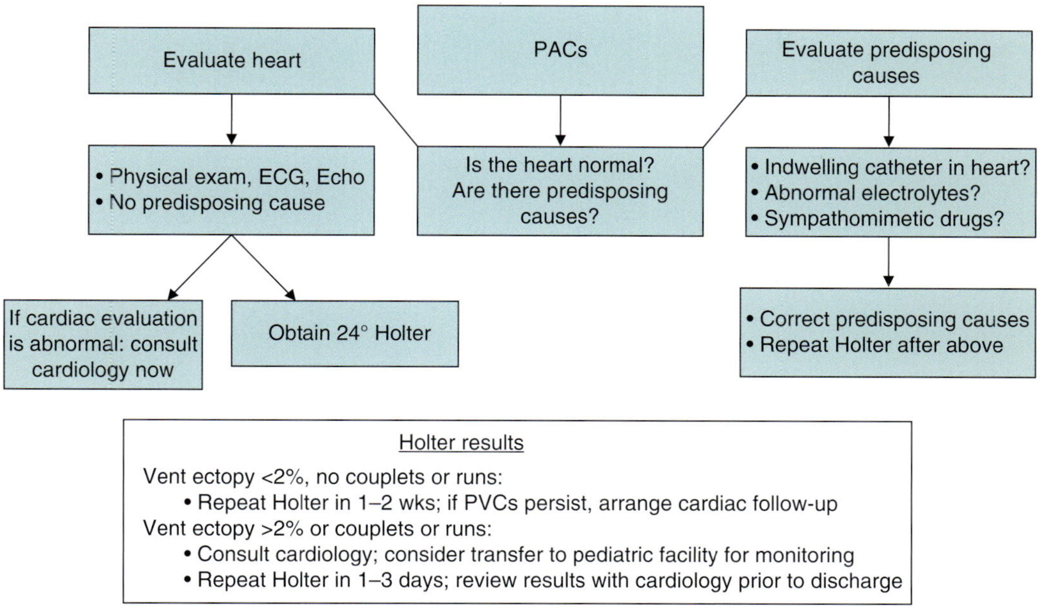

Figure 62.8 PVC management algorithm.

if PVCs persist, follow-up with cardiology is advised. In babies with >2% ventricular ectopy or complex ectopy, transfer to a cardiac intensive care unit or careful consultation with a cardiologist is usually advised. Assuming the baby remains healthy and asymptomatic, outpatient follow-up in the cardiology department occurs at relatively short intervals in the first months of life.

Frequency of PVCs <25% of total beats on Holter monitoring is unlikely to be associated with ventricular dysfunction. However, frequent PVCs, usually >35% on Holter monitoring, over a period of time can indicate left ventricular dilation or dysfunction [11]. When the frequency of PVCs is >35% of beats in 24 hours, periodic echocardiograms are advised to monitor ventricular size and function. In patients who have signs of left ventricular dilation or dysfunction, antiarrhythmic medication may be given to reduce the amount of ventricular ectopy in an effort to reverse left ventricular dilation and/or dysfunction.

In the infant without identified ion channelopathy, structural or functional cardiac disease, the natural history of isolated PVCs in the newborn favors gradual resolution. The complexity and amount of premature beats, and cardiac function, determines the frequency of follow-up. However, complete resolution of premature beats can occur over a period of years. A very small minority of such infants develop more significant or sustained arrhythmia requiring antiarrhythmic medication or intervention.

References

1 Southall DP, Richards J, Mitchell P, *et al.* (1980) Study of cardiac rhythm in healthy newborn infants. *Br Heart J*, **43**, 14–20.

2 Southall DP, Vuillamy DG, Davies MJ, *et al.* (1976) A new look at the neonatal electrocardiogram. *BMJ*, **2**, 615–618.

3 Southall DP, Orrell MJ, Talbot JF, *et al.* (1977) Study of cardiac arrhythmias and other forms of conduction abnormality in newborn infants. *BMJ*, **2**, 597–599.

4 Southall DP, Johnson AM, Shinebourne EA, Johnston PG, Vulliamy DG. (1981) Frequency and outcome of disorders of cardiac rhythm and conduction in a population of newborn infants. *Pediatrics*, **68** (1), 58–66.

5 Strasburger JF, Cheulkar B, Wichman HJ. (2007) Perinatal arrhythmias: diagnosis and management. *Clin Perinatol*, **34** (4), 627–644.

6 Hildreth V, Anderson RH, Henderson DJ. (2009) Autonomic innervation of the developing heart: origins and function. *Clin Anat*, **22**, 36–46.

7 Frassica JJ, Orav EJ, Walsh EP, Lipshultz SE. (1994) Arrhythmias in children prenatally exposed to cocaine. *Arch Pediatr Adolesc Med*, **148**, 1163–1169.

8 Laurent G, Saal S, Amarouch MY, *et al.* (2012) Multifocal ectopic Purkinje-related premature contractions: a new SCN5A-related cardiac channelopathy. *J Am Coll Cardiol*, **60** (2), 144–156.

9 Mitchell JL, Cuneo BF, Etheridge SP, *et al.* (2012) Fetal heart rate predictors of long QT syndrome. *Circulation*, **126**, 2688–2695.

10 De Rosa G, Butera G, Chessa M, *et al.* (2006) Outcome of newborns with asymptomatic monomorphic ventricular arrhythmia. *Arch Dis Child Fetal Neonatal Ed*, **91**, F419–422.

11 Kakavand B, Ballard HO, Diessa TG. (2010) Frequent ventricular premature beats in children with a structurally normal heart: a cause for reversible left ventricular dysfunction? *Pediatr Cardiol*, **31**, 986–990.

Part VI

Special Issues in the Newborn

63

Balloon Atrial Septostomy

Neil D. Patel[1] *and Damien Kenny*[2]

[1] *Children's Hospital of Los Angeles, Los Angeles, CA, USA*
[2] *Our Lady's Children's Hospital, Crumlin, Dublin, Ireland*

Balloon atrial septostomy (BAS) was introduced by Rashkind in 1966 as a non-surgical alternative to the Blalock–Hanlon technique to provide palliation for patients with transposition of the great arteries (TGA) until they reached the optimal age for complete correction [1]. It has evolved as a palliation for congenital heart defects that require an unrestricted atrial communication for survival and indications guidelines have been recently published [2]. Patients with TGA require mixing of systemic and pulmonary venous blood because they have parallel circulations. Additionally, patients with right-sided obstructive lesions such as tricuspid atresia require a non-restrictive atrial communication to decompress the right side of the heart and augment systemic cardiac output. Likewise, patients with left-sided obstructive lesions such as mitral stenosis and other forms of hypoplastic left heart syndrome can require a BAS to decompress the left atrium and increase cardiac output. Patients with total anomalous pulmonary veins require an atrial communication to allow for pulmonary and systemic venous blood to enter the systemic circulation. Finally, patients who are on extracorporeal membrane oxygen support with hypertensive left atrium may require decompression of the left atrium. Blade atrial septostomy or stenting of the septum is required when the atrial septum is thick and resistant to BAS [2].

Traditionally, BAS in neonates has been performed in the catheterization laboratory; however, nowadays it is mostly performed at the bedside under echocardiography guidance. Access is obtained via the umbilical or femoral veins, and an appropriate-sized sheath is used (usually 6 Fr). There are a number of catheters currently available for BAS; however, the most commonly used are the Fogarty™ Dilation Atrioseptostomy Catheter (Edwards Lifesciences, Irvine, CA), and the Z-5™ Atrioseptostomy catheter (NuMED Inc., Hopkinton, NY). The NuMED catheter has an end hole, which allows the catheter to pass over a wire and have its location confirmed by injecting contrast into the left atrium [2]. The NuMED balloon is available in two sizes: one for full-term neonates with large/normal sized left atrium with a capacity of 1.2 mL and a smaller one for premature infants or smaller left atrium with a capacity of 1 mL.

Once the balloon is positioned in the left atrium, and confirmed by echocardiography and/or fluoroscopy, it is inflated with saline (and contrast) to the appropriate volume. A rapid jerk is applied to the catheter, pulling the balloon through the atrial septum to the right atrium–inferior vena cava junction. The balloon is then deflated, and this procedure is repeated until the balloon passes through the defect without any resistance (Figures 63.1 and 63.2) [2].

There are a several potential complications with BAS: balloon rupture, failure of balloon deflation, abnormal balloon position resulting in cardiac perforation or mitral valve injury, or avulsion of the pulmonary veins or inferior vena cava [2]. Rarely, there have been reports of balloon separation from the shaft of the catheter. The potential for increased risk of brain injury is a controversial topic with BAS in the setting of TGA. McQuillen *et al.* [3] initially reported a significant increase in rates of brain injury associated with BAS. However, others have reported that brain injury is associated with lower pO2 levels and longer time to surgery, but not with BAS [4]. A meta-analysis found no association between BAS and brain injury [5]. There are no definitive data to discourage the use of BAS in the setting of TGA.

Visual Guide to Neonatal Cardiology, First Edition. Edited by Ernerio T. Alboliras, Ziyad M. Hijazi, Leo Lopez, and Donald J. Hagler.

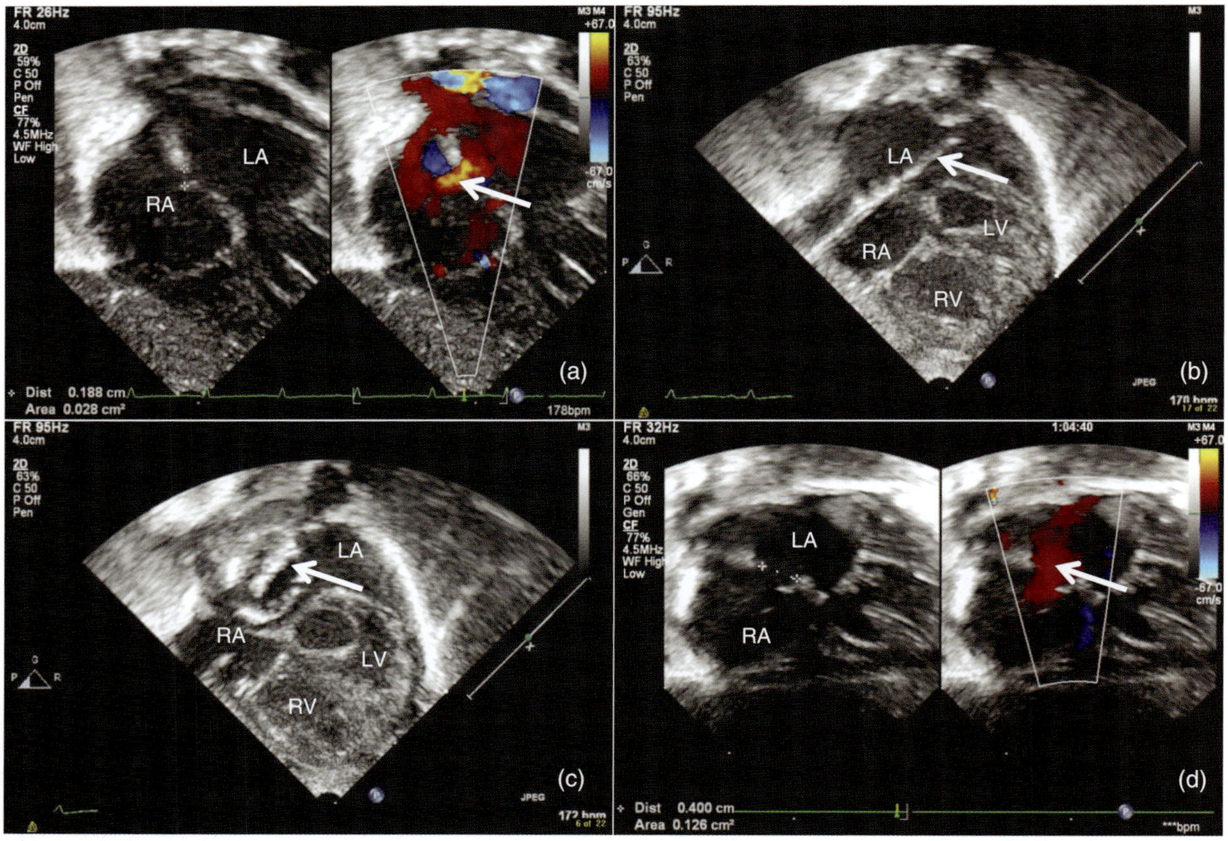

Figure 63.1 Balloon atrial septostomy (BAS) performed under echocardiography guidance in a preterm newborn weighing 1 kg with D-transposition of the great arteries: (a) atrial communication with restrictive flow (arrow); (b) NuMED Z-5™ Atrioseptostomy Catheter seen crossing the atrial septum over a 0.014 inch Sparta wire with the tip (arrow) in the left atrium; (c) balloon (inflated to 0.5 mL) seen in left atrium (arrow); (d) unrestricted flow (arrow) across atrial septum following BAS. LA, left atrium; LV, left ventricle; RA, right atrium; RV, right ventricle.

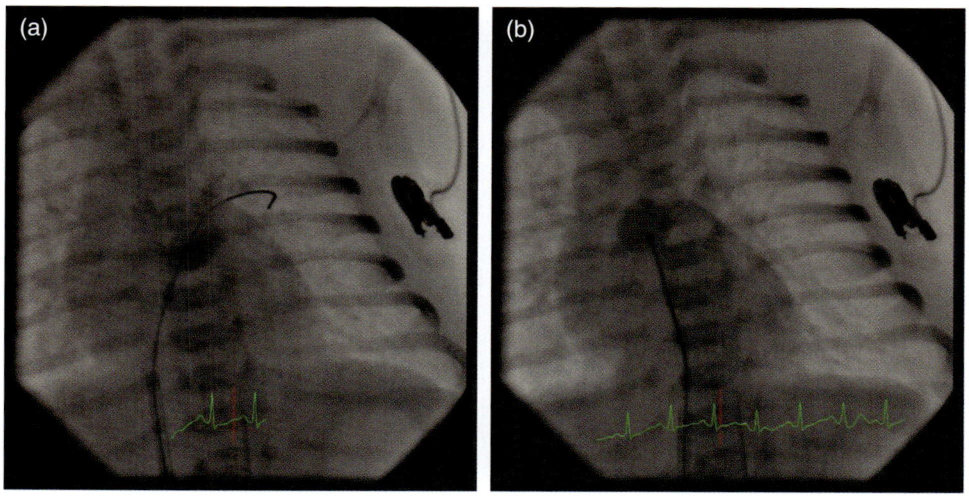

Figure 63.2 BAS performed under fluoroscopy in a newborn fullterm male infant with D-transposition of the great arteries. (a) Inflated balloon in the left atrium with tip of the wire in the left upper pulmonary vein. (b) The wire has been removed and the inflated balloon has been directed towards the roof of the left atrium, allowing for a more direct pullback course across the atrial septum, away from the mitral valve. (c) Demonstrates the balloon being forcefully jerked towards the atrial septum. (d) Balloon deformation (arrow) while being pulled through the atrial septum. (e) The balloon has been pulled through the atrial septum and is situated towards the right atrium–inferior vena cava junction.

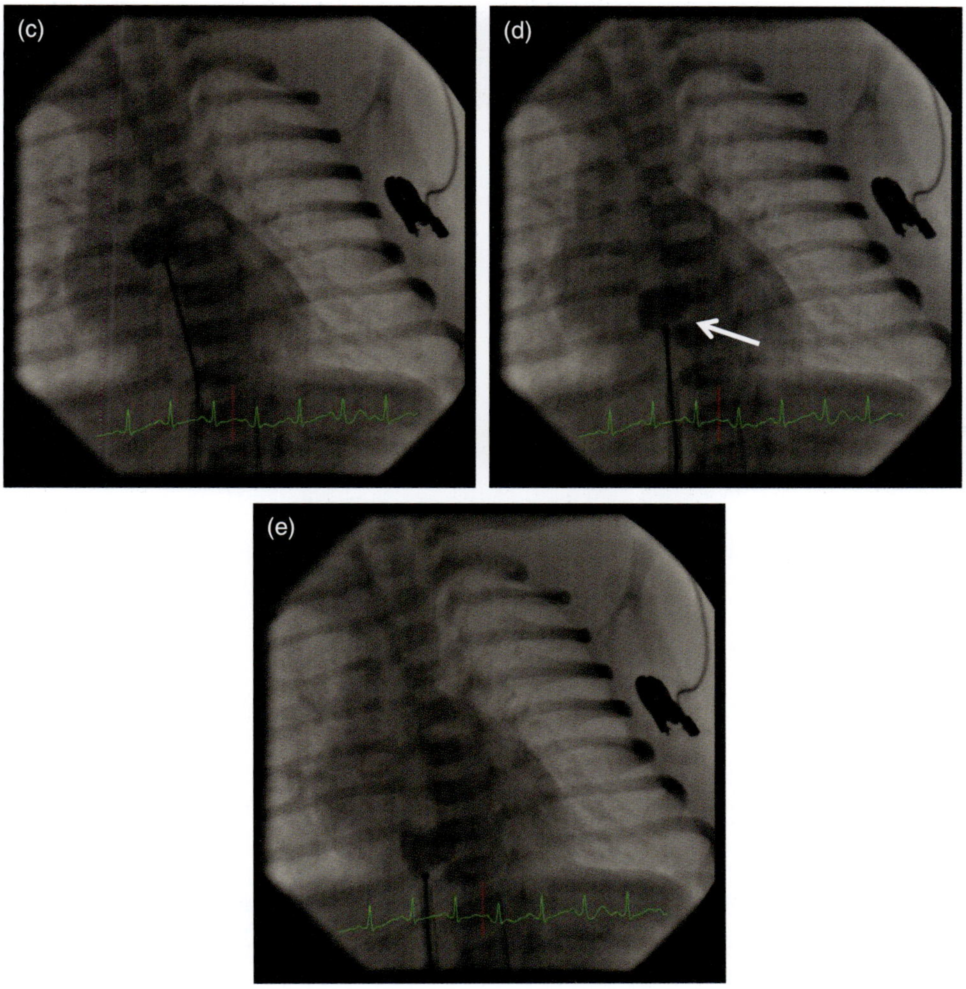

Figure 63.2 (*Continued*)

References

1 Rashkind WJ, Miller WW. (1966) Creation of an atrial septal defect without thoracotomy: a palliative approach to complete transposition of the great arteries. *JAMA* **196**, 991–992.
2 Feltes TF, Bacha E, Beekman RH, *et al.* (2011) Indications for cardiac catheterization and intervention in pediatric cardiac disease: a scientific statement from the American Heart Association. *Circulation*, **123**, 2607–2652.
3 McQuillen PS, Hamrick SE, Perez MJ, *et al.* (2006) Balloon atrial septostomy is associated with preoperative stroke in neonates with transposition of the great arteries. *Circulation*, **113**, 280–285.
4 Petit CJ, Rome JJ, Wernovsky G, *et al.* (2009) Preoperative brain injury in transposition of the great arteries is associated with oxygenation and time to surgery, not balloon atrial septostomy. *Circulation*, **119**, 709–716.
5 Polito A, Ricci Z, Fragasso T, Cogo PE. (2012) Balloon atrial septostomy and pre-operative brain injury in neonates with transposition of the great arteries: a systematic review and a meta-analysis. *Cardiol Young*, **22**, 1–7.

64

Interventional Therapeutic Procedures in the Newborn

Salwa Gendi[1], Qi-Ling Cao[2], and Ziyad M. Hijazi[2]

[1] University of Mississippi Medical Center, Jackson, MS, USA
[2] Sidra Medical and Research Center, Doha, Qatar

Therapeutic cardiac catheterization in the newborn is being applied to patients as an alternative to cardiovascular surgery or when the patient is a very high surgical risk.

As a result of significant advances in non-invasive imaging, diagnostic cardiac catheterization is only needed for specific indications: assessment of pulmonary vascular resistance and its reversibility; in cases of pulmonary atresia with intact septum to delineate the coronary arteries; to determine if there is RV-dependent coronary circulation; and in patients with tetralogy of Fallot with pulmonary atresia and multiple collaterals to delineate the exact anatomy prior to surgical correction of the defect.

The objective of this chapter is to give a general overview of the state of the art in interventional therapeutic procedures in the neonate:

1) *Opening of atrial communications:* atrial septostomy and atrial septal stenting.
2) *Balloon dilation of cardiac valves:* pulmonary, aortic, mitral, and tricuspid valves.
3) *Balloon angioplasty and/or stent placement:* in native coarctation and recoarctation, pulmonary artery angioplasty, systemic and pulmonary veins balloon angioplasty, patent ductus arteriosus (PDA) stenting.
4) *Transcatheter vascular occlusion:* PDA, aorto-pulmonary collateral vessels, coronary artery fistula,

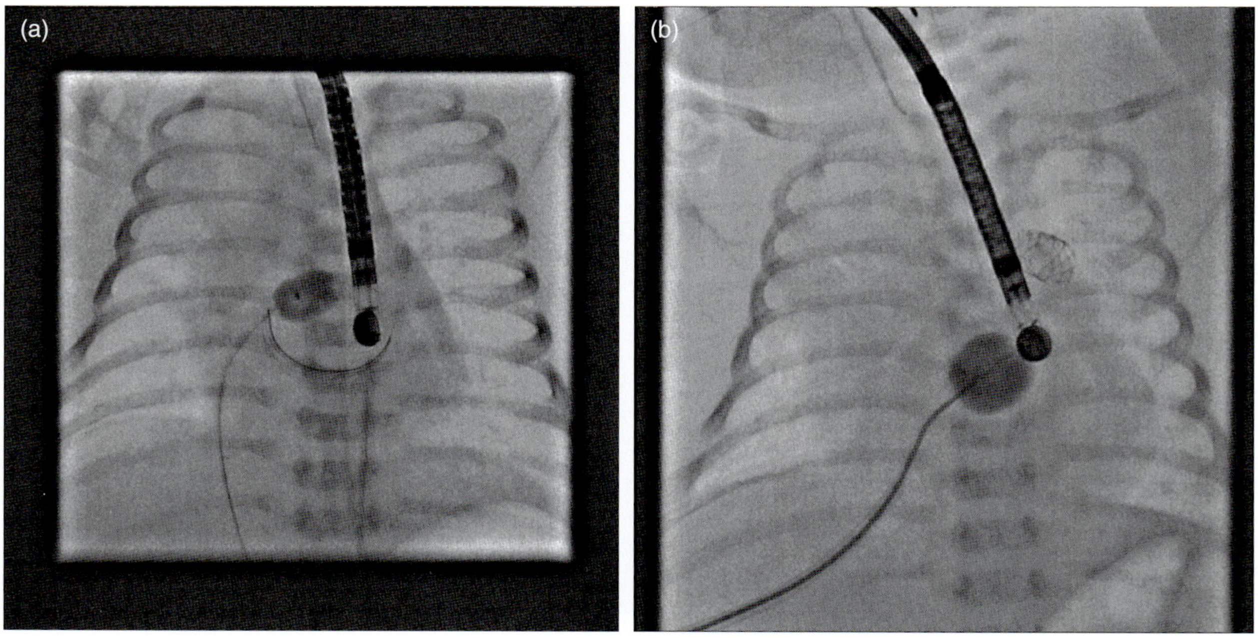

Figure 64.1 (a) Anteroposterior (AP) view showing a Rashkind balloon inflated in the left atrium (LA) through the umbilical venous (UV) catheter. (b) Rashkind balloon inflated in LA via a transhepatic approach.

Visual Guide to Neonatal Cardiology, First Edition. Edited by Ernerio T. Alboliras, Ziyad M. Hijazi, Leo Lopez, and Donald J. Hagler.

pulmonary arteriovenous malformations, venovenous channels.

5) *Closure of communications:* atrial septal defect (ASD), ventricular septal defect (VSD).

Opening of Atrial Communication

Atrial Septostomy

Atrial septostomy is needed when there is a restricted communication between the right and left atria. Few techniques have been developed to create the interatrial communication: balloon atrial septostomy; blade atrial septostomy; static balloon dilation of the septum; and radiofrequency perforation or trans-septal puncture to create the communication and then enlarge it using one of the above techniques. Stent implantation in the septum may provide a more durable solution [1].

Atrial septostomy can be performed in the cardiac catheterization laboratory or at the bedside under echocardiographic guidance. Once the balloon is positioned in the left atrium, the balloon is inflated, and a forceful jerk or pull is applied to the catheter to bring the balloon to the junction of the right atrium and inferior vena cava (Figures 64.1 and 64.2). There are possible complications: transient rhythm disturbances which may

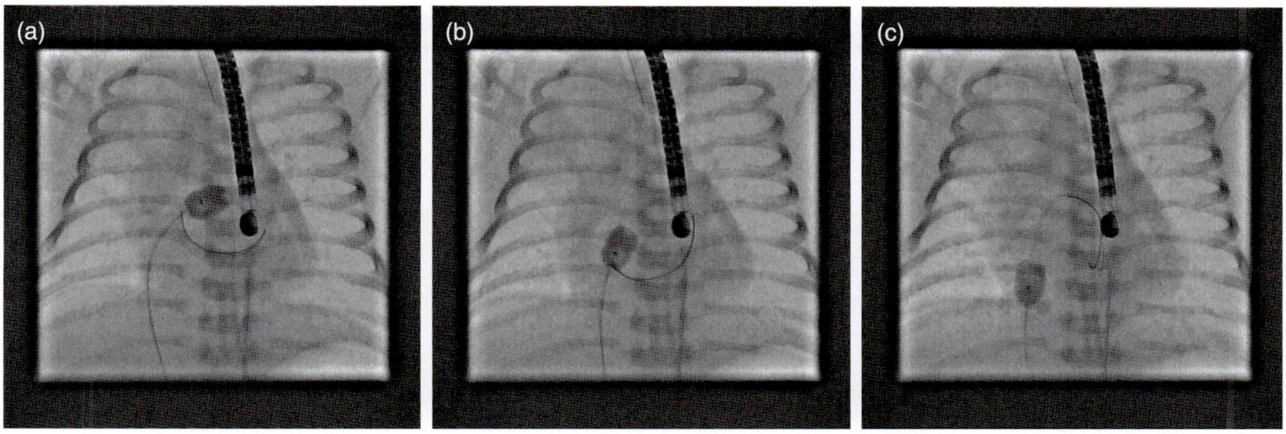

Figure 64.2 (a) AP view showing an inflated Rashkind balloon that has crossed the atrial septum and is in the LA. (b) The Rashkind balloon has crossed the atrial septum and is in right atrium (RA). (c) The Rashkind balloon is pulled further into the inferior vena cava (IVC)–RA junction.

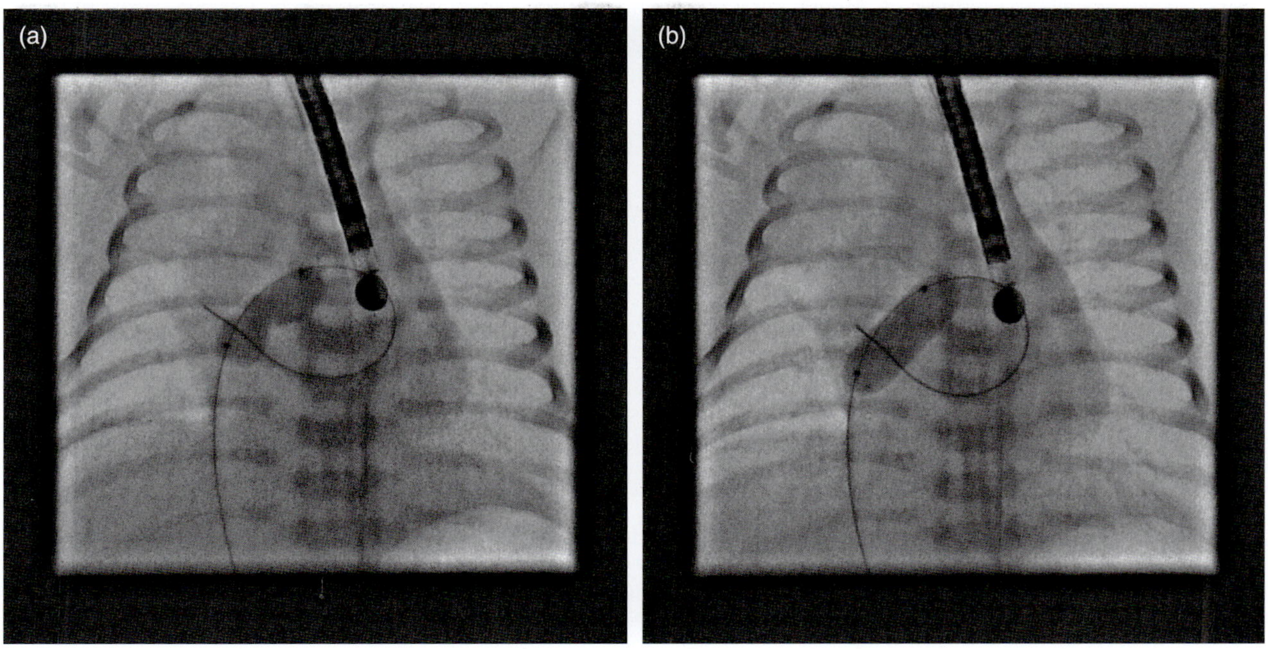

Figure 64.3 (a) AP view of static balloon dilatation showing catheter course from IVC to RA to LA across the patent foramen ovale (PFO). The dilated balloon shows a waist at the PFO site being dilated. (b) Same AP view of static balloon that has been fully dilated and with a disappearance of the "waist" in the PFO level.

be permanent or even fatal; failure to create adequate atrial communication; balloon fragment embolization; and laceration of the atrioventricular valves, systemic or pulmonary veins.

Blade Atrial Septostomy and Static Balloon Dilation

In neonates with thick or intact atrial septum, blade septostomy is needed prior to balloon septostomy. However, currently, most centers rely on static balloon (regular balloon or cutting balloon) to enlarge the communication as it is very effective when a controlled diameter of the opening is desired (Figure 64.3).

Atrial Septal Stenting

Atrial septal stenting is indicated in cases of thick septum subject to recoil. Also, if the opening is required for a longer period of time, stenting the defect can offer this benefit (Figure 64.4).

Transcatheter Balloon Dilation of Cardiac Valves

Pulmonary Valvuloplasty

Balloon valvuloplasty remains the treatment of choice for valvar pulmonary stenosis at all ages (Figure 64.5). Isolated valvar pulmonary stenosis represents 8–10% of all patients with congenital heart disease [1]. Critical pulmonary stenosis can be lethal in neonates without intervention (Figure 64.6). Indications for pulmonary valvuloplasty include symptomatic patient, asymptomatic patient with systolic gradient $\geq$40 mmHg across the pulmonary valve, right ventricular hypertrophy and dysfunction, and as a palliative procedure in a patient with complex cyanotic heart disease including some rare cases of tetralogy of Fallot [2]. The main complication of the procedure is pulmonary regurgitation which could present at a later stage during longer term follow-up.

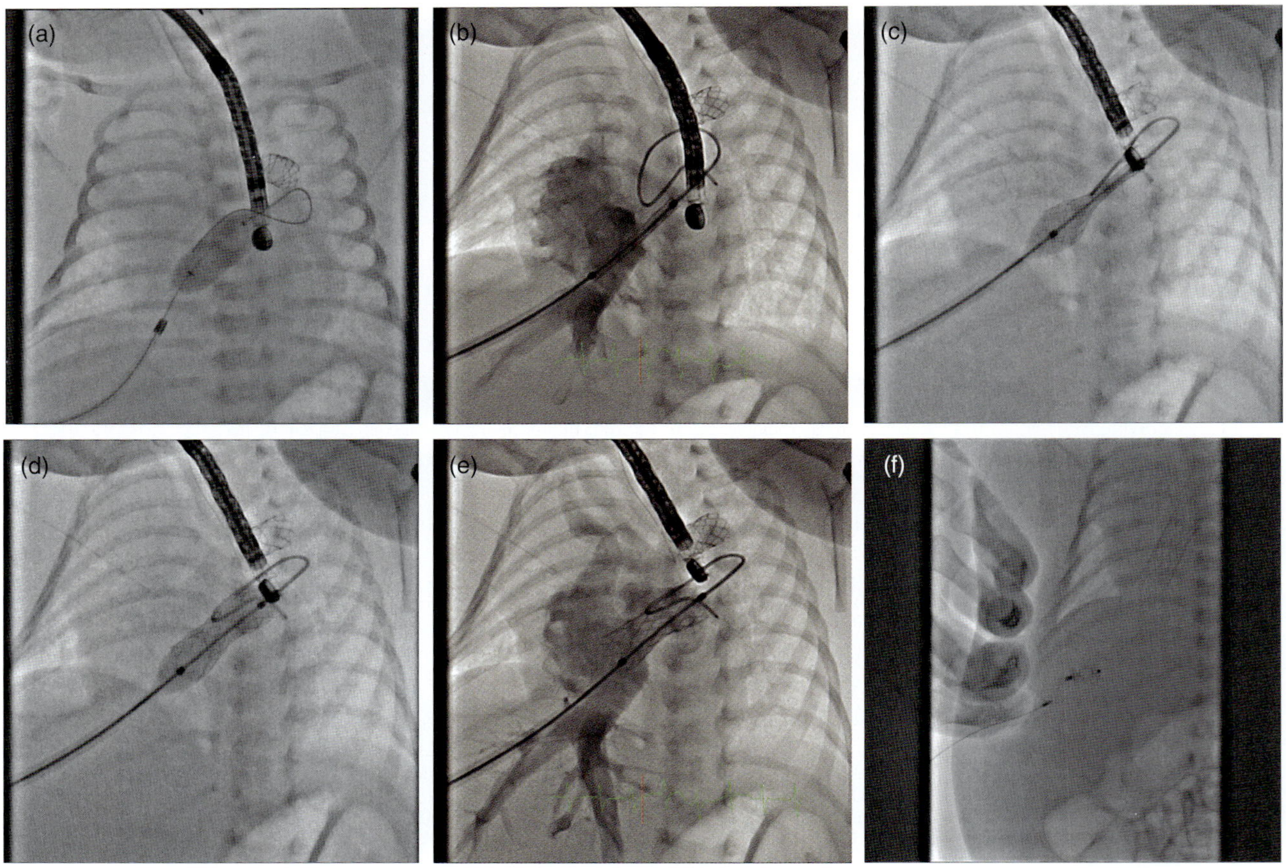

Figure 64.4 (a) Atrial septal stenting using the transhepatic approach from an AP view. The catheter course is from the transhepatic area to RA, across PFO and to LA. The balloon is inflated to measure the size of the defect. (b) A stent is passed over the deflated balloon and mounted across the interatrial septum (IAS). (c) The balloon is being expanded with resultant beginning of expansion of the stent across the IAS. (d) The stent is expanded further with further inflation of the balloon. (e) With further inflation of the balloon, the stent is fully expanded in the PFO with disappearance of the waist. (f) A vascular occluder is released in liver for hemostasis.

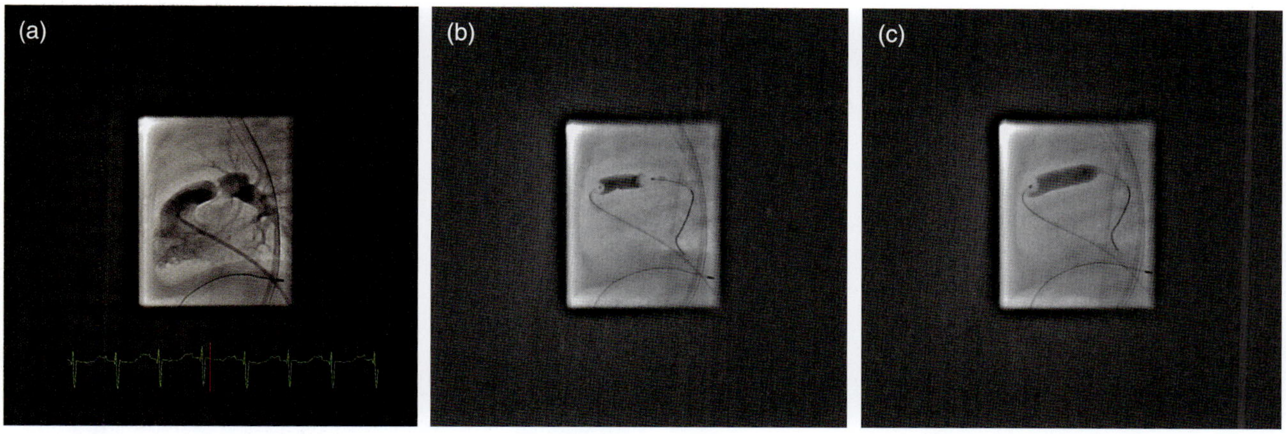

Figure 64.5 (a) Lateral view angiogram with contrast injection at the right ventricular outflow tract (RVOT) showing valvar pulmonary stenosis (PS) with thickening and doming of the valve cusps. (b) Same patient as in (a) with a partially inflated balloon that has crossed the stenotic pulmonary valve (PV). There is "waisting" of the balloon at the cusp level. (c) The balloon is fully expanded with a loss of the "waist" and consequent relief of obstruction across the PV.

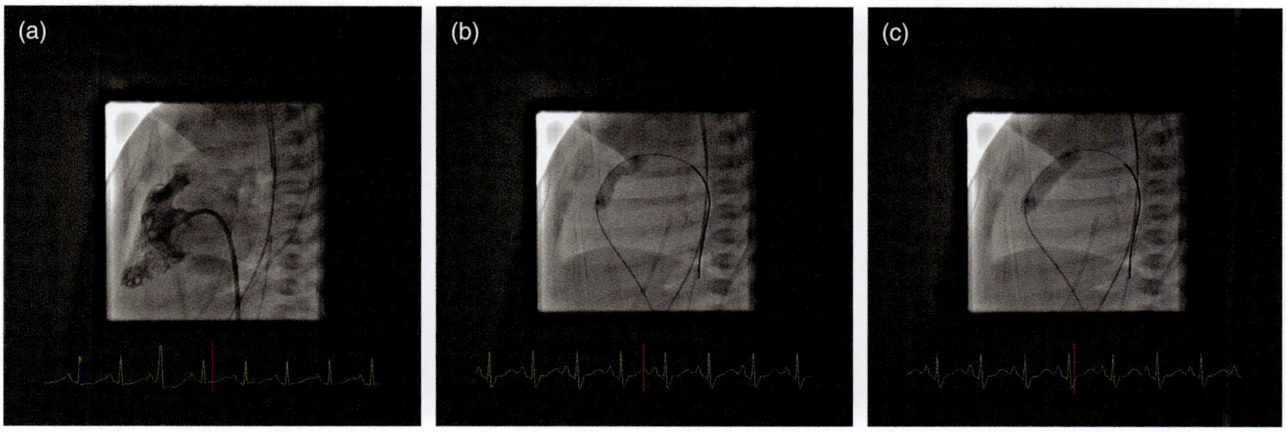

Figure 64.6 (a) Lateral view of an angiogram with injection in the RVOT in a neonate with critical pulmonary stenosis. Note the presence of only a little antegrade flow across a thick PV. (b) Same patient with critical PS with a partially inflated balloon that has crossed the stenotic PV, showing a "waist" at the site of stenosis. (c) Same patient with critical PS. With full expansion, there is straightening of the balloon profile and disappearance of the "waist."

To decrease the risk of pulmonary regurgitation, it is better to use smaller balloon to annulus ratio than the previously recommended (120–140%). In selected cases with pulmonary atresia, multiple techniques have been used to perforate the valve such as using the stiff end of the guidewire, laser, and, most commonly, radiofrequency wires. Complications encountered include perforation of the RV outflow tract leading to pericardial effusion and tamponade. A group that clearly needs to be excluded from this procedure are patients with RV-dependent coronary circulation [1, 3].

Aortic Valvuloplasty

Balloon aortic valvuloplasty has become a safe and effective treatment of valvar aortic stenosis (AS). It is indicated in the newborn with isolated critical valvar stenosis defined as ductal dependent circulation with congenital AS [4]. It is also indicated in isolated valvar AS with depressed LV function, with congestive heart failure or shock, or with a peak to peak gradient of ≥50 mmHg [1, 4]. The initial balloon chosen should be 85–90% of the aortic annulus measured by angiography. An optimal result is achieving an at least 50% reduction in the gradient with no increase in aortic regurgitation, or having a residual gradient of less than 35 mmHg and absence of regurgitation (Figure 64.7). Complications of the procedure include suboptimal relief of the obstruction, creation of moderate or severe aortic incompetence, femoral artery injury, thromboembolic stroke, injury to the mitral valve, or perforation of the myocardium [1].

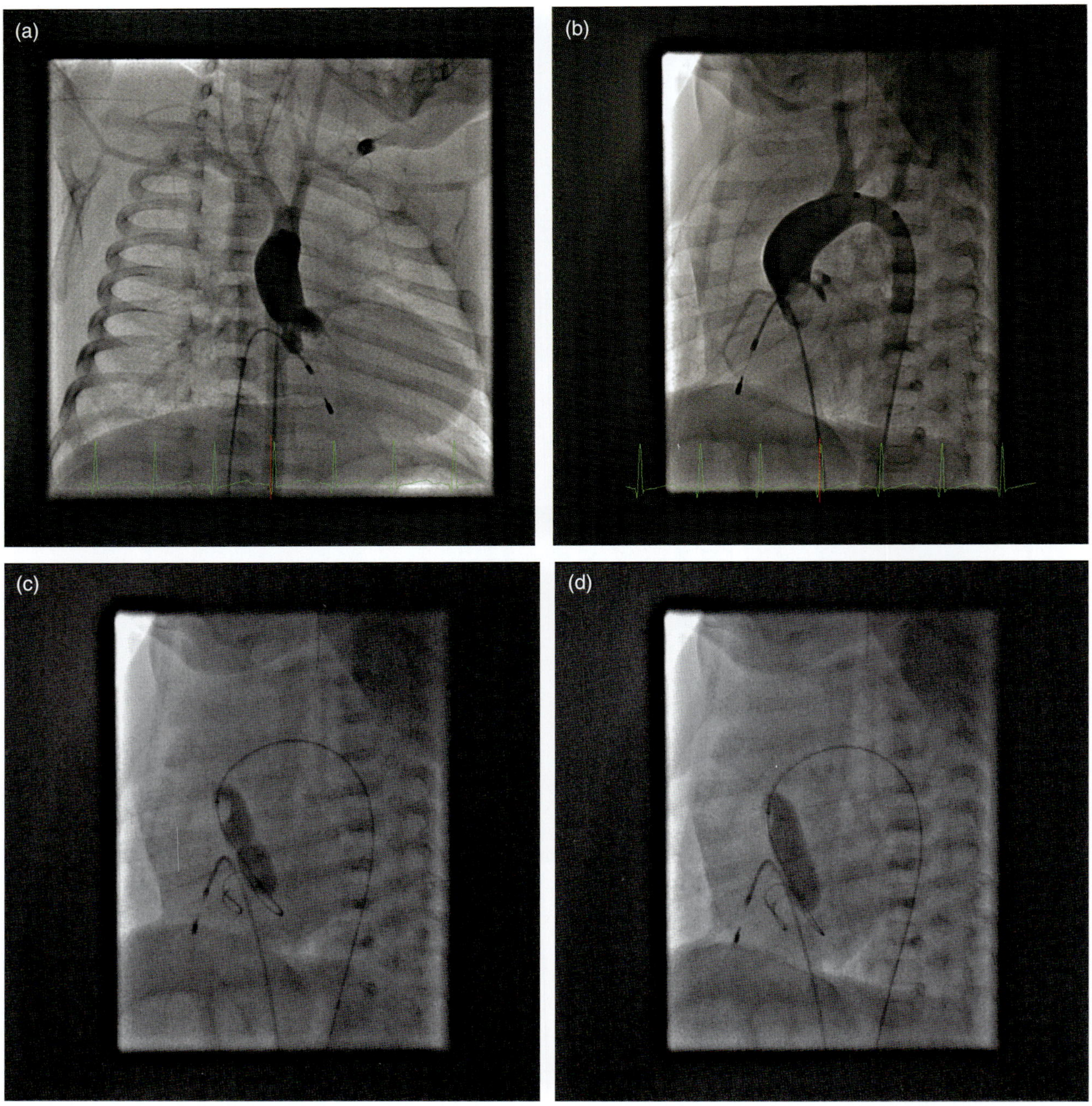

Figure 64.7 (a) AP view of an aortic angiogram showing doming of the aortic valve in a neonate with aortic valve stenosis. (b) Left anterior oblique (LAO) view of the same aortogram likewise demonstrating the doming of the aortic valve. (c) LAO view of the aortogram showing a partially inflated balloon across the AV stenosis showing a balloon "waist" at the valve level. (d) Same patient with aortic valve stenosis demonstrating a full inflation of the balloon and disappearance of the "waist" indicative of a successful valvuloplasty. (e) Simultaneous catheterization pressure tracing of LV and descending showing a pre-balloon peak to peak gradient of 50 mmHg. (f) Catheterization pressure tracing after balloon dilatation of the AV showing a marked decrease of gradient to only 10 mmHg.

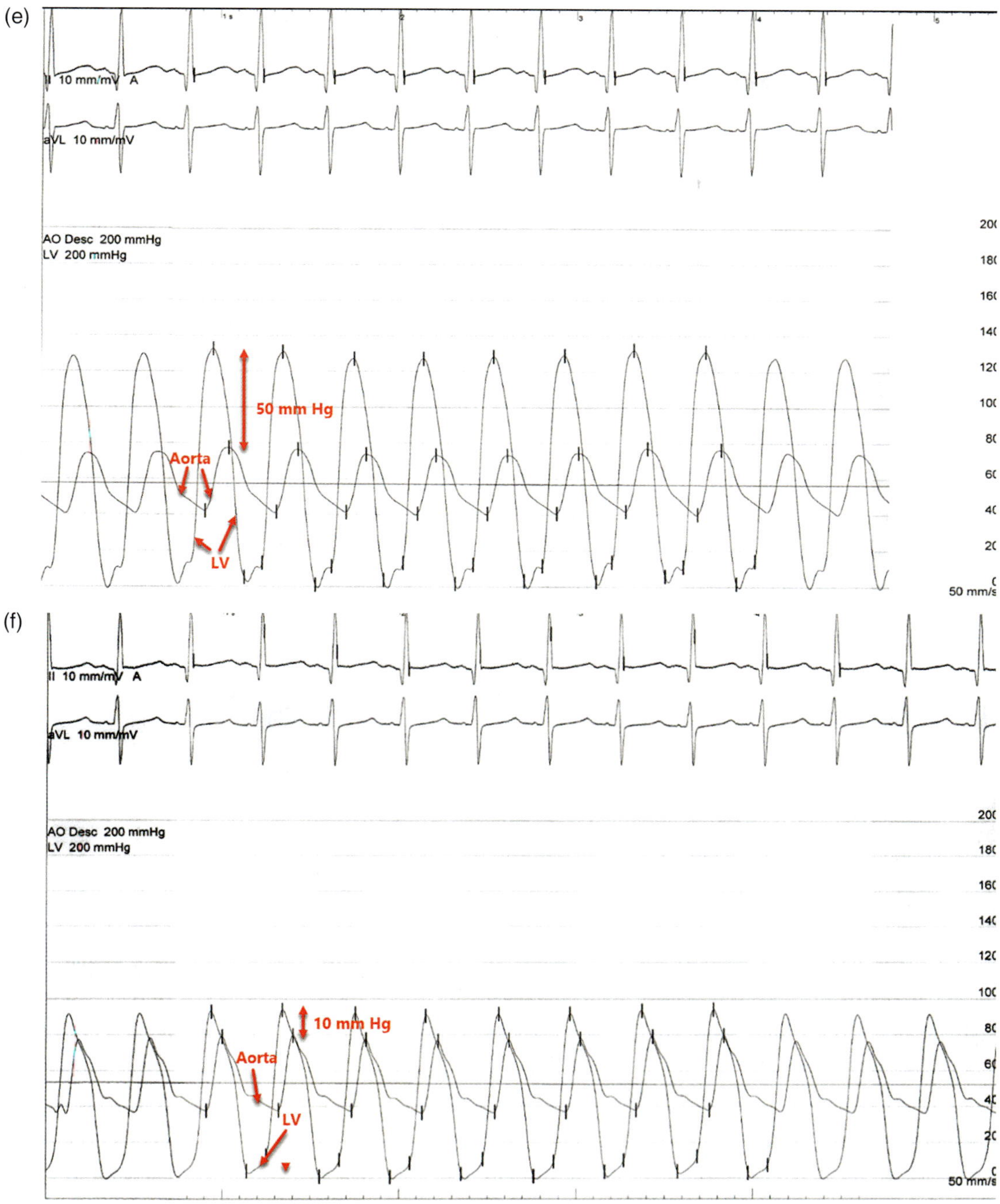

Figure 64.7 (*Continued*)

Mitral Balloon Valvuloplasty

Congenital mitral stenosis encompasses a broad spectrum of anatomic variants, including the typical variants with thickened leaflets, shortened chordae, and decreased interchordal spaces (mitral arcade); supramitral valve ring; double mitral orifices, parachute mitral valve, and the hypoplastic mitral valve associated with hypoplastic left heart syndrome (HLHS). Balloon valvuloplasty is rarely performed for mitral stenosis. Torn leaflets and chordal attachments and papillary muscle rupture are the most common cause of regurgitation after dilation [1].

Balloon Angioplasty and/or Stent Placement

Native Coarctation of the Aorta and Recoarctation

Coarctation of the aorta accounts for 6–8% of all cardiac defects. The usual location of caorctation is juxtaductal,

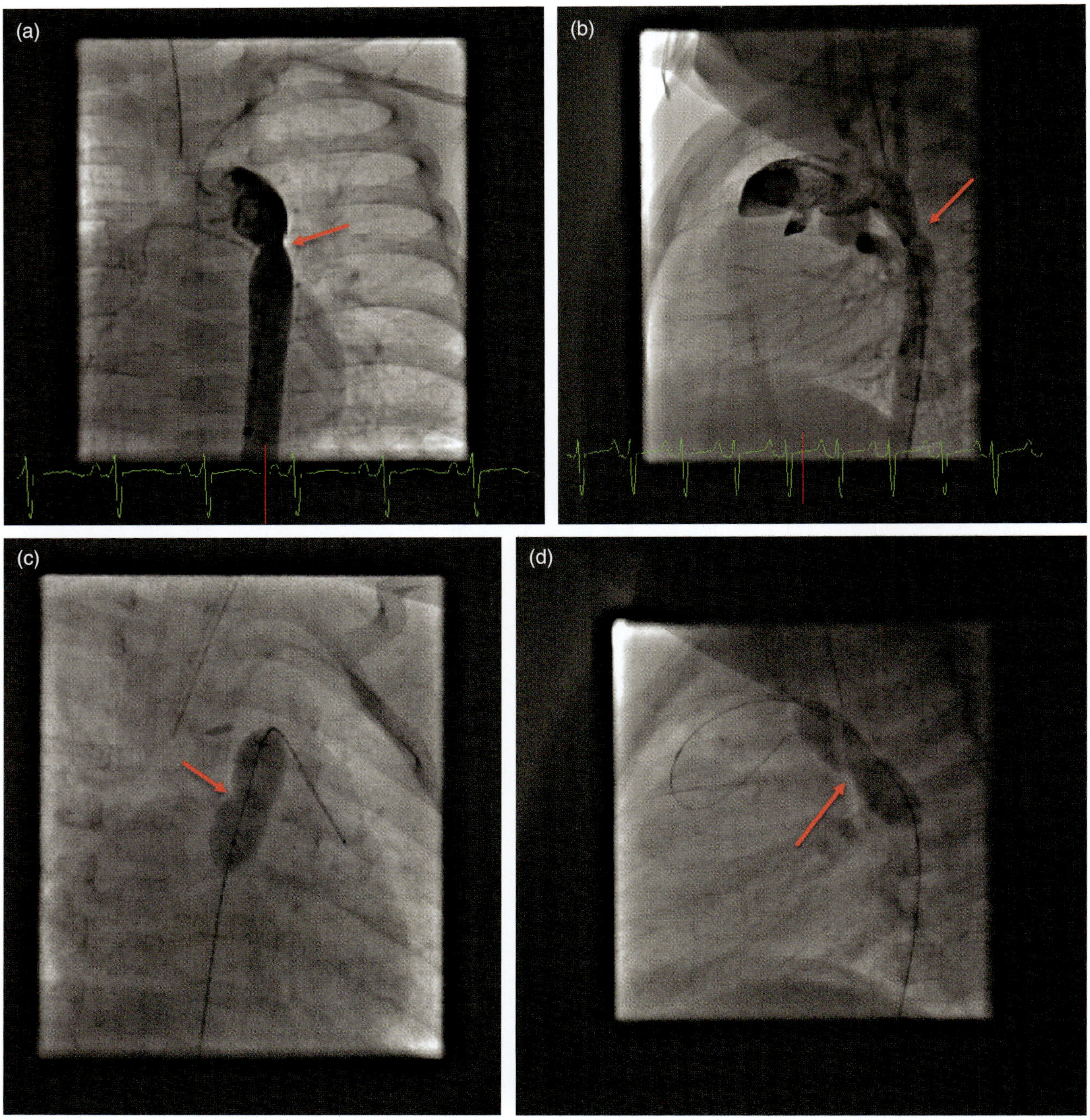

Figure 64.8 (a) AP view of an aortogram showing a coarctation of the aorta (red arrow) with narrowing in the isthmus. (b) Lateral view of the same aortogram demonstrating the coarctation of aorta (red arrow). (c) Right anterior oblique view (RAO) of the aortogram showing an inflated balloon with a "waist" created by the coarctation (red arrow). (d) AP view of the same aortogram showing an inflated balloon with a "waist" created by the coarctation (red arrow).

just distal to the left subclavian artery. Neonates present with signs and symptoms of low cardiac output and shock as the ductus arteriosus closes. A pressure gradient between upper and lower limbs and weak femoral pulse are suggestive of coarctation.

In recent years, balloon angioplasty has emerged as an alternative, less invasive option to the gold standard surgical therapy in infants with discrete narrowing and with no evidence of arch hypoplasia, and in cases of recoarctation after surgery or dilatation (Figure 64.8). The complications of the procedure are mainly recurrence of stenosis and a small but important incidence of aortic aneurysm. Stent implantation for native coarctation or recoarctation of the aorta has also emerged as a beneficial therapeutic option for patients who can receive a stent that can be expanded to an adult size [1, 3].

Pulmonary Artery Stenosis

The overall frequency of peripheral arterial stenosis is 2–3%. It is either an isolated lesion or associated with other defects or part of a syndrome. Severe pulmonary arterial stenosis is obvious when a pressure gradient of >20–30 mmHg is found or the elevation of RV or proximal main pulmonary artery pressure is greater than half to two-thirds of systemic pressure secondary to the more distal obstruction or when there is relative flow discrepancy between the two lungs of 35%/65% or worse [1, 2].

Treatment of pulmonary artery stenosis depends on the site of the stenotic segments. Percutaneous pulmonary angioplasty is suitable for distal lesions unreachable by surgery. Techniques of percutaneous treatment include balloon angioplasty, cutting balloon angioplasty, and intravascular stent placement (Figure 64.9) [2]. The major risk of pulmonary angioplasty is vessel perforation.

Systemic and Pulmonary Veins Balloon Angioplasty

Systemic venous stenosis occurs as a congenital defect, subsequent to surgery, from indwelling lines in the veins, or from external compression. No significant gradient could be detected because of the low-pressure system. Surgery of systemic venous stenosis is difficult and unrewarding. Balloon dilation, with or without stent implantation, has proved effective with little morbidity and mortality.

Pulmonary vein stenosis can be a congenital lesion or acquired after corrective surgery or lung transplantation. The treatment modalities include surgery, balloon angioplasty, use of cutting balloon and, as last resort, stenting in older babies. Restenosis rates after angioplasty and stent are high and particularly worse for congenital pulmonary vein stenosis. Potential complications include vessel dissection, stent malposition, and embolization. There is a high rate of restenosis that can make the procedure almost futile [3].

PDA Stenting

PDA stenting is indicated in cases where circulation is duct dependent. It is one of the important milestones in management of major congenital heart lesions in the neonatal period. Blalock–Taussig shunt remains the most common procedure; however, in the neonatal period, it carries a significant risk of morbidity and mortality. Feasibility of PDA stenting is affected by the morphology of the PDA and its relationship to the aorta and pulmonary artery. Flexible pre-mounted stents designed for coronary artery use are used for ductal stenting. The stent should cover the whole length of the duct to prevent restenosis. If needed, the use of two overlapping stents can be implanted. In neonates, a stent of 3–4 mm generally provides adequate palliation of pulmonary blood flow without leading to excessive pulmonary flow [1]. Neonates with hypoplastic left heart syndrome undergoing hybrid stage 1 palliation will require larger stents. In general, for a fullterm neonate (weight 3–4 kg), a stent diameter of about 8 mm is needed. Again, the entire length of the ductus has to be covered, otherwise restenosis can occur. In our laboratory, we generally use balloon expandable stents of 8 mm diameter and 18–20 mm long (Figure 64.10).

Transcatheter Vascular Occlusion

PDA Occlusion

Occlusion of PDA is indicated when neonates are symptomatic because of circulatory overload. Since the early successful trial of PDA occlusion, a variety of devices and innovative techniques have been used for transcatheter occlusion of PDA. Coils are used for PDA occlusion, and their use in small PDA of <3 mm in diameter has become the treatment of choice. In larger ducts, many devices are used to close such PDAs. Potential risks include inadvertent device embolization into the pulmonary or systemic artery, device obstruction to aortic or pulmonary flow especially in small infants, transient left ventricular systolic dysfunction, hemolysis, and recanalization (Figure 64.11).

Aortopulmonary Collateral Vessels

Aortopulmonary collateral vessels can be found in association with various congenital heart disease including pulmonary atresia, VSD, tetralogy of Fallot, and scimitar syndrome. They can be arterial or venous, and shunt left to right or right to left. As they are often difficult for the surgeon to access, they may be occluded with coils or occluder devices. The risks for occluding aortopulmonary collaterals are related to inadvertent device embolization into an important systemic artery. To decrease the risk, it is important to select a device that can be accommodated by the collateral vessel (Figure 64.12).

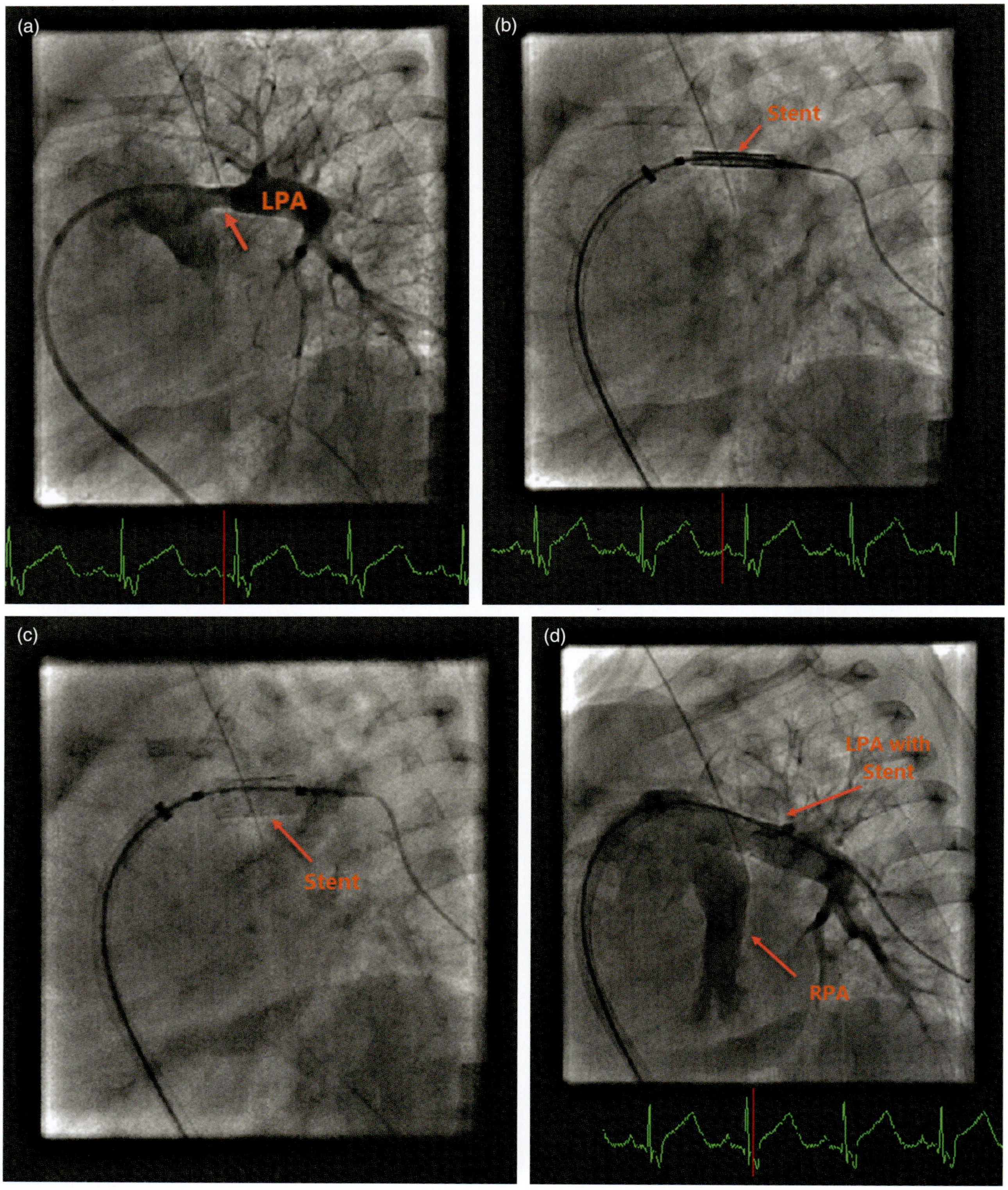

Figure 64.9 (a) Right anterior oblique view (RAO) showing an angiogram of the left pulmonary artery (LPA) with a proximal stenosis (red arrow). (b) Same RAO view of the patient with LPA stenosis with a stent mounted by a balloon in the stenotic area. (c) The same patient with a dilated stent. (d) Same RAO view of the patient with an angiogram of the LPA demonstrating the straightened stent with disappearance of the stenosis.

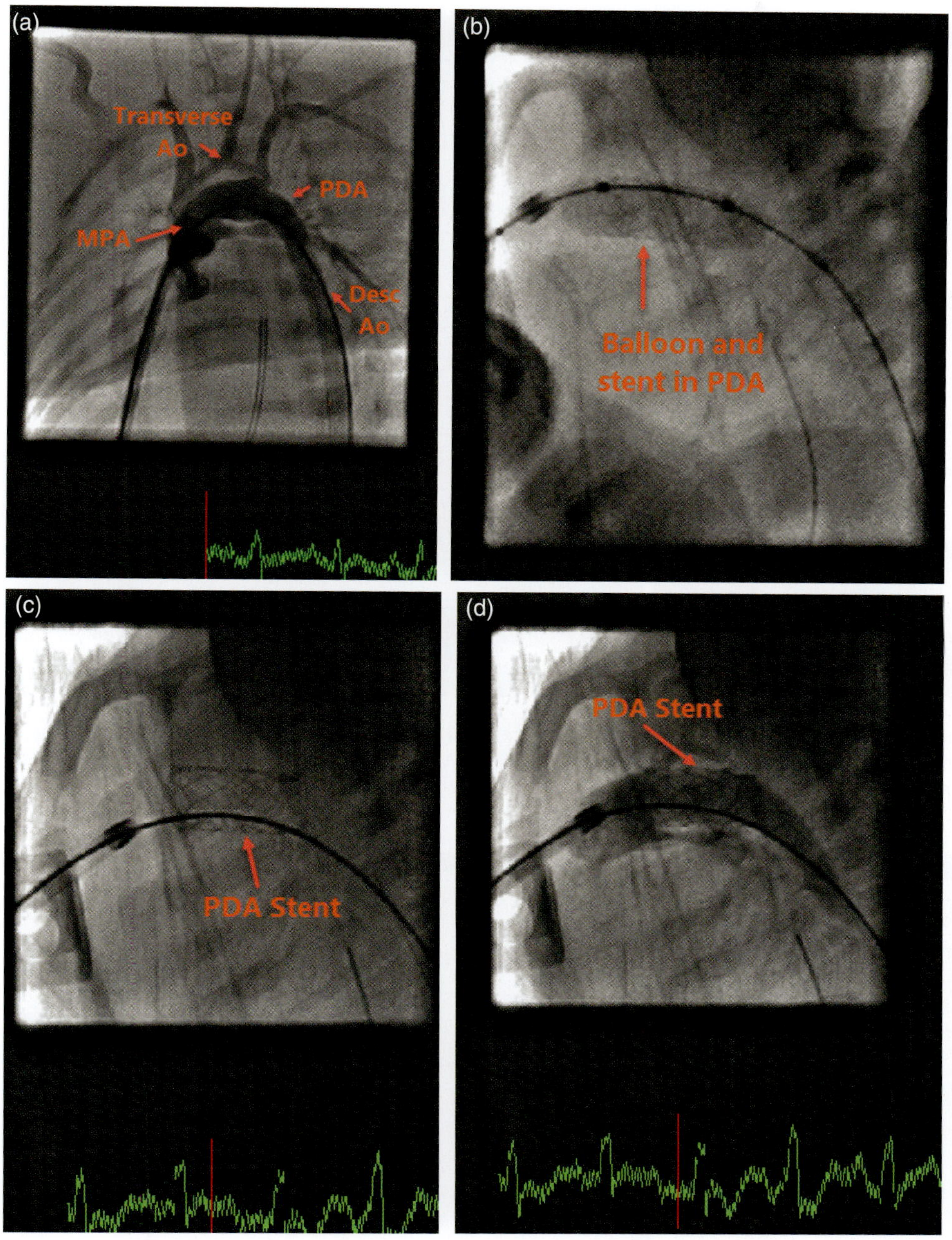

Figure 64.10 (a) Patient with hypoplastic left heart syndrome undergoing the Hybrid operation with plan to stent the PDA to maintain ductal patency. The figure is an AP view showing an angiogram of the great vessels with a hypoplastic aortic arch and a large PDA. (b) A stent was mounted by a balloon in the PDA. The figure demonstrates the stent dilated by the balloon. (c) Lateral view showing the PDA stent in full expansion. (d) Angiogram to demonstrate proper placement of the stent in the PDA.

Closure of Intracardiac Communications (ASD, VSD)

Many new devices are available for transcatheter closure of ASD and muscular VSD. These devices can rarely be used in neonates.

Closure of an ASD in neonates is rarely necessary. Some neonates with critical aortic valve stenosis or severe coarctation of the aorta require the ASD to be closed after treatment of the primary lesion. If such neonates continue to have congestive heart failure resulting from the left to right shunt, we resort to closing such defects. Figure 64.13 depicts a hybrid closure of a secundum ASD in a neonate with also a large muscular VSD.

Neonates with large muscular VSD and congestive heart failure can undergo hybrid closure [5] of their defects (Figure 64.14). The procedure is safe and proven to be effective.

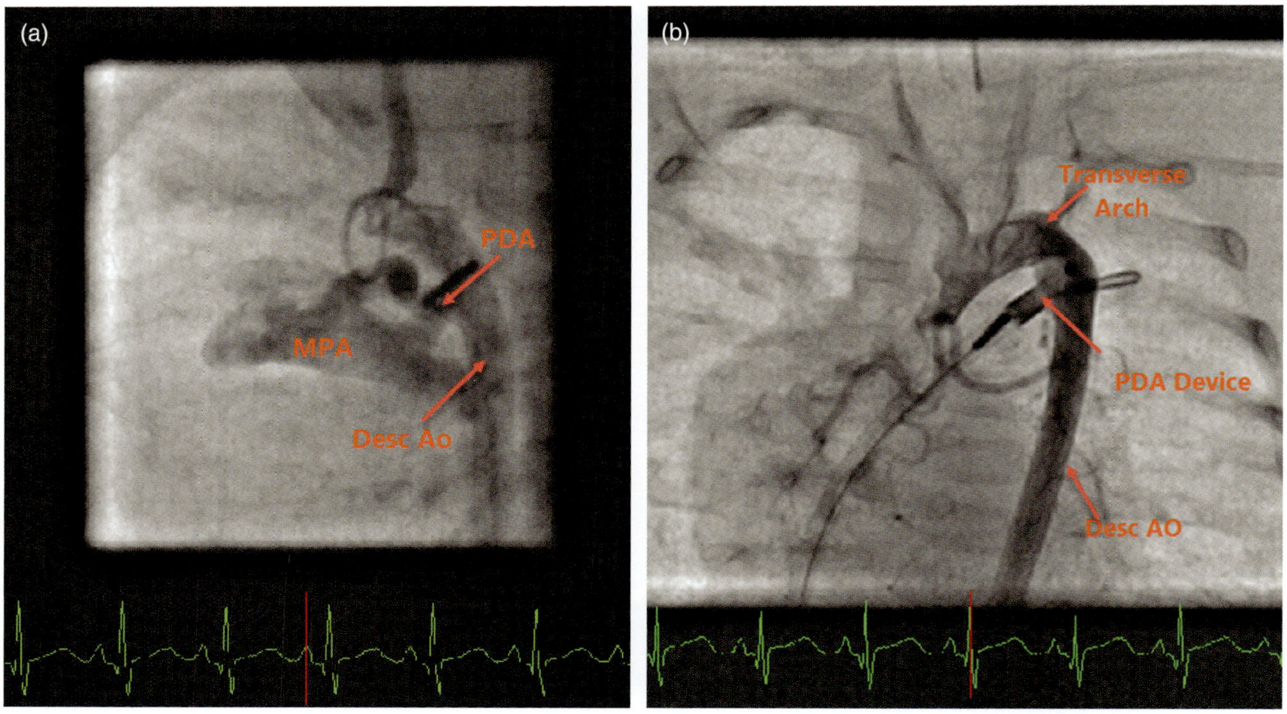

Figure 64.11 (a) Lateral view showing an angiogram of a moderate to large sized residual PDA after attempted surgical repair. Contrast was injected in the aorta showing residual left to right shunt with opacification of the PDA, MPA, and LPA. (b) Same patient with device in place and prior to release. There is no more residual left to right shunt with only the aorta having been opacified.

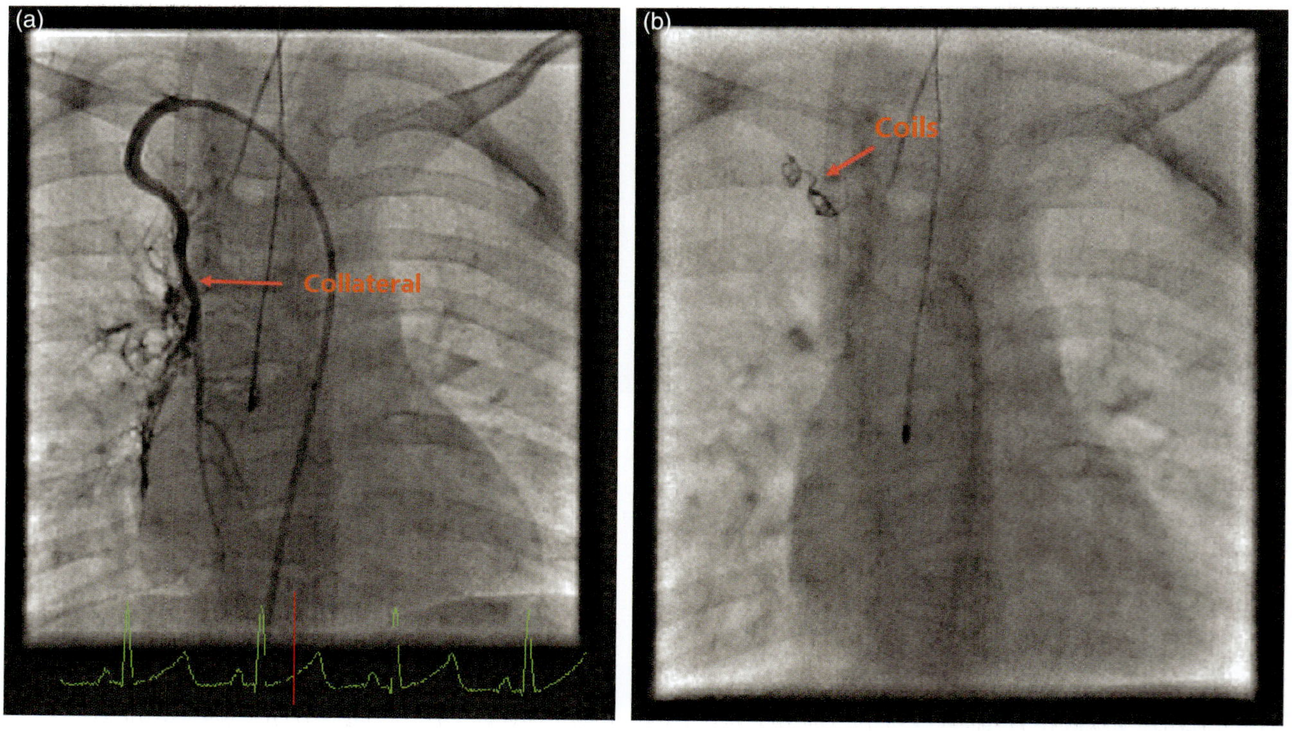

Figure 64.12 (a) AP view showing aortopulmonary collateral. (b) Coils were placed and released in the collateral.

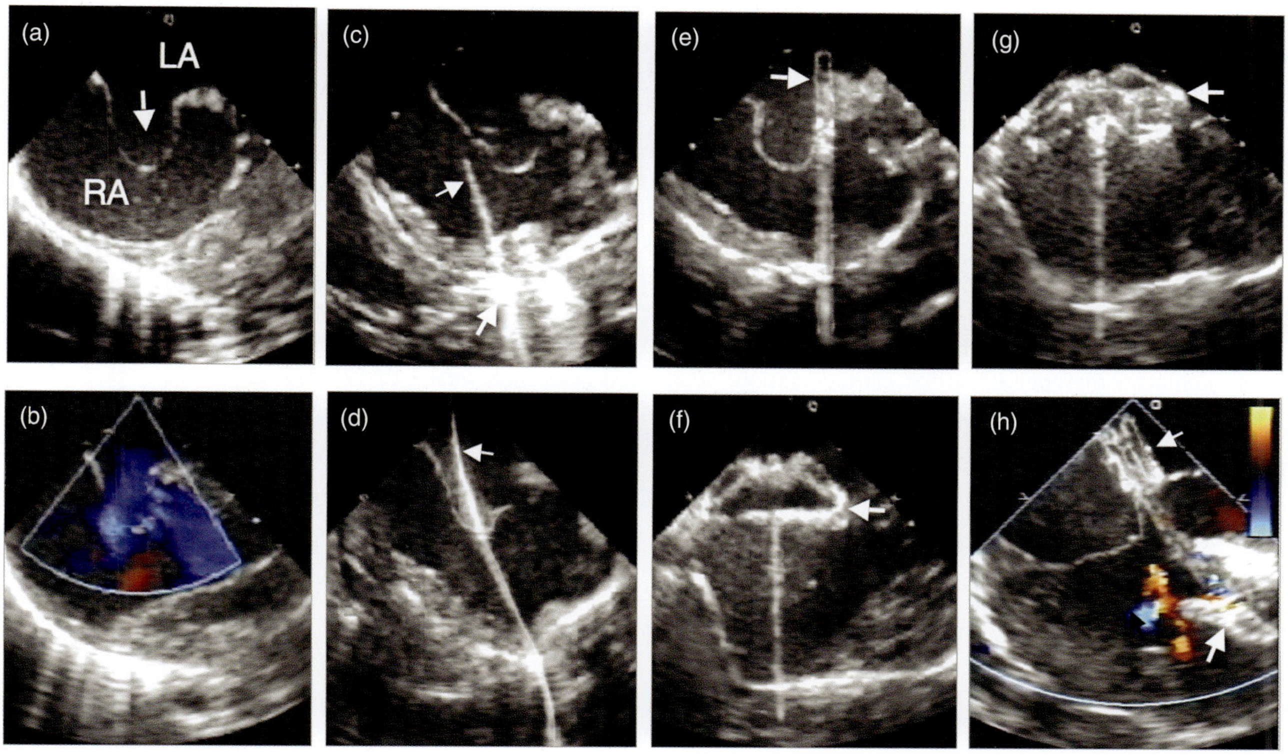

Figure 64.13 (a) TEE showing aneurysmal IAS bulging into RA. (b) Color flow Doppler across IAS showing fenestrated septum with left to right shunt. (c) Transatrial wire crossing the RA wall into RA. (d) Wire crossing the IAS into LA. (e) Delivery sheath crossing RA wall, passing through RA, IAS and into LA. (f) Delivery of LA disc. (g) Both discs have been delivered on both sides of the IAS. (h) Release of the device well-applied to the IAS and with no residual shunt.

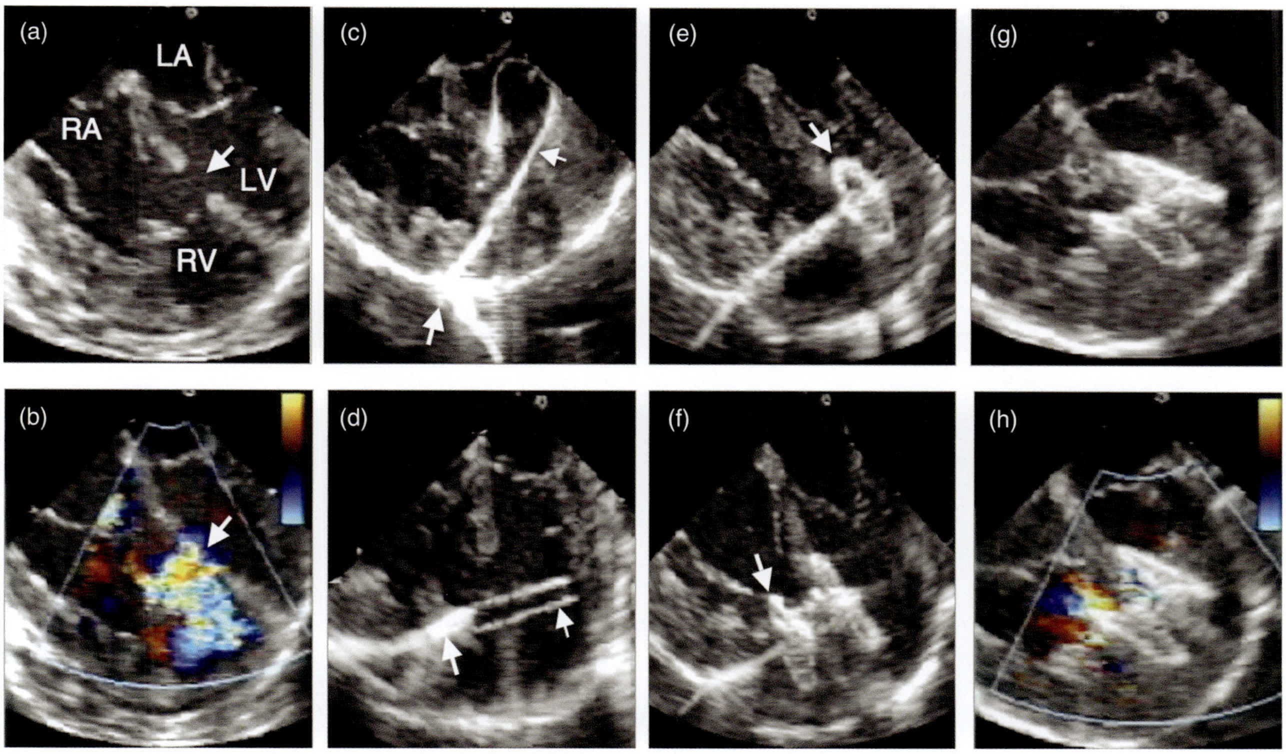

Figure 64.14 (a) Transesophageal echocardiogram four-chamber view showing a large mid-muscular VSD (white arrow). (b) Color flow across the VSD showing left to right shunt. (c) Transventricular wire crossing the anterior wall of the RV into LV through the VSD. (d) Delivery sheath crossing the anterior wall of the RV into LV through the VSD. (e) Delivery of LV disc. (f) Delivery of RV disc. (g) Release of the device into the VSD. (h) Color flow showing no residual shunt.

References

1 Feltes TF, Bacha E, Beekman RH, *et al.* (2011) Indications for cardiac catheterization and intervention in Pediatric Cardiac Disease: a scientific statement from the American Heart association. *Circulation*, **123**, 2606–2652.

2 Hijazi ZM, Awad SM. (2008) Pediatric cardiac interventions. *JACC Cardiovasc Interv*, **1**, 603–611.

3 Qureshi SA, Redington AN, Wren C, *et al.* (2000) Recommendations of the British Pediatric cardiac association for therapeutic cardiac catheterization in congenital heart disease. *Cardiol Young*, **10** (6), 649–667.

4 Cowley CG, Dietrich M, Mosca RS, *et al.* (2001) Balloon valvuloplasty versus transventricular dilatation for neonatal critical aortic stenosis. *Am J Cardiol*, **87**, 1125–1127.

5 Michel-Behnke I, Ewert P, Koch A, *et al*; Investigators of the Working Group Interventional Cardiology of the German Association of Pediatric Cardiology. (2011) Device closure of ventricular septal defects by hybrid procedures: a multicenter retrospective study. *Catheter Cardiovasc Interv*, 77 (2), 242–251.

65

The Hybrid Procedure

Ralf J. Holzer[1,2]

[1] *Division of Pediatric Cardiology, New York-Presbyterian/Weill Cornell Medical Center*
[2] *The Komansky Children's Hospital, New York, NY, USA*

Hybrid procedures encapsulate the procedural cooperation between interventional cardiologist and cardiothoracic surgeon. These procedures are performed for a variety of conditions, frequently complementing the standard surgical or interventional approaches. This chapter describes Hybrid procedures that are required during the neonatal period, and includes stage I palliation of hypoplastic left heart syndrome, perventricular closure of muscular ventricular septal defects (VSD), and Hybrid balloon aortic or pulmonary valvuloplasty.

Hybrid Palliation of Hypoplastic Left Heart Syndrome

Background

The overall outcome of conventional surgical palliation of hypoplastic left heart syndrome (HLHS) has remained poor. A recent randomized, multicenter, single ventricle trial documented a 12-month transplantation-free survival of 74% after Sano type palliation, and 64% after Norwood type palliation [1]. The main concept behind this Hybrid approach is to replace an early high-risk surgical procedure with a lower risk Hybrid intervention, thereby allowing the neonate to mature and grow before undergoing a more complex surgical intervention later in the first year of life. The hallmark of this Hybrid palliation is the combination of bilateral pulmonary artery (PA) banding as well as patent ductus arteriosus (PDA) stent placement and creation of a non-restrictive atrial communication during the neonatal period [2, 3]. Beyond the neonatal period, at the age of about 5 months, this is then followed by a comprehensive surgical palliation, which combines a bidirectional Glenn, with PA band and PDA stent removal, aortic arch reconstruction, as well as a Damus–Kay–Stansel connection. Fontan completion is then followed at about 2 years of age.

Stage I Hybrid Palliation

While Hybrid palliation has enhanced the spectrum of therapeutic options available to patients with HLHS, not all patients are suitable for this therapeutic strategy. Placing a stent across the retrograde aortic arch has the potential of limiting the flow to brain and coronary arteries. This is especially of concern in patients with aortic atresia, who do not have any other source of blood supply to these vital organs. Therefore it is crucial to rule out any pre-existing retrograde aortic arch obstruction (RAAO), which would be a contraindication to Hybrid palliation (Figure 65.1).

The procedure can be performed either in a dedicated Hybrid operating room or Hybrid catheterization laboratory, or in a conventional operating room with the aid of a portable c-arm. The procedure is commenced by the cardiothoracic surgeon who performs bilateral PA banding (Figure 65.2). While a PDA stent could theoretically be placed using a percutaneous approach, performing this at the time of PA banding has the advantage of avoiding the need for stiff wires and long sheaths, which often lead to hemodynamic instability in these patients. After successful bilateral band placement, PDA stenting is performed using a per main pulmonary artery (MPA) approach (Figures 65.3 and 65.4). Unless the PDA is stenotic or very short, an appropriate-sized self-expandable stent is chosen, most frequently being about 8 mm in diameter for a normal-sized neonate.

Creating a Non-Restrictive Atrial Communication

Creating a non-restrictive atrial level communication forms an integral part of the Hybrid palliation of HLHS. Its timing is crucial. After delivery, the left atrium in the majority of infants with HLHS is often very small, but

Visual Guide to Neonatal Cardiology, First Edition. Edited by Ernerio T. Alboliras, Ziyad M. Hijazi, Leo Lopez, and Donald J. Hagler.

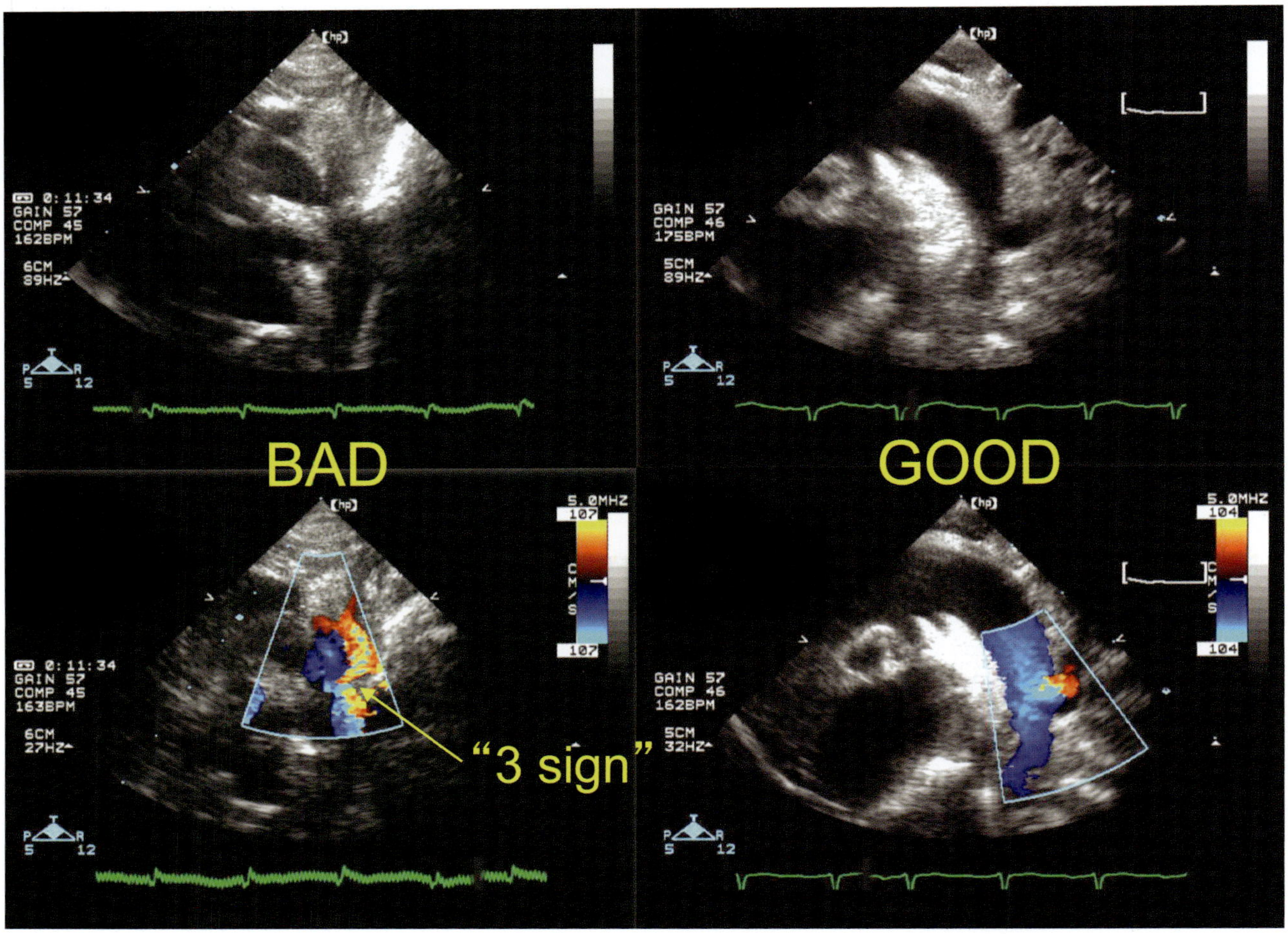

Figure 65.1 It is essential to evaluate the retrograde aortic arch prior to considering Hybrid palliation, which is particularly important in patients with aortic atresia. Echocardiography is the initial diagnostic technique of choice to image retrograde aortic arch (RAA), with the suprasternal views providing the best images. In patients with a concern for retrograde aortic arch obstruction (RAAO), the RAA is often "pinched in" at its ductal insertion (3-sign) with flow acceleration across the RAA, as shown on the left-hand image (unsuitable for Hybrid palliation). On the right-hand image, the RAA has a wider origin without being pulled in and less flow acceleration (suitable for Hybrid palliation). Where echocardiography does not clearly delineate the RAA, other diagnostic methods such as CT scanning should be considered.

increases in size over the first 1–2 weeks of life because of the increased volume loading when compared with fetal life. Therefore, performing the procedure too early at the time of Hybrid palliation often increases the technical challenges in creating a non-restrictive and lasting atrial communication, as frequently smaller balloon varieties have to be used during the procedure. In contrast, holding the atrial septal intervention until a clinically significant restriction develops can create other problems. The atrial septal thickness increases over the first few weeks of life, and what could have been an easy atrial septostomy at 1 week of age, becomes a more cumbersome and less successful intervention when performed on a thickened atrial septum a few weeks later. Predicting which infant will develop an atrial level restriction can be difficult, and therefore it is beneficial to perform the atrial septal intervention 1–2 weeks after Hybrid palliation, when the patient has recovered sufficiently to be discharged.

The physiologic changes that occur after this procedure should not be underestimated, and while the procedure itself is usually well tolerated, the most crucial time for the neonate is the first 24–48 hours after the procedure. This is because the PA bands are still very "loose" early after Hybrid palliation, and any sudden decrease in atrial level restriction can result in a sudden increase in flow across the pulmonary vascular bed, at the expense of systemic cardiac output. While the body adjusts to these physiologic changes, kidney and gut are at highest risk of untoward side effects, such as necrotizing enterocolitis. Patients should therefore be observed and monitored carefully in an intensive care environment and feeding introduced slowly. While creating tighter PA bands may alleviate those problems,

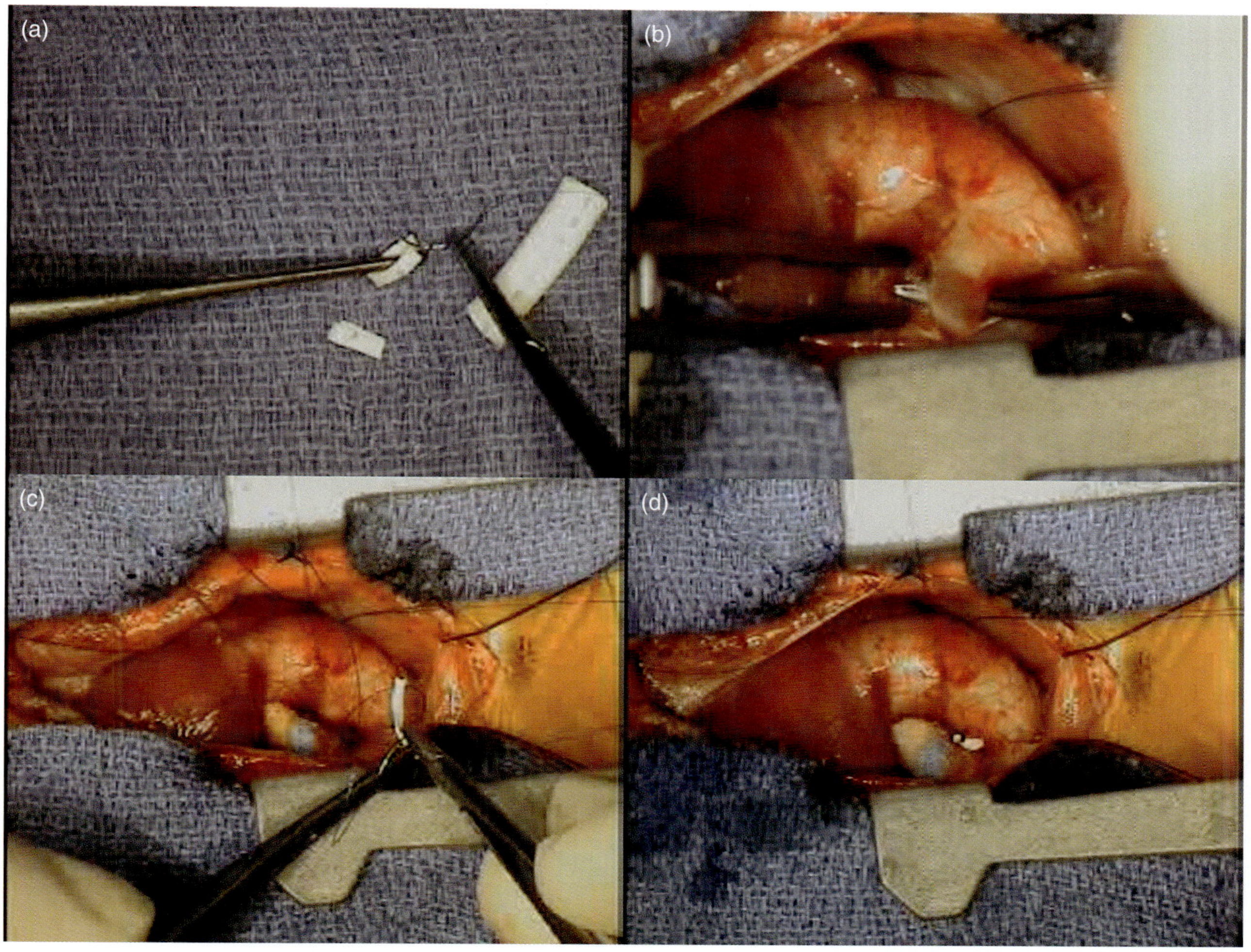

Figure 65.2 Bilateral pulmonary artery banding is performed initially during Hybrid Stage I palliation through a midline sternotomy. Pulmonary artery bands are fashioned by using 1 mm wide cut off ends from a 3.5 mm Gore-Tex tube graft. It is important to place the bands first, as a patent ductus arteriosus (PDA) stent would interfere with ability to place those bands easily. The left pulmonary artery (LPA) band is usually placed at the origin, while the right pulmonary artery (RPA) band is placed between the aorta and superior vena cava (SVC). (a) 1 mm wide cut off end from Gore-Tex tube graft; (b) right angle around LPA; (c) band being placed around the LPA; (d) completed LPA band. Placing the pulmonary artery bands usually leads to a small drop in saturations and an increase in systemic blood pressure of about 10 mmHg.

it will also lead to those bands becoming too tight before the patient reaches the ideal age of about 5 months for comprehensive stage II palliation.

From a technical perspective, evaluating the hemodynamic and angiographic results of Hybrid Stage I palliation during the same procedure is frequently the only transcatheter evaluation needed prior to comprehensive stage II palliation (Figure 65.5). The atrial septal intervention is usually performed after the hemodynamic and angiographic assessment towards the end of the procedure. In most patients, a 2 mL non-compliant septostomy catheter can be used, with the diameter of the fully inflated balloon being 13.5 mm (B. Braun Medical, Bethlehem, PA). Other techniques sometimes have to be employed, either alone or in combination, such as static septoplasty with or without radiofrequency perforation of the atrial septum (Figure 65.6), or stent placement across the septum [4]. In very small infants, a 1 mL septostomy balloon (B. Braun Medical, Bethlehem, PA), which has an outer diameter of 9.5 mm, may be more appropriate.

The Interstage Period

The main problems encountered during the interstage period that require transcatheter therapy are RAAO and stenosis across the PDA stent. Careful surveillance after Hybrid Stage I palliation is essential to identify any potential problems sufficiently early before impacting more severely on right ventricular function, with a low threshold of taking a patient to the catheterization laboratory.

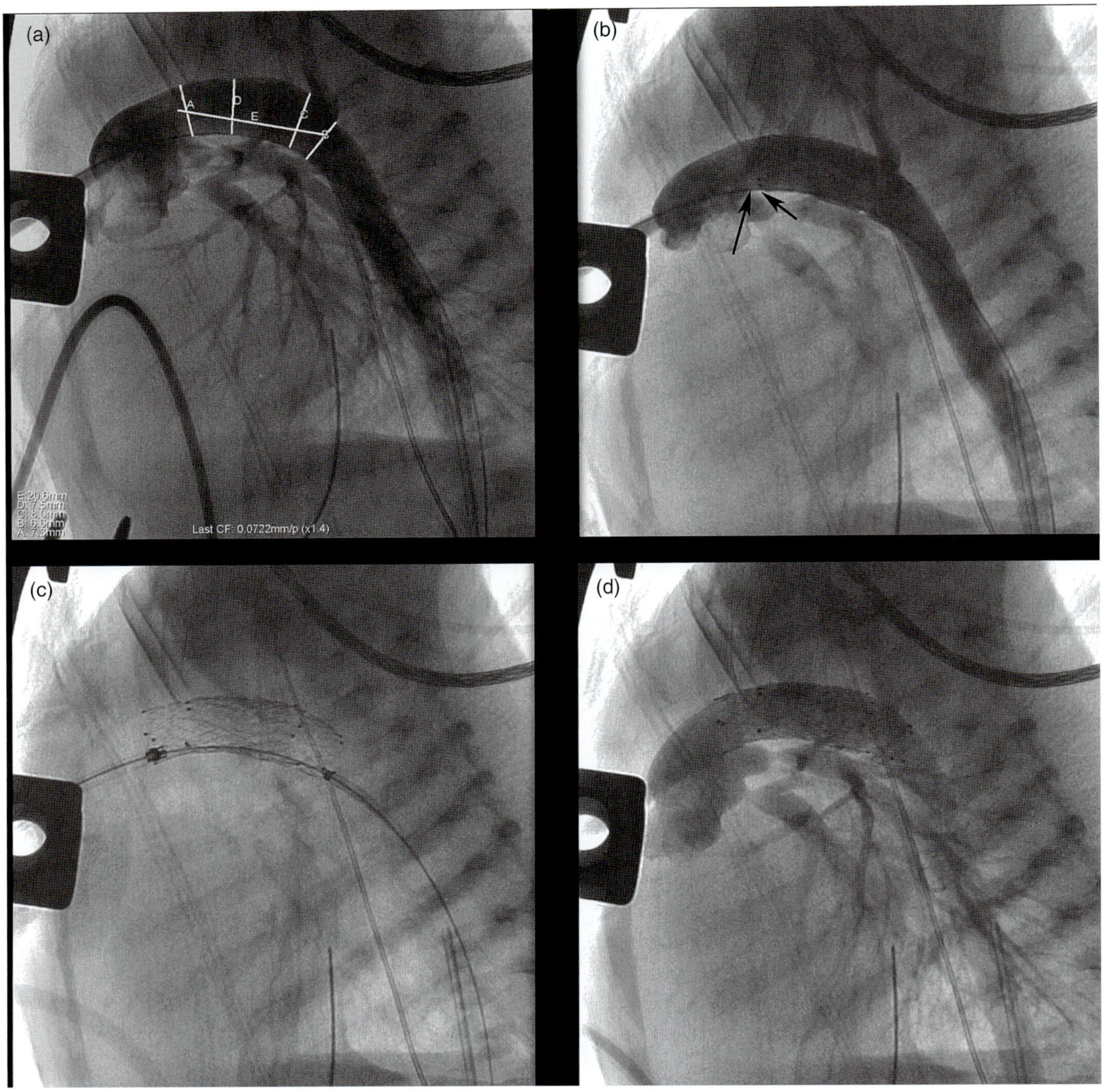

Figure 65.3 Hybrid PDA stent placement is performed using a per main pulmonary artery (MPA) approach. For this purpose a short 6 Fr sheath is placed through a purse string suture in the MPA just above the pulmonary valve. A silk suture is placed 2 mm from the tip and the dilator pulled back, thereby avoiding to inadvertently advancing the sheath or dilator into the MPA. With the surgeon holding the sheath in place from the head-end of the patient, a slightly stiffer 0.018 inch wire (V18, Boston Scientific, Natick, MA) is advanced under fluoroscopic guidance across the PDA into the descending aorta, followed by an angiography through the side arm of the 6 Fr sheath using a hand injection of contrast in standard lateral projection (a). Once an appropriately sized stent is chosen, it is advanced over the wire until it reaches the aorta just distal to the PDA, usually overlapping the RAA. An esophageal temperature probe serves as a great landmark during deployment of the stent. The stent is deployed (uncovered) at its appropriate distal position, bearing in mind that during deployment the stent can be pulled back slightly, but once part of the stent is uncovered it cannot and should not be pushed forward. An angiography is then performed to confirm stent positioning (b). If the stent is too short to cover the entire length of the PDA (b), a second stent can be deployed using the same technique, preferably avoiding to "double-cover" the origin of the RAA (c). This is followed by a final angiography to confirm appropriate stent positioning (d).

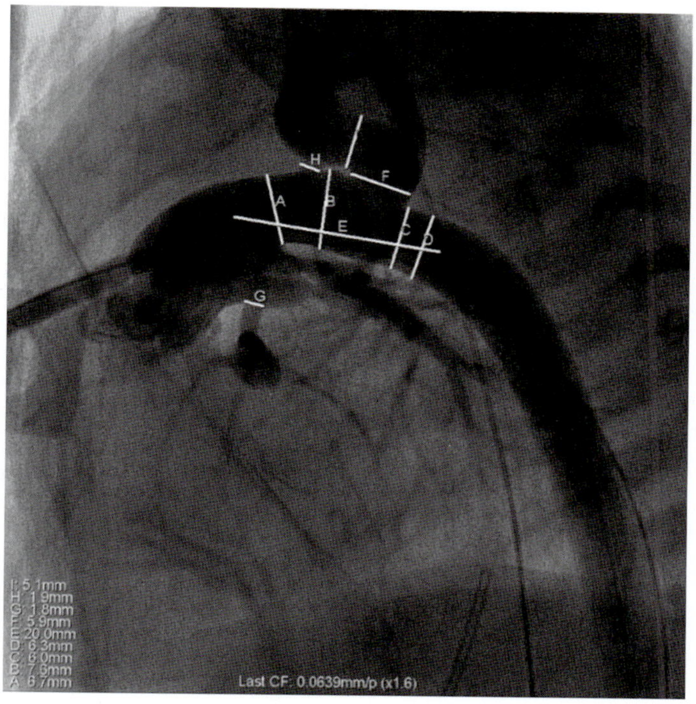

Figure 65.4 Important measurements that should be taken include the maximum and minimum diameter of the PDA, the diameter of the PDA at the aortic and pulmonary end, the size of the descending aorta, as well as the length of the PDA. In addition, the diameter and orientation of the RAA can be evaluated, as well as the position of the PA bands.

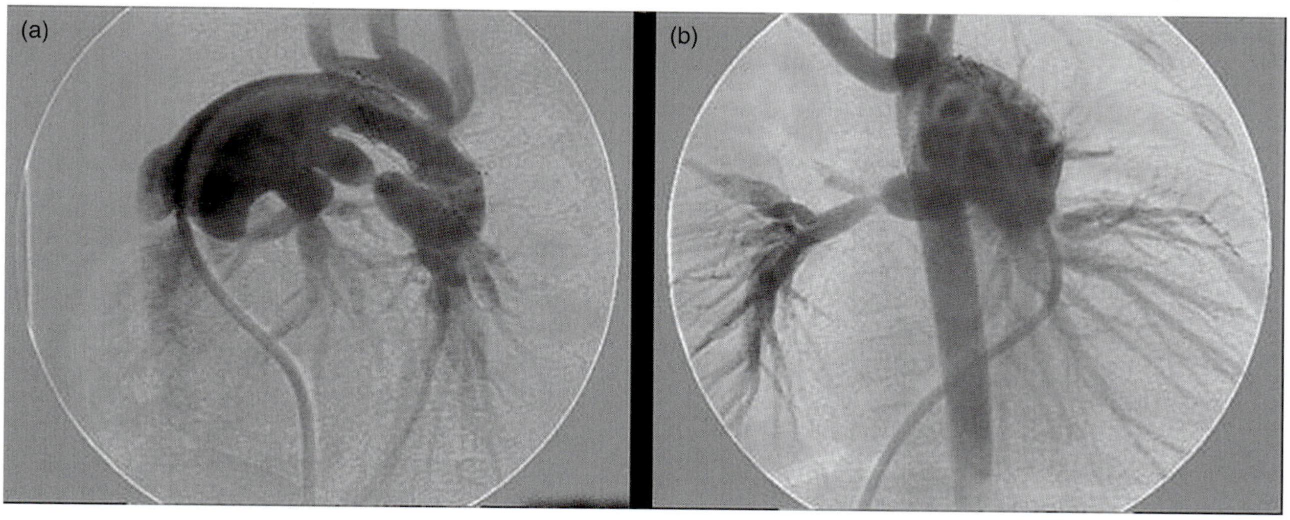

Figure 65.5 Prior to discharge, patients that have undergone Hybrid Stage I palliation are taken to the catheterization laboratory for a diagnostic evaluation as well as creation of a non-restrictive atrial communication. Using an antegrade femoral venous approach combined with an arterial monitoring cannula is the basic set-up for this procedure. The combination of a standard Judkins right coronary catheter with a pressure wire allows obtaining pressure recordings across the atrial septum, the bilateral pulmonary artery bands, the PDA stent, as well as the retrograde aortic arch. In some patients, manipulation of the pressure wire across the retrograde aortic arch can be facilitated through the arterial monitoring cannula. Angiographies should be performed in the MPA and the proximal portion of the PDA stent (usually as hand injections), delineating the pulmonary artery bands, the PDA stent, as well as the (retrograde) aortic arch.

Eagan *et al.* [5] reported that RAAO occurs in as many as 29% of patients after stage I palliation. This is an Achilles'heel of the Hybrid approach, especially in patients with aortic atresia, where cerebral and coronary blood flow depend solely on the flow delivered through the retrograde aortic arch. Even a subtle increase in tricuspid regurgitation or a mild decrease in right ventricular function should prompt an evaluation in the catheterization laboratory. The Doppler gradient across the retrograde arch, while a useful complementary

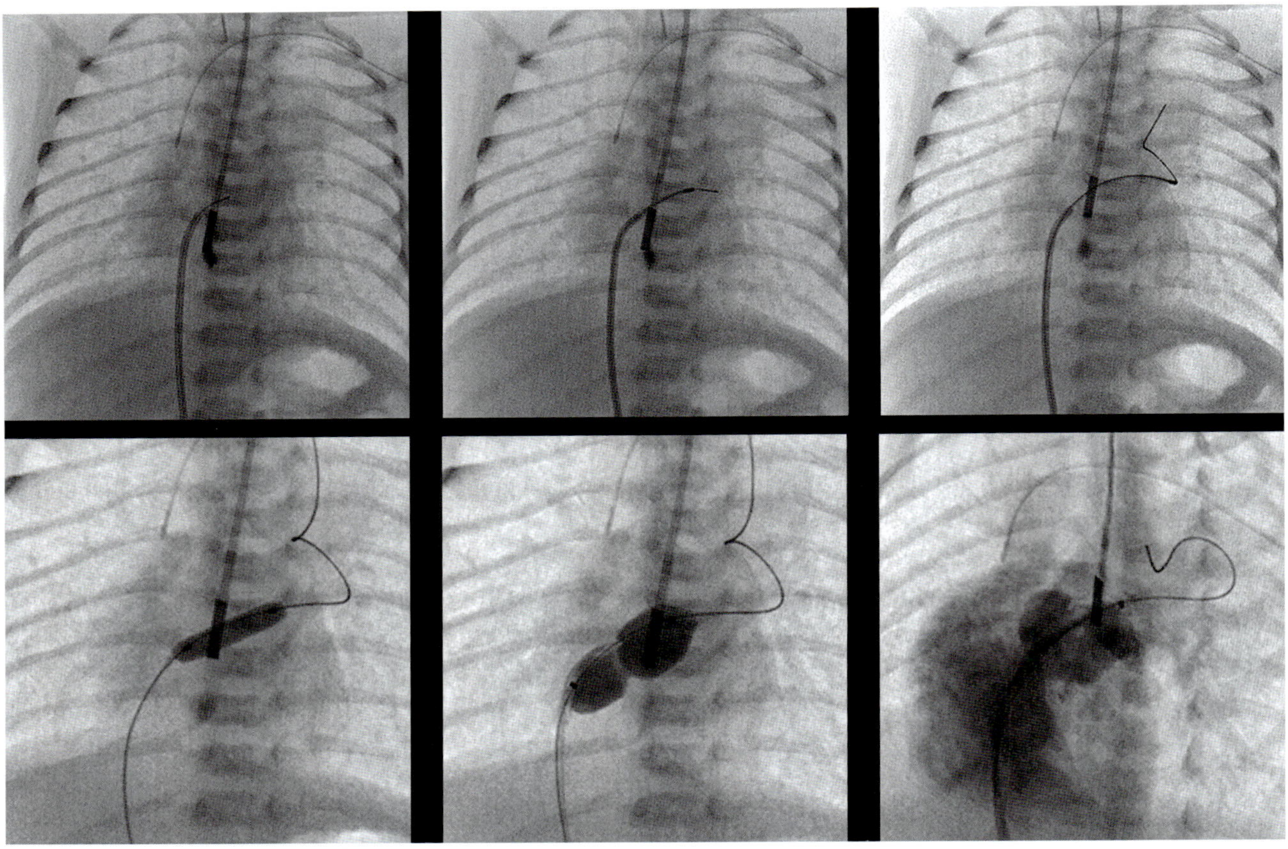

Figure 65.6 Some neonates are not suitable for direct balloon atrial septostomy. This is an example of a neonate with hypoplastic left heart syndrome and an intact atrial septum with a decompressing vein. RF perforation of the atrial septum is best performed using transesophageal echocardiographic (TEE) guidance. For this purpose, in small infants an intracardiac echocardiography probe can be used in the esophagus to delineate the atrial septum. A 5 French Judkins right coronary catheter is used and RF perforation performed, usually using about 5–7.5 for 2 s. Once the RF wire has crossed the atrial septum, a coaxial catheter can be tracked over the wire (top middle image), which then facilitates advancing a 0.014 inch coronary wire into the left atrium (top right image). This is then followed by cutting balloon catheter using initially a small (4 mm or less) cutting balloon, followed by static septoplasty using a larger 8–12 mm balloon (bottom middle image). The result is confirmed through pressure recordings, echocardiography, as well as an LA angiogram (bottom right image). Stent placement may be required in patients with a very thick and restrictive atrial septum and is best performed under TEE guidance, using premounted stents (frequently about 6 mm in diameter).

measure, is not sufficient alone to rule out the need for transcatheter evaluation.

RAAO rarely responds to balloon angioplasty alone. However, stent placement is not without problems, and in-stent stenosis tends to develop over the first 4–8 weeks after the procedure. Therefore, placing a stent too early in the first 3 months of life can lead to recurrence of the RAAO at a time when the patient is not yet ready or mature enough for comprehensive Stage II palliation. Therefore, the decision to place a stent should be made in conjunction with the surgical team, and a plan outlined on what to do if or when recurrence of RAAO occurs (Figure 65.7).

In contrast to stenting the RAAO, which is performed via a retrograde approach, placing an additional stent across the PDA, either for in-stent stenosis or for any residual or recurrent obstruction, is usually performed antegradely (Figure 65.8). Treating a combination of PDA in-stent stenosis and RAAO is a particular challenge, especially if the PDA in-stent stenosis involves the adjacent segment around the orifice of the RAAO (Figure 65.9). Placing a PDA stent first often limits the flow through the already stenotic retrograde aortic arch even further, potentially leading to a catastrophic hemodynamic deterioration (cardiac arrest). However, treating the RAAO first often prevents the subsequent placement of an additional PDA stent. In general, if both levels of obstruction are present, usually it is more important to treat the RAAO, allowing the patient's ventricular function to recover, and then embarking on an early surgical option, which includes an early Stage II, or a conversion to a classic Norwood type palliation, as well as other surgical modifications.

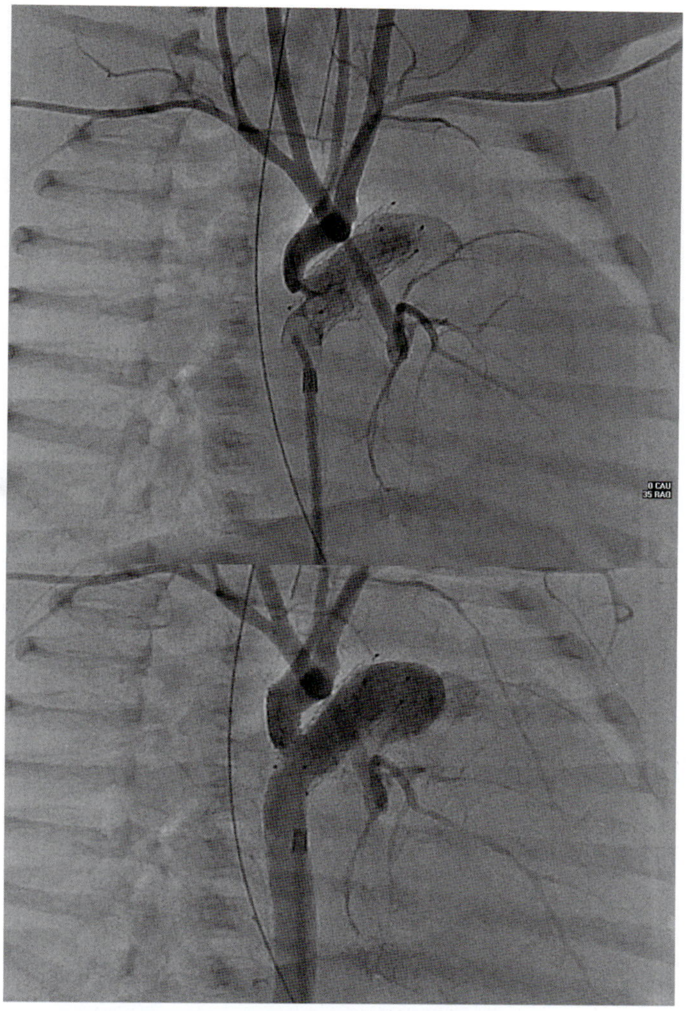

Figure 65.7 Stenting of the retrograde aortic arch is usually performed via a retrograde approach using a 4 French long sheath with a reasonably small outer diameter. Alternatively a short sheath can be used but care has to be taken when crossing the cells of the PDA stent. It is important to expect and be prepared for sudden hemodynamic deterioration and have epinephrine ready. In the presence of RAAO even an initial hand injection at the origin of the RAA can lead to cardiac arrest, which often does not resolve until the RAA has been stented. Usually, a 4–4.5 mm premounted coronary stent is used to stent the RAA. The top image (RAO projection) documents a tight stenosis of the RAA with the patient becoming asystolic following the hand injection at the mouth of the RAA. The subsequent stent delivery was performed under CPR with the in situ PDA stent serving as a roadmap. Once the stent was delivered (bottom image) spontaneous cardiac output recovered.

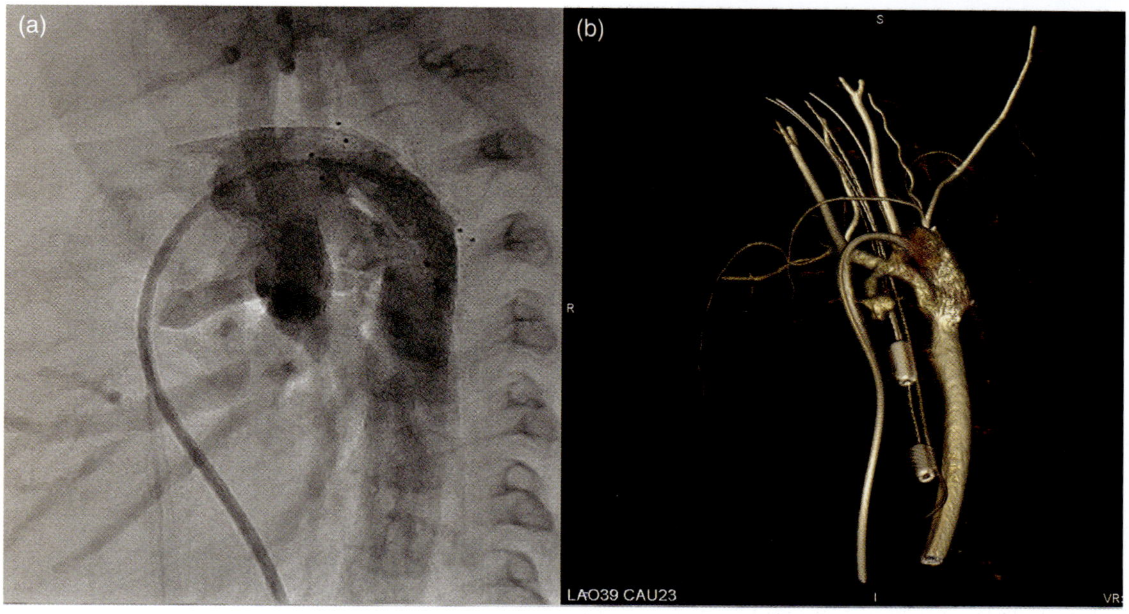

Figure 65.8 A stenosis of the PDA (either in stent stenosis, or recurrent or residual stenosis) is treated using an antegrade approach with a soft wire without the use of a long sheath and ideally a fairly soft wire, to avoid splinting open the tricuspid and pulmonary valve. An additional catheter can be placed retrograde for angiographic monitoring. Wherever possible, the length of the stent should be chosen as not to overlap the RAA, thereby avoiding a double-layer of stents across this orifice. (a) A residual stenosis distal to the PDA stent, which was not visible on a standard lateral projection. (b) 3D reconstructions of a rotational angiography performed under rapid transesophageal pacing documented that the initial PDA stent had not reached the origin of the RAA, leaving some part of the PDA uncovered. (c) These 3D reconstructions were used to obtain a 2D image using LAO and caudal angulation, which documented the area of narrowing. (d) The result after placement of an additional PDA stent.

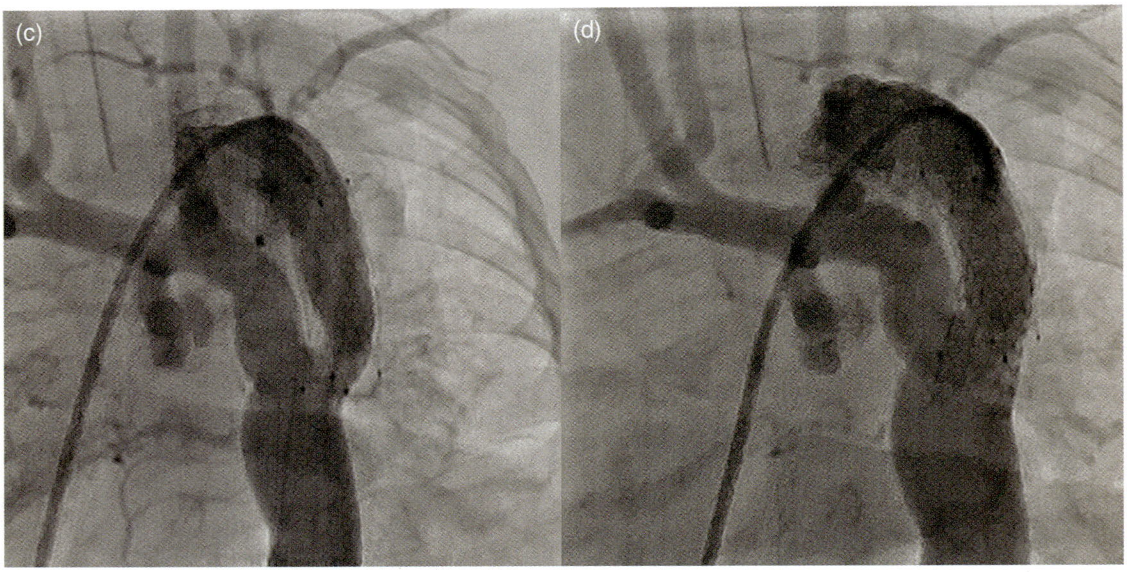

Figure 65.8 (*Continued*)

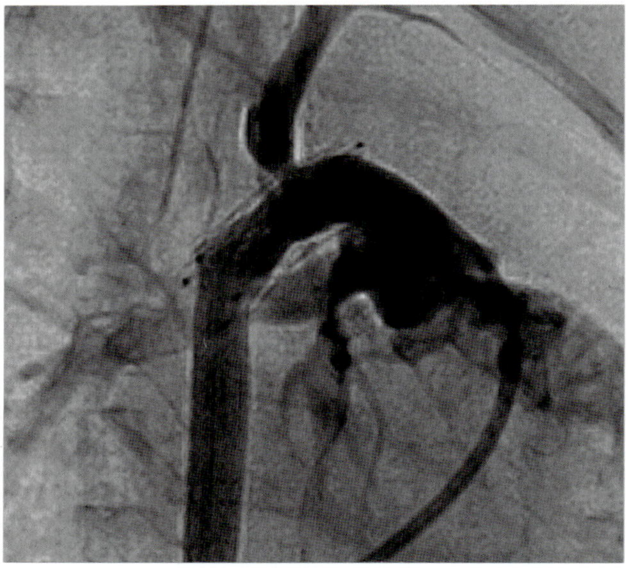

Figure 65.9 Three-month-old infant with a combination of RAAO as well as PDA in-stent stenosis.

Perventricular Closure of Ventricular Septal Defects

The majority of muscular VSDs are small to medium in size, and do not require any form of intervention in the neonatal period. The defects tend to become smaller with time, often eliminating the need for any form of surgical or transcatheter therapy. Occasionally, however, a large muscular VSD develops with signs and symptoms of heart failure once the pulmonary vascular resistance drops. In this situation, closure of the defect is indicated.

A surgical approach requires cardiopulmonary bypass. Closure of these defects can be challenging, with defects frequently hidden in the muscular right ventricular trabeculations, associated with a higher incidence of residual shunts and higher procedural risk. While VSDs can be closed percutaneously, disadvantages of this approach in neonates and infants include the need for an arteriovenous loop, as well as the fairly large and stiff delivery systems in relation to patient size. Studies have shown a significantly higher incidence of adverse events, lower procedural success, and a higher incidence of residual shunts when transcatheter closure of muscular VSD is performed in infants with a weight below 10 kg [6].

Perventricular closure of VSD is an off-pump Hybrid technique utilized to deploy an Ampatzer muscular VSD device across a VSD [7]. It is performed using either a median sternotomy or a limited subxiphoid incision, with a device being deployed using a short sheath placed through a purse string of the RV free wall across the VSD (Figure 65.10).

If a VSD cannot be crossed easily from the RV side, it may be beneficial to place a femoral arterial sheath and advance a catheter into the left ventricle with fluoroscopic guidance using a portable c-arm. An LV angiogram can be very helpful outlining the VSD and serving as a roadmap to cross the VSD using a left-sided transcatheter approach. Once a wire has been passed into the PA, a perventricular approach can be used to snare the wire, thereby creating an arterial-per-ventricular loop, which facilitates advancing the short sheath across the VSD into the LV.

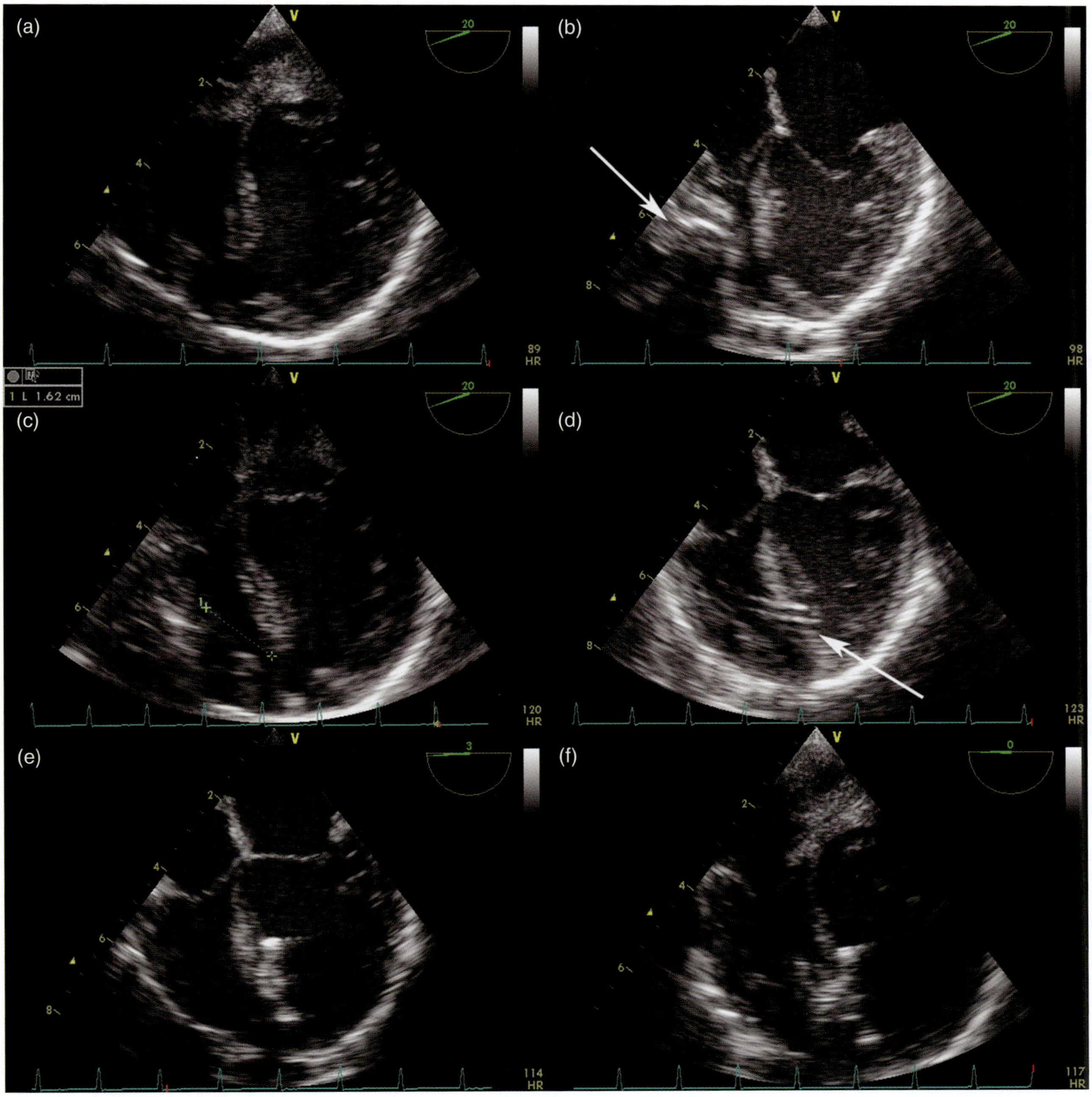

Figure 65.10 Perventricular closure of a muscular ventricular septal defect (VSD) in a 5-week-old infant. Once the RV free wall is exposed, the VSD is profiled (a) and the ideal access point to the VSD is determined using gentle manual pressure under transesophageal echocardiography guidance (b). This should be perpendicular to the VSD with sufficient distance between VSD and free wall to allow deployment of a device. The distance between RV free wall and VSD should be measured as to avoid advancing the sheath too far across the VSD (c). Once the access point has been chosen, a purse-string suture is placed and an 18 Gauge needle advanced through the purse string and directed towards the VSD. An 0.35 angled glidewire should be directed across the VSD under TEE guidance, followed by advancing a 7 Fr short sheath over the wire across the VSD, but not too far distally into the LV (d). The chosen device size should usually be about 2 mm larger than the size of the VSD. Its deployment is performed under TEE guidance where the device usually can readily be visualized crossing the sheath. The LV disk should be deployed just distal to the ventricular septum (e), taking care not to push the device against the LV free wall, or to entangle the mitral valve apparatus. This is followed by deploying the RV disk, and releasing the device after echocardiography confirmed an accurate device position as well as absence of interference with AV valves (f).

Hybrid Balloon Aortic or Pulmonary Valvuloplasty

In most neonates, balloon aortic valvuloplasty can be performed safely using a percutaneous approach with a 3 or 4 French arterial sheath. However, particularly in small and premature infants, this sheath size is too large for the femoral arterial vasculature. In this situation, a carotid cutdown is warranted. Once the cutdown has been performed, the hemostatic sheath is introduced and the remainder of the procedure performed in usual fashion. Using a carotid cutdown often facilitates crossing the aortic valve through a better approach coming from the neck. After the procedure the entry site is repaired surgically.

A Hybrid approach for balloon pulmonary valvuloplasty is rarely needed, as even in premature neonates the vein is usually sufficiently distensible to allow a percutaneous approach when needed. Exceptions are those patients with a very low weight and significantly depressed RV function. In these patients, the manipulations required to advance a wire across the pulmonary valve may be poorly tolerated, and a Hybrid approach can serve as a better tolerated alternative procedure (Figure 65.11) [8].

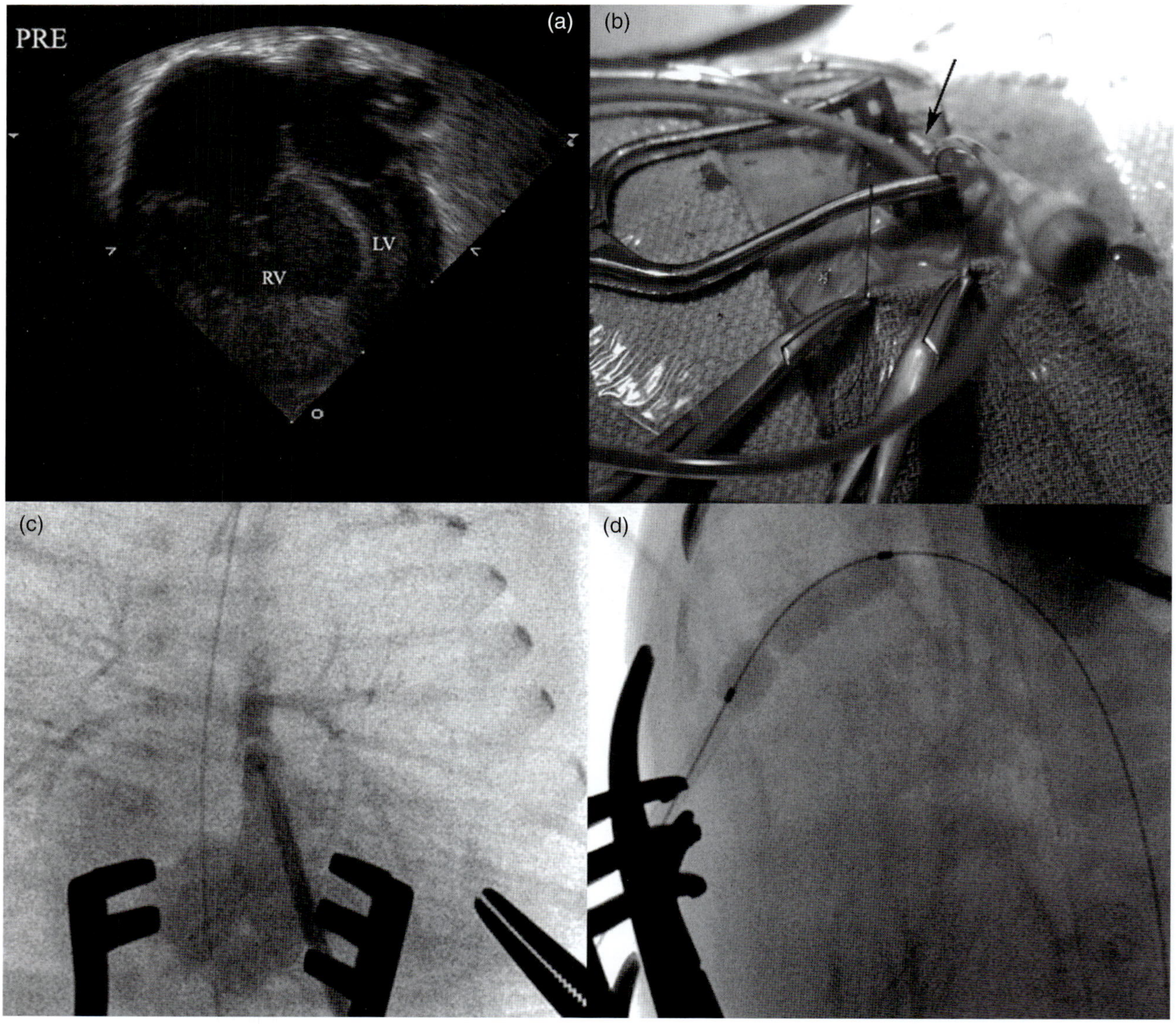

Figure 65.11 Four-week-old (700 g) infant born prematurely at 24 weeks' gestation with pulmonary valve stenosis and poor right ventricular function with a dilated RV (a). Given the size of the patient and the poor RV function a Hybrid approach to balloon pulmonary valvuloplasty was chosen. For this purpose a sub-xiphoid incision was performed and a purse string placed at the RV free wall in sufficient distance from the pulmonary valve to allow advancing a balloon through a sheath across the valve (b). A brief hand-injection through the side arm of the sheath was performed to determine the diameter of the valve annulus (c), and a wire readily advanced across the valve in one of the branch pulmonary arteries, followed by balloon valvuloplasty (d).

References

1 Ohye RG, Sleeper LA, Mahony L, *et al.* (2010) Comparison of shunt types in the Norwood procedure for single-ventricle lesions. *N Engl J Med*, **362** (21), 1980–1992.

2 Galantowicz M, Cheatham JP. (2005) Lessons learned from the development of a new hybrid strategy for the management of hypoplastic left heart syndrome. *Pediatr Cardiol*, **26** (2), 190–199.

3 Akintuerk H, Michel-Behnke I, Valeske K, *et al.* (2002) Stenting of the arterial duct and banding of the pulmonary arteries: basis for combined Norwood stage I and II repair in hypoplastic left heart. *Circulation*, **105** (9), 1099–1103.

4 Holzer RJ, Wood A, Chisolm JL, *et al.* (2008) Atrial septal interventions in patients with hypoplastic left heart syndrome. *Catheter Cardiovasc Interv*, **72** (5), 696–704.

5 Egan MJ, Hill SL, Boettner BL, *et al.* (2011) Predictors of retrograde aortic arch obstruction after hybrid palliation of hypoplastic left heart syndrome. *Pediatr Cardiol*, **32** (1), 67–75.

6 Holzer R, Balzer D, Cao QL, Lock K, Hijazi ZM. (2004) Amplatzer muscular ventricular septal defect I: device closure of muscular ventricular septal defects using the Amplatzer muscular ventricular septal defect occluder: immediate and mid-term results of a US registry. *J Am Coll Cardiol*, **43** (7), 1257–1263.

7 Bacha EA, Cao QL, Galantowicz ME, *et al.* (2005) Multicenter experience with perventricular device closure of muscular ventricular septal defects. *Pediatr Cardiol*, **26** (2), 169–175.

8 Holzer RJ, Sisk M, Phillips A. (2008) Hybrid balloon pulmonary valvuloplasty in a 700-g infant: thinking outside the box. *Catheter Cardiovasc Interv*, **72** (1), 93–96.

66

Neonatal Cardiac Surgical Procedures

Harold M. Burkhart

Division of Cardiovascular and Thoracic Surgery, University Health Sciences Center, Oklahoma City, OK, USA

The number of congenital heart surgeries performed in the USA is increasing every year with decreasing mortality. Based on the Society of Thoracic Surgeons database, 34 995 congenital heart surgeries were performed in 2012, with an operative mortality of 3.2%. Among these, 20% (6883 patients) were performed in neonates, with an operative mortality of 4.0%. The percentage of neonatal heart surgery performed in the USA has remained constant even in the face of as increasing number of congenital heart surgeries.

The most common primary cardiac conditions needing intervention during the neonatal period are patent ductus arteriosus (PDA) (14.2%), hypoplastic left heart syndrome (HLHS) (12.0%), coarctation (6.9%), transposition of great vessels (TGA) (6.5%), aortic arch hypoplasia (2.3%), pulmonary atresia with ventricular septal defect (2.3%), truncus arteriosus (2.1%), total anomalous pulmonary venous connection (1.7%), and interrupted aortic arch (1.4%). The most commonly performed neonatal cardiac surgical operative procedures are the Norwood procedure (11.4%), arterial switch operation (7.1%), modified Blalock–Taussig shunt (6.5%), coarctation repair (6.1%), total anomalous pulmonary venous connection repair (4.0%), aortic arch repair (3.3%), truncus arteriosus repair (1.8%), and surgical PDA ligation (1.4%). This chapter highlights the surgical principles of these commonly performed neonatal heart surgeries. The chapters on specific congenital cardiac lesions demonstrate further their surgical management in the neonate.

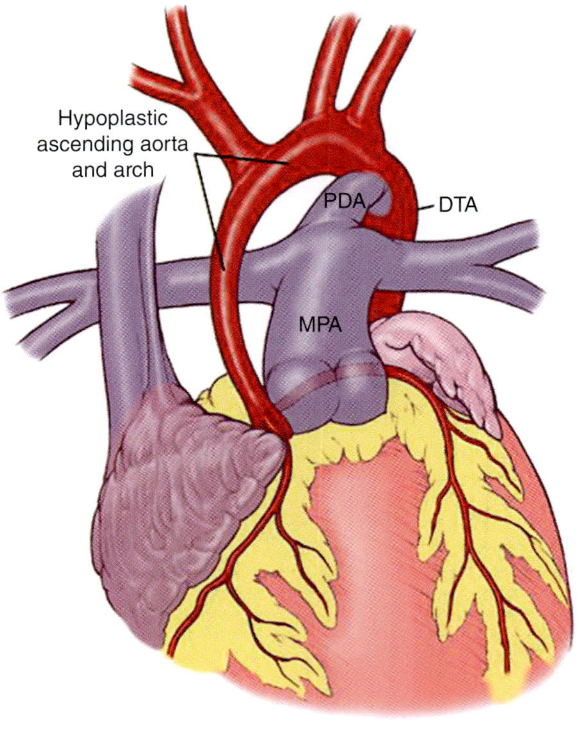

Figure 66.1 The classic anatomy of hypoplastic left heart syndrome (HLHS) consistent with a hypoplastic left ventricle, aortic root, ascending aorta and arch. A large patent ductus arteriosus (PDA) continues as the descending thoracic aorta (DTA). MPA, main pulmonary artery.

Hypoplastic Left Heart Syndrome (Figure 66.1)

Surgical intervention is indicated in almost all patients with HLHS. Prematurity (<35 weeks), low birth weight (<1000 g), presence of severe extracardiac anomalies, severe tricuspid and pulmonary regurgitation are relative contraindications for surgery. The Norwood procedure is usually undertaken in the first week of life in almost all patients with HLHS. We prefer to wait at least 24–48 hours after birth for transition from fetal circulation. Aggressive resuscitation is needed while waiting for surgery. Maintenance of ductal patency with prostaglandin infusion (PGE-1) is very important for distal body perfusion. Atrial balloon septostomy is rarely

Visual Guide to Neonatal Cardiology, First Edition. Edited by Ernerio T. Alboliras, Ziyad M. Hijazi, Leo Lopez, and Donald J. Hagler.

indicated before the surgery because the most patients will have an adequate patent foramen ovale (PFO). Systemic malperfusion with renal or liver dysfunction should be addressed prior to surgery to reduce surgical mortality. Small dose dopamine (3–5 μg/kg/min) or dobutamine are the preferred inotropic agents. Epinephrine is generally avoided because it increases the systemic vascular resistance. Preoperative intubation may be necessary to allow for manipulation of the pulmonary vascular resistance with low Fio2 (17–21%) and relative hypercarbia (Paco2: 45–50%). On occasion, it may be necessary to undertake surgery immediately after birth in neonates with an intact atrial septum or evidence of ductal closure resulting in systemic hypoperfusion.

Procedure: Norwood Procedure with Sano Modification (Figures 66.2, 66.3, and 66.4)

After midline sternotomy, the thymus is excised. The anatomy of HLHS is confirmed. The ascending aorta typically looks very small (2–3 mm in size) and is shifted to the right side by the large main pulmonary artery which also continues as the descending aorta through

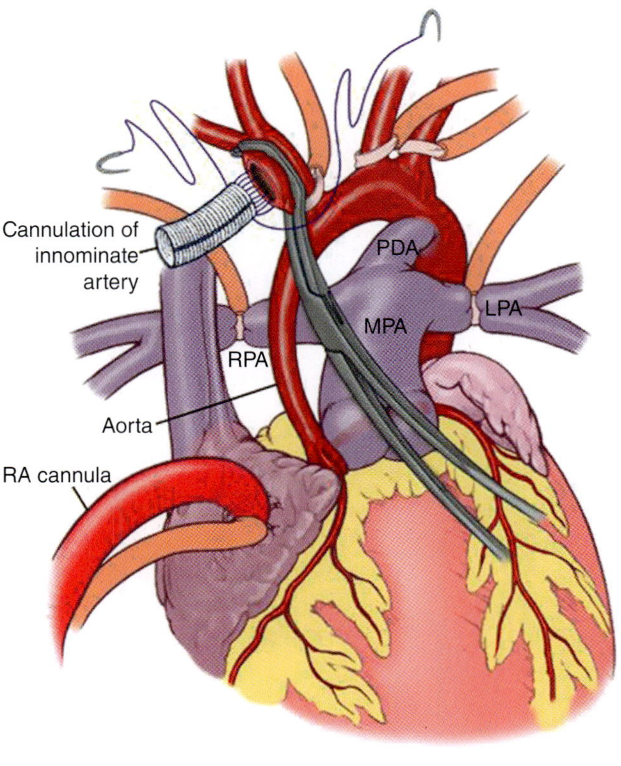

Figure 66.2 Cannulation method for cardiopulmonary bypass (CPB) with arterial cannula into innominate artery with synthetic graft and right atrium (RA) venous drainage cannula. Note that both branch pulmonary arteries (PAs) are controlled with tourniquet before going on CPB in order avoid pulmonary flooding and also to improve systemic perfusion. LPA, left pulmonary artery; RPA, right pulmonary artery.

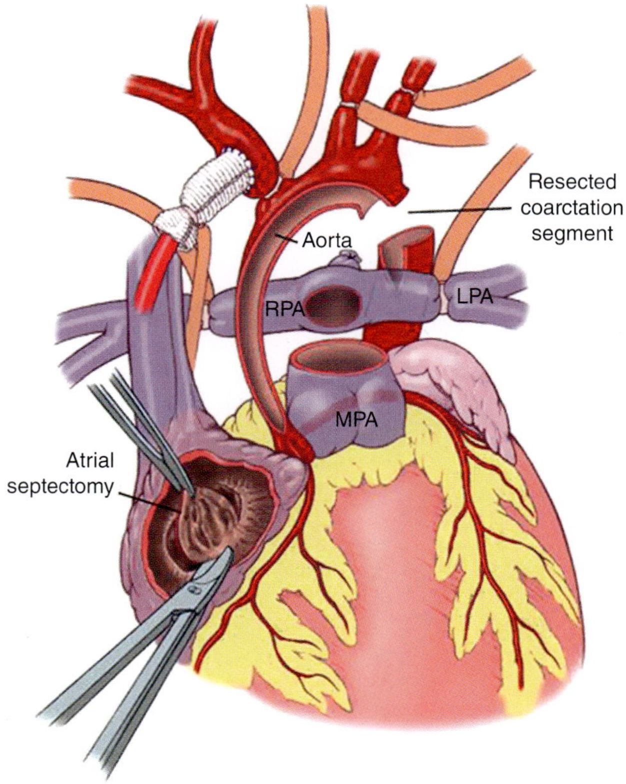

Figure 66.3 Snared arch vessels with wide open ascending aorta and arch. The PDA is ligated and the coarctation segment is resected. Atrial septectomy is carried out with antegrade cerebral perfusion and cardiotomy sucker bypass.

the large ductus. Surgery is usually undertaken in three stages, the first one being the Norwood procedure.

The aim of first stage (Norwood procedure) is to:

1) Establish systemic blood flow without any obstruction from the single functioning right ventricle through pulmonary valve (aortic arch and ascending aorta reconstruction with division of the PDA);
2) Establish pulmonary blood flow from the right ventricle using a valveless conduit (Sano shunt); and
3) Complete mixing of pulmonary venous return at the atrial level (atrial septectomy).

The aortic arch vessels (innominate artery, left common carotid, and left subclavian artery) are dissected and controlled. Our preferred approach for arch reconstruction is deep hypothermia with antegrade cerebral perfusion through the innominate artery. A 3.5 mm Gore-Tex graft is sutured to the innominate artery. The graft is cannulated with the arterial cannula, and the right atrial appendage is cannulated with the venous cannula. Cardiopulmonary bypass (CPB) is instituted and the pulmonary arteries are controlled.

The patient is cooled to 18°C. Complete dissection of the aortic arch vessels, coarctation, and descending aorta are performed. Care is taken to avoid damage to the

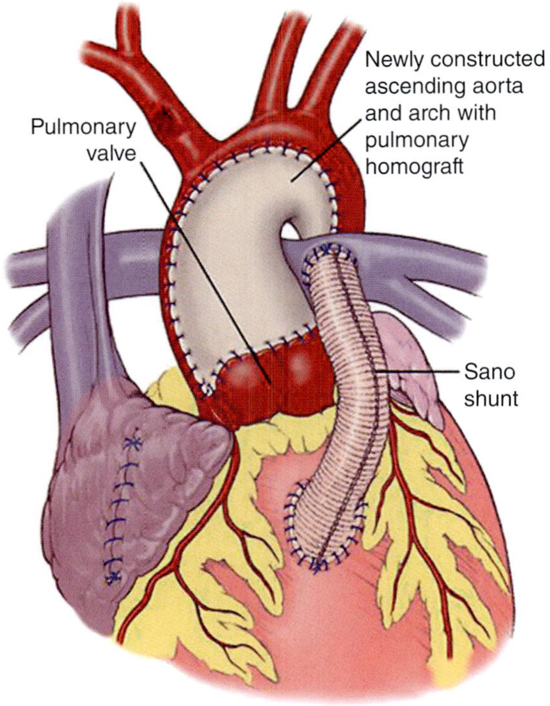

Figure 66.4 Completed Norwood procedure with reconstructed aortic arch and ascending aorta utilizing the pulmonary valve to provide systemic. The Sano shunt provides the pulmonary blood flow.

recurrent laryngeal nerve while dissecting the descending aorta. After adequate cooling, the PDA is divided. Next, the main pulmonary artery is divided above the commissural level. A 6 mm Gore-Tex graft is utilized for the Sano shunt (right ventricle to distal main pulmonary artery shunt) in most patients. The distal anastomosis of the Sano shunt is performed at this point in the surgery.

At this time the temperature would have reached 18°C. The aortic arch vessels are controlled and CPB flow is decreased to provide antegrade cerebral perfusion (10 mL/kg/min; CPB flow) through the innominate artery. The PDA and coarctation are completely excised. The aortotomy is extended proximally into the arch all the way to the sinotubular junction of the ascending aorta. The heart is arrested with direct cardioplegia into the hypoplastic aortic root.

The distal aortic arch and descending thoracic aorta are sutured together posteriorly. A fin-shaped pulmonary artery homograft patch is utilized to reconstruct the hypoplastic arch and ascending aorta anteriorly up to the sinotubular junction incorporating the pulmonary root into the reconstruction. Next, an atrial septectomy is performed. At this time, full CPB is re-instituted and the patient is rewarmed. The proximal Sano shunt anastomosis is performed during rewarming and the baby is weaned from bypass.

Transposition of the Great Arteries (Figure 66.5)

TGA is a conotruncal abnormality in which atria connect normally to their corresponding ventricle (AV concordance) but the ventricles connect to the wrong great arteries (VA discordance). Circulation in TGA is parallel with deoxygenated blood continuously circulating in the body and oxygenated blood recirculating in the lungs. Mixing of blood via a defect in the atrial septum is essential for survival. In children with TGA without any intracardiac shunt, balloon atrial septostomy and maintenance of ductal patency with prostaglandin infusion has an important role in preoperative stabilization.

Surgical Correction (Figures 66.6, 66.7, and 66.8)

The diagnosis of TGA is itself an indication for surgery. Patients with TGA with an intact ventricular septum typically undergo surgery within the first week of life, while those with a large VSD wait longer if needed.

The arterial switch operation (ASO) is considered the anatomic repair for children with TGA because the left ventricle is maintained as a systemic ventricle after correction. Earlier atrial switch operations (Senning and

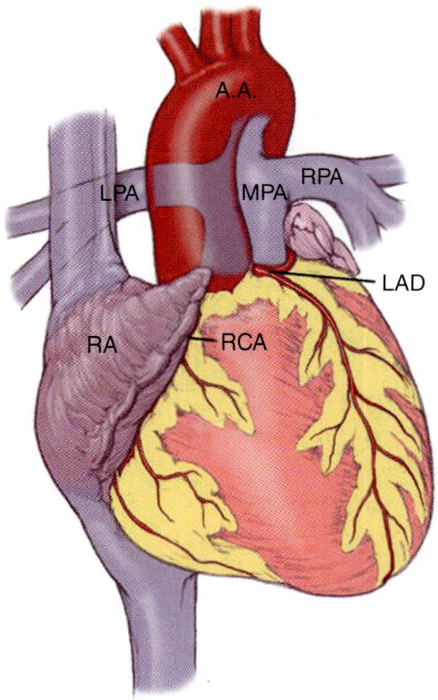

Figure 66.5 The anatomy in patients with D-transposition of the great arteries (D-TGA); AV concordance with VA discordance. The aorta is situated anterior and right of the pulmonary artery. The coronary arteries and its sinuses in the aorta face the corresponding sinuses in the pulmonary artery. AA, ascending aorta; LAD, left anterior descending coronary artery; RA, right atrium; RCA, right coronary artery.

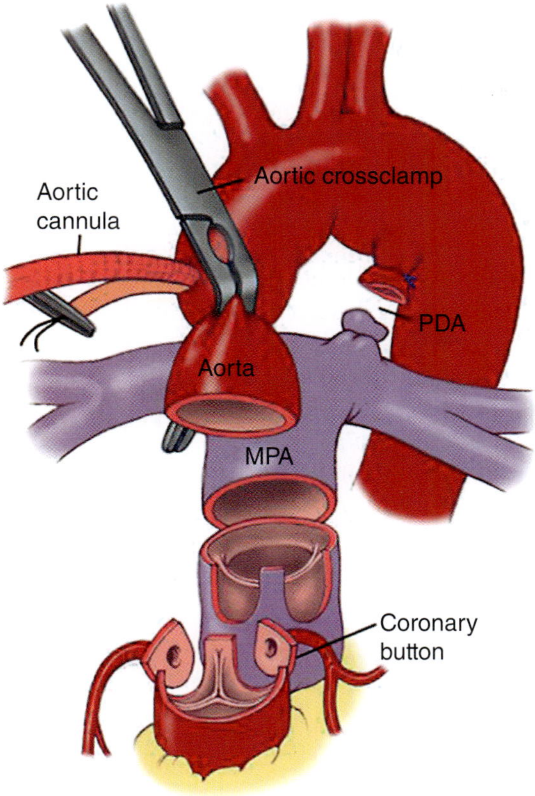

Figure 66.6 Completely divided ascending aorta and main pulmonary artery with harvested coronary arteries from the native aorta. Possible coronary reimplantation sites on the neo-aortic are demonstrated.

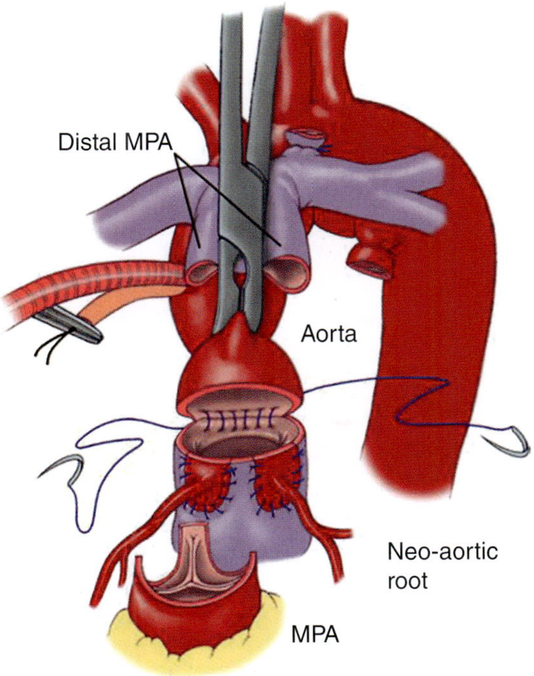

Figure 66.7 The newly constructed neo-aortic root with partially completed anastomosis between the neo-aortic root and distal ascending aorta. The LeCompte maneuver with the anteriorly placed pulmonary artery is also shown.

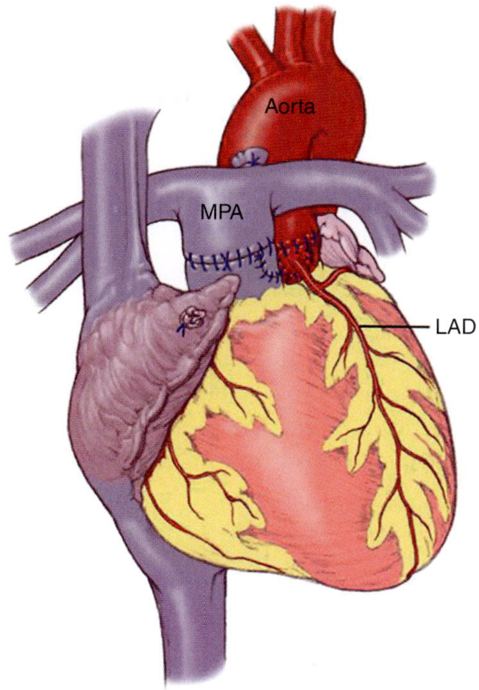

Figure 66.8 Completed arterial switch operation (ASO) with newly constructed outflow tracts, transferred coronaries, and the Lecompte maneuver.

Mustard) with rerouting of systemic and pulmonary venous circulations are considered physiologic because the right ventricle is maintained as the systemic ventricle after correction. The problem of late right ventricular failure with the atrial switch operation is avoided with the ASO procedure.

The basic principles of the ASO include switching of the great arteries to the corresponding morphologic ventricle and reconstruction of the ventricular outflow tracts to the appropriate distal vessel. In addition, the coronary arteries are transferred to the great vessel arising from the left ventricle and the pulmonary artery is transposed anterior to the aorta (LeCompte maneuver).

Procedure

After midline sternotomy, the anterior pericardium is harvested. The pulmonary artery branches are mobilized hilum to hilum to allow for the LeCompte maneuver. CPB is instituted and the ductus arteriosus is ligated and divided.

With moderate hypothermia, the heart is arrested with antegrade cold blood cardioplegia. Any associated intracardiac shunts are closed through a right atriotomy. Both the aorta and pulmonary artery are divided and the LeCompte maneuver is performed. Both coronary ostia are harvested along with aortic wall and adequate mobilization to prevent kinking or stretching is carried out. Taking the coronary ostium as a large button along with native aorta avoids late coronary ostial stenosis.

The harvested coronary buttons are transferred to the corresponding sinuses of the proximal main pulmonary artery (neo-aortic root). The right coronary artery is often implanted usually at a higher level than the left coronary artery in the neo-aortic root. Next, the distal segment of the ascending aorta is anastomosed to the neo-aortic root.

The neo-pulmonary root is reconstructed with large pantaloon-shaped patch of autologous pericardium. The distal main pulmonary artery is then anastomosed to the newly reconstructed neo-pulmonary root. After de-airing the left side of the heart, the aortic cross-clamp is released and the child is weaned from CPB.

Systemic to Pulmonary Artery Shunt (Figure 66.9)

On occasion, newborns with decreased pulmonary blood flow require a systemic artery to pulmonary artery shunt. Currently, these shunts are carried out as a palliative procedure prior to complete repair in a cyanotic neonate (e.g., tetralogy of Fallott, pulmonary atresia, or single ventricle anatomy) or in combination with another procedure (Norwood procedure). The most common shunt utilized is the modified Blalock–Taussig shunt (mBTS). The construction of this shunt involves connecting a small polytetrafluoroethylene (PTFE) graft from the innominate or subclavian artery to the pulmonary artery (PA). The procedure can be performed via thoracotomy or midline sternotomy. Advantages of a midline sternotomy approach include:

1) Both lungs can be ventilated through the entire procedure in unstable infants;
2) The shunt can be performed more centrally on the branch PAs which may avoid pulmonary artery branch stenosis;
3) Other cardiac procedures such as ligation of a patent ductus arteriosus, PA plasty or atrial septectomy can be performed at the same time;
4) Establishment of CPB can be performed easily if the situation demands;
5) Avoidance of musculoskeletal deformities caused by lateral thoracotomy; and
6) Avoids an extra scar during complete repair.

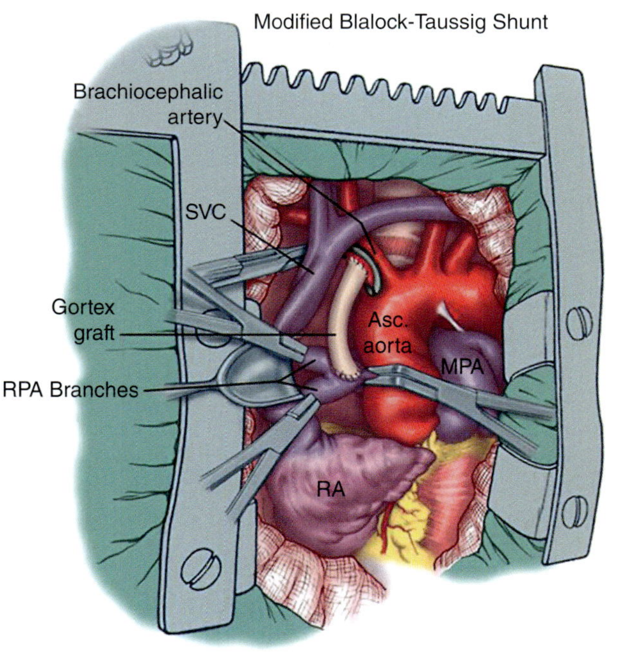

Figure 66.9 After a midline sternotomy, the innominate artery and right PA are exposed. The vessels are controlled and a modified Blalock–Taussig shunt is performed by suturing the graft to the inferior aspect on the innominate artery and the superior aspect of the right PA.

Procedure

After a median sternotomy is performed, the innominate artery is exposed up to its bifurcation and the presence of normal arch vessel anatomy is confirmed. The pericardium is opened and the right PA is identified. Heparin is administered and a side-biting vascular clamp is placed on the right subclavian–innominate artery junction.

The size of the graft is decided by the body weight of the child. As a general rule, infants with a body weight of 2.5–3.5 kg are better served with 3.5 mm graft and those weighing 4–5 kg with a 4 mm graft. The innominate artery is incised and the PTFE tube graft is sutured using a fine non-absorbable monofilament suture. The right PA is isolated using vascular clamps and the graft is sutured to the superior aspect of the artery. Patency of the graft is confirmed by increase in the oxygen saturation in the pulse oximetry (75–85%) with drop in the diastolic blood pressure. The chest is closed with a mediastinal drain after obtaining good hemostasis without protamine administration.

It is important to reduce the Fio2 on the ventilator to as close to atmospheric level 21% when possible, because oxygen is a pulmonary vasodilator that could lead to pulmonary edema and low cardiac output. As long as bleeding is not an issue, we consider starting the child on a heparin infusion. Antiplatelet agents are added from the day after surgery.

Neonatal Repair of Coarctation

Neonates with critical coarctation usually present with signs of shock. The preoperative optimization in neonates with critical coarctation involves maintaining ductal patency with PGE-1, with optimization of pulmonary and systemic vascular resistance.

Extended End-To-End Resection and Anastomosis (Figures 66.10, 66.11, 66.12, and 66.13)

Although various surgical techniques are available, resection and end-to-end anastomosis is the preferred mode of treatment in neonates with coarctation. In neonates with critical coarctation, ductal patency is maintained with PGE-1 which is continued until surgical repair. All acid–base imbalances are aggressively corrected. In the operating room in order to reduce the incidence of paraplegia, the infant is allowed to cool (34–35°C) and hypotension is avoided.

If possible, right radial and femoral artery monitoring lines are placed. The femoral line will provide the distal aortic pressure at the time of aortic clamping and will also help to monitor the gradient across the coarctation repair. The child is positioned with the left side up with left arm supported at the level of the head. A small left posterior thoracotomy with sparing of serratus anterior is carried out. The skin incision is made just below the tip of the scapula extending towards the spine. The chest is entered over the fourth rib and the left lung is retracted out of the way. After the mediastinal pleura over the descending aorta is opened, the PDA and nearby discrete aortic coarctation are identified.

While dissecting out the PDA, the left recurrent laryngeal and vagus nerve are identified and kept from harm.

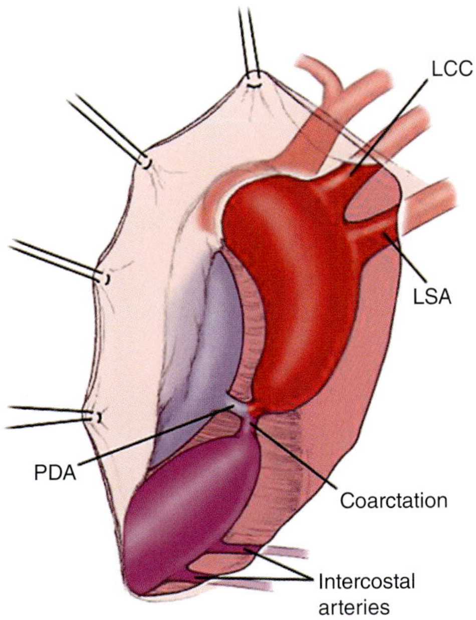

Figure 66.10 After a left thoracotomy, the discrete aortic coarctation and patent ductus arteriosus (PDA) are identified. LCC, left common carotid artery; LSA, left subclavian artery.

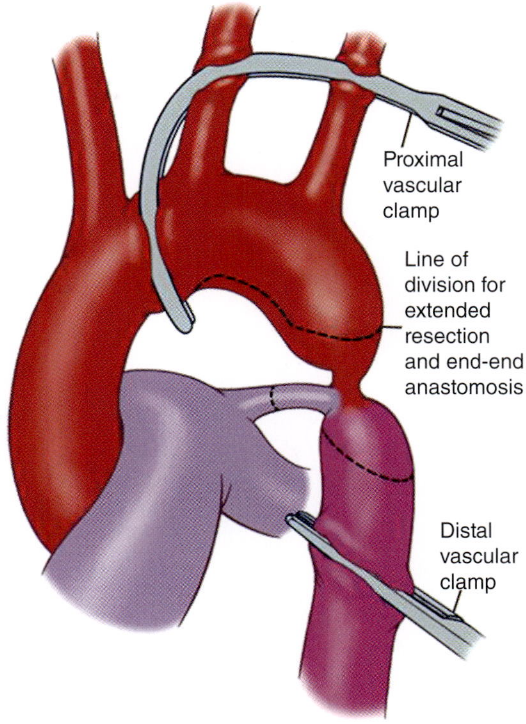

Figure 66.11 Dotted lines show the proposed site of excision of the coarctation segment and ductus. Please note that the proximal anastomosis is on the lesser curvature of arch just opposite the left common carotid artery. This not only allows a bigger anastomosis, but augments the aortic arch as well.

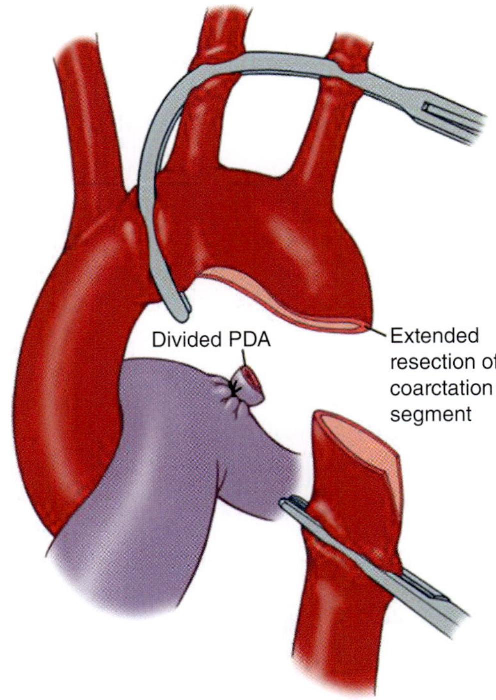

Figure 66.12 The extended resection of the coarctation segment with division of ductus arteriosus.

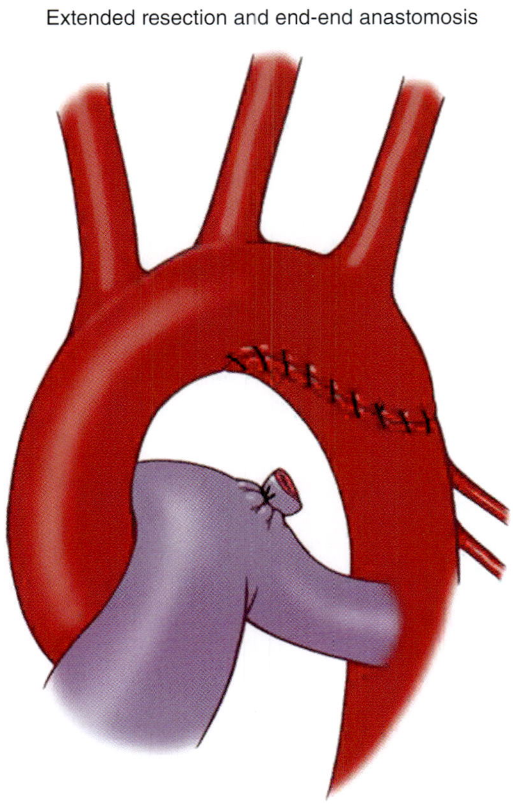

Figure 66.13 Completed coarctation excision with extended end-to-end anastomosis.

Both the aortic arch and descending aorta are mobilized on either side of coarctation in order to construct the anastomosis on the lesser curvature of arch just opposite the left common carotid artery. Adequate mobilization is essential for a tension free end-to-end anastomosis. Sometimes, ligating the ductus early will help to mobilize the aorta at this stage of surgery. The left subclavian and left common carotid arteries are defined prior to clamping the aortic arch. After heparin is administered, the ductus is ligated and divided and aortic clamps are placed above and below the coarctation.

Although the risk of paraplegia in neonates undergoing coarctation repair is very small, it is important to take a few precautions. Allowing the baby to cool, avoiding hypotension, keeping adequate blood pressure in the distal aorta while clamping the aorta, correcting acid–base imbalances and avoiding prolonged aortic clamping minimize the chances of paraplegia.

Complete excision of coarctation segment is necessary in order to reduce the chances of recurrent coarctation. An end-to-end anastomosis is fashioned using continuos fine monofilament suture with an option for interrupted suture in the anterior portion. The anesthesia team should be informed prior to releasing the aortic clamp to be prepared for possible hypotension resulting from lactic acidosis. Hypotension resulting from lactic acidosis can typically be managed with intravenous fluids and possibly intravenous sodium bicarbonate.

After closing the mediastinal pleura, the chest is closed with a single chest tube placed. A gradient of less than 10 mmHg across the repair site is preferred. Note that in time the gradient will improve as the vasoconstriction in the lower extremity induced by clamping and hypothermia resolves.

Total Anomalous Pulmonary Venous Connection

The presentation and clinical picture of total anomalous pulmonary venous connection (TAPVC) is determined by the presence of pulmonary venous obstruction and the size of the atrial septal defect (ASD). Neonates with obstructed TAPVC (stenosis of vertical vein or restrictive ASD) usually present with severe cyanosis, metabolic acidosis, and respiratory distress immediately after birth. Obstructed TAPVC in neonates is a true surgical emergency.

Surgical Correction of Supracardiac TAPVC (Figures 66.14, 66.15, and 66.16)

After a median sternotomy is performed, the anatomy is confirmed. If hemodynamics permit, the vertical vein is identified prior to going on CPB. The baseline PA pressure is often measured directly as well.

After instituting CPB, the ductus arteriosus is ligated. The vertical vein is controlled with a vessel loop. The right pleural space is opened in order to accommodate

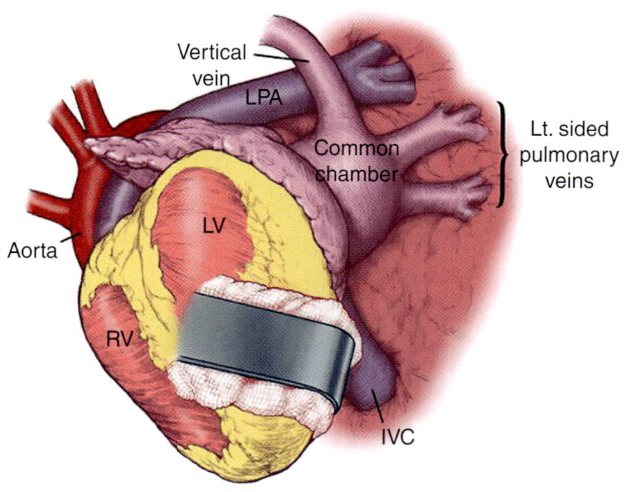

Figure 66.14 Supracardiac total anomalous pulmonary venous connection (TAPVC) is demonstrated. The left ventricular apex is lifted in order to see the pulmonary venous confluence posterior to the left atrium. IVC, inferior vena cava.

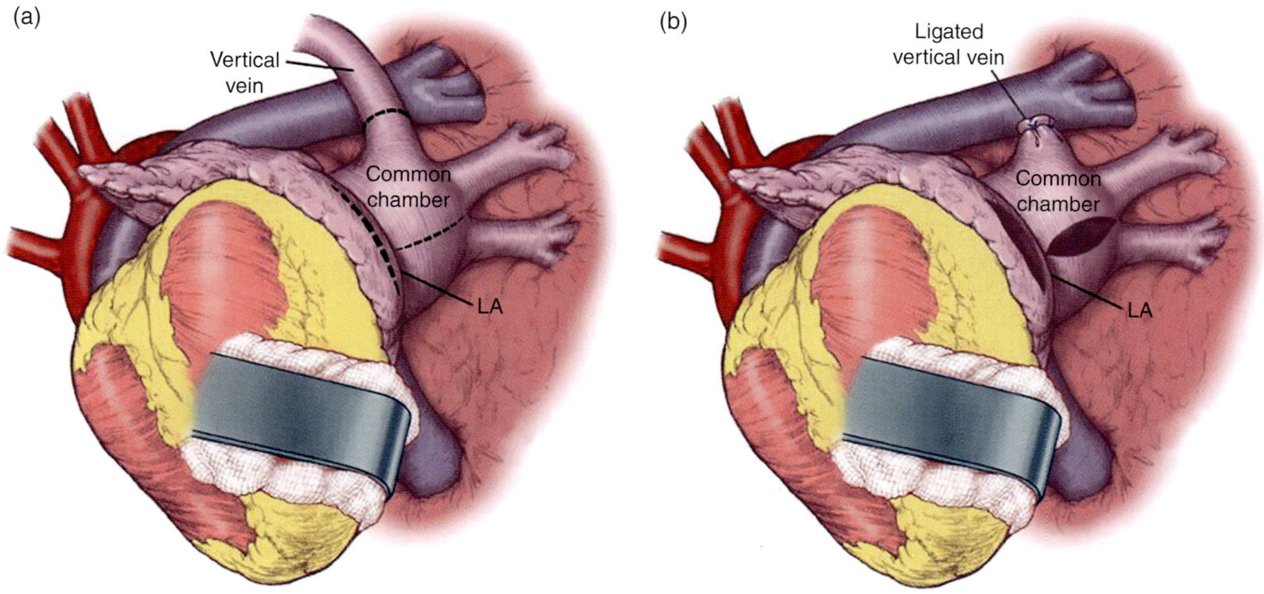

Figure 66.15 The incision in the pulmonary venous confluence with the corresponding oblique incision in the left atrium. The vertical vein is ligated.

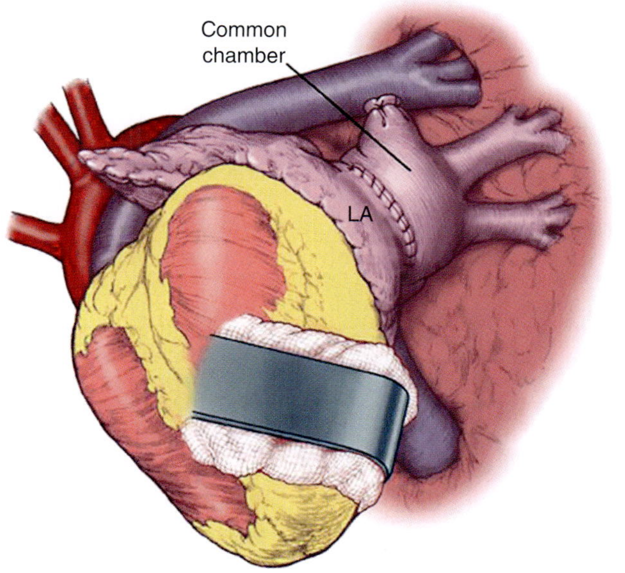

Figure 66.16 The completed anastomosis between the left atrium and the pulmonary venous confluence with divided vertical vein.

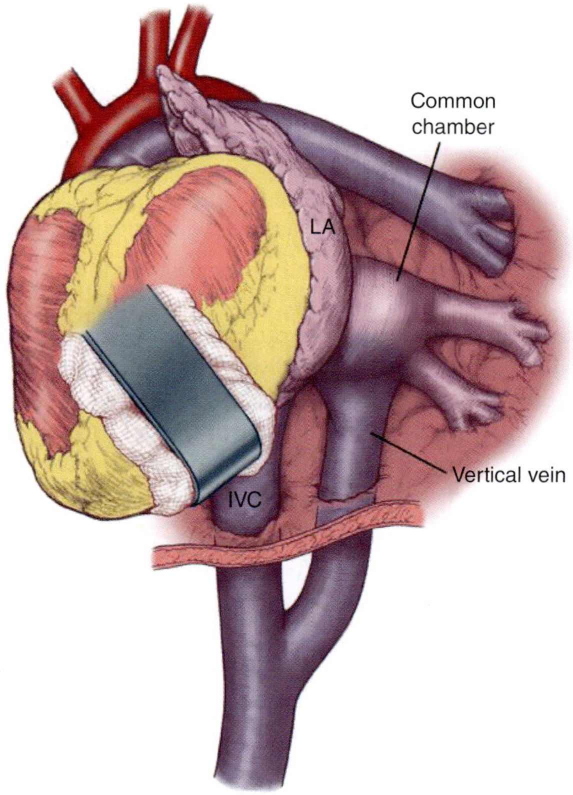

Figure 66.17 Infracardiac type TAPVC with descending vertical vein.

the heart while carrying out the left atrial to pulmonary vein anastomosis. The heart is arrested with cold antegrade blood cardioplegia and the apex of the heart is lifted rotated into the right pleural cavity. Now the pulmonary vein confluence and the posterior surface of the left atrium will come into view. The pulmonary vein confluence and left atrium are incised opposite to each other. A large tension-free anastomosis using fine monofilament suture is made between the left atrium and pulmonary vein confluence. If there is a small pulmonary venous confluence or concerns for stenosis, a sutureless technique can be employed. This involves

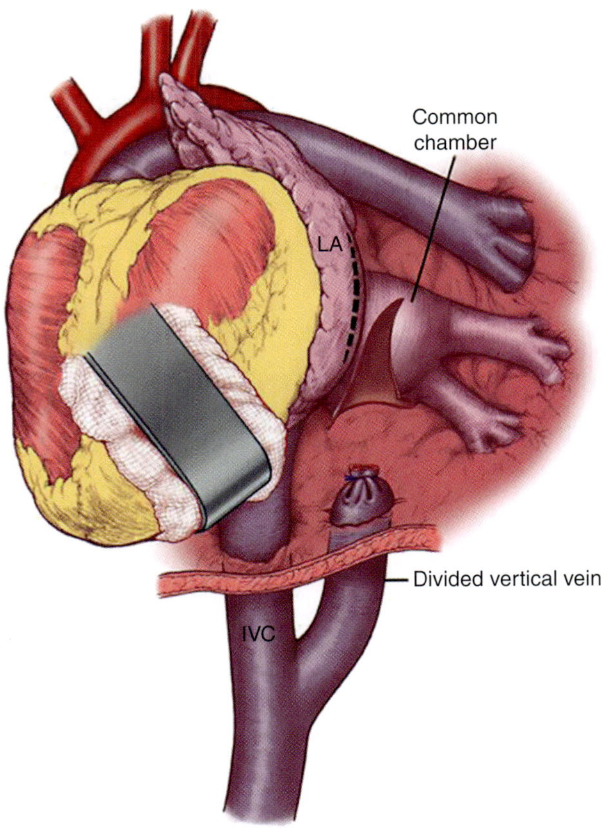

Figure 66.18 Ligation of the descending vertical vein at the level of the diaphragm. The diagram also shows the vertical incision on the pulmonary venous confluence and the corresponding incision on the left atrium.

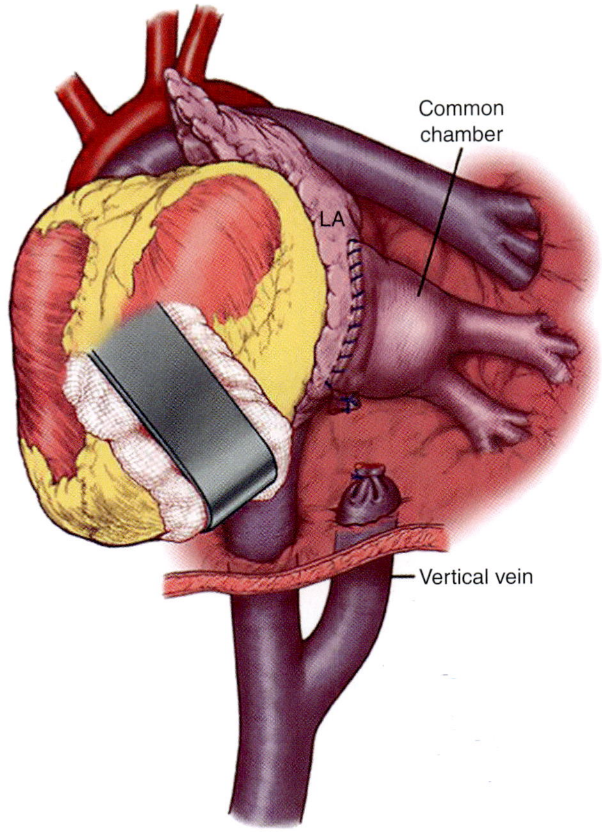

Figure 66.19 Completed anastomosis in the infracardiac type TAPVC with ligation of descending vertical vein.

suturing the left atrium to surrounding pericardium and avoiding direct suture to the venous confluence. The ASD is closed through a right atrial incision. After weaning CPB, the vertical vein is typically ligated.

After weaning from CPB, transesophageal echocardiography is utilized to assess the anastomosis. The pulmonary artery pressure is measured directly. Nitric oxide and milrinone infusion are mandatory irrespective of pulmonary artery pressure because pulmonary artery hypertensive crisis is one of the most common complications after repair in TAPVC.

Infracardiac TAPVC (Figures 66.17, 66.18, and 66.19)

Neonates with infracardiac TAPVC will present earlier in view of the high incidence of obstruction of the pulmonary venous drainage. Again, TAPVC with pulmonary venous obstruction should be considered a surgical emergency in neonates. The repair is similar to supracardiac TAPVC with a median sternotomy, posterior approach, and pulmonary confluence to left atrium anastomosis.

Interrupted Aortic Arch (Figures 66.20 and 66.21)

Neonates with interrupted aortic arch need to be stabilized medically and all multiorgan dysfunction corrected prior to undergoing surgical repair. A PDA is mandatory for the child to survive. The lower two-thirds of the body are dependent on ductal patency for perfusion, so maintenance of ductal patency is key in the medical stabilization. PGE-1 infusion is the mainstay of therapy for maintaining an open ductus. Mechanical ventilation is the next step in medical optimization. Positive pressure ventilation will alleviate the concern of respiratory depression caused by PGE infusion. Lower body perfusion can also be improved by manipulating pulmonary vascular resistance. Respiratory alkalosis and high Fio2 need to be avoided. Metabolic acidosis, renal dysfunction, and hepatic dysfunction need to be aggressively treated.

Surgery should be carried out on semi-urgent basis as soon as all metabolic dysfunction is reversed. The principles of the surgery remain the same in all types of interrupted aortic arch. Surgical intervention typically includes aortic arch reconstruction as well as correcting any associated intracardiac lesions.

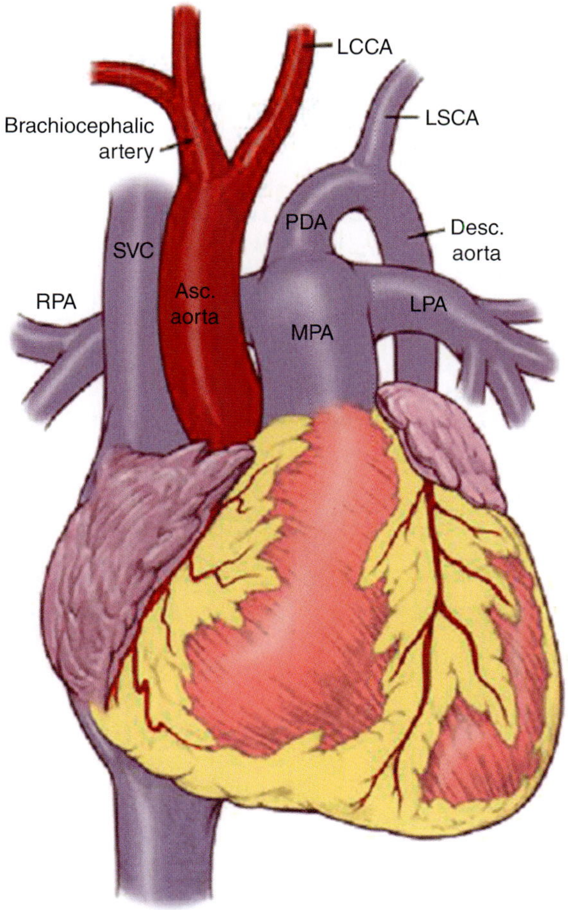

Figure 66.20 Type B interrupted aortic arch (most common type) with complete separation of the aortic arch between the left common carotid and left subclavian artery. A large PDA is giving rise to descending thoracic aorta.

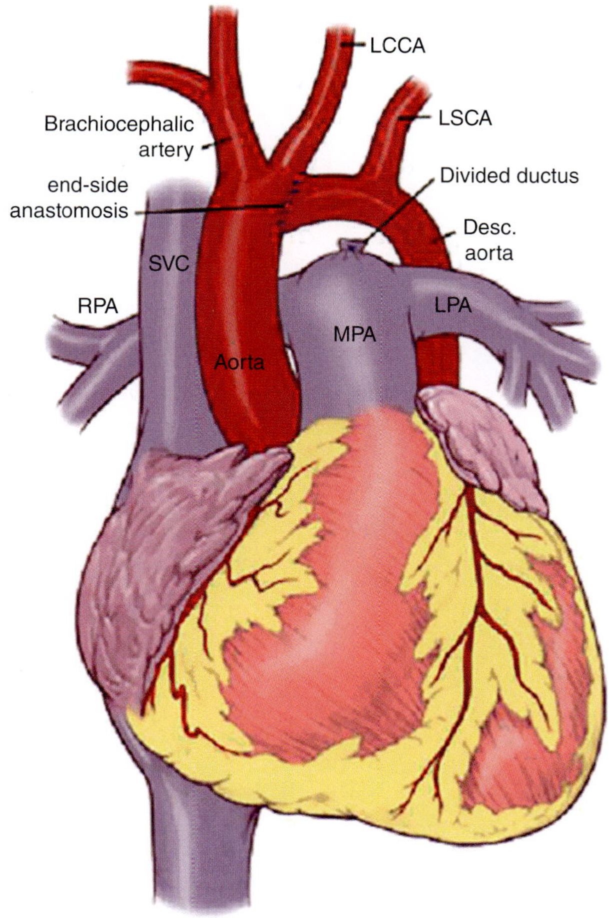

Figure 66.21 Post repair of interrupted aortic arch with direct end-to-side anastomosis and ligation of the PDA. LCCA, left common carotid artery; LSCA, left subclavian artery.

A median sternotomy is the preferred approach for single-stage repair. Dissection of the ascending aorta and associated branches and the main pulmonary artery is carried out while avoiding hemodynamic compromise. All aortic and pulmonary artery branches need to be identified and controlled. Dissection around the ductus and descending aorta is carried out after instituting CPB. The arterial cannula is inserted into a graft sutured to the innominate artery and bicaval venous cannulation is utilized. The patient is cooled on CPB to a core temperature of 18°C. When the core temperature reaches 18°C, circulatory arrest or low flow cerebral perfusion is established. The ductus is ligated and divided at its junction with the descending aorta. The descending aorta is well mobilized and is brought up to the level of left innominate artery. A tension-free anastomosis is performed between the ascending and descending aorta. On occasion, a patch is utilized to augment the anastomosis. Next, full CPB is reinstituted and any associated intracardiac lesions, such as a ventricular septal defect, can be closed during rewarming with aortic cross in place.

Truncus Arteriosus (Figures 66.22, 66.23, 66.24, and 66.25)

Once the diagnosis of truncus arteriosus is made, the baby should be stabilized and prepared for early surgery. The timing of surgery is preferably within the first week of life before the fall in pulmonary resistance. Without surgical correction, approximately 40% of patients will die within first month of life and 90% during infancy. Patients with severe truncal valve regurgitation and severe congestive cardiac failure are better served with surgical intervention within 24–48 hours. Patients with poor hemodynamics may need to be intubated. The Fio2 should be kept at 17–21% and relative hypercarbia (PaCo245–50%) maintained in order to keep the pulmonary resistance high. A heart rate of 120–140 beats per minute and diastolic blood pressure above 25 mmHg is preferred to avoid coronary ischemia from diastolic runoff.

Surgical correction is performed via midline sternotomy. Moderate hypothermia is normal, with deep

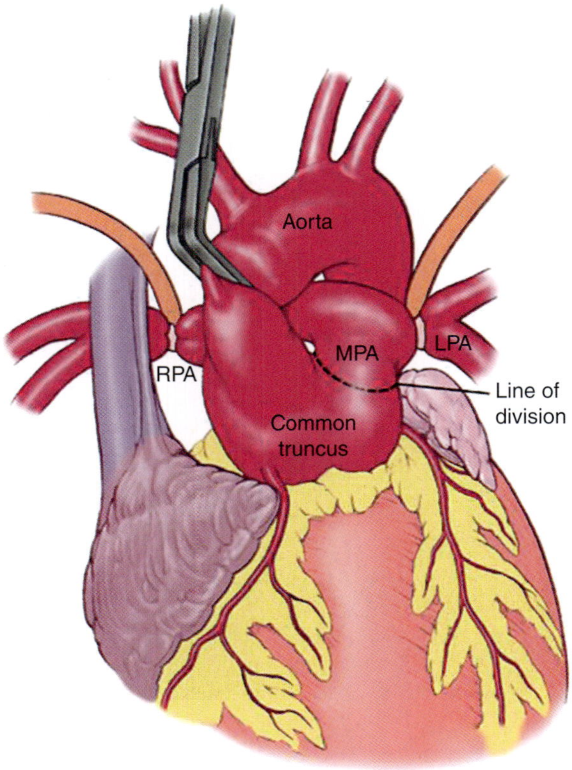

Figure 66.22 Type 1 truncus with snares on both pulmonary arteries, aortic cross-clamp in place, and the line of division on the truncus.

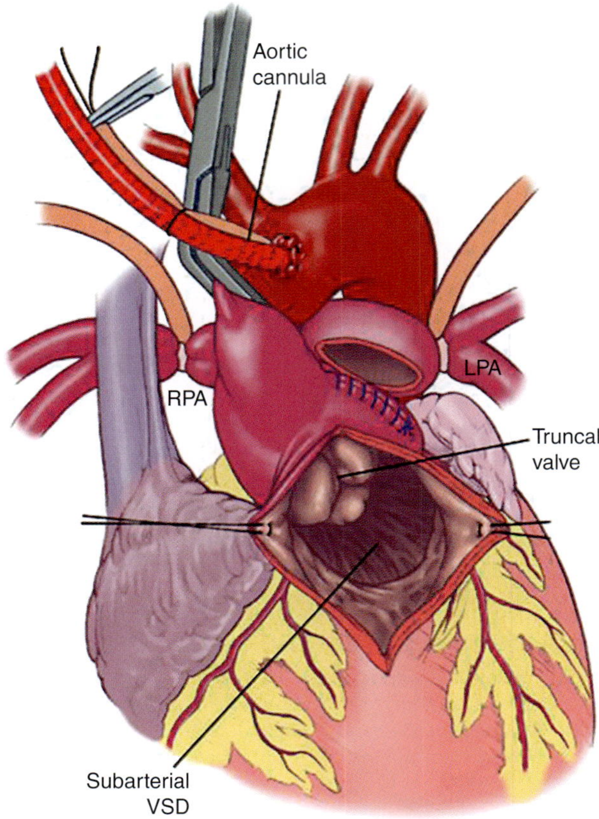

Figure 66.23 The pulmonary artery trunk has been divided from the truncus and the defect closed. The subarterial ventricular septal defect is well visualized through a right ventriculotomy. Note the close proximity of the truncal valve to the ventricular septal defect.

hypothermia and circulatory arrest being reserved for children with more complex forms of truncus or if there is associated interrupted aortic arch. The pulmonary arteries are controlled when instituting CPB to improve coronary artery perfusion and avoid perioperative myocardial ischemia from diastolic runoff into the pulmonary arteries. The aorta is cross-clamped as distally as possible to provide access to the pulmonary artery ostia. After cardiac arrest, the aorta is opened taking care to avoid the truncal valve, coronary origins, and pulmonary ostia. In patients with type 1 Collett and Edwards, in which origin of the truncus is well away from the left main coronary artery, the pulmonary arteries with a small rim of truncal wall are mobilized. The defect on the truncal root is then closed primarily or with a patch.

A right ventriculotomy is made in the infundibulum avoiding the coronary arteries ans well as the truncal valve. The subarterial ventricular septal defect is closed with a large bovine pericardial patch. The risk of heart block is small because the subarterial ventricular septal defect is separated from conduction system by the septal band.

After ventricular septal defect closure, the truncal valve is assessed and repaired if neccesary. After releasing the aortic cross-clamp, an appropriately sized cryopreserved pulmonary allograft is utilized for reconstruction of the pulmonary outflow tract. The distal anastomosis of the allograft is performed at the level of confluence of the pulmonary arteries. The proximal posterior aspect of the allograft is then approximated to the superior portion of the right infundibulotomy directly. A bovine pericardial patch is used anteriorly to augment the allograft to right ventricle connection.

Patent Ductus Arteriosus (Figures 66.26 and 66.27)

Indications

The presence of a PDA is not in itself an indication for surgery in the neonate because spontaneous closure will occur in most children. Heart failure in combination with a PDA with significant left to right shunt is an indication for surgery. In premature babies, the presence of a PDA, regardless of its size, produces significant hemodynamic deterioration from diastolic runoff. Invariably, in all premature babies with a PDA, the spontaneous closure of

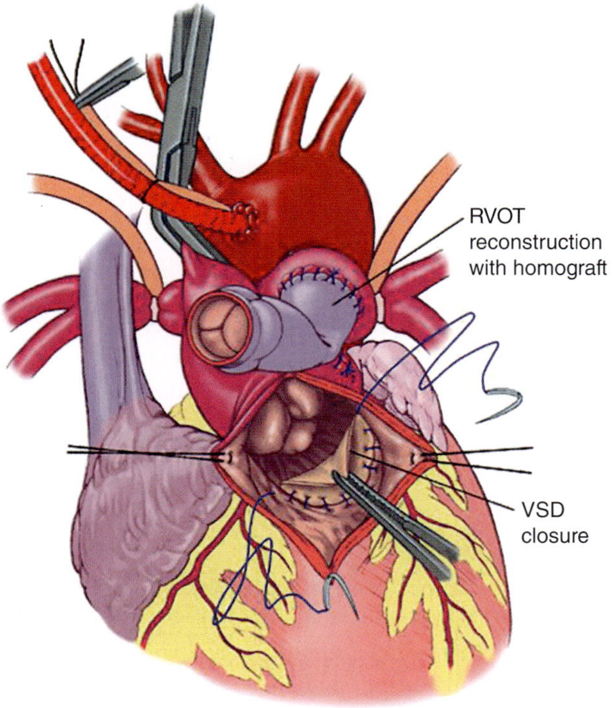

Figure 66.24 The ventricular septal defect (VSD) is closed with a patch. Note the completed proximal anastomosis between the homograft and pulmonary arteries. RVOT, right ventricular outflow tract.

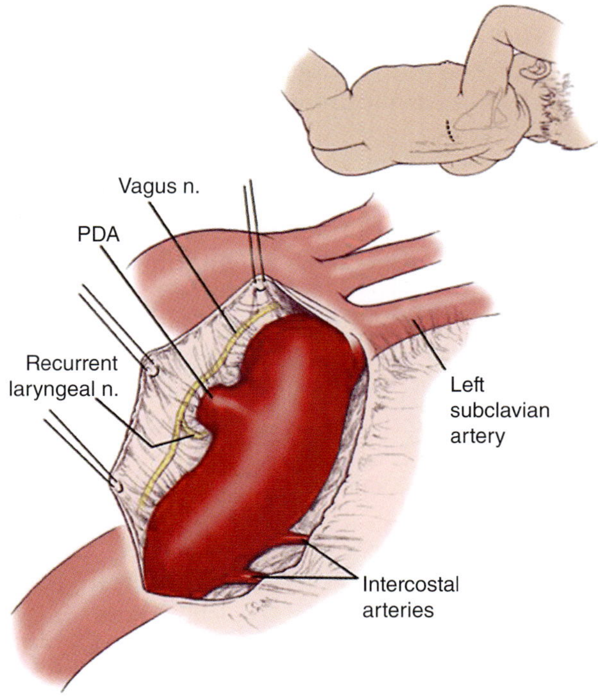

Figure 66.26 The left lateral position with left arm elevation showing skin incision site. Reflection of mediastinal pleura showing PDA, vagus nerve, left recurrent laryngeal nerve, left subclavian artery, aortic arch, and descending aorta.

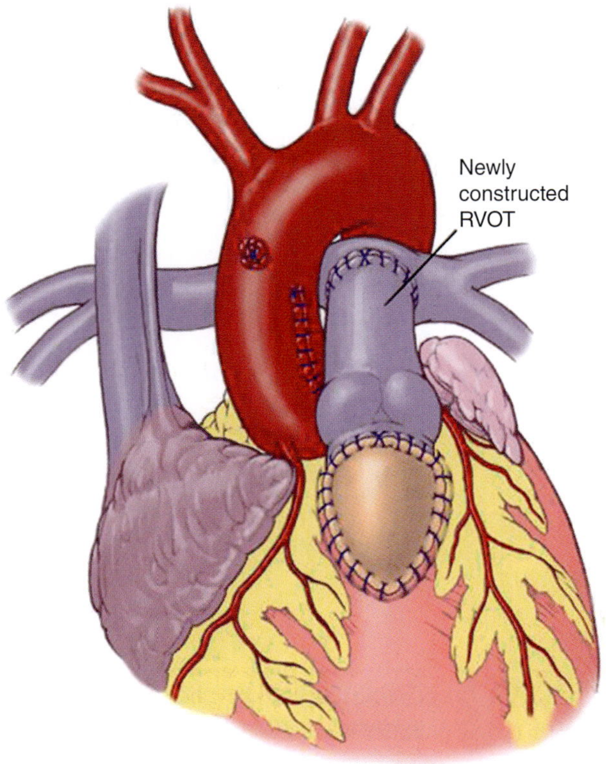

Figure 66.25 The completed surgical repair of truncus arteriosus.

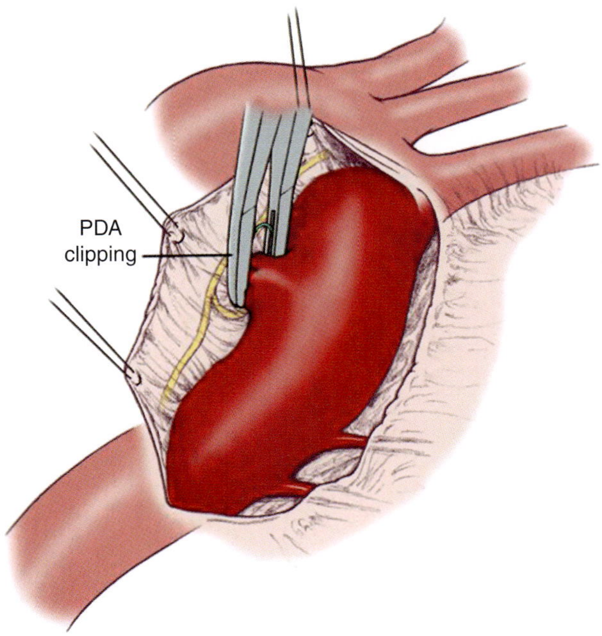

Figure 66.27 Application of a clip to the PDA.

ductus is impaired because of insensitivity of oxygen to insufficient smooth muscle on the ductus wall. Failure of medical therapy (indomethacin) to close the PDA in premature babies is an indication for surgical closure.

Procedure

The surgical ligation of a PDA in preterm infants is usually carried out in the neonatal intensive care unit. However, the surgery can be carried out in the cardiac operating room in the stable neonate. Transferring a preterm baby with mechanical ventilation and inotropic support requires a great team effort and necessitates particular attention to the inspired oxygen (Fio2) and body temperature.

Pulse oximetry or an invasive arterial line in the lower extremities is utilized. The patient is positioned with the left side of the chest up with left arm supported above the level of the head to elevate the scapula. A small left posterior thoracotomy (1.5–2 cm skin incision) is made just below the tip of the scapula extending towards the spine. The chest is entered through third intercostal space and the left lung is retracted. The mediastinal pleura over the descending aorta is divided after cauterizing the overlying left superior intercostal vein.

After the aortic arch, left subclavian artery and descending aorta are identified, careful dissection of the ductus is carried out. The size of the PDA is typically similar to the aortic arch or even larger in some infants. The appropriate vascular clip is applied across the entire PDA. This will result in an increase in diastolic and mean arterial pressures as a result of stopping the diastolic runoff through PDA. At the same time, the femoral arterial line or pulse oximetry are observed to confirm that the descending aorta remains patent. Care should be taken to not apply the clip too close to the aorta to avoid creating an aortic coarctation. A small size chest tube is placed and the chest is closed in the standard manner. Advantages of PDA clipping in the neonate include limited dissection and less trauma to the fragile ductus.

67

Extracorporeal Membrane Oxygenation and Ventricular Assist Devices

Vikas Sharma[1], Gregory J. Schears[2], and Joseph A. Dearani[2]

[1] *University of Utah Health Care Hospital and Clinics, Salt Lake City, UT, USA*
[2] *Mayo Clinic, Rochester, MN, USA*

Heart failure represents an important disorder in children, with increasing hospitalization rates and high morbidity and mortality [1]. The majority of these patients have related severe congenital heart diseases and debilitating cardiomyopathies, which usually present during first year of life [2]. There has been a progressive increase in the rates of heart transplant, especially in infants, but the limited availability of donor hearts for children prolongs the waiting period [3], resulting in increased rates of death while waiting [4].

The availability of mechanical circulatory support (MCS) systems for children is more limited than for adults, especially for infants and neonates. Extracorporeal membrane oxygenation (ECMO) remains the predominant technology for circulatory support in neonates and infants but extraordinary progress has been made in the field of mechanical pediatric circulatory support with the inception of the National Heart, Lung, and Blood Institute's Pediatric Circulatory Support Program (PCSP) [5], Pumps for Kids, Infants, and neonates (PumpKIN program) [6], and FDA approval for the Excor Pediatric ventricular assist device (Berlin Heart). The important milestones in pediatric circulatory support are shown in Table 67.1.

Table 67.1 Important advances in pediatric circulatory support.

Advance	Date
First successful use of ECMO in neonate	1974
Application of ECMO for respiratory failure in 45 newborns	1982
NHLBI Pediatric Circulatory Support Program	2004
Micro Med DeBakey VAD Child receives Humanitarian Device Exemption	2004
Pediatric INTERMACS enrollment	2006
Berlin Heart VAD US clinical Trial	2007
PumpKIN contact awarded	2010
Approval of Berlin Heart EXCOR by FDA	2011

ECMO, extracorporeal membrane oxygenation; FDA, Food and Drug Administration; INTERMACS, Interagency Registry for Mechanically Assisted Circulatory Support; NHLBI, National Heart, Lung, and Blood Institute; PumpKIN, Pumps for Kids, Infants, and Neonates; VAD, ventricular assist device.

Indications for Circulatory Support

The initiation of MCS in neonates and infants in most cases is either as a bridge to myocardial recovery or to transplant. More than 80% of these patients are post cardiotomy for complex congenital heart disease and cardiomyopathies or myocarditis, most of which develop in the first year of life [7]. Indications for MCS are listed in Box 67.1.

Types of Mechanical Circulatory Support Devices

The various options for MCS in children are listed in Table 67.2. In pediatric practice, the choice of MCS is influenced by the size and gestational age of the child, the type of support (cardiac or cardiopulmonary), and the expected duration. ECMO is an attractive and commonly used option because of its ability to support even the smallest of neonates and infants, but the thromboembolic, bleeding, and septic complications may limit its use to short duration [8]. Configuration of system components may also preclude effective rehabilitation. Centrifugal pumps (e.g., BioMedicus CentriMag,

Visual Guide to Neonatal Cardiology, First Edition. Edited by Ernerio T. Alboliras, Ziyad M. Hijazi, Leo Lopez, and Donald J. Hagler.

Box 67.1 Indications for mechanical circulatory support

Bridge to recovery

- Preoperative cardiac failure
- Postoperative cardiac failure
- Failure to wean from CPB post cardiac surgery
- Myocarditis/cardiomyopathy
- Post cardiac arrest support
- Respiratory failure
- Pulmonary hypertension
- Electively after staged repair for HLHS

Bridge to transplant

Bridge to bridge (short to long-term support)

CPB, cardiopulmonary bypass; HLHS, hypoplastic left heart syndrome.

Table 67.2 Types of mechanical circulatory support in infants.

Short-term support	
ECMO • Veno-arterial • Veno-venous	Usually >1.6 kg, >34 weeks' gestation Peripheral or central cannulation Non-pulsatile No patient mobility
Centrifugal pumps • Biopump • Pedimag	Usually >1.6 kg, >34 weeks' gestation Central cannulation Similar set-up to ECMO Less anticoagulation than ECMO Non-pulsatile No patient mobility
Long-term support	
Paracorporeal	
Thoratec PVAD (pneumatic)	
Thoratec HeartMate XVE LVAD[a] (electromechanical) (Thoratec Laboratories, Pleasanton, CA)	
Toyobo (pneumatic) (National Cardiovascular Center, Tokyo, Japan)	
Abiomed BVS 5000 (pneumatic) (Abiomed, Danvers, MA)[a]	
Abiomed AB5000 (pneumatic) (Abiomed, Danvers, MA)	
Berlin Heart EXCOR VAD (pneumatic) (Berlin Heart AG, Berlin, Germany)[b]	Pulsatile flow Univentricular or biventricular support Ambulation possible
MEDOS HIA VAD (pneumatic) (MEDOS Medizintechnik AG)	
Intracorporeal	
MicroMed DeBakey VAD (axial) (MicroMed Technologies)[a]	BSA >0.7 Left ventricular support
Jarvik 2000 Flowmaker (axial) (Jarvik Heart, New York, NY)	
Berlin Heart Incor. (axial) (Berlin Heart AG)	
Thoratec HeartMate II LVAD (axial) (Thoratec Laboratories, Pleasanton, CA)[a]	

BSA, body surface area; ECMO, extracorporeal membrane oxygenation; VAD, ventricular assist device.

a) Federal Drug Administration (FDA) approved, ventricular assist devices, suitable for children (BSA >0.7 m^2).

b) Federal Drug Administration (FDA) approved, ventricular assist devices, suitable for neonates (>2.4 kg).

Levitronix, Zurich, Switzerland; Capiox, Terumo, Ann Arbor, MI) can be used as a univentricular or biventricular support devices but can also be used to construct ECMO with an oxygenator. Centrifugal ventricular assist devices (VADs) differ from roller pumps in that the flow in centrifugal pumps depends on preload and afterload apart from pump speed, while in roller pumps output depends solely on displacement volumes and rotations

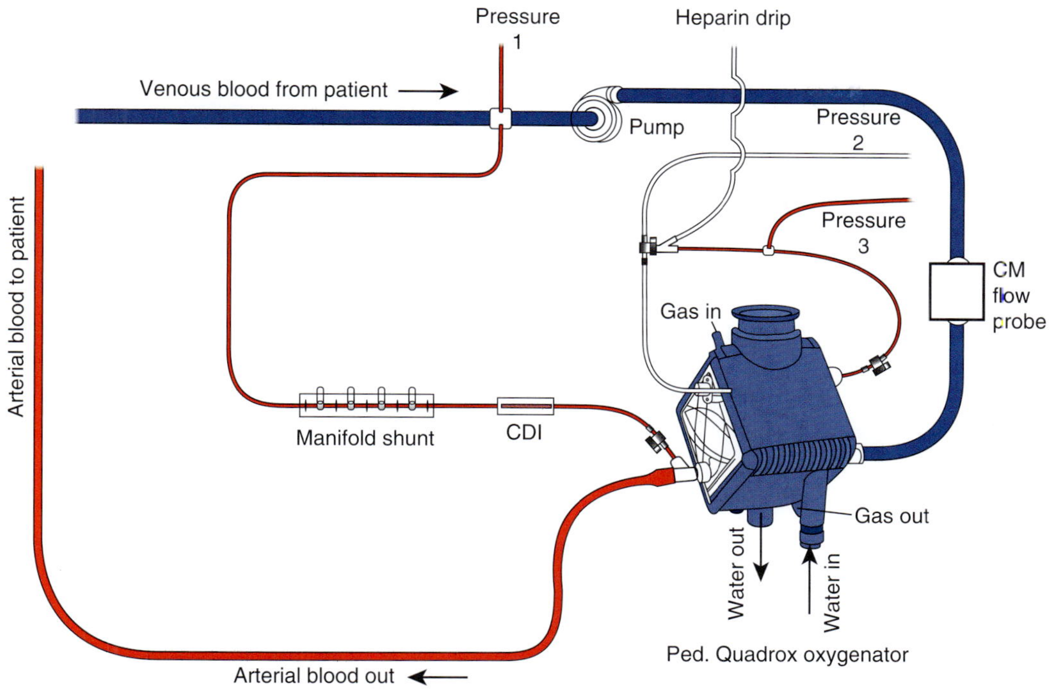

Maximum BF (range)	Oxygenator	Pump Head	Tubing Size
0.8-0.9 L/min	Quadrox iD	PediMag	3/16" A; 1/4" V
1.3-1.5 L/min	Quadrox iD	PediMag	1/4" A; V
2.0-2.22 L/min	Quadrox iD	CentriMag	1/4" A; V

Figure 67.1 Extracorporeal membrane oxygenation circuit (ECMO) for neonates and infants.

per minute (rpm). Compared with "traditional" ECMO, they have faster set-up time and lower anticoagulation requirements but still only provide a limited duration of support (Figure 67.1).

The pediatric VADs can provide a longer duration of support as a bridge to transplant but are limited by the lack of commercial availability for use in small children. In the USA, the DeBakey VAD Child (MicroMed Technology Inc, Houston, TX; Figure 67.2a), designed for use in children over 5 years and with a body surface area (BSA) greater than 0.7 m^2, and the Berlin Heart EXCOR (Berlin Heart, Berlin, Germany; Figure 67.2b) have been approved in the US by the FDA under a Humanitarian Device Exemption for neonates and infants <0.7 m^2 BSA. In recognition of existing devices for pediatric mechanical support, a family of devices is being developed by the PCSP (Figure 67.2c) [9].

Cannulation Techniques and Circuit Designs

Cannulation site is dependent on clinical situation (i.e., post cardiotomy, post CPR, or respiratory failure) and the size of the child. In infants, this is usually a central cannulation via right atrium and aorta–innominate artery and internal jugular for venoarterial ECMO (Figure 67.3a,b) or right internal jugular cannulation via a single lumen cannula for veno-venous ECMO (Figure 67.3c).

The cannulation strategies for VAD depend upon whether the child requires an isolated left ventricular or biventricular support (Figure 67.3d).

Management During Circulatory Support

The goals of ECMO are adequate cardiac decompression with good cardiac output for adequate body perfusion [10]. During ECMO, the central venous pressure remains low if adequate drainage is being achieved. The most common cause of inadequate venous return is faulty canula position [11]. The left atrial pressure should be low and the left ventricle (LV) should be decompressed. Increased left atrial pressure indicates inadequate LV unloading requiring placement of left ventricular vent. The mean arterial pressure should be maintained at a level appropriate for child's weight and is usually a function of peripheral vascular resistance, which can be pharmacologically controlled. Although ECMO provides full respiratory support, minimal ventilation is recommended: to prevent atelectasis, minimize lung injury, and provide adequate myocardial oxygenation.

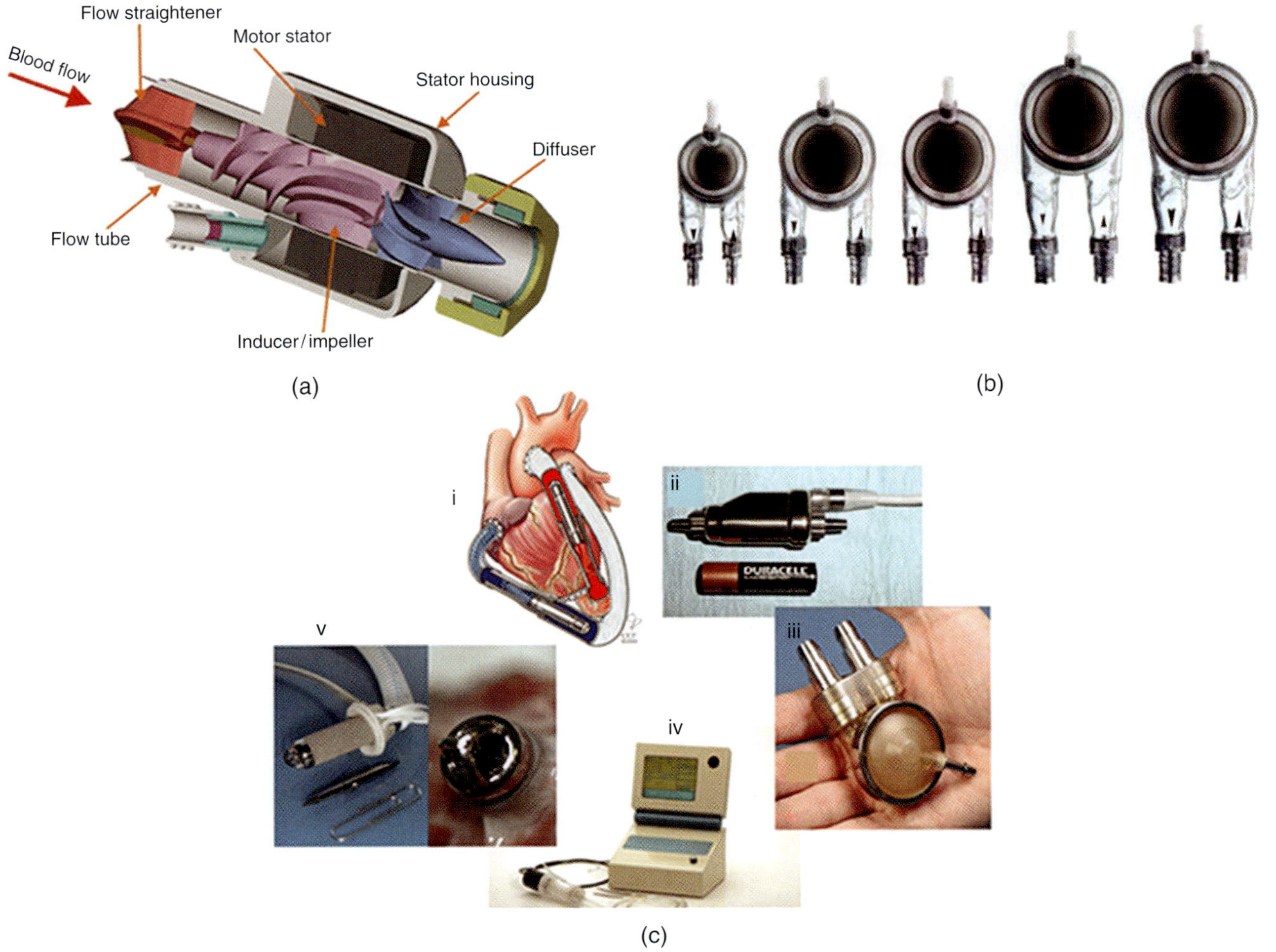

Figure 67.2 Types of ventricular assist devices (VAD). (a) DeBakey VAD Child (MicroMed Technology Inc, Houston, TX). (b) Berlin Heart EXCOR (Berlin Heart, Berlin, Germany). (c) The family of devices developed under the Pediatric Circulatory Support Program: (i) PediPump Ventricular Assist Device showing application for biventricular support; (ii) PediaFlow Ventricular Assist System; (iii) Penn State Infant VAD; (iv) Ension's pCAS system with prototype controller console; and (v) infant sized Jarvik 2000 showing thrombus-free bearings after 5 weeks in lamb animal model.

The basic principles of VAD are adequate preload and good LV decompression. Adequate left ventricular assist device (LVAD) performance requires good right ventricle output, to provide adequate preload. Right ventricular failure, arrhythmias, pulmonary hypertension, and tamponade can hamper VAD performance [12]. Serial echocardiograms to evaluate volume status, right heart function, and left ventricle unloading should be carried out.

Anticoagulation

Appropriate management of anticoagulation is essential in the pediatric population on MCS because of the high risk of hemorrhagic and thromboembolic complications. The protocols for management of anticoagulation differ from institution to institution; however, the general strategies for management of bleeding and thrombosis complications are shown in Box 67.2. The simplification of the circuit with fewer connectors and the use of a manifold shunt line are strategies for minimizing clot formation in the circuit.

In the absence of an oxygenator in the circuit, anticoagulation requirements are not as stringent on VAD as on ECMO and their activated clotting time (ACT) are maintained at 140–180 s. Children on the Berlin EXCOR device need to be started on aspirin and dipyridamole along with heparin infusion after the first week of initiation of MCS [13].

Nutrition and Fluid/Electrolyte Management

There is a need to maintain intravascular volume and electrolyte balance because of increased inflammatory response and increased capillary permeability, blood product usage, and hemolysis on MCS. Maintenance of adequate nutrition is essential for long-term success. These children should be supported with parenteral or enteral nutrition as soon as feasible. However, excessive

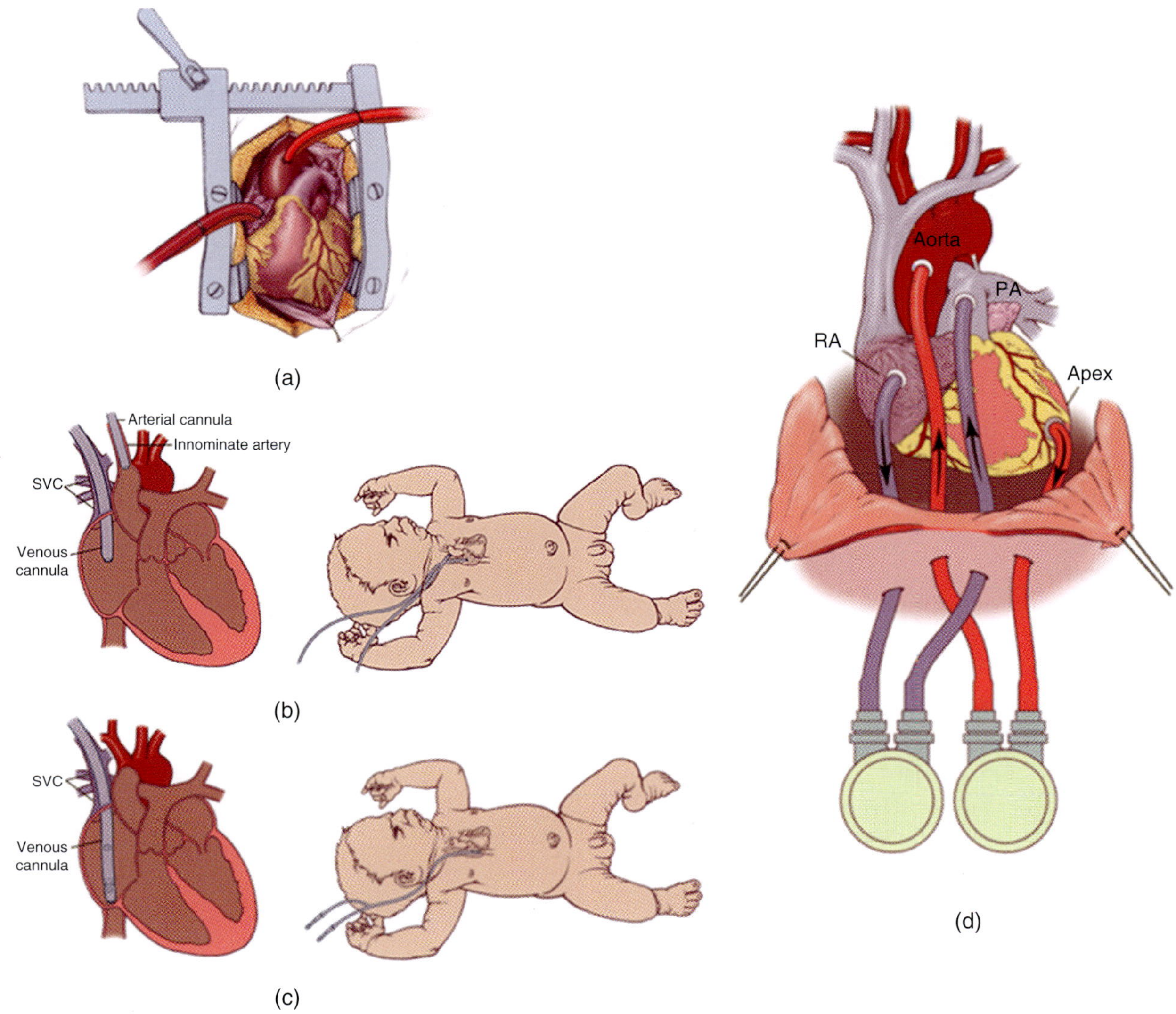

Figure 67.3 Cannulation strategies: (a) central veno-arterial extracorporeal membrane oxygenation circuit (ECMO); (b) peripheral veno-arterial extracorporeal membrane oxygenation circuit (ECMO); (c) veno-venous extracorporeal membrane oxygenation circuit (ECMO); (d) Berlin Heart Ventricular Assist Device (VAD).

Box 67.2 Measures to reduce bleeding and thrombosis on mechanical circulatory support

1) **In operating theatre**
   - Aggressive hemostasis in operating theatre
   - Reverse heparin partially at first to avoid circuit thrombosis
   - Normalize coagulation to distinguish medical from surgical bleeding
   - Begin laboratory tests in operating theatre
2) **Circuit design**
   - Simplify circuitry to minimize irregular surfaces and prothrombotic connectors
   - Use coated surface circuits
   - Use oxygenators and pumps with low thrombogenicity
3) **In ICU**
   - Transparent approach to coagulation management goals with care team
   - No delay in washouts if excessive bleeding (>2 mL/kg/hour) persists
   - No heparin until bleeding <1–2 mL/kg/hour
   - Limit anticoagulation for 1–2 days
   - Lower transfusion threshold to <9 g/dL if tolerated
   - Monitor for development of circuit thrombus formation

Table 67.3 Complications of ECMO (Extracorporeal Life Support Registry Report 2013 for International Complications).

Complication	Neonatal (%)	30 days–1 year (%)
Oxygenator failure	7.3	8
Raceway rupture	0.3	0.6
Tubing rupture	0.4	0.6
Pump failure	1.6	2.1
Air in circuit	3.2	9.5
Clots in circuit		
Oxygenator	11	7.4
Bridge	4.2	3.4
Bladder	6.2	4.4
Hemofilter	4.3	3.8
Canula malpositions	6	5.5
Heat exchanger malfunction	0.6	0.3
Hemorrhagic		
Gastrointestinal hemorrhage	0.9	1.9
Cannulation site bleeding	10.9	12
Hemolysis	11.1	9.8
DIC/consumption coagulopathy	3.8	3.3
Neurologic		
Brain death clinically determined	1.1	3.3
Neurologic seizure clinically determined	7.2	8.9
EEG determined seizures	2.7	3.1
CNS infarction	3.5	4.2
CNS hemorrhage	11.1	5.9
Infections		
Culture proven	7.4	11.4
WBC <1500	1.4	1.3
Renal		
Cr 1.5–3	4.7	2.5
Cr >3	1.4	3.8
Dialysis	3.8	6.9
Others		
Pulmonary hemorrhage	2.8	17.6
Cardiac tamponade	0.5	0.6
Infection (culture proven)	4.7	8.8

CNS, central nervous system; Cr, creatinine; ECMO, extracorporeal membrane oxygenation; EEG, electroencephalography; DIC, disseminated intravascular clotting; WBC, white blood cells.

calorie intake should be avoided as it leads to increased amino acid and protein breakdown and longer duration of ECMO [14].

Complications

Complications of MCS can be broadly classified into: mechanical complications, hemorrhagic or hemolysis, infectious, and end organ (i.e. neurological or renal; Table 67.3).

Experience with Berlin Heart EXCOR

A prospective, multicenter, single-group cohort study [15] comparing children who underwent implantation of the Berlin Excor Pediatric VAD as a bridge to transplantation with a historic control group of children who received circulatory support with ECMO showed that survival rates were significantly higher with the VAD than with ECMO. However, serious adverse events, including infection, stroke, and bleeding, occurred in a majority of study participants. A multicenter prospective cohort study involved all children implanted with the Berlin Heart EXCOR Pediatric VAD at 47 centers included 204 children supported with the EXCOR, with a median duration of support of 40 days (range, 1–435 days), demonstrated that survival at 12 months was 75%, including 64% who reached transplantation, 6% who recovered, and 5% who were alive on the device. Neurologic dysfunction occurred in 29% and was the leading cause of death.

A recent multicenter prospective cohort study showed that use of the Berlin Heart EXCOR has risen dramatically over the past decade. The EXCOR has emerged as a new treatment standard in the USA for a bridge to transplantation in pediatric patients [15].

Conclusions

Berlin Heart EXCOR Pediatric VAD has emerged as an alternative to ECMO for long-term support, especially in bridging children to transplantation. However, further efforts to improve the safety and survival of children supported with these devices through the development of the next generation of pediatric VAD is required.

The Future

There is a palpable sense of momentum in the field of mechanical circulatory support, especially with the contributions by the PCSP in 2004. Since then, as is evident in this update, the five participating contractors have made outstanding technical advancements toward the ultimate goal of providing safe and effective devices for circulatory support in infants, neonates, and young children with advanced severe heart disease. The size and flow characteristics of the devices and the various in vitro and in vivo test results reveal that the goals of the PCSP have been achieved in large part. The science and technologies developed through the program, such as the animal models, new assays, virtual fitting methodologies, and the novel bearings and biocompatible coatings, are poised to benefit the broader fields of MCS.

References

1. Rossano JW, Kim JJ, Decker JA, *et al.* (2012) Prevalence, morbidity, and mortality of heart failure-related hospitalizations in children in the United States: a population-based study. *J Card Fail*, **18**, 459–470.
2. Andrews RE, Fenton MJ, Ridout DA, Burch M. (2008) New-onset heart failure due to heart muscle disease in childhood: a prospective study in the United Kingdom and Ireland. *Circulation*, **117**, 79–84.
3. Aurora P, Edwards LB, Kucheryavaya AY, *et al.* (2010) The Registry of the International Society for Heart and Lung Transplantation: thirteenth official pediatric lung and heart–lung transplantation report, 2010. *J Heart Lung Transplant*, **29**, 1129–1141.
4. Department of Health and Human Services (2011) *Report of US organ procurement and transplantation network and scientific registry of transplant recipients, 1999–2011*. Department of Health and Human Services, Health Resources and Services Administration, Rockville, MD.
5. Baldwin JT, Borovetz HS, Duncan BW, *et al.* (2006) The National Heart, Lung, and Blood Institute Pediatric Circulatory Support Program. *Circulation*, **113**, 147–155.
6. National Heart, Lung, and Blood Institute (NHLBI) (2008) *RFP NHLBI-HV-09-14; Request for Proposals for the NHLBI Pumps for Kids, Infants, and Neonates (PumpKIN) Program.*
7. Fraser CD Jr,, Jaquiss RD, Rosenthal DN, *et al*; Berlin Heart Study Investigators. (2012) Prospective trial of a pediatric ventricular assist device. *N Engl J Med*, **367**, 532–541.
8. Paden ML, Conrad SA, Rycus PT, Thiagarajan RR; ELSO Registry (2013) Extracorporeal Life Support Organization Registry Report 2012. *ASAIO J*, **59**, 202–210.
9. Baldwin JT, Borovetz HS, Duncan BW, *et al.* (2011) The National Heart, Lung, and Blood Institute Pediatric Circulatory Support Program: a summary of the 5-year experience. *Circulation*, **123**, 1233–1240.
10. Subramaniam K, Boisen M, Shah PR, Ramesh V, Pete A. (2012) Mechanical circulatory support for cardiogenic shock. *Best Pract Res Clin Anaesthesiol*, **26**, 131–146.
11. Zwischenberger JB, Cilley RE, Hirschl RB, *et al.* Life-threatening intrathoracic complications during treatment with extracorporeal membrane oxygenation. *J Pediatr Surg*, **23**, 599–604.

12 Yuki K, Sharma R, DiNardo J. (2012) Ventricular-assist device therapy in children. *Best Pract Res Clin Anaesthesiol*, **26**, 247–264.

13 Almond CS, Buchholz H, Massicotte P, *et al.* (2011) Berlin Heart Excor Pediatric ventricular assist device investigational device exemption study: study design and rationale. *Am Heart J*, **162**, 425.e6–435.e6.

14 Shew SB, Keshen TH, Jahoor F, Jaksic T. (1999) The determinants of protein catabolism in neonates on extracorporeal membrane oxygenation. *J Pediatr Surg*, **34**, 1086–1090.

15 Almond CS, Morales DL, Blackstone EH, *et al.* (2013) Berlin Heart EXCOR Pediatric Ventricular Assist Device for bridge to heart transplantation in US Children. *Circulation*, **127**, 1702–1711.

68

Neonatal Cardiac Transplantation

Stephen Pophal[1], *Justin Ryan*[1], *and John J. Nigro*[2]

[1] Phoenix Children's Hospital, Phoenix, AZ, USA
[2] Rady Children's Hospital-San Diego, San Diego, CA, USA

History

Heart transplantation for the neonate and infant is an exceptionally powerful tool in the treatment of children with heart failure. The technique of heart transplantation was developed in the laboratory and the first human-to-human heart transplant was performed in December 3, 1967 on an adult by Dr. Christiaan Barnard in South Africa (Box 68.1). Several days later, on December 6, 1967, the first heart transplant in North America was performed on an 18-day-old infant with a fatal heart defect from an anencephalic baby by Dr. Adrian Kantrowitz at Maimonedes Medical Center in Brooklyn. Early attempts at transplantation were limited by the diagnosis and medical management of rejection.

Heart transplantation was brought into the modern era by the development of endomyocardial biopsy which allowed accurate diagnosis of rejection, and by the development of the immunosuppressant cyclosporine. Dr. Leonard Bailey and the team at Loma Linda made world headlines in 1984 by transplanting a baboon heart into baby Fae. The infant (Figure 68.1a,b) initially survived transplantation but died of immune-related multisystem organ dysfunction 20 days post-transplant. Baby Fae's transplant brought public attention to infant heart transplantation and this attention resulted in greater donor awareness and donation. The next infant transplant at Loma Linda was performed on Baby Moses in 1985 with a human donor (Figure 68.1c). He obtained prolonged survival and is still alive 25 years post transplant with the original heart graft [1].

Infant transplantation subsequently grew dramatically during the late 1980s and early 1990s, but reached a plateau in the mid 1990s. This plateau is likely related to limited number of donors and to improved surgerical results for single ventricle palliation.

Demographics of Transplant

Transplantation within the first year of life has always been a major component of pediatric heart transplantation (Figure 68.2) [2]. The International Society of Heart Lung Transplantation (ISHLT) registry data indicates that, while overall pediatric heart transplantation has grown since 2003, the number of infants transplanted remains relatively constant at about 100 infants per year [2]. Factors that have increased overall pediatric heart transplantation over the past 10 years likely include: the increased use of mechanical support; a renewed recognition of the utility of transplantation; the evolution of ABO incompatible transplantation; and continued efforts to expand donor pool with donor awareness.

Epidemiology

Box 68.2 lists the indications for infant heart transplantation. Evolution in the care of neonates with congenital heart disease has resulted in a progressive change in the indications for infant heart transplantation. The majority of infant transplants were initially performed for congenital heart disease (75%). Because of improvements in surgical outcomes for complex neonatal heart surgeries and development of alternative therapies, the number infant heart transplants for cardiomyopathy now equal those for congenital heart disease.

Post-Transplant Survival

While the initial risks of infant transplantation are higher than older age transplants (likely because of operative risk), the longitudinal survival is better. Infants have a survival at 20 years post-transplant of greater than 50%.

Visual Guide to Neonatal Cardiology, First Edition. Edited by Ernerio T. Alboliras, Ziyad M. Hijazi, Leo Lopez, and Donald J. Hagler.

Box 68.1 Pediatric heart transplantation history

1950–1960s: Animal experimentation
1967: Human to human transplant
1967: Pediatric heart transplant
1972: Endocardial biopsy
1981: Cyclosporine
1985: Infant heart transplant Loma Linda
2000: Berlin Heart
2001: ABO incompatible transplants

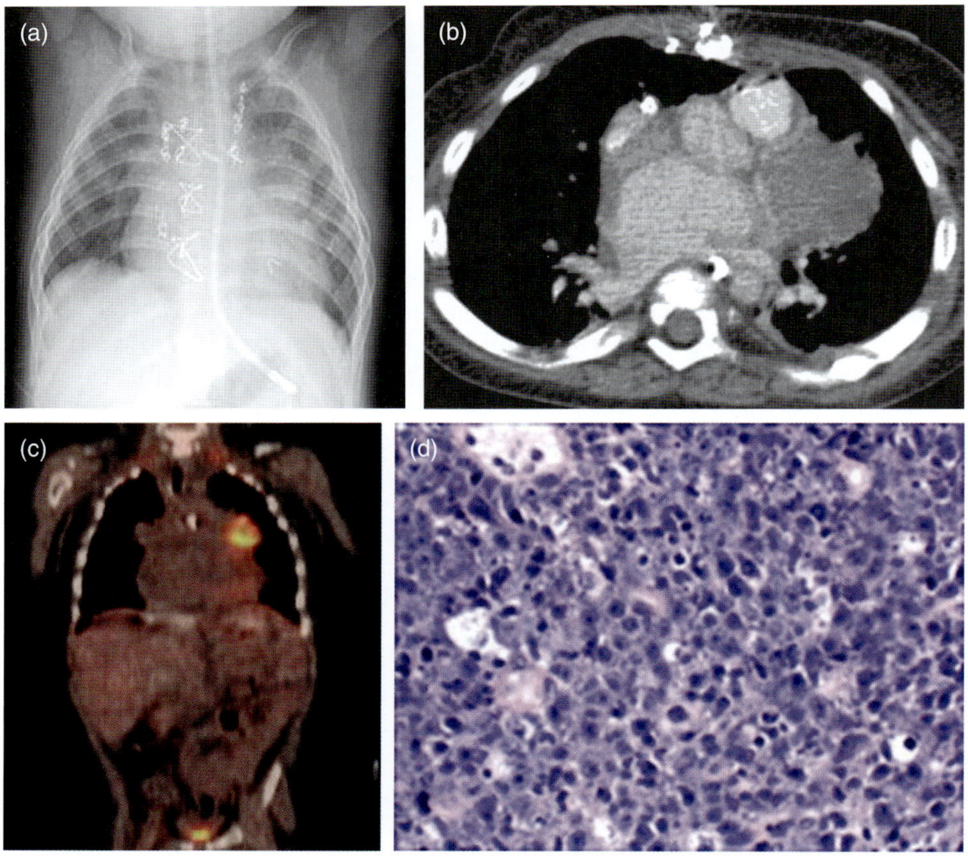

Figure 68.1 (a) Left hilar mass in a chest X-ray for a patient post infant heart transplantation. (b) The mass is more clearly seen on chest CT scan. (c) PET scanning reveales uptake in hilar mass. (d) Histology consistent with B-cell lymphoma/PTLD.

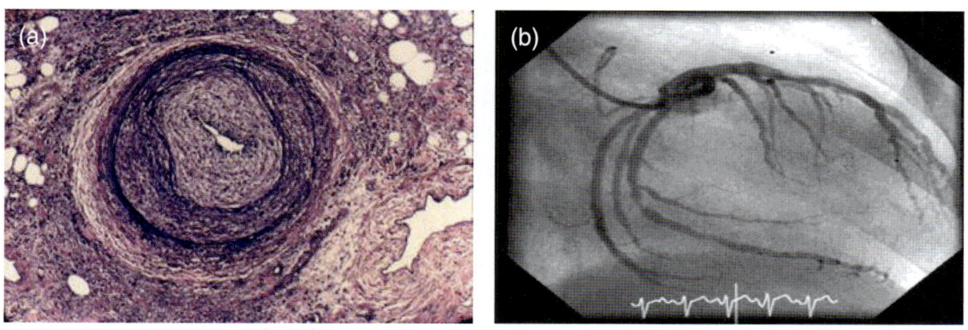

Figure 68.2 (a) Cross-sectional H&E staining of a coronary artery that demonstrates smooth muscle proliferation and near occlusion consistent with post-transplant coronary artery vasculopathy. (b) Coronary angiogram reveals diffuse abnormalities and narrowing of the coronary arteries in a patient with post-transplant coronary vasculopathy.

Box 68.2 Indications for infant heart transplantation

Congenital heart disease

- Otherwise lethal congenital heart disease, not ameliorated with medical therapy, inoperable, or with extremely high surgical risk
- Congenital heart disease that would provide a low quality of life or with high risk of profound residual heart failure, marked cyanosis, or irreversible pulmonary hypertension

Cardiomyopathy

- Progressive decrease in left ventricular function or functional status despite optimal medical therapy
- Uncontrollable malignant ventricular arrhythmias
- Symptomatic heart failure requiring continuous inotropic support, mechanical ventilation, or mechanical device support
- Increasing irreversible pulmonary vascular resistance not amenable to medical or surgical therapy that would preclude subsequent transplantation at a later date

Conditional survival analysis of all infants who survive heart transplant past 1 year indicates that more than 50% will be alive beyond 25 years (Figure 68.6b). The Loma Linda experience indicates that neonatal transplants have a graft survival advantage relative to other infants, with a 59% graft survival rate at 25 years post neonatal heart transplant [1].

Post- transplant survival for infants is affected by the underlying diagnosis, with congenital heart disease having an increased risk of mortality compared to those post-transplant for cardiomyopathy. Stratifying survival by era indicates that more recent transplantation provides better initial survival. This is likely related to improvements in perioperative care and to a lower operative mortality rate, which will result in better longitudinal survival.

Quality of Life

The majority of patients post infant heart transplant (>85%) have no activity limitations and have an excellent functional status post-transplant. However, this does not come without morbidity.

Immunosuppression

All heart transplant patients require immunosuppression to prevent rejection and this is based on classic (adult) triple-drug therapy. These protocols include the use of steroids, antiproliferative agents (azathioprine, mycophenolate), and calcineurin inhibitors (tacrolimus and cyclosporine), and are evolving with the introduction of new medications. There is an growing recognition that neonates likely require less aggressive immunosuppression than older heart transplant patients [3]. A common strategy utilizes induction therapy with anti-thymocyte globulin (rabbit) (Thymoglobulin®) followed by steroids, mycophenolate and tacrolimus. Maintenance immunosuppression is weaned aggressively in infants to mono or dual therapy with a calcineurin inhibitor (cyclosporine or tacrolimus) with or without mycophenolate or azathioprine.

Morbidity

Data from the ISHLT and Loma Linda indicates that approximately 20% of infants require treatment for acute rejection within the first year of life [1, 2, 4]. Furthermore, close to 20% of infant heart transplant patients develop post-transplant lymphoproliferative disease (PTLD) (Figure 68.1). PTLD is a hematogenous (B-cell lymphoma) malignancy, likely related to Epstein–Barr virus infection, which provides post solid organ transplant patients with significant morbidity. In addition, 30–35% of infants develop post-transplant coronary artery vasculopathy (CAV). CAV is a vasculopathy characterized by intimal hyperplasia with progressive occlusion of the graft coronary arteries. It is thought to be a manifestation of chronic rejection and is related to cytomegalovirus infection. CAV ultimately limits the long-term survival of the graft. Relative to other ages, infants have a slower onset of CAV over time, with a 65–70% freedom from CAV at 10 years (Figure 68.2).

Waitlist Mortality

Infant heart transplant waitlist mortality has been reported to be as high as 20–25%, providing the highest mortality for any solid organ waitlist [5]. Recent advances, including recognition that infant transplants can be performed across blood type [3] and advances in mechanical support (such as the Berlin Heart) have improved the effective donor pool and may decrease waitlist mortality. Data from Loma Linda and Great Ormond Street have also indicated that better donor utilization can be obtained by using a wider range of donors including undersized donors that weigh 75% of the recipient's weight and oversized donors of 400% of recipient's weight [1, 4, 6, 7]. The Loma Linda data also suggest that graft ischemic time can be safely extended above 4 hours for infant donors [6, 8] which allows for longer travel times and, potentially, extends donor availability and utilization.

Benefits

The favorable long-term outcome following neonatal heart transplantation has led some to believe that infants have a relatively naïve immune system that makes the neonatal period an ideal time to perform heart transplantation [3]. This unique time can present a window of opportunity for optimal transplant decision-making relative to other operative strategies.

Transplantation and Hypoplastic Left Heart Syndrome

The origins of neonatal and infant heart transplantation are closely tied to hypoplastic left heart syndrome (HLHS). With the evolution of the Norwood procedure and multistage single ventricle palliation, heart transplantation has changed from a primary procedure for HLHS to a supportive role reserved for highly selected neonates with HLHS or after failed single ventricle palliation. The recent Single Ventricle Reconstruction (SVR) trial indicated that there was a 65% transplant-free survival at 14 months post Norwood procedure combined with multistage single ventricle palliation as a primary strategy for neonates with HLHS [9]. Analysis of the original Loma Linda series for infant heart transplantation suggests a survival after listing for transplant of 68% at 1 year and 61% at 5 years [4]. The SVR trial and the Loma Linda Series are not equivalent groups, but comparison of these data suggests that primary transplantation does not represent an inferior strategy for neonates with HLHS who are at high risk for Norwood procedure (such as those with severe tricuspid regurgitation). Transplantation would likely provide equivalent or better intermediate survival, good functional capacity, good quality of life, and likely long-term graft survival [9].

Heart Transplant Technique

The technique for implantation is dependent on the underlying cardiac condition, with HLHS requiring the addition of an arch reconstruction [10]. Infant heart transplant is performed via a median sternotomy and cardiopulmonary bypass. Hypothermia can facilitate both myocardial protection and operative exposure by allowing lower flow rates (and pulmonary venous return), and allow for circulatory arrest to complete arch reconstruction. Remote aortic cannulation via placement of a tube graft to the innominate artery allows for selective cerebral perfusion if arch reconstruction is required. Biatrial reconstruction, as described by Lower and Shumway, is generally performed [10, 11], although a bicaval technique can be utilized if the cava are large enough to avoid the potential risks of caval stenosis. If required, the arch is reconstructed utilizing the donor aortic graft to augment the arch.

Conclusions

Infant and neonatal heart transplantation is a highly effective treatment for end-stage heart disease. It has been associated with excellent long-term survival and quality of life relative to older patients and other treatment alternatives. Long-term outcome following neonatal and infant heart transplantation suggests that neonates have a relatively naïve immune system that may provide for an optimal timing for heart transplantation. This treatment is limited by supply of donors and waitlist mortality. Long-term morbidities include PTLD and coronary artery vasculopathy. Donor awareness, ABO incompatible transplantation, evolution in mechanical support, and use of extended donor criteria can expand the donor pool to allow further growth of this treatment strategy.

References

1 Chinnock RE, Bailey LL. (2011) Heart Transplantation for congenital heart disease in the first year of life. *Curr Cardiol Rev*, **7** (2), 72–84.
2 Dipchand AI, Kirk R, Edwards LB, *et al*; International Society for Heart and Lung Transplantation. (2013) The Registry of the International Society for Heart and Lung Transplantation: Sixteenth Official Pediatric Heart Transplantation Report—2013; Focus Theme: Age. *J Heart Lung Transplant*, **32** (10), 979–988.

3 West LJ. (2011). ABO-incompatible hearts for infant transplantation. *Curr Opin Organ Transplant*, **16** (5), 548–554.

4 Razzouk AJ, Chinnock RE, Gundry SR, *et al.* (1996) Transplantation as a primary treatment for hypoplastic left heart syndrome: intermediate-term results. *Ann Thorac Surg*, **62** (1), 1–8.

5 Almond CSD, Thiagarajan RRM, Piercey GE, *et al.* (2009) Waiting list mortality among children listed for heart transplantation in the United States. *Circulation*, **119** (5), 717–727.

6 Bailey LL, Gundry SR, Razzouk AJ, *et al.* (1993) Bless the babies: one hundred fifteen late survivors of heart transplantation during the first year of life. The Loma Linda University Pediatric Heart Transplant Group. *J Thorac Cardiovasc Surg*, **105** (5), 805–814; discussion 814–815.

7 Kanani M, Hoskote A, Carter C, *et al.* (2012) Increasing donor-recipient weight mismatch in pediatric orthotopic heart transplantation does not adversely affect outcome. *Eur J Cardiothorac Surg*, **41** (2), 427–434.

8 Scheule AM, Zimmerman GJ, Johnston JK, *et al.* (2002). Duration of graft cold ischemia does not affect outcomes in pediatric heart transplant recipients. *Circulation*, **106** (12 Suppl 1), 163–167.

9 Ohye RG, Sleeper LA, Mahony L, *et al*; Pediatric Heart Network Investigators (2010) Comparison of shunt types in the Norwood procedure for single-ventricle lesions. *N Engl J Med*, **362** (21), 1980–1992.

10 Backer CL, Idriss FS, Zales VR, Mavroudis C. (1990) Cardiac transplantation for hypoplastic left heart syndrome: a modified technique. *Ann Thorac Surg*, **50** (6), 894–898.

11 Lower RR, Shumway NE. (1960) Studies on orthotopic homotransplantation of the canine heart. *Surg Forum*, **11**, 18–19.

69

Postoperative Care of the Newborn

Anthony F. Rossi[1] *and Enrique Oliver Aregullin*[2]

[1] *Nicklaus Children's Hospital, Miami, FL, USA*
[2] *Helen DeVos Children's Hospital (Congenital Heart Center CVTS), Grand Rapids, MI, USA*

General Principles

Postoperative care of the newborn after congenital heart surgery has evolved from being based on stabilization and maintenance of critical organ function to proactive management of oxygen delivery. Goal-directed medical care based on objective indices of cardiovascular well-being has a proven track record of improving outcomes. Anticipatory care based on evidence and institutional experience has resulted in prevention rather than management of adverse events. The development of checklists to guide the clinical team throughout the patient's hospital course from the preoperative state to discharge was inspired by mandatory checklists for aviation safety. Clinical pathways are an excellent tool to ensure that an individual patient remains on track for an excellent recovery. The focus today is not only on preventing postoperative mortality in the neonatal period, but also on favorably impacting the overall well-being of the baby and reducing complications that would impact the life of the child.

Optimum outcomes after newborn heart surgery require a comprehensive multidisciplinary team of specialists (Box 69.1). There has been debate over which type of intensive care unit these babies should be placed for postoperative recovery: a neonatal intensive care unit, a pediatric intensive care unit, or a pediatric cardiac intensive care unit. If the unit has an appropriately staffed team, optimum results can be achieved.

The best cardiovascular results begin with appropriate evaluation and stabilization of the preoperative patient. Diagnostic evaluation of most neonates can be completed non-invasively at the bedside. Occasionally, additional information such as cardiac catheterization or magnetic resonance imaging studies are required. Stabilization of the critically ill newborn includes restoration of perfusion and oxygen delivery to vital organs, including the brain. Babies presenting in extremis should be allowed to recover from the presenting condition if possible and show signs of end-organ recovery before surgery. There are exceptions to this general rule and those patients should undergo surgery without delay. These exceptions include patients presenting with severe cyanosis from obstructed total anomalous pulmonary venous connection and hypoplastic left heart syndrome (HLHS) with a severely restrictive or intact atrial septum. For other neonates, once there is evidence that adequate end-organ function has improved, there is no need to delay surgery.

Box 69.1 Recommended members of a comprehensive multidisciplinary team caring for the newborn after heart surgery

- Pediatric cardiologist
- Pediatric cardiac surgeon
- Pediatric cardiac intensivist
- Pediatric intensivist
- Neonatologist
- Pediatric neurologist
- Geneticist
- Pediatric critical care/cardiac critical care nursing
- Respiratory therapist
- Nutritionist
- Occupational/speech therapy
- Social worker
- Pharmacist

Visual Guide to Neonatal Cardiology, First Edition. Edited by Ernerio T. Alboliras, Ziyad M. Hijazi, Leo Lopez, and Donald J. Hagler.

Postoperative management begins with a comprehensive handover of the baby from the anesthesia and transport team to the critical care team. Standardized preprinted forms are highly recommended for recovering babies after complex procedures. Handoffs between these teams can be optimized by the use of checklists (Box 69.2). A typical checklist includes all the relevant data regarding the patient's intraoperative course including which anesthetics were used, at what dosage, and how the patient responded. A description of the operation is essential along with details of expected and unexpected findings. Perfusion records should provide data on duration of cardiopulmonary bypass, circulatory arrest, and aortic cross-clamp times. It is mandatory that key members of the baby's medical, surgical, and nursing teams are present at the time of these handoffs and that each member has a well-defined task. Having standard checklists for initial postoperative ICU orders (Figure 69.1) and daily rounds (Figure 69.4) are very important for effective intensive care delivery. Daily checklists for ICU rounds can prevent errors and improve outcomes. It it strongly suggested that checklists such as these be implemented into everyday practice in the ICU.

In the postoperative care of the newborn cardiac patient, the goal is to optimize the relationship between oxygen delivery and oxygen consumption through increasing oxygen delivery, decreasing oxygen consumption, or both. Critically ill patients who can achieve a normal level of oxygen delivery have been shown to have lower mortality, better end organ function, and shorter length of hospital stay. Unfortunately, measuring oxygen delivery or consumption in the postoperative neonate is difficult and not routinely performed clinically. The mixed venous oxygen saturation actually defines this relationship, but will not give the clinician any data regarding the primary aberration. When the A-V O2 difference is increased, clinical expertise is needed to decide whether oxygen delivery is diminished or oxygen consumption is increased. For certain patients, such as a baby recovering after the Norwood palliation, oxygen consumption can be pathologically elevated, even in the sedated and intubated neonate. Use of dopamine in the postoperative period can also increase oxygen consumption.

Even a skilled clinician can miscalculate the degree of oxygen delivery in a critically ill child. Intermittent or continuous measurement of mixed venous oxygen saturation can give a more accurate assessment of the degree of hemodynamic derangement. It has been shown that near-infrared spectrometry (NIRS), which measures regional oxygenation, is a safe non-invasive technique to assess cardiovascular well-being. Intermittent serial blood lactate monitoring can also be used to evaluate the

Box 69.2 Miami Children's Hospital Standardization of OR to CICU Hand-off Protocol

- Surgical hand-off by primary surgeon to ICU attending and receiving team (RN, RT, Fellows, ARNPs):
  - Patient history
  - Congenital defect
  - Operative procedure performed
  - Any complications and interventions done
  - Cardiopulmonary bypass time, deep hypothermic circulatory arrest time, aortic cross-clamp time
  - Off pump difficulties (i.e., arrhythmias, bleeding, hypotension, etc.)
  - Plan of care recommendations and clinical status alerts (for first post-op 24 hours):
- Hand-off by Anesthesia to receiving ICU team:
  - Lines (size)
  - Catheters
  - EET size and placement
  - Ventilation complications
  - EBL
  - Amount of blood products given in OR
  - Urine output
  - Medications given
  - Temp off pump
  - Current temp
  - Temp goal
- Hand-off by Perfusionist to receiving ICU team if patient return from OR on CPS
  - Flow measures
  - Volume
  - Size and site of cannulation catheters
  - CPS settings
- Receiving attending/Fellows/ARNP/RN able to ask questions of surgeon
- After all questions asked and answered, intra-op RN proceeds with hand-off
- Intra Op RN proceeds with hand-off to ICU RN:
  - Patient positioning
  - Intra Op V/S
  - Lines, drains, catheters
  - Blood product coming and available
  - When blood hanging due to expire
- Take back monitor; assure that all questions from surgical team have been answered and all information needed by receiving team obtained.
- Take back monitor states hand-off complete and surgical team released.

  Surgeon initials: ______________

  ICU Attending initials: ______________

Date: Time: Weight: Height__________

1. DIAGNOSIS: ____

2. PROCEDURE: ____

3. Allergies: ____________________________

4. Admit to CICU Dr. ________________________.

5. Notify Referring, Dr. ______________ of arrival to CICU.

6. Vital signs per CICU routine & ______ upper & lower extremity BP every a.m.

7. Urine output every hour, I & O, weigh daily, NPO.

8. NG or OG tube to appropriate suction (continuous or intermittent), irrigate with saline/air as needed per patient condition

9. Maintain normothermia______ or maintain rectal temperature ______.

10. Chest tube drainage system to 20 cm water suction. Milk chest tube as needed and record drainage with vital signs.

11. Chest X-ray after arrival, then every morning (6 a.m.) until extubated and after chest tube removal.

12. LAB WORK:
    a.______On arrival: CBC with differential, Profile 8, PT/PTT, iSTAT CG4+ (arterial) CRP
    b.______Daily: CBC with differential, Profile 8
    c.______Every 12 hours until: iSTAT CHEM 8+
    d.______Every Monday liver profile while on Parenteral Nutrition (PN)
    e.______PT, PTT, platelet count at 4 am prior to intracardiac line removal &/or prior to chest closure
    f.______iSTAT CG3+ (ABG) with ventilator change & as needed.
    g.______iSTAT CG4+ (ABG/Lactate) every ______ hours until less than 2.2, then daily
    h.______Daily CRP for 3 days post-op
    i.______ Keep 2 units PRBC available x 24 hours

13. RESPIRATORY CARE:
    a. Initial ventilator settings: FI02: _____ IMV:_____ Tidal Vol:_____
       PIP: _____ PEEP: _____
    b. Elevate head of bed to 30 degrees, midline, unless contraindicated (hypotension, severe shock, post-op repair).
    c. Oral care: perform and document oral care every 4 hours with Chlorhexidine 0.12% oral rinse (patient older than 2 months)
    d. Rotate and change patent's position as per nursing protocol
    e. Suction ETT with aerosolized pulmonary treatments and as needed. Do not use saline for suction unless indicated (example: thick secretions, etc).
    f. Change Yankauer and Ballard every 24 hours (day shift)
    g. Wean FI02 to keep 02 sat greater than 70% for single ventricle and 95% two ventricles)
    h. Other: ______________________________
    i. Suctioning every _____ hours & prn for ____________
    j. Ambu Bag every _______ hours with suctioning
    k. Pulmonary hypertensive precautions: Ambu bag with 100% Fi02; sedation prior to suctioning or painful stimuli.
    l. Single ventricle physiology guidelines: Ambu bag with 21% Fi02 or ventilator setting Fi02 only
    m. Nitric Oxide _____ parts per million
    n. Met hemoglobin every 6 hours
    o. Call MD for Nitric Oxide greater than 3 parts per million
    p. Call MD for Met hemoglobin greater than 5 %
    q. Ballard in –line suction set-up while on Nitric Oxide therapy

14. FLUIDS:
    a. Total hourly IV fluids today (2/3 maintenance)
    b. Total hourly IV fluids beginning at ______ post-op day #1 (full maintenance)

Figure 69.1 Sample postoperative ICU admission orders for neonate after cardiac surgery.

Total fluids: Calculation: (For first 1–10 kg = 4 mL/kg/hr; for next 11–20 kg= additional 2 mL/kg/hr; for next 21 + kg = additional 1 mL/kg/hr)

c. Maintenance: ______D10W 0.2 NS + 2 meq KCL/100 mL (less than 1 month of age)
_____ D5W 0.2 NS + 2 meq KCL/100 mL (1–3 months of age)
_____ D5W 0.3 NS + 2 meq KCL/100 mL (3 months to 3 years of age)
_____ D5W 0.45 NS + 2 meq KCL/100 mL (greater than 3 years of age)
Other:________________

d. ART line: Normal Saline with 2 units of Heparin/mL at 1 mL/hr.
e. CVP line: Normal Saline with 2 units of Heparin/mL at 1 mL/hr
f. PICC line:________________________________ with 1 unit of Heparin/mL at _____ mL/hr.
g. UVL/UAL: Normal Saline with 2 units of Heparin/mL at 1 mL/hr
h. Calcium can only be given via central line.
i. Drips: D10W
j. Transfuse blood products via peripheral IV

15. PARAMETERS TO NOTIFY MD/NURSE PRACTITIONER/PHYSICIAN ASSISTANT :

a. HR less than_____ beats per minute or greater than _____ beats per minute
b. Arterial BP(mean/systolic) less than_____ mmHg or greater than _____ mmHg
c. CVP/Right Atrial/Common Atrial less than _____ mmHg or greater than _____ mmHg
d. Left Atrial Pressure less than _____ mmHg or greater than _____ mmHg
e. 02 Sat less than _____ % or greater than _____ % or Sv02 less than _____ % or greater than_____ %
f. Lactate greater than 2.2 or greater than previously recorded values
g. Temperature greater than 101.5 F or 38.5 C, Hematocrit less than 36, K+ less than 3.4 or greater than 4.8, ICa ++ less than 1 or greater than 1.4
h. Chest tube drainage greater than 3 mL/kg/hr for first 4 hr; then 2 mL/kg/hr.
i. Any arrhythmias, signs of agitation or pain.
j. Urine output less than 1mL/kg/hr x 2 hours.
k. Single ventricle guidelines.
l. Pulmonary hypertension guidelines.

16. CARDIAC RHYTHM PARAMETERS:

a. Twelve lead EKG on arrival.
b. PACEMAKER SETTINGS:

MODE:_______________RATE:________________ AV INTERVAL:__________
OUTPUT: Atrial:_______________ Ventricle:_________________
SENSITIVITY: Atrial:_______________ Ventricle:________________

17. OPEN CHEST:

EKG after chest closed.
Chest tubes to suction x ____hours, then to waterseal. When chest closed, chest tubes to 20 cm water suction.
Do not change sternotomy or chest tube site dressings when chest is open.

18. WOUND CARE: (START 24 HOURS AFTER CHEST CLOSED)

Remove sternotomy/thoracotomy dressing on post-op day #1. Clean with chlorhexidine every day. Reapply dry sterile gauze/tegaderm only if there is drainage and change every day or as needed.
Clean chest tube sites with betadine or chlorehexidine every day. If chest tubes remains in greater than 24 hours, change dressing with sterile gauze and tegaderm every 3 days or as needed.

19. Social Work Consult: YES/NO
20. Other:____
21. MEDICATIONS:

a. Furosemide ____milligrams IV every____hrs (1–2 milligrams/kg/dose, every 6 hrs to every 24 hrs);
or Furosemide ______milligrams/kg/hr continuous IV drip (0.1 milligrams/kg/hr–0.4 milligrams/kg/hr)
b. Cefazolin : ______milligrams IV every ____hrs x 48 HOURS
(25 milligrams/kg/dose every 8 hr if greater than 7 days old, every 12 hr. if less than 7 days old)
Last dose given in OR at__________
c. Vancomycin _____milligrams IV every ____hours
(15–20 milligrams/kg/dose every 24 hours, less than 34 weeks of age)
(15–20 milligrams/kg/dose every 12 hours if greater than 34 weeks gestation and less than 2 months old)
(15–20 milligrams/kg/dose every 8 hours if greater than 2 months old)
______Vancomycin trough level prior to fourth dose
d. Ceftazidime ______ milligrams IV every _____ hours
(50 milligrams/kg/dose every 8 hours if greater than 1 month old)
(50 milligrams/kg/dose every 12 hours if less than 1 month old) (Cautious use if allergic to penicillin)

IF ALLERGIC TO PENICILLIN OR CEPHALOSPORINS USE :
Clindamycin ____milligrams IV every ______ hrs x 48 HOURS
Last dose given in OR at ________________

Figure 69.1 (*Continued*)

(greater than 1 month; 25 milligrams/kg/day, divided every 8 hrs)
(less than 1 month; 20 milligrams/kg/day, divide every 8 hrs)
e. Lacrilube to both eyes as needed during paralysis
f. Ranitidine ______milligrams IV every 8 hrs (1 – 2 milligrams/kg/dose)
g. Dopamine _____ micrograms/kg/minute IV continuous drip (2 – 10 micrograms/kg/minute)
h. Milrinone ______micrograms/kg/minute IV continuous drip (0.25 – 1 micrograms/kg/minute)
i. Epinephrine______ micrograms/kg/minute IV continuous drip (0.01 – 0.2 micrograms/kg/minute)
j. Calcium gluconate _____milligrams/kg/ hr IV(10 – 20 milligrams/kg/hr)
k. Heparin drip: Loading Dose:_____ units (50 – 100 units/kg) IV over 10 – 60 min.
Maintenance:_____ units/kg/hr (20 – 25 units/kg/hr) IV
_____PT/PTT prior to starting drip and every 4 hours. Goal PTT: ____________(Per protocol)
l. I.V. Potassium Chloride, Magnesium Sulfate and Calcium Gluconate replacement per CICU protocol
m. Other medication____

22. PAIN/SEDATION MANAGEMENT:

a. Vecuronium IV drip _____milligrams/kg/hr (0.03 – 0.05 milligrams/kg/hr)
Vecuronium IV______milligrams/kg/dose every hour prn noxious stimuli
(0.03 – 0.05 milligrams/kg/dose).Total dose ___________.
b. Rocuronium IV drip _____ milligrams/kg/hr (0.25 – 1 milligram/kg/hr)
Rocuronium IV _____ milligrams/kg/dose every hour prn noxious stimuli
(0.25 – 1 milligram/kg). Total dose ________.
c. Ketorolac _____milligrams IV every 6 hr prn moderate to severe pain (0.5 milligrams/kg/dose every 6 hr) x total of 5 days. May start on _____ (greater than 3 months old, platelets greater than 100,000, no active bleeding).
d. Acetaminophen (Tylenol) _________milligrams PO/PR every 4 hr prn temperature greater than 101.5 For (38.5 C) mild to moderate pain (10 – 15 milligrams/kg/dose)
e. Fentanyl IV drip _______micrograms/kg/hr (1 – 10 micrograms/kg/hr)
Fentanyl dose IV______ microgram/kg/dose every______ hrs prn prior to suctioning or noxious stimuli
(1 – 5 micrograms/kg/dose). Total dose ________________.
f. Morphine_______ milligrams IV every_____hrs prn severe pain while INTUBATED
(0.1 milligrams/kg/dose)
Morphine________milligrams IV every _____ hrs prn severe pain while WEANING from ventilator or when EXTUBATED (0.05 milligrams/kg/dose)
g. Midazolam (Versed) IV drip __________milligrams/kg//hr (0.05 – 0.1 milligrams/kg/hr)
Midazolam (Versed) IV bolus _____ milligrams/kg/dose every hour prn agitation
(0.05–0.1 mg/kg/dose).
Total dose _____________.
h. Lorazepam (Ativan) IV _______milligrams prn agitation every 4 hr (0.05 – 0.1 milligrams/kg/dose)
i. Chloral Hydrate ____milligrams PO/NG every 4 hrs prn sedation (25 – 50 milligrams/kg/dose)
MAXIMUM: 2 grams/24 hr

Print Name: ________________________ Signature ____________________________
Date: __________ Time: _____

Figure 69.1 (*Continued*)

clinical status of a postoperative neonate. Blood lactate monitoring has proven to be an excellent prognosticator of outcomes in the critically ill (Figure 69.3). Monitoring of serial systemic venous O2, NIRS, and serial lactate can be used as guides for goal-directed medical therapy, where therapy is targeted at specific end points that are usually considered indices of oxygen delivery.

Hyperthermia in postoperative patients is a well-described phenomenon. While the etiology for postoperative hyperthermia can vary, the detrimental effects are consistent. Hyperthermia will always increase oxygen consumption and the immediate postoperative period is the patient's most vulnerable period, with the cardiovascular system recovering from the trauma of surgery and adjusting to new physiologic demands. The ability of the cardiovascular system to meet the needs of these increased demands may be extremely limited. Resultant physiologic derangement can be manifested by a decrease in SvO2 or an increase in blood lactate. Data supporting proactive use of hypothermia are lacking. Active cooling can be difficult to achieve in the critically ill neonate. Overcooling to a dangerously low core body temperature has been reported to result in bleeding or even ventricular fibrillation.

CICU ROUNDING CHECKLIST (DATE: ________)

☐ Name ________________________________ Age ______ Weight ______

☐ Diagnosis ______________________ Post Op day #______ Operative Procedure ________________________________

____

☐ Significant events: Intra-operative? Initial 12–24 hours post op? Run of CPS?

- Significant post-operative issues/sequelae?

- Bedside Nurse: Clinical information update/ last 12 hours ? Any current patient/nursing issues or concerns

☐ Lines

- o Intra cardiac? How many days? Can we remove?
- o Central Lines? How many days? Can we remove? Can we change to PICC?

☐ Current Lab results?

- o Concerns? Labs to be ordered? Drugs levels? Can we discontinue? Decrease any labs? Cluster any labs?

☐ Systems:

- o Cardiac:

  Rhythm? EKG? Perfusion? Lactate? SVO2? NIRS? QP/QS?

  Inotropes? Open chest? Closure? HCT/HGB? Coags?

  Residual Lesions? Last ECHO results / Need an echo? Need a Cath?

  I's/O's: Urine output? Lytes: K+? Ca+ ? Mg + ? Foley?

  Heart Failure meds? Diuretics?

- o Respiratory:

  Intubated? How many days? Extubate today?

  Last CXR? Last ABG/CBG? FiO2 needs? Effusion? Atelectasis?

  Chest tube drainage: Worrisome/ No concerns? Can we remove chest tube?

  Concerns: PHN? Vocal Cord paralysis? Diaphragm paralysis? Subglottic stenosis?

- o GI:

  Feed? NG/ PO? / TPN? Tolerating Feeds/Vomiting/Reflux? Total Kilo cals? Gaining wt?

  Need to plan for G-Tube? Speech Therapy? Swallow study needed?

  Stooling? Colace/Glycerine suppository?

- o Integumentary

  Any areas of concern for pressure sores? RIK Mattress / Z-Flo?

  Surgical site? Chest tube site? Central Line site? A-Line site? IV infiltrates? G-Tube site?

Figure 69.2 CICU Rounding Checklist (Miami Children's Hospital/Nicklaus Children's Hospital).

- o Neuro

  Pupils? Moving all fours limbs? Recent MRI/US/CT results?

- o Pain

  Pain controlled? Sedation adequate? Can drips be changed to NG/PO? Withdrawal concerns?

☐ Current medications?

- o Wean / switch any medications from IV to po? Cluster any medications to decrease line entry?

☐ Bedside Nurse: Parental/Social information update

☐ Discharge Plan: Please Review Discharge Planning Checklist on other side of this Rounding Checklist

☐ **REVIEW/DETERMINE DAILY PLAN/GOALS**

- o TEAM LEADER: ANY ADDITIONAL COMMENTS FROM TEAM? ASK BEDSIDE RN: ANY ADDITIONAL ORDERS NEEDED/TO BE DISCHARGED?

☐ **ANNOUNCE ROUNDS ARE CONCLUDED ON PATIENT AND ANNOUNCE THE NEXT PATIENT'S NAME / ROOM NUMBER**

Figure 69.2 (*Continued*)

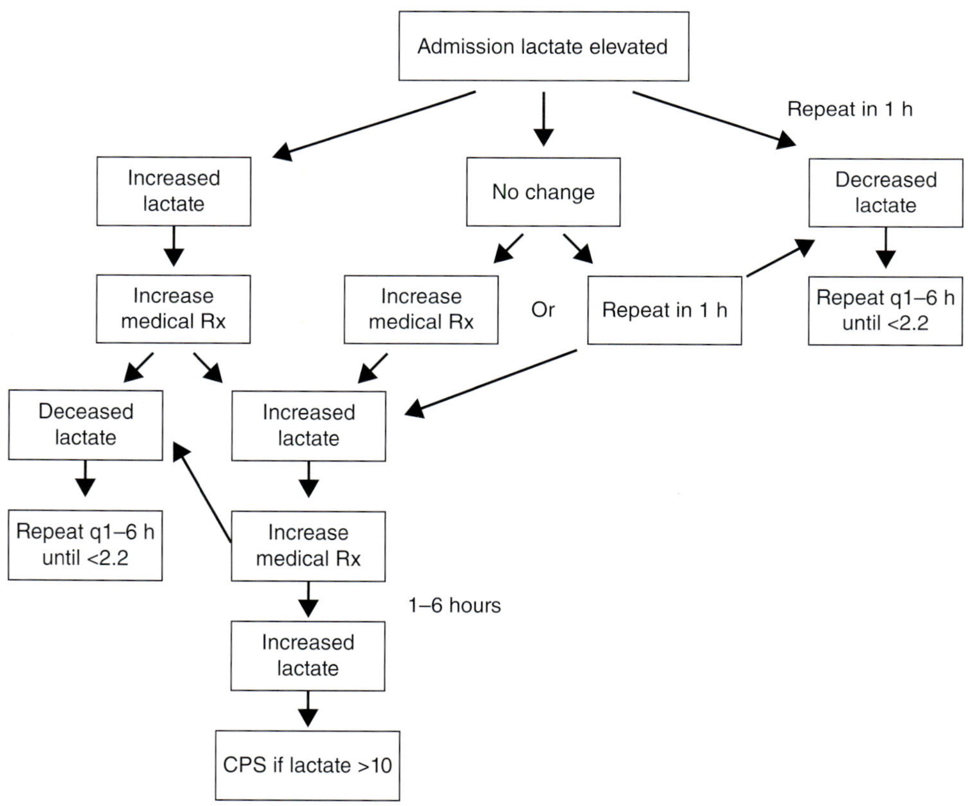

Figure 69.3 Algorithm directing postoperative care based on serial lactate measurements.

Inotropic Support of the Postoperative Patient

Low cardiac output syndrome (LCOS) is a common phenomenon that many neonates experience after congenital heart surgery (Figure 69.4). LCOS leads to diminished oxygen delivery and an increase in systemic vascular resistance (SVR). The increase in SVR can lead to worsening of the low cardiac output state by worsening ventricular function directly or indirectly. Increased SVR can result in increased pulmonary blood flow in patients with systemic to pulmonary artery shunts, causing a pathologic increase in ventricular loading conditions. For the failing ventricle recovering after heart surgery, the cornerstone of medical management is the use of afterload-reducing agents. This principle applies to those patients who have failing left ventricles, right ventricles, or single ventricles. Afterload reduction of systemic ventricles can be accomplished with the use of milrinone, sodium nitroprusside, or phenoxybenzamine. Afterload reduction of the right ventricle is aimed at lowering pulmonary vascular resistance and includes avoiding acidosis and hypercapnia or adding supplemental oxygen or nitric oxide. For patients with failing systemic ventricles, we target a systemic organ perfusion pressure of 40–50 mmHg (organ perfusion pressure = MAP–RAP or CVP). We suggest pushing the afterload-reducing agents to the maximum tolerated dosage and titrating the blood pressure up with the judicious use of a combination of inotropic agents and pressors.

The inodilator milrinone, a phosphodiesterase 3 inhibitor, has been shown to prevent or mitigate low cardiac syndrome in children recovering after congenital heart surgery. In most centers milrinone has become a first line drug for managing LCOS after congenital

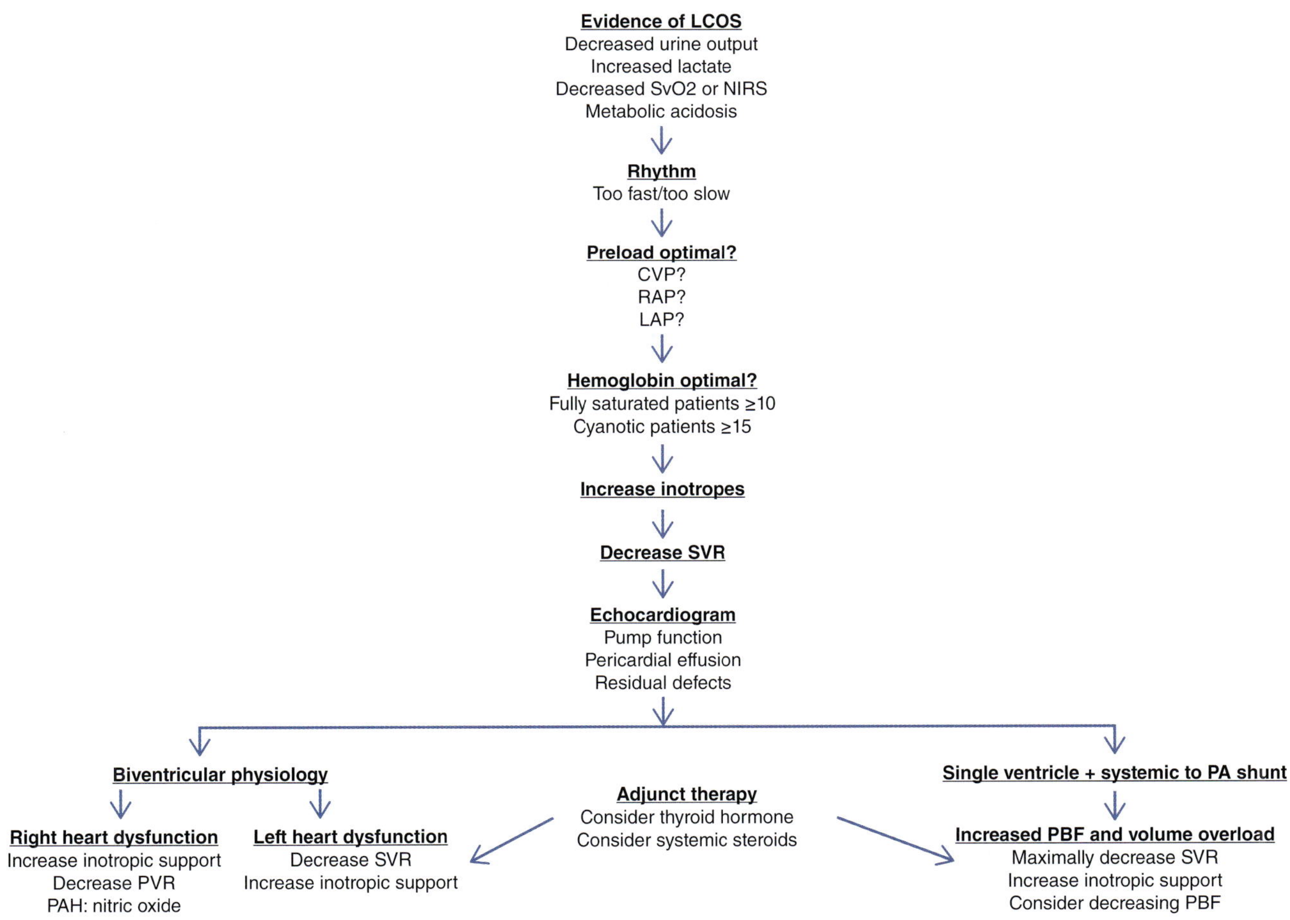

Figure 69.4 Management of low cardiac output syndrome (LCOS). CVP, central venous pressure; LAP, left atrial pressure; NIRS, near-infrared spectrometry; PAH, pulmonary artery hypertension; PVR, pulmonary vascular resistance; RAP, right atrial pressure; SVR, systemic vascular resistance.

heart surgery. The primary hemodynamic effects of milrinone are to increase ventricular contractility and to decrease systemic vascular resistance through arterial vasodilatation. The drug can also improve ventricular lusitropy or diastolic relaxation. There is also a mild but significant vasodilatory effect on the pulmonary vasculature. There are a few caveats to the clinical use of milrinone. The first is that it has a much longer half-life than most intravenous inotropic agents agents. The half-life has been estimated to be 2–4 hours in children but may be over 10 hours in the preterm infant. To achieve a steady state level in a clinically acceptable period of time, a bolus loading dose is needed prior to the start of the continuous infusion. A general rule of thumb is that a bolus of 10 μg/kgwill give the equivalent of an infusion of 0.1 μg/kg/min. So if one was planing to give an infusion rate of 0.5 μg/kg/min, the loading dose should be 50 μg/kg. It is our practice at Miami Children's Hospital that all neonates are given a large milrinone bolus (in the range of 100–200 μg/kg) as they are being weaned from cardiopulmonary bypass. Milrinone is primarily excreted by the kidneys and should be used cautiously in patients with renal dysfunction. Toxicity is manifested by vasodilatation and hypotension. For patients who experience milrinone toxicity, the drug is discontinued and if the patient remains hypotensive we add a low dose vasopressin infusion.

Epinephrine is a beta-adrenergic drug that possesses beta-1 and beta-2 properties. These effects are manifested by an increase in contractility and heart rate. At lower doses (less than 100 ng/kg/min) it is primarily a vasodilator. At higher doses it can produce systemic vasoconstriction via its effect on alpha receptors. It should be used cautiously (or avoided when possible) in patients with elevated pulmonary artery resistance because it is a potent pulmonary artery constrictor. In many centers epinephrine has replaced dopamine as the beta-adrenergic drug of choice in neonates recovering after congenital heart surgery.

Dopamine is a beta-adrenergic drug that is a systemic vasoconstrictor. Its effects are similar to epinephrine. Its use in neonates is diminishing for two reasons. First, it is clear that dopamine increases systemic oxygen consumption in some neonates after surgery while epinephrine does not. Second, its use has been linked to the development of postoperative junctional ectopic tachycardia.

Arginine vasopressin is a potent pressor agent used in a variety of vasodilatory shock conditions. Cardiopulmonary bypass can be associated with the development of vasodilatory hypotension often refractory to other pressor agents. Vasopressin can increase blood pressure under those conditions and improve systemic organ perfusion. Vasopressin does not increase heart rate and this is of considerable benefit for some neonates already pushed to their maximum heart rates. Also, as opposed to other pressors routinely used postoperatively, vasopressin does not increase pulmonary vascular resistance.

Mechanical Support of the Failing Heart After Surgery

Mechanical support of the neonate's heart after cardiac surgery is primarily used as a bridge towards myocardial recovery. Acute myocardial injury and low cardiac output states are not uncommon after neonatal surgery and for those patients refractory to medical therapy, mechanical support is a viable option. We have found lactate trending to be extremely useful in predicting survival after congenital heart surgery. A lactate of 10 or greater that does not begin to diminish in a predictable pattern strongly suggests the patient will not survive without support. It is acceptable to consider mechanical support if the amount of inotropic support is excessive. Drugs such as epinephrine have been shown to cause cardiac apoptosis at high doses.

For neonates recovering after congenital heart surgery, mechanical support is traditionally initiated with an extracorporeal membrane oxygenation (ECMO) type circuit. At this time, implantable ventricular assist devices, such as the Berlin Heart (Berlin GmbH, Berlin, Germany), are restricted for use in those patients being bridged to transplant. Despite the ability to improve tissue oxygenation, mechanical support is associated with a number of serious complications including neurologic injury and bleeding. Discontinuation of support should be attempted as soon as clinically possible. The likelihood of sufficient myocardial recovery to maintain acceptable hemodynamics decreases after 7–10 days. Discussions regarding end of life care or transplant should begin at this point if they have not started earlier.

Patients with congenital heart disease and their unique anatomic and physiologic differences can pose challenges not usually faced when using ECMO support in patients with structurally normal hearts. Patients with single ventricle physiology and systemic to pulmonary artery shunts have to perfuse both the pulmonary and systemic circulations through the arterial cannula. The required flow rates of the mechanical circuit are higher than flow rates required in those patients with two ventricles. Also, oxygenated blood from the ECMO circuit can further decrease pulmonary vascular resistance and potentially steal blood from the systemic circulation. If possible, ECMO should be used as a ventricular assist device and the oxygenator removed from the circuit.

Sedation, Analgesia, and Neuromuscular Blockade

Postoperatively, the priority is to create a pain-free environment for the newborn, but secondary goals include diminishing circulating catecholamines and minimizing VO2 in the baby's vulnerable postoperative state. Postoperative sedation is accomplished with a combination of drugs. Most centers use a combination of low dose opiate and a benzodiazepine. The opiate infusions are usually discontinued within 24–48 hours after surgery and the benzodiazapam infusions continued until just prior to extubation or occasionally until right after extubation. We try to avoid excessive agitation and irritability during the extubation period. Dexmedetomidine, an alpha-2 adrenergic agnostic, has sedative, anxiolytic, and analgesic properties. It has also been shown to provide neuroprotection under ischemic conditions. Dexmedetomidine is short acting and can be given as a continuous infusion (0.1–1 μg/kg/hour) or as a bolus for brief procedures (1–1.5 μg/kg). It can be given to intubated patients, be continued as the patient is bridged through extubation, and even after extubation. It is relatively hemodynamically safe, with bradycardia being the major cardiovascular effect. Its effects in the conduction system have made it a useful drug for the management of postoperative tachyarrhythmia. While experience in newborns has been limited, it is a useful drug in the postoperative period and may become a cornerstone of postoperative management in the future.

Postoperative Arrhythmias

Arrhythmias in patients recovering after congenital heart surgery are not infrequent, although their incidence appears to be decreasing. Postoperative arrhythmias are associated with significant increases in morbidity, length of hospital stay, and mortality. Mitigating the causative factors associated with postoperative arrhythmias and recognizing and treating them promptly and correctly will have a positive impact on postoperative outcomes. For neonates recovering after congenital heart surgery, complete heart block is the most common slow heart rhythm seen in the ICU, although sinus node dysfunction also occurs. Junctional ectopic tachycardia (JET) and ventricular tachycardia are the most prevalent tachyarrhythmias followed by supraventricular tachycardia (SVT).

Postoperative tachycardias occur in a number of different cardiac repairs and the incidence and severity is directly related to type of repair, surgical technique, hemodynamic status, electrolyte imbalances, agitation, pain, and temperature of the postoperative patient. Fever and increased circulating catecholamines (intrinsic or iatrogenic) can result in tachyarrhythmias. Once the patient has arrived in the critical care unit, the focus should be on optimizing hemodynamics and reducing oxygen demand along with maintaining normal electrolyte values.

JET is the most common arrhythmia seen the the postoperative period and its incidence is in the range of 0.8–8.5%. A narrow complex tachycardia with atrioventricular (AV) dissociation is pathognomonic for JET, although occasionally retrograde ventriculoatrial (VA) conduction may be present. It is often difficult to diagnose JET on a single monitored lead. However, if right atrial pressure or central venous pressure are being displayed on the bedside monitor, patients in JET with AV dissociation will exhibit intermittent cannon waves on these tracings. JET is self-limiting so, given time, it will resolve. For most neonates, if the JET rate is below 160 bpm, hemodynamics will not be seriously affected.

The management of these patients should begin with eliminating any postoperative fever. If the patient is normothermic, one can consider cooling the patient slowly. Our recommendations are to decrease the baby's temperature to about 35°C. This can usually be accomplished by turning off an infant's warmer. Drug therapy is begun if mild cooling and elimination or decreasing the catecholamines being administered has not resulted in a significant decrease in heart rate. Intravenous amiodarone is an effective treatment of postoperative JET. Its administration has been associated with hypotension but this can usually be managed by slowing the infusion rate or giving a bolus of calcium. Some have advocated utilizing a continuos infusion of amiodarone although in our center we give 2-3 mg/kg/hour until the arrhythmia has been adequately controlled. We can often discontinue this infusion within 1 or 2 hours. The maximum dose is 15–20 mg/kg/day. This regimen minimizes the total amount of amiodarone a patient receives and so helps to diminish some of the side effects of amiodarone.

SVTs are not uncommon after congenital heart surgery. The most common type of SVT is an AV reciprocating tachycardia. There can be atrial flutter or atrial ectopic tachycardia in patients with pre-existing atrial pathology, such as neonates with Ebstein anomaly or in neonates who have had extensive surgery involving the atrium, such as total anomalous pulmonary venous connection. It can be difficult to distinguish SVT from sinus tachycardia even with a 12-lead ECG, and an atrial electrogram, taken from atrial pacing wires or from an esophageal electrode, is helpful. Reviewing the heart rate trend can be diagnostic for re-entrant arrhythmias. The rapid onset and termination of re-entrant arrhythmias can often be clearly distinguished in the graphic trends.

While usually well tolerated in an otherwise healthy baby, hemodynamics can be significantly adversely affected by SVT in the postoperative period. Management requires prompt recognition and treatment. Adenosine is the cornerstone of treatment of SVT in otherwise well patients. It is recommended that adenosine is used with caution in the postoperative patient. Conversion from a hemodynamically stable rhythm to a more malignant one is well documented in the literature. Atrial overdrive pacing (via atrial pacing wires or a transesophageal pacing wire) or electrical cardioversion might be reasonable alternatives or even the preferred treatment of choice in the most unstable patients.

Sustained ventricular tachycardia is uncommon in the postoperative period. The hemodynamics are almost always adversely affected by this rhythm, although at slower rates ventricular tachycardia can be tolerated for some time. The incidence of ventricular tachycardia increases with operations that include coronary surgery, such as arterial switch and the Ross procedure, and those operations that include ventriculotomies. Management is somewhat determined by the degree of hemodynamic instability. The most ill patients require urgent cardioversion followed by medical therapy. Lidocaine bolus followed by a continuos infusion can be used, although treatment with procainamide or amiodarone can be more efficacious.

Postoperative bradyarrhythmias frequently include sinus node disfunction or complete heart block. Sinus node dysfunction can be well tolerated and requires no treatment. For those patients who experience hemodynamically significant changes related to decreased heart rate, pharmacologic treatment with a catecholamine is usually sufficient. Complete heart block can be seen in operations that include ventricular septal defect (VSD) closure. Treatment always requires pacing. In our experience, VVI pacing is well-tolerated and improves hemodynamics sufficiently so that more complicated pacing modes, such as DDD, are unnecessary. Temporary atrial pacing wires notoriously fail to sense atrial activity efficiently.

Special Considerations

Patients With Pulmonary Hypertension

Patients with pulmonary hypertension (PHTN) are at higher risk for pulmonary hypertensive episodes or crises, especially in the immediate postoperative period or during sedation (Boxes 69.3 and 69.4; Tables 69.1 and 69.2). Endotracheal suctioning is a frequent trigger for pulmonary vasoconstriction events. As the resistance to blood flow through the pulmonary vessels rises, the right ventricle (RV) begins to fail, leading to less pulmonary blood flow, cyanosis, impaired cardiac output, and a drop in arterial BP (PHTN crisis). Perioperative care focuses on avoiding factors that can trigger further PHTN. Ventilation needs to be optimized, as well as sedation, medication, and pain management.

Preterm or Low Birth Weight Children

Management of the neonate with congenital heart disease and comorbidity of either prematurity or low birth weight remains challenging (Figure 69.5). Issues regarding timing of surgery lack clinical consensus. A strong case can be made for allowing time to pass to achieve somatic growth in low birth weight babies and to allow for brain maturation in those patients who are born preterm. However, aberrant physiologic conditions, such as ventricular volume overload conditions or

Box 69.3 Precautions in suctioning to avoid pulmonary hypertension (PHTN) crisis/event

1) Must *bolus* with fentanyl IV prior to suctioning (when mechanically ventilated; as ordered)
2) Manual hyperventilation 100% oxygen (before and after each suction pass)
3) If nitric oxide has been ordered, this must be used when bagging patient
4) Monitor clinical status for signs and symptoms of PHTN event or crisis

Box 69.4 Management of pulmonary hypertensive crisis

1) Manual hyperventilation 100% oxygen, check chest motion, auscultate and MD notified
2) PRN fentanyl bolus. IV fluid bolus, chemical paralysis and add sedation, prn – each as ordered
3) Monitor clinical status for signs and symptoms of improvement perfusion and pressures, serial lactate measurements
4) New interventions including: ventilator adjustments, higher IV or PO vasodilator doses, inhaled nitric oxide

Table 69.1 Strategies for treatment of pulmonary hypertension.

Avoid	Encourage
Factors that raise PVR or pulmonary vasoconstriction	Factors that lower PVR by pulmonary vasodilatation
Hypoxia	Oxygen
Acidosis/hypercarbia	Alkalosis/hypocarbia
Agitation/pain/excessive stimuli	Sedation/anesthesia
Excessive hematocrit	Normal to low hematocrit
Hyperinflation	Normal functional residual capacity
Atelectasis, hypoventilation	Nitric oxide

PVR, pulmonary vascular resistance.

severe cyanosis, make waiting for surgical correction or palliation dangerous or impractical. Also, patients who are unable to be weaned from mechanical ventilation are unlikely to benefit from waiting for somatic growth. The decision to operate or wait on the preterm or low birth weight neonate needs to be made on a case-by-case basis. A risk–benefit equation should be developed for all low birth weight babies balancing the risks of operating on small and sometimes more immature babies against waiting for significant somatic growth to occur under less than optimal physiologic conditions.

Issues on Postoperative Care in the Newborn for Specific Lesions (see also chapters on specific cardiac defects)

Surgery for Hypoplastic Left Heart Syndrome

Stage 1 palliation of HLHS was originally described in 1981 for babies with HLHS. Variations of this operation are used to palliate a number of neonates who have in common severe aortic outlet obstruction, hypoplasia of the left heart, and hypoplasia of the transverse aortic arch associated with distal coarctation.

Since the time of Norwood's original report for this universally fatal disease, there have been a number of surgical approaches to this problem which have resulted in varying degrees of success: primary neonatal heart transplantation, the Sano modification which substitutes a conduit from the right ventricle to the pulmonary arteries for systemic to pulmonary artery shunt, and, most recently, the Hybrid palliation.

Timing of Surgery

Palliation of HLHS should be performed as soon as the patient is hemodynamically stable.

Norwood Operation

Objectives of the Norwood operation include creating unobstructed blood flow from the RV to the systemic circulation, augmenting the aortic arch to eliminate ascending aortic and transverse arch hypoplasia, eliminating distal aortic coarctation, insertion of a systemic to pulmonary artery shunt, and ensuring unobstructed egress of pulmonary venous blood flow to the RV with resection of the atrial septum. This circulation is inherently inefficient and results in significant hemodynamic derangement in the early postoperative period for many infants.

The placement of a systemic to pulmonary artery shunt can result in the "steal" of blood from the systemic and coronary circulations into the pulmonary vascular bed. Even under optimal circumstances, these infants are subjected to ventricular volume overload. The degree of ventricular volume overload is directly related to the the amount of pulmonary blood flow, which can change at any given time under different physiologic conditions. Factors that determine the amount of pulmonary blood flow include the size of the shunt, anatomically where the shunt originates from the systemic side, and the ratio

Table 69.2 Differentiating pulmonary hypertensive event from crisis.

Condition	Pulmonary hypertensive event	Pulmonary hypertensive crisis
Definition	Acute rise in PAP pressure with a stable arterial blood pressure	Paroxysmal event: PAP systolic pressures match or exceed systemic pressures, resulting in RV failure and immediate fall in arterial blood pressure
Heart rate	Stable or decreased	Decreased
O2 saturation	Stable or elevated	Elevated
CVP or right atrial pressure	Elevated	Elevated
Pulmonary artery pressure	Stable	Decreased
Left atrial pressure	Decreased	Severely decreased
Cardiac output	Decreased	Severely decreased
	Stable	Decreased prior to BP collapse

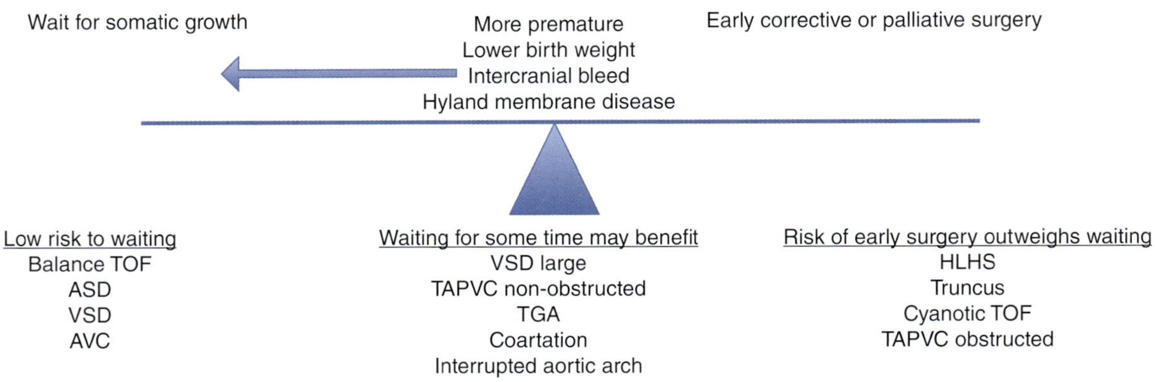

Figure 69.5 Surgical decision-making in premature or low birth weight infants with cardiac defects. ASD, atrial septal defect; AVC, atrioventricular canal defect; HLHS, hypoplastic left heart syndrome; TAPVC, total anomalous pulmonary venous circulation; TGA, transposition of the great arteries; TOF, tetralogy of Fallot; VSD, ventricular septal defect.

of the systemic to pulmonary artery resistances. The amount of pulmonary blood flow or, more appropriately, the amount of pulmonary blood flow as it is related to the systemic blood flow, is defined by the pulmonary to systemic blood flow ratio (Qp/Qs). Managing these babies has focused on "balancing the circulation" to optimize the amount of systemic blood flow and oxygen delivery. Mathematical models have predicted that the optimal Qp/Qs ranges somewhere between 0.7 and 1. It has become clear that the optimal Qp/Qs is that ratio associated with the highest systemic cardiac output and the highest arterial oxygen saturation. Balancing the circulation historically focused on minimizing the amount of pulmonary blood flow to enhance systemic blood flow by trying to alter the pulmonary vascular resistance utilizing inspired gases. However, pulmonary blood flow is most affected by the fixed obstruction at the level of the shunt and judicious use of systemic vasodilators is a much more effective way to augment systemic blood flow.

An effective postoperative management strategy is to maximize systemic vasodilation and then increase systemic vascular resistance if necessary. Systemic vasodilatation can be accomplished with a number of vasodilators including phenoxybenzamine, milrinone, and sodium nitroprusside. A reasonable clinical goal would be to have a pink, warm baby who has adequate coronary and organ perfusion pressures. In our practice, we recommend a diastolic blood pressure of 30 mmHg or greater, and a mean arterial blood pressure of 40–50 mmHg.

Early complications include the development of LCOS, acute cardiovascular collapse later in the postoperative course, injury to the recurrent laryngeal nerve with resultant vocal chord injury and dysphagia, development of necrotizing enterocolitis, and late arch obstruction secondary to recoarctation.

Sano Modification

Postoperatively, infants recovering after the Sano operation for HLHS appear to have a much simpler management paradigm in the ICU that those recovering after the traditional Norwood operation. Because the aortic to pulmonary artery shunt has been eliminated, balancing the systemic and pulmonary circulations is not necessary. Coronary perfusion is inherently improved as diastolic blood pressure is usually higher in patients without a shunt. Goals in the postoperative period are similar to those of patients with biventricular physiology. Patients typically have an arterial oxygen saturation of 75–85%. Early cyanosis secondary to obstruction in the newly created right ventricular outflow tract can occur.

Hybrid Procedure (see also Chapter 65)

Hybrid palliation of HLHS consists of creating a pathway for unobstructed systemic blood flow by using a metal stent to maintain ductal patency, diminishing the pulmonary blood flow and protecting the pulmonary vascular bed in preparation for a later cavopulmonary artery shunt with the use of bilateral pulmonary artery bands, and performing an atrial septostomy or placing a stent in the atrial septum. The postoperative recovery is quite straightforward. Cardiopulmonary bypass is avoided in the neonatal period. Retrograde arch obstruction resulting in impaired coronary blood flow leading to ventricular dysfunction has been reported in almost 30% of patients undergoing the Hybrid procedure.

Heart Transplantation (see also Chapter 68)

Primary heart transplantation for HLHS is now mostly of historical interest, with few programs offering this as a primary therapy. Transplantation gained popularity in the late 1980s and early 1990s. Survival post transplant was excellent, but about 25% of recipients waiting for transplant died on the transplant list because of the scarcity of donor hearts.

Surgery for Complete Transposition of the Great Arteries

The arterial switch operation (ASO) for infants with complete transposition of the great arteries (D-TGA) was introduced in the early 1980s as an alternative to the atrial switch (Mustard and Senning) operations. The ASO offered an anatomic correction that could be performed early in the neonatal period. This would spare these cyanotic infants the morbidity and mortality associated with waiting for the ASO. For babies with D-TGA with intact ventricular septum or D-TGA with associated VSD, the ASO is now accepted as the procedure of choice.

Timing of Surgery

The timing of the ASO varies depending on the baby's clinical condition. Babies born with an adequate atrial communication may have acceptable levels of oxygenation and can undergo surgery electively in the first few days of life. Those patients who present with more severe degrees of cyanosis should undergo a balloon atrial septostomy, be allowed to stabilize, and then undergo the ASO within a few days. PGE-1 should be used cautiously in patients with D-TGA, especially those who have not undergone a balloon atrial septostomy. PGE-1 infusions in these babies have been associated with closure or restriction at the level of the patent foramen ovale secondary to increased flow and pressure in the left atrium as a consequence of augmented pulmonary blood flow.

Postoperative care of the infant after an ASO is focused on improving left ventricular performance. High doses of inotropic infusions are rarely required. Inotropic support consists of dopamine or low dose epinephrine combined with a systemic arterial dilator such as milrinone. Sodium nitroprusside can be substituted for milrinone. During the period of time that the left ventricle is recovering from the trauma of surgery, we recommend using the maximum amount of systemic vasodilator the infant can tolerate, maintaining mean arterial blood pressure in the 40–50 mmHg range. Prolonged time on the ventilator is unwarranted and patients should be extubated when their hemodynamics permit.

About 10% of patients with D-TGA present in the newborn period with pulmonary artery hypertension (PAH) preoperatively. These patients are usually profoundly cyanotic. Our practice suggests that prompt surgical correction, restoring normal physiology and arterial oxygenation, and then managing postoperative PAH is superior to a preoperative ECMO run while awaiting for the PAH to resolve.

Neonatal Tetralogy of Fallot Repair

Postoperative management of the neonate after tetralogy repair can be challenging. LCOS is not uncommon and is usually secondary to right ventricular dysfunction. In the neonate with a large incision in the right ventricular outflow tract, both systolic and diastolic function can be significantly depressed. A transannular patch across the pulmonary valve annulus will result in severe pulmonary regurgitation, further compromising right ventricular function. Modest amounts of inotropic support are required during the early postoperative period. A milrinone infusion is added for all of the neonates and may have the added advantage of improving right ventricular diastolic function. It is strongly recommended that the surgeon leave the foramen ovale open. This allows right to left shunting and maintains systemic cardiac output as the right ventricle recovers.

Timing of Surgery

We advocate for complete neonatal repair of tetralogy of Fallot in symptomatic patients and only in rare circumstances would we see the need for surgical palliation.

Part VII

Neonatal Formulary

70

Drugs

Enrique Oliver Aregullin[1] *and Anthony F. Rossi*[2]

[1] *Helen DeVos Children's Hospital (Congenital Heart Center CVTS), Grand Rapids, MI, USA*
[2] *Nicklaus Children's Hospital, Miami, FL, USA*

The medication armamentarium available to the clinicians involved in the care of children with heart disease is expanding because survival of patients has lengthened. Patients with pulmonary hypertension secondary to several forms of congenital heart disease can now be effectively managed. Newborns with increased pulmonary blood flow often require long-term use of heart failure anticongestive medications until more definitive interventional or surgical procedures are performed. The use of these medications, particularly inotropic agents and diuretics, has a pivotal role during the postoperative period in the intensive care unit setting. Currently, children are undergoing surgical intervention at an increasingly younger ages, with excellent results aided by advanced anesthetic and postoperative care. However, this has led to cardiac patients with prolonged hospitalizations who often require pain and sedation management strategies according to their underlying condition. A knowledge of the anticoagulation management of critically ill neonates is also very important for

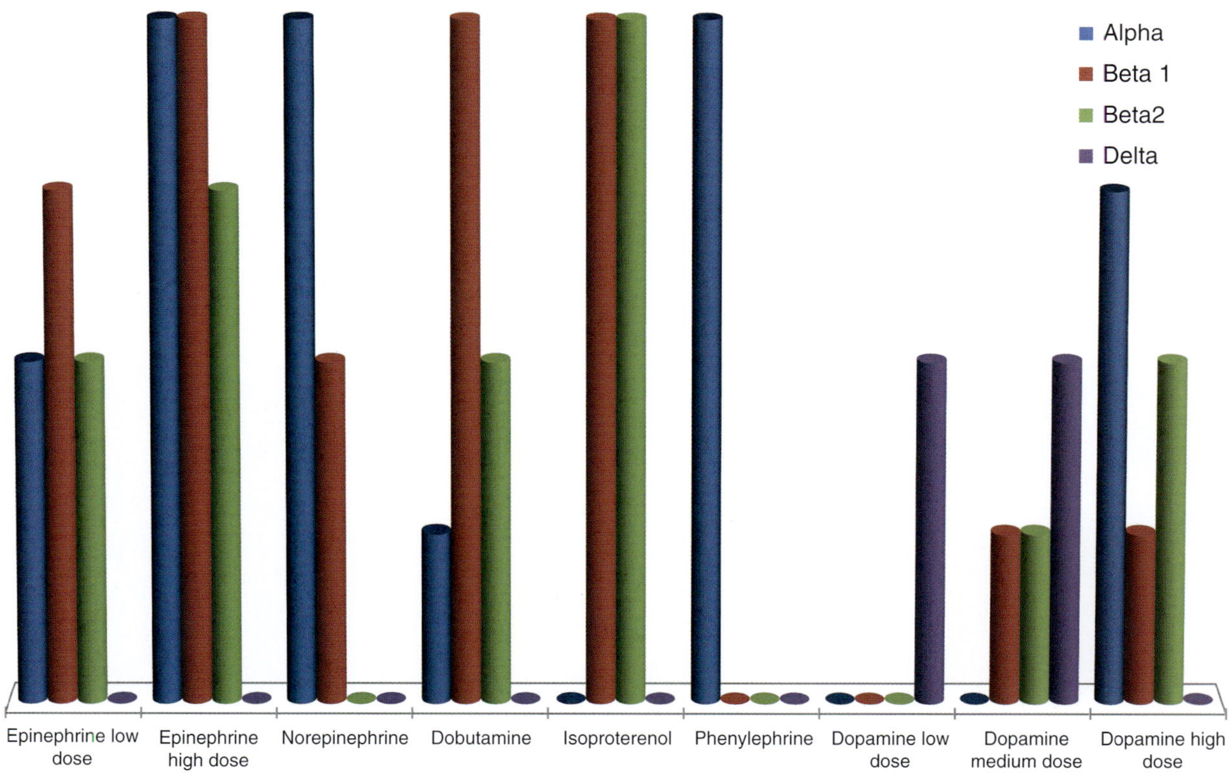

Figure 70.1 Relative effects of catecholamines on receptors.

Visual Guide to Neonatal Cardiology, First Edition. Edited by Ernerio T. Alboliras, Ziyad M. Hijazi, Leo Lopez, and Donald J. Hagler.

Table 70.1 Common medications used in the management of neonates with cardiac conditions.

Low cardiac output					
Drug	Pharmacology	Use	Dose	Side effects	Precautions
Milrinone	Myocardial cAMP Phosphodiesterase inhibitor; lowers both systemic and pulmonary vascular resistance	Low cardiac output, including postoperative	IV Loading dose: 50–75 μg/kg over 15 minutes, continuous infusion of 0.5–0.75 μg/kg/minute	Hypotension, arrhythmia	Avoid use in severe obstructive aortic or pulmonic valvular disease, renal dysfunction
Epinephrine	Dose dependent stimulates alpha 1, beta 1, beta 2 receptors	Low cardiac output, including postoperative, depressed ventricular function, cardiac arrest	IV: 0.01–0.03 mg/kg (0.1–0.3 mL/kg of 1:10,000 solution) every 3–5 min. Continuous infusion of 0.05–2 μg/kg/min	Arrhythmia, hypertension, vasoconstriction, ventricular ectopy	Caution in patients taking MAO inhibitors and TCA
Norepinephrine	Alpha and beta adrenergic receptor agonist resulting in significant vasoconstriction	Shock that persists after adequate fluid volume replacement; cardiogenic shock	Initial: 0.05–0.1 μg/kg/minute, titrate to desired effect; maximum dose: 1–2 μg/kg/minute	Arrhythmias, bradycardia, peripheral ischemia	Volume depletion should be corrected before therapy
Dopamine	Precursor of norepinepherine; dose-dependent stimulation of DA1, DA2, B1, and alpha	Increase cardiac output in shock which persists after adequate fluid volume replacement; low dosage to increase renal perfusion	Continuous IV infusion: 1–20 μg/kg/minute; Low dosage: 1–5 μg/kg/minute, increased renal blood flow Intermediate dosage: 5–15 μg/kg/minute, increased renal blood flow, heart rate, cardiac output High dosage: >15 μg/kg/minute, vasoconstriction, increased blood pressure	Hypertension, tachycardia, vasoconstriction, arrhythmia	Volume depletion should be corrected before therapy
Dobutamine	Stimulates beta 1 adrenergic receptors (minimal beta 2 and alpha), resulting in increase myocardial contractility and heart rate	Management of patients with cardiac decompensation	Continuous IV infusion: 2–20 μg/kg/minute; titrate to desired response	Hypertension, increased ventricular ectopic activity	Hypovolemia should be corrected prior to use
Phenylephrine	Alpha adrenergic receptors agonist resulting in potent vasoconstriction	Hypotension and vascular failure in shock	Continuous IV infusion: 0.1–0.5 μg/kg/minute, titrate to desired effect	Arrhythmia, hypertension, severe peripheral and visceral vasoconstriction	Not a substitute for replacement of blood extravasation; may cause severe necrosis
Vasopressine	Binds to AVPR1 receptors resulting in increased intracellular Ca levels; vasoconstriction	Pulseless arrest, ventricular fibrillation or tachycardia, asystole/pulseless electrical activity; vasodilatory shock unresponsive to fluid resuscitation	Continuous IV infusion: 0.17–10 milliunits/kg/minute (0.01–0.6 units/kg/hour) have been used	Arrhythmia, hypertension, vasoconstriction	Caution in vascular and renal disease

Calcium chloride	Enhances contractility through regulation of action potential	Hypocalcemia; cardiac disturbances of hyperkalemia or hypocalcemia; hypermagnesemia	Cardiac arrest in the presence of hyperkalemia or hypocalcemia, hypermagnesemia, or calcium channel blocker toxicity: IV, IO: 20 mg/kg; may repeat in 10 minutes if necessary; if effective, consider IV infusion of 20–50 mg/kg/hour	Arrhythmia, bradycardia, hypotension, vasodilation, hypercalcemia	Caution in chronic renal failure
Calcium gluconate	Enhances contractility through regulation of action potential	Hypocalcemia cardiac disturbances secondary to hyperkalemia	Cardiac arrest in the presence of hyperkalemia or hypocalcemia, hypermagnesemia, or calcium channel blocker toxicity: Dosage expressed in mg of calcium gluconate: IV, IO: 60–100 mg/kg/dose; may repeat in 10 minutes if necessary; if effective, consider IV infusion	Arrhythmia, bradycardia, hypotension, vasodilation, hypercalcemia	Caution in severe hypokalemia
Digoxin	Inhibition of Na–K pump resulting in increase Ca intracellular influx. Decreases conduction through AV and sinus nodes by inhibiting ATPase	Mild to moderate heart failure; chronic atrial fibrillation. To slow ventricular rate in supraventricular tachyarrhythmias	Heart failure, atrial dysrhythmias: injection, oral solution; loading dose: 1st half initially administered followed by 1/4 of calculated dose q8 × 2 doses Preterm, oral: 20–30 μg\kg. IV: 15–25 μg\kg Full-term neonates, oral: 25–35 μg\kg. IV: 20–30 μg\kg Maintenance dosage, equal divided doses every 12 hours: Preterm neonates, oral 5–7.5 μg\kg. IV 4–6 μg\kg Full-term neonates, oral: 8–10 μg\kg. IV: 5–8 μg\kg	Accelerated junctional rhythm, atrial tachycardia, heart block, PR prolongation	Total digitalizing dose should be decreased by 50% in end-stage renal disease. Caution in patients with an accessory bypass tract during an episode of atrial fibrillation or flutter

Vasodilators and antihypertensives

Drug	Pharmacology	Use	Dose	Side effects	Precautions
Captopril	Angiotensin converting enzyme inhibitor	Hypertension, heart failure, left ventricular dysfunction	Premature neonates: Oral: Initial: 0.01 mg/kg/dose every 8–12 hours; titrate dose Term neonates, PNA ≤7 days: Oral: Initial: 0.01 mg/kg/dose every 8–12 hours; titrate dose Term neonates, PNA >7 days: Oral: Initial: 0.05–0.1 mg/kg/dose every 8–24 hours; titrate dose upward to maximum of 0.5 mg/kg/dose given every 6–24 hours	Angioedema, hypotension, tachycardia, renal failure	Use lower listed initial dose in hyponatremia, hypovolemia

(Continued)

Table 70.1 (Continued)

Drug	Pharmacology	Use	Dose	Side effects	Precautions
Vasodilators and antihypertensives					
Enalapril	Angiotensin converting enzyme inhibitor	Management of mild to severe hypertension, CHF	Oral: Initial: 0.04–0.1 mg/kg/day every 24 hours; titrate to effect as required every few days; maximum dose: 0.27 mg/kg/day	Hypotension, worsening of renal function	Use lower listed initial dose in hyponatremia, hypovolemia
Carvedilol	Alpha and beta antagonist	Mild to severe chronic heart failure; hypertension	Oral: dose not established: initial 0.08 mg/kg/dose BID. Doses had been increased as tolerated q2 wks to a mean maintenance dose of 0.46 mg/kk/dose BID	AV block, bradycardia, edema, hypotension, anaphylactoid reaction	Caution in mild to moderate hepatic impairment; may mask the signs of hypoglycemia
Phenoxybenzamine	Non-specific, long-acting, irreversible alpha adrenergic antagonist-potent peripheral vasodilator	Hypertension. Has been used in the management of HLHS	Oral, initial: 0.2 mg/kg once daily; maximum dose: 10 mg/dose; increase every 4 days by 0.2 mg/kg/day increments; usual maintenance dose: 0.4–1.2 mg/kg/day every 6–8 hours; maximum doses of up to 2–4 mg/kg/day have been recommended	Hypotension, tachycardia	Use with caution in renal dysfunction
Nitroprusside	Peripheral vasodilator	Management of hypertensive crises; used for controlled hypotension	Continuous IV infusion: start 0.3–0.5 µg/kg/minute, titrate to effect; maximum dose: 8–10 µg/kg/minute	Bradycardia, ECG changes, hypotension, tachycardia. Cyanide toxicity	Caution in severe renal impairment, increased intracranial pressure

Drug	Pharmacology	Use	Dose	Side effects	Precautions
Antiarrhythmics					
Adenosine	Slows conduction time through the A-V node.	Paroxysmal supraventricular tachycardia, including that associated with accessory bypass tracts (e.g., WPW)	Paroxysmal supraventricular tachycardia: Rapid IV: Initial dose: 0.05–0.1 mg/kg; if not effective within 1–2 minutes, increase dose by 0.05–0.1 mg/kg increments every 1–2 minutes to a maximum single dose of 0.3 mg/kg	AV block, hypotension, ST segment depression, transient new arrhythmia	Caution in underlying dysfunction of sinus or A-V node, cardiac postoperative patients
Amiodarone	Class III, inhibits alpha and beta adrenergic receptors, prolongs action potential and refractoriness	Oral: Management of life-threatening recurrent ventricular arrhythmias IV: Management and prophylaxis of recurrent VF and unstable VT. Supraventricular arrhythmias	SVT: Oral: Loading dose: 10–20 mg/kg/day in 2 divided doses for 7–10 days; dosage should then be reduced to 5–10 mg/kg/day once daily IV: Loading dose: 5 mg/kg given over 60 minutes; may repeat initial loading dose to a maximum total initial load: 10 mg/kg; do not exceed total daily bolus of 15 mg/kg/day	AV block, bradycardia, arrhythmia, hypotension, hyperthyroidism, hypothyroidism, pulmonary fibrosis, optic neuritis	Bolus infusion rates of 60 minutes to avoid hypotension

Atenolol	Class II antiarrhythmic agent, long- acting selective beta blocker	Supraventricular and ventricular arrhythmias; hypertension	Initial, Oral: 0.5–1 mg/kg/day given once daily or divided in 2 doses per day; titrate dose to effect; usual range: 0.5–1.5 mg/kg/day; maximum dose: 2 mg/kg/day; do not exceed 100 mg/day	Edema, hypotension, bradycardia,second- or third-degree AV block	Caution in renal impairment, bronchospasm, and hyperthyroidism
Esmolol	Class II Selective beta 1 blocker	Supraventricular tachycardia, perioperative tachycardia, and hypertension	Term neonates: PNA 0–7 days: Initial: 50 μg/kg/minute; titrate dose by 25–50 μg/kg/minute every 20 minutes Term neonates: PNA 8–28 days: Initial: 75 μg/kg/minute; titrate dose by 50 μg/kg/minute every 20 minutes Maximum dose: 1000 μg/kg/minute	Hypotension, peripheral ischemia	Caution in hyper-reactive airway disease
Flecainide	Class Ic antiarrhythmic agent, sodium channel blocker, cell membrane depression	Life-threatening ventricular arrhythmias, symptomatic supraventricular tachycardias	Oral: Supraventricular tachycardia: Initial: 2 mg/kg/day every 12 hours; titrate to clinical response	Edema, proarrhythmic, sinus node dysfunction	Caution in sick sinus syndrome, myocardial dysfunction
Lidocaine	Class Ib antiarrhythmic agent, sodium channel blocker, local anesthetic depressing myocardial irritability	Ventricular arrhythmias; PALS guidelines recommend lidocaine when amiodarone is not available for cardiac arrest with pulseless VT or VF	Antiarrhythmic: Ventricular tachycardia, ventricular fibrillation : IV, IO: Loading dose: 1 mg/kg/dose; follow with continuous infusion; may repeat bolus; Continuous IV infusion: 20–50 μg/kg/minute; use lower dose for neonates with shock, hepatic disease, cardiac arrest, or CHF	Arrhythmia, bradycardia, heart block, hypotension, seizure	Hepatic dysfumction should receive 1/2 the usual loading dose
Propranolol	Beta-blocker, class II anti-dysrhythmic agent	Oral: Management of hypertension, tetralogy of Fallot cyanotic spells IV: Supraventricular arrhythmias, ventricular tachycardias	Oral: Initial: 0.25 mg/kg/dose every 6–8 hours; increase slowly as needed to maximum of 5 mg/kg/day IV: Initial: 0.01 mg/kg slow IV push over 10 minutes; may repeat every 6–8 hours as needed; increase slowly to maximum of 0.15 mg/kg/dose every 6–8 hours	Bradycardia, hypotension, impaired myocardial contractility, bronchospasm	May block hypoglycemia-induced tachycardia
Sotalol	Combined b adrenergic blocking and class III antiarrhythmic	Treatment of life-threatening ventricular arrhythmias. Maintenance of sinus rhythm in symptomatic atrial fibrillation and atrial flutter	Oral: 2 mg/kg/day divided every 8 hours; if needed, increase dosage gradually by 1–2 mg/kg/day increments	Bradycardia, hypotension, proarrhythmia, QTc interval prolongation	Baseline QTc interval must be determined prior to initiation

(Continued)

Table 70.1 (Continued)

Ductal management

Drug	Pharmacology	Use	Dose	Side effects	Precautions
Ibuprofen	Non-steroidal anti-inflammatory agent Prostaglandin synthesis inhibitor	Closure of PDA	IV: Treatment of PDA: Initial dose: 10 mg/kg, followed by two doses of 5 mg/kg at 24 and 48 hours after the initial dose	Edema, renal failure, aplastic anemia, erythema multiforme, GI hemorrhage	Caution in decreased hepatic function and coagulation disorders
Indomethacin	Prostaglandin synthesis inhibitor	Closure of PDA	IV: PDA, treatment: Initial: 0.2 mg/kg/dose, followed by 2 doses depending on postnatal age (PNA): PNA at time of first dose <48 hours: 0.1 mg/kg at 12- to 24-hour intervals PNA at time of first dose 2–7 days: 0.2 mg/kg at 12- to 24-hour intervals PNA at time of first dose >7 days: 0.25 mg/kg at 12- to 24-hour intervals	Edema, renal failure, aplastic anemia, erythema multiforme, GI hemorrhage	Caution in cardiac dysfunction, hypertension, renal impairment, coagulation disorders
Prostaglandin E1	Direct effect on vascular smooth muscles causing pulmonary, systemic, and ductus arteriosus vasodilatation	Maintenance of patency of ductus arteriosus	Continuous IV infusion: 0.05–0.1 μg/kg/minute	Bradycardia, hypotension, tachycardia, fever, apnea	If hypotension or fever, the infusion rate should be reduced

Anticoagulation

Drug	Pharmacology	Use	Dose	Side Effects	Precautions
Acetylsalicylic acid (Aspirin)	Inhibits prostaglandin synthesis and formation of platelet aggregating thromboxane A2	Antiplatelet, anti-inflamatory	Oral: Full-term neonate: Antiplatelet effects: 1–5 mg/kg/dose once daily	Anemia, coagulopathy, thrombocytopenia. Gastrointestinal ulceration, interstitial nephritis	Caution in renal impairment and coagulopathy
Clopidrogel	Irreversibly modifies ADP platelet receptor thereby inhibiting ADP-dependent platelet aggregation	Antiplatelet, antiinflamatory	Oral: Safety and efficacy have not been established in neonatal patients: 0.2 mg/kg/dose once daily	Anemia, coagulopathy, thrombocytopenia. Gastrointestinal ulceration, interstitial nephritis	Caution in platelet disorders, coagulopathy, or hepatic impairment
Heparin (unfractionated heparin)	Potentiates antithrombin III which inactivates clotting factors XIIa, XIa, IXa, Xa, IIa and prevents the conversion of fibrinogen to fibrin	Prophylaxis and treatment of thromboembolic disorders	IV infusion: Initial loading dose: 75 units/kg given over 10 minutes; then initial maintenance dose: 28 units/kg/hour; adjust dose to maintain APTT of 60–85 seconds	Bleeding, immunologically mediated heparin-induced thrombocytopenia	Caution in coagulopathy, renal and liver dysfunction

Enoxaparin	Potentiate the effect of antithrombin III and inactivates coagulation factor Xa and IIa	Prophylaxis and treatment of thromboembolic disorders	Subcutaneous: Prophylaxis: 0.75 mg/kg/dose every 12 hours Treatment: 1.5 mg/kg/dose every 12 hours.	Bleeding is the major adverse effect	Caution in coagulopathy, renal and liver dysfunction
Warfarin	Inhibits hepatic synthesis of vitamin K-dependent factors (II, VII, IX, X)	Prophylaxis and treatment of thromboembolic disorders and thromboembolic complications in prosthetic heart valves or atrial fibrillation	Oral: loading dose: 0.2 mg/kg. Subsequent doses are dependent upon patient's INR. Usual maintenance dose: ~0.1 mg/kg/day	Bleeding is the major adverse effect	Close monitoring for drug–drug and drug–dietary interactions

Diuretics

Drug	Pharmacology	Use	Dose	Side Effects	Precautions
Acetazolamide	Carbonic anhydrase inhibitor, diuretic	Diuretic. Bicarbonaturia produces metabolic acidosis	Oral, IV: 5 mg/kg/dose. Daily. Maximum single dose = 375 mg	Hypokalemia, acidosis, renal calculi	Caution in respiratory acidosis, renal impairment
Bumetanide	Loop diuretic, prevent re-absorption of Cl at ascending loop of Henle	Edema secondary to heart failure or renal disease	Oral, IM, IV: 0.01–0.05 mg/kg/dose every 12–24 hours	Hypotension, hypokalemia, hyponatremia, hypochloremia, metabolic alkalosis	Sulfonamide hypersensitivity
Chlorothiazide	Inhibits renal tubular reabsorption of Na at distal tubule	Edema secondary to heart failure or renal disease. Hypertension	Oral: 20–40 mg/kg/day in 2 divided doses IV: 5–10 mg/kg/day in 2 divided doses; doses up to 20 mg/kg/day have been used	Hypokalemia, hypochloremia, alkalosis, hypotension	Sulfonamide hypersensitivity
Ethacrynic acid	Potent loop diuretic, prevent re-absorption of Cl at ascending loop of Henle	Edema secondary to CHF or renal disease; hypertension	Oral: 1 mg/kg/dose once daily, increase at intervals of 2–3 days to a maximum of 3 mg/kg/day IV: 1 mg/kg/dose; repeat doses are not routinely recommended, however if indicated, repeat doses every 8–12 hours	Hypovolemia, hypokalemia, hypochloremic alkalosis, hypotension, hyponatremia, ototoxic	Avoid in severe renal dysfunction
Furosemide	Loop diuretic, prevent re-absorption of Cl at ascending loop of Henle	Edema secondary to CHF or renal disease; hypertension	Oral: 1 mg/kg/dose 1–2 times/day. IV: 1–2 mg/kg/dose every 12–24 hours Continuous IV infusion: 0.2 mg/kg/hour, increase in 0.1 mg/kg/hour; maximum infusion rate 0.4 mg/kg/hour	Hypovolemia, hypokalemia, hypochloremia, hypochloremic metabolic alkalosis	Prolonged use may cause nephrocalcinosis
Metolazone	Blocks sodium re-absorption at distal renal tubules	Edema in CHF, and impaired renal function; hypertension	Oral: 0.2–0.4 mg/kg/day divided every 12–24 hours	Hepatic dysfunction, calcium retention, hypokalemia, hypochloremic metabolic alkalosis,	Hepatic disease, sulfonamide cross-sensitivity

(Continued)

Table 70.1 (Continued)

Diuretics					
Drug	**Pharmacology**	**Use**	**Dose**	**Side effects**	**Precautions**
Spironolactone	Aldosterone blocker	Potassium-sparing diuretic. Edema in CHF, and impaired renal function; hypertension	Oral: Diuretic: 1–3 mg/kg/day divided every 12–24 hours	Potassium retention, gynecomastia, hyperchloremic metabolic acidosis	Hyperkalemia when used with other potassium sparing drugs
Pulmonary Medications					
Drug	**Pharmacology**	**Use**	**Dose**	**Side Effects**	**Precautions**
Bosentan	Endothelin receptor antagonist	Treatment of pulmonary arterial hypertension	Oral: 1 mg/kg/dose twice daily short-term use (2–16 days)	Significant hepatic dysfunction	Caution in anemia; may cause edema
Epoprostenol	IV: Direct vasodilator of systemic and pulmonary arterial vascular beds; Inhaled: Direct vasodilator of pulmonary vascular bed.	Treatment of pulmonary arterial hypertension	Expressed in nanograms (ng)/kg/minute. Continuous IV infusion: 2 ng/kg/minute slowly titrated to 20 ng/kg/minute Doses as high as 60 ng/kg/minute have been used Inhalation: 5 ng/kg/min by continuous inhalation increase by 1–2 ng/kg/min q15 min	Hypotension, tachycardia	Abrupt withdrawal can result in rebound pulmonary hypertension
Nitric oxide	Direct vasodilator of pulmonary arterial vascular bed increases cyclic guanosine monophosphate leading to decreased intracellular calcium and subsequent smooth muscle relaxation	Treatment of hypoxic respiratory failure with pulmonary hypertension	Inhalation: 10–40 ppm	Methemoglobinemia, acute lung injury (oxidative product NO2)	Doses of INO > 20 ppm do not appear to be more effective in improving oxygenation and are associated with increased adverse effects
Sildenafil	Inhibits phosphodiesterase 5 increasing cGMP; vasodilator pulmonary vascular bed	Persistent pulmonary hypertension of the newborn refractory to treatment with inhaled nitric oxide; facilitation of weaning from nitric oxide; pulmonary hypertension following cardiac surgery	Oral: 0.5–3 mg/kg/dose every 6–12 hours IV: GA >34 weeks and PNA <72 hours: PPHN: 0.4 mg/kg loading dose administered over 3 hours followed by continuous infusion of 1.6 mg/kg/day	Hypotension, arrhythmias, hypertonia	The FDA recommends against the use of sildenafil for treatment of PAH in children and adolescents; the mortality risk of long-term use in neonates is unknown
Sedative, Analgesics, Muscle relaxants					
Drug	**Pharmacology**	**Use**	**Dose**	**Side Effects**	**Precautions**
Chloral hydrate	CNS depressant	Short-term sedative and hypnotic prior to non-painful therapeutic or diagnostic procedures	Oral, rectal: 25 mg/kg/dose for sedation prior to a procedure	GI irritation, laryngospasm if aspirated Myocardial and respiratory depressant	Drug and metabolites can accumulate with repeated use

Clonidine	Central alpha-2-adrenergic agonist	Neonatal abstinence syndrome, management of hypertension	Neonatal abstinence syndrome (opioid withdrawal): Limited information: Oral: 0.5–1 μg/kg/dose every 4–6 hours	Dry mouth, arrhythmia, hypotension	Do not discontinue abruptly
Dexmedeto-midine	Selective alpha-2-adrenoceptor agonist	Sedation of mechanically ventilated patients in an intensive care setting. Studies have shown neuroprotective and antiarrhythmic properties	IV continous infusion: Loading dose: 0.5–1 μg/kg; followed by a maintenance infusion of 0.2–0.75 μg/kg/hour, doses as high as 1 μg/kg/hour have been used	Bradycardia, respiratory depression, nausea	Caution in heart block, severe ventricular dysfunction, hypovolemia
Etomidate	Non-barbiturate hypnotic through enhanced GABA at the limbic system	Sedation for short procedures in the setting of diminished cardiovascular function	IV: 0.1–0.3 mg/kg	Myoclonus	Caution in renal and hepatic failure
Fentanyl	Semisynthetic opiate analgesic	Sedation; relief of pain; preoperative medication; adjunct to general anesthesia	IV: 1–4 μg/kg/dose; may repeat every 2–4 hours Continuous I.V. infusion: 1–5 μg/kg/hour	Respiratory depression, chest wall rigidity	Caution in bradycardia, hepatic, renal disease, increased ICP
Ketamine	Dissociative anesthesia by direct action on the cortex and limbic system	Anesthesia, short surgical procedures; has been used for rapid sequence intubation	IV: Limited data available; dose not established: 0.5–2 mg/kg/dose, every 2 hrs PRN	Hypertension, tachycardia, respiratory depression, laryngospasm, hypersalivation	Caution in elevated ICP
Ketorolac	NSAID, inhibits cyclooxygenase. Centrally by triggering the release of endogenous opoids	Short-term management moderate to severe acute pain	IV: Dose not established; limited data available: 0.5 mg/kg/dose every 8 hours for up to 1–2 days	GI bleeding, impaired platelet aggregation, acute renal failure	Use with caution in hepatic or renal failure
Lorazepam	CNS depression through enhanced GABA at limbic system	Management of anxiety, preoperative sedation	IV, IM, PO: 0.05–0.1 mg/kg (max = 4 mg/ dose) every 4–8 hr PRN	Respiratory depression, hypotension, bradycardia, dependence	Care should be observed in the postoperative cardiac surgical patient, and with hemodynamic instability
Midazolam	CNS depression by inducing GABA at limbic system	Preprocedure sedation, anxiolysis, continuous IV sedation of mechanically ventilated patients	IV 0.05–0.1 mg/kg max 2.5 mg PRN IN 0.2 mg/kg PRN PO 0.3–0.75 mg/kg PRN IM 0.1–0.2 mg/kg PRN PR 0.5–1 mg/kg Continuous infusion IV: 0.03–0.1 mg/kg/hour	Respiratory depression, hypotension, bradycardia, myclonic jerking	Caution in heart failure, renal, hepatic dysfunction
Morphine sulfate	Strongest narcotic analgesic	Management of severe acute pain; aid with TOF spells	Oral: Oral solution: 0.08 mg/kg/dose every 4–6 hours, maximum dose: 0.2 mg/kg/dose for neonatal abstinence IM, IV, SC: 0.05–0.1 mg/kg/dose every 4–6 hours	Physical dependence, CNS and respiratory depression, bronchospam	Caution in biliary tract disease or acute pancreatitis
Rocuronium	Post-synaptic Acetylcholine receptor blocker	Facilitate endotracheal intubation and provide skeletal muscle relaxation during mechanical ventilation	IV: 0.6–1.2 mg/kg (1–1.2 mg/kg for rapid sequence induction) PRN Continous IV infusion: Infusion 0.5–1 mg/kg/h	Hypotension, arrhythmia, bronchospasm	Caution in hepatic impairment, neuromuscular disease

Table 70.2 Receptor locations and targets of vasoactive agents.

Target	Receptor location	Main actions
Alpha adrenergic	Arterioles	Vasoconstriction Increased afterload Bradycardia (baroflex) Increased cerebral blood flow Decreased renal and hepatosplenic perfusion
Beta adrenergic	Myocardium Conduction system Myocardial and skeletal muscle arterioles	Inotropic effect Chronotropic effect Vasodilatation Increased hepatosplenic perfusion
Alpha 1 receptors	Arterioles	Vasoconstriction
Alpha 2 receptors	Arterioles: coronary and renal	Vasoconstriction
Beta 1	Myocardium Conduction system Myocardial and skeletal muscle arterioles	Chronotropic effect Inotropic effect Vasodilatation
Beta 2	Myocardium Conduction system Myocardial and skeletal muscle arterioles	Chronotropic effect Inotropic effect Vasodilatation
D1	D1 Postsynaptic receptor in peripheral vasculature Vasodilatation	Vasodilatation
D2	D2 Presynaptic receptor in peripheral vasculature Vasodilatation	Vasodilatation

the caregiver. Advances in care have included management with Food and Drug Administration approved medications, as well as many "off-label "drugs. This chapter reviews selected medications currently used for treatment of perioperative low cardiac output, congestive heart failure, pulmonary hypertension, sedation, pain, and anticoagulation in neonates (Tables 70.1 and 70.2; Figure 70.1).

Further Reading

Severin PN, Awad S, Shields B, *et al.* (2013) The Pediatric Cardiology Pharmacopeia: 2013 Update. *Pediatr Cardiol*, **34**, 1–29.

Taketomo CK, Hodding JH, Kraus DM. (2012) *Pediatric and Neonatal Dosage Handbook*, 19th edn, Lexi-Comp, Hudson, OH.

71

Nutrition

Nicole Sutton

Albert Einsein College of Medicine; Children's Hospital at Montefiore, Bronx, NY, USA

Nutrition is a vital consideration in children with heart disease. Congenital heart disease (CHD) and heart failure can cause malnutrition, and there is evidence that malnutrition can delay or complicate corrective surgery. Congenital heart surgery can cause metabolic and nutritional changes, so that mitigating the stress response to surgery and optimizing the nutritional status of a postoperative patient can lead to better outcomes.

Stress Response to Surgery or Shock

With hypoperfusion, the metabolic rate decreases. When perfusion is restored, the metabolic state becomes hypermetabolic and this can last for days to weeks. The hypermetabolic state starts with a catabolic state and then becomes anabolic. A prolonged stress response leads to a prolonged and irreversible catabolic state [1]. In this catabolic state, there is release of mediators of the stress response including endocrine mediators and pro-inflammatory cytokines, such as tumor necrosis factor α, and interleukin 6 (IL-6). High levels of IL-6 and low levels of insulin-like growth factor-1 have been associated with hyper-metabolism and increased morbidity and mortality in critically ill infants [2]. Cardiac output increases, peripheral vascular resistance decreases, capillaries leak, ventilation and carbon dioxide production increase, the hepatic synthesis of procoagulants increase, and the production of albumin decreases. Gluconeogenesis from the breakdown of smooth and skeletal muscle and lipolysis fuels this process. The nervous system controls this process, and there is evidence that adequate analgesia attenuates this stress response [1]. Protein turnover in children is increased in even mild stress and outstrips new protein synthesis [3]; this is correlated with the severity of illness [4].

The normal newborn's metabolic balance is delicate. The newborn only has modest stores of carbohydrates, protein, and fat, and is therefore poorly prepared to deal with the severe metabolic demands of critical illness or surgery. During cardiac surgery there is a surge of epinephrine that leads to increased lipolysis and glucagon release. These effects are mitigated by the use of high dose narcotics. Controlling the stress response through surgery or critical illness decreases catabolism and improves outcomes, including mortality [5–7].

Metabolic Needs in Uncorrected CHD

The neonate with uncorrected CHD has an increased metabolic need when compared to a normal neonate. Studies have shown varying rates of growth failure in children with unrepaired CHD. Studies have tried to correlate these finding with the presence or absence of cyanosis, heart failure, pulmonary hypertension, or the type of shunting (right to left or left to right) but these correlations have not been found, and it seems most likely that it is the degree of cardiovascular compromise that is related to the failure to thrive and poor weight gain [8]. The poor weight gain of the neonate with CHD appears to be multifactorial. Many children with CHD have chromosomal anomalies associated with poor growth and/or feeding difficulties. In addition, they can be hypermetabolic. They can also have malabsorption or inadequate oral intake because of breathlessness and fatigue.

In a study of children who underwent a biventricular repair at 5 days, excluding patients with facial, gastrointestinal, neurologic abnormalities, chromosomal anomalies, or birth weight less than 2500 g, the median weight for age z score (WAZ) at surgery was −0.2, and by discharge it had dropped to −1.2. Delayed postoperative nutrition and reintubation following initial postoperative extubation were significantly and independently associated with decrease in WAZ. The length of stay was also correlated with worse average daily weight gain. There was also a trend towards association between lack of intake preoperatively and poor postoperative growth [9].

The Pediatric Heart Network Infant Single Ventricle Trial was a randomized placebo controlled trial of

Visual Guide to Neonatal Cardiology, First Edition. Edited by Ernerio T. Alboliras, Ziyad M. Hijazi, Leo Lopez, and Donald J. Hagler.

the angiotensin-converting enzyme (ACE) inhibitor enalapril in infants with single ventricle physiology. A total of 1245 neonates were screened for entry to the trial: 16% were born prematurely vs. 12% in normal neonates; 18% had low birth weight <2.5 kg vs. 8% in normal neonates; 22% were small for gestational age vs. 10% in the control population; and 8% had a genetic syndrome. Some 49% had hypoplastic left heart syndrome (HLHS), but there was no difference in the size of patients with HLHS and those with other single ventricles physiologies [10]. The primary outcome of the trial was the WAZ at 14 months of age. The trial showed that there was no growth benefit for children treated with enalapril. Serial growth data were systematically collected. The trial excluded patients born <35 weeks, small for gestational age (<10th percentile), and patients with chromosomal anomalies. Average WAZ decreased from birth to study enrollment from −0.15 to −1.27. HLHS was not a risk factor for poor growth compared with other forms of single ventricle physiology. From data after the Glenn operation, earlier age at the Glenn and greater daily caloric intake were associated with better growth [11]. In addition, the study found that lower height z scores in early infancy were associated with neurodevelopmental disability [12].

Further studies have shown that not only is there weight loss between the first and second stage palliations for single ventricles, but also that this is associated with poor outcomes from the Glenn operation. A study by Anderson *et al.* [13] looked at 100 infants with single ventricles that underwent the Glenn operation at their institution. They found a decrease in the WAZ from birth to the admission for the Glenn operation, from −0.04 to −1.3. Postoperative hospital stays were longer for the patients with lower WAZ at the time of the surgery, younger age, and having an arch reconstruction. In addition, it has been reported that lower WAZ at the time of the Fontan operation is associated with an increased risk of infection and a longer hospital stay [14].

Feeding

For full-term and preterm infants, the recommended feedings should be with breast milk if available. The Global Neonatal Consensus Symposium on feeding the preterm infant stresses the importance of aggressive enteral and parental nutrition immediately after birth to prevent the development of nutritional deficiencies, improve growth and neurodevelopmental outcomes in the long term [15]. In general, oral feeds should be started shortly after birth to promote oral skills as in patients without CHD if the patients are clinically stable.

The benefits of enteral feeding for neonates are well known, but the risks of feeding neonates with CHD, especially prostaglandin-dependent neonates, are not clear and studies have shown a wide variation in hospital practice, with providers outside of the USA more likely to feed patients on prostaglandin (PGE) with or without umbilical arterial catheter (UAC) lines [16]. Recent studies have shown that it is safe to feed preoperative neonates on PGE enterally even with a UAC or umbilical venous catheter (UVC) [17, 18].

Studies have looked at differences in the style of Norwood Stage I and its relation to gastrointestinal complications and growth. There were no differences in interstage weight gain, necrotizing enterocolitis (NEC), or feeding intolerance between the patients with a Blalock–Taussig shunt (BTS) or a Sano shunt [19]. In addition, patients with Norwood Stage I operations have been compared with patients who have undergone Hybrid Stage I operations, and both have increased incidences of vocal cord palsy with abnormal oral feeding evaluations (70% abnormal) and barium swallow studies (81% abnormal), and an inability to feed orally at hospital discharge [20]. In studies in which patients undergo routine postoperative fiberoptic endoscopic evaluation of swallowing and vocal cord function after Norwood operation, there is a high incidence of vocal cord dysfunction (23%), but this seems to be somewhat dependent on the style of the aortic arch dissection and can be decreased with different surgical arch reconstruction techniques [21]. Vocal cord and swallowing difficulties often lead to gastrostomy tube (GT) placement. Some centers have advocated routine GT placement in patients with HLHS. This was thought to decrease length of stay, improve interstage growth, and increase survival to bidirectional Glenn operation. Studies have not shown a relationship to shorter hospitalization or to better interstage growth, but one study did show better survival to Glenn [22]. Studies have shown that nasogastric tubes (NGT) are safe to use in patients with a single ventricle [23] in the interstage period. About 30–50% of patients are able to eat orally on discharge. Full oral intake seems to be related to the time between surgery and the first oral intake, the amount taken with the first feeding, as well as longer cross-clamp time, longer ventilator time, and genetic anomalies [24]. The mode of feeding does not lead to significantly different average daily weight gains in the interstage period, and patients who are only on oral feeds may stop gaining weight sooner than the patients who are tube fed (NGT or GT) [25].

Studies have also shown that the use of an enteral feeding protocol in postoperative patients with HLHS decreases the time to full feeds, the length of stay in the hospital, and the incidence of NEC when compared with prior time periods not using a protocol [26, 27].

In 2003, the Joint Council on Congenital Heart Disease (JCCHD) was formed to increase communication between societies that represent pediatric cardiologists, congenital cardiac surgeons, and adult congenital heart disease specialists, such as the American College of

Cardiology, American Heart Association, American Academy of Pediatrics, American Board of Pediatrics, Congenital Heart Surgery Society, and so on. They developed a quality improvement (QI) project to allow pediatric cardiologists to satisfy the ABP requirements for recertification that would focus on significantly improving the outcome of care for children with congenital heart disease. The task force chose to focus on children with HLHS during the interstage period with the goal of improving the quality of life and decreasing the mortality between Norwood operation and the bidirectional Glenn operation. They defined three key drivers, one of which was optimizing nutritional status [28]. This was based on studies showing that interstage monitoring of weight and saturations after the Norwood operation improved interstage mortality [29, 30]. The home monitoring programs are now part of the interstage care in the centers participating in the JCCHDQI collaborative. In the home monitoring programs, parents are instructed on how to feed patients (i.e. what type of feeds, NGT, GT, or oral; how many calories; what volume, and how often) and record daily weights and saturations. They are instructed in "red flags" for which they should call their cardiologist, which include weight loss >30 g/day, failure to gain at least 100 g in 3 days, or poor intake, changes in saturation, and so on. These trigger an outpatient visit to look for a treatable problem.

A recent study [31] looked at 148 patients at one center in an interstage monitoring program after Stage I that showed improved growth velocity during the interstage period with an average of 26 ± 8 g/day. In addition, even though there was a decrease on the WAZ from birth (−0.4 ± 0.9) to hospital discharge from Stage I (−1.3 ± 0.9), there was an improvement during the interstage period to the time of the bidirectional Glenn operation (−0.9 ± 1). The JCCHD QI collaborative has recently reported the growth of 132 infants from 16 different sites. They found that sites that used a specific feeding protocol after the Stage I prior to discharge, and that monitored for specific red flag criteria related to growth in the interstage period had significantly better growth than those that did not [32]. They defined growth failure as less than 20 g/day weight gain and/or a decrease >2 major weight for length percentiles [33].

The JCCHDQI put together a Feeding Working Group to make recommendations for feeding patients with HLHS from birth to the bidirectional Glenn operation [34]. They reviewed the literature as well as feeding practices in in the collaborative. In the preoperative stage, they recommend starting total parenteral nutrition (TPN) early, and enteral feeding in patients who are hemodynamically stable. Enteral feeds are started with breast milk if available, and can be performed with UAC or PGE. Postoperatively, they recommend that enteral feeding should be started as early as possible when the patient is hemodynamically stable. Oral feeding should be initiated following a feeding evaluation. In the interstage period, they recommend close monitoring of weight gain. When growth failure is identified, changes in nutritional management should be made, and a dietitian should be involved in assessment and management of growth in each visit in the interstage period and, as needed, the use of red flags associated with feeding.

Our center joined the JCCHDQI Collaborative in 2009, and as part of our ongoing QI projects we have developed our own feeding protocols using the above reference papers, and updating them as new data have come to light. We currently use these feeding protocols for all neonates with CHD. The first protocol was developed for intubated patients (Figure 71.1). We use this protocol for all neonates >36 weeks, >2 kg, without a history of NEC or other gastrointestinal abnormalities. The patient should have evidence of stable cardiac output (i.e., stable vital signs and good peripheral perfusion). We start with NGT feeds when intubated, and switch to nasoduodenal tube (NDT) only if there are significant issues with vomiting or reflux. We feed with a UAC or UVC in place, and on PGE. Feeding can be started and/or advanced on milrinone, dopamine, dobutamine, and epinephrine ≤0.02 μg/kg/min. We do not feed enterally on epinephrine >0.02 μg/kg/min, vasopressin or norepinephrine at any dose. We discuss whether to start feeds every day on rounds, and when the patient is thought to be ready to start feeds we discuss the goal feeds, which are generally a volume of 6 mL/kg/hour and calories of 120–150 kcal/kg/day. Feeds are started with expressed breast milk or 20 calorie house formula. The abdominal girth and feeding tube position are documented prior to starting feeds. Feeds are stated at 1 mL/kg/hr for 4 hours. If there is abdominal distention, vomiting, nausea, or diarrhea, feeds are held for 1 hour, and then restarted at 1 mL/kg/hour for 4 hours. If there is no abdominal distention, vomiting, nausea, or diarrhea, feeds are increased to 2 mL/kg/hour. There is a stepwise progression in the feeding volume until the goal volume of feeds. After the goal volume is achieved and tolerated for 24 hours, the calories are increased from 20 to 24, to 27, and up to 30 calories daily as needed to reach the goal calories/kg/day. When the goal calories are achieved, the feeds are compressed to 2 hours, 1.5 hours, 1 hour, and 30 minutes. The TPN should be decreased for the enteral feeding after the patient is tolerating 2 mL/kg/hr.

We also developed guidelines for patients that are extubated (Figure 71.2). We do not start oral feeds in patients that are on continuous positive airway pressure (CPAP), bilevel positive airway pressure (BiPAP), high flow nasal cannula (NC), or NC ≥3 L; instead, we continue to use the intubated protocol with NGT or NDT feeds until infants are off respiratory support. We then determine if the patients are high or low risk or oral feeding. High risk is defined as intubated >5 days, aortic arch surgery (HLHS, interrupted arch repair,

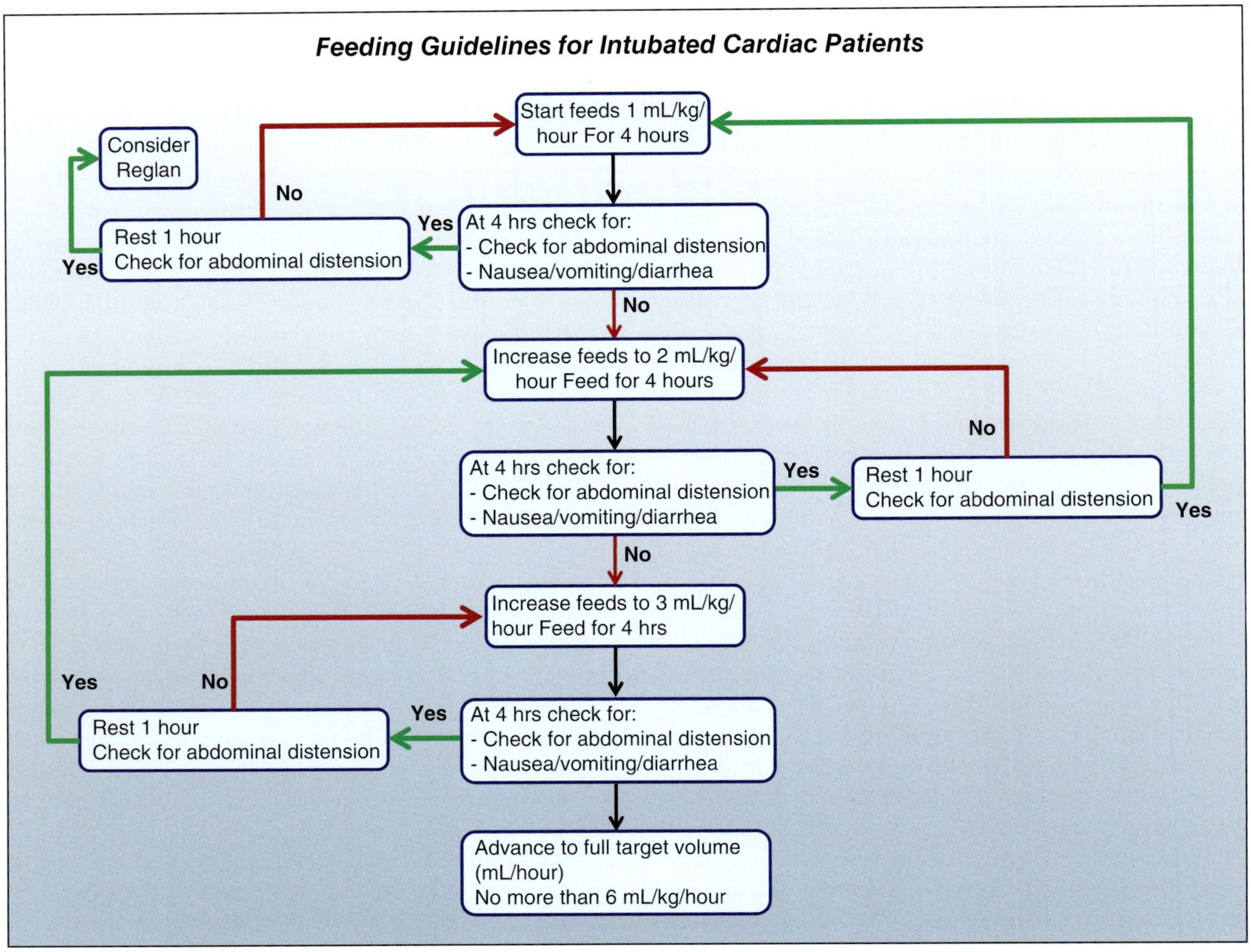

Figure 71.1 Feeding guidelines for intubated cardiac patients. CPAP, continuous positive airway pressure; BiPAP, bilevel positive airway pressure; HLHS, hypoplastic left heart syndrome; NC, nasal cannula; NDT, nasoduodenal tube; NGT, nasogastric tube; PO, oral (per os); WOB, work of breathing.

hypoplastic arch repairs, but not coarctation repairs), history of aspiration and/or dysphagia, and patients who did not tolerate NDT feeds. Low-risk patients are defined as patients who do not meet any of the high-risk criteria, extubated within 72 hours, tolerating current feeds, and/or successfully orally fed prior to surgery. High-risk patients are not fed orally until they are seen for swallowing and feeding disorders and undergo a full evaluation to see if it safe to feed them orally. After this evaluation, feeding should be performed as per their recommendations. The low-risk patients are assessed for increased work of breathing (WOB), increased respiratory rate, and/or hoarse voice/cry prior to starting feeds orally. If they have any of these symptoms, they should also be evaluated for swallowing and feeding disorders prior to oral feeding. If they do not have any of these signs, they are allowed to eat orally. They are fed for 20–30 minutes and observed to evaluate oral effort, energy effort, reflux symptoms, desaturations with feeds, and WOB to determine if they are successful oral feeders. If they are successful, the goal oral feeds are slowly adjusted and they can attempt breastfeeding. If they are not successful, swallowing and feeding disorders may be diagnosed.

The feeding protocols at our institution have been very successful with patients, nursing and medical staff. We also give the families with infants with single ventricles feeding instructions for home that include the type of formula, the calories, and how to much to feed, and at what interval. The families record each feeding on special sheets, and record a daily saturation and weight. Patients with single ventricles are followed up weekly and total feeds adjusted as necessary to keep within the goal calories/kg/day. In addition, the families are instructed about "red flag" criteria prior to discharge and at each weekly visit, which include temperature >100.5°F, increased WOB, cyanosis, low saturations, weight gain of less than 100 g, or being very fussy or consolable. We have found this to be a very easy to understand system for the families.

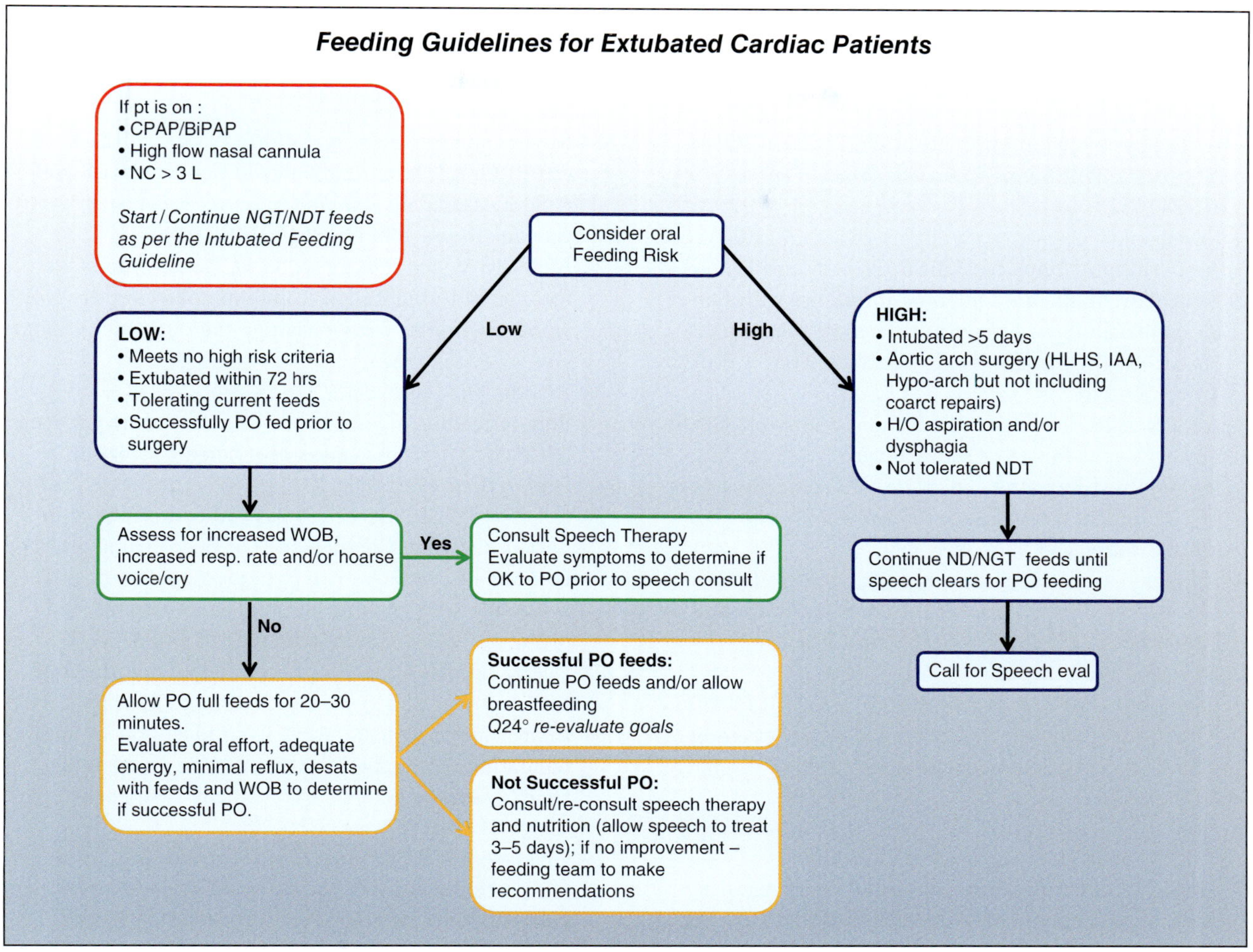

Figure 71.2 Feeding guidelines for extubated cardiac patients.

References

1 Zuckberg AL, Lefton-Greif MA. (2006) Nutrition and metabolism in the critically ill child with cardiac disease, in, *Critical Heart Disease In Infants and Children*, 2nd edn (eds DG Nichols, RM Ungerleider), Mosby, Philadelphia.

2 van den Berghe G, de Zegher F, Bouillon R. (1998) Clinical review 95: acute and prolonged critical illness as different neuroendocrine paradigms. *J Clin Endrocrinol Metab*, **83**, 1827–1834.

3 Tomkins AM, Garlick PJ, Schofield WN, Waterlow JC. (1983) The combined effects of infection and malnutrition on protein metabolism in children. *Clin Sci*, **65** (3), 313–324.

4 Cogo PE, Carnielli VP, Rosso F, *et al.* (2002) Protein turnover, lipolysis and endogenous hormonal secretion in critically ill children. *Crit Care Med*, **30** (1): 65–70.

5 Anand KJ, Brown MJ, Bloom SR, Aynsley-Green A. (1985) Studies on the hormomal regulation of fuel metabolism in the human newborn infant undergoing anesthesia and surgery. *Horm Res*, **22**, 115–128.

6 Anand KJ, Hansen DD, Hickey PR. (1990) Hormonal-metabolic stress responses in neonates undergoing cardiac surgery. *Anesthesiology*, **73** (4), 661–670.

7 Anand KJ, Sippell WG, Aynsley Green A. (1987) Randomized trial of fentanyl anaesthesia in preterm babies undergoing surgery: Effects on the stress response. *Lancet*, **329**, 62–66.

8 Mitchell IM, Logan RW, Pollock JCS, Jamieson MPG. (1995) Nutritional status of children with congenital heart disease. *Br Heart J*, **73**, 277–283.

9 Anderson JB, Marino BS, Irving SY, *et al.* (2011) Poor post-operative growth in infants with two-ventricle physiology. *Cardiol Young*, **21**, 421–429.

10 Williams RV, Ravishankar C, Zak V, *et al.* (2010) Birth weight and prematurity in infants with single ventricle physiology: pediatric heart network infant

single ventricle trial screened population. *Congenit Heart Dis*, **5** (2), 96–103.

11 Williams RV, Zak V, Ravishankar C, *et al.* (2011) Factors affecting growth in infants with single ventricle physiology: a report from the Pediatric Heart Network Infant Single Ventricle Trial. *J Pediatr*, **159**, 1017–1022.

12 Ravishankar C, Zak, V, Williams IA, *et al.* (2013) Association of Impaired Linear Growth and Worse Neurodevelopmental Outcome in Infants with Single Ventricle Physiology: a report from the Pediatric Heart Network Infant Single Ventricle Trial. *J Pediatr*, **162**, 250–256.

13 Anderson JB, Beekman RH, Border WL, *et al.* (2009) Lower weight-for-age z score adversely affects hospital length of stay after bidirectional Glenn procedure in 100 infants with a single ventricle. *J Thorac Cardiovasc Surg*, **138**, 397–404.

14 Anderson JB, Kalkwarf HJ, Kehl JE, Eghtesady P, Marino BS. (2011) Low weight-for-age z-score and infection risk after the Fontan Procedure. *Ann Thorac Surg*, **91**, 1460–1466.

15 Lapillonne A, O'Connor D, Wang D, Rigo J. (2013) Nutritional recommendations for the later preterm infant and the preterm infant after hospital discharge. *J Pediatr* **162**, S90–100.

16 Howley LW, Kaufman J, Wymore E, *et al.* (2012) Enteral feeding in neonates with prostaglandin-dependent congenital heart disease: international survey on current trends and variations in practice. *Cardiol Young*, **22**, 121–127.

17 Natarajan G, Reddy Anne S, Aggarwal S. (2010) Enteral feeding of neonates with congenital heart disease. *Neonatology*, **98**, 330–336.

18 Willis L, Thureen P, Kaufman J, *et al.* (2008) Enteral feeding in prostaglandin-dependent neonates: is it a safe practice? *J Pediatr*, **153**, 867–869.

19 Johnson JN, Ansong AK, Li JS, *et al.* (2011) Celiac artery flow pattern in infants with single right ventricle following the norwood procedure with a modified Blalock–Taussig or right ventricle to pulmonary artery shunt. *Pediatr Cardiol*, **32** (4), 479–486.

20 Davies RR, Carver SW, Schmidt R, *et al.* (2013) Gastrointestinal complications after Stage I Norwood versus hybrid procedures. *Ann Thorac Surg*, **95**, 189–196.

21 Averin K, Uzark K, Beekman RH, *et al.* (2012) Postoperative assessment of laryngopharyngeal dysfunction in neonates after Norwood Operation. *Ann Thorac Surg*, **94**, 1237–1261.

22 Garcia X, Jaquiss RDB, Imamura M, *et al.* (2011) Preemptive gastrostomy tube placement after Norwood Operation. *J Pediatr*, **159**, 602–607.

23 Hebson CL, Oster ME, Kirshbom PM, *et al.* Association of feeding modality with interstage mortality after single-ventricle palliation. *J Thorac Cardiovasc Surg*, **144**, 173–177.

24 Sables-Baus S, Kaufman J, Cook P, da Cruz EM. (2012) Oral feeding outcomes in neonates with congenital cardiac disease undergoing cardiac surgery. *Cardiol Young*, **22**, 42–48.

25 Uzark K, Wang Y, Rudd N, *et al.* (2012) Interstage feeding and weight gain in infants following the Norwood operation: can we change the outcome? *Cardiol Young*, **22**, 520–527.

26 Braudis NJ, Curley MAQ, Beaupre K, *et al.* (2009) Enteral feeding algorithm for infants with hypoplastic left heart syndrome status post stage I palliation. *Pediatr Crit Care Med*, **10** (4), 460–466.

27 Del Castillo SL, Mc Culley ME, Khemani RG, *et al.* (2010) Reducing the incidence of necrotizing enterocolitis in neonates with hypoplastic left heart syndrome with the introduction of an enteral feed protocol. *Pediatr Crit Care Med*, **11** (3), 373–377.

28 Kugler JD, Beekman RH, Rosenthal GL, *et al.* (2009) Development of a Pediatric Cardiology Quality Improvement Collaborative: from inception to implementation. From the Joint Council on Congenital Heart Disease Quality Improvement Task Force. *Congenit Heart Dis*, **4**, 318–328.

29 Ghanayem NS, Hoffman GM, Mussatto KA, *et al.* (2003) Home surveillance program prevents interstage mortality after the Norwood procedure. *J Thorac Cardiovasc Surg*, **126**, 1367–1377.

30 Srinivasan C, Sachdeva R, Morrow WR, *et al.* (2009) Standardized management improves outcomes after the Norwood Procedure. *Congenit Heart Dis*, **4**, 329–337.

31 Hehir DA, Rudd N, Slicker J, *et al.* (2012) Normal interstage growth after the Norwood Operation associated with interstage home monitoring. *Pediatr Cardiol*, **33**, 1315–1322.

32 Anderson JB, Iyer SB, Schidlow DN, *et al.* (2012) Variation in growth of infants with a single ventricle. *J Pediatr*, **161**, 16–21.

33 Iyer SB, Anderson JB, Slicker J, Beekman RH, Lannon C. (2011) Using statistical process control to identify early growth failure among infants with hypoplastic left heart syndrome. *World J Pediatr Congenit Heart Surg*, **2**, 576–585.

34 Slicker J, Hehir DA, Horsely M, *et al.* (2013) Nutrition algorithms for infants with hypoplastic left heart syndrome: birth through the first interstage period. *Congenit Heart Dis*, **8** (2), 89–102.

Index

Note: Page numbers in *italic* denote figures and boxes, those in **bold** denote tables.

Visual Guide to Neonatal Cardiology, First Edition. Edited by Ernerio T. Alboliras, Ziyad M. Hijazi, Leo Lopez, and Donald J. Hagler.

d

u

v